**Epidemiology and Environmental Hygiene
in Veterinary Public Health**

Epidemiology and Environmental Hygiene in Veterinary Public Health

Edited by

Tanmoy Rana, M.V.Sc & PhD
Assistant Professor, Department of Veterinary Clinical Complex
West Bengal University of Animal & Fishery Sciences
Kolkata, India

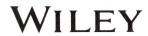

Copyright © 2025 by John Wiley & Sons, Inc. All rights reserved, including rights for text and data mining and training of artificial intelligence technologies or similar technologies.

Published by John Wiley & Sons, Inc., Hoboken, New Jersey.
Published simultaneously in Canada.

No part of this publication may be reproduced, stored in a retrieval system, or transmitted in any form or by any means, electronic, mechanical, photocopying, recording, scanning, or otherwise, except as permitted under Section 107 or 108 of the 1976 United States Copyright Act, without either the prior written permission of the Publisher, or authorization through payment of the appropriate per-copy fee to the Copyright Clearance Center, Inc., 222 Rosewood Drive, Danvers, MA 01923, (978) 750-8400, fax (978) 750-4470, or on the web at www.copyright.com. Requests to the Publisher for permission should be addressed to the Permissions Department, John Wiley & Sons, Inc., 111 River Street, Hoboken, NJ 07030, (201) 748-6011, fax (201) 748-6008, or online at http://www.wiley.com/go/permission.

The manufacturer's authorized representative according to the EU General Product Safety Regulation is Wiley-VCH GmbH, Boschstr. 12, 69469 Weinheim, Germany, e-mail: Product_Safety@wiley.com.

Trademarks: Wiley and the Wiley logo are trademarks or registered trademarks of John Wiley & Sons, Inc. and/or its affiliates in the United States and other countries and may not be used without written permission. All other trademarks are the property of their respective owners. John Wiley & Sons, Inc. is not associated with any product or vendor mentioned in this book.

Limit of Liability/Disclaimer of Warranty: While the publisher and author have used their best efforts in preparing this book, they make no representations or warranties with respect to the accuracy or completeness of the contents of this book and specifically disclaim any implied warranties of merchantability or fitness for a particular purpose. No warranty may be created or extended by sales representatives or written sales materials. The advice and strategies contained herein may not be suitable for your situation. You should consult with a professional where appropriate. Further, readers should be aware that websites listed in this work may have changed or disappeared between when this work was written and when it is read. Neither the publisher nor authors shall be liable for any loss of profit or any other commercial damages, including but not limited to special, incidental, consequential, or other damages.

For general information on our other products and services or for technical support, please contact our Customer Care Department within the United States at (800) 762-2974, outside the United States at (317) 572-3993 or fax (317) 572-4002.

Wiley also publishes its books in a variety of electronic formats. Some content that appears in print may not be available in electronic formats. For more information about Wiley products, visit our web site at www.wiley.com.

Library of Congress Cataloging-in-Publication Data Applied for:

Hardback ISBN: 9781394208159

Cover Design: Wiley
Cover Images: Courtesy of Tanmoy Rana

Set in 9.5/12.5pt STIXTwoText by Straive, Pondicherry, India

SKY10099721_031025

Contents

List of Contributors *ix*
Preface *xv*
Acknowledgments *xvii*

Section 1   Impacts of Epidemiology *1*

1   **Epidemiology: Principles, Aims and Scope, Methods, Components and Application** *3*
Ismail A. Odetokun, Aminu Shittu, Akeem Adebola Bakare, Oluwadamilola
Olawumi Abiodun-Adewusi, and Nma Bida Alhaji

2   **Factors Influencing Livestock Diseases and Animal Productivity** *33*
Negin Esfandiari and Mohammadreza Najafi

3   **Determinants of Disease, Adjustment of Rates, Trends and Emergence** *41*
Kollannur Davis Justin and Kadankandath Athira

4   **Transmission, Maintenance of Infection, and Consequences of Disease** *67*
Shriya Rawat, Parul, Nishant Sharma, Barkha Sharma, Udit Jain, and Vipul Thakur

5   **Ecology of Diseases, Hypothesis, and Life Table Technique and Its Application** *81*
Samuel U. Felix, Samuel C. Maureen, Simpson Monya, and Eshun A. Ama

6   **Measures of Occurrence of Disease Pattern and Association** *99*
Amitava Roy and Tanmoy Rana

7   **Animal Disease Surveillance, Survey Systems, and Associate Indices** *107*
Amitava Roy and Tanmoy Rana

8   **Epidemiological Studies, Measures of Disease Frequency, and Mortality** *117*
Samuel U. Felix, Samuel C. Maureen, Simpson Monya, Mariam Yakubu, and Njideka Adeniyi

9   **Animal Disease Alerts and Forecasting** *135*
Amitava Roy and Tanmoy Rana

10   **Strategies of Disease Management: Prevention, Control, and On-farm Biosecurity** *145*
Harshit Saxena, Akhilesh Kumar, Varun Kumar Sarkar, Manav Kansal, and Kartikey Verma

11   **Economic Impact on Animal Diseases** *155*
Justin Davis K, Athira K, and Javed Jameel A

vi | Contents

12 **International Laws and Regulations on Controlling Livestock Diseases** *177*
Bhavanam Sudhakara Reddy, Sirigireddy Sivajothi, and Kambala Swetha

13 **Role of OIE in Global Trade in Animals and Animal Products** *185*
Somu Yogeshpriya and Tanmoy Rana

14 **Comparative Epidemiological Studies** *191*
Maninder Singh and Jay P. Yadav

15 **Clinical Trials, Diagnostic Testing, and Risk Analysis** *197*
Negin Esfandiari and Mohammadreza Najafi

16 **Observational Studies** *207*
Ashemi Yusuf, Amitava Roy, and Tanmoy Rana

17 **Nature of Data, Data Collection, and Management** *215*
Abbas Rabiu Ishaq

18 **Systematic Reviews in Epidemiological Studies** *229*
Pratistha Shrivastava and Raghvendra Mishra

19 **Statistical and Mathematical Modeling** *245*
Ashish C. Patel

20 **Health Schemes and Its Importance** *251*
Sabhyata Sharma, Abhishek Pathak, Abhinav Meena, and Sandeep Kumar

21 **Animal Health, Management, and Nutritional Epidemiology** *261*
Amitava Roy, Tanmoy Rana, and Arkaprabha Shee

22 **Vaccines and Vaccination** *271*
J. Jyothi and M. Bhavya Sree

Section 2 **Impact of Environmental Hygiene in Veterinary and Public Health** *277*

23 **Aims, Scope, Administration, and Importance of Veterinary Public Health** *279*
Chandra Shekhar

24 **Role of Veterinarians in Public Health** *287*
Pratistha Shrivastava, Simant Kumar Sahoo, and K.M. Venkatesh

25 **One Health Concept and Initiatives in Veterinary Public Health** *299*
Naveen Kumar, Amit Kumar, Dinesh Mittal, and Manesh Kumar

26 **Sources and Hazardous Effects of Environmental Contaminants** *309*
Atul Kumar and Anil Patyal

27 **General Aspects of Environmental Hygiene** *321*
*Udit Jain, Faizan ul Haque Nagrami, Vijay Laxmi Tripathi, Parul, Barkha Sharma,
Shweta Sharma, Parul Singh, and Shikhar Karan Verma*

Contents | vii

28 Natural Resources: Definition, Types, Examples, Uses, and Abuses *329*
Udit Jain, Faizan ul Haque Nagrami, Barkha Sharma, Priyambada, Parul, and Uma Sharma

29 Epidemiology and Environmental Health in Veterinary Medicine *339*
J. Jyothi and M. Bhavya Sree

30 Precision Livestock Farming and Its Advantage to the Environment *343*
Amitava Roy and Tanmoy Rana

31 Biodiversity: Concept, Pattern, Importance, Threats, and Conservation *349*
Jitendrakumar Nayak, Varun Asediya, Santanu Pal, and Pranav Anjaria

32 Definition, Scope, Characteristics, and Importance of Ecosystems *365*
Udit Jain, Faizan ul Haque Nagrami, Barkha Sharma, Parul, and Uma Sharma

33 Environmental Pollution: Air, Water, Soil, Marine, and Thermal Pollution *385*
Parul, Udit Jain, Barkha Sharma, Anuj Kumar, Renu Singh, and Sanjay Bharti

34 Environmental Pollution Effect on Animal and Human Health *393*
Goverdhan Singh, Balram Yadav, and Vivek Agrawal

35 Rural and Urban Pollution *405*
Mona Abdelghany Nasr and Nourhan Eissa

36 Global Warming and Green House Effect: Impact of Climate Change, Protocol, Treaties and Convention *415*
Baleshwari Dixit, Sulochana Sen, and Rajesh Kumar Vandre

37 Environmental Enrichment and Welfare of Animals *427*
Deepak Nelagonda, Ramadevi Pampana, and Manoj Kumar Karanam

38 Basics of Water Supply, Quality, and Purification *439*
Nourhan Eissa and Mona Abdelghany Nasr

39 Type, Cause, Effects, Control Methods of Noise Pollution *451*
Baleshwari Dixit, Sapna Sharma, Ranvijay Singh, and Serlene Tomar

40 Environmental Contamination and Food Chain Bioaccumulation *461*
Kaushik Satyaprakash, Annada Das, Dipanwita Bhattacharya, and Souti Prasad Sarkhel

41 Principles and Issues of Environmental Protection *477*
Baleshwari Dixit, Neelam Kurmi, Sapna Sharma, Serlene Tomar, and Yamini Verma

42 Challenges of Emergency Animal Management During Disasters *487*
Javed Jameel A, Justin Davis K, and Athira K

43 Sources of Air Pollution in Animal Houses and Its Consequences *497*
Parul Singh, Barkha Sharma, Udit Jain, Renu Singh, Sanjay Bharti, and Meena Goswami

44 Farm Waste and Sewage Disposal *505*
Jaysukh B. Kathiriya and Bhavesh J. Trangadia

viii *Contents*

45 **Biomedical Waste Management** *523*
Gungi Saritha

46 **General Hygiene, Sanitation, and Disinfection of Animal Housing and Hospital Environment** *537*
Jay P. Yadav, Sivakumar Mani, and Maninder Singh

47 **Management of Stray, Fallen Animals and Carcass Disposal** *551*
Poornima Gumasta, Narendra Kumar, Mahmuda Malik, and Diptimayee Sahoo

48 **Vector and Reservoir Control in Veterinary Public Health** *557*
Jitendrakumar Nayak, Santanu Pal, Pranav Anjaria, and Varun Asediya

49 **Principles of General Disease Prevention and Control Measures** *569*
Jitendrakumar Nayak, Manasi Soni, Pranav Anjaria, and Manubhai N. Brahmbhatt

50 **Accident Prevention for Animal Well-being** *581*
Abbas Rabiu Ishaq

51 **Maintenance of Industrial Hygiene** *593*
Mona Abdelghany Nasr and Nourhan Eissa

52 **Environmental Planning, Monitoring, and Management** *599*
Jaysukh Kathiriya and Bhavesh J. Trangadia

Index *615*

List of Contributors

Javed Jameel A
Department of Veterinary Clinical Medicine, Ethics and Jurisprudence, College of Veterinary and Animal Sciences, Kerala Veterinary and Animal Sciences University, Pookode, India

Oluwadamilola Olawumi Abiodun-Adewusi
Department of Health Sciences and Social Work Western Illinois University, Macomb, IL, USA, 61455

Eshun A. Ama
Department of Food and Animal Science Alabama A&M University, Normal, AL, USA

Njideka Adeniyi
Department of Food and Animal Science Alabama A&M University, Normal, AL, USA

Vivek Agrawal
Department of Veterinary Parasitology, College of Veterinary Sciences & Animal Husbandry, Nanaji Deshmukh Veterinary Science University, Mhow, Indore, India

Nma Bida Alhaji
Department of Veterinary Public Health and Preventive Medicine, University of Abuja, Abuja, FCT, Nigeria, 900105

Pranav Anjaria
College of Veterinary Science and Animal Husbandry Kamdhenu University, Anand, India

Varun Asediya
M. B. Veterinary College, Dungarpur, India

Akeem Adebola Bakare
Division of Epidemiology, Department of Environmental and Public Health Sciences, University of Cincinnati Cincinnati, OH, USA, 45221

Sanjay Bharti
College of Veterinary & Animal Sciences, DUVASU Mathura, India

Dipanwita Bhattacharya
Faculty of Veterinary and Animal Sciences, Institute of Agricultural Sciences, Banaras Hindu University Mirzapur, India

Manubhai N. Brahmbhatt
College of Veterinary Science and Animal Husbandry Kamdhenu University, Anand, India

Annada Das
Department of Livestock Products Technology West Bengal University of Animal and Fishery Sciences Kolkata, India

Baleshwari Dixit
Department of Veterinary Public Health & Epidemiology College of Veterinary Science & Animal Health, 486001, Rewa, NDVSU, Jabalpur, Madhya Pradesh, India
and
Department of Livestock Products Technology College of Veterinary Science and Animal Husbandry Rewa, NDVSU, Jabalpur, Madhya Pradesh, India

Nourhan Eissa
Department of Animal Hygiene and Zoonoses, Faculty of Veterinary Medicine, University of Sadat City, Sadat City, Egypt

Negin Esfandiari
Department of Food Hygiene and Quality Control Division of Epidemiology, Faculty of Veterinary Medicine University of Tehran, Tehran, Iran

List of Contributors

Samuel U. Felix
Faculty of Veterinary Medicine, National Animal Production Research Institute, Ahmadu Bello University, Zaria, Nigeria
Department of Food and Animal Science, Alabama A&M University, Normal, AL, USA

Meena Goswami
College of Veterinary & Animal Sciences, DUVASU Mathura, India

Poornima Gumasta
College of Veterinary and Animal Sciences, Bihar Animal Sciences University, Patna, Bihar, India

Abbas Rabiu Ishaq
Paws and Claws Specialist Veterinary Clinic, Riyadh, KSA

Udit Jain
College of Veterinary & Animal Sciences, DUVASU Mathura, India

J. Jyothi
Department of Veterinary Medicine, P.V. Narasimha Rao Telangana Veterinary University, Hyderabad, India

Athira K
Department of Veterinary Epidemiology and Preventive Medicine, College of Veterinary and Animal Sciences Kerala Veterinary and Animal Sciences University Pookode, India

Justin Davis K
Department of Veterinary Epidemiology and Preventive Medicine, College of Veterinary and Animal Sciences Kerala Veterinary and Animal Sciences University Pookode, India

Manav Kansal
ICAR-IVRI, Izatnagar, Bareilly, India

Manoj Kumar Karanam
Department of Veterinary Surgery and Radiology, College of Veterinary Science, Garividi, India

Jaysukh B. Kathiriya
Department of Veterinary Public Health & Epidemiology College of Veterinary Science & Animal Husbandry Kamdhenu University, Junagadh, India

Akhilesh Kumar
Division of Medicine, ICAR-IVRI, Izatnagar, Bareilly, India

Amit Kumar
Department of Veterinary Surgery and Radiology, Lala Lajpat Rai University of Veterinary and Animal Sciences Hisar, India

Anuj Kumar
College of Veterinary & Animal Sciences, DUVASU Mathura, India

Atul Kumar
Department of Veterinary Public Health and Epidemiology, CSK HP Agricultural University Palampur, India

Manesh Kumar
Department of Veterinary Public Health and Epidemiology, Lala Lajpat Rai University of Veterinary and Animal Sciences, Hisar, India

Narendra Kumar
College of Veterinary and Animal Sciences, Bihar Animal Sciences University, Patna, Bihar, India

Naveen Kumar
Department of Veterinary Public Health and Epidemiology, Lala Lajpat Rai University of Veterinary and Animal Sciences, Hisar, India

Sandeep Kumar
Cluster University of Jammu, Jammu and Kashmir, India

Neelam Kurmi
Department of Animal Husbandry and Dairying Sagar, India

Mahmuda Malik
College of Veterinary and Animal Sciences, Bihar Animal Sciences University, Patna, Bihar, India

Sivakumar Mani
Department of Veterinary Public Health and Epidemiology, Veterinary College and Research Institute,Tamil Nadu Veterinary and Animal Sciences University, Theni, India

Samuel C. Maureen
JayCare Medical Centre, Crestwood Medica Center, Huntsville, AL, Kaduna, Nigeria

List of Contributors | xi

Abhinav Meena
Department of Veterinary Parasitology,
Apollo College of Veterinary Medicine, Jaipur, Rajasthan,
302031, India

Raghvendra Mishra
Department of Veterinary Public Health, M.B. Veterinary
College, Dungarpur, India

Dinesh Mittal
Department of Veterinary Public Health and
Epidemiology, Lala Lajpat Rai University of Veterinary
and Animal Sciences, Hisar, India

Simpson Monya
Department of Food and Animal Science, Alabama A&M
University, Normal, AL, USA

Faizan ul Haque Nagrami
College of Biotechnology, DUVASU, Mathura, India

Mohammadreza Najafi
Department of Pathobiology, Faculty of Veterinary
Medicine, Urmia University, Urmia, Iran

Mona Abdelghany Nasr
Department of Anatomy and Embryology, Faculty of
Veterinary Medicine, University of Sadat City, Sadat
City, Egypt

Jitendrakumar Nayak
College of Veterinary Science and Animal Husbandry
Kamdhenu University, Anand, India

Deepak Nelagonda
Department of Poultry Science, SNK AH Polytechnic
College, Anantapur, India

Ismail A. Odetokun
Department of Veterinary Public Health and Preventive
Medicine, University of Ilorin, Ilorin, Kwara State,
Nigeria, 240003

Santanu Pal
ICAR – Indian Veterinary Research Institute, Izatnagar
Bareilly, India

Ramadevi Pampana
Department of Veterinary Parasitology, College of
Veterinary Science, Garividi, India

Parul
College of Veterinary & Animal Sciences, DUVASU
Mathura, India

Ashish C. Patel
Veterinary College, Kamdhenu University, Anand, India

Abhishek Pathak
Department of Veterinary Parasitology, Apollo College of
Veterinary Medicine, Jaipur, Rajasthan, India

Anil Patyal
Department of Veterinary Public Health and
Epidemiology, Dau Shri Vasudev Chandrakar Kamdhenu
Vishwavidyalaya, Durg, India

Priyambada
College of Biotechnology, DUVASU, Mathura, India

Tanmoy Rana
Department of Veterinary Clinical Complex, West Bengal
University of Animal & Fishery Sciences, Kolkata, India

Shriya Rawat
College of Veterinary & Animal Sciences, SVPUAT
Meerut, India

Bhavanam Sudhakara Reddy
College of Veterinary Science, Sri Venkateswara
Veterinary University, Proddatur, Andhra Pradesh, India

Amitava Roy
Department of Livestock Farm Complex, West Bengal
University of Animal & Fishery Sciences, Kolkata, India

Diptimayee Sahoo
College of Veterinary and Animal Sciences, Bihar Animal
Sciences University, Patna, Bihar, India

Simant Kumar Sahoo
Veterinary Officer, Odisha State Government,
Gajapati, India

Gungi Saritha
Department of Veterinary Medicine, Sri Venkateswara
Veterinary University, Tirupati, India

Varun Kumar Sarkar
Division of Medicine, ICAR-IVRI, Izatnagar,
Bareilly, India

Souti Prasad Sarkhel
Faculty of Veterinary and Animal Sciences, Institute of Agricultural Sciences, Banaras Hindu University Mirzapur, India

Kaushik Satyaprakash
Faculty of Veterinary and Animal Sciences, Institute of Agricultural Sciences, Banaras Hindu University, Mirzapur, India

Harshit Saxena
Division of Medicine, ICAR-IVRI, Izatnagar, Bareilly, India

Sulochana Sen
Department of Animal Genetics and Breeding, College of Veterinary Science & Animal Health, Rewa, India

Barkha Sharma
College of Veterinary & Animal Sciences, DUVASU Mathura, India

Nishant Sharma
College of Veterinary & Animal Sciences, GBPUAT Pantnagar, India

Sabhyata Sharma
Department of Veterinary Parasitology, Apollo College of Veterinary Medicine, Jaipur, Rajasthan, India

Sapna Sharma
Department of Public Health & Epidemiology Post Graduate Institute of Veterinary Education and Research College, 302031, Jaipur, India

Shweta Sharma
College of Biotechnology, DUVASU, Mathura, India

Uma Sharma
College of Biotechnology, DUVASU, Mathura, India

Arkaprabha Shee
Subject Matter Specialist (Animal Sci.), Dhaanyaganga Krishi Vigyan Kendra, Sargachi, Murshidabad, India

Chandra Shekhar
Department of Veterinary Public Health & Epidemiology College of Veterinary Science & Animal Husbandry Acharya Narendra Deva University of Agriculture & Technology, Ayodhya, India

Aminu Shittu
Division of Quantitative Epidemiology, Department of Theriogenology and Production, Usmanu Danfodiyo University, Sokoto, Sokoto State, Nigeria, 840004

Pratistha Shrivastava
Department of Veterinary Parasitology, Institute of Veterinary Sciences and Animal Health, SOADU Bhubaneswar, India

Goverdhan Singh
College of Veterinary and Animal Science Navania, Vallabhnagar, Udaipur, RAJUVAS, Bikaner, India

Maninder Singh
Department of Veterinary Public Health and Epidemiology, College of Veterinary Science, Guru Angad Dev Veterinary and Animal Sciences University, Rampura Phul, India

Parul Singh
College of Veterinary & Animal Sciences, DUVASU, Mathura, India

Ranvijay Singh
Department of Veterinary Public Health and Epidemiology College of Veterinary Science and A.H. NDVSU 482001, Jabalpur, Madhya Pradesh, India

Renu Singh
College of Veterinary & Animal Sciences, DUVASU Mathura, India

Sirigireddy Sivajothi
College of Veterinary Science, Sri Venkateswara Veterinary University, Proddatur, Andhra Pradesh, India

Manasi Soni
College of Veterinary Science and Animal Husbandry Kamdhenu University, Anand, India

M. Bhavya Sree
P.V. Narasimha Rao Telangana Veterinary University Hyderabad, India

Kambala Swetha
College of Veterinary Science, Sri Venkateswara Veterinary University, Proddatur, Andhra Pradesh, India

Vipul Thakur
College of Veterinary & Animal Sciences, SVPUAT
Meerut, India

Serlene Tomar
Department of Livestock Products Technology,
College of Veterinary Science and Animal Husbandry,
Rewa, NDVSU, Jabalpur, Madhya Pradesh, India

Bhavesh J. Trangadia
Department of Veterinary Pathology, College of Veterinary
Science & Animal Husbandry, Kamdhenu University
Junagadh, India

Vijay Laxmi Tripathi
College of Biotechnology, DUVASU, Mathura, India

K.M. Venkatesh
Veterinary Practitioner, Tamil Nadu, India

Kartikey Verma
CoVSc & AH, SVPUAT, Mathura, India

Shikhar Karan Verma
College of Veterinary & Animal Sciences, DUVASU
Mathura, India

Yamini Verma
Department of Veterinary Pathology, College of Veterinary
Science & Animal Health, Jabalpur, India

Rajesh Kumar Vandre
Department of Animal Genetics and Breeding, College of
Veterinary Science & Animal Health, Rewa, India

Balram Yadav
College of Veterinary and Animal Science Navania,
Vallabhnagar, Udaipur, RAJUVAS, Bikaner, India

Jay P. Yadav
Department of Veterinary Public Health and
Epidemiology, College of Veterinary Science, Guru Angad
Dev Veterinary and Animal Sciences University, Rampura
Phul, India

Mariam Yakubu
Department of Food and Animal Science, Alabama A&M
University, Normal, AL, USA

Somu Yogeshpriya
Department of Veterinary Medicine, Veterinary College
and Research Institute, Tamil Nadu Veterinary and
Animal Sciences University, Orathanadu, India

Ashemi Yusuf
World Bank Regional Disease Surveillance System
Enhancement Project, Abuja, Nigeria

Preface

Veterinary epidemiology deals with a close association between adverse effects with a selected potential causative factor/cause of interest, such as exposure to a chemical or a disease agent. The basic principle of veterinary epidemiology is that disease occurs seldom in a population, but it may be more likely to happen in certain groups of a population, at certain times, and also in specific locations with a specific pattern. Veterinary epidemiology can play a major role in emerging disease outbreaks, denoting the understanding of the etiological factors as a good prevention of infections with a zoonotic significance. On the other hand, environmental hygiene generally covers all the practical preventive and control strategies used for the improvement of the basic environmental conditions affecting animal health and is in relation to various diseases. Various environmental conditions including purity of water, the status of animal waste disposal as well as food from contamination are the most provoking indices for the occurrence of diseases with zoonotic concern. Various pollutants and waste materials are hazardous to animal health. The book provides a target-organ-oriented presentation of environmental hazards, with a detailed discussion of selected exposures of asbestos, radon, lead, and indoor and outdoor air pollutants. The book also designs observational studies, validity in epidemiological studies, systematic reviews, and statistical modeling, to deliver more advanced material for the students actively involved in the epidemiological study. The full scope of epidemiology, with chapters covering causality, disease occurrence, determinants, disease patterns, disease ecology, and much more are elaborately described in this book. The book features updated information regarding current resources on the subject of veterinary epidemiology, surveillance, and diagnostic test validation and performance. The book describes the logical progression in relation to epidemiological concepts and methods for the developments in research and teaching. This book also expands risk, statistical and economic analyses, and surveillance for various diseases. The contamination of diseases largely depends on environmental indices. pollutants and all of which interact to affect health. Transmission of germs, viruses, and vectors may increase due to inadequate routine cleaning of the environment. The book entitled "Epidemiology and Environmental Hygiene in Veterinary Public Health" 1e will provide a current resource on the subject of veterinary epidemiology and environmental hygiene. Both aspects are essential for the spreading of diseases. The book is a reference for veterinary general practitioners, government veterinarians, agricultural economists, and members of other disciplines interested in animal diseases. It is also very essential reading for epidemiology as well as veterinary public health students at both the undergraduate and postgraduate levels. The book chapters are systematically arranged for the epidemiological significance and environmental hygiene in veterinary public health. The book is designed to intensify the current thoughts and scientific modules for the betterment of understanding for the readers. The book will be designed interestingly by providing color figures, line figures, and tables. The book will also be helpful for students, researchers, academicians, industry sectors, milk producer's unions, veterinarians, and farm managers as a reference book. The book will be of primary importance for audience/readers involved in epidemiological as well as public health research. The management of environmental hygiene with epidemiological forecasts will be discussed elaborately by emphasizing the degree of severity of diseases. The book was structured on the thoughts and understanding of the readership globally in such a fashion that every epidemiology professional/Veterinary Medicine faculty/Territory Veterinary Professional will gather knowledge and will be expertise in Veterinary Epidemiology and Environmental hygiene all in one in the book. Moreover, the epidemiology and spreading/contamination of diseases largely depend on environmental indices. Environmental hygiene is the most important prevention to protect against contamination of any disease. The proposed book will relate the correlation between epidemiology and environmental hygiene nicely. In my opinion, the book is stronger, more powerful, and more relevant for the readership. The impact of environmental hygiene and its effect on animal health is elaborately described in a lucrative manner. This book provides useful information about the man–environmental–health interrelationships with a strong basic background in the environmental health discipline. This book elaborately describes the nature of environmental hazards with the great relationship between the environment and the health of man. The final aspect of the book deals with the overall prospects for the planning and management of the environmental hygiene. This book is a valuable resource for individuals working in the environmental health sciences.

Dr. Tanmoy Rana
West Bengal University of Animal & Fishery Sciences
Kolkata, India

Acknowledgments

I want to thank Dr. Rituparna Bose, Acquisition Editor, Editor, Health and Life Sciences, Academic Publishing Group (APG), Bhavya Boopathi, Managing Editor, Health Professions & Vet Medicine, Susan Engelken, Baskaran, Keerthana, Support Service Administrator, Wiley, and Other members for their continual guidance and support during preparing this book. I would like to convey my sincere thanks to all contributors who are the pillar of the book and write the manuscript within the stipulated time. I would also like to acknowledge my colleagues, friends, and others who help me to edit such a valuable book. I also convey my sincere gratitude to the Hon'ble Vice Chancellor, West Bengal University of Animal & Fishery Sciences, Kolkata, India for providing me the opportunity and making a platform to edit an international book. I must also recognize the contributions of the many precious veterinary practitioners as well as researchers whose works are highly cited profusely throughout the text of the book. Last but not the least; I am also indebted to my family who bears me to edit this work.

Dr. Tanmoy Rana
West Bengal University of Animal & Fishery Sciences
Kolkata, India

Section 1

Impacts of Epidemiology

1

Epidemiology: Principles, Aims and Scope, Methods, Components and Application

Ismail A. Odetokun[1], Aminu Shittu[2], Akeem Adebola Bakare[3], Oluwadamilola Olawumi Abiodun-Adewusi[4], and Nma Bida Alhaji[5]

[1] *Department of Veterinary Public Health and Preventive Medicine, University of Ilorin, Ilorin, Kwara State, Nigeria, 240003*
[2] *Division of Quantitative Epidemiology, Department of Theriogenology and Production, Usmanu Danfodiyo University, Sokoto, Sokoto State, Nigeria, 840004*
[3] *Division of Epidemiology, Department of Environmental and Public Health Sciences, University of Cincinnati, Cincinnati, OH, USA, 45221*
[4] *Department of Health Sciences and Social Work, Western Illinois University, Macomb, IL, USA, 61455*
[5] *Department of Veterinary Public Health and Preventive Medicine, University of Abuja, Abuja, FCT, Nigeria, 900105*

1.1 Introduction

1.1.1 Definition of Veterinary Epidemiology

Veterinary epidemiology is a dynamic scientific field focused on the in-depth analysis of disease patterns, their geographical distribution, and the multifaceted determinants of diseases and health-related events within animal populations (Toma et al. 1999; Doherr and Audigé 2001). Drawing heavily from the principles and methodologies of epidemiology, the field of veterinary epidemiology extends these concepts to the domain of animal health and well-being (Thrusfield et al. 2018). Veterinary epidemiologists wield a diverse array of investigative tools and techniques to rigorously monitor, analyze, and interpret data about a wide spectrum of animal diseases and health-related challenges (Martin et al. 1987). Veterinary epidemiology is fundamentally concerned with the systematic exploration of how diseases manifest and propagate within animal populations. This approach is crucial for effective disease control, prevention, and safeguarding of both animal and public health (Salman 2009a).

1.1.2 Importance of Veterinary Epidemiology in Safeguarding Animal and Public Health

Veterinary epidemiology is a discipline with profound significance in safeguarding both animal and public health. Its role encompasses a wide range of critical aspects, each contributing to the well-being of animals and humans. Let's explore its importance in greater detail:

1) **Preventing Zoonotic Diseases:** One of the paramount roles of veterinary epidemiology is to monitor and control animal diseases, which is essential in preventing zoonotic diseases. Zoonotic diseases are those that can be transmitted from animals to humans. By identifying and addressing diseases in animal populations, veterinary epidemiologists play a crucial part in reducing the risk of such diseases spilling over to humans. For instance, by controlling diseases in livestock, they minimize the risk of zoonotic pathogens entering the food supply and affecting human health (Heymann 2015; Thrusfield et al. 2018).

2) **Early Detection and Containment of Disease Outbreaks:** Veterinary epidemiology contributes significantly to the early detection and containment of disease outbreaks in animal populations. By implementing surveillance systems and conducting regular monitoring, it enables the rapid identification of diseases. Early detection is vital for implementing control measures that can help prevent the rapid spread of diseases within animal populations. This, in turn, helps to avert economic losses in the livestock industry (Salman 2009a).

3) **Economic Impact and Livestock Industry:** The economic implications of animal diseases are substantial. Disease outbreaks in livestock can result in significant financial losses for the livestock industry, which can affect food

Epidemiology and Environmental Hygiene in Veterinary Public Health, First Edition. Edited by Tanmoy Rana.
© 2025 John Wiley & Sons, Inc. Published 2025 by John Wiley & Sons, Inc.

production, trade, and livelihoods. Veterinary epidemiology plays a critical role in minimizing these economic losses by controlling and preventing diseases. This benefits both animal agriculture and the broader economy (Rushton 2008).

4) **Ensuring Food Safety:** The discipline of veterinary epidemiology contributes to food safety by ensuring the health of animals within the food production chain. Healthy animals are more likely to produce safe food products, whether it's meat, dairy, or other animal-derived products. Monitoring and controlling diseases in animals are integral to preventing the contamination of food products, which can lead to foodborne illnesses in humans. It helps in maintaining the integrity of the food supply and public trust in food safety (Doherr and Audigé 2001).

5) **Assessment of Veterinary Interventions:** Veterinary epidemiology aids in the assessment of the efficacy and safety of veterinary interventions, including vaccines and treatments. By conducting studies and analyzing data, veterinary epidemiologists help determine the effectiveness of various interventions in preventing or treating diseases in animals. This ensures that the products and practices used in animal health management are safe and efficient (Martin et al. 1987).

Veterinary epidemiology is vital for safeguarding animal and human health, from preventing zoonotic diseases to enabling early detection and control of animal disease outbreaks. The economic benefits, food safety, and the assessment of veterinary interventions underscore its significance in maintaining the health and well-being of both animal populations and the broader public.

1.2 Principles of Veterinary Epidemiology

1.2.1 Understanding Disease Patterns

1.2.1.1 Descriptive Epidemiology
Descriptive epidemiology is a foundational principle of veterinary epidemiology that serves as the initial step in understanding disease patterns in animal populations. This approach involves the systematic collection and analysis of data to characterize the patterns and distribution of diseases among animals (Dohoo et al. 2009). Descriptive epidemiology is crucial for identifying key factors such as time, place, and affected populations, providing a fundamental understanding of disease occurrence (Thrusfield et al. 2018). In this chapter, we'll explore the significance of descriptive epidemiology in veterinary medicine, provide examples, and suggest references for further reading.

Significance of Descriptive Epidemiology
Descriptive Epidemiology is Essential for a Multitude of Reasons, Including:

a) **Identifying Temporal Trends:** One of the primary objectives of descriptive epidemiology is to recognize temporal patterns in disease occurrence. By analyzing data over time, it helps determine when diseases are more likely to occur, whether they exhibit seasonality, and whether there are long-term trends (Martin et al. 1987; Magnet and Izquierdo 2023). For example, in a study of foot-and-mouth disease in cattle, descriptive epidemiology may reveal that outbreaks tend to peak during certain seasons, such as the rainy season.

b) **Mapping the Geographic Distribution:** Another critical aspect of descriptive epidemiology is mapping the geographical distribution of disease cases. It helps identify specific regions or areas where diseases are concentrated or where clusters of cases occur (Elliott et al. 2000; Pfeiffer et al. 2008). In the context of a brucellosis outbreak in a country, descriptive epidemiology can highlight areas with the highest prevalence of the disease and regions where control measures should be prioritized.

c) **Characterizing Affected Populations:** Descriptive epidemiology delves into the characteristics of the populations affected by the disease. This includes data on species, age, sex, and other relevant attributes of the animals involved. For instance, in the study of avian influenza in poultry, descriptive epidemiology may reveal whether the disease primarily affects certain species, such as ducks or chickens, or whether it impacts birds of a particular age group (Nguyen et al. 2014; Islam et al. 2023).

d) **Early Detection of Outbreaks:** By regularly monitoring and analyzing disease data, descriptive epidemiology enables the early detection of outbreaks (Al-Hemoud et al. 2021). This is particularly crucial for rapid response and the implementation of control measures. For example, in the context of African swine fever (ASF) outbreak, monitoring temporal and geographic patterns can help identify emerging outbreaks in specific pig populations (Kim et al. 2021).

Tools in Descriptive Epidemiology

Descriptive epidemiology employs a range of tools and techniques to explore the distribution and patterns of diseases within animal populations. Among these, two key tools are disease mapping and spatial analysis. These tools play a critical role in understanding the geographic dimensions of disease occurrence.

a) **Disease Mapping:** Disease mapping is a powerful tool that allows epidemiologists to visualize and analyze the geographic distribution of disease cases. It involves plotting the locations of disease cases on a map, creating a spatial representation of the outbreak (Cromley and McLafferty 2012). Disease mapping typically involves collecting data on the geographic coordinates (latitude and longitude) of disease cases. These coordinates are then used to place points on a map, with each point representing a reported case. The map can also incorporate various symbols, colours, or shading to differentiate between affected and unaffected areas. Disease mapping provides a clear, visual representation of disease distribution, making it easier to identify areas with higher disease incidence and clusters of cases (Elliott et al. 2000; Pfeiffer et al. 2008). This spatial visualization is crucial for decision-making, as it helps authorities and epidemiologists target control measures, allocate resources efficiently, and implement interventions in areas with the greatest need.

b) **Spatial Analysis:** Spatial analysis is a statistical examination of the spatial distribution of disease cases. It involves the application of various analytical techniques to explore the geographic patterns of disease incidence, assess clustering, and understand spatial relationships (Elliott et al. 2000; Pfeiffer et al. 2008). Spatial analysis employs statistical methods to evaluate the spatial arrangement of disease cases in their geographic locations. Techniques may include spatial autocorrelation (examining the degree of similarity between neighbouring locations), cluster analysis (identifying disease clusters), and point pattern analysis (assessing the arrangement of cases) (Pfeiffer et al. 2008). Spatial analysis is essential for determining whether disease cases are randomly distributed, clustered, or exhibit spatial patterns. This knowledge aids in identifying high-risk areas, understanding disease transmission dynamics, and tailoring interventions. For instance, spatial analysis might reveal that cases of bovine tuberculosis tend to cluster in specific counties or regions within a country, which can inform targeted surveillance and control strategies (Shittu et al. 2013; Tembo et al. 2020).

1.2.1.2 Analytical Epidemiology

Analytical epidemiology is a crucial branch of veterinary epidemiology that goes beyond describing disease patterns. It focuses on investigating the causes of diseases by exploring the relationships between potential risk factors or exposures and disease outcomes. The primary goal of analytical epidemiology is to establish a causal relationship between these exposures and disease occurrence. This is achieved through a range of research methods and statistical techniques. Let's delve into analytical epidemiology, its significance, and the common methods used.

Understanding Analytical Epidemiology

Analytical epidemiology is a pivotal branch of veterinary epidemiology that delves deep into understanding the causes of diseases in animal populations. It aims to answer the fundamental question: "Why does a disease occur in certain animals or populations?" This form of epidemiology investigates the role of various risk factors, exposures, or interventions in disease causation (Dohoo et al. 2009). By identifying causal relationships between these factors and disease occurrence, analytical epidemiology provides critical insights that are indispensable for disease prevention and control strategies.

Common Methods in Analytical Epidemiology

1) **Case-Control Studies:** Case-control studies are a fundamental method in analytical epidemiology (Filardo et al. 2011). These observational studies are designed to compare animals or groups with a specific disease (cases) to those without the disease (controls). The primary objective of case-control studies is to identify factors associated with the disease's occurrence. This method is widely used in veterinary epidemiology for investigating various diseases and risk factors (Dohoo et al. 2009; Thrusfield et al. 2018).

   Analytical epidemiology holds significant importance in veterinary medicine for several reasons:

   - **Evidence-Based Decision-Making:** It provides a scientific basis for understanding the causes of diseases. This, in turn, helps in making evidence-based decisions regarding disease prevention and control measures (Haimerl et al. 2013).
   - **Disease Intervention:** It aids in pinpointing the factors contributing to disease occurrence and spread. This information is vital for developing targeted interventions, control measures, and management practices (Salman 2009b).

- **Evaluating Interventions:** It plays a key role in assessing the effectiveness of interventions such as vaccines, treatments, and management practices. By conducting analytical studies, veterinary epidemiologists can determine whether these interventions are achieving their desired outcomes (Nuvey et al. 2022).
- **Preventing Outbreaks:** It is valuable in identifying high-risk factors and populations. This knowledge can be instrumental in preventing disease outbreaks and ensuring the health and well-being of animal populations (Morse et al. 2012; Halasa et al. 2020; Todd 2020).

2) **Cohort Studies:** Cohort studies are a vital method in analytical epidemiology, particularly when researchers aim to study the long-term effects of exposures on disease outcomes (Bhopal 2016a). These studies involve following a group of animals with a common exposure over time to assess how that exposure affects their health.
3) **Statistical Modeling:** Statistical modelling is a powerful method in analytical epidemiology that involves the use of mathematical and statistical techniques to analyze data and assess the relationships between risk factors and disease outcomes (Grassly and Fraser 2008; Yadav and Akhter 2021). These models enable researchers to quantify the strength of associations and make predictions about disease occurrence. In the context of veterinary epidemiology, statistical modelling plays a crucial role in understanding and managing diseases. Here's an example:

1.2.2 Causation and Association

Causation in veterinary epidemiology involves establishing a cause-and-effect relationship between a particular factor (exposure) and a disease outcome. It implies that the factor is responsible for the occurrence of the disease (Thrusfield et al. 2018). Demonstrating causation is a complex process that requires thorough investigation and adherence to specific criteria.

Association, on the other hand, signifies a statistical relationship between a factor (exposure) and a disease outcome. An association does not necessarily imply causation. While an association suggests that there is a connection between the factor and the disease, it could be due to various factors, including confounding variables or chance (Koepsell and Weiss 2009; Thrusfield et al. 2018).

Veterinary epidemiologists employ various criteria to assess causation, helping distinguish true causation from mere association. Some of these criteria include:

1) **Temporality:** The exposure must precede the disease outcome in time. This criterion ensures that the exposure is a potential cause rather than a result of the disease. For example, if vaccination against a specific disease precedes a decrease in disease incidence, this suggests a temporal relationship (Dohoo et al. 2009).
2) **Strength of Association:** A strong association between the exposure and the disease outcome is more suggestive of causation. A weak association is less likely to be causal. The strength of association is often quantified using measures like the relative risk or odds ratio (Dohoo et al. 2009; Shimonovich et al. 2021).
3) **Dose-Response Relationship:** A dose-response relationship implies that as the level or intensity of exposure increases, the risk of the disease outcome also increases (Kilcoyne et al. 2013; Pettygrove 2016). For example, if higher levels of pesticide exposure are associated with a higher incidence of a specific health condition in domestic dogs and their owners (Wise et al. 2022), this suggests a dose-response relationship.
4) **Consistency:** Consistency means that the observed association is consistent across different studies and populations. If multiple studies in various settings consistently show an association between a factor (e.g., a specific toxin) and a disease (e.g., toxic-related symptoms), it adds strength to the argument for causation (Gad 2024).

1.2.3 Population Approach

The population approach in veterinary epidemiology is centred on the health and well-being of entire animal populations, rather than just individual cases (Bhopal 2016b). It recognizes that the health of a group of animals is influenced by a complex interplay of factors and that controlling diseases at the population level is often more effective in preventing and managing health issues (Dohoo et al. 2009). This approach emphasizes preventive measures and interventions that benefit the larger population.

Reasons for the Population Approach in Veterinary Epidemiology:
The population approach is crucial in veterinary epidemiology for several reasons:

1) **Disease Control:** The population approach is instrumental in controlling the spread of diseases within animal populations. By focusing on entire groups of animals, epidemiologists can implement strategies that reduce the risk of disease outbreaks and minimize the associated economic losses (Salman 2009b).

2) **Preventive Measures:** The population approach places a strong emphasis on preventive measures, including vaccination campaigns, biosecurity measures, and surveillance systems (Salman 2009a). These measures are vital for maintaining and improving the health of animal populations by reducing the risk of disease introduction and spread.
3) **Public Health:** Many diseases that affect animals are zoonotic, meaning they can be transmitted to humans. Controlling these diseases in animal populations is essential for safeguarding public health. Preventing zoonotic diseases at the population level reduces the risk of human infection (Rahman et al. 2020).

1.3 Aims and Scope of Veterinary Epidemiology

The main goal of Veterinary Epidemiology is to gain insights into how animal diseases spread and what factors contribute to their occurrence as well as how they evolve. This knowledge plays a role in devising measures for preventing, controlling, and eradicating diseases. Veterinary Epidemiology covers a range of areas including diseases, zoonoses (diseases that can be transmitted between animals and humans) population dynamics, and the impact of environmental factors on animal health. It also delves into the ramifications of diseases on both animal industries and society. Veterinary Epidemiology is a field for comprehending, averting, and managing animal diseases. Its extensive scope and interdisciplinary approach offer insights into disease patterns, transmission dynamics, and risk factors. Applying principles researchers and practitioners contribute towards enhancing animal health, public health, and the sustainability of animal industries (Noah 2023).

1.3.1 Surveillance of Animal Diseases

Monitoring animal diseases involves continuous tracking as well as gathering data about the occurrence, distribution, and characteristics of diseases within populations of animals. This comprehensive process serves as a tool for disease management and control by enabling the detection of outbreaks by analyzing disease trends promptly and developing well-informed strategies to mitigate the impact, on both animal welfare and human health (Drewe et al. 2011). Surveillance encompasses components such as gathering data, analyzing information, detecting early signs, assessing trends, and risks reporting findings, and facilitating communication (Drewe et al. 2011).

1.3.1.1 Types of Surveillance
- **Passive Surveillance**
  Passive surveillance relies on the reporting of disease cases by veterinarians, farmers, or diagnostic laboratories. It is a process that provides data without the need for specific data collection efforts.
- **Active Surveillance**
  Active surveillance involves efforts to collect data often focusing on target populations or regions. This method is particularly useful for monitoring diseases or populations at risk.
- **Syndromic Surveillance**
  Syndromic surveillance emphasizes monitoring signs or symptoms rather than confirmed disease diagnoses. It plays a role in the detection of emerging diseases and can be implemented in real-time surveillance systems.

1.3.1.2 Monitoring Disease Outbreaks
Monitoring and managing animal disease outbreaks is important in veterinary medicine. By monitoring and promptly responding to these outbreaks, we can effectively prevent the spread of diseases and safeguard both animal and human populations. To monitor animal disease outbreaks systematically and comprehensively, a multi-faceted approach is adopted involving surveillance to gather and analyze data on disease occurrences while also investigating suspected cases (Drewe et al. 2011). Various sources of information are used, including laboratory tests, clinical observations, and reporting systems. These tools help veterinarians and public health officials spot patterns and trends making it easier to detect diseases early and respond appropriately (Drewe et al. 2011).

Furthermore, advancements in technology have revolutionized disease monitoring. Geographical Information Systems (GIS) are employed to map the occurrence of diseases, helping identify high-risk areas. Additionally, modern techniques like Polymerase Chain Reaction (PCR) have improved capabilities, enabling accurate detection of pathogens. By monitoring and working together collaboratively we can protect the well-being of animals and human health while minimizing the impact of disease outbreaks on our society (Drewe et al. 2011).

1.3.1.3 Identifying Emerging Diseases

Emerging diseases are novel infectious diseases that have recently appeared or are increasing rapidly in frequency. Identifying and understanding these diseases is crucial for prevention, control, and management (Drewe et al. 2011). A comprehensive approach is needed to address these challenges. Firstly, surveillance systems play a role in detecting emerging diseases. Early identification allows for responses and containment measures. Effective surveillance involves monitoring disease patterns and analysing data thoroughly while promptly reporting any trends or outbreaks. Secondly, laboratory diagnostics are essential for identifying and characterizing emerging diseases (Drewe et al. 2011). Cutting-edge technologies and methodologies are utilized to identify pathogens or genetic material which greatly assists in the diagnosis of diseases and conducting investigations. However, scientists, healthcare professionals, and policymakers must collaborate and share information. International cooperation, research networks, and open data platforms play a role in facilitating the exchange of knowledge and expertise thus enabling a response to emerging diseases (Salman 2009a). Adopting an approach encompassing surveillance, diagnostics, and collaboration is essential for recognizing and comprehending emerging diseases (Salman 2009). By remaining vigilant and fostering cooperation among nations we can effectively combat these threats to global health.

1.3.2 Disease Control and Prevention

In the field of epidemiology, disease control, and prevention play a role. It is crucial to have strategies in place to manage outbreaks and ensure the well-being of animals and humans. Disease control and prevention are important for maintaining the health of animal populations with vaccination programs and quarantine measures being components (Perez 2015). These strategies not only help contain the spread of diseases but also prevent the emergence of ones.

1.3.2.1 Vaccination Programs

Vaccination is an aspect of disease control. Its purpose is to protect animals against diseases. Vaccination programs offer benefits from safeguarding animals to protecting entire populations. The basic idea behind vaccination is to stimulate an animal system so that it develops resistance against pathogens. This is achieved by introducing an inactive version (or sometimes just a part) of the pathogen into the animal's body. As a result, the immune system produces a targeted response, including creating memory cells that "remember" the pathogen. This enables a more efficient response if the animal encounters the pathogen, in the future (Robertson 2020).

Hence vaccination programs play a role, in controlling and preventing diseases. It is crucial to customize vaccination programs according to the needs of animal populations, known as targeted strategies. This involves considering factors such as disease prevalence, population density, and the vulnerability of species. The primary objective of any vaccination program is to cover the targeted population or achieve herd immunity (Robertson 2020). Herd immunity occurs when a sufficient proportion of the population becomes immune reducing the transmission of agents and safeguarding individuals. Understanding vaccination principles, including vaccine selection and administration protocols is vital for achieving success (Robertson 2020).

1.3.2.2 Quarantine Measures

On the other hand, quarantine measures are another aspect of disease control in veterinary epidemiology. They are typically implemented when there is suspicion or confirmation of a disease outbreak within a population (Drewe et al. 2011). During the quarantine period, infected animals are isolated from ones throughout the incubation phase (Robertson 2020). This also applies to animals before introducing them to an existing population. These measures aim to prevent disease spread and allow time for interventions to be implemented. These interventions may include testing, treatment options, and in cases where necessary, euthanasia (Drewe et al. 2011).

The successful implementation of quarantine measures depends on adherence, to protocols. These guidelines involve identifying animals at risk, providing isolation facilities, and closely monitoring for signs of illness. Since many infectious diseases are global, it is crucial to have cooperation for the implementation of quarantine measures. This includes sharing information between countries following protocols and enabling trade with risk of disease transmission (Drewe et al. 2011).

Controlling and preventing diseases requires a collaborative approach. This involves maintaining surveillance, implementing targeted vaccination programs, and enforcing quarantine measures (Robertson 2020). These combined efforts contribute to the health and well-being of animal populations. By adhering to these principles veterinary professionals can effectively address the challenges posed by agents thus safeguarding the health of both animals and humans (Robertson 2020).

1.3.3 Research and Investigation

In the field of epidemiology conducting research and thorough investigations are crucial for understanding diseases. This extensive exploration focuses on the methods used to study disease outbreaks and pinpoint risk factors. It sheds light on the role these activities play in controlling and preventing diseases well as studying health conditions that affect animal populations (Drewe et al. 2011).

The essence of research in this field lies in comprehending the patterns, causes, and impacts of health and disease conditions within groups of animals. It is essential for gaining insights into diseases and implementing control measures. Through research, we unravel the complexities of disease dynamics, identify factors that contribute to risks, and develop targeted interventions. This empirical approach enhances our ability to protect animal populations, preserve biodiversity, and mitigate threats that can be transmitted between animals and humans. In our pursuit of knowledge, veterinary epidemiological research serves as a cornerstone for ensuring the well-being of both animals and humans in an interconnected world.

On the other hand, investigation in Veterinary Epidemiology involves an examination of disease outbreaks, to control them effectively while preventing their recurrence. Employing investigation techniques can help determine the cause behind an outbreak, understand its mode of transmission, and identify steps to prevent future incidents.

1.3.3.1 Investigating Disease Outbreaks

Investigating outbreaks of diseases in the field of epidemiology is a process that plays a vital role in controlling diseases. Epidemiologists employ methodologies to trace the origin, transmission pathways, and factors contributing to outbreaks. This relies on a surveillance system that constantly monitors and gathers data on animal populations allowing for detection of abnormalities in disease patterns (Drewe et al. 2011). Advanced diagnostic tools help identify pathogens quickly aiding in intervention. Epidemiological studies, such as case-control analyses provide insights into the dynamics of outbreaks. These investigations are crucial for devising targeted interventions and preventive measures to ensure the health and resilience of animal populations when faced with challenges (Salman 2009).

1.3.3.2 Identifying Risk Factors

Identifying risk factors is a pursuit in epidemiology to understand disease dynamics better. Systematic assessments involve scrutinizing elements like animal demographics, environmental variables, and management practices to pinpoint sources of disease (Perez 2015). In-depth, case-control studies meticulously compare unaffected groups to determine the variables contributing to disease outbreaks and devise interventions (Robertson 2020). Spatial and temporal analyses reveal patterns and correlations that shed light on risk factors while enhancing our understanding of disease spread. Mapping the distribution of cases over space and time provides insights into dynamics aiding in identifying environmental or geographical risk factors (Thrusfield and Christley 2018).

In addition, it is crucial to highlight the significance of reservoirs and vector surveillance as their role extends beyond the primary host species. To effectively identify transmission pathways and implement measures that disrupt the disease cycle it becomes essential to conduct thorough surveillance of potential reservoirs and vectors (Thrusfield and Christley 2018). This meticulous investigation provides insights for professionals enabling them to develop targeted interventions that proactively mitigate risks and safeguard the health of animal populations (Robertson 2020).

1.4 Methods in Veterinary Epidemiology

1.4.1 Data Collection

Introduction: Data collection in veterinary epidemiology is defined as gathering, recording, and analyzing information about animal health and diseases. The data collection procedure is an integral part of animal population health studies; hence, it is critical for comprehending disease dynamics and developing effective health management strategies (Drewe et al. 2011).

Scope and Relevance: Traditional data collection activities include everything from documenting individual disease cases to conducting large-scale surveys. However, recent trends in data management and information technology have upscaled the process to include database management, big data analysis, machine learning, data simulation, and mathematical modelling (Drewe et al. 2011). Ultimately, gathering and analyzing data in veterinary epidemiology is critical for identifying disease patterns, comprehending epidemiological trends, and making sound decisions in animal health management. Some of the importance of data collection include the following.

1) **Surveillance and Early Detection:** In veterinary epidemiology, data collection enables continuous surveillance of animal health; thereby, helping in identifying and tracking disease trends over time. Continuous monitoring is critical for the early detection of emerging or re-emerging diseases. Additionally, real-time data collection is crucial for understanding the spread and severity of the disease, especially in cases of an outbreak (Perez 2015). Information garnered can often guide the immediate response, including quarantine measures, vaccination campaigns, and other control strategies (Salman 2009).
2) **Understanding Disease Dynamics**: Data collection helps veterinary epidemiologists to understand the nitty-gritty of a disease outbreak, right from the first observable clinical sign to all prevention and control strategies deployed to contain the outbreak (Perez 2015). Furthermore, the collected data can also be deployed to predict and prevent future outbreaks.
3) **Research and Policy Development**: Data collected from a disease investigation can serve as a critical resource for epidemiological research and the development of public health policies while also helping to improve veterinary clinical practices (Salman 2009).

1.4.2 Methods of Data Collection

1.4.2.1 Case Reporting
Case Reporting: In the field of veterinary epidemiology, case reporting serves as a vital mechanism for understanding and managing animal health and disease outbreaks. It involves the systematic documentation of individual animal disease cases by veterinarians or animal health workers, as well as all treatment and control strategies deployed to handle the disease. Timely documentation of cases is essential for the early detection of disease outbreaks; hence, enabling quick and effective response measures to mitigate the spread (Drewe et al. 2011).

Furthermore, case reports offer invaluable insights into the progression and characteristics of diseases within individual animals and populations. Case reporting can be mandatory in cases of diseases with significant public health or economic implications, with specific reporting pattern platforms from national and international regulations while voluntary reporting albeit not legally required is critical for tracking emerging diseases or less common health issues. Consequently, mandatory reporting ensures the systematic tracking of major diseases, whereas voluntary reporting is critical for identifying emerging health threats (Drewe et al. 2011).

Often, case data is entered into specialized databases or disease registries with the use of electronic systems or epidemiological software. Subsequently, data access report data is analyzed to determine disease trends, patterns, and potential outbreak hotspots (Drewe et al. 2011). This information is critical for epidemiological research, disease control strategies, vaccination programs, and public health policies. accuracy and completeness are critical, necessitating regular data quality checks and validation procedures (Robertson 2020).

1.4.2.2 Sampling
Sampling: Sampling forms a crucial part of data collection in veterinary epidemiology, offering insights into disease prevalence, risk factors, and the overall health status of animal populations. It involves taking a sizable number of animals from the overall population; especially since it is difficult to conduct any reasonable study with the whole animal population (Thrusfield and Christley 2018).

Principles of Sampling Design: The first step in survey design is to clearly define the objectives. This includes determining what information is needed, such as disease prevalence, risk factors, or general health indicators. The strength of any survey is to represent the population of interest as much as possible, it is therefore critical to select the appropriate target population (Drewe et al. 2011). This decision affects the survey results' relevance and applicability to the general population. Various data collection methods, ranging from questionnaires and interviews to physical examinations and laboratory testing, can be used depending on the survey objectives. Additionally, effective execution necessitates meticulous planning, which includes logistics coordination, resource allocation, and personnel training (Robertson 2020).

Overview of Sampling Methods

Random Sampling: In this method, every member of the population has an equal chance of being included in the sample. This method is ideal for obtaining a representative sample.

Stratified Sampling: The population is divided into subgroups (strata), and samples are taken from each subgroup. This method is useful when the population is diverse, and the researcher is interested in specific subgroups.

Cluster Sampling: Used when random sampling is impractical or costly. The population is divided into clusters (like farms or regions), and a sample of clusters is selected (Drewe et al. 2011).

The choice of sampling technique depends on the objectives of the survey, the nature of the population, and the resources available. Selecting the appropriate sampling method is crucial to minimizing bias and ensuring the representativeness of the sample.

Challenges in Conducting Sampling: Determining the right sample size and achieving a high response rate are fundamental for obtaining reliable results. Additionally, ensuring the accuracy and quality of the data collected is a significant challenge, requiring rigorous methodology and careful data handling. Some sampling in remote locations can suffer logistical challenges due to poor accessibility and limited resources. Since sampling in veterinary epidemiology often requires direct and invasive contact with the animals, they must be conducted ethically, respecting the welfare of animals and the rights of owners (Drewe et al. 2011).

Conclusively, sampling is an indispensable tool in veterinary epidemiology, providing essential data for understanding and managing animal health. Despite the challenges, a well-designed and executed sampling, coupled with appropriate techniques, yields invaluable insights that drive effective disease control strategies and inform public health policies. The success of these endeavours' hinges on meticulous planning, execution, and overcoming the various challenges inherent in the process (Drewe et al. 2011).

Challenges of Data Collection in Veterinary Epidemiology

While data collection is essential in veterinary epidemiology, it is fraught with various challenges and considerations. This section explores the logistical hurdles, resource constraints, and issues related to data quality and integrity that researchers and practitioners face in the field.

Access to Populations: Accessing animal populations in remote or underserved areas poses significant logistical challenges due to geographical barriers, lack of infrastructure, and limited accessibility (Drewe et al. 2011).

Resource Constraints: Budget constraints can constrain the breadth and depth of data collection efforts. This frequently has an impact on the equipment's quality, the number of personnel, and the scope of the study. Skilled personnel are required for efficient data collection. Shortages of trained veterinarians, epidemiologists, and data analysts can stymie these efforts significantly (Drewe et al. 2011). A lack of sophisticated technological tools for data collection, analysis, and storage can also be a constraint.

To conduct an efficient sampling despite the challenge, the veterinary epidemiologist must follow the following steps:

Ensuring Accuracy and Reliability: Potential reporting and sampling biases such as selection bias, reporting bias, and measurement bias must be identified and mitigated. Hence, implementing data validation and cross-verification procedures is critical for maintaining accuracy and reliability (Drewe et al. 2011).

Data Management and Security: Data management entails organizing, storing, and maintaining data in a way that allows it to be easily retrieved and analyzed. It is critical to ensure the security and confidentiality of collected data, especially when dealing with sensitive information (Drewe et al. 2011). This includes secure storage, restricted access, and compliance with data protection laws and regulations.

Ethical Issues in Data Collection: A major ethical concern is ensuring the welfare of animals during data collection. This includes reducing distress and following ethical research practices. In cases where data collection requires interaction with animal owners or caregivers, informed consent is required.

Legal Compliance: It is critical to follow local, national, and international regulations governing animal research and data protection. Legal considerations extend to the sharing and publication of collected data, ensuring that it is done legally and ethically.

1.4.3 Statistical Analysis

1.4.3.1 The Importance of Statistical Analysis

In the field of veterinary epidemiology, data are continuously generated from case reports to survey results and beyond. Hence, making sense of this data necessitates a robust, albeit technical, approach, which statistical analysis provides. Statistical methods in veterinary epidemiology perform several important tasks:

- **Interpreting Data**: Statistics provide the tools to extract meaning from numbers, whether it's understanding the prevalence of a disease in a population or the efficacy of a new vaccine (Drewe et al. 2011).
- **Unveiling Patterns and Trends**: Statistical analysis, in addition to interpretation, is critical in uncovering hidden patterns and trends within data. It enables epidemiologists to see beyond the obvious, revealing variations that would otherwise go unnoticed.
- **Establishing Relationships**: Identifying relationships between variables is one of the most important roles of statistical analysis. For example, understanding how environmental factors influence disease spread or the impact of genetic predispositions on health outcomes can be assessed by some statistical techniques.
- **Informing Decision-Making:** Statistical analysis influences real-world animal health management decisions and strategies, ranging from local farm interventions to national disease control strategies.
- **Enhancing Disease Surveillance and Response**: Accurate statistical analysis strengthens disease surveillance systems, allowing for faster and more effective responses to outbreaks, emerging health threats, and disease control policies (Thrusfield and Christley 2018).

Key Statistical Methods and Their Applications

Several statistical methods are used in veterinary epidemiology, each tailored to different types of data and research questions. These methods are more than just analytical tools; they are how complex data is made understandable and actionable.

Descriptive Statistics:
- **Purpose**: These are the most basic statistics used to describe and summarize the basic characteristics of data sets. Additionally, descriptive statistics provide a quick overview of the data, allowing a snap-short detail about the datasets.
- **Common Measures:** In statistical analysis, it is common to find averages (means), which show central trends, medians (central values), and modes (most common values). Additionally, variability can also be measured through range (difference between extremes) and standard deviation (extent of data dispersion), which give you a full picture of how the data is distributed.
- **Uses**: Descriptive statistics are frequently used as the first step in data analysis, providing a broad picture of disease occurrence, treatment efficacy, or animal population health (Drewe et al. 2011).

Inferential Statistics:
- **Purpose**: Based on a sample of data, inferential statistics are used to draw conclusions or make predictions about a population. These methods are critical for determining the likelihood that findings are due to chance.
- **Key Techniques:** In epidemiology, hypothesis testing, confidence intervals, and regression analysis help to draw meaningful conclusions from samples within populations and show how variables are related. These methods enhance understanding of data patterns and underpin robust, evidence-based conclusions in public health research.
- **Uses:** inferential statistics help researchers conclude disease rates, risk factors, and the effectiveness of interventions in a larger population, not just from the specific data samples they study.

Multivariate Analysis:
- **Purpose**: Multivariate analysis is essential when dealing with complex data involving multiple variables. It enables the investigation of the concurrent effects of multiple variables.
- **Techniques Used**: Methods such as multiple regression analysis, factor analysis, and cluster analysis fall under this category.
- **Uses:** Multivariate analysis is used to investigate complicated connections, like how different genetic, environmental, and behavioural factors work together to affect the spread of a disease or the effectiveness of treatment.

1.4.3.2 Variables

Variables are measurable factors that play pivotal roles in the field of veterinary epidemiology, as they are essential factors utilized to investigate the patterns of health and disease within animal populations. Variables can be demographic factors such as age, breed, and sex; environmental factors such as climate and housing, as well as genetic factors, can influence animal health and diseases. Other factors that influence the transmission and control of diseases are behavioural patterns, the characteristics of pathogens, and management practices. These variables collectively contribute to the comprehension and control of animal health and disease by epidemiologists, which is crucial for the preservation of both animal and public health (Drewe et al. 2011).

Types of Variables:

- **Categorical Variables**: These include nominal variables (e.g., breed, gender) and ordinal variables (e.g., disease severity scored as mild, moderate, or severe). Analyzing these often involves chi-square tests, logistic regression, or non-parametric tests like Kruskal-Wallis (Drewe et al. 2011).
- **Continuous Variables**: These are numeric variables that can take any value within a range (e.g., age, weight). These variables can be analyzed using linear regression, ANOVA, and Pearson's correlation are typically used.
- **Discrete Variables**: These are count variables, such as the number of cases of a disease in a population. Poisson regression and other count data models are appropriate for discrete variables (Drewe et al. 2011).
- **Time-to-Event Variables:** These are very important in survival analysis (for example, how long it takes to get better or die). These variables can be analyzed using Cox proportional hazards models and Kaplan-Meier curves.

Choosing the Right Statistical Test:

- **Match Test to Variable Type**: The type of variable dictates the statistical test. For instance, comparing the means of a continuous variable across groups requires a t-test, or ANOVA, while comparing the proportions of a categorical variable requires a chi-square test (Dohoo et al. 2010).
- **Consideration of Data Distribution**: The choice of parametric or non-parametric tests depends on whether the data distribution meets certain assumptions, like normality (Dohoo et al. 2010).

Application of Statistics in Veterinary Epidemiology

1) Disease Prevalence and Incidence Analysis

   Descriptive Statistics: Fundamental descriptive statistical methods, such as the computation of means and rates, are crucial in comprehending the prevalence (the proportion of a population affected at a specific point in time) and incidence (the occurrence of new cases over a given period) of diseases. The acquisition of this data is crucial to assess the magnitude and dissemination of diseases within animal populations (Drewe et al. 2011).

   Application in Surveillance Programs: These calculations are integral to disease surveillance and monitoring programs. They help in identifying trends, assessing the impact of interventions, and planning future control measures.

2) Risk Factor Analysis

   Regression Analysis: Sophisticated regression methodologies, such as logistic regression and multivariate regression models, are utilized to ascertain and measure risk factors. This entails the examination of how various factors, such as age, breed, and environmental conditions, influence the occurrence and frequency of diseases.

   Application in Intervention Strategies: The identification of risk factors is crucial for developing targeted interventions. For instance, if a particular breed is found to be at higher risk for a disease, specific health monitoring protocols can be developed.

3) Epidemiological Modeling

   Logistic and Poisson Regression Models: These models have proven to be highly valuable in the prediction of disease outbreaks and the comprehension of infection dynamics. A framework is offered by these models to assess the likelihood of disease incidences and the anticipated quantity of cases (Dohoo et al. 2010).

   Resource Allocation and Policy Making: Predictive models are critical in informing resource allocation during outbreaks and guiding policy development for disease prevention.

4) Survival Analysis

   Cox Proportional Hazards Model: The model is extensively employed in the field of veterinary epidemiology to conduct time-to-event analyses. The measurement of time until an event, such as death or disease occurrence, plays a significant role in studying disease progression and evaluating the impact of treatments (Thrusfield and Christley 2018).

Application in Clinical Trials and Longitudinal Studies: Survival analysis is particularly important in clinical trials and longitudinal studies, where understanding the time dynamics of disease is crucial.

5) Data Quality and Management

Handling Missing Data and Biases: Sophisticated statistical techniques are utilized to tackle challenges such as incomplete data, inaccuracies in measurements, and biases in reporting. These methodologies are implemented to ascertain the dependability and credibility of the study's outcomes (Oyama et al. 2018).

Data Management Strategies: Effective data management, including robust data cleaning and validation techniques, is crucial for accurate statistical analysis. This ensures the integrity and reliability of epidemiological data.

6) Advanced Statistical Methods

Multivariate Analysis and Data Reduction: Methods such as principal component analysis (PCA) and factor analysis are commonly employed to mitigate the complexity of data and discern latent patterns within extensive datasets.

Machine Learning in Epidemiology: The advent of machine learning and artificial intelligence has introduced new possibilities in data analysis, from pattern recognition in large datasets to predictive modelling.

Ethical Considerations in Data Analysis

Ethical Implications of Data Use: The ethical considerations in the use of epidemiological data are paramount, especially when they influence public health policies and animal welfare decisions.

Transparency and Accountability: Ensuring transparency in methodology and interpretation is essential for maintaining the integrity of epidemiological research. This includes acknowledging limitations and potential biases in statistical methods.

Challenges and Future Directions in Statistical Analysis

Complex Data Sets: The increasing complexity of epidemiological data, including genomic and environmental data, requires sophisticated statistical approaches for accurate interpretation.

Advancements in Technology: The integration of advanced technologies like big data analytics and bioinformatics poses both challenges and opportunities. These technologies enable the handling of large, complex datasets but also demand advanced statistical expertise (Thrusfield et al., 2018).

Zoonotic Diseases: The rise of zoonotic diseases, which transfer between animals and humans, underscores the importance of robust statistical analysis in identifying risk factors and transmission patterns.

Global Health Challenges: Climate change, globalization, and changing land use patterns are contributing to emerging health challenges. Statistical analysis is crucial in modelling these changes and predicting their impact on animal and human health.

Data Visualization and Communication

Why visualization is important: Using good visualization techniques is a key part of turning complicated statistical results into formats that are easy to understand. This encompasses the utilization of graphical representations, diagrams, and interactive visual aids (Thrusfield et al., 2018).

Communicating Findings: Clear communication of statistical findings is essential for informing public health decisions, policy formulation, and community engagement.

1.4.3.3 Statistical Software and Tools in Veterinary Epidemiology

Software Applications: Efficient data analysis is facilitated through the utilization of specialized statistical software packages. Prominent software tools encompass R, SAS, and SPSS, each presenting distinct functionalities tailored to various forms of analysis (Thrusfield et al., 2018).

Emerging Tools: The development of new software and applications, including those incorporating machine learning and AI, is enhancing the capabilities of epidemiologists in data analysis and interpretation.

1.4.3.4 Spatial and Temporal Analysis in Veterinary Epidemiology

Introduction: Veterinary epidemiology is the study of how diseases spread in animals over large and small areas of land and time. This section provides a comprehensive examination of the intricate aspects of these analyses, including their methodologies, applications, and implications for the comprehension and management of animal health and disease dynamics.

Fundamentals of Spatial Analysis in Epidemiology

Defining Spatial Analysis: Spatial analysis in veterinary epidemiology primarily focuses on the investigation of the geographic patterns and dissemination of diseases within animal populations. The objective of this study is to investigate the impact of geographical elements, including topography, climate, and interactions between humans and animals, on the patterns of diseases (Ward 2007). Geographic Information Systems (GIS) and spatial statistics play a pivotal role in this analysis by facilitating the visualization and examination of data concerning its geographical context (Ward 2007).

Spatial Data Types and Sources: Spatial data in the field of veterinary epidemiology is commonly obtained from a wide range of sources, encompassing veterinary clinics, wildlife surveys, remote sensing techniques, and public health records (Ward 2007). The data can be classified into three categories: point data, area data, and continuous data. Point data refers to exact locations; area data represents data aggregated over specific regions, and continuous data denotes data that exhibit continuous variation across space (Ward 2007).

Spatial Statistics and Modeling Techniques: Key techniques in spatial statistics include point pattern analysis, cluster detection (e.g., Ripley's K-function), and spatial autocorrelation (e.g., Moran's I). These methods help identify disease clusters and hotspots. Spatial modelling involves creating predictive models of disease spread, incorporating factors like animal movement patterns, environmental conditions, and sociodemographic factors (Thrusfield and Christley 2018).

Temporal Analysis in Epidemiology: Temporal analysis is a field of study that focuses on comprehending the development and chronology of diseases. This entails the identification of patterns, fluctuations based on seasons, and possible cyclic patterns associated with diseases. Additionally, methods such as time-series analysis and epidemic curve analysis are utilized to monitor the occurrence of diseases over a period and evaluate the effectiveness of interventions (Ward 2007).

Analyzing Time-to-Event Data in Veterinary Studies: In epidemiology, survival analysis, which includes tools like Kaplan-Meier estimators and Cox proportional hazards models, is very important for looking at time-to-event data (Annibale Biggeri et al. 2016). This analysis helps in understanding the duration until an event (e.g., recovery, death, disease outbreak) occurs. These techniques are particularly relevant in longitudinal studies, where individual animals or populations are monitored over extended periods (Ward 2007).

Combining Spatial and Temporal Dimensions: The integration of spatial and temporal data enables a comprehensive understanding of disease dynamics. The application of spatio-temporal analysis allows for the examination of the evolving patterns of diseases across different periods and geographical areas (Annibale Biggeri et al. 2016). Hence, to forecast the dissemination of diseases and their spatial and temporal interactions, researchers utilize spatio-temporal models such as Bayesian hierarchical models and spatio-temporal autocorrelation models.

Applications in Real-World Epidemiology: The utilization of spatio-temporal analysis is a common approach in veterinary epidemiology case studies, as it allows for the examination of outbreaks, disease progression, and the assessment of control measures' efficacy. These analyses play a crucial role in shaping public health policies by identifying high-risk areas and periods, facilitating the efficient allocation of resources, and enabling proactive measures to be taken in anticipation of potential future outbreaks.

Emerging Techniques and Tools: The utilization of sophisticated spatial analysis techniques, such as machine learning algorithms and artificial intelligence, has become more prevalent in disease studies for pattern recognition and predictive modelling. The utilization of remote sensing technologies and satellite imagery enables the acquisition of extensive spatial data with high resolution, thereby augmenting the potential for conducting comprehensive epidemiological investigations on a large scale (Pfeiffer and Stevens 2015).

Challenges in Spatio-Temporal Analysis: The examination of spatio-temporal data is inherently intricate, necessitating advanced statistical techniques and computational resources (Annibale Biggeri et al. 2016). The challenges encompassed in this domain consist of effectively managing extensive datasets, resolving data quality concerns, and navigating the intricate nature of integrating spatial and temporal components. The accurate understanding of spatio-temporal data and models is of utmost importance, as incorrect interpretations can result in ineffective or detrimental disease control strategies (Annibale Biggeri et al. 2016).

Ethical Implications: The ethical aspects related to data privacy, confidentiality, and the responsible utilization of predictive models should be considered when dealing with spatial and temporal data in the field of veterinary epidemiology. Maintaining privacy and promoting public health are crucial considerations when utilizing data, particularly when it pertains to specific geographical areas or sensitive information.

Implementing Analysis in Field Settings: The implementation of spatial and temporal analysis in field studies necessitates meticulous planning of data collection, which entails considering various factors, including sampling strategies, geographical coverage, and temporal resolution (Annibale Biggeri et al. 2016). The translation of the findings obtained from these analyses into implementable strategies necessitates effective communication with various stakeholders, encompassing policymakers, veterinarians, and the broader public.

Global Disease Monitoring and Epidemiological Networks: Spatial and temporal analysis are of utmost importance in the field of global health, as they serve as vital tools for monitoring transboundary and zoonotic diseases. It facilitates comprehension of the patterns of disease transmission across various countries and continents (Pfeiffer and Stevens 2015). Epidemiological networks and global surveillance systems depend on these analyses to monitor the spread of diseases, anticipate areas at risk of outbreaks, and facilitate international collaboration in response initiatives (Annibale Biggeri et al. 2016).

One Health Approach and Integrative Analysis: Spatial and temporal analysis greatly enhances the efficacy of the One Health approach, which acknowledges the interdependence of human, animal, and environmental health. By incorporating data from various domains, a comprehensive comprehension of the dynamics of health and disease is attained. In this context, the utilization of spatial and temporal analysis can effectively elucidate the interconnections between different domains, such as the influence of environmental degradation on disease patterns, specifically the heightened risk of zoonotic diseases.

Adapting to Emerging Diseases and Climate Change: As the emergence of novel diseases and the evolution of existing ones are influenced by various factors, such as climate change and habitat alteration, it becomes imperative for spatial and temporal analysis to undergo adaptation and evolution (Oyama et al. 2018). This entails the integration of novel data sources and modelling methodologies to comprehend the evolving dynamics. The integration of climate change projections into predictive models can offer significant value in terms of anticipation and preparedness for future disease risks.

Technological Advancements and Data Integration: Technological advancements have been consistently contributing to the progress of spatial and temporal analysis, encompassing enhanced Geographic Information System (GIS) tools, advanced modelling software, and increased computational capabilities to effectively manage large datasets (Pfeiffer and Stevens 2015). The incorporation of emerging data sources, such as mobile phone data, social media analytics, and citizen science initiatives, presents novel prospects for comprehending and controlling the dissemination of diseases.

Developing Expertise in Spatial and Temporal Analysis: The increasing demand for focused training programs and workshops aimed at veterinary epidemiologists and public health professionals is driven by the recognition of the distinct expertise necessary for spatial and temporal analysis. Collaborative research endeavours and partnerships among academic institutions, governmental entities, and international organizations have the potential to foster the exchange of knowledge and the development of expertise in these analytical methodologies (Oyama et al. 2018).

Promoting interdisciplinary collaboration: The resolution of intricate health issues through the utilization of spatial and temporal analysis necessitates the establishment of interdisciplinary cooperation, which involves the integration of knowledge and skills from various fields such as epidemiology, geography, environmental science, and data science. The establishment of collaborative environments and networks that facilitate the cooperation of professionals from various disciplines is crucial for the progress of applying these analyses in the field of veterinary epidemiology (Thrusfield and Christley 2018).

Informing Policy and Public Health Decision Making: The utilization of spatial and temporal analysis yields invaluable insights that can effectively inform the development of public health policies and facilitate decision-making processes (Thrusfield and Christley 2018). These factors have the potential to guide the allocation of resources, planning for emergency responses, and formulating long-term strategies for disease control. It is imperative to establish communication and collaboration with policymakers and public health officials to effectively convey intricate analytical findings in a comprehensible and practical manner, which is essential for the successful management of diseases.

1.4.4 Modelling and Simulation

1.4.4.1 Definition and Purpose of Modeling and Simulation in Veterinary Epidemiology

Modelling and simulation in veterinary epidemiology constitute a powerful approach to understanding the dynamics of diseases within animal populations (de Jong 1995). At its core, modelling involves the creation of mathematical or computational representations that simulate the complexities of disease spread, providing valuable insights into potential outcomes and facilitating evidence-based decision-making (Keeling and Rohani 2008). Simulation, on the other hand, involves the execution of these models to mimic real-world scenarios, allowing researchers to observe and analyze the behaviour of diseases under various conditions (Huang et al. 2010). An example of this is discussed by Premashthira et al. (2011) on models simulating FMD outbreaks under different control strategies and the use of spatial analysis to evaluate FMD spread and control outcomes. The primary purpose of modelling and simulation in veterinary epidemiology is to enhance our understanding of disease dynamics, predict future trends, and assess the effectiveness of control measures (Kirkeby et al. 2021; Zohdi 2023). By creating virtual representations of disease processes, researchers can explore hypothetical scenarios, identify risk factors, and design targeted interventions, ultimately contributing to the improvement of animal health, public health, and economic outcomes (Rushton 2008; Huang et al. 2010; Kirkeby et al. 2021).

1.4.4.2 Historical Evolution and Significance

The use of models and simulations in veterinary epidemiology has evolved, parallel to advancements in computational technologies and epidemiological methodologies (Kirkeby et al. 2021). Early models were often simplistic, focusing on basic disease spread patterns. With the advent of more sophisticated computational tools, models have become increasingly complex, incorporating a range of factors such as animal demographics, environmental conditions, and intervention strategies (Keeling and Rohani 2008; Jalali et al. 2021).

Historical Milestones:
- **Pre-computational Era:** Initial models were theoretical and lacked computational capabilities, relying on mathematical equations to represent disease dynamics (Kopec et al. 2012; Chen 2014).
- **Computational Era:** The introduction of computers in the mid-twentieth century enabled the development of more intricate models, allowing for simulations and the consideration of multiple variables. This era saw an increased focus on simulating real-world scenarios and incorporating a broader range of variables (Chen 2014; Deichmann 2019; Anon 2023).
- **Interdisciplinary Integration:** Modern models benefit from collaboration between epidemiologists, statisticians, and computer scientists, fostering a multidisciplinary approach to problem-solving. This interdisciplinary approach ensures that models are both scientifically robust and practically applicable (Chen 2014; Deichmann 2019; Overton et al. 2020; Anon 2023).

Modelling and simulation have significantly contributed to the advancement of veterinary epidemiology by providing a platform to test hypotheses, refine theories, and guide empirical research. They offer a complementary perspective to traditional epidemiological methods, allowing for the exploration of complex systems that may be challenging to study directly.

1.4.4.3 Relationship with Traditional Epidemiology

Modelling and simulation do not replace traditional epidemiology but rather complement it, offering a set of tools to address specific challenges and questions. Traditional epidemiology relies on observational studies, field investigations, and statistical analyses to understand disease patterns and risk factors. In contrast, modelling provides a synthetic environment where researchers can manipulate variables and observe outcomes under controlled conditions.

Complementary Roles:
- **Traditional Epidemiology:** Observes and analyzes real-world data, identifies associations, and generates hypotheses (Frérot et al. 2018).
- **Modeling and Simulation:** Tests hypotheses, predicts future scenarios, and assesses the impact of interventions in a controlled environment (Zohdi 2023).

By integrating both approaches, researchers can leverage the strengths of each to gain a more comprehensive understanding of disease dynamics, ultimately contributing to improved animal and public health outcomes.

1.4.4.4 Mathematical Modeling

Mathematical modelling in veterinary epidemiology involves the use of mathematical equations to represent the dynamics of disease spread within animal populations. These models provide a quantitative framework for understanding, predicting, and controlling diseases (Dohoo et al. 2009).

Overview of Mathematical Models:
- **Differential Equations:** Many mathematical models in veterinary epidemiology are expressed as systems of differential equations. These equations describe how the number of animals in different disease compartments changes over time (Keeling and Rohani 2008; Fournié et al. 2011).

- **Agent-Based Models:** Another approach involves individual-based or agent-based models, where each animal is represented individually, allowing for a more detailed exploration of interactions (Fournié et al. 2011; Roche et al. 2011; Lanzas and Chen 2015).

Types of Mathematical Models:

Deterministic versus Stochastic Models:
- **Deterministic Models:** These models assume that the future is entirely determined by the current state of the system. They are characterized by fixed parameters and produce a single predicted outcome for a given set of initial conditions. They are well-suited for scenarios where the population structure and disease parameters are well-defined and stable (Keeling and Rohani 2008; Brauer et al. 2019).
- **Stochastic Models:** In contrast, stochastic models incorporate randomness into the modelling process. They account for uncertainties in disease transmission, making them suitable for scenarios where chance plays a significant role. They are useful when uncertainties and random events play a significant role, reflecting the inherent variability in disease transmission (Keeling and Rohani 2008; Brauer et al. 2019).
- **Compartmental Models (e.g., SIR Models):** Compartmental models divide the population into compartments based on disease status. One of the most widely used compartmental models is the Susceptible-Infectious-Recovered (SIR) model (Keeling and Rohani 2008; Brauer et al. 2019).

Deterministic versus Stochastic Models in Veterinary Epidemiology:

Example: In a deterministic model of avian influenza spread, the transmission rate between susceptible and infectious birds remains constant. In a stochastic model, this rate may vary, reflecting the inherent randomness in disease transmission (Rao and Upadhyay 2013).

Compartmental Models (e.g., SIR Models): Compartmental models classify individuals into compartments based on their disease status. The SIR model, for instance, includes compartments for susceptible (S), infectious (I), and recovered (R) individuals (Keeling and Rohani 2008; Brauer et al. 2019; Hunter and Kelleher 2022).

Application to Veterinary Epidemiology: In a poultry population facing an outbreak of avian influenza, the SIR model can depict how the number of susceptible birds decreases over time as more become infected, leading to an increase in the recovered compartment (Malek and Hoque 2022).

Advantages and Limitations: Compartmental models simplify complex systems but may overlook individual-level variations. They are valuable for gaining insights into disease dynamics and assessing the impact of interventions (Siegenfeld et al. 2022).

Extensions: Models can be extended to include additional compartments (e.g., exposed, vaccinated) to capture more nuances in disease spread.

Mathematical modelling serves as a cornerstone in veterinary epidemiology, allowing researchers to explore the intricacies of disease spread, evaluate control strategies, and contribute to evidence-based decision-making.

1.4.4.5 Predictive Modelling

Predictive modelling in veterinary epidemiology involves the use of advanced mathematical and computational techniques to anticipate and forecast future disease patterns based on historical data, current conditions, and relevant parameters (Halasa et al. 2020). The primary goal is to move beyond understanding past trends and instead predict future disease patterns, allowing for proactive and strategic decision-making in disease prevention and control.

Techniques and Approaches:

Time Series Analysis: Time series analysis is a fundamental tool in predictive modelling, involving the examination of data collected over successive time intervals to identify patterns and trends (Montgomery et al. 2015). In veterinary epidemiology, time series analysis is crucial for understanding the seasonality of diseases, identifying periodic patterns, and making predictions based on historical data (Ward et al. 2020; Punyapornwithaya et al. 2022).

Machine Learning Algorithms: Machine learning algorithms, a subset of artificial intelligence, have gained prominence in predictive modelling. These algorithms can identify complex patterns within large datasets and make predictions based on learned patterns (Sarker 2021; Rahman et al. 2023; Santangelo et al. 2023; Taye 2023). In veterinary epidemiology, machine learning is employed to analyze diverse data sources, including animal health records, climate data, and demographic information. Machine learning models can handle complex interactions between variables and adapt to changing conditions (Gouda et al. 2022; Guitian et al. 2023). For instance, ensemble methods like Random Forests can integrate information from diverse sources, providing robust predictions.

Spatial Modeling: Predictive modelling often incorporates spatial components, especially in diseases with geographical variations. Spatial models consider the spatial distribution of cases, environmental factors, and host populations to predict disease spread and identify high-risk areas.

Benefits:

- **Early Warning Systems:** Predictive models contribute to early detection by highlighting potential disease hotspots before outbreaks occur (Meckawy et al. 2022).
- **Resource Allocation:** These models assist in optimizing resource allocation by directing interventions to areas at higher risk of disease occurrence (Ren et al. 2022).

Challenges and Considerations:

Data Quality and Availability: The effectiveness of predictive models depends largely on the quality and availability of data; incomplete or inaccurate data can undermine the accuracy of predictions (Nugroho 2023).

Dynamic Nature of Diseases: Veterinary diseases often exhibit dynamic characteristics influenced by various factors (Roberts et al. 2021). Predictive models must adapt to changing conditions and incorporate real-time data for accurate predictions.

Applications of Modeling and Simulation

Disease Spread and Dynamics   Modelling and simulation play a pivotal role in veterinary epidemiology, particularly in understanding the spread and dynamics of diseases within animal populations. This section explores the diverse applications of modelling and simulation in deciphering transmission patterns and evaluating control measures.

Understanding Transmission Patterns:

1) **Transmission Dynamics Modeling:** Transmission dynamics models, such as compartmental models (e.g., SIR - Susceptible, Infected, Recovered), are instrumental in simulating how diseases propagate through animal populations over time (Keeling and Rohani 2008).
2) **Spatial Spread Modeling:** Spatial models assess how diseases move geographically, aiding in identifying high-risk areas and understanding the impact of spatial factors on transmission (White et al. 2018; Lin and Wen 2022).

Evaluating Control Measures:

1) **Vaccination Strategies:** Modeling allows the assessment of different vaccination scenarios, including target populations, vaccination coverage, and timing, to optimize strategies for disease prevention (Nuraini et al. 2021; Ferreira et al. 2022).
2) **Biosecurity Measures:** Simulation models assess the impact of biosecurity measures, such as quarantine and movement restrictions, on disease spread and provide insights into their efficacy (Léger et al. 2017).
3) **Antimicrobial Usage Impact:** Simulation models explore the consequences of antimicrobial use on disease dynamics, considering factors like resistance development and treatment efficacy (Li et al. 2017; Hillock et al. 2022).

Challenges and Considerations:

1) **Data Requirements:** Obtaining accurate and comprehensive data for model input remains a challenge, and model outcomes are only as reliable as the data used for calibration and validation (Li and Mahadevan 2016).
2) **Complexity versus Simplicity Trade-off:** Striking a balance between model simplicity and complexity is essential, as overly intricate models may require extensive data and computational resources (Aragonés et al. 2006).

Public Health and Zoonotic Disease Modeling

In veterinary epidemiology, modelling and simulation play an important role in safeguarding public health, particularly concerning zoonotic diseases. Zoonotic diseases, which can be transmitted between animals and humans, necessitate a comprehensive understanding of their dynamics to assess risks and formulate effective intervention strategies.

Assessing Risks to Human Health: Modeling and simulation serve as indispensable tools for assessing the risks posed to human health by zoonotic diseases (Rees et al. 2021; Esposito et al. 2023). These models consider various factors, such as the prevalence of the disease in animal populations, the nature of human-animal interactions, and environmental influences (Rees et al. 2021). For instance, in the case of avian influenza, models may evaluate the potential for transmission from birds to humans, taking into account factors like migratory patterns, poultry farming practices, and genetic variations in the virus (Millman et al. 2015). This assessment aids in quantifying the risk of disease spillover and informs preventive measures.

Intervention Strategies: The application of modelling in public health extends to the development and evaluation of intervention strategies for managing zoonotic diseases. Models can simulate different scenarios to assess the impact of various interventions, such as vaccination campaigns, changes in animal husbandry practices, or enhanced surveillance measures (Sims 2013). For example, in the context of a zoonotic disease transmitted from livestock to humans, a model may explore the efficacy of vaccinating specific animal populations or implementing biosecurity measures on farms (Carpenter et al. 2022). These simulations provide valuable insights into the potential outcomes of different strategies, enabling policymakers to make informed decisions on the most effective interventions to safeguard public health.

The integration of modelling and simulation in the domain of public health and zoonotic disease modelling offers a robust framework for risk assessment and intervention planning. By providing insights into the dynamics of diseases that can affect both animals and humans, these models contribute to the development of proactive measures aimed at preventing and mitigating the impact of zoonotic diseases on public health.

Decision Support Systems

In the context of veterinary epidemiology, the integration of modelling and simulation culminates in the development and deployment of Decision Support Systems (DSS). These systems represent a sophisticated application of computational models designed to assist stakeholders, policymakers, and veterinary professionals in making informed decisions regarding disease prevention, management, and control.

Supporting Policy and Management Decisions: DSS in veterinary epidemiology serve as invaluable aids in the formulation of policies and the execution of effective management strategies. These systems assimilate vast datasets, leveraging mathematical models to simulate various scenarios and project potential outcomes (Lanzas and Chen 2015). This aids decision-makers in understanding the consequences of different interventions, resource allocations, or policy implementations. For example, in the context of a contagious livestock disease outbreak, a DSS may simulate the impact of different culling strategies, vaccination campaigns, or movement restrictions (Capon et al. 2021). Decision-makers can then use these simulations to identify the most effective and ethically sound strategies to mitigate the spread of the disease. The development and utilization of DSS not only underscore the synergy between modelling and real-world applications but also mark a paradigm shift in veterinary epidemiology (Ezanno et al. 2020). These systems provide a dynamic platform for evidence-based decision-making, allowing stakeholders to navigate the complexities of disease control with a better understanding of potential outcomes.

Technological Advances: The landscape of DSS continues to evolve with advancements in technology. Integration with artificial intelligence, machine learning algorithms, and real-time data streams enhances the capabilities of these systems (Xu et al. 2021). The ability to adapt to changing conditions, incorporate emerging data, and provide timely insights positions DSS as dynamic tools in the arsenal of veterinary epidemiologists.

The integration of modelling and simulation into DSS represents a pinnacle in the evolution of veterinary epidemiology. By providing decision-makers with the ability to explore diverse scenarios and assess the potential impact of interventions, these systems contribute significantly to the development of robust, effective, and ethically sound strategies for disease prevention and control.

Challenges and Limitations in Modeling and Simulation in Veterinary Epidemiology

Modelling and simulation have become indispensable tools in veterinary epidemiology, offering valuable insights into disease dynamics and informing decision-making processes. However, like any scientific approach, they come with inherent challenges and limitations that warrant careful consideration (Reeves et al. 2011; Heesterbeek et al. 2015).

Data Limitations and Quality: One of the primary challenges in veterinary epidemiological modelling is the availability and quality of data. Accurate simulations rely on robust datasets, including information on disease prevalence, environmental factors, and animal demographics (Mazzucato et al. 2023). In many cases, data may be incomplete, outdated, or subject to biases. Addressing this challenge requires ongoing efforts to enhance data collection methods, promote data sharing across institutions, and invest in surveillance systems that provide real-time, high-quality information for robust modelling.

Complexity and Assumptions: Modeling real-world scenarios in veterinary epidemiology often involves simplifications and assumptions to make simulations computationally feasible. The challenge lies in striking the right balance between model complexity and usability. Overly complex models may lead to challenges in interpretation, while overly simplistic models may fail to capture the intricacies of disease dynamics (Lanzas and Chen 2015). Researchers and modellers must be transparent about the assumptions made and continually validate models against real-world data to ensure their accuracy and reliability.

Ethical Considerations: The use of modelling and simulation in public health raises ethical considerations (Bak 2022), particularly when decisions based on these models have significant implications for animals, ecosystems, and human populations (Kiani et al. 2022). Ethical challenges may include the potential for unintended consequences, the allocation of resources based on model predictions, and the impact on stakeholders, including farmers, policymakers, and the public (Brock and Wikler 2006). Ensuring transparency in modelling methodologies, engaging stakeholders in the modelling process, adhering to ethical guidelines, and prioritising transparency to build trust in the modelling outcomes are crucial in navigating these challenges.

Adaptive Modeling and Advances: As challenges emerge, ongoing advancements in modelling techniques and technologies offer solutions. Adaptive modelling, incorporating real-time data, allows for dynamic adjustments to changing circumstances. Machine learning algorithms and artificial intelligence contribute to refining models and overcoming some data limitations (Aldoseri et al. 2023). Collaborative efforts among researchers, veterinarians, and policymakers ensure a multidisciplinary approach to tackling challenges and continuously improving modelling practices.

Future Trends

Modelling and simulation in veterinary epidemiology are poised for exciting developments, driven by emerging trends that promise to enhance the precision and scope of these tools.

Integration of Molecular Epidemiology: The integration of molecular epidemiology into veterinary modelling is a transformative trend with substantial implications for disease control (Muellner et al. 2011). Molecular techniques, such as whole-genome sequencing and phylogenetic analysis, allow researchers to trace the genetic evolution of pathogens (Brown 2002; Quainoo et al. 2017). This not only enhances our ability to identify sources and transmission routes but also aids in predicting potential mutations that could affect virulence or resistance to interventions. For example, in the context of antimicrobial resistance in veterinary medicine, molecular epidemiology can provide insights into the genetic mechanisms behind resistance, guiding more effective strategies for prudent antibiotic use (Palma et al. 2020).

Moreover, the integration of molecular data enables the development of spatiotemporal models that incorporate genetic information (Clegg et al. 2011; Muellner et al. 2011; Chen et al. 2016; Camilo et al. 2021). This allows researchers to map the spread of specific pathogen strains with unprecedented precision. Understanding the genetic diversity within pathogen populations becomes crucial for tailoring control measures, such as vaccines, to the circulating strains, thereby optimizing their effectiveness. The future holds the promise of a comprehensive One Health approach, where genomic data from animals, humans, and the environment are integrated to offer a unified understanding of disease dynamics and transmission pathways (Chakraborty and Barbuddhe 2021; Waddington et al. 2022; Djordjevic et al. 2023).

Advancements in Computational Power: The relentless progress in computational power is reshaping the landscape of veterinary epidemiology. High-performance computing not only facilitates the execution of more sophisticated models but also enables the handling of vast datasets (Espinal-Enríquez et al. 2017) generated by molecular and spatial technologies. This evolution empowers researchers to conduct detailed simulations that consider various scenarios and factors influencing disease dynamics.

Furthermore, advancements in machine learning algorithms are enhancing the predictive capabilities of models. Machine learning techniques, such as neural networks and deep learning, can discern complex patterns within data, uncovering novel insights that may not be apparent through traditional modelling approaches (Alowais et al. 2023). These technologies hold immense potential for identifying subtle relationships between variables, predicting emerging disease trends, and optimizing intervention strategies.

As computational power becomes more accessible, the democratization of modelling tools is underway. User-friendly interfaces and cloud-based platforms enable a broader community (Bachmann et al. 2022), including veterinary practitioners and policymakers, to engage with modelling and simulation. This democratization fosters collaboration and knowledge exchange, democratizing the benefits of modelling beyond academic and research settings (Shum et al. 2012).

Interdisciplinary Collaboration: Interdisciplinary collaboration (Seidl 2015; Ribeiro et al. 2019) emerges as a critical trend, acknowledging that the intricate challenges of veterinary epidemiology require diverse expertise (Grant et al. 2016). For example, understanding the dynamics of vector-borne diseases necessitates collaboration between entomologists, ecologists, and epidemiologists (Høye et al. 2021). Integrating ecological factors, such as habitat changes or climate variations, into models enhances their predictive accuracy (Beugnet and Chalvet-Monfray 2013; Caminade et al. 2019; Rocklöv and Dubrow 2020; Jabeen et al. 2022; Mojahed et al. 2022). By combining insights from diverse fields, researchers can develop more holistic models that account for the interconnected factors influencing disease transmission. This collaborative approach not only enriches the modelling process but also contributes to a more comprehensive understanding of the intricate relationships between animals, their environments, and the pathogens they harbour.

Public health researchers contribute valuable insights, especially in zoonotic disease modelling. Collaboration between veterinary and human health experts ensures a unified understanding of diseases that affect both animals and humans (Degeling et al. 2015; Prata et al. 2022; Sharan et al. 2023). This holistic approach considers the interconnectedness of ecosystems and recognizes that disease emergence and transmission transcend disciplinary boundaries.

Moreover, interdisciplinary collaboration (Seidl 2015; Ribeiro et al. 2019) extends to stakeholder engagement. Involving farmers, policymakers, and local communities in the modelling process enhances the relevance and applicability of models. This participatory approach not only integrates local knowledge but also fosters a sense of ownership and responsibility (Gonsalves et al. 2005) for disease control measures.

1.5 Components of Veterinary Epidemiology

The study of veterinary epidemiology is crucial for understanding and addressing animal health challenges as well as ensuring food safety and protecting human health from zoonotic diseases. In this section, we will explore the components of veterinary epidemiology that lay the foundation for comprehending and managing these health concerns. By monitoring diseases, veterinary epidemiology helps identify patterns using the concept of "agent, host, and environment." This approach examines risk factors, and transmission pathways, and enables the development of control strategies (National Research Council 2013).

1.5.1 Agent, Host, and Environment

In veterinary epidemiology, it is essential to grasp the dynamic interplay between agents (disease-causing factors) hosts (animals affected by these factors), and the environment in which they interact. These three components form the core pillars on which disease transmission study and prevention are based. A comprehensive understanding of agents, hosts, and their environment known as the Triad of disease causation plays a role in exploring their roles and interactions within veterinary epidemiology.

1.5.1.1 Triad of Disease Causation
The triad of disease causation is a fundamental concept in the field of veterinary epidemiology. It is also known as the epidemiologic triangle, which consists of three key components that interact to determine the occurrence and transmission of diseases in animal populations. Understanding these elements is crucial for veterinarians and epidemiologists in analyzing and managing disease outbreaks.

Disease Causation Triad: The concept of the epidemiological triad of disease is fundamental and well-established in veterinary epidemiology. The "Triad of Disease Causation" suggests that the interaction of three key factors—the agent, the host, and the environment—causes diseases. Consequently, understanding the dynamics of these components can greatly aid in disease management and control in animal populations. We can look at these components.

Firstly, the agent is an important component of the triad since it represents the actual cause of the disease. Agents, in most cases, refer to the microorganism or pathogen that causes the disease condition. Hence, they include many organisms, including bacteria, prions, viruses, parasites, fungi, and other entities that can cause diseases. Various factors, including how a disease spreads, its strength, and its ability to adapt to different surroundings all play a role in the cause of the disease. Pathogenicity (the ability to make people sick), virulence (the severity of the illness caused), infectivity (the ability to infect others), and immunogenicity (the ability to make the immune system react) are all ways to measure how well an agent can make people sick. Furthermore, understanding the agent's properties, lifecycle, and modes of transmission is critical for developing disease prevention and control strategies. For example, knowing how a virus replicates and attaches to the host cells can aid in developing antiviral drugs or vaccines (Perez 2015).

Secondly, the host is the biological organism attached to the agents. The host refers to the animal species that can be affected by a disease. The host-agent relationship is critical to the occurrence and progression of the disease. Various host factors, such as genetic makeup, age, sex, nutritional status, and immune system competence, all play a role in disease dynamics. These factors can influence the host's susceptibility to the agent and the course of the disease. Additionally, the natural behaviour and reaction of the host to the presence of an agent can also have a significant impact on the disease transmission dynamics within and between populations. Most hosts often move from one place to another and can play an important role in the geographical spread of disease. A typical example is migratory birds, which often move hundreds of kilometres and spread agents such as avian influenza viruses. Different species may have genetic and physiological factors that influence their susceptibility to specific diseases. For example, certain dog breeds may be more prone to developing types of cancer while certain bird species may be more vulnerable to avian influenza. Additionally, factors such as age, sex, and overall health status can also play a role in determining an animal's susceptibility to diseases (Carlson et al. 2022).

Thirdly, the environment includes all external factors that affect the interaction between the host and the agent. These factors include physical factors such as temperature, rainfall, and humidity and biological factors such as the presence of other animals or vectors. Recently, management and socioeconomic factors, such as the availability of veterinary services, as well as management practices, such as hygiene and housing conditions, have been included in the environmental context. The environment can help or hinder the agents' ability to spread and cause diseases, including persistence and survival outside the host, and affect the host's susceptibility and recovery. For example, favourable environmental conditions such as wet and warm climates can promote the spread of mosquito-borne diseases such as malaria in animals. The environment also includes social factors such as animal population density, animal movement/trade, and human behaviours that contribute to the spread of diseases.

To make effective plans to stop, control, or eliminate diseases in veterinary epidemiology, we need to have a deep understanding of these triads. A comprehensive approach considering agent, host, and environmental factors allows for a more nuanced understanding of disease dynamics, ultimately benefiting animal and public health.

1.5.1.2 Ecological Perspectives

Ecological Perspectives: In veterinary epidemiology, the ecological perspective of diseases focuses on how the agent, the host, and the environment interact in complex ways. It encourages a complete understanding of how diseases spread in ecological systems. These perspectives can arise through interaction between the disease triads or ecological balance in nature. Veterinary epidemiologists also utilize ecological perspectives to gain a comprehensive understanding of disease dynamics. The concept of interaction is central to ecological perspectives. It highlights the multidimensional exchanges between the agent, host, and environment. These interactions are important in determining the onset, spread, and manifestation of diseases within animal populations. The interaction can be an agent-host **interaction**, which defines the host's susceptibility and response to the agent. This interaction includes the mechanisms of infection, host immune responses, and sequala of diseases (Escobar 2020).

Another one is the **agent-environment interaction**, where the environment, as previously mentioned, can have a significant impact on the agent's survival, proliferation, and transmission. Certain pathogens, for example, may thrive in specific environmental conditions, such as warm, humid climates, or may require specific vectors for transmission. Lastly, the **host-environment interaction** is also important since the environment can influence the host's susceptibility to disease. This can be done by modifying the physiology, behaviour, and pattern of host exposure to agents. Typically, environmental stressors such as extreme temperatures and precipitation can impair the host's immune system, making it more susceptible to infections.

The simultaneous interaction of agent, host, and environment is a complex dynamic that frequently defines disease epidemiological patterns. Understanding this three-way interaction is critical for forecasting disease outbreaks and developing effective control strategies. For example, the concept of the "One Health" approach acknowledges the interconnectedness between animal and environmental health. This approach emphasizes the importance of collaboration and communication across fields to tackle complex health challenges. By embracing the One Health perspective veterinary epidemiologists acknowledge that diseases affecting animals can have consequences for human health and vice versa (Escobar 2020). This comprehensive viewpoint guides the development of integrated strategies that not only safeguard animal populations but also protect public health (Gibb et al. 2020).

Balance: Balance emphasizes the equilibrium or disequilibrium states that can mitigate or exacerbate disease occurrence among the agent, host, and environment. When there is a balance, the system may exhibit a stable state in which diseases occur at a predictable, often manageable level. For example, endemic diseases can persist at a low level without causing major outbreaks (Escobar 2020).

A disequilibrium state, which often results from changes in one or more of the triad components, can disrupt the balance, resulting in disease outbreaks. These can result from introducing a new, virulent agent, changes in host population density, or adverse environmental changes. Understanding and pursuing a balance among the three components can be an important strategy in veterinary epidemiology (Gibb et al. 2020).

Animal disease prevention strategies may include interventions aimed at reducing the virulence of the agent, improving host resistance, or changing the environment to prevent disease transmission. Veterinary epidemiologists can better understand how complicated disease systems are by looking at them from an ecological point of view. This understanding helps them develop more effective and long-lasting ways to stop and control diseases.

1.5.2 Disease Transmission

Understanding disease transmission modes is critical in veterinary epidemiology because it informs the design of disease prevention and control strategies in animal populations. In the field of epidemiology, a crucial aspect revolves around comprehending how diseases are transmitted. By investigating the mechanisms through which infectious agents propagate, veterinary professionals can develop strategies to control and prevent their dissemination. Transmission modes are broadly classified as direct and indirect transmission (Benson et al. 2021).

1.5.2.1 Direct Transmission

Direct Transmission: A direct transfer of infectious agents from an infected host to a susceptible host occurs without the involvement of intermediaries. This is a common transmission mode for diseases that spread through close or physical contact (Lange et al. 2016). The following are some examples of direct transmission mechanisms: Diseases can be spread through touch or contact with bodily fluids. Skin-to-skin contact, for example, can spread ringworm infections among animals. **Droplet Transmission:** Respiratory droplets released by an infected host while coughing or sneezing can transmit pathogens to a susceptible host. Droplet transmission spreads diseases such as influenza and kennel cough in dogs (Filippitzi et al. 2017). Vertical transmission occurs when a mother passes her genes to her offspring, either in utero, during birth, or through breastfeeding. The bovine leukaemia virus, for example, can be passed from infected cows to their calves via milk. Pathogens can be introduced into the host's body directly through bites, scratches, or other skin or mucous membrane penetration (Benson et al. 2021).

1.5.2.2 Indirect Transmission

Indirect Transmission: When an infectious agent is transferred to a susceptible host via an intermediary agent or a specific vehicle, this is called indirect transmission. Susceptible hosts can inhale infectious agents transported in dust or droplet nuclei suspended in the air. In birds, diseases such as aspergillosis are frequently transmitted via airborne transmission. In **waterborne pathogen transmission,** pathogens can spread through contaminated water. Waterborne transmission of diseases such as leptospirosis is common in various animal species (Lange et al. 2016). Additionally, **foodborne disease transmission** is seen when animals consume contaminated food which can result in the transmission of diseases such as salmonellosis to animals. **vector-borne transmission** is seen where pathogens can be transferred from an infected host to a susceptible host via insects or other vectors. For instance, mosquito bites spread heartworm disease. Inanimate objects or materials, such as bedding, feeders, or surgical instruments, can harbour pathogens and aid in their transmission to susceptible hosts. Lastly, **soilborne transmission** is common where pathogenic organisms in soil can infect animals when they encounter or ingest the contaminated soil (Benson et al. 2021).

1.5.3 Risk Factors

Risk factors are characteristics or exposures that increase the likelihood of the occurrence of a disease in an animal population. Risk factors encompass a range of influences that contribute to the occurrence and spread of diseases. Understanding these risk factors is critical for veterinary epidemiologists when predicting and managing outbreaks of diseases (Oyama et al. 2018). These factors are broadly classified as biological and environmental:

Biological Factors: Biological factors are characteristics of the host that are either inherent or acquired thereby influencing their susceptibility or response to infectious agents (Cappai et al. 2018). **Genetic** predispositions are the genetic makeup of an animal which can greatly influence its susceptibility to certain diseases. For example, due to their genetic backgrounds, certain dog breeds are more prone to specific genetic disorders or diseases. Also, **the age** of an animal can impact its immune competence and infection susceptibility. Animals that are young or geriatric may have weakened immune systems, making them more susceptible to disease (Matteo Mazzucato et al. 2023). Additionally, some diseases have **sex biases** due to hormonal differences or other sex-related biological factors. For example, mammary tumours may be more common in female animals, whereas urinary blockages may be more common in male animals.

The **immune status** of the host can be changed by previous exposure to pathogens, vaccinations, or other related infections; simultaneously, it is very important in determining how susceptible and responsive they are to infectious agents (Cappai et al. 2018).

Environmental Factors: Environmental factors are outside elements that can help or hinder disease transmission and manifestation (Matteo Mazzucato et al. 2023).

Climatic conditions can impact the survival and spread of infectious agents. Warm and humid climates, for example, may favour mosquito breeding, facilitating the spread of vector-borne diseases such as heartworm disease. Likewise, **poor hygiene** can increase the risk of infection; hence, adequate cleaning and disinfection practices in animal housing facilities are critical for disease prevention (Gardner et al. 2002; Tonozzi 2022). **Management conditions** such as overcrowding, poor ventilation, and inadequate shelter can cause stress, promote the spread of infectious agents, and increase disease susceptibility (Tonozzi 2022).

1.6 Challenges and Future Trends

1.6.1 Emerging Infectious Diseases

Livestock epidemics can have significant economic, social, and welfare impacts, with emerging and re-emerging pathogens often causing localized outbreaks. Emerging infectious diseases (EIDs), such as COVID-19, MERS, anthrax, and Ebola, are rapidly spreading or newly appearing in populations. Ecological, environmental, and demographic changes increase human exposure to unfamiliar microbes, promoting disease spread. As these factors grow more prevalent, along with the evolution of pathogens and drug resistance, the emergence of new infections is likely to continue, underscoring the need for effective surveillance and control.

A large portion (60.3%) of EIDs are zoonotic, with 71.8% originating from wildlife, such as the Nipah virus in Malaysia and SARS-CoV-2 in China. The rise of wildlife-derived EIDs, now 52.0% of recent cases, highlights their growing threat to global health. Understanding the factors that increase human-wildlife contact is crucial for predicting disease emergence (Jones et al. 2008). Epidemiology focuses on analyzing the dynamics and causes of EIDs to develop strategies that prevent, mitigate, or eliminate their impact on vulnerable populations (Pfeiffer 2002).

The history of infectious diseases is marked by microbes exploiting favorable conditions to spread and thrive. The same historical processes that have led to the emergence of "new" infections continue today, now intensified by modern life. Factors driving disease emergence are more widespread, and the rapid pace of travel and global connectivity, as seen in influenza outbreaks (Morse 1995) and the recent COVID-19 pandemic, further accelerates the spread of these diseases.

Understanding the factors driving disease emergence is crucial for directing resources to the most critical areas and developing effective prevention strategies. The initial step in combating emerging diseases is establishing robust global disease surveillance systems that provide early warnings of new infections. This system should be integrated with national health efforts and supported by rapid response mechanisms. However, global surveillance capabilities are severely lacking (Morse 1995), as demonstrated by the challenges faced during the recent COVID-19 pandemic.

EIDs continue to pose a significant challenge, claiming millions of lives each year despite recent progress. New, more virulent pathogens regularly emerge due to various human, social, political, environmental, technological, microbial, and ecological factors. Addressing EID threats effectively requires anticipating these challenges, with the One Health approach offering the most comprehensive solution.

1.6.2 Data Collection and Analysis Technologies

Analysing data is complex but crucial for enhancing disease preparedness and minimizing future losses. Effective data collection, storage, and distribution are vital for epidemiological studies. Veterinary epidemiological data are collected through observation, questionnaires, and documentary sources, with observation being key. Robust database management systems, such as GIS, GPS, and remote sensing, are essential for managing and reporting data, with GIS specializing in integrating and displaying spatial information.

Advancements in information technologies are revolutionizing the collection, analysis, and sharing of animal health data, improving disease management and surveillance. Despite their potential, these technologies are underused globally for early disease detection and response. Key technologies include mobile health (mHealth) tools, wireless sensors, biosensors, crowdsourced data, and electronic health (eHealth) systems. While challenges remain, there are significant opportunities to develop these technologies for near real-time data analysis, benefiting both developing and developed countries. To better integrate animal and human health data, international data standards and mechanisms are needed, with the One Health approach enhancing coordination and disease response at the human-animal interface.

Artificial intelligence (AI), including machine learning and deep learning, is set to revolutionize veterinary epidemiology by improving predictive analytics and diagnostic performance. Unlike in human epidemiology, veterinary AI tools lack premarket screening, raising ethical and legal concerns, particularly with uncertain outcomes. Techniques like random forest use multiple classification trees to estimate variable relationships and validate predictions. AI also helps build models to explore connections between variables, such as gene expression and disease risk, and complex molecular interactions. Veterinary informatics enhances data management and analysis to improve health outcomes.

Veterinary epidemiologic informatics is a fast-evolving field that integrates information technology, communications, social and behavioural sciences, and veterinary medicine to enhance human and animal health.

1.6.3 One Health Approach

In our increasingly globalized world, health challenges are shared across humans, animals, and their environments, driven by rapid population growth and changes in farming and urbanization. These developments have led to more forest encroachment, ecosystem alterations, and closer interactions between humans, food animals, and wildlife, increasing global animal trade. This interconnectedness exposes humanity to numerous challenges that require sustainable global management. One major issue is the spread of emerging and re-emerging infectious diseases at the animal-human-environment interface, which entails significant medical, social, economic, and environmental costs. Addressing these issues effectively requires interdisciplinary and multisectoral approaches, with the One Health framework offering a comprehensive strategy for human, animal, and environmental health organizations and policymakers at local, regional, and global levels.

1.7 Conclusion

Epidemiology serves as a vital discipline in public health, encompassing a comprehensive set of principles, aims, and methodologies. Its scope extends beyond the mere study of disease occurrence to the intricate analysis of factors influencing health patterns within populations. The multifaceted components of epidemiology, from surveillance and data collection to statistical analysis and interpretation, converge to provide a holistic understanding of health phenomena. As a result, epidemiological insights not only contribute to the identification and mitigation of health threats but also inform the development of targeted interventions for disease prevention and control. This dynamic field continuously evolves to adapt to emerging challenges, employing innovative methods and technologies to enhance its effectiveness. Through its diverse applications, epidemiology remains an indispensable tool for shaping public health policies, promoting community well-being, and advancing our collective efforts to safeguard global health.

References

Aldoseri, A., Al-Khalifa, K.N., and Hamouda, A.M. (2023). Re-thinking data strategy and integration for artificial intelligence: concepts, opportunities, and challenges. *Applied Sciences* 13 (12): 7082. https://doi.org/10.3390/app13127082.

Al-Hemoud, A., AlSaraf, M., Malak, M. et al. (2021). Analytical and early detection system of infectious diseases and animal health status in Kuwait. *Frontiers in Veterinary Science* 8: 676661. https://doi.org/10.3389/fvets.2021.676661.

Alowais, S.A., Alghamdi, S.S., Alsuhebany, N. et al. (2023). Revolutionizing healthcare: the role of artificial intelligence in clinical practice. *BMC Medical Education* 23: 689. https://doi.org/10.1186/s12909-023-04698-z.

Anon 2023. Computational modeling. https://www.nibib.nih.gov/science-education/science-topics/computational-modeling (accessed 22 December 2023).

Aragonés, E., Gilboa, I., Postlewaite, A., et al. 2006. Accuracy vs. simplicity: a complex trade-off. 2006. 47 p. Working papers; https://ddd.uab.cat/record/45134 (accessed 23 December 2023).

Bachmann, N., Tripathi, S., Brunner, M., and Jodlbauer, H. (2022). The contribution of data-driven technologies in achieving the sustainable development goals. *Sustainability* 14 (5): 2497. https://doi.org/10.3390/su14052497.

Bak, M.A. (2022). Computing fairness: ethics of modeling and simulation in public health. *Simulation* 98 (2): 103–111. https://doi.org/10.1177/0037549720932656.

Benson, L., Davidson, R.S., Green, D.M. et al. (2021). When and why direct transmission models can be used for environmentally persistent pathogens. *PLoS Computational Biology* 17 (12): e1009652. https://doi.org/10.1371/journal.pcbi.1009652.

Beugnet, F. and Chalvet-Monfray, K. (2013). Impact of climate change in the epidemiology of vector-borne diseases in domestic carnivores. *Comparative Immunology, Microbiology and Infectious Diseases* 36 (6): 559–566. ISSN 0147-9571, https://doi.org/10.1016/j.cimid.2013.07.003.

Bhopal, R.S. (2016a). Epidemiological study designs and principles of data analysis: A conceptually integrated suite of methods and techniques. In: *Concepts of Epidemiology: Integrating the Ideas, Theories, Principles, and Methods of Epidemiology*, 3e (ed. R.S. Bhopal). Oxford: Oxford Academic), https://doi.org/10.1093/med/9780198739685.003.0009, (accessed 21 December 2023).

Bhopal, R.S. (2016b). The epidemiological concept of population. In: *Concepts of Epidemiology: Integrating the Ideas, Theories, Principles, and Methods of Epidemiology*, 3e (ed. R.S. Bhopal). Oxford: Oxford Academic), https://doi.org/10.1093/med/9780198739685.003.0002, (accessed 21 December 2023).

Biggeri, A., Catelan, D., Conesa, D., and Vounatsou, P. (2016). Spatio-temporal statistics: applications in epidemiology, veterinary medicine and ecology. *Geospatial Health* 11 (1): https://doi.org/10.4081/gh.2016.469.

Brauer, F., Castillo-Chavez, C., and Feng, Z. (2019). *Mathematical Models in Epidemiology*. Springer https://doi.org/10.1007/978-1-4939-9828-9.

Brock, D.W. and Wikler, D. (2006). Ethical issues in resource allocation, research, and new product development. In: *Disease Control Priorities in Developing Countries*, 2nde (ed. D.T. Jamison, J.G. Breman, A.R. Measham, et al.), 86–89. Washington (DC): The International Bank for Reconstruction and Development/The World Bank; New York: Oxford University Press.

Brown, T.A. (2002). *Genomes*, 2nde. Oxford: Wiley-Liss.

Camilo, T.A., Mendonça, L.P., dos Santos, D.M. et al. (2021). Spatial distribution and molecular epidemiology of Babesia vogeli in household dogs from municipalities with different altitude gradients in the state of Rio de Janeiro, Brazil. *Ticks and Tick-borne Diseases* 12 (5): 101785. https://doi.org/10.1016/j.ttbdis.2021.101785.

Caminade, C., McIntyre, K.M., and Jones, A.E. (2019). Impact of recent and future climate change on vector-borne diseases. *Annals of the New York Academy of Sciences* 1436 (1): 157–173. https://doi.org/10.1111/nyas.13950.

Capon, T.R., Garner, M.G., Tapsuwan, S. et al. (2021). A simulation study of the use of vaccination to control foot-and-mouth disease outbreaks across Australia. *Frontiers in Veterinary Science* 8: 648003. https://doi.org/10.3389/fvets.2021.648003.

Cappai, S., Rolesu, S., Coccollone, A. et al. (2018). Evaluation of biological and socio-economic factors related to persistence of African swine fever in Sardinia. *Preventive Veterinary Medicine* 152: 1–11. https://doi.org/10.1016/j.prevetmed.2018.01.004.

Carlson, C.J., Albery, G.F., Merow, C. et al. (2022). Climate change increases cross-species viral transmission risk. *Nature* 607: 1–1. https://doi.org/10.1038/s41586-022-04788-w.

Carpenter, A., Waltenburg, M.A., Hall, A. et al. (2022). The vaccine preventable zoonotic disease working group. vaccine preventable zoonotic diseases: challenges and opportunities for public health progress. *Vaccines (Basel)* 10 (7): 993. https://doi.org/10.3390/vaccines10070993.

Chakraborty, T. and Barbuddhe, S.B. (2021). Enabling One Health solutions through genomics. *The Indian Journal of Medical Research* 153 (3): 273–279. https://doi.org/10.4103/ijmr.IJMR_576_21.

Chen, D. (2014). Modeling the spread of infectious diseases: a review. In: *Analyzing and Modeling Spatial and Temporal Dynamics of Infectious Diseases* (ed. D. Chen, B. Moulin, and J. Wu), 19–42. Jones Wiley.

Chen, W.M., Zhou, Q.R., Wang, X.M. et al. (2016). Integration of spatial epidemiology and molecular epidemiology used for study on tuberculosis. *Zhonghua Liu Xing Bing Xue Za Zhi* 37 (12): 1683–1686. https://doi.org/10.3760/cma.j.issn.0254-6450.2016.12.024.

Clegg, S.R., Coyne, K.P., Parker, J. et al. (2011). Molecular epidemiology and phylogeny reveal complex spatial dynamics in areas where canine parvovirus is endemic. *Journal of Virology* 85 (15): 7892–7899. https://doi.org/10.1128/JVI.01576-10.

Cromley, E.K. and McLafferty, S.L. (2012). *GIS and Public Health*, 2nde. New York: Guilford Press.

Degeling, C., Johnson, J., Kerridge, I. et al. (2015). Implementing a One Health approach to emerging infectious disease: reflections on the socio-political, ethical and legal dimensions. *BMC Public Health* 15: 1307. https://doi.org/10.1186/s12889-015-2617-1.

Deichmann, U. (2019). From Gregor Mendel to Eric Davidson: mathematical models and basic principles in biology. *Journal of Computational Biology* 26 (7): 637–652. https://doi.org/10.1089/cmb.2019.0087.

Djordjevic, S.P., Jarocki, V.M., Seemann, T. et al. (2023). Genomic surveillance for antimicrobial resistance — a One Health perspective. *Nature Reviews. Genetics* 25: https://doi.org/10.1038/s41576-023-00649-y.

Doherr, M.G. and Audigé, L. (2001). Monitoring and surveillance for rare health-related events: a review from the veterinary perspective. *Philosophical Transactions of the Royal Society of London. Series B, Biological Sciences* 356 (1411): 1097–1106. https://doi.org/10.1098/rstb.2001.0898.

Dohoo, I., Martin, W., and Stryhn, H. (2009). *Veterinary Epidemiologic Research*. Prince Edward Island: VER Inc.

Dohoo, I., Martin, W. and Stryhn, H. (2010) *Veterinary Epidemiologic Research*. VER Inc., Charlottetown. Prince Edward Island, Canada.

Drewe, J.A., Hoinville, L., Cook, A.J.C. et al. (2011). Evaluation of animal and public health surveillance systems: a systematic review. *Epidemiology and Infection* 140: https://doi.org/10.1017/s0950268811002160.

Elliott, P., Wakefield, J.C., Best, N.G., and Briggs, D.J. (2000). *Spatial Epidemiology: Methods and Applications*. Oxford University Press.

Escobar, L.E. (2020). Ecological niche modeling: an introduction for veterinarians and epidemiologists. *Frontiers in Veterinary Science* 7: https://doi.org/10.3389/fvets.2020.519059.

Espinal-Enríquez, J., Mejía-Pedroza, R.A., and Hernández-Lemus, E. (2017). Chapter 13 - Computational approaches in precision medicine. In: *Progress and Challenges in Precision Medicine* (ed. M. Verma and D. Barh), 233–250. Academic Press https://doi.org/10.1016/B978-0-12-809411-2.00013-1.

Esposito, M.M., Turku, S., Lehrfield, L., and Shoman, A. (2023). The impact of human activities on zoonotic infection transmissions. *Animals (Basel)* 13 (10): 1646. https://doi.org/10.3390/ani13101646.

Ezanno, P., Andraud, M., Beaunée, G. et al. (2020). How mechanistic modelling supports decision making for the control of enzootic infectious diseases. *Epidemics* 32: 100398. https://doi.org/10.1016/j.epidem.2020.100398.

Ferreira, L.S., de Almeida, G.B., Borges, M.E. et al. (2022). Modelling optimal vaccination strategies against COVID-19 in a context of Gamma variant predominance in Brazil. *Vaccine* 40 (46): 6616–6624. https://doi.org/10.1016/j.vaccine.2022.09.082.

Filardo, G., Adams, J., and Ng, H.K.T. (2011). Statistical methods in epidemiology. In: *International Encyclopedia of Statistical Science* (ed. M. Lovric). Berlin, Heidelberg: Springer https://doi.org/10.1007/978-3-642-04898-2_547.

Filippitzi, M.E., Brinch Kruse, A., Postma, M. et al. (2017). Review of transmission routes of 24 infectious diseases preventable by biosecurity measures and comparison of the implementation of these measures in pig herds in six European countries. *Transboundary and Emerging Diseases* 65 (2): 381–398. https://doi.org/10.1111/tbed.12758.

Fournié, G., Walker, P., Porphyre, T. et al. (2011). Mathematical models of infectious diseases in livestock: concepts and application to the spread of highly pathogenic avian influenza virus strain type H5N1. *Health and Animal Agriculture in Developing Countries* 36: 183–205. https://doi.org/10.1007/978-1-4419-7077-0_11.

Frérot, M., Lefebvre, A., Aho, S. et al. (2018). What is epidemiology? Changing definitions of epidemiology 1978-2017. *PLoS One* 13 (12): e0208442. https://doi.org/10.1371/journal.pone.0208442.

Gad, S.C. (2024). Epidemiology. In: *Encyclopedia of Toxicology*, 4the (ed. P. Wexler), 313–318. Academic Press https://doi.org/10.1016/B978-0-12-824315-2.00902-7.

Gardner, I.A., Willeberg, P., and Mousing, J. (2002). Empirical and theoretical evidence for herd size as a risk factor for swine diseases. *Animal Health Research Reviews* 3 (1): 43–55. https://doi.org/10.1079/ahrr200239.

Gibb, R., Franklinos, L.H.V., Redding, D.W., and Jones, K.E. (2020). Ecosystem perspectives are needed to manage zoonotic risks in a changing climate. *BMJ* 371: https://doi.org/10.1136/bmj.m3389.

Gonsalves, J., Becker, T., Braun, A. et al. (ed.) (2005). *Participatory Research and Development for Sustainable Agriculture and Natural Resource Management: A Sourcebook. Volume 2: Enabling Participatory Research and Development*. Ottawa, Canada:

International Potato Center-Users' Perspectives With Agricultural Research and Development, Laguna, Philippines and International Development Research Centre.

Gouda, H.F., Hassan, F.A.M., El-Araby, E.E. et al. (2022). Comparison of machine learning models for bluetongue risk prediction: a seroprevalence study on small ruminants. *BMC Veterinary Research* 18: 394. https://doi.org/10.1186/s12917-022-03486-z.

Grant, C., Lo Iacono, G., Dzingirai, V. et al. (2016). Moving interdisciplinary science forward: integrating participatory modelling with mathematical modelling of zoonotic disease in Africa. *Infectious Diseases of Poverty* 5: 17. https://doi.org/10.1186/s40249-016-0110-4.

Grassly, N. and Fraser, C. (2008). Mathematical models of infectious disease transmission. *Nature Reviews. Microbiology* 6: 477–487. https://doi.org/10.1038/nrmicro1845.

Guitian, J., Arnold, M., Chang, Y., and Snary, E.L. (2023). Applications of machine learning in animal and veterinary public health surveillance. *Revue Scientifique et Technique* 42: 230–241. https://doi.org/10.20506/rst.42.3366.

Haimerl, P., Arlt, S., and Heuwieser, W. (2013). Entscheidungsfindung in der tierärztlichen Praxis [Decision making in veterinary practice]. *Tierarztliche Praxis Ausgabe K Kleintiere Heimtiere* 41 (4): 229–236.

Halasa, T., Græsbøll, K., Denwood, M. et al. (2020). Prediction models in veterinary and human epidemiology: our experience with modeling sars-CoV-2 spread. *Frontiers in Veterinary Science* 7: 513. https://doi.org/10.3389/fvets.2020.00513.

Heesterbeek, H., Anderson, R.M., Andreasen, V. et al. (2015). Modeling infectious disease dynamics in the complex landscape of global health. *Science* 347 (6227): aaa4339. https://doi.org/10.1126/science.aaa4339.

Heymann. (2015). *Control of Communicable Diseases Manual*, 20the. Washington, DC: American Public Health Association.

Hillock, N.T., Merlin, T.L., Turnidge, J. et al. (2022). Modelling the future clinical and economic burden of antimicrobial resistance: the feasibility and value of models to inform policy. *Applied Health Economics and Health Policy* 20: 479–486. https://doi.org/10.1007/s40258-022-00728-x.

Høye, T.T., Ärje, J., Bjerge, K. et al. (2021). Deep learning and computer vision will transform entomology. *Proceedings of the National Academy of Sciences* 118 (2): e2002545117. https://doi.org/10.1073/pnas.2002545117.

Huang, C.Y., Tsai, Y.S., and Wen, T.H. (2010). Simulations for epidemiology and public health education. *Journal of Simulation* 4 (1): 68–80. https://doi.org/10.1057/jos.2009.13.

Hunter, E. and Kelleher, J.D. (2022). Understanding the assumptions of an SEIR compartmental model using agentization and a complexity hierarchy. *Journal of Computational Mathematics and Data Science* 4: 100056. https://doi.org/10.1016/j.jcmds.2022.100056.

Islam, A., Islam, S., Flora, M.S. et al. (2023). Epidemiology and molecular characterization of avian influenza A viruses H5N1 and H3N8 subtypes in poultry farms and live bird markets in Bangladesh. *Scientific Reports* 13: 7912. https://doi.org/10.1038/s41598-023-33814-8.

Jabeen, A., Ansari, J.A., Ikram, A. et al. (2022). Impact of climate change on the epidemiology of vector-borne diseases in Pakistan. *Global Biosecurity* 4 (1): https://doi.org/10.31646/gbio.163.

Jalali, M.S., DiGennaro, C., Guitar, A. et al. (2021). Evolution and reproducibility of simulation modeling in epidemiology and health policy over half a century. *Epidemiologic Reviews* 43 (1): 166–175. https://doi.org/10.1093/epirev/mxab006.

Jones, K.E., Patel, N.G., Levy, M.A. et al. (2008). Global trends in emerging infectious diseases. *Nature* 451: 990–994. https://doi.org/10.1038/nature06536.

de Jong, M.C.M. (1995). Mathematical modelling in veterinary epidemiology: why model building is important. *Preventive Veterinary Medicine* 25 (2): 183–193. https://doi.org/10.1016/0167-5877(95)00538-2.

Keeling, M.J. and Rohani, P. (2008). *Modeling Infectious Diseases in Humans and Animals*. Princeton University Press. JSTOR, https://doi.org/10.2307/j.ctvcm4gk0 (accessed 21 December 2023).

Kiani, A.K., Pheby, D., Henehan, G. et al. (2022). Ethical considerations regarding animal experimentation. *Journal of Preventive Medicine and Hygiene* 63 (2 Suppl 3): E255–E266. https://doi.org/10.15167/2421-4248/jpmh2022.63.2S3.2768.

Kilcoyne, A., O'Connor, D., and Ambery, P. (ed.) (2013). Dose–response relationship. In: *Pharmaceutical Medicine*, Oxford Specialist Handbooks. Oxford: Oxford Academic https://doi.org/10.1093/med/9780199609147.003.0041, (accessed 21 December 2023).

Kim, Y.J., Park, B., and Kang, H.E. (2021). Control measures to African swine fever outbreak: active response in South Korea, preparation for the future, and cooperation. *Journal of Veterinary Science* 22 (1): e13. https://doi.org/10.4142/jvs.2021.22.e13.

Kirkeby, C., Brookes, V.J., Ward, M.P. et al. (2021). A practical introduction to mechanistic modeling of disease transmission in veterinary science. *Frontiers in Veterinary Science* 7: 546651. https://doi.org/10.3389/fvets.2020.546651.

Koepsell, T.D. and Weiss, N.S. (2009). Confounding and its control. In: *Epidemiologic Methods: Studying the Occurrence of Illness* (ed. T. Koepsell). New York: Oxford Academic, https://doi.org/10.1093/acprof:oso/9780195150780.003.0011, (accessed 21 December 2023).

Kopec, J.A., Edwards, K., Manuel, D.G., and Rutter, C.M. (2012). Advances in microsimulation modeling of population health determinants, diseases, and outcomes. *Epidemiology Research International* 2012: 584739. https://doi.org/10.1155/2012/584739.

Lange, M., Kramer-Schadt, S., and Thulke, H.-H. (2016). Relevance of indirect transmission for wildlife disease surveillance. *Frontiers in Veterinary Science* 3: https://doi.org/10.3389/fvets.2016.00110.

Lanzas, C. and Chen, S. (2015). Complex system modelling for veterinary epidemiology. *Preventive Veterinary Medicine* 118 (2–3): 207–214. https://doi.org/10.1016/j.prevetmed.2014.09.012.

Léger, A., De Nardi, M., Simons, R. et al. (2017). Assessment of biosecurity and control measures to prevent incursion and to limit spread of emerging transboundary animal diseases in Europe: an expert survey. *Vaccine* 35 (44): 5956–5966. https://doi.org/10.1016/j.vaccine.2017.07.034.

Li, C. and Mahadevan, S. (2016). Role of calibration, validation, and relevance in multi-level uncertainty integration. *Reliability Engineering & System Safety* 148: 32–43. https://doi.org/10.1016/j.ress.2015.11.013.

Li, J., Xie, S., Ahmed, S. et al. (2017). Antimicrobial activity and resistance: influencing factors. *Frontiers in Pharmacology* 8: 364. https://doi.org/10.3389/fphar.2017.00364.

Lin, C.-H. and Wen, T.-H. (2022). How spatial epidemiology helps understand infectious human disease transmission. *Tropical Medicine and Infectious Disease* 7 (8): 164. https://doi.org/10.3390/tropicalmed7080164.

Magnet, A. and Izquierdo, F. (2023). Epidemiology of wildlife infectious diseases. *Veterinary Sciences* 10 (5): 332. https://doi.org/10.3390/vetsci10050332.

Malek, A. and Hoque, A. (2022). Mathematical modeling of bird flu with vaccination and treatment for the poultry farms. *Comparative Immunology, Microbiology and Infectious Diseases* 80: 101721. https://doi.org/10.1016/j.cimid.2021.101721.

Martin, S. W., Meek, A. H., & Willeberg, P. 1987. Veterinary epidemiology: principles and methods. Originally published 1987 by Iowa State University Press I Amas.

Mazzucato, M., Marchetti, G., Barbujani, M. et al. (2023). An integrated system for the management of environmental data to support veterinary epidemiology. *Frontiers in Veterinary Science* 10: https://doi.org/10.3389/fvets.2023.1069979.

Meckawy, R., Stuckler, D., Mehta, A. et al. (2022). Effectiveness of early warning systems in the detection of infectious diseases outbreaks: a systematic review. *BMC Public Health* 22 (1): 2216. https://doi.org/10.1186/s12889-022-14625-4.

Millman, A.J., Havers, F., Iuliano, A.D. et al. (2015). Detecting spread of avian influenza A(H7N9) virus beyond China. *Emerging Infectious Diseases* 21 (5): 741–749. https://doi.org/10.3201/eid2105.141756.

Mojahed, N., Mohammadkhani, M.A., and Mohamadkhani, A. (2022). Climate crises and developing vector-borne diseases: a narrative review. *Iranian Journal of Public Health* 51 (12): 2664–2673. https://doi.org/10.18502/ijph.v51i12.11457.

Montgomery, D.C., Jennings, C.L., and Kulahci, M. (2015). *Introduction to Time Series Analysis and Forecasting*, 2nde. John Wiley & Sons, Inc.

Morse, S.S. (1995). Factors in the emergence of infectious diseases. *Emerging Infectious Diseases* 1 (1): 7–15.

Morse, S.S., Mazet, J.A., Woolhouse, M. et al. (2012). Prediction and prevention of the next pandemic zoonosis. *Lancet* 380 (9857): 1956–1965. https://doi.org/10.1016/S0140-6736(12)61684-5.

Muellner, P., Zadoks, R.N., Perez, A.M. et al. (2011). The integration of molecular tools into veterinary and spatial epidemiology. *Spat Spatiotemporal Epidemiol* 2 (3): 159–171. https://doi.org/10.1016/j.sste.2011.07.005.

National Research Council (2013). Veterinarians in wildlife and ecosystem health. In: *Workforce Needs in Veterinary Medicine*, 128–156. Washington, DC: The National Academies Press, Edited by Alan Kelly.

Nguyen, L.V., Stevenson, M., Schauer, B. et al. (2014). Descriptive results of a prospective cohort study of avian influenza in the Mekong River Delta of Viet Nam. *Transboundary and Emerging Diseases* 61 (6): 511–525. https://doi.org/10.1111/tbed.12055.

Noah, D. L. 2023. Basic principles of epidemiology. MSD Veterinary Manual. URL https://www.msdvetmanual.com/public-health/principles-of-epidemiology/basic-principles-of-epidemiology

Nugroho, H. (2023). A review: data quality problem in predictive analytics. *IJAIT International Journal of Applied Information Technology* 7 (02): 79–91. <//journals.telkomuniversity.ac.id/ijait/article/view/5980>. Date (accessed 23 December 2023). https://doi.org/10.25124/ijait.v7i02.5980.

Nuraini, N., Sukandar, K.K., Hadisoemarto, P. et al. (2021). Mathematical models for assessing vaccination scenarios in several provinces in Indonesia. *Infectious Disease Modelling* 6: 1236–1258. https://doi.org/10.1016/j.idm.2021.09.002.

Nuvey, F.S., Arkoazi, J., Hattendorf, J. et al. (2022). Effectiveness and profitability of preventive veterinary interventions in controlling infectious diseases of ruminant livestock in sub-Saharan Africa: a scoping review. *BMC Veterinary Research* 18: 332. https://doi.org/10.1186/s12917-022-03428-9.

Overton, C.E., Stage, H.B., Shazaad, A. et al. (2020). Using statistics and mathematical modelling to understand infectious disease outbreaks: COVID-19 as an example. *Infectious Disease Modelling* 5: 409–441. https://doi.org/10.1016/j.idm.2020.06.008.

Oyama, M.A., Shaw, P.A., and Ellenberg, S.S. (2018). Considerations for analysis of time-to-event outcomes subject to competing risks in veterinary clinical studies. *Journal of Veterinary Cardiology* 20 (3): 143–153. https://doi.org/10.1016/j.jvc.2018.03.001.

Palma, E., Tilocca, B., and Roncada, P. (2020). Antimicrobial resistance in veterinary medicine: an overview. *International Journal of Molecular Sciences* 21 (6): 1914. https://doi.org/10.3390/ijms21061914.

Perez, A.M. (2015). Past, present, and future of veterinary epidemiology and economics: one health, many challenges, no silver bullets. *Frontiers in Veterinary Science* 2: https://doi.org/10.3389/fvets.2015.00060.

Pettygrove, S. 2016. "dose-response relationship". Encyclopedia Britannica, 23 September, https://www.britannica.com/science/dose-response-relationship (accessed 21 December 2023).

Pfeiffer D. (2002). Veterinary epidemiology–an introduction. http://www.panaftosa.org.br/Comp/MAPA/431857.pdf accessed Dec 31, 2023.

Pfeiffer, D.U. and Stevens, K.B. (2015). Spatial and temporal epidemiological analysis in the Big Data era. *Preventive Veterinary Medicine* 122 (1–2): 213–220. https://doi.org/10.1016/j.prevetmed.2015.05.012.

Pfeiffer, D.U., Robinson, T.P., Stevenson, M. et al. (2008). *Spatial Analysis in Epidemiology*. Oxford University Press.

Prata, J.C., Ribeiro, A.I., and Rocha-Santos, T. (2022). Chapter 1 - An introduction to the concept of One Health. In: *One Health* (ed. J.C. Prata, A.I. Ribeiro, and T. Rocha-Santos), 1–31. Academic Press https://doi.org/10.1016/B978-0-12-822794-7.00004-6.

Premashthira, S., Salman, M.D., Hill, A.E. et al. (2011). Epidemiological simulation modeling and spatial analysis for foot-and-mouth disease control strategies: a comprehensive review. *Animal Health Research Reviews* 12 (2): 225–234. https://doi.org/10.1017/S146625231100017X.

Punyapornwithaya, V., Mishra, P., Sansamur, C. et al. (2022). Time-series analysis for the number of foot and mouth disease outbreak episodes in cattle farms in Thailand using data from 2010–2020. *Viruses* 14 (7): 1367. https://doi.org/10.3390/v14071367.

Quainoo, S., Coolen, J.P.M., van Hijum, S.A.F.T. et al. (2017). Whole-genome sequencing of bacterial pathogens: the future of nosocomial outbreak analysis. *Clinical Microbiology Reviews* 30 (4): 1015–1063. https://doi.org/10.1128/CMR.00016-17.

Rahman, M.T., Sobur, M.A., Islam, M.S. et al. (2020). Zoonotic diseases: etiology, impact, and control. *Microorganisms* 8 (9): 1405. https://doi.org/10.3390/microorganisms8091405.

Rahman, S.Z., Senthil, R., Ramalingam, V., and Gopal, R. (2023). Predicting infectious disease outbreaks with machine learning and epidemiological data. *Journal of Advanced Zoology* 44 (S4): 110–121. https://doi.org/10.17762/jaz.v44iS4.2177.

Rao, V.S.H. and Upadhyay, R.K. (2013). Modeling the spread and outbreak dynamics of avian influenza (H5N1) virus and its possible control. *Dynamic Models of Infectious Diseases* 2: 227–250. https://doi.org/10.1007/978-1-4614-9224-5_9.

Rees, E.M., Minter, A., Edmunds, W.J. et al. (2021). Transmission modelling of environmentally persistent zoonotic diseases: a systematic review. *The Lancet Planetary Health* 5: https://doi.org/10.1016/S2542-5196(21)00137-6.

Reeves, A., Salman, M.A., and Hill, A.E. (2011). Approaches for evaluating veterinary epidemiological models: verification, validation and limitations. *Revue Scientifique et Technique* 30 (2): 499–512. https://doi.org/10.20506/rst.30.2.2053.

Ren, J., Liu, M., Liu, Y., and Liu, J. (2022). Optimal resource allocation with spatiotemporal transmission discovery for effective disease control. *Infectious Diseases of Poverty* 11 (1): 34. https://doi.org/10.1186/s40249-022-00957-1.

Ribeiro, C.S., van de Burgwal, L.H.M., and Regeer, B.J. (2019). Overcoming challenges for designing and implementing the One Health approach: a systematic review of the literature. *One Health* 7: 100085. https://doi.org/10.1016/j.onehlt.2019.100085.

Roberts, M., Dobson, A., Restif, O., and Wells, K. (2021). Challenges in modelling the dynamics of infectious diseases at the wildlife–human interface. *Epidemics* 37: 100523. https://doi.org/10.1016/j.epidem.2021.100523.

Robertson, I.D. (2020). Disease control, prevention and on-farm biosecurity: the role of veterinary epidemiology. *Engineering* 6 (1): 20–25. https://doi.org/10.1016/j.eng.2019.10.004.

Roche, B., Drake, J.M., and Rohani, P. (2011). An Agent-Based Model to study the epidemiological and evolutionary dynamics of Influenza viruses. *BMC Bioinformatics* 12: 87. https://doi.org/10.1186/1471-2105-12-87.

Rocklöv, J. and Dubrow, R. (2020). Climate change: an enduring challenge for vector-borne disease prevention and control. *Nature Immunology* 21: 479–483. https://doi.org/10.1038/s41590-020-0648-y.

Rushton, J. (ed.) (2008). *The Economics of Animal Health and Production*. CAB International 2009.

Salman, M.D. (ed.) (2009a). *Animal Disease Surveillance and Survey Systems: Methods and Applications*. John Wiley & Sons.

Salman, M.D. (2009b). The role of veterinary epidemiology in combating infectious animal diseases on a global scale: the impact of training and outreach programs. *Preventive Veterinary Medicine* 92 (4): 284–287. https://doi.org/10.1016/j.prevetmed.2009.09.004.

Santangelo, O.E., Gentile, V., Pizzo, S. et al. (2023). Machine learning and prediction of infectious diseases: a systematic review. *Machine Learning and Knowledge Extraction* 5 (1): 175–198. https://doi.org/10.3390/make5010013.

Sarker, I.H. (2021). Machine learning: algorithms, real-world applications and research directions. *SN Computer Science* 2: 160. https://doi.org/10.1007/s42979-021-00592-x.

Seidl, R. (2015). A functional-dynamic reflection on participatory processes in modeling projects. *Ambio* 44 (8): 750–765. https://doi.org/10.1007/s13280-015-0670-8.

Sharan, M., Vijay, D., Yadav, J.P. et al. (2023). Surveillance and response strategies for zoonotic diseases: a comprehensive review. *Science in One Health* 2: 100050. https://doi.org/10.1016/j.soh.2023.100050.

Shimonovich, M., Pearce, A., Thomson, H. et al. (2021). Assessing causality in epidemiology: revisiting Bradford Hill to incorporate developments in causal thinking. *European Journal of Epidemiology* 36: 873–887. https://doi.org/10.1007/s10654-020-00703-7.

Shittu, A., Clifton-Hadley, R.S., Ely, E.R. et al. (2013). Factors associated with bovine tuberculosis confirmation rates in suspect lesions found in cattle at routine slaughter in Great Britain, 2003-2008. *Preventive Veterinary Medicine* 110 (3–4): 395–404. https://doi.org/10.1016/j.prevetmed.2013.03.001.

Shum, S.B., Aberer, K., Schmidt, A. et al. (2012). Towards a global participatory platform: democratising open data, complexity science and collective intelligence. *The European Physical Journal Special Topics 214* (1): 109–152. https://doi.org/10.1140/epjst/e2012-01690-3.

Siegenfeld, A.F., Kollepara, P.K., and Bar-Yam, Y. (2022). Modeling complex systems: a case study of compartmental models in epidemiology. *Complexity* 2022: https://doi.org/10.1155/2022/3007864.

Sims, L.D. (2013). Intervention strategies to reduce the risk of zoonotic infection with avian influenza viruses: scientific basis, challenges and knowledge gaps. *Influenza and Other Respiratory Viruses* 7 (Suppl. 2): 15–25.

Taye, M.M. (2023). Understanding of machine learning with deep learning: architectures, workflow, applications and future directions. *Computers* 2023 (12): 91. https://doi.org/10.3390/computers12050091.

Tembo, N.F.P., Muma, J.B., Hang'ombe, B., and Musso, M. (2020). Clustering and spatial heterogeneity of bovine tuberculosis at the livestock/wildlife interface areas in Namwala District of Zambia. *Veterinary World* 13 (3): 478–488. https://doi.org/10.14202/vetworld.2020.478-488.

Thrusfield, M. and Christley, R. (2018). Describing disease occurrence. In: *Veterinary Epidemiology*, 4the (ed. M. Thrusfield), 58–85. Blackwell Science Ltd https://doi.org/10.1002/9781118280249.ch4.

Thrusfield, M., Christley, R., Brown, H. et al. (2018). *Veterinary Epidemiology*, 4the. Wiley & Sons https://doi.org/10.1002/9781118280249.ch3.

Todd, E. (2020). Food-borne disease prevention and risk assessment. *International Journal of Environmental Research and Public Health* 17 (14): 5129. https://doi.org/10.3390/ijerph17145129.

Toma, B., Vaillancourt, J.-P., Dufour, B. et al. (1999). *Dictionary of Veterinary Epidemiology*. Wiley-Blackwell.

Tonozzi, C. C. (2022). Canine influenza (Flu) - respiratory system. [online] Merck Veterinary Manual. https://merckvetmanual.com/respiratory-system/respiratory-diseases-of-small-animals/canine-influenza-flu (accessed 21 December 2023).

Waddington, C., Carey, M.E., Boinett, C.J. et al. (2022). Exploiting genomics to mitigate the public health impact of antimicrobial resistance. *Genome Medicine* 14: 15. https://doi.org/10.1186/s13073-022-01020-2.

Ward, M.P. (2007). Spatio-temporal analysis of infectious disease outbreaks in veterinary medicine: clusters, hotspots and foci. *Veterinaria Italiana* 43 (3): 559–570. https://pubmed.ncbi.nlm.nih.gov/20422535/ (accessed 21 December 2023).

Ward, M.P., Iglesias, R.M., and Brookes, V.J. (2020). Autoregressive models applied to time-series data in veterinary science. *Frontiers in Veterinary Science* 7: 604. https://doi.org/10.3389/fvets.2020.00604.

White, L.A., Forester, J.D., and Craft, M.E. (2018). Dynamic, spatial models of parasite transmission in wildlife: their structure, applications and remaining challenges. *Journal of Animal Ecology* 87 (3): 559–580.

Wise, C.F., Hammel, S.C., Herkert, N.J. et al. (2022). Comparative assessment of pesticide exposures in domestic dogs and their owners using silicone passive samplers and biomonitoring. *Environmental Science & Technology* 56 (2): 1149–1161. https://doi.org/10.1021/acs.est.1c06819.

Xu, Y., Liu, X., Cao, X. et al. (2021). Artificial intelligence: a powerful paradigm for scientific research. *The Innovation* 2 (4): 100179. https://doi.org/10.1016/j.xinn.2021.100179.

Yadav, S.K. and Akhter, Y. (2021). Statistical modeling for the prediction of infectious disease dissemination with special reference to COVID-19 spread. *Frontiers in Public Health* 9: 645405. https://doi.org/10.3389/fpubh.2021.645405.

Zohdi, T.I. (2023). *Modeling and Simulation of Infectious Diseases; Microscale Transmission, Decontamination and Macroscale Propagation*. Springer Cham https://doi.org/10.1007/978-3-031-18053-8.

2

Factors Influencing Livestock Diseases and Animal Productivity

Negin Esfandiari[1] and Mohammadreza Najafi[2]

[1] *Department of Food Hygiene and Quality Control, Division of Epidemiology, Faculty of Veterinary Medicine, University of Tehran, Tehran, Iran*
[2] *Department of Pathobiology, Faculty of Veterinary Medicine, Urmia University, Urmia, Iran*

2.1 Factors Influencing Livestock Diseases

Disease does not develop spontaneously. It happens when the host (an animal), the agent (like a virus), and the environment (like a tainted water source) interact. Although some diseases have a predominantly hereditary basis, almost all diseases are caused by a combination of genetic and environmental variables, with the precise ratio varying depending on the condition. Using communicable diseases as a model, it is possible to more clearly illustrate many of the underlying concepts driving the spread of disease. Numerous elements, such as genetic origin, food habits, and immunological traits, influence vulnerability.

Numerous factors, such as earlier exposure to both natural illness and immunization, affect an individual's immunological status. Biological, physical, and chemical components can all contribute to the development of disease, as well as less obvious ones like stress. Both direct and indirect transmission of diseases are possible.

As an example, direct contact between animals can result in the direct transfer of a disease. A common means of transmission, such as tainted air or water, or a vector like the mosquito, might result in indirect transmission. The ability of a particular organism to spread and cause outbreaks thus depends on the properties of the organism, such as its rate of development and the method by which it is transmitted from one animal to another. Different organisms also spread in different ways.

The introduction of a harmful organism into a host can lead to the development of an infectious disease. Infectious agents are only able to prolong their existence if they can successfully transmit the pathogen to a susceptible host, cause the host to get infected, and then replicate within the host in order to keep the infection cycle going. This is true regardless of whether or not the pathogen causes disease. The full course of infection that an infectious agent causes is referred to as its life cycle.

Only clinical disease is immediately noticeable. Even though they are not clinically evident, infections without symptoms play a crucial role in the web of disease transmission, especially in veterinary medicine as subclinical disease plays an important role in reducing productivity.

2.1.1 Clinical and Subclinical Disease

It is essential to have an accurate understanding of the varied manifestations of disease severity. Only symptoms of clinical disease are immediately noticeable. However, infections that do not manifest themselves clinically are still significant, particularly in the chain of events that lead to disease transmission, even though they are not visible to the naked eye. Inapparent cases can still transmit the disease; therefore, it is necessary to identify such cases in order to contain the disease's spread. It would appear that severity is connected to both the virulence of the organism (that is, how effective the organism is at creating disease) and the location in the body where the organism multiplies. It is necessary to have an understanding of all these components, as well as characteristics of the host such as the immunological response, in order to understand how disease might travel from one individual to another.

Epidemiology and Environmental Hygiene in Veterinary Public Health, First Edition. Edited by Tanmoy Rana.
© 2025 John Wiley & Sons, Inc. Published 2025 by John Wiley & Sons, Inc.

Over the course of time, not only has our clinical and biological knowledge expanded, but so has our capacity to differentiate between the various stages of disease. Among these are clinical diseases as well as nonclinical diseases.

- *Clinical disease*: clinical disease is characterized by signs and symptoms.
- *Subclinical disease*: the following are examples of conditions that could be considered nonclinical.

  1) Preclinical disease: disease in an early stage. A disease that is not yet manifest in a clinical setting but has the potential to develop into a clinical condition in the future.
  2) Subclinical disease: a disease that is not clinically obvious and is not likely to become clinically apparent in the foreseeable future. The majority of the time, a serological (antibody) response or culture of the organism is used to diagnose this kind of sickness.
  3) Chronic disease: disease that lasts for a long time. The infected animal is unable to "shake off" the disease and it stays with the animal for years, often for the rest of its life. The development of symptoms many years after an illness was assumed to have been treated is an interesting reaction that has been occurring more frequently in recent years. As a result, these conditions have developed into cases of clinical disease, even if they are substantially distinct from the initial illness.
  4) Latent disease: an infection that does not result in the active multiplication of the agent, such as the infection that occurs when viral nucleic acid is integrated into the nucleus of a cell as a provirus. In contrast to persistent infection, just the genetic message is present in the host, not the viable organism. This is because the host has been rendered incapable of supporting the infection. One definition of a latent infection is one that continues to be present in an animal in the absence of any obvious clinical manifestations. As a result, it is difficult to differentiate between the states of latency, chronic infection, and carrier status. Transmission to other susceptible animals may or may not occur concurrently with latency depending in the circumstances. There is a delicate equilibrium that develops between the host and the infectious agent in cases of persistent bacterial infections, such as tuberculosis. This equilibrium allows the bacterium to multiply but the disease may not advance for a very long period. Persistence is not typically associated with obvious replication of the infectious agent in cases of viral and rickettsial infections, unless the latter is reactivated. The likelihood of an infectious disease remaining latent in a host might vary not just with the specific infectious agent and host species, but also with the age of the host at the time of infection. The control of disease can be hampered by unidentified latent infection.

2.1.2 Carrier State

The term "carrier" is frequently employed to refer to a variety of contexts. A carrier is, in the most general definition, any animal that sheds an infectious agent but does not demonstrate clinical indications of having the infection. Therefore, an animal that is just subclinically or inapparently sick may nevertheless be a carrier of the agent, and may shed it either constantly or sporadically. There is a wide range of times during which an animal can be a carrier of an infection; nonetheless, during these times, carriers can be important sources of infection for susceptible animals. The state of being a carrier might be temporary or chronic, meaning that it can linger for months or even years. Animals that excrete the pathogen during the disease's incubation are considered to be incubatory carriers. Animals that are convalescent carriers shed the pathogen when they are healing from a disease, and the shedding may then last for a very long time.

2.1.3 Herd Immunity

Herd immunity is the resistance of a group of animals to a disease to which a large proportion of the group members are immune. If a significant portion of the population have immunity, then it is quite likely that the entire population, and not just those who possess immunity, will be protected. Why does immunity in the whole population develop? This occurs in any community where there are animals because disease can transmit from one animal to another. When a sufficient number of animals in a community have acquired immunity to a disease, the probability that an infected animal would come into contact with a susceptible animal to which it can pass on the virus decreases significantly. Instead, the diseased animal will have more contacts with animals that are immune to the disease. It is less likely that an infected animal will spread disease to a susceptible member of the community if there is a sizable percentage of immune animals in the population.

Why is it so critical to understand the notion of herd immunity? When we carry out vaccination campaigns, it is possible that it will not be essential to attain vaccination rates of 100% in order to successfully immunize the population. By immunizing a significant portion of the population, we may obtain a level of protection that is quite effective; the remaining portion of the population will be protected as a result of herd immunity.

Certain requirements need to be satisfied before there can be herd immunity. It is necessary for the infectious agent to be confined to a single host species within which transmission can take place, and for this transmission to be relatively straightforward from one member of the host species to another. If we have a reservoir in which the organism may exist outside the human host, then herd immunity will not work since there will be other ways for the disease to be transmitted. In addition, infections need to generate a robust immune response. If immunity is only acquired in part, we will not be able to cultivate a sizable population of animals that are immune within the society.

In order for herd immunity to take effect, the risk of an infected person coming into contact with every other member of the community must be equal. This is referred to as "random mixing." However, if an animal is infected and only interacts with other animals that are susceptible to the disease (meaning that there is no random mixing of the population), then it is likely that the diseased animal would spread the disease to other species that are vulnerable to it. When populations are consistently interacting with one another, herd immunity functions at its highest level.

2.1.4 Incubation Period

The time that passes between an individual becoming infected and the beginning of obvious symptoms of their sickness is referred to as the incubation period. If infection occurred today, the symptoms of the disease that an animal has may not manifest for a few days or weeks after it became sick. During this time, also known as the incubation phase, the animal continues to exhibit no signs of the disease and feels fully well.

Why does it take so long for symptoms of disease to appear once an infection has taken place? What factors contribute to the length of the incubation period? It could be a reflection of the amount of time required for the organism to replicate adequately up to the point where it reaches the critical mass required for clinical illness to develop. It is likely also related to the location within the body where the organism duplicates – whether it replicates superficially, close to the surface of the skin, or deeper within the body. The amount of the infectious agent that an animal was exposed to at the time of infection may also have an effect on how long it takes for symptoms to appear after infection. It is possible that a higher dose will make the incubation time shorter.

2.1.5 Modes of Transmission

When a pathogenic organism successfully invades a host, the result is infectious illness. Successful transmission to a susceptible host, induction of infection within the host, and replication of the agents to perpetuate the cycle of infection are essential to the continuing survival of infectious agents, with or without the development of disease. The life cycle of an infectious agent is the full cycle of infection it causes.

Transmission can take place in either a vertical or horizontal (lateral) direction. Infections that spread horizontally through a population might move from any part of the population to any other part of the population. Infections that are passed vertically from one generation to the next occur when the embryo or fetus gets infected while it is still in the uterus (in mammals) or while it is still in the egg (in birds, reptiles, amphibians, fish, and arthropods). Vertical transmission is the most common type of infection transmission. Some people also regard the transmission of diseases from mother to child through breast milk to be vertical. Many people think of air-borne transmission of infectious agents as indirect because of the distances required, but this type of transmission is actually direct because no intermediary vehicle is used.

2.2 Determinants of Disease

Disease is caused by a variety of factors, called disease determinants. A determinant is any trait that influences a population's health. Knowledge of determinants aids in the identification of animal species that are predisposed to illness development. As a result, it is required for illness prevention and serves as a tool for differential diagnosis. This chapter explores the many types of determinants and their interactions.

Disease determinants can be classified in various ways but here we focus on those associated with host, agent, or environment. These three groups of factors are sometimes called the triad (Figure 2.1).

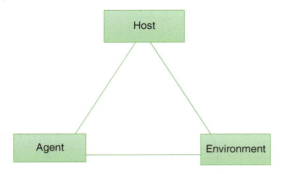

Figure 2.1 The determinants of disease triad.

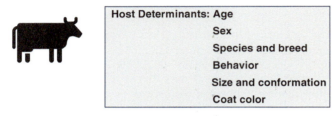

Figure 2.2 Host determinants of animal disease.

Investigations into diseases and epidemics take advantage of the interplay between and interdependence of agent, host, time, and environment. The host is an organism that typically carries the disease; the agent is what causes the disease to occur. Time considers incubation periods, the life expectancy of the host or the pathogen, and the length of the course of the illness or condition. Environments are the surroundings and situations that are external to the human or animal that cause or permit disease transmission.

2.2.1 Host Determinants

The host is a plant, animal, or arthropod that has the potential to become infected with an infectious agent and consequently provides nutrition to that agent when it does so. The host is where the agent will typically replicate or develop, depending on the case.

The sensitivity (or vulnerability) and infectiousness of a host are the primary factors that determine that host's capacity to transfer infection. There is a possibility that susceptibility to infection is restricted to a particular species or group of species. Within a species, susceptibility can vary greatly, and this variation may be related to age or the selection of genetically resistant animals after being exposed to an infectious agent (Figure 2.2).

2.2.1.1 Age

Numerous diseases have a clear relationship with aging. Many bacterial and viral illnesses, for example, are more likely to affect young animals than older ones and to be fatal, because the animals either lack acquired immunity (especially if they are not given colostrum) or have inadequate nonimmunological host resistance. In contrast, several protozoan and rickettsial illnesses cause softer reactions in children than in adults.

2.2.1.2 Sex

Hormonal, occupational, behavioral, and genetic factors may all have a role in the varied occurrence of disease in different sexes. The effects of sex hormones may predispose animals to disease.

When animal use is equated with occupation, sex-associated occupational hazards, though more relevant to human disease than animal disease, can occasionally be detected in animals.

There are three ways that sex might affect, limit, or relate genetic differences in disease occurrence. Sex-linked inheritance, which is frequently referred to as Mendelian inheritance, happens when the DNA causing a disease is present on either the X or Y chromosome. When a disease's DNA does not reside in the sex chromosomes but only manifests in one sex – as in the case of cryptorchidism in dogs – sex-limited inheritance occurs. When the threshold for the overt expression of a trait is lower in one sex than the other, it is called sex-influenced inheritance, leading to an excess incidence in one sex over the other.

2.2.1.3 Species and Breed

Different species and breeds play varied roles in the spread of disease due to differences in their sensitivity and responses to various infectious agents.

2.2.1.4 Behavior

The risk of a disease spreading from one species to another can be influenced by behavior.

2.2.1.5 Size and Conformation

Size has been found to be a disease factor, independent of specific breed relationships. Similarly, animals' conformation may make some diseases more likely to develop.

2.2.1.6 Coat Color

Predisposition to some diseases is associated with coat color, which is heritable and a risk indicator.

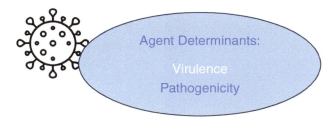

Figure 2.3 Agent determinants of animal disease.

2.2.2 Agent Determinants

Infectivity, virulence, and stability are three critical features of pathogens that affect the propagation of infectious agents (Figure 2.3). The amount of a certain organism that is needed to start an infection is referred to as that organism's infectious potential. There is a wide range of infectious potential among different kinds of organisms. Infectivity can differ between various strains of the same organism, and can also be influenced by factors such as mode of transmission of the infection, age of the host, and their natural defenses. When an infectious agent may infect more than one species, the degree to which it is infectious for each of those species' respective hosts is typically rather varied. The level of virulence also has an effect on transmission and can vary. It is common for repeated passage through the same species of animal to enhance virulence for that species, while at the same time decreasing virulence for the animal that served as the natural host in the first place. The stability of an organism can be defined as the amount of time that it can survive outside its host and still be infectious. Some creatures are only able to endure for short periods of time; in other words, they are highly fragile. Other species, on the other hand, are more resilient.

2.2.2.1 Virulence and Pathogenicity

The capacity of various infectious agents to infect and cause disease in animals varies. The potential for infection depends on the host's innate susceptibility and whether the host is immune. Pathogenicity and virulence are two characteristics that describe an agent's capacity to cause disease. The ability of an infectious agent to inflict disease on a specific host, in terms of severity, is known as virulence. Case fatality is an indicator of virulence when death is the only outcome. Pathogenicity is sometimes used interchangeably with virulence, with virulence reserved for differences in the disease-inducing capability of various strains of the same organism. However, the term "pathogenicity" refers to the effectiveness of disease induction.

Pathogenicity or virulence can be achieved by changing an agent's antigenic composition to one to which the host is neither genetically nor immunologically resistant. However, antigenic alterations are not usually the cause of pathogenicity changes. They could simply be indications of such changes, with the determinants linked to the generation of inhibitory, poisonous, or other chemicals, as well as the immune-mediated harm that may result.

Different genotypic changes can occur in infectious agents, the most important ones being mutation, recombination, conjugation, transduction, and transformation.

2.2.3 Environmental Determinants

The environment consists of location, climate, and husbandry (Figure 2.4). Environmental determinants of disease have received special attention in livestock enterprises because intensive production systems expose animals to unnatural settings.

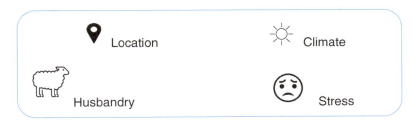

Figure 2.4 Environmental determinants of animal disease.

2.2.3.1 Location

The natural spatial distribution of animals and disease is influenced by local geological formations, vegetation, and climate. Urban living, proximity to gas and oil sites, and noise, which is associated with location and may also be deemed to be related to "occupation" and husbandry, can all have an impact on animal disease. Because of the seasonal influences of climate, the temporal distribution of disease is also affected by location.

2.2.3.2 Climate

There are two types of climates: macroclimate and microclimate. The *macroclimate* consists of the usual weather components to which animals are exposed: rainfall, temperature, sun radiation, humidity, and wind, all of which can have an impact on health. The macroclimate can also have an impact on the stability of infectious agent.

A climate that exists in a constrained area is called a *microclimate*. This could be as small as a few millimeters of a plant or animal's surface or as big as a pig pen or calves' housing. Microclimate can be either terrestrial (like that found over the surface of leaves) or biological (like that found over the surface of a host's body). Arthropods and helminths both have their development influenced by the terrestrial environment. During a disease, the biological microclimate might alter, aiding in its spread.

2.2.3.3 Climate Change

The effects of climate change on frequency and distribution of disease in both humans and animals are currently causing widespread concern. These effects can be either direct (such as rising temperatures or more extreme events) or indirect (such as through water scarcity, famine, and coastal flooding). This effect is "bidirectional," meaning that both increases and decreases in illness incidence may be a result of climate change.

For some time, there has been conjecture that one of the main factors could be global warming, which is caused by an increase in the greenhouse effect brought on by the large industrial output of carbon dioxide emissions.

2.2.3.4 Husbandry

2.2.3.4.1 Housing

The significance of properly constructed ventilation in an animal housing is obvious. The structure of bedding materials and surfaces also plays a role in the health and productivity of animals.

2.2.3.4.2 Diet

Diet has a clear impact on disorders caused by a lack of energy, protein, vitamins, and minerals. Sometimes the impacts are less obvious. Feeding regimens may also be a factor.

2.2.3.4.3 Management

Stocking density and production policy are determined by management. Increased densities make microbial infections more difficult to combat. Internal replacement policies (i.e., maintaining a "closed" population) are less likely to introduce viruses than policies involving the purchase of animals from outside the herd.

2.2.3.5 Stress

There is no broadly recognized comprehensive theory of stress. It is used in human medicine to characterize emotional conflicts and unhappiness. In veterinary medicine, it is frequently attributed to variables such as weaning, overcrowding, transportation, dietary changes, and other environmental issues such as severe heat. These are called stressors or stimuli.

Among the causes of stress are low temperatures, inadequate ventilation, a lack of adequate room for feeding and watering, and excessive use of medication.

Variables such as plasma cortisol are observed to change in response to a variety of psychological stimuli; some of them may be painful while others may be enjoyable. Changes in biological function in reaction to a stressor can be enough to eliminate the threat. When the response is prolonged and extensive, however, some aspects of biological function may be affected, leaving the animal vulnerable to negative effects; for example, endocrine events critical for reproductive success may be disrupted and immune function may be altered, resulting in susceptibility to infectious disease and abnormal behavior.

The way in which animals react to stressors varies greatly. Certain individuals may respond to certain stimuli while others may not, and certain animals may respond to the same stressor in radically different ways when compared to other animals. Experience, genetics, and "coping style" will influence whether an animal interprets a stimulus as a stressor, as well as the sort of biological reaction launched by the animal in response to the stimulus.

Evidence for the significance of stress as a disease determinant has typically been presented in the context of specific management situations, rather than in relation to a well-understood, unequivocal physiological response.

Overall, determinants linked with the host, agent, or environment do not operate in isolation but rather interact to cause disease. The interdependent operation of components that produce, prevent, control, mediate, or otherwise influence the occurrence of an event is referred to as interaction.

2.3 Factors Influencing Animal Productivity

Livestock systems cover approximately 30% of the planet's ice-free terrestrial surface area, and this sector is increasingly organized in long market chains, employing approximately 1.3 billion people worldwide and directly supporting the livelihoods of 600 million smallholder farmers in developing countries.

As a result, livestock production is an important component of global agriculture. In fact, human populations around the world rely heavily on domestic animals for a variety of purposes, including the production of meat, fat, milk, and other dairy products, eggs, and fibers such as wool or cashmere, as well as transportation, draft, and fertilizer provision, particularly in developing countries.

It is generally agreed that large ruminants are the most important species of domestic livestock anywhere in the world. The extensive range of items that they offer is illustrative of the significance of the organization. In wealthy countries, their contributions are primarily limited to commercial products like meat and milk. This is not the case in less developed countries where they are a source of food, notably protein for human diets, but also provide revenue, employment, transport, and can act as a store of wealth. Additionally, they provide draft power and organic fertilizer for the growing of crops in impoverished nations. It is consequently of the utmost significance that these areas achieve maximum potential in terms of their animal output.

In such a scenario, livestock productivity is critical for farmers' revenue, livelihoods, and, ultimately, the survival of entire populations and cultures that rely on animal production. A variety of factors influence livestock productivity and production. Climate, nutrition, and health are the most important considerations.

Climate and geographic location are without a doubt the two most important aspects in livestock production. In fact, climatological factors such as average temperature and patterns of precipitation have a significant impact on the availability cycle of pasture and food resources throughout the course of the year, as well as the sorts of disease and parasite outbreaks that occur among animal populations.

One of the most significant elements that has a negative impact on the production and productivity of livestock is the presence of diseases and parasites. Animal diseases have a significant influence on worldwide food supply, as well as on trade, commerce, and human health. Over the course of the past few decades, there has been a general decrease in the burden caused by cattle diseases. This decline is a direct result of the increased availability of effective medications and vaccines, as well as advancements in diagnostic technology.

It is expected that future diseases will be efficiently handled by the technology used for disease surveillance and control. At the same time, new diseases have emerged and will continue to spread because of the movement of animals and animal products across international borders.

Many diseases affect livestock productivity. It is a significant obstacle when it infects draft animals during the plowing season and limits their ability to perform, which occurs in underdeveloped nations where livestock are exposed to a variety of diseases that influence output. This results in a reduction in the amount of land that can be cultivated with staple food crops and a drop in the income that farmers receive from the rental of draft animals. They also pose a health risk to humans, which adds another layer of complexity to the situation.

Around one billion cattle, the vast majority of which are found in tropical regions, are at risk from a variety of tick species, tick-borne illnesses, and worms, all of which have the potential to inflict large productivity losses. Other diseases that can influence livestock production include but are not limited to foot and mouth disease, brucellosis, blue tongue, bovine tuberculosis, salmonellosis, and bovine viral diarrhea.

Ruminant diseases caused by parasitic gastrointestinal nematode infections have the biggest influence on animal health and productivity. Production losses arise from decreased food intake, increased endogenous protein loss, inefficient utilization of dietary energy for tissue deposition, and impairment of bone formation.

Diseases that affect livestock are primarily an economic burden for the owners and farmers who raise animals for a living. Infectious diseases that lower production, productivity, and profitability relate to high treatment costs, disruption of local markets and international trade, and an increase in the severity of poverty in rural, local, and regional populations. On a biological level, infections compete with one another for the productive potential of animals, which decreases the portion of that potential that may be utilized for human uses.

Revenue can be lost because of livestock diseases in two ways: directly, because of deaths, stunting, reduced fertility, and changes in herd structure; and indirectly, as a result of additional costs for drugs and vaccines, added labor costs, and profit losses due to denied access to better markets and the use of suboptimal production technology.

The importance of genetic diversity in livestock in terms of disease resistance is underscored by the fact that organisms that cause disease are constantly adapting and developing resistance to the treatments that are available. Today's livestock production is highly reliant on the application of antimicrobial agents and anthelmintics for the purpose of preventing and treating illnesses and parasites, respectively.

When raising animals, natural resistance to illnesses and parasites is not typically chosen as a desirable trait but evidence shows that it might be of importance as, for example, some native livestock are less susceptible to the effects of some diseases than imported livestock.

Man-made elements such as religion and culture substantially impact animal species or breed selection. Additionally, economic constraints, marketing options, and access to infrastructures like highways, docks, and trains also affect livestock welfare and production.

It is vital to establish mitigation methods at local, regional, national, and international levels in order to reduce the effect of all the negative aspects that have been stated thus far on the productivity of farm animals. It is essential that these initiatives center on the study and utilization of local genetic resources that show a high level of adaptation to the most critical problem for that particular location, whether that problem is climate, disease, or nutrition induced.

Further Reading

Dohoo, I.R., Martin, S.W., and Stryhn, H. (2009). *Veterinary Epidemiologic Research*. Charlotte: VER Inc.

Gordis, L. (2013). *Epidemiology E-Book*. St Louis: Elsevier Health Sciences.

Lamy, E., Van Harten, S., Baptista, E. et al. (2012). Factors influencing livestock productivity. In: *Environmental Stress and Amelioration in Livestock Production* (ed. V. Sejian, N. SMK, T. Ezeji, et al.), 19–51. Berlin: Springer.

Smith, R.D. (2020). *Veterinary Clinical Epidemiology: From Patient to Population*. Boca Raton: CRC Press.

Thrusfield, M. and Christley, R. (2018). *Veterinary Epidemiology*. Hoboken: Wiley.

3

Determinants of Disease, Adjustment of Rates, Trends and Emergence

Kollannur Davis Justin and Kadankandath Athira

Department of Veterinary Epidemiology and Preventive Medicine, College of Veterinary and Animal Sciences, Thrissur, Kerala Veterinary and Animal Sciences University, Mannuthy, Kerala, 680651, India

3.1 Introduction

The study of disease dynamics, patterns, causes, and effects of health and disease conditions in populations is termed as *epidemiology*. It helps to understand the patterns of disease occurrence in populations for potential preventive and control measures. The basic essence of epidemiology is that disease is not a random event. Each individual in a population has a unique set of characteristics and exposures to risk factors, that determine their probability of disease. Clinical medicine is the branch of medicine that is focused on the health of the individual whereas epidemiology and veterinary public health targets the assessment of risk factors at the community level. Studies on the assessment of risk factors helps the veterinarians and stakeholders to develop policies and interventions for disease control and prevention. The *One Health concept* is in par with the principles of epidemiology because exposures for many diseases occur at the interface between humans, animals and the environment. Failure to consider the interactions between them may result in failure of the public health policies to effectively control disease and protection of the environment (Johnson-Walker & Kaneene, 2018).

The livestock sector accounts for half of the global agricultural economy and the new era of globalization are characterized by unrestricted movements of people, animal products and by-products, exchange of money, technology and information. We had witnessed the livestock revolution that had made tremendous changes in the diet of people from a cereal-based diet to a diet based on proteins (Cartin-Rojas, 2012). Infections that have either appeared in a population newly or rapidly increasing in incidence in a new geographic range is termed as emerging infectious diseases. The recent animal health emergencies have highlighted the vulnerability of livestock industry to epizootic episodes caused by infectious diseases. The spread of diseases to new places that were not endemic occurs through the large-scale movement of animals (Beverelli & Ticku, 2023). Sixty percent of emerging diseases that affect humans are zoonotic and about 75% of them are from the wildlife. Recently, there is an increasing trend in the occurrence of novel infectious diseases in human subjects and animals. It is clear that infections will continue to emerge, and that many of these infections will be zoonotic. This emphasizes the importance of close co-operation between the veterinary and human health communities, in working together and exchanging information on a regular basis (Morse, 2004).

3.2 Determinants of Disease

Any factor that influences the health of a population is referred to as a determinant. Determinants in this context refer to any characteristic that effect the incidence and distribution of diseases (Tadesse et al., 2019). Information of determinants facilitate identification of groups of animal that are at particular risk of developing disease. It is an integral part of disease diagnosis, prevention and control. Determinants can be grouped in three ways namely, primary and secondary; intrinsic and extrinsic and those associated with Epidemiological triads (host, agent or environment). The three classifications can be summarized as shown in Box 3.1.

Epidemiology and Environmental Hygiene in Veterinary Public Health, First Edition. Edited by Tanmoy Rana.
© 2025 John Wiley & Sons, Inc. Published 2025 by John Wiley & Sons, Inc.

Box 3.1 Classification of Determinants

1) **Primary and Secondary Determinants:**
   - **Primary Determinants:** These are the fundamental factors directly responsible for the occurrence of a disease. For example, the presence of a specific pathogen in a particular environment might be a primary determinant.
   - **Secondary Determinants:** These are factors that influence the primary determinants. They may not directly cause the disease but can exacerbate or mitigate the impact of the primary determinants. For instance, climate conditions or the availability of vectors can be secondary determinants.
2) **Intrinsic and Extrinsic Determinants:**
   - **Intrinsic Determinants:** These are internal factors related to the host organism. It could include genetic predispositions, age, sex, immune status, and physiological conditions.
   - **Extrinsic Determinants:** These are external factors that exist outside the host organism. Examples include the presence of specific vectors, environmental conditions, and the characteristics of the infectious agent.
3) **Determinants Associated with Epidemiological Triads:**
   - **Host Determinants:** Factors related to the host organism, such as genetic susceptibility, immunization status, age, and overall health.
   - **Agent Determinants:** Characteristics of the infectious agent, including its virulence, ability to survive in the environment, and mode of transmission.
   - **Environment Determinants:** External factors in the environment that can influence disease transmission, such as climate, geographical location, presence of vectors, and sanitation conditions.

Understanding these determinants is crucial in disease diagnosis, prevention, and control. It helps in identifying high-risk groups, implementing targeted preventive measures, and developing strategies to control the spread of diseases. Additionally, this knowledge assists in designing effective vaccination programs, managing environmental factors, and predicting disease outbreaks.

3.2.1 Primary and Secondary Determinants

Knowledge regarding the distinction between primary and secondary determinants is crucial for a comprehensive assessment of disease dynamics. It allows for targeted interventions and preventive measures that address the root causes (primary determinants) and contributing factors (secondary determinants) associated with the development and spread of diseases in animal populations. The essence of these determinants can be related from Box 3.2.

Some of the primary and secondary determinants of a disease are shown in the Figure 3.1.

Box 3.2 Primary and Secondary Determinants Characteristics

Primary determinants	**Definition**: Factors whose differences make a major effect in inducing disease **Characteristics**: Often necessary causes, meaning that the presence or variation of the primary determinant is essential for the disease to occur. **Example**: Exposure to parvovirus is a primary determinant of canine parvoviral enteritis. Genetic factors, such as the rate of aging of valves, may also be primary determinants associated with the development of certain conditions, such as valve incompetence, and may vary with the breed.
Secondary determinants	**Definition**: Correspond to enabling, predisposing, and reinforcing factors. **Characteristics**: These factors may not be directly responsible for causing the disease but influence its occurrence, severity, or distribution. **Example**: In the context of canine heart valve incompetence, sex is a secondary determinants where Male dogs are more likely to develop incompetence (Toker et al., 2011). Sex, in this case, is a factor that influences the occurrence of the disease but is not the direct cause.

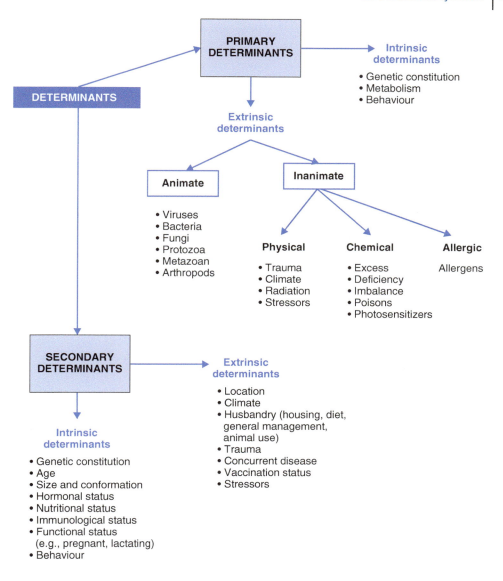

Figure 3.1 Classification of determinants of disease.

3.2.2 Intrinsic and Extrinsic Determinants

Whether the determinants are intrinsic or extrinsic is critical for developing effective disease control and prevention strategies. Intrinsic determinants often involve the host's inherent characteristics, and interventions may need to focus on genetic selection, breeding practices, or individual health management. Extrinsic determinants, on the other hand, may require environmental or management changes to reduce the risk of disease. By considering both intrinsic and extrinsic determinants, veterinarians and researchers can develop holistic approaches to disease management that address the complex interplay between host factors, environmental conditions, and external influences. This comprehensive understanding is essential for promoting health of animals and preventing the transmission of diseases. Some of the characters of intrinsic and extrinsic determinants (Box 3.3) of canine pruritus and haemolysis are described in Tables 3.1 and 3.2 respectively.

3.2.3 Determinants Associated with Host, Agent and Environment

It's fascinating how the understanding of disease causation has evolved, moving from a focus on microbes as primary causes to a broader consideration of host, agent, and environmental factors, often referred to as the triad. The recognition of management and husbandry as a distinct group highlights the complexity of factors influencing disease in intensive animal enterprises. The distinction between "simple" diseases, where the infectious agent is the main determinant, and

3 Determinants of Disease, Adjustment of Rates, Trends and Emergence

---

Box 3.3 Character of Intrinsic and Extrinsic Determinants

Intrinsic Determinants (Endogenous):	**Nature**: Factors within the host organism. **Examples**: **Genetic Composition**: The genetic makeup of the host, like aberrant genes, which can be main causes of genetic disorders. **Species, Breed, and Sex**: Intrinsic characteristics that vary among individuals and can influence susceptibility or resistance to certain diseases.
Extrinsic Determinants (Exogenous):	**Nature**: External factors outside the host organism. **Examples**: **Transportation**: An extrinsic factor that can lead to weight loss and physical trauma in animals, potentially resulting in bruising of carcasses (Huertas et al., 2010) **Environmental Conditions**: Factors such as climate, geography, and the presence of vectors that are external to the host but can significantly impact disease transmission.

Table 3.1 Some determinants of canine pruritus (Logas, 2003; Tater, 2012; Sousa, 2013).

Intrinsic determinants		Extrinsic determinants				
Host characteristics	Internal disease	Chemicals	Environment	Diet	End-ecto Parasites	Bacteria, fungi and yeasts
Breed	Neoplasia: Mast cell tumor cutaneous T-cell lymphoma (CTCL)	Irritant contact dermatitis	Solar dermatitis	Adverse food reactions	Hookworm dermatitis	Bacterial folliculitis
Age	Immune-mediated disorders: Systemic lupus erythematosus	Calcinosis cutis			Pelodera dermatitis	
					Schistosomiasis	Deep pyoderma
					Dirofilariosis	
		Adverse drug reactions			Scabies	Dermatophytosis
					Pediculosis	
					Demodicosis	Malassezia dermatitis
					Otodectes cyanotis	
					Trombiculiasis	
	Hormonal: Hypersensitivity				Cheyletiellosis	

"complex" diseases, where a multifactorial nature prevails, underscores the diverse dynamics in disease causation. Examples like "environmental" mastitis and the potential influence of trace elements on prion diseases highlight the intricate interactions between hosts, agents, and environmental factors. Thus, "environmental" mastitis involves an interaction between specific infectious agents (*Escherichia coli* or *Streptococcus uberis*), environmental factors such as milking machine faults and poor hygiene, and host susceptibility, with cows being most susceptible in early lactation. Another example involves the claim that the binding of trace elements (copper and manganese) seen in the soil to prion proteins may influence the onset of diseases like scrapie and other transmissible spongiform encephalopathies.

The complexity of a multifactorial disease often hinges on how it is defined, especially when considering clinical signs presented by animal owners. For instance, pruritus in a dog may stem from various lesions, each with distinct sufficient causes. Defining a "disease" in terms of a loss of production, such as "reproductive failure" in a pig herd, adds layers of complexity, involving factors like fertility, infections in males and metabolic derangement of the sow or foetus during pregnancy. The interplay of these elements contributes to the intricate causal web. Reproductive failure in pigs encompasses genetic, nutritional, infectious, toxic, environmental, and management factors, providing a detailed breakdown within the broader categories of agent, host, and environmental determinants. Genetic factors involve issues in both parents and

3.2 Determinants of Disease | 45

Table 3.2 Causes of haemolysis (Adapted from Fleischman, 2012).

Intrinsic determinants			Extrinsic determinants		
Congenital RBC abnormalities	**Immune-mediated**	**Haemophagocytic syndrome**	**Fragmentation/physical damage to RBC membrane (microangiopathy)**	**Infections**	**Drugs, toxins, chemical damage to RBC membrane**
Defects of haeme synthesis	Autoimmune		Mechanical (disseminated intravascular coagulation, caval syndrome, glomerulonephritis, haemolytic uremic syndrome)	Haemotropic mycoplasmosis	Zinc toxicosis (ingestion of pennies minted after 1983 or of zinc-containing ointments)
	Primary/ idiopathic IMHA		Abnormal endothelium (hemangiosarcoma, vasculitis, splenic torsion, hepatic disease)		
	Neonatal isoerythrolysis		Thermal injury (severe burns, heatstroke)		
	Incompatible blood transfusions		Osmotic injury (freshwater near-drowning)		
Membrane defects (stomatocytosis, increased osmotic fragility, nonspherocytic anaemia)	Secondary				
	Infections			Ehrlichiosis	Severe snake envenomation (crotalids)
	Neoplasia				Oxidants (ingestion of onion or onion products, garlic, acetaminophen, propylene glycol, vitamin K, benzocaine, methylene blue, naphthalene moth balls)
	Drug effects (penicillins, cephalosporins, sulfonamides, methimazole)				
Enzyme defects (pyruvate kinase deficiency, phosphofructokinase deficiency)	Vaccination adverse reaction			Babesiosis Cytauxzoonosis FeLV Septicemia	Severe hypophosphatemia

offspring, such as abnormal genitalia or inherited predispositions. Inadequate supply of specific micronutrients can lead to decreased litter sizes, embryonic death, and delayed puberty, emphasizing the importance of nutrition. The plane of nutrition also plays a role, with diet restriction potentially delaying puberty, while strategic feeding practices like 'flushing' before ovulation can enhance reproductive performance in gilts.

The environment's impact on reproduction involves climatic, social, and structural components, where high temperatures, for instance, can induce infertility in male pigs. Management factors, including herd age, boar: sow ratio, heat detection efficiency, and breeding policies, also play crucial roles. These factors contribute to the multifactorial nature of disease, and the three classification schemes – host, agent, and environment – are not mutually exclusive. The third classification system further delineates determinants into those associated with the host, agent, or environment, providing a comprehensive perspective on the complexities of reproductive challenges in pig herds.

The three determinant classification schemes – host, agent, and environment – are not mutually exclusive, providing distinct perspectives on the multifactorial nature of disease (Figure 3.2). Schwabe et al. (Schwabe et al., 1977), Martin et al. (Martin et al., 1987), and Smith (Smith, 2005) have adopted a similar system, as has Reif (Reif et al., 1983) in his

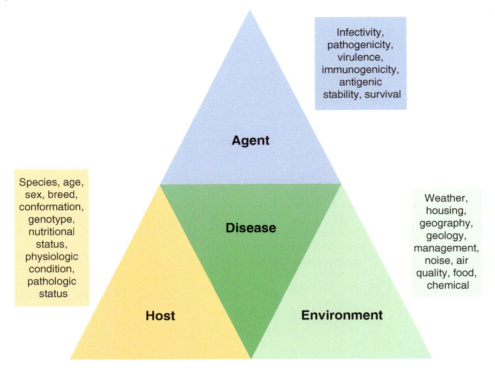

Figure 3.2 The classic epidemiological triad comprising of agent, host and environment. "The classic epidemiological triad," the three components of epidemiological system: agent, host and environment (Thrusfield et al., 2018; Pfeiffer, 2002).

examination of determinants in diseases of dogs and cats. This classification helps in understanding and analyzing the intricate interplay of factors influencing the occurrence and dynamics of animal diseases.

The One Health approach underscores the interconnectedness of human, animal, and environmental health. Instances like Sea Turtle Egg Fusariosis (STEF) disease highlight common intersecting points, where fungi reservoirs in plumbing, hospital water, and air distribution systems pose risks for both humans and sea turtles. Environmental sources, such as Fusarium-contaminated soil or plant material, can lead to risks like keratitis following traumatic inoculation, emphasizing the shared vulnerabilities and the importance of a holistic perspective in addressing health challenges (Figure 3.3) (Saenz et al., 2020).

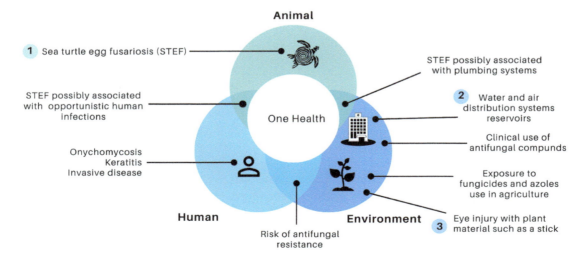

Figure 3.3 Animal, environment, and human interaction: a One Health perspective. *Animal, environment, and human interaction: a One Health perspective.* The One Health triad of humans, animals, and the environment is analogous with the other triads that epidemiologists use to describe disease dynamics within a population. The host, agent, environment triad is used to describe the interplay between these three key components of infectious disease transmission. Changes in any of these components alters the probability of disease (Saenz et al., 2020 / MDPI / CC BY 4.0).

3.2.3.1 Host Determinants

3.2.3.1.1 Genotype

The genotype, or genetic constitution, of a host plays a pivotal role in certain diseases, where alterations in gene structure significantly impact pathogenesis and can be inherited. Conditions like haemophilia A and B in dogs exemplify genetic diseases with a pronounced genetic cause. In contrast, simple infectious diseases often have minimal genetic components. Many diseases, including bovine foot lameness and mastitis, fall between these extremes, reflecting a complex interplay of genetic and environmental factors in their development.

3.2.3.1.2 Age

The occurrence of numerous diseases demonstrates a clear association with age. Bacterial and viral diseases are often more likely to occur and be fatal in young animals due to a lack of acquired immunity or low non-immunological host resistance (Quinn et al., 2011). Conversely, many protozoan and rickettsial infections induce milder responses in the young compared to the old (Zintl et al., 2005). Assessing the impact of a disease in a specific age range requires considering the proportions of each age group in the total population, as the absolute number of cases alone may not accurately reflect the disease's overall impact.

3.2.3.1.3 Sex

Sexual differences in disease occurrence can be influenced by various factors:

- **Hormonal Determinants**: Sex hormones, such as those in bitches, may contribute to diseases like diabetes mellitus, with signs often appearing after oestrus (Fall et al., 2007). Neutering can decrease the likelihood of mammary carcinoma, potentially influenced by the effect of oestrogens on tumor development (Beauvais et al., 2012).
- **Occupational Determinants**: While more relevant to humans, sex-associated occupational hazards can occasionally be identified in animals. For example, the increased risk of male dogs contracting heartworm infection may be linked to heightened "occupational" exposure during hunting.
- **Social and Ethological Determinants**: Behavioral patterns, like bite wound abscesses being more common in male cats, can impact disease occurrence. Behavior also influences the likelihood of disease transmission between species, as seen with opossums in New Zealand increasing the chance of tuberculosis transmission to cattle through confrontational behavior, contrasting with badgers in the UK, which are more likely to retreat and reduce aerosol transmission risk.
- **Genetic Determinants:** Contribute to differences in disease incidence, with inheritance patterns falling into categories such as sex-linked, sex-limited, or sex-influenced.
  Sex-linked Inheritance: Associated with Mendelian inheritance, it occurs when the DNA responsible for a disease is on the X or Y sex chromosomes. Canine haemophilia A and B, linked to the X chromosome, exemplify this, inherited recessively with a higher prevalence in males.
  Sex-limited Inheritance: Disease-related DNA is not on the sex chromosomes, but the disease is expressed in only one sex, as seen in cryptorchidism in dogs.
  Sex-influenced Inheritance: The threshold for overt expression of a characteristic is lower in one sex, leading to excess incidence in that sex. Canine patent ductus arteriosus is an example.

Some diseases may exhibit apparent sex associations, like epilepsy, melanoma, and pharyngeal fibrosarcoma predominantly in male dogs (Kearsley-Fleet et al., 2013; Bronden et al., 2009). However, the genetic component might not be clearly identified or the inheritance method established. Notably, apparent sex associations in certain diseases may actually be related to gender-associated factors, as seen in the increased mortality rate in male dairy calves, primarily linked to husbandry practices rather than a direct genetic influence.

3.2.3.1.4 Species and Breed

Variations in susceptibility and responses to infectious agents exist among species and breeds, influencing their roles in disease transmission. For instance, Dogs do not develop heartwater, illustrating species-specific resistance to certain infectious agents. Pigs exhibit greater resistance to FMD virus via the respiratory tract compared to cattle and sheep (Donaldson & Alexandersen, 2001). Cattle, with their extreme susceptibility and higher respiratory tidal volume, are more likely to be infected through airborne spread between farms. Pigs are less susceptible to airborne virus due to lower tidal volume and indoor housing practices, reducing the likelihood of encountering sufficient virus for clinical disease initiation. However, if infected, pigs can excrete significant quantities of airborne virus, making them substantial sources during epidemics, given their often-large population sizes.

Breed-specific variations in disease susceptibility are evident across species includes, Rottweilers and Dobermann Pinschers react more severely to this virus compared to other breeds. Boxers appear more susceptible to mycotic diseases like coccidioidomycosis than other breeds. Different breeds of poultry exhibit varying susceptibility to various viruses (Hassan et al., 2004). Monkeys are not susceptible to poliovirus due to the absence of the 'right' cell receptors. Introduction of species or breeds to new ecosystems can lead to apparently new diseases. For example, exposure of European breeds of sheep to bluetongue virus in South Africa resulted in severe disease in imported Merino sheep but not in indigenous sheep (Coetzee et al., 2012). Non-infectious diseases also show breed variations. British breeds of sheep have a higher frequency of intestinal carcinoma, Hereford cattle are more prone to ocular squamous cell carcinoma, and there is considerable breed predisposition variation in canine and feline skin tumors. Genetic relationships can contribute to disease patterns; for instance, Boston terriers and bull terriers share a high risk of developing mastocytoma due to their common origin (London & Thamm, 2013). However, the risk of a breed developing a specific disease may vary between countries, indicating different genetic pools, environments, or management practices.

3.2.3.1.5 Behavior

Behavioral patterns and cultural habits significantly influence the likelihood of infection transmission between species. In New Zealand, opossums' tendency to stand their ground when confronted by cattle increases the chance of aerosol transmission, highlighting the impact of behavior on disease dynamics. Mutual grooming behavior in Meerkats may be favorable for the spread of tuberculosis (Drewe et al., 2010). Similarly, in domestic animals, the higher incidence of bite wound abscesses in male cats compared to females is attributed to their behavioral patterns, emphasizing the role of behavior in shaping the risk of infection. Understanding these behavioral aspects is crucial for effective disease management and prevention strategies.

3.2.3.1.6 Other Host Determinants

Size, conformation, and coat color can significantly influence disease predisposition:

- ❖ **Size and Conformation**: Diseases like hip dysplasia and osteosarcoma are more common in larger breeds of dogs (LaFond et al., 2002), and this trend extends to large children for osteosarcoma. The conformation of animals, such as a small pelvic outlet in certain cows, can predispose them to dystocia. Conformation can indirectly affect health, for example, when calves are unable to suckle due to large teats, leading to hypogammaglobulinemia and an increased risk of fatal colibacillosis.
- ❖ **Coat Color**: Predisposition to certain diseases is associated with coat color, which is heritable and serves as a risk indicator. For instance, white cats have a higher risk of cutaneous squamous cell carcinoma due to the lack of pigment, which normally protects the skin from the sun's ultraviolet radiation. On the contrary, canine melanomas are more prevalent in deeply pigmented animals. Additionally, white cats often have a genetic defect linked to deafness, and Dalmatians with white coat color may be associated with congenital deafness. Understanding these associations is crucial for preventive care and health management in different animal populations.

3.2.3.2 Agent Determinants

3.2.3.2.1 Virulence and Pathogenicity

Infectious agents exhibit variations in their ability to infect and induce disease in animals, with factors like inherent host susceptibility and immunity playing crucial roles. The terms virulence and pathogenicity help characterize an agent's disease-causing potential: *Virulence* is the ability of an infectious agent to cause disease in a host, often expressed in terms of severity. Quantitatively, it may be defined as the ratio of clinical cases to the number of animals infected (Last, 2001; Porta, 2014). Case fatality, when death is the only outcome, serves as an indicator of virulence. Newcastle disease virus is virulent to poultry, but majority of the infections in wild birds are not virulent (Miller & Koch, 2013).

Pathogenicity: Sometimes used interchangeably with virulence, but specifically refers to the quality of disease induction. For example, the pathogenicity of *Naegleria fowleri* is influenced by environmental conditions, being pathogenic in warm water but not in cold water. Pathogenicity can also be quantified as the ratio of individuals developing clinical illness to those exposed to infection (Last, 2001; Porta, 2014). These characteristics are intrinsic to infectious agents and can be phenotypically or genotypically conditioned. Pathogenicity and virulence are determined by a variety of host and agent characteristics, which may be either unique to specific pathogens or conserved across several different species (Wilson et al., 2002). Determinants of bacterial virulence and pathogenicity include factors like toxin and adhesin production, along with invasion strategies and resistance to host defense mechanisms. Changes in antigenic composition may contribute to pathogenicity, but not always; they can also be indicators of underlying changes associated with the production of inhibitory or toxic substances, such as exotoxins and endotoxins, leading to immune-mediated damage.

3.2.3.2.2 Gradient of Infection

The concept of a "gradient of infection" encapsulates the diverse responses of an animal to a challenge by an infectious agent (Table 3.3). It reflects the combined impact of the agent's pathogenicity and virulence, as well as host characteristics such as susceptibility, and the ensuing pathological and clinical reactions. This gradient influences the availability of the agent for further transmission to susceptible animals and affects the veterinarian's ability to detect, treat, and control the infection. In cases where an animal is insusceptible or immune, significant replication and shedding of the infectious agent typically do not occur. As a result, such animals play a less significant role in the transmission of infection to others (Thrusfield, 2007).

3.2.3.2.3 Outcome of Infection

Clinical disease can lead to various outcomes, including the development of a *long-standing chronic clinical infection, recovery, or death*. Each outcome has implications for the potential of an animal to act as a source of infection. Animals with chronic infections can serve as potential sources of infectious agents. In most cases, death removes an animal as a source of infection. However, exceptions exist, such as with *Trichinella spiralis* and anthrax infections, where carcasses can contaminate the soil. Successful recovery may result in sterile immunity, achieved through an effective host response that

Table 3.3 Gradient of infection: the various responses of an animal to challenge by an infectious agent (Thrusfield, 2007 / with permission of John Wiley & Sons).

Gradient of infection	Definition	Example
Inapparent (silent) infection	Infection of a susceptible host without clinical signs. The infection may run a similar course to that which produces a clinical case, with replication and shedding of agent. The inapparently infected animal poses a considerable problem to the disease controller because it is impossible to detect without auxiliary diagnostic aids such as antigen detection or serology.	Sheep may show either no or transient clinical signs of infection with foot-and-mouth disease virus, although they may excrete virus and serology is recommended for the diagnosis of the infection (Kitching & Hughes, 2002; Donaldson, 2000).
Subclinical infection	Occurs without overt clinical signs	Hypomagnesaemia in animals produce no clinical signs.
Clinical infection	A clinical infection causes noticeable symptoms. If the disease is mild, and the symptoms are too vague for a clear diagnosis, it is called an abortive reaction	The response to foot-and-mouth disease virus in sheep can be so mild that it makes the disease hard to diagnose (Kitching & Hughes, 2002; Ayres et al., 2001).
	Severe disease, known as a frank clinical reaction, occurs when symptoms are strong enough for a clear diagnosis. The most extreme reaction can lead to death. Interestingly, in some infections, death serves as a way for the infectious agent to be released and spread to other animals.	E.g. In sheep, the clear clinical signs of FMD are seen periods of stress like parturition (Brown et al., 2002; Reid, 2002; Tyson, 2002); Infection with *Trichinella spiralis*, which is transmitted exclusively by flesh eating.

Increasing severity of disease

			Clinical signs		
Signs in animal	No signs	No signs (Subclinical disease)	Mild disease	Severe disease	Death
Type of infection	No infection	Inapparent infection	Overt infection		
Status of animal	Insusceptible or immune	Susceptible			

eliminates all infectious agents from the body. Animals with sterile immunity no longer pose a threat to susceptible populations. The two important states to consider are the *carrier state* and *latent infections*. In the carrier state, some animals may become carriers, harboring and shedding infectious agents without showing clinical signs. Carriers can play a significant role in the transmission of diseases. In latent infections, the infectious agent persists in the body without causing clinical signs. Reactivation of latent infections can occur, contributing to disease spread.

3.2.3.3 Environmental Determinants

The environment, encompassing factors like location, climate, and husbandry practices, plays a crucial role in determining disease outcomes. In livestock enterprises, especially in intensive production systems like chicken battery houses, animals are exposed to unnatural environments, warranting careful consideration of environmental determinants. Similarly, in human medicine, social and occupational exposures, such as exposure to smoke in relation to lung cancer, highlight the impact of the environment on health. Moreover, the health and welfare of captive wild animals can also be significantly influenced by their environment (Kirkwood, 2007). Table 3.4 classifies the environmental determinants based on the location, climate, husbandry and stress parameters.

Determinants associated with the host, agent, and environment do not act in isolation; instead, they interact with each other. The term "interaction" refers to the interdependent operation of these factors, working together to produce or prevent a particular effect, such as the induction of disease. In the case of hypomagnesemia, factors leading to a net

Table 3.4 Classification of environmental determinants (Thrusfield, 2007 / with permission of John Wiley & Sons).

Environmental determinants		
Determinants	**Variants**	**Impact**
Location	Local geological formations Vegetation Noise	➤ The occurrence of jaw tumors in sheep is linked to areas where bracken grows, highlighting the usefulness of maps in identifying disease causes. ➤ Non-specific Chronic lung disease in middle-aged and older dogs has been linked to living in urban areas in the US, where urban residence is associated with higher levels of air pollution.
Climate	Macroclimate	The normal weather conditions animals are exposed to – such as rainfall, temperature, solar radiation, humidity, and wind – can all impact their health: ➤ **Temperature**: Low temperatures can cause hypothermia, especially in newborn animals. Wind and rain can increase heat loss, making animals more vulnerable to cold stress. ➤ **Cold Stress**: This can lead to health issues, like reducing digestion efficiency, which may increase the risk of diseases such as infectious enteritis. ➤ **Geographical Limitations**: The spread of certain parasites, like the French heartworm (*Angiostrongylus vasorum*), is restricted by cold temperatures (Jeffery et al., 2004). ➤ **Wind**: It can carry infectious agents, like the foot-and-mouth disease virus, and insect vectors, such as *Culicoides* species carrying bluetongue virus, over long distances. ➤ **Solar Radiation**: Ultraviolet radiation from the sun can act as a primary factor in causing health issues, like skin cancer (cutaneous squamous cell carcinoma).
	Microclimate	A microclimate is a climate that exists within a small, specific area. ➤ **Terrestrial Microclimate**: Influences the growth and development of arthropods and helminths. ➤ **Biological Microclimate**: Can change during a disease, aiding in its spread. For example, in malaria, sweating during the parasitaemic phase increases skin humidity, attracting more mosquitoes when the protozoon is abundant. ➤ **Stable Dust**: Linked to respiratory hypersensitivity and non-allergic lung disease, and can also carry microorganisms. ➤ **Ammonia Levels**: High levels can cause keratoconjunctivitis in hens and turbinate atrophy in pigs. ➤ **Poor Ventilation**: Associated with chronic respiratory disease in horses. ➤ **Household Humidity**: High humidity levels are linked to increased levels of canine mite allergens.

Table 3.4 (Continued)

		Environmental determinants
Determinants	**Variants**	**Impact**
Husbandry	Housing	➢ **Claw Lesions**: Pigs raised on aluminium slats tend to have more frequent and severe claw lesions compared to those raised on steel or concrete slabs, or on soil. ➢ **Limb Lesions**: Pigs raised on concrete floors are more likely to develop limb lesions than those on asphalt-based floors. Additionally, hoof lesions and vulva biting, which is linked to aggression, are common issues among group-housed sows. ➢ **Floor Slope**: Excessive floor slope can increase the risk of rectal prolapse in pigs due to the greater effect of gravity (Smith & Straw, n.d.).
	Diet	➢ **Dietary Deficiencies**: Diseases caused by deficiencies in energy, protein, vitamins, and minerals are clearly affected by diet. ➢ **Biotin**: Higher dietary levels of biotin can reduce the occurrence of foot lesions in sows. ➢ **Gastric Torsion**: In sows kept in stalls, gastric torsion is linked to once-a-day feeding rather than twice-a-day feeding. This suggests that eating a large amount of food at once may be a contributing factor.

	Management	➢ **Management**: Management practices set the stocking density and production policies.
		➢ **Stocking Density**: Higher stocking densities increase the risk of microbial infections.
		➢ **Animal Occupation**: The type of work or role an animal has can influence disease occurrence. For example:
		  • **Equine Limb Injuries**: These are relatively common among hunters.
		  • **Hump-Sore**: Also known as "yoke gall," is more common in draught zebus compared to non-working cattle.

Stress		➢ **Factors Influencing Health**: Weaning, overcrowding, transportation, changes in diet, and other environmental conditions can all impact animal health. ➢ **Stress and Disease**: Stress can be a primary factor in conditions such as post-capture myopathy syndrome and porcine stress syndrome.

decrease in magnesium intake interact with those causing a net increase in magnesium loss, resulting in the condition. Parasitism increases the demand for amino acids in the alimentary tract, leading to protein deficiency, which, in turn, affects the development and maintenance of immunity. Bovine alimentary papillomas caused by a papilloma virus can transform the papillomas into carcinomas in areas where bracken fern is common, indicating an interaction between the infectious agent (virus) and the environment (bracken fern). There is also an example of interaction between a gene (host factor) and stressors (environmental factors) leading to the porcine stress syndrome.

3.3 Adjustment of Rates, Trends and Emergence

Epidemiology is the study of how health-related states, conditions, or events are distributed and determined within populations, and how these findings can be used to control health problems (Last, 1988). It is a quantitative science that looks at how disease processes occur, the factors influencing their occurrence, and the host's response to infectious agents (Evans, 1979). While clinicians focus on disease, epidemiologists examine both infection and disease. Since infections can occur without causing disease, studying only clinical illness provides an incomplete view and is less effective for control and prevention efforts (Evans, 2009).

One key aspect of epidemiological analysis is the comparison of basic health indicators. This approach helps in identifying risk areas, defining needs, and documenting health inequalities across different populations, subgroups, or over time within a single population. Crude rates – whether they relate to mortality, morbidity, or other health events – serve as summary measures of population experiences, making comparative analysis possible. However, using crude rates for comparison can be problematic when population structures differ in terms of factors such as age, sex, or socioeconomic status. These factors can significantly affect the magnitude of crude rates and potentially lead to misleading interpretations due to a phenomenon known as confounding.

To avoid certain confounding factors, specific rates are calculated within well-defined subgroups of a population. For instance, age-specific rates can reveal how diseases impact different age groups, allowing for a more detailed analysis of health patterns and facilitating more accurate rate comparisons. However, working with numerous subgroups can be impractical, especially if the subgroups are small, which can lead to imprecise specific rates.

To address these challenges, the standardization (or adjustment) of rates is employed. This classic epidemiological method removes the confounding effects of variables, such as age, that may differ between populations being compared. Standardization provides a summary measure that simplifies data interpretation for users, like decision-makers, who prefer synthetic health indices.

Age is the most commonly adjusted factor in practice. Age-standardization is particularly useful in comparative mortality studies because age structure significantly influences overall mortality rates. For instance, in countries with moderate mortality rates, an older population will generally show higher crude mortality rates compared to a younger population.

There are two primary methods of standardization:

Direct Method: This involves applying age-specific rates from the populations being studied to a standard age distribution. This method adjusts for differences in age structure between populations by using a common age distribution as a reference.

Indirect Method: This method uses a standard set of age-specific rates (usually from a standard population) and applies them to the age distribution of the populations being studied. It provides a summary measure by comparing observed rates to expected rates based on the standard.

Both methods aim to facilitate more accurate and meaningful comparisons across populations by accounting for differences in age structure or other confounding variables

In the direct standardization method, we calculate the rate we would expect in populations if they had the same composition according to the variable we wish to adjust or control (such as age or socioeconomic status). This is done by applying the age-specific rates from the populations under study to a "standard" population that has a fixed distribution for the variable being adjusted. This method provides the number of "expected" cases for each stratum if the populations had the same composition. The adjusted or "standardized" rate is then calculated by dividing the total number of expected cases by the total population of the standard group.

An important aspect of this method is choosing an appropriate standard population. The value of the adjusted rate depends on the standard population used. Although the choice of the standard can be somewhat arbitrary, it's essential to select a standard that is not radically different from the populations being compared. The standard population can be derived from the study population (e.g. its sum or average) or from an external source. However, care must be taken to ensure that the size of the standard population does not unduly influence the adjusted rates.

When comparing adjusted rates, one can calculate the absolute difference, ratio, or percentage difference between them. This comparison is only valid if the same standard was used for calculating the adjusted rates. If the standard population changes (as occurred in the United States in 1999 when the standard was updated), it is necessary to recalculate the time series to maintain consistency. For international comparisons, organizations like WHO and PAHO use the "old" standard population defined by Waterhouse.

The direct method is frequently used but requires specific rates for all relevant population strata, which are not always available or may be imprecise if based on small numbers. In such cases, the indirect standardization method may be more suitable.

Indirect Method

The indirect standardization method differs in approach and interpretation from the direct method. In this method, instead of using the standard population's structure, we apply the specific rates of the standard population to the populations being compared, which are stratified according to the variable being controlled (such as age or socioeconomic status). This process generates a total of expected cases for each population.

The Standardized Mortality Ratio (SMR) is then calculated by dividing the total number of observed cases by the total number of expected cases. The SMR helps compare each population to the standard population. An SMR greater than one (or 100% if expressed as a percentage) indicates that the observed population has a higher risk of dying compared to the standard population. Conversely, an SMR less than one (or 100%) suggests a lower risk of dying in the observed population compared to the standard.

Additionally, the actual adjusted rates can be derived by multiplying the crude rates of each population by their respective SMRs. This approach yields a single adjusted value for each population, which, while still a synthetic measure, accounts for differences in population composition.

SMRs are commonly used in epidemiology for comparing different study groups because they are straightforward to calculate and offer a relative risk estimate between the standard and the studied populations. However, this method may not be appropriate if the rates vary significantly between strata across different groups. Despite this, comparing each group to the standard population remains valuable, and SMRs for different causes can be calculated using the same standard.

3.3.1 Epidemics and Their Investigation

Epidemics or outbreaks are often classified based on the source of infection. Common-source outbreaks occur when a group of individuals is exposed to a single source of infection, which is often called a common vehicle. Common-source outbreaks can be further classified into point-source outbreaks, where exposure to the common source occurs at a specific point in time. This is exemplified in many foodborne outbreaks. The epidemic curve in such cases is sharply defined and limited, typically occurring within the incubation period of the disease. Propagated or progressive outbreaks is characterized by the multiplication and spread of the infectious agent from one host to another. It is often referred to as contact spread and can occur through direct contact, indirect contact, or respiratory droplets. The spread is person-to-person, but it could involve animal or arthropod intermediates. The epidemic curve in propagated outbreaks depends on several factors, including the number of susceptible individuals, the degree of contact with infected individual, the incubation period, the transmission, the portal of entry, and the infectiousness of the agent.

3.3.1.1 Pathogenesis of an Outbreak

An outbreak of an infectious disease necessitates the convergence of three fundamental elements: the presence or introduction of an infectious agent, whether from an infected human, animal, bird, or vector, or its occurrence in environmental reservoirs such as air, water, food, soil, or on fomites; the existence of a sufficiently large population of susceptible individuals; and the availability of an effective transmission mechanism that facilitates the interaction between the infectious agent and the susceptible hosts.

Epidemics tend to arise under a set of specific and interrelated circumstances, such as when a previously unexposed group of susceptible individuals is introduced into a setting where a particular disease is endemic, thereby creating an environment ripe for transmission. Additionally, when a novel source of infection penetrates an area from which the microbial agent had been previously absent, a situation exacerbated by factors like the return of travellers from foreign locales, the influx of new immigrants, or the contamination of food, water, or other resources by an unfamiliar agent, the risk of an epidemic is significantly heightened. Furthermore, epidemics may be precipitated when changes in social, behavioral, sexual, or cultural practices facilitate effective contact between a preexisting infection of low endemicity and a vulnerable population. This risk is compounded when there is an increased susceptibility to infection or disease, whether through immunosuppression or other factors that compromise the host's immune response, such as preceding viral infections, nutritional disorders, immunosuppressive drug treatments, or the presence of chronic diseases. Lastly, an epidemic may be triggered by a sudden increase in the virulence or dosage of the microbial agent, thereby amplifying its capacity to spread and cause disease among susceptible individuals.

3.3.1.2 Investigation of an Outbreak

The first step in the investigation of an outbreak is to determine if an epidemic or outbreak actually exists. This involves recognizing an unusual increase in the number of cases of a particular disease. Once the outbreak is confirmed, efforts are made to assess the extent of the problem. This includes identifying the number of cases, the affected population, and any commonalities among those affected. Investigating the time, place, and person involved in the outbreak is crucial. Understanding where and when the cases occurred and identifying common characteristics among affected individuals can help pinpoint the source and mode of transmission. Understanding how the disease is spreading is essential for effective control measures. This involves identifying potential vectors, modes of transmission, and risk factors contributing to the spread of the disease. Once key information is gathered, strategies for controlling the outbreak are implemented. This may include isolation of affected individuals, quarantine measures, vaccination campaigns, or other preventive measures. Health authorities at various levels need to be notified promptly. Collaboration with national or state disease control agencies is often necessary for a coordinated response. Timely communication and information sharing are crucial. Written reports detailing the findings and actions taken during the investigation are essential. These reports serve as a reference for future outbreaks and contribute to the body of knowledge on disease epidemiology. Public communication is a critical aspect of outbreak management. News releases should be prepared to inform the public without causing unnecessary

54 | *3 Determinants of Disease, Adjustment of Rates, Trends and Emergence*

Table 3.5 The steps in epidemic investigations (Adapted from Evans, 2009).

Steps in the investigation of an Epidemic

1) Determine that an epidemic or outbreak actually exists by comparing with previous data on the disease

2) Establish an etiologic diagnosis if possible; if not, define the condition epidemiologically and clinically. Collect materials for isolation and serological test, and data from sick and well-exposed animals

3) Investigate the extent of the outbreak by a quick survey of hospitals, physicians, and other sources and its basic epidemiological characteristics in terms of time, place, person, probable method of spread, and the spectrum of clinical illness. Prepare a spot map of cases and an epidemic curve.

4) Formulate a working hypothesis of the source and manner of spread as a basis for further study

5) Test the hypothesis by determining infection and illness rates in animals exposed or not exposed to putative source(s) of infection by questionnaire, interview, and laboratory tests. Try to isolate the agent from the putative source(s)

6) Extend epidemiological and laboratory studies to other possible cases or to animals exposed but not ill

7) Analyze the data and consider possible interpretations

8) On the basis of the analysis, initiate both short- and long-term control measures

9) Report the outbreak to appropriate public health officials

10) Inform veterinarians, other health officials, and the public of the nature of the outbreak and the ways to control it

panic. Clear and transparent communication helps build trust and compliance with control measures. The investigation involves collaboration among various experts, including epidemiologists, clinicians, and laboratory professionals. Each plays a unique role in analyzing and managing the outbreak (Table 3.5).

3.4 Major Trends in Disease Dynamics

The twenty-first century has been marked by a series of severe infectious disease outbreaks. Among these, the COVID-19 pandemic stands out as a defining global health crisis, with profound effects on health, economies, and daily life. Other notable outbreaks include the 2003 SARS coronavirus outbreak, the 2009 swine flu pandemic, the 2012 MERS coronavirus outbreak, the 2013–2016 Ebola virus epidemic in West Africa, and the 2015 Zika virus epidemic, all of which resulted in significant morbidity and mortality, spreading across borders and affecting multiple countries. Concurrently, the last few decades have seen an era of unprecedented technological, demographic, and climatic changes: airline flights have doubled since 2000, more people have lived in urban than rural areas since 2007, populations continue to grow, and climate change poses an increasing threat to society (Baker et al., 2022).

The challenges in interpreting animal disease trends due to biases in detection and reporting suggests a correlation between the centuries-long improvement in human wealth and health and a parallel decline in infectious diseases in animals, marking a shift to noncommunicable diseases – a phenomenon termed the *second epidemiological transition*. Radostits highlights innovations in veterinary medicine, contributing to improved health through effective drugs, vaccines, diagnostic technologies, and preventive measures. Over the past decades, there have been significant advancements in controlling and managing various endemic diseases in intensive dairy, pig, and poultry production. Key areas of improvement include tackling mastitis, infectious causes of infertility, gastrointestinal parasitism in dairy; addressing erysipelas and classical swine fever in pig farming; and managing diseases like Newcastle disease in intensive poultry production. For example, it has been estimated that, in the United Kingdom, the number of cases of clinical mastitis decreased by more than 70% between the 1960s and late 1990s (Perry et al., 2013).

In the developing world, particularly in Africa, the distribution and impact of livestock diseases have seen limited changes, attributed to the distinctive development context. Notably, the successful control of rinderpest, with global eradication anticipated by 2011, stands out as a significant achievement. Additionally, the widespread adoption of veterinary drugs, often against official policies, has brought benefits to animal health and human livelihoods. However, this comes with the trade-off of increased drug resistance due to less rational use. Understanding the drivers of disease is crucial for prediction and management. Climate change and trade in livestock were identified as key factors influencing disease patterns, with demographic, social, economic, and environmental drivers also playing roles. However, inequality and foreign land purchase were not deemed significant in this context (Figures 3.4–3.6 and Table 3.6) (Grace et al., 2015).

3.4 Major Trends in Disease Dynamics | 55

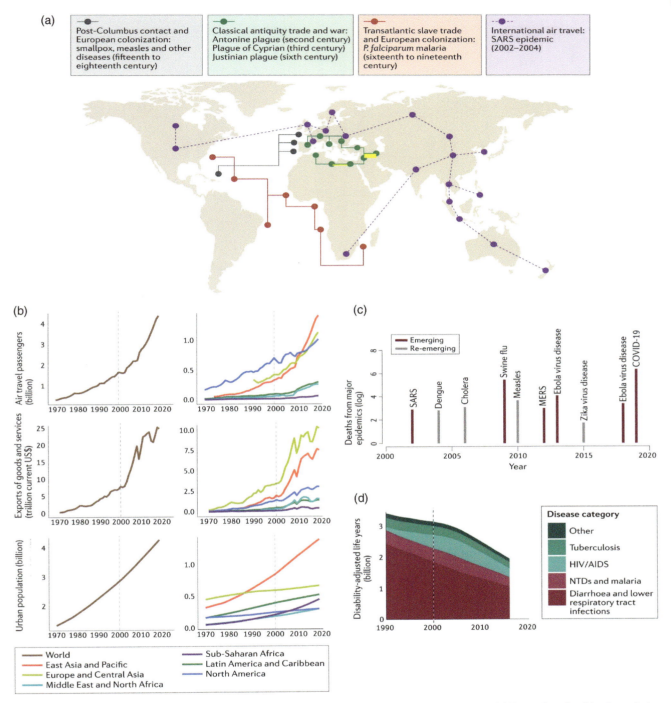

Figure 3.4 Examples of epidemic periods associated with different eras of human transportation. (a) **Examples of epidemic periods associated with different eras of human transportation (land, maritime and air travel) are shown**. *Overland trade networks and war campaigns are thought to have contributed to multiple epidemics in the Mediterranean in late classical antiquity (green), beginning with the Antonine plague, which reportedly claimed the life of the Roman emperor Lucius Verus. Maritime transportation (red and gray) leading to European contact with the Americas and the subsequent Atlantic slave trade resulted in the importation of Plasmodium falciparum malaria and novel viral pathogens. In modern times, air travel (purple) resulted in the importation of severe acute respiratory syndrome (SARS) coronavirus to 27 countries before transmission was halted. (b) In recent years, increases in air travel, trade and urbanization at global (left) and regional (right) scales have accelerated, indicating ever more frequent transport of people and goods between growing urban areas. (c) Log deaths from major epidemics in the twenty-first century. (d) Disability-adjusted life years lost from infectious diseases. MERS, Middle East respiratory syndrome; NTD, neglected tropical disease* (Baker et al., 2022 / with permission of Springer Nature).

56 | *3 Determinants of Disease, Adjustment of Rates, Trends and Emergence*

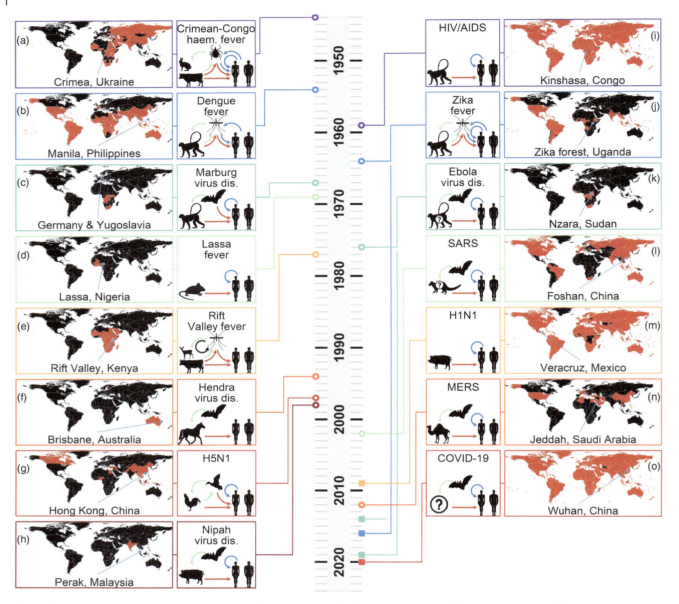

Figure 3.5 Major diseases of animal-origin affecting human health (Dharmarajan et al., 2022 / ScienceOpen / CC BY 4.0) ***A timeline of emergence of diseases of animal-origin which are considered to be a threat to global health or which require urgent research as identified by the World Health Organization***, including: (a) Crimean-Congo hemorrhagic fever; (b) Dengue fever; (c) Marburg virus disease; (d) Lassa fever; (e) Rift Valley fever; (f) Hendra virus disease; (g) Highly Pathogenic Asian Avian Influenza A subtype H5N1; (h) Nipah virus disease; (i) HIV/AIDS; (j) Zika fever; (k) Ebola virus disease; (l) Sudden Acute Respiratory Syndrome (SARS); (m) Influenza A virus subtype H1N1; (n) Middle East Respiratory Syndrome (MERS); (o) Coronavirus Disease 2019 (COVID-19).

For each disease the year of initial identification (round symbols on time line) or declaration of a public health emergency of international concern (square symbols on time line) are shown. The spatial extent of each disease is also given as a map highlighting with areas where transmission is reported (red areas) and the location from where the pathogen was first reported (blue symbol). Also, depicted are the major routes of transmission in the zoonotic source population (green arrows), primary zoonotic event (red arrows) and mode of maintenance in the human population (green arrows). Diseases include those that are strictly zoonotic and maintained in the human population only through transmission from a vertebrate animal host (e.g. Rift Valley fever and Hendra virus disease), diseases that are primarily maintained by zoonotic spillover but which can also be transmitted directly between humans (e.g. Ebola/Marburg virus diseases and MERS), and diseases of animal-origin which

3.4 Major Trends in Disease Dynamics

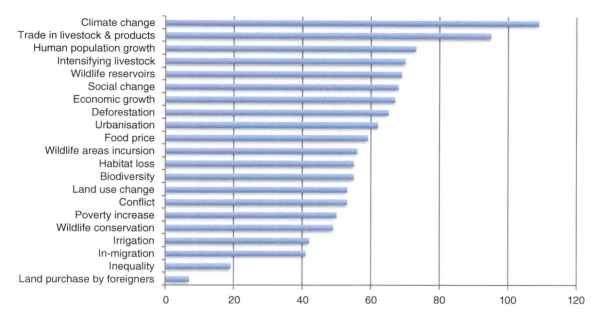

Figure 3.6 Drivers of change in disease dynamics (Grace et al., 2015).

Table 3.6 Current trends in the distribution of some infectious diseases of animals (Thrusfield, 2007; Bardhan et al., 2020; Jost et al., 2021)

Disease	Host and risk factors	Trends or impact of note
Anthrax	All animals, particularly devastating in cattle	World-wide range, now contracting to mainly tropics and sub-tropics
Avian influenza (AI)	Wild-domestic bird mixing	Over the past decade, significant epidemics have included the H5N8 avian influenza outbreaks, notably the 2014–2015 epidemic in the United States and the 2016–2017 epidemic in Europe. The latter outbreak impacted both domestic and wild bird populations across 30 countries, highlighting the widespread nature of these epidemics and their considerable impact on wildlife and agriculture
African swine fever (ASF)	Spillover/spill back – wild and domestic suids	Severe losses to pig production in China after 2018 detection, and significant increase in pork price; spread to many other countries in Asia and the Pacific
Aujeszky's disease	Pigs	Spreading, recently entered Japan
Bluetongue	Sheep	Spreading for past 100 years
Bovine brucellosis	Cattle	Eradicated from many developed countries in recent decades
Contagious bovine pleuropneumonia	Cattle	Eradicated from much of Europe
Middle East respiratory syndrome (MERS)	Human and other ruminant contact with infected camels	Negligible clinical impacts on camels; Approximately 2500 human cases to date and 850 deaths since first detection in 2012; US$ 12 billion in losses from human introduction into the Republic of Korea
Glanders	Horses	Mostly eradicated from developed countries
Johne's disease	Cattle, sheep, goats	World-wide distribution with increasing prevalence in some countries, and spreading in Europe
Lumpy skin disease	Cattle	Extending from Africa to the Middle East

(Continued)

Table 3.6 (Continued)

Disease	Host and risk factors	Trends or impact of note
Nipah	Swine or human contact with infected bat secretions	Over 1 million pigs lost to control; >100 human deaths; US$ 671 million in losses
Rabies	All mammals, some birds	Eradication is problematic. Geographically isolated areas (including some island masses) are generally free, although most countries experience rabies to some extent
Rift valley fever	Cattle, sheep, goats, man	Extending from Africa to the Middle East
Rinderpest	Artiodactyls	Only a few pockets of infection remaining. Global mass vaccination ended
Sheep pox	Sheep	Eradicated from Europe in 1951. Present in Africa, Middle East and India
Swine vesicular disease	Pigs	Decreased significance since 1982
Tuberculosis	Many species, especially serious in cattle	Eradication has proved problematic but some success has been achieved. No country is totally free of tuberculosis

show very efficient human-to-human transmission (e.g. HIV infection, H5N1/H1N1 influenza). Several diseases are suspected to be of zoonotic origin but the vertebrate animal reservoir remains unconfirmed (e.g. Ebola virus disease, SARS and COVID-19).

3.4.1 The Burden Pyramid of Infectious Disease

At the community level, depicting the true epidemic curves of any infectious disease are always challenging. The overall burden of directly transmitted infectious diseases involves multiple stages, including infections, healthcare-seeking behavior, hospitalization, severity (including admission to the intensive care unit), and mortality (Figure 3.7). The syndromic information on the morbidity and mortality of these diseases is not free from biases and is often underestimated. The available data represent only the visible part of the total infections in the community, likened to the tip of an iceberg. Epidemiological analyses are described as highly data-driven, and the quality and comprehensiveness of the data collected

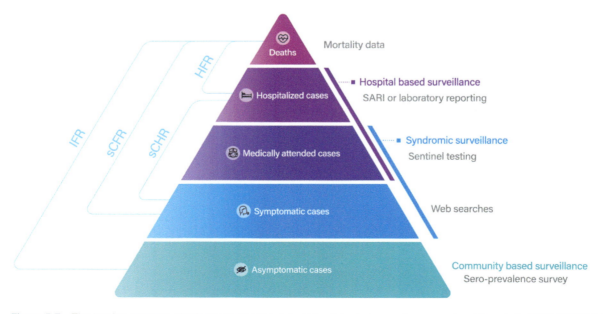

Figure 3.7 The burden pyramid of infectious disease and epidemiological severity parameters (Ryu et al., 2022 / MDPI / CC BY 4.0). *The clinical spectrum of infectious diseases and the possible surveillance system at each level. Note: SARI, severe acute respiratory infection; IFR, infection fatality rate; sCFR, symptomatic cases fatality rate; sCHR, symptomatic hospitalization rate; and HFR, hospitalization fatality rate.*

significantly influence the outcomes of these analyses. Advancements in data observation, surveillance systems, integration, and assimilation techniques, along with enhanced methods for data retrieval and reconstruction, are essential for gaining a comprehensive understanding of disease characteristics and transmission dynamics. Accurate estimation of the proportion of asymptomatic infections, evolving case definitions over time, and nowcasting true infection rates are critical steps that can enable the generation of real-time epidemiological curves (epi-curves) for any disease. These improvements contribute significantly to more effective and timely public health responses (Ryu et al., 2022).

3.5 Climate Sensitive Diseases, Neglected Tropical Diseases (NTDs), Emerging and Re-emerging Diseases

3.5.1 Climate Sensitive Livestock Diseases

Climate change may affect livestock disease through direct and indirect pathways. There is a link between the climate and the distribution of infectious diseases, timing, intensity of disease outbreaks and factors such as pathogens, vectors, hosts (animals and humans) and ecosystem services (Grace et al., 2015).

- **Pathogens**: Higher temperatures and increased humidity generally accelerate the development of parasites and pathogens that have life stages outside the host. Changes in wind patterns can influence the spread of pathogens, while extreme climate events like flooding can create conditions suitable for water-borne pathogens. Drought and desiccation are detrimental to most pathogens.
- **Vectors**: Vector-borne diseases are especially vulnerable to the effects of climate change, as alterations in rainfall patterns and temperature can significantly influence the distribution and abundance of disease vectors. These environmental changes can expand or shift the habitats of vectors such as mosquitoes, ticks, and other carriers, potentially leading to the spread of diseases into new regions and affecting the incidence and severity of outbreaks.
- **Hosts**: Livestock may be exposed to new pathogens and vectors as their ranges expand due to climate change. Climate stress, such as heat and inadequate food/water, can compromise the immunity of hosts.
- **Ecosystem Services**: Climate change has the potential to significantly alter ecosystem structure and function, which can, in turn, impact disease transmission. Changes in biodiversity driven by climate change may reduce the capacity of ecosystems to dilute the transmission of diseases, thereby increasing the risk of outbreaks. The Intergovernmental Panel on Climate Change (IPCC) estimates that if global mean temperatures rise by 2–3 °C, 20–30% of the world's vertebrate species could face an increasingly high risk of extinction, which would profoundly affect ecosystem dynamics and the balance of disease transmission within these environments.
- **Humans**: Climate change can influence human behavior in ways that may significantly affect how animals are kept, which in turn can increase their exposure or vulnerability to pathogens or vectors. While the drivers of disease are varied, the impacts resulting from changes in human behavior – such as shifts in farming practices, land use, and animal husbandry – can be considerably more pronounced than those occurring through biological pathways. These behavioral changes can lead to conditions that facilitate the spread of diseases, underscoring the complex interplay between climate change, human actions, and animal health.

The effects of climate change on health might be counterbalanced by advancements in wealth and technology, which can enhance disease control. However, the increasing prevalence of climate-related food-borne, water-borne, and vector-borne diseases adds complexity to this issue (Intergovernmental Panel on Climate Change (IPCC), 2023).

Most diseases, whether affecting humans or animals, tend to be more prevalent in areas characterized by hot, wet climates and lower socio-economic conditions. Tropical regions that are economically prosperous, such as Singapore and Hong Kong, show disease levels comparable to non-tropical, wealthy countries. This suggests that improved living standards, healthcare, public awareness, and infrastructure play crucial roles in disease prevention and control. Improved living standards, health care, and socio-economic conditions are cited as factors contributing to the elimination of vector-borne diseases in the United States (Gubler et al., 2001) and the eradication of malaria in Finland. Socio-economic factors like household size and living standards are considered (Hulden & Hulden, 2009). It is challenging to develop credible estimates of the impact of animal disease under different climate scenarios due to the multifaceted nature of disease dynamics. Scenarios that suggest greater wealth, peace, and knowledge sharing are expected to result in less disease, including climate-sensitive diseases. The impact of climate change on non-vector-borne diseases and livestock diseases has received relatively little attention. There is a lack of detailed information on the likely impact of these diseases under different climate scenarios. The need to identify livestock diseases that are likely to be sensitive to climate change as a crucial first step. Understanding the potential impacts of climate change on these diseases is essential for developing effective mitigation and adaptation strategies.

The climate sensitive diseases are particularly important for individuals involved in livestock keeping. Gastroenteritis caused by Salmonella species is a major concern, with an estimated 94 million cases occurring globally each year, resulting in 155000 deaths. The majority of these cases (81 million) are foodborne. Campylobacteriosis is also noted as a significant concern, primarily being foodborne (Majowicz et al., 2010). The burden to human health associated with campylobacter infection is even higher than that caused by Salmonella. Parasitic endemic diseases are identified as a priority, particularly those that impose a high burden on productivity. E.g. water-transmitted leptospirosis and soil-associated anthrax.

Predicting the impact of global environmental change on infectious diseases is not a straightforward process. It involves understanding the complex interactions among pathogens, vectors, hosts, and their environment within ecosystems. Merely plotting the predicted rise in temperature and imputing changes in temperature-sensitive pathogen development is not sufficient. The impact of environmental change on infectious diseases involves a multitude of factors and processes. Within complex ecosystems, processes related to pathogens, vectors, hosts, and the environment can be up- or down-regulated. Additionally, ecosystems may undergo phase transitions, marked by abrupt changes in dynamics. New evidence suggests that disease vectors, such as mosquitoes, may evolve in relatively short time frames, potentially within a decade, in response to changes in temperature (Egizi et al., 2015). This highlights the dynamic nature of vector populations and their ability to adapt to environmental shifts. Environmental change is dynamic and involves various interconnected factors, including climate change, land use changes, and alterations in ecosystems. These changes can have cascading effects on infectious disease dynamics. The ecological interactions and adaptive capacities of pathogens and vectors is crucial for accurate projections of disease patterns under global environmental change.

Mathematical models are described as powerful tools for understanding disease dynamics. These models provide a structured and quantitative framework for simulating and analyzing the complex interactions among pathogens, hosts, vectors, and the environment. Mathematical models have been successfully applied in the field of epidemiology, aiding in the understanding of disease spread, transmission dynamics, and the impact of various factors on disease outcomes. Statistical, process-based, and landscape-based models, are the main types of models used to forecast future climatic influences on infectious diseases.

Many emerging infectious diseases are zoonoses, meaning they can be transmitted between animals and humans. A significant portion of these diseases is classified as "neglected," indicating a lack of attention and resources for their prevention and treatment. Zoonoses pose a dual burden as they affect both humans and animals. This dual impact emphasizes the interconnectedness of human and animal health. Disability-Adjusted Life Year (DALY) is a metric that quantifies the burden of disease by combining both mortality and morbidity into a single measure (Di-Bari et al., 2023). DALYs are used to measure the impact of diseases on human health. The road map for neglected tropical diseases (NTDs) sets a target of a 75% reduction in DALYs by 2030 compared to 2020. As of 2019, data for 181 countries indicate an 11% reduction in NTD DALYs compared to 2015. Notable percentage reductions for specific NTDs include 36% for human African trypanosomiasis, 24.9% for foodborne trematodiases, 18.9% for soil-transmitted helminthiases, and varying reductions for other diseases like rabies, lymphatic filariasis, schistosomiasis, cysticercosis, leishmaniasis, and leprosy. The comparative analysis of DALYs reflects progress in reducing the burden of certain NTDs. However, the variations in reduction percentages indicate that challenges persist in achieving the overall 75% reduction target by 2030 (Figure 3.8).

3.5.2 Economically Important Diseases at the Wildlife–Livestock Interface

The order Chiroptera (bats) had perceived importance in the context of emerging infectious diseases, particularly zoonotic diseases that have been linked to bats. It provides examples of viruses, such as Nipah, Ebola Reston virus, and Middle East respiratory syndrome (MERS) coronavirus, that have been identified as having bat origins and have demonstrated the potential for spillover to livestock. These viruses that were originated in bats had spilled over to affect pigs (Nipah and Ebola Reston virus) and camels (MERS coronavirus). The trend of agricultural expansion and intensification of the wildlife interface, especially in tropical systems are associated with external economic and development pressures and a potential driver for the spillover and emergence of infectious diseases (Wiethoelter et al., 2015). The exclusion of coronaviruses from the list is identified as an important gap in animal health surveillance, suggesting a need for a more comprehensive understanding of the role of coronaviruses in wildlife and livestock diseases (Figure 3.9 and Table 3.7).

3.5 Climate Sensitive Diseases, Neglected Tropical Diseases (NTDs), Emerging and Re-emerging Diseases | 61

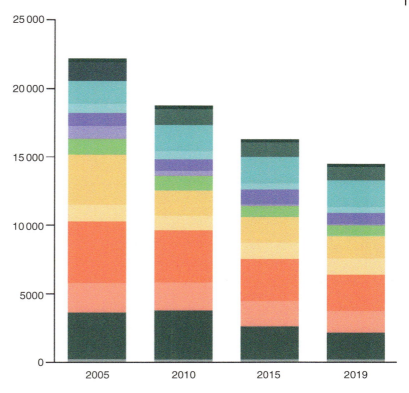

Figure 3.8 Burden of NTDs assessed using DALYs (in thousands) during 2005–2019 (World Health Organization, 2023).

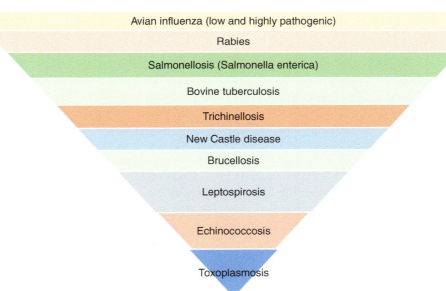

Figure 3.9 The top ten diseases at the wildlife–livestock interface (Adapted from Wiethoelter et al., 2015).

Table 3.7 Top three wildlife–livestock interfaces including the five predominant diseases (Adapted from Wiethoelter et al., 2015).

Wildlife	Livestock	Diseases
Birds	Poultry	Avian influenza, Newcastle disease, salmonellosis, avian chlamydiosis, poxvirus infections
Artiodactyls	Cattle	Bovine tuberculosis, brucellosis, malignant catarrhal fever, foot and mouth disease, theileriosis
Carnivores	Cattle	Rabies, bovine tuberculosis, echinococcosis, leptospirosis, salmonellosis

3.5.3 Some of the Key Challenges and Knowledge Gaps

Some key challenges and knowledge gaps in the control of livestock sensitive diseases are paucity of information, complexity of disease dynamics, multi-host disease systems and joint occurrence of climate sensitive diseases in common landscapes (Grace et al., 2015).

- **Paucity of Information:** One major challenge is the lack of epidemiological and ecological observations on animal diseases in the poorest countries (Grace et al., 2015). This scarcity of data hinders the development of a comprehensive understanding of climatfe-sensitive diseases. Current surveillance systems are limited in their ability to detect a significant proportion of diseases. Additionally, there is a lack of effective linkage between livestock disease surveillance and the surveillance of diseases in humans and wildlife.
- **Complexity of Disease Dynamics:** The dynamics of climate-sensitive diseases are complex, involving numerous pathways, both direct and indirect, through which climate can influence disease transmission and prevalence. These drivers of disease are not all equal, and the impacts mediated through changes in human population and behavior may have effects that are orders of magnitude greater than those mediated through biological factors.
- **Multi-host Disease Systems**: Many climate-sensitive diseases affect multiple host species, including livestock, wildlife, and sometimes humans. The presence of multiple hosts makes the transmission dynamics of these diseases more stable. The implication is that prevention and control measures for these diseases must be highly effective across various host species to achieve the intended outcomes.
- **Joint Occurrence of Climate Sensitive Diseases in Common Landscapes:** There is a phenomenon of climate-sensitive livestock diseases co-occurring in common areas. This suggests that the emergence and transmission of these diseases are influenced by similar ecological factors. Understanding the common landscapes where these diseases overlap is crucial for developing targeted and effective strategies for disease prevention and control.

3.6 Factors and Determinants of Disease Emergence

Emerging infectious diseases are defined as infections that have either newly appeared in a population or are rapidly increasing in incidence or expanding in geographic range (Morse, 2004). This definition highlights the dynamic nature of certain diseases. Zoonotic diseases are described as global health threats that result from the complex interactions between humans, animals, and the environment. Of the approximately 1415 species of infectious agents pathogenic to humans, nearly 60% are zoonotic. This indicates that a significant proportion of diseases affecting humans have origins in animals. There is a 75 per cent prevalence of newly appearing or rapidly increasing emerging pathogens with a zoonotic nature. Food-borne diseases and antimicrobial resistance (AMR), both contribute to the burden on existing health systems and national economies. The One Health concept recognizes the interdependence of human, animal, and environmental health and emphasizes a collaborative, interdisciplinary approach to address health challenges. Early detection, prevention, and control of zoonotic diseases in animals not only protect animal health but also contribute to safeguarding human health (Kumar et al., 2021).

The World Health Organization (WHO) estimates that around one-third of the annual global deaths – approximately 20 million – are due to infectious diseases. The majority of these deaths are caused by acute respiratory infections, gastrointestinal infections, tuberculosis, and malaria. This pattern of illness and mortality has remained largely unchanged over the past century. In the United States, infectious diseases rank as the third leading cause of death, following heart disease and cancer. Globally, they are the second leading cause of death and the leading cause of disability-adjusted life-years (DALYs), with one DALY representing one lost year of healthy life.

The dynamics of infectious disease emergence involve both the introduction of a pathogen to a new host population and its subsequent dissemination. Often, this stems from existing pathogens seizing opportunities to infect new hosts. Occasionally, a new pathogen variant can evolve, leading to the emergence of a novel disease. The process, termed "microbial traffic," describes how infectious agent cross species or move from isolated groups to new populations, contributing to disease spread. Increased microbial traffic, often linked to various activities, can facilitate the emergence of diseases, sometimes with epidemic consequences. Notably, many emerging infections originate in specific geographic locations before spreading to new areas (Figure 3.10).

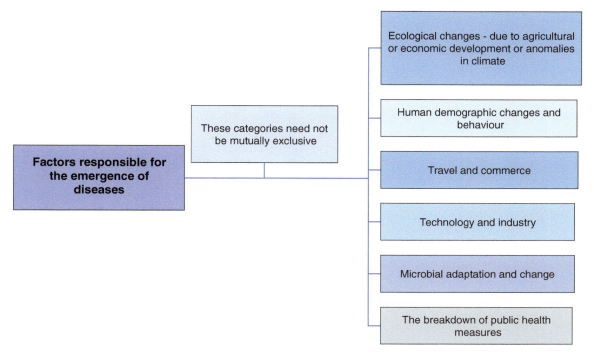

Figure 3.10 Factors responsible for the emergence of diseases (Adapted from Morse, 2004).

3.7 Future Global Health Challenges

The significant presence of livestock in the global economy, particularly in developing countries, underscores its importance for rural livelihoods. With approximately 38 billion livestock worldwide in 2013, the sector plays a vital role, especially for around one billion impoverished farmers, many of whom are women. Climate change adds complexity, as its indirect impacts on animal diseases may surpass direct effects, emphasizing the need for comprehensive strategies in managing both economic and environmental aspects of livestock farming (Grace et al., 2015).

While significant strides in basic healthcare have enhanced global well-being, upcoming decades pose challenges. Population growth, urbanization, and the escalating threat of antimicrobial resistance (AMR) are key concerns. The misuse of antibiotics in both livestock and human medicine contributes to rising global resistance. With drug-resistant infections causing over half a million deaths yearly, the economic toll is substantial, projected to potentially reach $100 trillion by 2050 due to productivity losses and the expensive nature of prolonged hospital stays and treatments. Addressing these challenges requires concerted efforts in healthcare management and antibiotic stewardship National Intelligence Council (2021).

Over the next two decades, the tangible impacts of climate change, including higher temperatures, sea level rise, and extreme weather events, will affect every nation. The developing world is poised to bear a disproportionate share of the costs and challenges, amplifying risks to food, water, health, and energy security amid environmental degradation. Meeting the Paris Agreement's goal of limiting warming to 1.5°C will necessitate intensified efforts to reduce greenhouse gas emissions. However, as the world approaches this threshold – likely within the next 20 years – calls for geoengineering research and potential deployment may rise, even with concerns about potential adverse consequences. Striking a balance between mitigation, adaptation, and ethical considerations becomes increasingly crucial in navigating the complex landscape of climate change responses National Intelligence Council (2021).

The ongoing acceleration of historical processes leading to the emergence of new infections is driven by modern life conditions. Factors like the speed of travel and global interconnectedness contribute to the increased prevalence of elements responsible for disease emergence (Morse, 2004). The recent example of the COVID-19 pandemic highlights the rapid access of microbes to new populations in today's interconnected world. Anticipating future challenges, it becomes imperative to proactively address the conditions fostering the emergence of new infections and strengthen global preparedness for potential health threats.

3.8 Conclusion

The link between livestock growth and epidemic disease risk underscores the need for urgent global action. Anthropogenic changes driving wildlife spillover demand heightened disease surveillance, particularly in situations fostering human-animal contact. The shift from extensive to intensive livestock systems and global movement through weakly secured value chains adds complexity. Recognizing infectious diseases' global impact, stemming from pathogen emergence and population mobility, emphasizes the urgency to address common infections, including HIV, in the developing world. A comprehensive strategy is crucial, focusing on disease hotspots, robust surveillance, and effective control measures to tackle the complexity of current and future infectious disease challenges. Indeed, the interconnectedness of our world demands a coordinated global effort to address the challenges posed by infectious diseases. Prioritizing early detection, surveillance, and effective control measures at the intersection of human and animal interaction is crucial for a comprehensive strategy. Time-sensitive action and collaboration across borders are essential to mitigate the impact of emerging infectious threats.

References

Ayres, E., Cameron, E., Kemp, R. et al. (2001). Oral lesions in sheep and cattle in Dumfries and Galloway. *Veterinary Record* 148: 720–723.

Baker, R.E., Mahmud, A.S., Miller, I.F. et al. (2022). Infectious disease in an era of global change. *Nature Review. Microbiology.* 20: 193–205.

Bardhan, D., Satyapal, Kumar, N. et al. (2020). Trends and patterns of major animal diseases in India. *International Journal of Current Microbiology and Applied Sciences* 2020 (9): 453–471.

Beauvais, W., Cardwell, J.M., and Brodbelt, D.C. (2012). The effect of neutering on the risk of mammary tumours in dogs – a systematic review. *Journal of Small Animal Practice* 53: 314–322.

Beverelli, C. and Ticku, R. (2023). Global livestock trade and infectious diseases. Working paper. RSC 2023/09. Robert Schuman Centre for Advanced Studies Global Governance Programme. 2023. 494.

Bronden, L.B., Eriksen, T., and Kristensen, A.T. (2009). Oral malignant melanomas and other head and neck neoplasms in Danish dogs – data from the Danish Veterinary Cancer Registry. *Acta Veterinaria Scandinavica* 51: 54.

Brown, L.D., Cai, T.T., and Das, G.A. (2002). Confidence intervals for a binomial proportion and asymptotic expansions. *The Annals of Statistics* 30: 160–201.

Cartin-Rojas, A. (2012). Chapter 7: Transboundary animal diseases and international trade. In: *International Trade from Economic and Policy Perspective*, 143–166. Intech.

Coetzee, P., Stokstad, M., Venter, E.H. et al. (2012). Bluetongue: a historical and epidemiological perspective with the emphasis on South Africa. *Virology Journal* 9: 198.

Dharmarajan, G., Li, R., Chanda, E. et al. (2022). The animal origin of major human infectious diseases: what can past epidemics teach us about preventing the next pandemic? *Zoonoses* https://doi.org/10.15212/zoonoses-2021-0028.

Di-Bari, C., Venkateswaran, N., Fastl, C. et al. (2023). The global burden of neglected zoonotic diseases: current state of evidence. *One Health* 17: 100595. https://doi.org/10.1016/j.onehlt.2023.100595.

Donaldson, A.I. (2000). The role of sheep in the epidemiology of foot-and-mouth disease and proposals for control and eradication in animal populations with a high density of sheep. *Report of the session of the research group of the standing technical committee of the European commission for the control of Foot-and-Mouth disease*, pp. 107–116, Borovets, Bulgaria (5–8 September 2000). AGA: EUFMD/RG/00. Food and Agriculture Organization of the United Nations, Rome.

Donaldson, A.I. and Alexandersen, S. (2001). Relative resistance of pigs to infection by natural aerosols of FMD virus. *Veterinary Record* 148: 600–602.

Drewe, J.A., Eames, K.T.D., Madden, J.R., and Pearce, G.P. (2010). Application of epidemiological tools to the investigation of a wild disease. Society for Veterinary Epidemiology and Preventive Medicine, Proceedings, Nantes, pp. 53–66 (24–26 March 2010). Alban, L. (ed.) Kelly, LA.

Egizi, A., Fefferman, N.H., and Fonseca, D.M. (2015). Evidence that implicit assumptions of 'no evolution' of disease vectors in changing environments can be violated on a rapid timescale. *Philosophical Transactions of the Royal Society of London. Series B, Biological Sciences.* 370: 1665.

Evans, A.S. (1979). Definitions of epidemiology [letter]. *American Journal of Epidemiology* 109: 379–381.

Evans, A.S. (2009). Epidemiological concepts. In: *Bacterial Infections of Humans* (ed. A.S. Evans and P.S. Brachman). Springer Science, Business Media, LLC.

Fall, T., Hamlin, H.H., Hedhammar, A. et al. (2007). Diabetes mellitus in a population of 18000 insured dogs: incidence, survival, and breed distribution. *Journal of Veterinary Internal Medicine* 21: 1209–1216.

Fleischman, W. (2012). Anemia: Determining the cause. *Compendium: Continuing Education for Veterinarians*. Vetlearn.com. 34 (6): E1–E9.

Grace, D., Bett, B., Lindahl, J., and Robinson, T. (2015). Climate and livestock disease: assessing the vulnerability of agricultural systems to livestock pests under climate change scenarios. CCAFS Working Paper no. 116. Copenhagen, Denmark: CGIAR Research Program on Climate Change, Agriculture and Food Security (CCAFS).

Gubler, D.J., Reiter, P., Ebi, K.L. et al. (2001). Climate variability and change in the United States: potential impacts on vector- and rodent-borne diseases. *Environmental Health Perspectives* 109: 223–233.

Hassan, M.K., Afify, M.A., and Aly, M.M. (2004). Genetic resistance of Egyptian chickens to infectious bursal disease and Newcastle disease. *Tropical Animal Health and Production* 36: 1–9.

Huertas, S.M., Gil, A.D., Piaggio, J.M., and van Eerdenberg, F.J.C.M. (2010). Transportation of beef cattle to slaughterhouses and how this relates to animal welfare and carcass bruising in an extensive production system. *Animal Welfare* 19: 281–285.

Hulden, L. and Hulden, L. (2009). The decline of malaria in Finland--the impact of the vector and social variables. *Malaria Journal* 8: 94.

Intergovernmental Panel on Climate Change (IPCC) (2023). Summary for policymakers. In: *Climate Change 2023: Synthesis Report. Contribution of Working Groups I, II and III to the Sixth Assessment Report of the Intergovernmental Panel on Climate Change* [Core Writing Team, H. Lee and J. Romero (eds.)]. 2023. IPCC, Geneva, Switzerland, pp. 1–34, https://doi.org/10.59327/IPCC/AR6-9789291691647.001.

Jeffery, R.A., Lankester, M.W., McGrath, M.J., and Whitney, H.G. (2004). *Angiostrongylus vasorum* and *Crenosoma vulpis* in red foxes (*Vulpes vulpes*) in Newfoundland, Canada. *Canadian Journal of Zoology* 82: 66–74.

Johnson-Walker, Y.J. and Kaneene, J.B. (2018). Epidemiology: science as a tool to inform one health policy. In: *Beyond One Health: From Recognition to Results*, 1e (ed. J.A. Herrmann and Y.J. Johnson-Walker), 3–29. US: John Wiley & Sons.

Jost, C.C., Machalaba, C., Karesh, W.B. et al. (2021). Epidemic disease risks and implications for veterinary services. *Revue Scientifique et Technique* 40: 497–509.

Kearsley-Fleet, L., O'Neill, D.G., Volk, H.A. et al. (2013). Prevalence and risk factors for canine epilepsy of unknown origin in the UK. *Veterinary Record* 172: 338.

Kirkwood, J.K. (2007). Welfare, husbandry and veterinary care of wild animals in captivity; changes in attitudes, progress in knowledge and techniques. In: *International Zoo yearbook 38* (ed. O. PJS and F.A. Fiskin), 124–130. London: The Zoological Society of London.

Kitching, R.P. and Hughes, G.J. (2002). Clinical variation in foot and mouth disease: sheep and goats. *Revue Scientifique et Technique, Office International des Epizooties* 21: 505–512.

Kumar, H.B.C., Hiremath, J., Yogisharadhya, R. et al. (2021). Animal disease surveillance: its importance & present status in India. *Indian Journal of Medical Research* 153: 299–310.

LaFond, E., Breur, G.J., and Austin, C.C. (2002). Breed susceptibility for developmental orthopedic diseases in dogs. *Journal of the American Animal Hospital Association* 38: 467–477.

Last, J.M.E. (1988). *A Dictionary of Epidemiology*, 2e. New York: Oxford University Press.

Last, J.M. (2001). *A Dictionary of Epidemiology*, 4e. New York: Oxford University Press.

Logas, D. (2003). An approach to pruritus. In: *BSAVA Manual of Small Animal Dermatology*, 2e (ed. A.P. Foster and C.S. Foil), 37–42. Cloucester: British Small Animal Veterinary Association.

London, C.A. and Thamm, D.H. (2013). Mast cell tumours. In: *Withrow and Mac Ewe's Small Animal Clinical Oncology*, 5e (ed. S.J. Withrow, D.M. Vail, and R.L. Page), 335–355. Elsevier Saunders, St. Louis.

Majowicz, S.E., Musto, J., Scallan, E. et al. (2010). The global burden of nontyphoidal Salmonella gastroenteritis. *Clinical Infectious Disease*. 2010 50 (6): 882–889.

Martin, S.W., Meek, A.H., and Willeberg, P. (1987). *Veterinary Epidemiology: Principles and Methods*. Ames: Iowa State University Press.

Miller, P.G. and Koch, G. (2013). Newcastle disease. In: *Diseases of Poultry*, 13e (ed. D.E. Swayne), 89–107. Ames: Wiley-Blackwell.

Morse, S.S. (2004). Factors and determinants of disease emergence. *Revue scientifique et technique (International Office of Epizootics)* 23: 443–451.

National Intelligence Council, 2021. Global Trends 2040: A More Contested World, Office of the Director of National Intelligence, March, https://www.dni.gov/index.php/gt2040-home (accessed 15 April, 2024).

Perry, B.D., Grace, D., and Sones, K. (2013). Current drivers and future directions of global livestock disease dynamics. *Proceedings of the National Academy of Sciences of United States of America* 110: 20871–20877. https://doi.org/10.1073/pnas.1012953108.

Pfeiffer, D.U. (2002). Basic concepts of veterinary epidemiology. In: *Veterinary Epidemiology – An introduction*, 62. United Kingdom: Royal veterinary college.

Porta, M. (2014). *A Dictionary of Epidemiology*, 6e. Oxford: Oxford University Press.

Quinn, P.J., Markey, B.K., Leonard, F.C. et al. (2011). *Veterinary Microbiology and Microbial Diseases*, 2e. Chichester: Wiley-Blackwell.

Reid, H.W. (2002). FMD in a parturient sheep flock (Letter). *Veterinary Record* 150: 791.

Reif, J.S., Schweitzer, D.J., Ferguson, S.W., and Benjamin, S.A. (1983). Canine neoplasia and exposure to uranium mill tailings in Mesa County, Colorado. Epidemiology Applied to Health Physics. *Proceedings of the 16th Midyear Topical Meeting of the Health Physics Society*, Albuquerque, New Mexico, pp. 461–469 (9–13 January 1983). Rio Grande Chapter of the Health Physics Society.

Ryu, S., Chun, J.Y., Lee, S. et al. (2022). Epidemiology and transmission dynamics of infectious diseases and control measures. *Viruses* 14: 2510. https://doi.org/10.3390/v14112510.

Saenz, V., Alvarez-Moreno, C., Le Pape, P. et al. (2020). A one health perspective to recognize fusarium as important in clinical practice. *Journal of Fungi* 6: 235. https://doi.org/10.3390/jof6040235.

Schwabe, C.W., Riemann, H., and Franti, C. (1977). *Epidemiology in Veterinary Practice*. Philadelphia: Lea and Febiger.

Smith, K.D. (2005). *Veterinary Clinical Epidemiology*, 3e. Boca Raton: CRC Press.

Smith, W.J. and Straw, B.E. (n.d.). Prolapses. In: *Diseases of Swine*, 9e (ed. B.E. Straw, J.J. Zimmerman, S. D'Allaire, and D.J. Taylor), 965–970. Oxford: Blackwell publishing.

Sousa, C.A. (2013). Diagnostic approach to the itchy dog. *In Practice* 35 (S1): 2–6.

Tadesse, B., Molla, W., Mengsitu, A., and Jemberu, W.T. (2019). Transmission dynamics of foot and mouth disease in selected outbreak areas of northwest Ethiopia. *Epidemiology and Infection* 147 (e189): 1–6. https://doi.org/10.1017/S0950268819000803.

Tater, K.C. (2012). An approach to pruritus. In: *BSAVA Manual of canine and Feline Dermatology*, 3e (ed. H. Jackson and R. Marsella), 37–45. Quedgeley: British Small Animal Veterinary Association.

Thrusfield, M. (2007). Chapter 5. Determinants of disease. In: *Veterinary Epidemiology*, 3e. Iowa: Blackwell publishing.

Thrusfield, M., Christley, R., Brown, H. et al. (2018). *Veterinary Epidemiology*, 4e. USA: Wiley Blackwell, John Wiley and Sons, Ltd.

Toker, M., Sen, Y., Kaya, M. et al. (2011). Mitral valve prolapse in dogs: a 12 year long retrospective study by echocardiography. *Revue de Medecine Veterinaire* 162: 352–357.

Tyson, J.D. (2002). FMD in a parturient sheep flock (Letter). *Veterinary Record* 151: 127.

Wiethoelter, A.K., Beltran-Alcrudo, D., Kock, R., and Siobhan, M.M. (2015). Global trends in infectious diseases at the wildlife–livestock interface. *Proceedings of the National Academy of Sciences of United States of America* www.pnas.org/lookup/suppl/doi:10.1073/pnas.

Wilson, J.W., Schurr, M.J., LeBlanc, C.L. et al. (2002). Mechanisms of bacterial pathogenicity. *Postgraduate Medical Journal* 78: 216–224.

World Health Organization (2023). *Global Report on Neglected Tropical Diseases 2023*. Geneva: World Health Organization https://www.who.int/publications/i/item/9789240067295.

Zintl, A., Gray, J.S., Skerrett, H.E., and Mulcahy, G. (2005). Possible mechanisms underlying age-related resistance to bovine babesiosis. *Parasite immunology.* 27: 115–120.

4

Transmission, Maintenance of Infection, and Consequences of Disease

Shriya Rawat[1], Parul[2], Nishant Sharma[3], Barkha Sharma[2], Udit Jain[2], and Vipul Thakur[1]

[1] *College of Veterinary & Animal Sciences, SVPUAT, Meerut, India*
[2] *College of Veterinary & Animal Sciences, DUVASU, Mathura, India*
[3] *College of Veterinary & Animal Sciences, GBPUAT, Pantnagar, India*

4.1 Introduction

Infectious diseases are illnesses that are caused by organisms, usually microscopic in nature like bacteria, viruses, parasites, and fungi that may be transmitted from one infected animal to another susceptible host. As per WHO estimates in 2022, communicable diseases cause nearly 26% of deaths globally with respiratory tract infections, diarrheal diseases, malaria, and tuberculosis among the top contributors (GBD 2015 Disease and Injury Incidence and Prevalence Collaborators 2016). Two of these conditions, respiratory tract infections and diarrheal ailments, were included in the WHO top 10 deadliest diseases of the world in 2019. The burden of infectious disease in India in 2019 was round 80.77 million DALYs by one estimate (Roser et al. 2021). Though the impact of infectious diseases is considerable, there has been a substantial decrease in deaths due to control measures including vaccination, awareness, development of new therapeutics, and government initiatives.

No control can be effective until the epidemiology and natural history of an agent are understood. Thorough knowledge of the chain of transmission, primary and secondary host, reservoir, methods of transmission, agent susceptibility, environmental factors favoring or suppressing an agent, all with reference to time and space, can greatly affect the outcome of a control strategy. This chapter aims to delve into the basic concepts of transmission of an agent, how it survives both inside and outside a host, and what finally ensues.

4.2 The Classic Disease Triangle

The epidemiological triangle represents what occurs around us every day. It gives a holistic view of the disease process. Its three components – agent, host, and environment – influence each other and finally the outcome of a disease. Fluctuation in environmental conditions may affect the life cycle of mosquitoes, which changes the dynamics of vector-borne diseases. An extended winter may arrest the development of mosquitoes, prolonging their life cycle and thereby their availability to transmit an agent. However, an increase in rainfall above the normal with high temperature may accelerate the development and thereby the vector density in an area, increasing the occurrence of mosquito-borne disease like dengue, Japanese encephalitis, malaria, Zika, etc. Figure 4.1 represents an epidemiological triad for rabies and Kyasanur Forest disease (KFD).

4.2.1 Rotavirus Diarrhea

Rotavirus, a member of the double-stranded Reoviridae, causes diarrheal infection in the young of most mammalian species. The disease is known as winter diarrhea as it causes nearly 50% of pediatric hospital admissions during winters (Ghoshal et al. 2020). The agent here is the wheel-shaped virus, the host may be human (children <5 years of age), calf, piglet, lamb, or kid, and the environment includes the feces containing the virus, the food and water contaminated by the feces containing the virus, the temperature, humidity, etc.

Epidemiology and Environmental Hygiene in Veterinary Public Health, First Edition. Edited by Tanmoy Rana.
© 2025 John Wiley & Sons, Inc. Published 2025 by John Wiley & Sons, Inc.

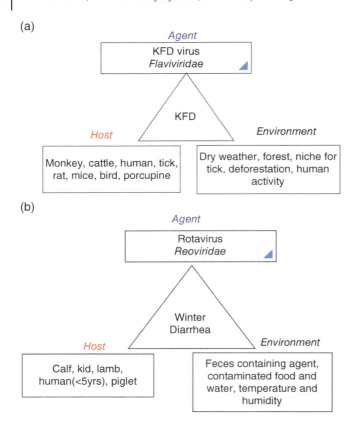

Figure 4.1 Epidemiological triad for (a) KFD, (b) winter diarrhea.

4.2.2 Kyasanur Forest Disease

The agent here is the KFD virus belonging to the family Flaviviridae. The disease generally occurs in monkeys in the Kyasanur Forest area in the Shivmoga district of Karnataka, India. The host here is the monkeys though accidental infection may occur in cattle and humans who venture into the forest to graze their animals. The disease is transmitted by means of the tick *Haemaphysalis spinigera* in which transovarian transmission has also been observed. Porcupines, rats, mice, forest birds, ticks, and small mammals act as reservoir hosts. The disease generally occurs in the dry months when tick activity is at its peak.

4.3 Factors Affecting the Spread of Disease

The mere presence of host, agent, and environment in a setting does not lead to a disease. For example, students in a classroom may be exposed to a respiratory virus by the coughing and sneezing of their tutor. But all do not get disease and in those who get the disease, the intensity may vary. Also, variations may be observed in morbidity and mortality rates with strains of the same pathogen. The recent SARS-CoV-2 virus is an apt example of this, with the Omicron variant being much milder than the Delta.

Factors affecting spread may be classified as:

- host factors: susceptibility and infectiousness
- agent factors: infectivity, pathogenicity, virulence, and stability
- effective contact.

4.3.1 Host Factors

Susceptibility is the innate and acquired ability of an individual to resist establishment of a pathogen. It may be affected by the genetic makeup, age, species, sex, previous exposure, and vaccination status of the host, to name a few. For example, Algerian sheep and dwarf pigs are resistant to anthrax infection while most other species of livestock are susceptible. Further susceptibility to a pathogen may be seen in a single (African swine fever, equine infectious anemia) or multiple species (anthrax, foot and mouth disease) which greatly affects its control.

Infectiousness refers to the time period when an animal is infective and to the amount of infectious agent a host can transmit (Thrusfield and Christley 2018). The time from when an agent enters the body of an individual to the first appearance of clinical signs is known as its incubation period. Also, an individual may shed an agent after a certain lapse of time during which the agent may resist the host immune system and replicate to reach sufficient numbers in order to be effective for transmission. This time lapse between entry of an agent and its shedding from a susceptible host is known as the eclipse, prepatent, or latent period for viruses, parasites, and bacteria, respectively. In silent or inapparent infections, there is always an eclipse period but no incubation period. The time lapse from infection to maximum infectiousness denotes the generation time.

In vector-borne diseases, a similar time is required before the biological vector becomes capable of transmitting the agent. This period is referred to as the extrinsic incubation period. For a vector to pick up an infection, the agent must be present in sufficient numbers inside the body of the host (threshold level). In Japanese encephalitis, the *Culex* mosquito may pick up the infection from infected pigs, which amplify the virus in their body, and transmit it to susceptible human population. But the reverse is not possible because the level of viremia is not sufficient in humans to infect mosquitoes. Therefore humans act as a dead end of the infection.

4.3.2 Agent Factors

The infectivity of an agent refers to its ability to infect a susceptible host, pathogenicity is its ability to cause disease, and virulence determines the extent of the disease caused. Infectivity is expressed in terms of the infective dose. The infective dose of *Coxiella* is a single bacterium (Jones et al. 2006), 500 organisms in case of *Campylobacter* and $106-10^{11}$ for *Shigella* (Janssen et al. 2008; van Seventer and Hochberg 2017). Levels below the minimum dose may not cause clinical infection. Virulence may vary with the strain of the agent, with repeated passage in natural and unnatural hosts leading to increase and decrease in virulence, respectively.

Stability is another factor which determines the outcome of a disease in an area. Though agents have devised methods by which they may evade the extremes of environmental conditions, they may be eliminated from an area due to their labile nature. Rabies virus is a highly lethal virus but it does not survive well outside its host and is susceptible to sunlight, desiccation, and pH <3 or >11 (Bleck 2006). Being an enveloped virus, it is easily inactivated by organic solvents like 70% alcohol, phenol, etc. However, anthrax bacilli can survive for years in the soil and on bones. Pathogens that have better survivability have greater chances of transmission and successful maintenance in a population and are not influenced by the vagaries of nature.

4.3.3 Effective Contact

An effective contact is required for transmission of an infectious agent. A host and agent may be present in an area but until and unless they are linked by any of the transmission portals, there will be no disease. Elimination of mosquito populations will decrease the cases of malaria though the parasite and host population may be present in adequate numbers.

4.4 Some Basic Concept Related to Disease Transmission

Before going into the details of transmission and disease, let's get acquainted with some basic concepts of disease.

4.4.1 Host

An individual animal or human which can provide lodgment and establishment of an infectious agent. Following establishment, the infectious agent can easily develop and multiply inside the host body.

4.4.1.1 Definitive Host

A host in which the infectious agent undergoes maturity or sexual development. *Plasmodium* spp. are important human parasites and associated with malaria throughout the world. The life cycle of *Plasmodium* involves mosquitoes which pick up the gametocytes from the infected individual which differentiate into macrogametocytes and microgametocytes and undergo sexual development to form the oocyte. The oocyte ruptures to release sporozoites that are injected into another susceptible human host by the infected mosquito. In the human, the parasite undergoes asexual multiplication through schizont, trophozoite, and gametocyte phases.

4.4.1.2 Primary/Natural/Maintenance Host

A host which is responsible for maintaining an infectious agent in its endemic area. The primary host is often thought of as the definitive host but this may not be true for parasites where a definitive host requires execution of the sexual phase of development. Horses are the primary host for Hendra virus infection in Australia.

4.4.1.3 Secondary Host

A host which maintains an infectious agent outside the endemic area.

4.4.1.4 Accidental Host

A host which is generally not involved in the natural life cycle of the agent, but can acquire the infection on exposure. Such hosts generally do not pass on the infection to other susceptible hosts and are therefore called dead-end hosts or culs-de-sac. Japanese encephalitis virus causes a distinct disease entity with considerable morbidity and mortality in children below 15 years of age in eastern regions of India but humans are an accidental host for the flavivirus as the actual cycle involves pigs and mosquitoes in the domestic cycle and birds (egret/heron) and mosquitoes in the wild cycle. The virus is unable to elicit viremia of sufficient grade to infect the mosquitoes inside the human body.

4.4.1.5 Paratenic Host

A host which transmits the infectious agent mechanically without any development or multiplication. *Musca domestica* are efficient transmitters of various infectious agents. They pick up the agents from feces or other infected materials, carry them on the bristles of their body or in their saliva (vomit), and drop them off at the next available site. There is no development or multiplication in these nor is there any time lag in the transmission.

4.4.2 Reservoir

An animate organism or inanimate object which maintains an infectious agent and can act as source of infection to others. A primary host normally acts as the reservoir of infection for the susceptible population. The infectious agent may develop or multiply inside the reservoir (dog for rabies) or may remain dormant for years (spores of anthrax bacilli in soil can survive for decades). The reservoir may (fruit bat for Nipah virus) or may not (rodents for leptospira) show any symptoms.

4.4.3 Carrier

An individual that does not show any signs of disease though it may shed the infectious agent, transmitting the infection to others. Carriers can further be classified as incubatory, healthy, and convalescent. Incubatory carrier are those which shed the infectious agent during the incubation period of the disease. Examples include chickenpox and rabies. The rabies virus is shed in the saliva of infected dogs as early as five days before infection starts. A convalescent carrier sheds the infectious agent during its recovery period when its clinical signs have waned, for example SARS-CoV-2. Healthy carriers are individuals that are apparently healthy but shed pathogen. A famous example of this is Typhoid Mary (Mary Mallon), a cook who was a healthy carrier of *Salmonella typhi* and transmitted the infection to more than 50 unsuspecting individuals (Soper 1939).

4.4.4 Vector

An animate host, usually an arthropod, that transmits the infection by biting or by depositing infective material on the skin, on food or other objects. Vectors can be further classified as mechanical or biological.

4.4.5 Fomite

An inanimate object that be contaminated by the infectious agent and which aids in the transmission of infection to others.

4.5 Chain of Transmission

The stages an infectious agent goes through during its spread in a population make up the chain of transmission for that pathogen. There are six links in this chain: infectious agent, reservoir, portal of exit, mode of transmission, portal of entry, and susceptible host. In the process of disease transmission, a pathogen must leave its reservoir host via an exit portal (saliva, milk, respiratory, or conjunctival discharge, exudate from lesions or the feces) and be transmitted to a susceptible host through an entry portal (mouth, skin, nostrils, eye) to be maintained in nature.

Let us consider the example of rabies, the disease caused by Lyssavirus of the family Rhabdoviridae. The enveloped virus causes a highly fatal encephalitic disease in humans. Dogs are considered the primary reservoir though most mammals can harbor the virus. The virus multiplies in the brain of the affected dog and exits via the saliva. The disease is generally transmitted when an infected dog bites a susceptible host, the portal of entry in this case being the abraded skin although infections through the mucous membranes of eye, nose, and mouth are also reported. If there is a break in even one of these links, the transmission of rabies will not occur. Therefore, knowledge of the chain of transmission is vital before devising any control strategy. Figure 4.2 shows the chain of transmission for rabies.

4.6 Modes of Transmission

Every pathogen must adopt one or more mechanisms by which it is transmitted from one host to the next. It is vital to appreciate that a single pathogen may utilize more than one method of transmission in a single setting. Norovirus, an important cause of diarrhea worldwide, contributing 18% of the total share, is transmitted by four major routes: person to person, fomite borne, water borne, and food borne.

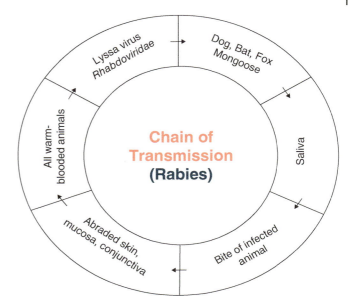

Figure 4.2 Chain of transmission for rabies virus.

Broadly, transmission can be classified as horizontal or vertical. When a pathogen is transmitted between individuals of the same generation, it is called horizontal. The recent SARS-CoV-2 infection originated in China and spread all over the globe, affecting most of the human population. When the pathogen is transmitted from an individual to its progeny, i.e., from one generation to the next, it is designated as vertical. Vertical transmission may be germinative when the infection involves the ovary or ovum (e.g., avian leukosis viruses), transplacental (e.g., feline panleukopenia virus), ascending from the lower genital canal to the placenta (e.g., *Staphylococccus* infection), acquired at the time of parturition (e.g., herpes simplex virus) or via the colostrum (e.g., bovine leukemia).

This horizontal and vertical flow of infectious agents may be achieved directly by contact between two hosts (direct transmission) or indirectly by means of some animate or inanimate (indirect transmission) agency. Figure 4.3 depicts the horizontal and vertical transmission of *Toxoplasma gondii*.

4.6.1 Direct Transmission

This involves the immediate transfer of infectious agents by physical contact with an individual or its secretions/excretions. Most sexually transmitted diseases are categorized as direct, where transmission occurs via the mucous membranes. Rabies transmitted by the bite of a rabid animal, toxoplasmosis transmitted vertically via the placenta, anthrax by contact with infected animal, and trichinosis by eating meat of pigs containing the larvae are all examples of direct transmission.

4.6.2 Indirect Transmission

This requires the involvement of an additional animate or inanimate object. These include fomite-borne, vector-borne and air-borne transmission.

Fomites are nonliving objects that become contaminated by the infectious agent which is later picked up by a susceptible host. Doorknobs, tires of vehicles, pens, brushes, clippers, clothing, blankets, etc. are some important examples of fomites that are contaminated on a daily basis. Food, water, and fomites can serve as important environmental reservoirs that help in the maintenance and spread of a disease. Fomites are important with regard to the spread of many fungal, bacterial, and viral agents. Gram-negative bacteria are known to survive for longer periods on fomites than their Gram-positive counterparts. Fomites are particularly important in healthcare settings and contribute a major share of hospital-acquired infections.

Vectors are arthropods such as mosquitoes, ticks, fleas, and flies that help in transmission of infectious agents. These may act as just a "pick up and drop service" (mechanical) or contribute to the multiplication and/or development of the

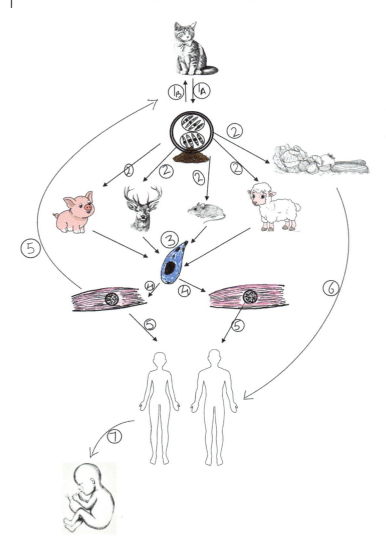

Figure 4.3 Life cycle of *Toxoplasma gondii*. 1A, 1B Eggs pass out in feces and become infectious after a few days in environment; cat is infected with eggs. 2 Eggs may contaminate food water and pass on to other animals. 3 Tachyzoites form inside host. 4 Tachyzoites change into cysts, present in nerves and muscle of host. 5 Transmission of infection to humans and cats through cysts in animal tissue. 6 Infection in humans may occur through eggs in food or water and by handling cat litter. 7 Vertical transmission of infection may occur through placenta.

pathogen (biological). *Musca domestica*, the common housefly, is one of the most robust examples of a mechanical vector, capable of transmitting nearly 100 diseases in humans and animals.

Biological transmission via a vector can be of three types.

- *Developmental*: when there is development only occurring inside the body of the vector, e.g., the larva of *Dirofilaria immitis* and *Wuchereria bancrofti* in mosquitoes.
- *Propagative*: when the infectious agent undergoes multiplication inside the vector, e.g., louping ill virus in ixodid ticks.
- *Cyclopropagative*: when development and multiplication both occur inside the arthropod, e.g., *Babesia* in ticks.

Air-borne transmission may be classified as direct when two individuals are in close contact but as indirect when the agent is transmitted via the wind to far-off locations, as in the case of FMD virus. When an individual expels an agent by coughing or sneezing, generally droplets are released. These are large particles of >10 μm which can travel short distances; due to environmental factors like desiccation, they may change to droplet nuclei which are <5 μm and can travel over 50 m. They also remain suspended in the air and so are important with regard to air-borne transmission. SARS-CoV-2, tuberculosis, and influenza are all examples of air-borne transmission. Table 4.1 and Figure 4.4 depict the important modes of transmission.

Table 4.1 Modes of transmission of pathogens.

		Mode of transmission	
1	Direct	Contact	HIV-AIDS, conjunctivitis, Ebola
		Bite	Rabies
		Transplacental (vertical)	Toxoplasmosis, brucellosis, Zika virus
		Droplet	Common cold
2	Indirect	Vector (biological)	Malaria, anaplasmosis
		Vector (mechanical)	Equine encephalitis, salmonellosis
		Fomite	Rhinovirus, SRAS
		Air-borne	FMD

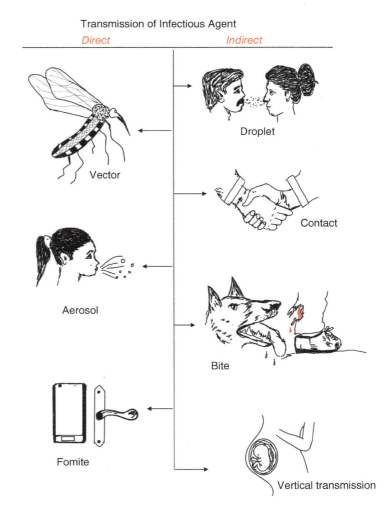

Figure 4.4 Modes of transmission of infectious agent. Direct: contact, bite, droplet, vertical transmission. Indirect: vector, aerosol, fomite.

4.7 Methods of Transmission

Direct and indirect transmission may occur by the following methods.

4.7.1 Ingestion

This is one of the most common methods of transmission. It occurs most frequently by means of an inanimate vehicle in which the pathogen may or may not multiply. Bacteria can multiply in milk whereas eggs of parasites do not multiply in feces. This method is also referred as to the fecal–oral route. Microorganisms are excreted in the feces and contaminate water or food, thus finding a way into a host. It is the most important method of transmission of brucellosis from cattle to humans.

4.7.2 Inhalation

This method involves aerosolization of the pathogen which enters the body via the nostrils. This method is generally adopted by respiratory pathogens, which exit the host by violent sneezing or coughing. Large droplets generally do not travel very far as they settle under gravity, and are transmitted to individuals in the vicinity of the source of infection. Smaller particles known as droplet nuclei do not settle and can travel long distances, infecting animals in different farms. *Mycobacterium tuberculosis* is an important air-borne infection.

4.7.3 Inoculation

This method involves arthropods that inject the disease-causing pathogen into the body of a host while taking a meal. Babesiosis, anaplasmosis, dengue, West Nile fever, and KFD are all acquired following inoculation by a vector.

4.7.4 Venereal

This method involves the sexual transmission of an agent. This method is seen in vertebrates and invertebrates. African swine fever virus is sexually transmitted from male to female *Ornithodoros* ticks (Plowright et al. 1974). HIV-AIDS, gonorrhea, herpes, and chlamydia are all examples of sexually transmitted diseases.

4.7.5 Contact

This involves transmission without the involvement of another factor. Direct contact may occur while treating infected patients in a healthcare setting. These include fungal infections, SARS-CoV-2, etc.

4.7.6 Iatrogenic

Infections that are acquired in a healthcare setting during medical procedures like vaccination, surgery, blood transfusion, and use of dirty equipment. *Toxoplasma* infections by blood or organ transfusion, hepatitis C and HIV-AIDS infection by blood transfusion, and extraneous virus in vaccines are examples of iatrogenic transmission.

4.7.6.1 Nipah Virus Encephalitis

Nipah virus encephalitis is an encephalitic disease caused by members of the family Paramyxoviridae. *Pteropus* fruit bats are the primary reservoir of infection. Infection can be acquired by pigs and humans and is often fatal. Transmission generally occurs by direct contact with infected animals, consuming contaminated food products or through close contact with an infected person. The first outbreak was reported in 1998–1999 in Malaysia and Singapore in pigs. The pigs were infected by bats roosting close to their farm by consumption of partially eaten fruits and contact with excretions/secretions of the bats. Human handlers also acquired the infection from pigs. In India, the first outbreak was reported in Siliguri (2001) and Nadia (2006) districts of West Bengal bordering Bangladesh (Pillai et al. 2020). In Bangladesh, the consumption of date palm sap was linked to disease. In the Siliguri outbreak, transmission was human to human. Figure 4.5 shows the transmission cycle of Nipah virus in nature.

Figure 4.5 Nipah virus modes of transmission. Ingestion: bat to pig via contaminated fruits. Bat to human via fruits and date palm sap. Inhalation: pig to pig/human to human. Nosocomial: human to human. Contact: bat to pig/bat to human/pig to pig/pig to human/human to human. Fomite: bat to human/pig to human/human to human/pig to pig.

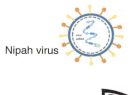
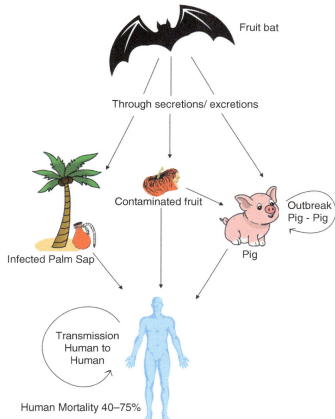

4.8 Maintenance of Infection

An infectious agent needs to be able to survive adverse environmental conditions both inside and outside the body of the host. A pathogen must overcome the onslaught of surface-active chemicals, specific reactive cells, acidic gastrointestinal conditions, antibodies, and phagocytes in order to establish itself inside the host. Over time, pathogens have evolved mechanisms that help them evade these barriers. The success of these pathogens is directly dependent on how successfully they mount this antiimmune response and thereby the final consequence of the infection.

Once a pathogen exits a host via any of the portals, it must face adverse conditions such as desiccation, varying temperatures, ultraviolet light, chemical disinfectants, etc. Every pathogen has a predilection for a specific temperature and relative humidity. Levels above or below these may retard its development and may also lead to death. The strategies used by pathogens in order to survive inside and outside the host are discussed below.

4.8.1 Hit and Run

The hit and run strategy is generally employed by viruses, and involves invasion of a host cell and rapid exit before the host can mount an immune response. These viruses are highly infectious, generally cytolytic, and destroy the host cell. Examples include the respiratory viruses like rhinovirus and influenza. These types of pathogens require a large population of susceptible individuals for maintenance and propagation of infection.

4.8.2 Resistant Form

Bacteria prepare themselves to bear the external stressor by changing into spore forms. These are the dormant stage of bacteria that revert back to vegetative forms on encountering favorable environmental conditions. They can resist temperatures ranging from 150 °C to absolute zero. They are also resistant to ethanol, ultraviolet radiation, pH gradients, desiccation, and nutrition depletion. Anthrax spores can survive in soil for decades without loss of viability. On encountering a susceptible host, they may reactivate and cause overt disease. Many fungus also sporulate when exposed to adverse environmental conditions. These spores can easily be blown by air over long distances and infect a new host.

4.8.3 Biofilm

Bacterial biofilms are clusters of bacteria that are attached to a surface or to one another and enclosed in a self-produced matrix (Vestby et al. 2020). The first biofilm was reported by Antonie van Leeuwenhoek in 1683 in his dental plaque. These protective forms are produced inside as well as outside the body of the host and help the bacteria to evade the host immune response and antibiotics. Biofilms cause persistent medical conditions associated with medical implants, chronic wounds, urinary tract infections, and recalcitrant typhoid fever, to name a few. Studies in recent decades have demonstrated that bacteria are generally present in the biofilm mode of growth with the single-celled planktonic stage only a transient phase (Ciofu and Tolker-Nielsen 2019). Biofilm of *Salmonella typhi* on gall stones has been observed in patients with recurring typhoid (Vestby et al. 2020).

4.8.4 Hit and Stay/Persistence Within Host

Many pathogens can survive inside the host by evading the host immune response. They develop strategies like immune suppression and tolerance. Immune suppression may involve interruption of the complement cascade, disrupting phagocytoses, etc. Tolerance is a means of presenting its antigen such that it is not recognized as foreign (molecular mimicry). Some bacteria like *Mycobacterium tuberculosis* avoid elimination by inhibiting apoptosis and inducing macrophage death. They recruit body cells as Trojan horses for wider dissemination of the pathogen. *Trypanosoma* species keep changing their surface antigen so by the time a host has developed antibodies against one antigen, it switches to another, thereby surviving in the host. *Pseudomonas aeruginosa* also forms a capsule around itself to prevent its elimination.

4.8.5 Extended Host Range

An agent may infect only one host or have an extended host range. The dynamics of disease propagation and control is different for single and multiple host pathogens. As per the CDC Yellow Book, nearly 60% of human infections are acquired from animals, i.e., they infect more than one species. Also, emerging and reemerging pathogens have a broad host range that often may cover several mammalian and nonmammalian species (Woolhouse and Gowtage-Sequeria 2005).

The extended host range limits the effectiveness of control strategies adopted. Rabies virus affects nearly all warm-blooded animals. Control of dog rabies does not signify the eradication of the disease as many wild mammals harbor the virus and may transfer it to humans and animals at the wildlife–human interface.

4.8.6 No Environmental Stage

Some pathogens avoid external stressors by avoiding any stage in the environment. Such pathogens devise mechanisms of transmission that do not require them to be exposed to the harsh external environment. These include venereal transmission (HIV-AIDS), vertical transmission (gonorrhea), vector-borne transmission (Chagas disease), and transmission by means of flesh eating. The adult of *Trichinella spiralis* is present in the gastrointestinal tract of pigs and the larval stage is present in the muscle. The parasite does not come out but passes to a new host on consumption of the muscle. The larva survives even in the decaying muscles of the host and may be picked up by other pigs which have a scavenging habit.

Some important mechanisms adopted by fungi to evade the immune response inside the host are discussed below. As soon as a fungus invades a new host, its immune system mounts a response against the cell wall components like chitin, glucans, polysaccharides (e.g., mannoproteins), waxes, and pigments. The beta-glucan of the cell wall is covered by mannoproteins for pathogenic fungi like *Candida* spp., hydrophobin RodA by *Aspergillus fumigatus,* polysaccharide capsule by

Cryptococcus neoformans, and a coat of alpha-1,3-linked glucans for *Histoplasma capsulatum* (Chai et al. 2009). They also secrete substances that reduce the amount of exposed beta-glucan on the cell surface. Another method of evasion by fungi like *Candida albicans* and *C. neoformans* is secretion of proteins that interfere with the complement system inside the host body.

4.9 Consequences of Disease

Invasion by an infectious agent does not always result in disease. Various factors discussed above determine the course of the invasion. An agent may invade, establish, and overcome the host immunity to cause overt disease or be eliminated by the host. We have tried to demarcate the various consequences of an infection in the text below, but readers must take note that one condition may overlap another. Figure 4.6 highlights the key consequences of invasion of a host by a pathogen.

4.9.1 Active Disease

4.9.1.1 Inapparent
An inapparent infection is characterized by multiplication and shedding of an infectious agent by a host but with no apparent clinical signs. The host appears healthy, thereby transmitting infection to other unsuspecting individuals.

4.9.1.2 Subclinical
As for inapparent infection, subclinical cases do not exhibit any clinical signs that may indicate the presence of a pathogen. But here production losses may be encountered. For example, in subclinical mastitis in bovines, the animal's udder and milk appear physically normal but there is a marked decrease in milk production. This decrease can be taken as a prompt to examine the milk of an animal for mastitis even with no apparent clinical signs.

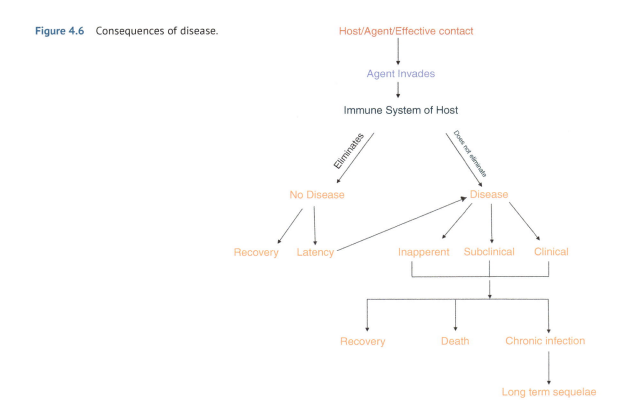

Figure 4.6 Consequences of disease.

4.9.1.3 Clinical/Overt

Clinical infection is marked by overt clinical signs that may range from mild to severe depending on the degree of infection. In clinical mastitis, the udder may show the cardinal signs of inflammation, such as redness, pain, swelling, and elevated body temperature followed by changes in the quantity and physical quality of the milk.

4.9.2 Latency

A latent infection is when a pathogen lies dormant in a host and does not multiply or cause any signs. The agent remains masked inside the host body and is not recognized as such. It is a characteristic of many viruses and bacteria. Bacteria like *Mycobacterium* and viruses like herpes are commonly associated with latent infection. The organism remains dormant in the body and may be activated when host immunity decreases or the host is taking immunosuppressive medication. Certain bacteria like *Salmonella* may remain in the gall bladder of the host after infection has cleared and may cause repeated incidences of disease.

4.9.3 Recovery

Following an infection, a host may itself or by external assistance (antibiotic/antiviral therapy) be able to eliminate an infectious agent. Once an individual recovers, it is believed that the infectious agent has been eliminated from the body but this is not always the case. An agent may go into hiding inside the host and persist even after all the diagnostic tests point to complete elimination. It is believed that once the host immunity wanes, the agent may again become active, causing overt symptoms; for example, *Salmonella* may reside in the gall bladder of the host post recovery and may cause repeated episodes of typhoid fever.

4.9.4 Death

Death marks the close of progression of infection and removes the host from the transmission chain.

4.9.5 Carrier Stage

Another outcome of invasion by a pathogen is the carrier stage. As discussed earlier, a carrier sheds infectious agent without showing any clinical signs. Carriers are particularly important in the transmission and maintenance of infectious agents in an area.

4.9.6 Chronic Stage

This stage of disease occurs when an active infection does not resolve for a long time. The pathogen persists in the body following primary infection, causing recurrence of disease.

References

Bleck, T.P. (2006). Rabies. In: *Tropical Infectious Diseases: Principles, Pathogens, and Practice*, 2e (ed. R.L. Guerrant, D.H. Walker, and P.F. Weller), 839–851. Philadelphia: Elsevier Churchill Livingstone.

Chai, L.Y.A., Alieke, M.G., Vonk, G., and Kullberg, B.J. (2009). Fungal strategies for overcoming host innate immune response. *Medical Mycology* 47 (3): 227–236.

Ciofu, O. and Tolker-Nielsen, T. (2019). Tolerance and resistance of Pseudomonas aeruginosa biofilms to antimicrobial agents-how P. aeruginosa can escape antibiotics. *Frontiers in Microbiology* 10: 913.

GBD 2015 Disease and Injury Incidence and Prevalence Collaborators (2016). Global, regional, and national incidence, prevalence, and years lived with disability for 310 diseases and injuries, 1990–2015: a systematic analysis for the Global Burden of Disease Study 2015. *Lancet* 388 (10053): 1545–1602.

Ghoshal, V., Das, R.R., Nayak, M.K. et al. (2020). Climatic parameters and rotavirus diarrhea among hospitalized children: a study of eastern India. *Frontiers in Pediatrics* 8: 573448.

Janssen, R., Krogfelt, K.A., Cawthraw, S.A. et al. (2008). Host–pathogen interactions in Campylobacter infections: the host perspective. *Clinical Microbiology Reviews* 21 (3): 505–518.

Jones, M.K., Nicas, M., Hubbard, A.E., and Reingold, A.L. (2006). The infectious dose of *Coxiella burnetii* (Q fever). *Applied Biosafety* 11 (1): 32–41.

Pillai, S.V., Krishna, G., and Veettil, V.M. (2020). Nipah virus: past outbreaks and future containment. *Viruses* 12 (4): 465.

Plowright, W., Perry, C.T., and Greig, A. (1974). Sexual transmission of African swine fever virus in the tick, *Ornithodoros moubata porcinus*, Walton. *Research in Veterinary Science* 17: 106–113.

Roser, M., Ritchie, H. and Spooner, F. (2021). Burden of disease. https://ourworldindata.org/burden-of-disease (accessed 20 January 2024).

van Seventer, J.M. and Hochberg, N.S. (2017). *Principles of Infectious Diseases: Transmission, Diagnosis, Prevention, and Control*, International Encyclopedia of Public Health, 2e, vol. 6. New York: Academic Press.

Soper, G.A. (1939). The curious career of Typhoid Mary. *Bulletin of the New York Academy of Medicine* 15: 698–712.

Thrusfield, M. and Christley, R. (2018). Transmission and maintenance of infection. In: *Veterinary Epidemiology*, 4e, 115–137. Oxford: Wiley-Blackwell.

Vestby, L.K., Grønseth, T., Simm, R., and Nesse, L.L. (2020). Bacterial biofilm and its role in the pathogenesis of disease. *Antibiotics* 9 (2): 59.

Woolhouse, M.E. and Gowtage-Sequeria, S. (2005). Host range and emerging and reemerging pathogens. *Emerging Infectious Diseases* 11 (12): 1842–1847.

5

Ecology of Diseases, Hypothesis, and Life Table Technique and Its Application

Samuel U. Felix[1,2], Samuel C. Maureen[3], Simpson Monya[2], and Eshun A. Ama[2]

[1] *Faculty of Veterinary Medicine, National Animal Production Research Institute, Ahmadu Bello University, Zaria, Nigeria*
[2] *Department of Food and Animal Science, Alabama A&M University, Normal, AL, USA*
[3] *JayCare Medical Centre, Crestwood Medica Center, Huntsville, AL, 35801, Kaduna, Nigeria*

5.1 Introduction

Disease ecology, a specialized area within ecology, focuses on understanding the processes of disease transmission through a quantitative lens. Unlike epidemiology, which primarily describes health patterns within populations, disease ecology emphasizes identifying the systems and mechanisms that drive these patterns (Wale and Duffy 2021). While epidemiology traditionally examines the distribution and determinants of health states and events, disease ecology delves into the underlying dynamics and mechanisms. As noted by Brandell et al. (2020), disease ecology is a rapidly growing field within ecology and evolutionary biology, integrating insights from various biological sciences. Building on the foundational population disease models developed by Anderson and May (1991), disease ecology has evolved to address both theoretical and practical questions across diverse systems, including human, animal, and plant health. This encompasses a wide range of topics from the emergence of zoonotic diseases to the impacts of crop diseases and livestock outbreaks, and the immunological dynamics in wholly anthroponotic systems (Taylor et al. 2019).

5.2 Disease Ecology and Factors in Emergence

Several authors have identified various causal factors of infectious disease emergence, such as land use change, human movement, encroachment, wildlife translocation, rapid transport, and climate change (Goldstein et al. 2022). These ecological factors are part of four major categories that also include social, political, and economic factors; genetic and biological factors; and physical environmental factors.

Our approach to understanding the interaction of these factors and their causal relationships differs by framing disease emergence as an ecological-evolutionary phenomenon influenced by human and animal interactions. We are particularly interested in how human and animal factors interact with natural processes, focusing on mechanisms that influence pathogen transmission and evolution, ultimately leading to regional and global impacts (Daszak et al. 2001). As an initial step, we differentiate between two broad categories of factors: "demographic and societal" and "disease intervention and policy," as previously suggested by Gubler (1998). This categorization distinguishes between factors related to specific environments or ecosystems and those involving biological and policy-related elements. However, both sets of factors can be understood within a single ecological framework that considers the interaction between natural systems and human-designed systems. Our focus is on the first category, examining how ecological concepts and principles can explain disease emergence.

Classic ecology, or natural history, has been foundational to infectious disease research since the establishment of "Koch's Postulates" and the subsequent advancements in microbiology and zoonotic disease epidemiology during the nineteenth and twentieth centuries (Will 2022). Early zoonotic disease research primarily involved this descriptive, empirical ecology, focusing on identifying the life cycles, transmission patterns, and incidental and natural hosts of pathogens. It also examined the demographic, life history, dispersal, and habitat attributes of reservoirs and vectors.

Epidemiology and Environmental Hygiene in Veterinary Public Health, First Edition. Edited by Tanmoy Rana.
© 2025 John Wiley & Sons, Inc. Published 2025 by John Wiley & Sons, Inc.

Although this empirical, field-based approach is crucial for designing effective prevention and control programs, it has been somewhat neglected in recent years (Chitimia-Dobler et al. 2019). Fortunately, theoretical disease ecology has seen significant growth, largely driven by the work of Anderson, May, and others. This development has led to a substantial synthesis, applying ecological and evolutionary biology principles to the study of infectious diseases.

Parallel to this, systems ecology has expanded its scope by incorporating complexity theory to address emerging infections, offering preliminary insights into its implications (Barwell et al. 2023). This advancement, along with decades of applying systems ecology to natural resources and economic development, has yielded crucial insights with significant potential for understanding zoonotic disease emergence as a cross-scale process. This field uses complex systems theory applied to coupled human-natural systems to explain how local phenomena can trigger a cascade of effects, eventually reaching global proportions. The findings suggest that this cross-scale behavior is governed by relatively few variables and is mitigated by social and ecological resilience. A loss of resilience in ecological systems is observed to lead inevitably to unpredictable events or the "surprises" typical of complex systems. This integration of social-ecological systems and resilience theory helps explain the unpredictability of disease emergence events (Ullah et al. 2015).

5.2.1 Population Ecology, Genetics, and Emergence Disease

The relevance to disease emergence lies in the theoretical insights from population biology, which explain how the size of a host population influences the persistence of a pathogen within that population (Kortessis et al. 2023). The collective findings suggest that there are specific thresholds, dependent on the pathogen and host population, below which a pathogen cannot be sustained. With the exponential growth of human and domestic host and vector populations worldwide, surpassing these thresholds can explain a significant portion of the increase in emerging infectious diseases (Shocket et al. 2023).

To elaborate, while zoonotic disease emergence is not exclusively a tropical phenomenon, it is predominantly associated with tropical developing regions undergoing rapid population growth and ecological changes. Before the post-World War II economic era, most ecosystems in the tropics were characterized by dispersed human settlements and a limited number of large cities (over 500 000) (Biswas et al. 2023). These were interspersed with extensive areas of cropland, pastureland, and relatively untouched forests. However, since then, this pattern has essentially reversed during what has been the most rapid period of large-scale ecological transformation in human history. The previously scattered settlements and sparse large cities have amalgamated into expansive megacities and their surrounding periurban settlements, with only remnants of undisturbed forest surviving amidst extensive cropland, scrub, and ecologically degraded lands. Consequently, the presence of density-dependent thresholds in population is highly pertinent to the emergence of diseases (Zhu and He 2023).

This phenomenon elucidates the abrupt transitions of urban diseases from nonpersistent to endemic states and from endemic to epidemic behaviors, which occur as population densities of susceptible humans, hosts, and vectors reach critical levels. A notable example is measles, whose transmission rate requires human settlements with populations exceeding 250 000 – numbers that surpass historical norms in most preindustrial states and even in many geographically isolated populations today (Björnstad 2018). As a result, many infectious diseases that are endemic on continents have failed to establish themselves on islands, despite occasional introductions and localized outbreaks. The same principles of mathematical ecology that explain threshold densities for diseases like measles also account for the considerably lower thresholds required for vector-borne diseases such as arboviruses (Prasad et al. 2022).

The theoretical demonstration particularly highlights that the pathogen's "reproductive rate" shows a quadratic increase with the density of vector populations (Figure 5.1) (Jervis et al. 2023). This means that threshold densities can be quickly surpassed as domestic and peridomestic hosts and vectors expand or reexpand their geographic ranges, leading to increased densities. This phenomenon helps explain the rapid reemergence of dengue and dengue hemorrhagic fever in the American tropics, as vector populations grew due to relaxed controls and new breeding habitats associated with urbanization (Gupte et al. 2023). An analogous situation can be seen with the accumulation of "dead and down" wood in forests with a history of fire suppression, where the build-up of fuel becomes an "accident waiting to happen," similar to how the proliferation of host or vector populations can lead to widespread infection from a single event.

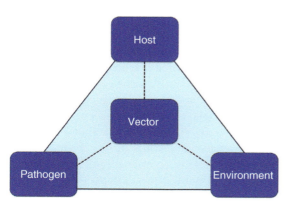

Figure 5.1 Disease epidemiological triad.

The significantly increased densities of humans, host reservoirs, and vectors result in a higher number of pathogen genomes. This increase in genetic variability, due to the larger population size and density, can accelerate microbial adaptation, including the evolution of pathogenesis and antimicrobial resistance. Genetic variability is augmented through various mechanisms, including mutation. The probability of producing more virulent variants increases not only with the size of the host population but also with crowding and the intermingling of different host species (Baker et al. 2022).

In a broader context, the dynamic interactions between parasites (pathogens) and hosts inherently involve a coadaptive and evolutionary "dance" along the pathogenicity threshold (Figure 5.2). This threshold is more frequently crossed due to unnatural anthropogenic disturbances, beyond the mere increase in population sizes and pathogen genetic diversity.

Exploring ecological communities and the associated "community ecology" theory reveals several principles and mechanisms that explain how both human disturbances and natural environmental variations contribute to these population-level factors (Singer et al. 2021). Several implications arise regarding zoonotic disease emergence, though most have not yet been thoroughly detailed within the medical, public health, or zoonotic disease literature.

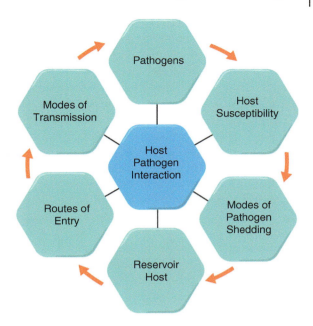

Figure 5.2 Cycle of pathogen infection.

A significant insight from ecology stems from the overarching principle of community assembly (Brandl et al. 2023). Research has illustrated that communities tend to organize according to "assembly rules," which govern the spatial distribution, composition, and abundance of species within ecological communities. These rules are influenced by interspecific interactions such as predation, competition, and parasitism. While density-independent factors like weather and natural disasters play a significant, though temporary, role in most ecosystems, the process of community assembly and disassembly has been extensively studied in insular ecosystems, the "species-area relationship," and the phenomenon of faunal collapse (Rayfield et al. 2023).

The ecological significance of this research body, initially framed in terms of "habitat fragmentation," highlights how human land and resource use contribute to species extinction as the primary mechanism. Despite initial debates, a substantial body of evidence now supports and widely accepts its relevance, particularly in tropical forest ecosystems (Figure 5.3).

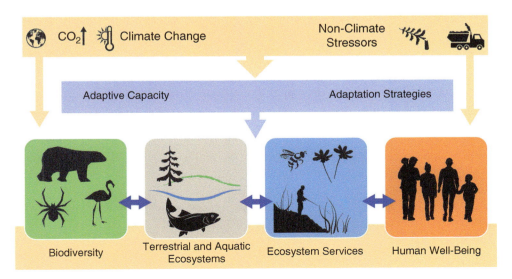

Figure 5.3 Ecological system of living things.

The critical importance of habitat fragmentation and related human disturbances in the context of disease emergence lies in their role in disrupting well-organized natural communities. Human activities such as deforestation, pesticide use, and various forms of pollution often result in the decline of predator populations. Notably, carnivorous mammals are frequently the first to disappear following forest fragmentation (Sivapalan and Blöschl 2015). Their local extinction disrupts natural "top-down" control within ecological communities, leading to increases in the abundance, or even "hyperabundance," of species like rodents and biting insects.

The process of community disassembly, coupled with the subsequent loss of natural population control mechanisms, is closely associated with the conversion of natural landscapes into urban and agricultural areas. The widespread use of broad-spectrum pesticides, habitat simplification, and fragmentation exacerbate these changes. Decreased species diversity contributes to "ecological release" among remaining species, as their predators, competitors, and parasites decline or disappear. Some of these species may already serve as zoonotic reservoirs or vectors. Consequently, ecological release may facilitate their proliferation, potentially explaining the prevalence of emerging zoonotic diseases in regions where recent human settlement and agricultural expansion have encroached into tropical forests (De Thoisy et al. 2021).

In developed regions, a parallel phenomenon occurs with the regrowth of forests, contributing to the emergence of zoonotic diseases. For instance, the reforestation observed in eastern North America over the past fifty years has created more suitable habitat for forest edge-adapted species like whitetail deer and white-footed mice. With few predators and competitors, the population of white-tailed deer, primary hosts for the adult tick Ixodes scapularis, has surged upon reinvading the area. This ecological shift is widely recognized as a significant factor in the emergence of Lyme disease in the region (Biswas et al. 2023).

Expanding on the concept of "ecological release," it has been proposed to explain the phenomenon of invasive species. This occurs when highly successful introduced species manage to evade their natural complement of parasites, predators, and competitors. This extended understanding of ecological release provides valuable insights into the success of invasive domestic species such as Rattus and Aedes species, which serve as hosts and vectors for some of the most challenging urban zoonotic diseases, both historically and currently.

In summary, the emergence of zoonotic infectious diseases can be partly understood as a consequence of disrupting natural ecological communities. This disruption dismantles the inherent predator-prey, competitive, and host-parasite relationships that typically regulate and stabilize species abundance. Such disruptions can result from the use of nonselective pesticides and changes in land use and cover that affect species distribution and abundance. Importantly, the disassembly of natural ecological communities due to habitat fragmentation is a gradual process, unlike exponential decay. Depending on factors such as habitat loss extent, sizes, shapes, and spatial relationships of remaining fragments, this process may extend over decades, centuries, or longer as communities gradually move toward a new equilibrium.

Consequently, the frequency of disease emergence is expected to follow a similar trajectory, initially peaking and then gradually declining as ecosystems stabilize. Shifting focus to systems ecology and disease emergence, systems thinking has been pivotal in ecological science since the 1960s. This approach emphasizes the ecosystem concept, with a significant focus on describing and understanding energy and nutrient flows across diverse ecosystems (Orlowski et al. 2023). Recent developments have also highlighted the human dimensions of global environmental change.

While global-scale ecosystem changes have been considered in relation to human and infectious diseases, a formal and systematic framework in this context has yet to be fully developed. Current evidence largely remains anecdotal.

However, the advancement and application of systems theory, operating somewhat independently of mainstream systems ecology, offer significant potential for establishing a more systematic interpretation of how ecosystem changes contribute to disease emergence (Walker and Cooper 2011). Recent developments have focused on applying the theory of "complex adaptive systems" to ecological systems, viewing ecosystems as self-organizing entities that are far from equilibrium, evolutionary, and nonlinear in nature. Key properties of complex systems, including organization, diversity, resilience, and the occurrence of "surprise" deviations from expected behaviors, are crucial features often associated with a healthy state.

These properties are critical in understanding the loss of ecosystem resilience and increased vulnerability. This vulnerability applies both to social systems attempting to manage and control natural variables (such as vectors and pathogens) and the ecosystems themselves, where changes in these variables can have profound impacts.

Human interventions altering natural disturbance patterns, such as flood control projects, often diminish ecosystem resilience. Additionally, secondary disturbances like wildfires, storms, floods, and earthquakes can trigger cascading effects due to their influence across different scales. For example, a localized thunderstorm igniting a fire might spread regionally due to accumulated fuel resulting from years of fire suppression practices. Environmental changes associated with population growth and development frequently overlook the necessity of preserving resilience, portraying ecosystems as "overconnected" or "brittle," potentially leading to unforeseen consequences.

In summary, while the relationship between ecosystem changes and disease emergence remains complex and multifaceted, systems theory offers a promising avenue for developing a structured framework to better understand and address these dynamics. Integrating these insights could enhance our ability to manage and mitigate the risks associated with emerging infectious diseases in an increasingly interconnected and dynamic world.

Floods, which are commonly linked to outbreaks of water-borne diseases, tend to increase in frequency and severity when natural systems lose resilience due to efforts aimed at "controlling" rather than managing natural variability (Batalini de Macedo et al. 2022). The transformation of upland forests into plantations or cropping systems for enhanced natural resource production, along with conventional agricultural practices, leads to a decrease in ecosystem heterogeneity. This reduction in diversity reduces the landscape's ability to act as a buffer against disease outbreaks, thereby facilitating their spread more easily across the homogeneous environment. This includes immunologically vulnerable domesticated species.

5.3 Ecological Monitoring

Ecological monitoring techniques are essential for generating data that can be used to:
Define the geographic boundaries of important diseases affecting humans and livestock.
Identify the causes of these boundaries and the factors that regulate them.
Predict the potential veterinary and medical implications of changes and trends in existing land use systems.
Ecological monitoring provides a range of ecosystem data, encompassing environmental, faunal, and socio-economic factors (Garcia-Bustos et al. 2023).

5.4 Environmental Factors

5.4.1 Permanent Attributes

5.4.1.1 Topography
Elevation plays a crucial role in influencing rainfall, maximum and minimum temperatures, and consequently, the distribution of potential wildlife disease reservoirs and arthropod vectors (Gebrezgiher et al. 2023). In regions with seasonal climates, there can be vertical movements of susceptible animals across contour lines. The interplay of vertical and horizontal air movements, driven by temperature changes and topographic features, can impact the spread of infectious agents and harmful chemicals. Consequently, many diseases exhibit altitudinal distributions.

For example, in Peru, anthrax is reported to be restricted to livestock in areas below 2000 m above sea level (masl). While most Peruvian livestock are found above this altitude, animals at higher elevations remain fully susceptible to experimental challenges. The ingestion of locoweed (Oxytropis sericea) by cattle, especially calves, significantly increases the prevalence and severity of congestive heart failure when consumed at high altitudes. At lower altitudes, animals only exhibit signs of locoweed poisoning. Elevation also influences the incidence of avian malaria in native birds in Hawaii, where the malarial parasite, mosquito vector, and native birds are distributed differently along an altitudinal gradient.

In Switzerland, rabies control has been effective through the aerial distribution of vaccine baits in valleys. Similar landscape epidemiology studies in Virginia, USA, have shown comparable findings. In France, rabies has been eradicated in foxes through systematic vaccine baiting. Beyond altitude, the aspect, or the direction a slope faces, can significantly influence disease agents and their vectors. For instance, tick fever virus activity and tick vectors in Colorado were concentrated on south-facing sunny slopes in montane areas where optimal conditions of soil type, moisture, and temperature prevail.

Soils
The bedrock and resulting soil type exert significant influence on the flora and fauna inhabiting a specific area. The chemical and physical composition of soil substrates can be linked to various diseases and deficiencies, such as fluorine, selenium, and arsenic poisoning, as well as deficiencies in iodine and copper. Certain soil types may also host plants that are toxic to domestic livestock and wildlife. Soil chemistry has been observed to affect the viability of Bacillus anthracis spores. In regions of the USA dominated by calcium-rich, neutral-to-alkaline soils, livestock mortality rates due to anthrax

during the period analyzed from 1945 to 1955 were over 21 times higher compared to losses in other areas (Smith et al. 2000). Soil structure can also limit the distribution of hookworms (Ancylostoma spp.) and other parasitic nematodes (Upshall et al. 1987).

Drainage, Waterholes, and Swamps

Swampy areas provide habitat for various species of aquatic rodents, some of which act as reservoir hosts for leptospirosis caused by Leptospira interrogans – a globally significant disease affecting domestic and wild animals, as well as humans. Additionally, these rodents and lagomorphs carry tularemia, caused by Francisella (Pasteurella) tularensis, which is a zoonotic disease with potential bioweapon implications. Springs, often feeding into swamps, can concentrate Johne's disease bacilli. Human-made alterations such as dams, irrigation systems, and canals can profoundly alter the ecology of pathogenic agents, their reservoirs, and vectors. As these features dry out, they often create ecological conditions – pH 7.5, water temperature of 27 °C, and high organic content – that are favorable for the incubation of anthrax bacilli. Marsh soil is also abundant with spores of Clostridium botulinum, which may be present in the digestive tracts of animals and birds in these areas.

Boreholes accessing underground water sources may contain toxic levels of heavy metals like lead and arsenic. Water from artificial boreholes, pipelines, and capped springs may be restricted to domestic livestock, potentially depriving wildlife of previously accessible water sources. Trampling around water sources significantly reduces water penetration by compacting the surface soil. When coupled with overgrazing, this intensifies runoff, which can have far-reaching consequences for adjacent pans and swamps. Overgrazing and trampling also affect vegetation and microclimates, making these areas concentration points for arthropod vectors and disease agents. Similarly, stock trails to and from water sources pose epidemiological risks.

Caves

Caves, found in diverse geological formations, serve as daytime roosts for bats, nocturnal roosts for diurnal birds, and shelters for mammals like hyenas (*Crocuta crocuta* and *Hyaena hyaena*). Bats and birds inhabiting caves provide a food source for soft ticks dwelling in crevices on cave roofs, which act as vectors for several avian diseases. In specific regions, bats and other cave-dwelling mammals are recognized as reservoirs for the rabies virus and, reportedly, the Marburg virus (Markotter et al., 2020). Ethiopian caves are home to hyraxes (*Procavia capensis*), identified as the confirmed animal reservoir for *Leishmania aethiopica* and its sandfly vector, *Phlebotomus pedifer*.

Static Animal Features

Termite mounds serve as shelters for snakes and viverrids, which are reservoirs for rabies, and they also provide breeding sites for sand flies of the Phlebotomus species, vectors of leishmaniasis. Additionally, termite mounds act as indicators of specific soil types and drainage patterns. Burrows created by warthogs (*Phacochoerus aethiopicus*) and aardvarks (*Orycteropus afer*) are often infested with soft ticks (*Ornithodorus moubata*), which are vectors of African swine fever and relapsing fever. Burrows of colonial rodents such as gerbils, susliks, springhares, and prairie dogs create habitats for soft ticks, hard ticks, mosquitoes, sandflies, and fleas, which can serve as vectors for diseases like relapsing fever, brucellosis, tick spirochaetosis, leishmaniasis, tularemia, listeriosis, toxoplasmosis, viral encephalitis, tick-borne rickettsiosis, Crimean-Congo hemorrhagic fever, and bubonic plague.

Bird roosts and nesting colonies often harbor soft ticks of the Argas group, which may carry viruses capable of causing diseases in humans. Tree cavities may hold water where mosquitoes breed; these mosquitoes feed on birds (and humans) and serve as vectors for avian malaria and numerous other blood-borne parasites.

5.4.2   Semipermanent Environmental Attributes

Plant physiognomy and landscape zones are often categorized based on vegetation types, which play a crucial role in influencing the geographical distribution of animal populations and the habitats of their pathogen vectors. The combination of soil type, climate, vegetation, and land use creates conditions that can promote the establishment of natural foci for certain infections and delineate the boundaries of plant toxicities and vector habitats (Poorter et al. 2023).

The composition of plant communities is closely associated with various wildlife diseases, often characterized by specific ecozones defined by distinct vegetation types. These vegetation types are dependent on soil characteristics, and microclimates influenced by plants and soil can significantly impact the occurrence of certain parasites. For example, the larval stages of hookworms (Ancylostoma spp.) cannot survive in well-drained sandy soils, and molluscan intermediate hosts of the meningeal worm (Parelaphostrongylus tenuis) of the white-tailed deer (*Odocoileus virginianus*) in the USA require suitable moist leaf litter to aestivate during hot, dry weather (Upshall et al. 1987). Thus, the distribution of parasites is closely tied to the ecological requirements of their intermediate hosts, which are influenced by vegetation, soil type, and climate.

Another example involves the gerbil (*Meriones shawi*), an important animal reservoir in endemic areas whose habitat does not overlap with Psammomys. Effective control of cutaneous leishmaniasis in Tunisia requires a comprehensive ecological and geographical approach. The habitats of Psammomys are strictly defined by the distribution of Atriplex, which is mechanically destroyed and replaced by planting Acacia cyanophylla. Gerbil populations are managed through the use of wheat/oil baits soaked in 3% zinc phosphate to control their numbers effectively.

Zoogenic features such as wallows and salt licks exhibit seasonal fluctuations and can serve as significant sites for disease transmission among wildlife. For instance, wallows in Uganda have been observed to harbor tuberculosis-infected African buffalo (*Syncerus caffer*), potentially contaminating the environment with infectious pathogens. Animal carcasses within these wallows provide ideal conditions for the production of Clostridium botulinum toxin, with the anaerobic environment of swamps or wallows facilitating botulism outbreaks.

The toxin produced can be transferred to birds through saprophagous fly larvae that feed on the carcasses and are subsequently consumed by the birds. Even a few larvae can contain enough toxin to be lethal to a bird. Additionally, droplet transmission can occur when social animals gather closely in wallows, facilitating diseases like bovine tuberculosis among African buffalo in Uganda. Wallows can also become infection foci for anthrax spores, as vultures that have fed on anthrax-infected carcasses may bathe and drink in these sites, spreading the disease.

Similarly, salt licks can concentrate animals, making them potential sites of infection transmission due to the close interaction among various species that visit them foci of infection due to the congregation of animals that visit them.

5.4.2.1 Distribution of Nonmigratory Mammals

The spatial distribution of non-migratory mammals plays a critical role in the ecology of both enzootic (animal-specific) and zoonotic (transmissible from animals to humans) diseases. In certain geographic landscapes, rodents such as gerbils (Rhombomys spp.) in Central Asia and prairie dogs (*Cynomys leucurus*) in the USA aggregate in large numbers, forming "villages" and "towns" respectively. These burrows not only provide habitats for the rodents but also serve as breeding grounds for sandflies, which act as vectors for diseases such as leishmaniasis affecting both the rodents and humans.

Prairie dogs, specifically, are reservoirs for plague (*Yersinia pestis*), transmitting the disease through fleas of the genus Oropsylla. Furthermore, fruit bats (Pteropus spp.) have been implicated in the emergence of several viruses, including Hendra and Nipah viruses, which belong to a new genus within the Paramyxoviridae family. Surveillance of wildlife, particularly bats, has been crucial in understanding the origin and spread of Nipah virus, which caused significant outbreaks among pigs and humans in the Malay Peninsula.

In Bangladesh, Nipah virus outbreaks resulted in the deaths of at least 89 people between 2001 and 2008, with mortality rates ranging from 40% to 100% in infected individuals. These outbreaks were linked to the consumption of fresh date palm sap contaminated by bats, highlighting contaminated food items and domestic animals as important transmission pathways for Nipah virus (Markotter et al., 2020).

5.4.2.2 Human Settlements, Villages, Roads, Farms, and Ranches

Old structures such as buildings, cemeteries, and abandoned human settlements serve as habitats for various potential reservoirs of wildlife diseases. These include hedgehogs (*Erinaceus europaeus*), rodents, tortoises, snakes, and lizards, which can attract and provide sustenance for *Ornithodorus* ticks and sand flies. Ornithodorus ticks are vectors of relapsing fever, while sand flies transmit leishmaniasis. In East Africa, abandoned kraals (livestock enclosures) and manyattas (traditional huts) are often infested with hungry fleas, primarily *Ctenocephalides felis*, and soft ticks such as *Ornithodorus moubata*. These environments facilitate the proliferation of these ectoparasites, contributing to the transmission of diseases among wildlife and potentially to humans as well.

5.4.2.3 Ephemeral or Seasonal Environmental Attributes

Meteorological data plays a crucial role in delineating climatic constraints that affect the distribution of animals and diseases. Parameters such as insolation, rainfall, air temperature, humidity, soil moisture, and soil temperature can be continuously monitored and recorded, providing insights into ecological and epidemiological dynamics. Extreme weather events can directly impact populations, causing mortality among vulnerable individuals such as the very young, elderly, and those compromised by malnutrition, parturition, or lactation. Variations in climatic factors can lead to shifts in epidemiological patterns, influencing the distribution of animals, parasites, and pathogens which are often constrained by specific climatic parameters

For instance, certain disease agents, like the Old World screw worm (*Chrysomya bezziana*), require specific humidity and temperature conditions during their life cycle stages to survive. Outside these optimal conditions, their survival is compromised. Similarly, parasitic nematodes and other pathogens exhibit narrow tolerances for temperature, humidity, and soil conditions. Viruses and bacteria also show preferences for particular environmental conditions; for example, the virus causing malignant catarrhal fever tends to persist longer in moist environments compared to dry ones, while avian influenza (H5N1) virus survives better in cold winter conditions.

Animals that hibernate or aestivate to avoid extreme climates can harbor pathogens during dormancy periods, potentially leading to disease outbreaks upon emergence. Hedgehogs (Erinaceus europaeus) in Europe and marmots (Marmota bobac) in Central Asia are examples of species that can carry diseases like foot-and-mouth disease virus and plague, respectively, through hibernation cycles (Woodford 2009). In regions like Tatarstan, Russia, the mild winter of 2007–2008 facilitated the high survival rate of rodents, which are natural reservoirs for hantaviruses causing hemorrhagic fever with renal syndrome (HFRS). This led to increased incidence of HFRS among humans engaged in activities like fishing and forestry.

5.4.3 Insolation

Insolation, or exposure to sunlight, serves as a natural disinfectant due to its intense ultraviolet (UV) irradiation, which is detrimental to many pathogens. This UV radiation is particularly effective in sterilizing surfaces and environments where pathogens may be present. Additionally, the infrared spectrum of sunlight also plays a role in affecting the viability of certain organisms, including parasitic nematodes. Even when embedded within dung pellets of hosts, the eggs of these nematodes can be negatively impacted by the infrared radiation, contributing to their reduced survival rates.

In natural ecosystems, carrion beetles play a beneficial role by burying dung pellets. This behavior not only aids in decomposition but also helps in the survival of some nematode eggs and larvae. By burying dung pellets and depositing their own eggs within them, carrion beetles create microenvironments that shield nematode eggs from direct sunlight, thereby increasing their chances of survival despite the UV and infrared radiation exposure.

5.4.4 Faunal Factors

In ecological and epidemiological contexts, observing declines in plant biomass can serve as an early warning sign of impending rodent outbreaks, which often precede outbreaks of diseases such as plague or viral encephalomyocarditis. This correlation underscores the ecological interconnectedness between vegetation dynamics and animal populations, particularly rodents that can act as disease reservoirs.

Moreover, the chemical composition of plants plays a critical role in influencing ecosystem health. Certain plants have the ability to concentrate elements like selenium or produce toxic compounds such as hydrogen cyanide under specific environmental conditions. For example, Kikuyu grass (*Pennisetum clandestinum*) is known to produce toxic levels of hydrogen cyanide under certain climatic circumstances. Similarly, plants like locoweed (Oxytropis spp.) in the United States contain toxic alkaloids that pose risks to grazing animals, with toxicity levels often exacerbated during dry periods.

In times of climatic variability, the energy content of food plants becomes particularly crucial. Extreme climatic conditions can affect nutrient availability in plants, impacting the ability of animals to obtain sufficient nutrition for reproduction and lactation. This highlights the intricate relationships between plant chemistry, climate variability, and animal health, emphasizing the importance of ecological monitoring and understanding these interactions in disease prevention and management strategies.

5.4.4.1 Mammal Productivity

Disease factors exert significant impacts on productivity, as demonstrated by the case of "yearling disease" (rinderpest) affecting young wildebeest (*Connochaetes taurinus*) on Tanzania's Serengeti Plains. This example illustrates how disease can disrupt population structures by disproportionately affecting susceptible age groups and exerting selective pressures on hosts of different species, ages, and genders. For instance, rinderpest did not uniformly impact all susceptible species and age groups; older animals that survived initial exposures often developed acquired immunity, which provided protection.

Seasonal movements of migratory species play a crucial role in the epidemiology of infectious diseases. For instance, the seasonal excretion of cell-free malignant catarrhal fever virus by parturient wildebeest in East Africa illustrates how wildlife movement patterns influence disease dynamics. In Sudan, visceral leishmaniasis is closely linked to traditional livestock grazing patterns, with transmission occurring seasonally in acacia forests along river borders.

Fire is another environmental factor that transiently alters landscapes and affects disease ecology. It can kill arthropod vectors, parasitic nematode eggs, and larvae, while also altering vegetation in ways that may favor the survival of certain disease agents over others. Additionally, the sudden removal of vegetative cover due to fire can impact the vulnerability of rodent reservoir hosts to predation.

Water bodies serve as critical habitats for many infectious disease agents, their hosts, and vectors. Water can act as a carrier for infectious diseases and may also transport toxic substances, both natural (e.g. mercury, fluoride) and anthropogenic (e.g. oil, pesticides). Temporary flooding events can sterilize large areas, affecting termites, certain tick species, small burrowing rodents, and specific plant species. The interfaces between flooded and surrounding landscapes often become epidemiologically significant zones, particularly in flood plains that regularly occur seasonally in arid and semi-arid regions. During dry seasons, these flood plains attract large numbers of wild and domestic animals to water sources, facilitating the transmission of infectious diseases among species that would otherwise be spatially separated.

This interplay between environmental factors, animal behaviors, and disease dynamics underscores the complexity of disease ecology and highlights the need for integrated approaches to understand and mitigate disease risks in diverse ecosystems.

5.4.5 Techniques for Ecological Monitoring

Several various methodologies are employed for collecting and processing data to generate maps and analyze surface trends. Three primary techniques include ground sampling, aerial surveys conducted through systematic reconnaissance flights, and remote sensing utilizing satellite imagery.

5.4.5.1 Ground Sampling

Data collected on the ground, whether by human technicians or automated methods, complements information gathered remotely through aerial surveys or remote sensing. While aerial and remote sensing provide broad data, ground-based observations ("ground truthing") offer greater precision. Permanent features such as topography, soils, drainage lines, water bodies, lakes, swamps, caves, and animal and bird colonies are meticulously examined for mineral presence, salinity levels, and the presence of mammal, bird, and reptile populations, along with their ectoparasites, molluscan hosts, arthropods, and insect vectors.

Various cultural and serological methods are employed to investigate animals, insects, and arthropods for the presence of potential disease agents. Vegetation cover and type are analyzed to detect habitats of disease reservoirs and vectors and their spatial distribution in relation to mapped vegetation. Areas inhabited by animals are surveyed using bacterial cultures to detect pathogens. Pathological evidence from slaughtered animals, along with blood, serum, and parasite samples, is further analyzed in base laboratories. Samples, including collections of arthropod vectors, are strategically gathered across habitats to precisely define pathogen, reservoir, and vector boundaries, while seasonal variations are closely monitored.

Predictions of disease outbreaks often hinge on monitoring reservoir, donor, and vector populations. For instance, the analysis of disgorged undigested food pellets from diurnal birds of prey can indirectly reveal shifts in rodent behavior influenced by plague infection. Outbreaks of epizootic diseases are considered indicative of ecological imbalance, whereas the presence of enzootic diseases suggests ecological stability. Monitoring "indicator species" helps forecast changes in disease patterns; for example, overgrazing leading to increased warthog populations, carriers of African swine fever, which pose risks to domestic pigs.

Similarly, local declines in predator populations like leopards can lead to an increase in baboon numbers in settled areas of Africa. Baboons, reservoirs of Schistosoma mansoni, contaminate water sources, facilitating the spread of bilharziasis. Monitoring parasites of wild and domestic animals yields insights into the presence of donors, vectors, and intermediate hosts within their ranges. For instance, finding a larval pentastome in a gazelle confirms the presence of its obligate final host in that herbivore's range. The load and variety of gastrointestinal nematodes can be linked to climatic conditions, host population density, and cropping practices, which can disrupt host-parasite balances.

5.4.5.2 Systematic Reconnaissance Flights

Low-altitude flights (approximately 100–150 m above ground level) using fixed-wing aircraft are employed to gather data on large animal populations and various ecological parameters. Trained observers visually document their observations, which are then mapped or stored digitally on tape or disk for analysis. Systematic digital photography, whether in black and white or false color, is also utilized to collect data that can be analyzed in the future. These methods are effective in capturing both permanent or semi-permanent attributes of ecosystems and transient phenomena.

For instance, low-level photography techniques have been utilized to monitor African elephant (*Loxodonta africana*) and Cape buffalo (*Syncerus caffer*) herds, enabling the assessment of recruitment age structures that can indicate the presence of diseases and conditions affecting reproductive efficiency (Croze 1972). Similar methods have been applied to monitor domestic herds and flocks, including the use of color photography before and after drought periods to evaluate mortality rates specific to different color morphs.

High-altitude photography, conducted at around 3000 m above ground level, provides valuable habitat information. It allows detection of overgrazing by large herbivores and irruptions of wild rodents, which can be identified using false color photographs. This information, combined with other indirect indicators of potential disease outbreaks, serves as an early warning system, facilitating timely implementation of preventive measures. These aerial monitoring techniques thus contribute significantly to ecological and epidemiological research by providing comprehensive data on ecosystem dynamics and potential health risks.

5.4.5.3 Remote Sensing

Satellite imagery provides a modern counterpart to traditional aerial photography, offering detailed visual data captured from space that rivals and often exceeds the quality of images obtained from low-flying aircraft in the past. Advancements in technology have significantly enhanced the utility of satellite images, making them not only comparable but sometimes superior to aerial photographs, while also being more cost-effective to acquire. Satellites can be programmed for repeated observations over specific areas at predetermined times, allowing for systematic monitoring and analysis.

False-color techniques are frequently employed to enhance specific features in satellite images, such as highlighting green vegetation or depicting changes in environmental conditions. For instance, areas undergoing drying processes might exhibit a color gradient ranging from vibrant red, indicating healthy vegetation, to bright pink, signifying drying or stressed vegetation.

In practical applications, satellite imagery has been instrumental in environmental studies, including in New Zealand where it was used to identify and map the preferred habitats of the brush-tailed possum (*Trichosurus vulpecula*), a small mammal that has become invasive and infected with bovine tuberculosis. To manage the possum population effectively, strategic poisoning campaigns have been implemented, with poison baits strategically placed in identified vegetational habitats to achieve optimal results while minimizing unintended ecological impacts (McKenzie et al. 2002).

5.4.5.4 Global Information Systems

The Global Information System (GIS) is a software platform designed to store, manage, analyze, and retrieve data based on spatial relationships, enabling automated map generation to visualize these spatial connections. It holds significant potential for epizootiological research, provided that disease-related data is formatted to integrate seamlessly with other datasets such as climate records, forest classifications, stream networks, topographical features, and human demographic information stored in separate databases. This integration allows researchers to explore complex spatial relationships and patterns crucial for understanding disease dynamics across various landscapes and environments.

5.4.6 Practical Application of Veterinary Data Acquired by Ecological Monitoring

The veterinary interpretation of routine ecological monitoring data is crucial not only for addressing issues related to human, domestic, and wild animal diseases but also for understanding the broader implications for human health, food security, and economic stability, particularly in relation to domestic livestock. It is essential to recognize that ecological monitoring should encompass not just zoonotic and emerging diseases but also the interconnectedness of animal health with human health, a perspective shared by medical professionals dealing with zoonoses and anthropo-zoonoses. This multidisciplinary approach extends the benefits of ecological data to inform policy-making across various sectors.

Utilizing foundational monitoring data, maps can be developed to delineate areas where diseases currently exist or where they may potentially emerge in the future. Over time, as monitoring continues, predictive models such as probability maps can be generated. For example, these maps might indicate that in Area X, there is an 80% likelihood of a foot-and-mouth disease outbreak within the next decade, while in Area Y, a rabies outbreak may occur once every 10 years. Such predictive insights are invaluable for implementing targeted control and preventive measures, which justify the significant investment and effort required for maintaining an ecological monitoring system.

Furthermore, fostering a comprehensive understanding among planning authorities about the implications drawn from ecological data can play a pivotal role in preventing ecological disasters. These disasters often stem from uninformed development practices that disrupt finely balanced and long-established ecological dynamics. Thus, integrating ecological insights into planning and decision-making processes is essential for sustainable development and mitigating risks associated with disease outbreaks and other ecological disturbances.

5.5 Life Table Techniques and Application

AA life table is a comprehensive record that tracks survival and reproductive rates across different age groups, sizes, or developmental stages within a population. This tool is widely utilized by ecologists and demographers alike to delve into mortality patterns, forecast population trends, and effectively manage endangered species (Teng et al. 2022).

In human population dynamics, life tables play a crucial role in predicting whether a population will grow or decline. This prediction hinges not only on the number of offspring individuals have and their lifespan, but also on the timing of childbirth. Surprisingly, the age at which people become parents significantly influences population growth or decline.

In conservation biology, life tables have proven indispensable, as exemplified by efforts to protect the loggerhead sea turtle population in the southeastern United States. Despite conservation measures aimed at safeguarding nesting beaches, the loggerhead population continued to decline, particularly due to high mortality rates among eggs and hatchlings. A detailed analysis using a life table revealed that reducing mortality among older turtles would likely have a more substantial impact on reversing the population decline. Consequently, conservation strategies shifted towards advocating for the installation of turtle exclusion devices on fishing nets to prevent drowning of older turtles (São Miguel et al. 2022).

This example underscores the utility of life tables not only in understanding demographic trends but also in guiding targeted conservation actions aimed at preserving vulnerable species.

5.5.1 Life Table Varieties

Life tables come in two varieties: cohort and static. **A cohort life table** follows the survival and reproduction of all members of a cohort from birth to death. A cohort is the set of all individuals born, hatched, or recruited into a population during a defined time interval. Cohorts are frequently defined on an annual basis (e.g. all individuals born in 2024), but other time intervals can be used as well.

A static life table records the number of living individuals of each age in a population and their reproductive output. The two varieties have distinct advantages and disadvantages, some of which we discuss below.

Life tables (whether cohort or static) that classify individuals by age are called age-based life tables. These treat age the same way we normally do: that is, individuals that have lived less than one full year are assigned age zero; those that have lived one year or more but less than two years are assigned age one; and so on. Life tables represent age by the letter x, and use x as a subscript to refer to survivorship, fecundity, and so on, for each age.

Size-based and stage-based life tables classify individuals by size or developmental stage, rather than by age. These types of tables are often more useful or practical for studying organisms that are difficult to classify by age, or whose ecological roles depend more on size or stage than on age.

5.5.2 Cohort Life Tables

To In constructing a cohort life table, such as for humans born in the United States in 1900, the process involves recording the initial number of individuals born in that year and tracking how many survive into subsequent years (e.g. 1901, 1902, etc.) until the cohort is no longer represented by survivors. This documented progression is formally known as the survivorship schedule.

In addition to survivorship, it is essential to compile a fecundity schedule, which details the number of offspring produced by individuals at each age. Typically, the total number of offspring is divided by the number of individuals in that age group, providing the average number of offspring per individual, termed per capita fecundity.

Many life tables focus exclusively on females and their female offspring. For species with equal numbers of males and females at each age, including both sexes in the analysis yields the same results. However, for organisms such as plants, hermaphroditic animals, and others where sex distinctions are absent or complex, adjustments may be necessary in life table calculations to account for these variations.

5.5.3 Static Life Tables

In population biology, a static life table resembles a cohort life table but introduces complexities, particularly for mobile animals with long lifespans where tracking entire cohorts throughout their lives is impractical. Instead, population biologists often opt to enumerate the number of individuals at each age group at a specific point in time. For instance, they count the population in the 0–1-year-old category, the 1–2-year-old category, and so on.

These age-specific counts serve as proxies for survivor counts in a cohort, enabling researchers to perform the same calculations as in cohort life tables. However, it's essential to acknowledge that this approach assumes age-specific survivorship and fertility rates have remained constant since the birth of the oldest individuals in the population. In reality, such rates typically vary over time, which can occasionally result in unexpected outcomes like negative mortality rates. To mitigate these issues, researchers often use averaging methods across multiple age groups or incorporate additional assumptions into their analyze.

5.5.4 Life Table Parameters

Survivorship and fecundity schedules serve as fundamental data points in constructing a life table. These schedules provide essential information from which various demographic parameters can be derived, such as age-specific survival rates, mortality rates, fecundity rates, survivorship curves, life expectancy, generation time, net reproductive rate, and intrinsic rate of increase. The specific quantities calculated from these schedules depend on the objectives and scope of the life table being constructed. Each of these metrics offers insights into different aspects of population dynamics and life history strategies, thereby facilitating a comprehensive understanding of species demographics and ecological interactions within populations.

5.5.4.1 Key Parameters

x and nx When conducting a study, these are the data generally collected on populations. We then calculate the rest of the life table from these data.

- **x** The first column represents the age classes. This column could represent days, minutes, or life stages (eggs, juveniles, adults, etc.).
- **nx** The number of individuals from the original cohort that are alive at the specified age, age class, or life stage (x).

From information on the number of individuals at each age, we can calculate a variety of survival and mortality rates.

- **dx** The difference between the number of individuals alive for any age class (nx) and the next older age class (nx + 1) is the number of individuals that have died during that time intervals. **dx** is a measure of age-specific mortality.
- **qx** The number of individuals that died during any given time interval (dx) divided by the number alive at the beginning of that interval (nx) provides an age-specific mortality rate.
- **Sx** The age-specific survival rate for age interval x is the proportion of individuals that survive during any given time interval.

Figure 5.4 A cohort of 3751 individuals tracked over time. The number alive at the beginning of each year is given in column B and the average number of offspring per female is given in column C. Columns D through G are calculated from information in columns A through C.

	A	B	C	D	E	F
1	Cohort Life Table: Fecundity Schedule and Population Growth					
2						
3	Age class (x)	S_x	b_x	l_x	$(l_x)(b_x)$	$(l_x)(b_x)(x)$
4	0	3751	0.00	1.0000	0.0000	0.0000
5	1	357	10.51	0.0952	1.0003	1.0003
6	2	159	0.00	0.0424	0.0000	0.0000
7	3	59	0.00	0.0157	0.0000	0.0000
8	4	57	0.00	0.0152	0.0000	0.0000
9	5	53	0.00	0.0141	0.0000	0.0000
10	6	29	0.00	0.0077	0.0000	0.0000
11	7	19	0.00	0.0051	0.0000	0.0000
12	8	17	0.00	0.0045	0.0000	0.0000
13	9	13	0.00	0.0035	0.0000	0.0000
14	10	7	0.00	0.0019	0.0000	0.0000
15	11	0		0.0000	0.0000	0.0000
16				Total	1.0003	1.0003
17	R_0	1.0003				
18	G	1.0000				
19	r est.	0.0003				

- **lx** The number of individuals surviving to any given life stage as a proportion of the original cohort size. **lx** represents the probability at birth of surviving to any given life stage.

Calculating life expectancy (Ex) requires calculating two additional parameters: Lx and Tx.

- **Lx** The number of individuals that are alive in the middle of the first age class – 0.5 years old or 1.5 years old.
- **Tx** The total years lived into the future by individuals in age class x. This value is calculated by summing the values of Lx cumulatively from age x to the end of the life table. The number of time units left for all individuals to live from age x onward is obtained by summing the Lxs.
- **Ex** The life expectancy for an individual of age x is age-specific life expectancy divided by number of individuals at age x. Life expectancy represents the average additional length of time that an individual will live once it has reached age x.

A typical life table is shown in Figure 5.4.

If we were to build a cohort life table for a population born during the year 2000, we would record how many individuals were born during the year 2000, and how many survived to the *beginning* of 2001, 2002, etc., until there were no more survivors. This record is called the **survivorship schedule**. We would also record the **fecundity schedule**: the number of offspring born to members of each age class. The total number of offspring is usually divided by the number of individuals in the age class, giving the average number of offspring per individual, which is represented by bx.

5.5.4.2 Calculating Key Parameters
Standardized Survival Schedule (lx).
Because In order to compare cohorts that start with different initial sizes, it is essential to standardize each cohort relative to its initial size at time zero, denoted as n_0. This standardization involves dividing each subsequent cohort size, n_x by n_0. The resulting proportion, representing the original number surviving to the beginning of each interval, is denoted as l_x and is calculated as follows:

$$I_x = n_x / n_0$$

We can also think of l_x as the probability that an individual survives from birth to the beginning of age x. Because we begin with *all* the individuals born during the year (or other interval), l_x always begins at a value of one (i.e. n_0/n_0), and can only decrease with time. At the last age, k, n_k is zero.

Age-specific Survivorship (S_x).
Standardized survivorship, l_x, gives us the probability of an individual surviving from birth to the beginning of age x. But what if we want to know the probability that an individual who has already survived to age x will survive to age $x+1$? We calculate this age-specific survivorship as $S_x = l_x + 1/l_x$, or equivalently:

$$S_x = n_{x+1}/n_x$$

Life Expectancy (E_x)
You may have heard another demographic statistic, life expectancy, mentioned in discussions of human populations. Life expectancy is how much longer an individual of a given age can be expected to live beyond its present age. Life expectancy is calculated in three steps.

First, we compute the proportion of survivors at the midpoint of each time interval (L_x – note the capital L here); that is:

$$L_x = (n_x + n_{x+1})/2$$

Second, we sum all the L_x values from the age of interest (n) up to the oldest age, k:

$$T_x = \sum_{x=1}^{\infty}(L_x)$$

Finally, we calculate life expectancy as:

$$E_x = T_x / n_x$$

Life expectancy is age specific – it is the expected number of time-intervals remaining to members of a given age. The statistic most often quoted (usually without qualification) is the life expectancy at birth (E_0).

Survivorship Curves
There are three classic survivorship curves, called Type I, Type II, and Type III (Figure 5.5). To understand survivorship curves, you can use survivorship schedules (S_x) to calculate and graph **standardized survivorship** (l_x), **age-specific survivorship** (g_x), and **life expectancy** (e_x).

5.5.4.3 Population Growth or Decline
We frequently want to know whether a population can be expected to grow, shrink, or remain stable, given its current age-specific rates of survival and fecundity. We can determine this by computing the **net reproductive rate** (R_0). To predict long-term changes in population size, we must use this net reproductive rate to estimate the intrinsic rate of increase (r).

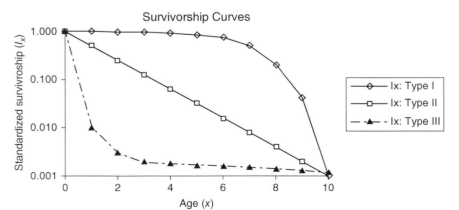

Figure 5.5 Hypothetical survivorship curves. Note that the y-axis has a logarithmic scale. Type 1 organisms have high survivorship throughout life until old age sets in, and then survivorship declines dramatically to 0. Humans are type 1 organisms. Type III organisms, in contrast, have very low survivorship early in life, and few individuals live to old age.

Net Reproductive Rate (R_0)

We calculate net reproductive rate (R_0) by multiplying the standardized survivorship of each age (l_x) by its fecundity (b_x), and summing these products:

$$R_0 = \sum_{x=0}^{k} l_x b_x$$

The net reproductive rate is the lifetime reproductive potential of the average female, adjusted for survival. Assuming survival and fertility schedules remain constant over time, if $R_0 > 1$, then the population will grow exponentially. If $R_0 < 1$, the population will shrink exponentially, and if $R_0 = 1$, the population size will not change over time. You may be tempted to conclude the $R_0 = r$, the intrinsic rate of increase of the exponential model. However, this is not quite correct because r measures population change in absolute units of time (e.g. years) whereas R_0 measures population change in terms of generation time. To convert R_0 into r, we must first calculate generation time (G) and then adjust $R0$.

Generation Time

Generation time is calculated as:

$$G = \frac{\sum_{x=0}^{k} l_x b_x x}{\sum_{x=0}^{k} l_x b_x}$$

For organisms that live only one year, the numerator and denominator will be equal, and generation time will equal to one year. For all longer-lived organisms, generation time will be greater than one year, but exactly how much greater will depend on the survival and fertility schedules. A long-lived species that reproduces at an early age may have a shorter generation time than a shorter-lived one that delays reproduction.

Intrinsic Rate of Increase

We exponential population growth and its implications for disease dynamics involves calculating the intrinsic rate of increase (r) using concepts such as the basic reproductive number (R0), as described by Gotelli (2001). The size of a population growing exponentially at time t can be expressed by the equation $N_t = N_0 \times e^{\wedge}(rt)$, where N_0 is the initial population size, e is the base of natural logarithms, and r represents the intrinsic rate of increase.

To illustrate the growth over one generation time, G, from time zero, the population equation becomes:

$$N_G = N_0 e^{rG}$$

Dividing both sides by N_0 gives us:

$$\frac{N_G}{N_0} = e^{rG}$$

We can think of N_G/N_0 as roughly equivalent to R_0; both are estimates of the rate of population growth over the period of one generation.

Substituting R_0 into the equation gives us:

$$R_0 \approx e^{rG}$$

Taking the natural logarithm of both sides gives us:

$$\ln\left(R_0\right) \approx rG$$

and dividing through by G gives us an estimate of r:

$$r \approx \frac{\ln\left(R_0\right)}{G}$$

Finally, we can use our estimate of r (uncorrected or corrected) to predict the size of the population in the future. This kind of analysis is done for human populations to predict the effects of changes in medical care and birth control programs. If we assume that all age groups are roughly equivalent in size, a similar analysis can be done for endangered species to determine what intervention may be most effective in promoting population growth. The same analysis can be applied to pest species to determine what intervention may be most effective in reducing population size.

5.5.5 Reproductive Value

The idea that different individuals have different "value" in terms of their contribution to future generations is called their *reproductive value* (Fisher 1930). As Caswell (2001) states, "The amount of future reproduction, the probability of surviving to realize it, and the time required for the offspring to be produced all enter into the **reproductive value** of an age-class."

The reproductive value of an individual of age x is designated at V_x, and is the number of offspring that an individual is expected to produce over its remaining lifespan (after adjusting for the growth rate of the population). Biologists are often interested in knowing the "value" of different individuals from a practical standpoint because knowing something about the reproductive value can suggest which individuals should be harvested, killed, transplanted, etc. from a conservation or management perspective.

The reproductive value of different ages is strongly tied to an organism's life history. Typically, reproductive value is low at birth, increases to a peak near the age of first reproduction, and then declines (Caswell 2001).

References

Anderson, R.M. and May, R.M. (1991). *Infectious Diseases of Humans: Dynamics and Control*. Oxford: Oxford University Press.

Baker, R.E., Mahmud, A.S., Miller, I.F. et al. (2022). Infectious disease in an era of global change. *Nature Reviews Microbiology* 20 (4): 193–205.

Barwell, L., Purse, B., and Hesketh, H. (2023). Invasive parasite bio-characteristics. In: *Parasites and Biological Invasions* (ed. J. Bojko, A. Dunn, and A. Blakeslee), 58–76. Wallingford: CABI.

Batalini de Macedo, M., Mendiondo, E.M., Razzolini, M.T.P. et al. (2022). Multi-stage resilience analysis of the nexus flood-sanitation-public health in urban environments: a theoretical framework. *Urban Water Journal* 20: 1–18.

Biswas, J.K., Mukherjee, P., Vithanage, M., and Prasad, M.N.V. (2023). Emergence and re-emergence of emerging infectious diseases (EIDs) looking at "One Health" through the lens of ecology. In: *One Health: Human, Animal, and Environment Triad* (ed. M. Vithanage and M. Prasad), 19–37. Hoboken: Wiley.

Björnstad, O.N. (2018). *Epidemics: Models and Data Using R*. New York: Springer International Publishing.

Brandell, E.E., Becker, D.J., Sampson, L. et al. (2020). The rise of disease ecology. BioRxiv. www.biorxiv.org/content/10.1101/2020.07.16.207100v1.full (accessed 16 April 2024).

Brandl, S.J., Lefcheck, J.S., Bates, A.E. et al. (2023). Can metabolic traits explain animal community assembly and functioning? *Biological Reviews* 98 (1): 1–18.

Caswell, H. (2001). *Matrix Population Models*, 2e. Sunderland: Sinauer Associates.

Chitimia-Dobler, L., Mackenstedt, U., and Petney, T.N. (2019). Transmission/natural cycle. In: *The TBE Book*, vol. 2 (ed. G. Dobler, W. Erber, M. Broker, et al.), 62–86. Singapore: Global Health Press.

Croze, H. (1972). A modified photogrammetric method for assessing the age structure of elephant populations and its use in Kidepo National Park. *East African Wildlife Journal* 10: 91–115.

Daszak, P., Cunningham, A.A., and Hyatt, A.D. (2001). Anthropogenic environmental change and the emergence of infectious diseases in wildlife. *Acta Tropica* 78: 103–116.

De Thoisy, B., Duron, O., Epelboin, L. et al. (2021). Ecology, evolution, and epidemiology of zoonotic and vector-borne infectious diseases in French Guiana: transdisciplinarity does matter to tackle new emerging threats. *Infection, Genetics and Evolution* 93: 104916.

Fisher, R.A. (1930). *The Genetical Theory of Natural Selection*. Oxford: Clarendon Press.

Garcia-Bustos, V., Cabañero-Navalon, M.D., Ruiz-Gaitán, A.C. et al. (2023). Climate change, animals, and *Candida auris*: insights into the ecological niche of a new species from a one health approach. *Clinical Microbiology and Infection* 29 (7): 858–7862.

Gebrezgiher, G.B., Makundi, R.H., Katakweba, A.A. et al. (2023). Arthropod ectoparasites of two rodent species occurring in varied elevations on Tanzania's second highest mountain. *Biology* 12 (3): 394.

Goldstein, J.E., Budiman, I., Canny, A., and Dwipartidrisa, D. (2022). Pandemics and the human–wildlife interface in Asia: land use change as a driver of zoonotic viral outbreaks. *Environmental Research Letters* 17 (6): 063009.

Gotelli, N.J. (2001). *A Primer of Ecology*, 3e. Sunderland: Sinauer Associates.

Gubler, D.J. (1998). Resurgent vector-borne diseases as a global health problem. *Emerging Infectious Diseases* 4: 442–450.

Gupte, P.R., Albery, G.F., Gismann, J. et al. (2023). Novel pathogen introduction triggers rapid evolution in animal social movement strategies. *eLife* 12: e81805.

Jervis, M.A., Kidd, N.A., Mills, N.J. et al. (2023). Population dynamics. In: *Jervis's Insects as Natural Enemies: Practical Perspectives* (ed. I. Hardy and E. Wajnberg), 591–667. Cham: Springer International Publishing.

Kortessis, N., Glass, G., Gonzalez, A. et al. (2023). Neglected consequences of spatio-temporal heterogeneity and dispersal: metapopulations, the inflationary effect, and real-world consequences for public health. bioRxiv. www.biorxiv.org/content/10.1101/2023.10.30.564450v1.full (accessed 16 April 2024).

Markotter, W., Coertse, J., De Vries, L., Geldenhuys, M., & Mortlock, M. (2020). Bat-borne viruses in Africa: a critical review. Journal of zoology, 311(2): 77–98.

McKenzie, J.S., Morris, R.S., Pfeiffer, D.U., and Dymond, J.R. (2002). Application of remote sensing to enhance the control of wildlife-associated *Mycobacterium bovis* infection. *Photogrammetric Engineering and Remote Sensing* 68: 153–159.

Orlowski, N., Rinderer, M., Dubbert, M. et al. (2023). Challenges in studying water fluxes within the soil-plant-atmosphere continuum: a tracer-based perspective on pathways to progress. *Science of the Total Environment* 881: 163510.

Poorter, L., Amissah, L., Bongers, F. et al. (2023). Successional theories. *Biological Reviews* 98 (6): 2049–2077.

Prasad, R., Sagar, S.K., Parveen, S., and Dohare, R. (2022). Mathematical modeling in perspective of vector-borne viral infections: a review. *Beni-Suef University Journal of Basic and Applied Sciences* 11 (1): 102.

Rayfield, B., Baines, C.B., Gilarranz, L.J., and Gonzalez, A. (2023). Spread of networked populations is determined by the interplay between dispersal behavior and habitat configuration. *Proceedings of the National Academy of Sciences* 120 (11): e2201553120.

São Miguel, R.A., Anastácio, R., and Pereira, M.J. (2022). Sea turtle nesting: what is known and what are the challenges under a changing climate scenario. *Open Journal of Ecology* 12 (1): 1–35.

Shocket, M.S., Caldwell, J.M., Huxley, P.J. et al. (2023). Modelling the effects of climate and climate change on transmission of vector-borne disease. In: *Planetary Health Approaches to Understand and Control Vector-Borne Diseases* (ed. K. Fornace, J. Conn, M. Mureb, et al.), 253–318. Wageningen: Wageningen Academic.

Singer, S.D., Laurie, J.D., Bilichak, A. et al. (2021). Genetic variation and unintended risk in the context of old and new breeding techniques. *Critical Reviews in Plant Sciences* 40 (1): 68–108.

Sivapalan, M. and Blöschl, G. (2015). Time scale interactions and the coevolution of humans and water. *Water Resources Research* 51 (9): 6988–7022.

Smith, K.L., de Vos, V., Bryden, H. et al. (2000). Bacillus anthracis diversity in the Kruger National Park. *Journal of Clinical Microbiology* 38: 3780–3784.

Taylor, R.A., Ryan, S.J., Lippi, C.A. et al. (2019). Predicting the fundamental thermal niche of crop pests and diseases in a changing world: a case study on citrus greening. *Journal of Applied Ecology* 56 (8): 2057–2068.

Teng, K.T.Y., Brodbelt, D.C., Pegram, C. et al. (2022). Life tables of annual life expectancy and mortality for companion dogs in the United Kingdom. *Scientific Reports* 12 (1): 6415.

Ullah, I.I., Kuijt, I., and Freeman, J. (2015). Toward a theory of punctuated subsistence change. *Proceedings of the National Academy of Sciences* 112 (31): 9579–9584.

Upshall, S.M., Burt, M.D.B., and Dilworth, D.G. (1987). Parelaphostrongylus tenuis in New Brunswick: the parasite in whitetailed deer (*Odocoileus virginianus*) and moose (*Alces alces*). *Journal of Wildlife Diseases* 23: 683–685.

Wale, N. and Duffy, M.A. (2021). The use and underuse of model systems in infectious disease ecology and evolutionary biology. *American Naturalist* 198 (1): 69–92.

Walker, J. and Cooper, M. (2011). Genealogies of resilience: from systems ecology to the political economy of crisis adaptation. *Security Dialogue* 42 (2): 143–160.

Will, R. (2022). Molecular epidemiology and evolution of Corynebacterium diphtheriae and *Vibrio cholerae*. Doctoral dissertation, University of Cambridge.

Woodford, M.H. (2009). Veterinary aspects of ecological monitoring: the natural history of emerging infectious diseases of humans, domestic animals and wildlife. *Tropical Animal Health and Production* 41 (7): 1023–1033.

Woodford, M.H. (2018). Veterinary aspects of ecological monitoring. In: *Routledge Revivals: Wildlife Management in Savannah Woodland (1979)* (ed. S. Ajayi and L. Halstead), 74–84. Oxford: Routledge.

Zhu, Z. and He, X. (2023). Rich and complex dynamics of a time-switched differential equation model for wild mosquito population suppression with Ricker-type density-dependent survival probability. *AIMS Mathematics* 8 (12): 28670–28689.

6

Measures of Occurrence of Disease Pattern and Association

Amitava Roy[1] and Tanmoy Rana[2]

[1] Department of Livestock Farm Complex, West Bengal University of Animal & Fishery Sciences, Kolkata, India
[2] Department of Veterinary Clinical Complex, West Bengal University of Animal & Fishery Sciences, Kolkata, India

6.1 Introduction

Concerns about animal health are very important in the cattle industry. Consequently, effective working relationships between farmers, veterinarians, government agencies, and international organizations have emerged over much of the world. The Food and Agriculture Organization (FAO) of the United Nations (www.fao.org) and the World Organisation for Animal Health (OIE: Office International des Épizooties) (www.oie.int) are the two most significant agencies concerned in animal health and international trade. Ensuring openness in the global animal disease situation is one of the OIE's main goals (including zoonotic illnesses). Zoonoses are a major category of newly developing infectious illnesses (Kahn 2006). The OIE is dedicated to characterizing the variables that contribute to the development of disease, evaluating the relative significance of each variable, and characterizing the scope and dispersion of the illness.

The FAO has a stake in zoonotic and emerging illnesses because it is the UN organization tasked with ensuring the safety and quality of food. The FAO Food and Nutrition Division's Food Quality and Standards Service oversees the FAO/World Health Organization Food Standards Program and is involved in all matters pertaining to food safety. Its tasks include supporting FAO member countries in problem solving, building infrastructure, encouraging standardization to ease trade, and defending the rights of consumers (Orriss 1997). Animal disease epidemics have caused significant economic losses in a number of nations and regions worldwide recently, despite significant advances in scientific knowledge and hygienic standards in livestock farming.

6.2 Definition of Disease

A change in the overall state of the body or in the states of any of its organs that prevents or interferes with the body's ability to perform its activities normally is referred to as a disease. Visual bodily symptoms are the most common way that the functional disruption presents itself. When it comes to cattle sickness, those who handle livestock notice these clinical symptoms. As a result, farmers and veterinarians frequently identify illness before others do. Diseases might originate from the inside or the outside (Table 6.1) and could result from several interrelated reasons. On the other hand, very little is understood about the underlying causes of intrinsic livestock diseases. These include neoplasms, autoimmune, metabolic and endocrine disorders, and age-related organ degradation. Some of these illnesses most likely have external origins as well. "Infectious diseases" are caused by live organisms like bacteria, viruses, or parasites. These are examples of external sources of disease.

Nonliving causes of disease include trauma, extremes of temperature, exposure to chemicals, and dietary deficiencies.

Numerous methods can be used to introduce infectious illnesses into a nation or area. According to Vose (1997), the primary danger of introduction is thought to be the (illegal) importation of animals and animal products (Table 6.2). Moreover, it is often recognized that wildlife serves as a significant reservoir for the spread of illnesses like hog cholera or classic swine

Epidemiology and Environmental Hygiene in Veterinary Public Health, First Edition. Edited by Tanmoy Rana.
© 2025 John Wiley & Sons, Inc. Published 2025 by John Wiley & Sons, Inc.

6 *Measures of Occurrence of Disease Pattern and Association*

Table 6.1 External factors that can cause illness.

Noncontagious	Contagious
Heat	Parasite
Intoxication	Bacteria
Irradiation	Fungi
Trauma	Virus
Food-related	Prion

Table 6.2 Primary hazards to biosecurity.

Hazards	Risk variables
Changes in vector competency or an expansion of the disease vector's range	Variations in the host population and the climate
Spread from animal to animal	Animal density in holdings and the variety of species found there
Avian migrants or other wild species	Interaction between cattle (e.g., free-range holdings) and wild birds or animals
Live animal imports as well as animal goods	Unauthorized traveler or food company imports or movements
Movement of livestock	Imports or movements of food companies or unauthorized travelers

fever (Frölich et al. 2002; Leighton 1995). It was discovered in 2005 that migratory birds were a major source of international transmission in relation to previous outbreaks of highly pathogenic avian influenza (HPAI) (Swayne and Suarez 2000).

However, there is still much disagreement on and a lack of understanding of the specifics of this spread. It was extremely rare and most likely unprecedented that over 6000 migratory birds died from the highly virulent H5N1 virus, which first appeared at the Qinghai Lake Nature Reserve in central China in late April 2005 (Liu et al. 2005). Concerns have been raised about the possibility of a chronic danger of virus introduction or reintroduction to domestic chicken flocks in countries situated along the migration routes of birds originating in central Asia (WHO 2006).

6.3 Pathways Through Which Pathogenic Pathogens Cause Livestock Diseases

Finding a sickness that precisely matches the traditional textbook definition is rare. In order to make an informed comparison and take into account all available alternatives when making a diagnosis, a successful investigator must therefore possess solid knowledge and comprehension of the possible behaviors of a disorder. A illness or production-limiting issue may be complex, so the investigator must acknowledge this and take into account environmental factors that could affect the disease's course (Neumann 1989). The following variables can affect an infectious disease's occurrence, spread, and characteristics.

- The features of the host population (such as genetics, animal demography, migratory patterns, interactions with wild animals, and animal use).
- The properties of the infectious agent and environmental conditions.

According to the Food and Agriculture Organization (FAO 2004a), there are two main ways in which infectious illnesses spread between vulnerable and infected hosts.

- Transfer via vehicle (horizontal or vertical) contact.
- Vector transmission, whether biological or mechanical.

When an infected person comes into direct or indirect physical touch with a susceptible host, the infectious agent is transmitted through contact. If the infectious agent was spread by aerosols, milk, feces, urine, or placental fluids, indirect contact would result. Contact transmission is further subdivided into two categories: vertical transmission between individuals and their progeny, and horizontal transmission between individuals by direct contact. During pregnancy or after delivery, the mother and her fetus are typically the sites of vertical transmission of infectious pathogens through colostrum. When an infected person comes into contact with a susceptible host through nonliving materials like water, food, bedding, medicines, veterinary supplies, shoes, tires, and other items, this is known as vehicular transmission. The infectious agent may survive in or on the vehicle for a long time and as a result, it may be able to spread over large distances for an extended amount of time (FAO 2004a). When an invertebrate host (vector) is used in vector transmission, the infectious agent is passed from the diseased person to the susceptible host. Either mechanically (without passing through a stage of development or multiplication) or biologically (going through a stage of development or multiplication), the vector can transfer the infectious agent.

Disease transmission models are a valuable resource for learning about the underlying causes of many diseases (Eisenberg et al. 2002). Selecting intervention and control techniques requires a thorough grasp of the underlying causes of various diseases. The OIE's list includes the majority of infectious illnesses that are significant to the livestock industry. To guarantee the hygienic safety of the global commerce in terrestrial and aquatic animals and their products, the OIE publishes the Animal Health Codes for terrestrial and marine environments. The following criteria for listing diseases are outlined in the Terrestrial Code.

- Emerging illnesses.
- Zoonotic potential.
- Considerable proliferation within naive populations.
- International dissemination.

The diseases in this list, with a few notable exceptions, all have a high morbidity and occasionally a high death rate. The latter is reliant on the host (immune status, genetic background), the virus's virulence, and additional variables. Numerous disease patterns can be caused by agents of animal disease. Typically, the illnesses are divided into two groups: "zoonotic" and "others." Traditional zoonotic illnesses like tuberculosis and anthrax continue to pose a major threat to public health but some latent zoonotic infections, including *Escherichia coli* O157:H7, have gained significant attention in industrialized nations. Novel ideas are required to prevent human infection because animals infected with several of these diseases only exhibit mild, temporary sickness, or no clinical indications at all.

6.4 Disease Incidence Patterns

The overall patterns of disease occurrence are a reflection of how randomly or nonrandomly they are distributed throughout time and geography. Counting cases is the first step toward figuring out how important distribution is through time and in space. Cases might be characterized by illnesses, fatalities, or other metrics. Conventional mapping techniques are typically useful in demonstrating the spatial grouping of illness occurrences. Epidemiologists can now map environmental elements linked to disease episodes because of the development of geographic information systems (GIS). According to Tran et al. (2004), these methods are now especially crucial for the surveillance of infectious and vector-borne illnesses. A traditional space–time analysis method called the Knox test allows for both prospective and retroactive detection of spatial and temporal grouping (Rogerson 2001).

The four descriptive terms discussed in the sections below, in general, can be used to characterize the temporal and space distribution of disease episodes in populations (Toma et al. 1999) (Figure 6.1).

6.4.1 Incidence of Sporadic Diseases

The occurrence of sporadic diseases can be viewed as random events without clustering; their distribution is uneven in terms of both time and space. Such a distribution is uncommon. Over the past 20 years, equine infectious anemia has been an intermittent illness occurrence in France.

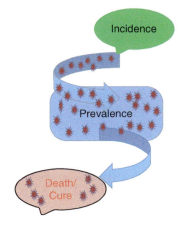

Figure 6.1 Incidence and prevalence (prevalence = incidence × average duration).

6.4.2 Incidence of Endemic Diseases

A clustering of instances in space but not in time is referred to as an endemic sickness. An endemic disease is one that persists throughout time in a population within a certain region, regardless of whether it manifests clinically. For instance, in many nations or areas, bovine tuberculosis is an endemic infectious illness that affects animals.

6.4.3 Incidence of Epidemic Diseases

An epidemic disease exhibits temporal and spatial grouping. This indicates that a greater number of people are affected by the disease than would be predicted in a given area at a given period. For instance, a disease is considered epidemic if, in a zone or compartment of a country, 2–3 disease outbreaks are typically anticipated during a given time of year and suddenly 40 or more outbreaks occur in the region in a few months.

6.4.4 Incidence of Pandemic Diseases

A pandemic is a widespread epidemic that affects multiple nations or even continents. Examples from the field of human medicine include the recent pandemic-scale HPAI outbreak and previous influenza pandemics.

6.5 Finding the Disease's Level

The sample chosen for testing should be representative of the target population and large enough to obtain an acceptable level of precision when designing surveillance to measure the level of disease in a population. For additional details on sample selection and sample size computation for surveys intended to measure immunity in a population to estimate vaccination coverage, for example, or to assess the degree of sickness in a population, see Cameron (2012).

To demonstrate how to calculate various illness frequency measures, the example below is given. Keep in mind that the herd is the unit of interest in this example, and a herd is considered infected when a farmer reports that one or more animals exhibit clinical signs of disease and subsequent laboratory testing confirms the diagnosis. Individual animals, individual pens inside a barn, herds or flocks, villages, etc. could potentially be the unit of interest.

6.5.1 Example A

Farmers in a particular province are requested to report cases of foot and mouth disease (FMD) in their herds, based on clinical indicators and a positive diagnosis from laboratory tests. The province has 50 herds in all, none of which had an infection before week 1. For the sake of this example, it is assumed that all farmers, should FMD be present in their herd, would detect and report clinical indicators of the disease. Additionally, it is expected that the herd will remain sick for the duration of the study once FMD has been reported. The outcomes are displayed as follows.

6.5.1.1 Accumulated Occurrence

This represents the percentage of disease-free units (individuals, pens, herds, etc.) that acquire a certain disease over a predetermined period of time, provided the unit does not pass away from any other disease during that time. For units to be included in the enumerator or denominator of this calculation, they must be free of disease at the start of the observation period (Pfeiffer 2002).

6.5.1.2 Density of Incidence

The instantaneous potential for change in disease status per unit of time at time t, compared to the size of the disease-free population at time t, is known as the incidence density (also called real incidence rate, hazard rate, force of morbidity or mortality). According to Pfeiffer (2002), the denominator is the total amount of time that all individuals have spent at risk (i.e., the population's time at risk), whereas the enumerator is the number of new cases over the observed period.

6.5.1.3 Prevalence

This is the percentage of a population that is afflicted with a disease at any certain period. It can be seen as the likelihood that a unit (individual, pen, herd, etc.) belonging to the same population at this particular moment has the illness (Pfeiffer 2002). The overall number of "cases" at any one period is what is measured by prevalence, not the age of the cases. The number of new instances and the length of the illness both have an impact on prevalence.

6.5.2 Example B

Over the course of a year, the FMD status of several villages in a province is described in this example. When FMD is confirmed in a specific village, that date marks the start of the red line; after 14 days, no new instances of FMD are observed in that village and the red line ends. Thus, it is assumed that the shaded line depicts the time-frame within which a specific town is designated as "FMD infected." The province consists of 20 settlements in total.

Using the village as the unit of interest, the aforementioned example allows us to determine the prevalence of FMD in the province at any given point in time (point prevalence) or period (period prevalence). Any town where FMD is present (i.e., has been reported and verified by laboratory testing) is considered a "case" in this instance.

6.5.2.1 Point Prevalence

The number of villages classified as infected in June divided by the total number of villages in the province yields the prevalence of FMD-infected villages in the province in June.

$$3 / 20 = 0.15 \text{ or } 15\%$$

6.5.2.2 Period Prevalence

The number of occurrences that are known to have happened within a given time-frame, such as a year (annual prevalence), is referred to as the period prevalence. According to Thrusfield (2007), it is the total of the point prevalence at the start of the period and the number of new instances that arise during it.

Therefore, the point prevalence at the start of the period (i.e., the prevalence of FMD in January) plus the number of new villages that become infected during this period (February to June), divided by the total number of villages in the province, is how the period prevalence for the first six months (January to June) is calculated:

$$\left(2 + 5\right) / 20 = 0.35 \text{ or } 35\%$$

This indicates that throughout a six-month period (January to June), 35% of the province's villages had FMD infections. Although the unit of interest in this example is villages, the same methods and computations are applied to determine disease frequency measurements at the animal level.

6.5.2.3 Rate of Attack

The number of new cases divided by the population at risk is the definition of attack rate. Even though it uses the same formula as cumulative incidence, this is typically used in situations where there is a brief danger period, like when cattle are fed tainted feed.

6.6 Correlation Between Incidence and Prevalence

In a cross-sectional survey, a long-lasting disease has a higher chance of being found than one with a short lifespan. As a result, the duration (D) and incidence rate (I) of a disease determine its prevalence (P). This indicates that a shift in incidence rate, a shift in the mean illness duration, or a shift in both incidence and duration may all contribute to a shift in prevalence. A disease can also be described by other helpful metrics, such as the morbidity rate, mortality rate, death rate, case fatality rate, etc. Although these metrics are extensively discussed in the literature, they are not included in this manual even though SEACFMD member countries may utilize them (OIE 2016). Further information and definitions of these measures can be found in any textbook on veterinary epidemiology.

6.7 Investigating Illness Outbreaks is Important

Finding the source of a disease is the main goal of an outbreak investigation, since it helps direct control strategies and stop the spread of the illness. The information acquired may also be utilized to assess current preventive tactics and determine new approaches to stop outbreaks in the future.

Three important pieces of information can be recorded during outbreak investigations.

- The rate at which the disease is spreading within a population of interest.
- The geographical distribution of both disease-positive and disease-negative enterprises.
- The traits or behaviors that are more prevalent in disease-positive enterprises than in disease-negative enterprises.

These three crucial pieces of knowledge enable the greatest possible adaptation of traditional disease control processes to the unique circumstances and surroundings, leading to more successful disease control measures.

6.8 Strategies for Controlling Animal Diseases

Numerous programs for the control of animal diseases are carried out by national veterinary services. Information on epidemiological surveillance, official control and eradication strategies for particular illnesses or disease complexes, and animal disease emergency preparedness are all included in current animal disease control programs (Pearson et al. 2005). Programs for the reliable control of animal diseases are also critical to global trade and food safety. The World Trade Organization (WTO), OIE, Codex Alimentarius Commission, European Union, and national governments have established the scientific underpinning for these projects. Guidelines for the international commerce of animals and animal products are provided by the OIE Terrestrial Animal Health Code (OIE 2005). A disease control strategy must always include surveillance, and a current evaluation of the state of animal health diseases is a crucial step in the process (Stärk et al. 2006). Both passive and active surveillance are possible in surveillance programs. The practice of continuously monitoring a population's endemic illness profile in order to identify any unexpected changes is known as passive surveillance.

In order to evaluate the prevalence of a disease in a given population or establish its absence with reliable evidence, active surveillance entails collecting data on that disease (FAO 2004b). In order to identify newly emerging, unusual clinical disorders, Vourc'h et al. described "syndromic surveillance" systems (Vourc'h et al. 2006). Diagnosing emerging diseases requires early identification of the unknown, unexpected, and abnormal clinical disease (CDC 1998). Instead of emphasizing clinical diagnosis, syndromic surveillance concentrates on clinical symptoms. As a result, clinical illness trends are tracked and categorized into syndromes. However, the experience of field veterinarians limits the ability to recognize cases of unusual diseases (Cuenot et al. 2003). According to Vourc'h et al. (2006), these surveillance systems need to be appealing enough to practitioners to keep them using them and motivated to turn in their case data. Syndromic surveillance can reveal anomalous occurrences that call for further action.

Many newly discovered illnesses are zoonotic, meaning they could pose a risk to both human and animal health in the future (Kahn 2006). To distinguish between well-known clinical disorders, uncommon disease occurrences, and developing diseases, a great deal of study is needed to ascertain the "normal" disease event (Grant and Olsen 1999). Therefore, the most difficult task is developing surveillance systems that are dependable and effective. Monitoring operations where the project intends to control a disease that is present in some zones or areas but missing from others that contain susceptible people may also be included in surveillance initiatives. The overall goal of this initiative is to identify issues and implement solutions (WHO 1989). A crucial component of any surveillance or control plan is laboratory testing (Schmitt 2003). The majority of nations have national laboratories that support national disease eradication initiatives and test for foreign animal diseases (FADs).

Nonetheless, extra consideration should be given to how laboratory test results are interpreted. To guarantee the accuracy of test results, numerous national and state laboratories are creating quality assurance programs (such as ISO 17025 accreditation). Veterinary services depend on the diagnostic proficiency of their laboratory system, which needs to be able to support surveillance programs for disease detection, provide testing for FAD control programs, and certify disease-free status (OIE 2006). Risk assessments utilize data from surveillance and monitoring programs. One part of risk analysis that calculates the hazards connected to a hazard is risk assessment. Hazard identification, risk management, and risk communication are the other parts of a risk analysis. Food safety and international trade are two areas where risk analyses are very crucial (Stärk and Salman 2001).

There are well-established, globally accepted standards for risk assessment and guidelines to ascertain the likely dangers with respect to a particular disease for diseases specified in the Terrestrial Animal Health Code. A herd that was previously deemed to be infected can now be declared "disease free" by using any one of a number of methods, either separately or in combination. Treatment, vaccination, "test and remove" (removing diseased animals one at a time) and "stamping out," or partial or complete depopulation, are some of these methods. The criteria for declaring a nation, region, or section free from illness or infection, with or without surveillance, are outlined in the Terrestrial Animal Health Code (OIE 2005). Cleaning and disinfection procedures go hand in hand with the aforementioned strategies (Stärk 2005). A nation's status as disease or pathogen free must be verified and protected. Strategies for monitoring and surveillance can be used to document the state.

Disease notification systems and clinical follow-up visits are examples of passive surveillance. To determine whether the disease is present or absent, active surveillance requires random sampling of the population. It is necessary to take statistical and epidemiological factors into account while designing random surveys. Import limitations, early warning systems, surveillance programs, and biosecurity measures at the farm level are all necessary for the long-term maintenance of the disease- or pathogen-free status. A disease control program may also include screening, zoning, mobility control within a nation, and management of wildlife reservoirs. These techniques have been crucial in limiting the most recent HPAI outbreaks (OIE 2006). Veterinary professionals and farmers alike need to be made more aware of unexpected clinical indications. Risk awareness declines when an agent or illness is missing from a herd or area for an extended period of time. Errors can happen when farmers, producers, importers, or veterinarians feel "safe," which raises the possibility of reinfection.

6.9 Conclusion

Livestock diseases can be brought on by a wide range of agents and circumstances. The OIE's list of animal diseases is the most significant for global trade. Animal disease agents can significantly affect the health and productivity of livestock, and zoonotic agents can spread diseases to humans in addition to animals. Furthermore, it is important to keep in mind that variations in the virulence of the causative agent may exist, leading to alterations in the disease's clinical characteristics. Animal health officials and field veterinarians must be knowledgeable about the clinical characteristics of the disease, the global distribution of the major diseases (especially classic swine fever, FMD, and other diseases that cause epidemics), and the countries that have recently experienced an outbreak of the disease as these are the most likely sources of infection, in order to protect their country's animal herds and flocks (Pearson et al. 2005).

Furthermore, data regarding current trade and tourism trends can be extremely valuable (Done 2003). The possibility of enacting a FAD has grown in the last few years. Furthermore, consumers' perception of the risk to public health has changed significantly and this needs to be addressed (Engle 2003). Consequently, it is necessary to have a capable group of experts on hand that may be called upon to help in the event that a notifiable animal disease epidemic occurs. Since illnesses have no territorial boundaries, international cooperation is just as important.

References

Cameron, A. (2012). *Manual of Basic Animal Disease Surveillance*. Nairobi: African Union Inter-African Bureau for Animal Resources (AU-IBAR).

Centers for Disease Control (CDC) (1998). Preventing emerging infectious diseases: a strategy for the 21st century. Overview of the updated CDC Plan. *MMWR Recomm Rep* 47: 1–14.

Cuenot, M., Calavas, D., Abrial, D. et al. (2003). Temporal and spatial patterns of the clinical surveillance of BSE in France, analyzed from January 1991 to May 2002 through a vigilance index. *Veterinary Research* 34: 261–272.

Done, S.D. (2003). *Foreign Animal Diseases. Lessons Learnt Regarding Practitioners in Animal Health Emergency Management*, 315–319. Perry: American Association of Swine Veterinarians.

Eisenberg, J.N.S., Brookhart, M.A., Rice, G. et al. (2002). Disease transmission models for public health decision making: analysis of epidemic and endemic conditions caused by waterborne pathogens. *Environmental Health Perspectives* 110 (8): 783–790.

Engle, M. (2003). *Monitoring Health of National and State Herds*, 361–370. Perry: American Association of Swine Veterinarians.

Food and Agriculture Organization (FAO) (2004a). *Epidemiology: Some Basic Concepts and Definitions*. Rome: FAO.

Food and Agriculture Organization (FAO) (2004b). *Surveillance and Zoning for Aquatic Animal Diseases*. Rome: FAO.

Frölich, K., Thiede, T., Kozikowski, T., and Jakob, W. (2002). A review of mutual transmission of important infectious diseases between livestock and wildlife in Europe. *Annals of the New York Academy of Sciences* 969: 4–13.

Grant, S. and Olsen, C.W. (1999). Preventing zoonotic diseases in immunocompromised persons: the role of physicians and veterinarians. *Emerging Infectious Diseases* 1 (5): 159–163.

Kahn, L.H. (2006). Confronting zoonoses, linking human and veterinary medicine. *Emerging Infectious Diseases* 12: 556–561.

Leighton, A. (1995). Surveillance of wild animal diseases in Europe. *Revue Scientifique et Technique* 14 (3): 819–830.

Liu, J., Xiao, H., Lei, F. et al. (2005). Highly pathogenic H5N1 influenza virus infection in migratory birds. *Science* 309 (5738): 1206.

Neumann, G.B. (1989). *Patterns of Animal Disease*. New Zealand: Massey University.

Office International des Épizooties (OIE) (2005). *Terrestrial Animal Health Code*, 14e. Paris: OIE.

Office International des Épizooties (OIE) (2006). Ensuring good governance to address emerging and re-emerging animal disease threats. In: *Beijing Conference*. Paris: OIE.

Office International des Épizooties (OIE) (2016). *3rd Edition of the SEACFMD Roadmap (2016–2020)*. Paris: OIE.

Orriss, G.D. (1997). Animal diseases of public health importance. *Emerging Infectious Diseases* 2 (4): 497–502.

Pearson, J., Salman, M.D., BenJebara, K. et al. (2005). *Global Risks of Infectious Animal Diseases*. Ames: Council for Agricultural Science and Technology.

Pfeiffer, D.U. (2002). *Veterinary Epidemiology – An Introduction*. London: Royal Veterinary College.

Rogerson, P.A. (2001). Monitoring point patterns for the development of space-time clusters. *Journal of the Royal Statistical Society. Series A* 164 (Part 1): 87–96.

Schmitt, B.J. (2003). Veterinary diagnostic laboratories and their support role for veterinary services. *Revue Scientifique et Technique* 22 (2): 533–536.

Stärk, K.D.C. (2005). Methods for population-based herd sanitation: an overview. *Deutsche Tierärztliche Wochenschrift* 112 (8): 292–295.

Stärk, K.D.C. and Salman, M. (2001). Relationships between animal health monitoring and the risk assessment process. *Acta Veterinaria Scandinavica* 94 (Suppl. 1): 71–77.

Stärk, K.D.C., Regula, G., Hernandez, J. et al. (2006). Concepts for risk-based surveillance in the field of veterinary medicine and veterinary public health: review of current approaches. *BMC Health Services Research* 6: 20.

Swayne, D.E. and Suarez, D.L. (2000). Highly pathogenic avian influenza. *Revue Scientifique et Technique* 19 (2): 463–482.

Thrusfield, M.V. (2007). *Veterinary Epidemiology*, 3e. Oxford: Blackwell Publishing.

Toma, B., Vaillancourt, J.P., Dufour, B. et al. (ed.) (1999). *Dictionary of Veterinary Epidemiology*, 1e. Ames: Iowa State University Press.

Tran, A., Deparis, X., Dussart, P. et al. (2004). Dengue spatial and temporal patterns, French Guiana, 2001. *Emerging Infectious Diseases* 10 (4): 615–621.

Vose, D. (1997). Risk analysis in relation to the importation and exportation of animal products. *Revue Scientifique et Technique* 16 (1): 17–29.

Vourc'h, G., Bridges, V., Gibbens, J. et al. (2006). Detecting emerging diseases in farm animals through clinical observations. *Emerging Infectious Diseases* 12 (2): 204–210.

World Health Organization (WHO) (1989). *Guide to Planning Health Promotion for AIDS Prevention and Control*. Geneva: WHO.

World Health Organization (WHO) (2006). Avian influenza ('bird flu') – fact sheet. WHO, Geneva.

7

Animal Disease Surveillance, Survey Systems, and Associate Indices

Amitava Roy[1] and Tanmoy Rana[2]

[1] *Department of Livestock Farm Complex, West Bengal University of Animal & Fishery Sciences, Kolkata, India*
[2] *Department of Veterinary Clinical Complex, West Bengal University of Animal & Fishery Sciences, Kolkata, India*

7.1 Introduction

Due to the shifting nature of international trade and growing worries about exotic infections, there has been a demand for animal disease surveillance systems in recent years (Stärk et al. 2006). In response, a variety of rubrics of surveillance modalities have emerged, ranging from risk-based surveillance (Stärk et al. 2006) to participatory disease surveillance (Jost et al. 2007) and targeted surveillance (DEFRA 2011). Research has synthesized these terminologies (Hoinville et al. 2013). Technical criteria related to risk and risk factors that underlie disease, as well as ways to improve disease searching and monitoring to better account for such criteria, have received a lot of attention in the veterinary epidemiology literature, with a focus on risk-based surveillance in particular (Stärk et al. 2006). In comparison, studies that concentrate on the surveillance equation's resource allocation side are far more constrained.

Cannon (2009) evaluated various metrics of surveillance resource optimization problems based on various decision-maker objectives (e.g., maximizing benefits from early detection, minimizing detection time, maximizing detection), and provided general examples for configuring each technique. Though they have not been widely used in the veterinary research, these optimization approaches to surveillance have been used in other related fields, including fisheries surveillance (Millar 1995) and invasive species management in the ecology literature (Hauser and McCarthy 2009). Instead, surveillance programs are typically examined more broadly, for example, as part of a benefit–cost analysis employing economic welfare indicators (producer and consumer surplus) (Moran and Fofana 2008) or as a part of a simulation analysis of disease mitigation alternatives (Bennett et al. 2010).

Häsler et al. (2012) computed the nett margin available for surveillance expenses in the context of bovine viral diarrhea (BVD) and bluetongue, respectively, by combining simulation tools on the benefits side with an accounting of alternative mitigation costs. Häsler et al. (2012) offered a theoretical explanation of the connection between intervention spending and surveillance. To maximize the nett benefits associated with prevented disease losses, the authors emphasized the need to simultaneously examine both types of expenditures, rather than concentrating just on the tradeoffs between surveillance and intervention. Prattley et al. (2007) used portfolio theory from the finance literature in the context of risk-based surveillance to create numerical indicators that offer recommendations for the distribution of surveillance resources depending on their risk elements.

Gilbert et al. (2013) created survey-based procedures to evaluate different farm and veterinary behavior factors and predictors that affect reporting and compliance in a probabilistic manner. The production system used, participation in the monitoring scheme, frequency of veterinarian contact, herd size, and farm-level record keeping were among the traits that were considered farm-level predictors. None of these risk-based strategies, meanwhile, specifically examined how to distribute resources in light of various risk variables.

A further, and crucial, omission from all these assessments is the consideration of risk factors in relation to the optimal distribution of resources, however that may be defined, as these variables may have a substantial impact on how well those resources mitigate disease. This is related to the fact that the nature of monitoring itself is dynamic, which is an important factor but seldom taken into account. The nature of surveillance programs will vary depending on the disease's setting, the effectiveness of disease control initiatives, and the personal aims and objectives of decision makers.

Epidemiology and Environmental Hygiene in Veterinary Public Health, First Edition. Edited by Tanmoy Rana.
© 2025 John Wiley & Sons, Inc. Published 2025 by John Wiley & Sons, Inc.

Although Hadorn and Stärk (2008) conducted a comparison between active and passive monitoring systems using a decision tree framework, their study failed to account for the possibility that these goals could alter over time in response to shifts in the success of controlling (or failing to control) disease. Häsler et al. (2011), in contrast, took into account surveillance in relation to the kind of disease and the phases at which diseases evolve over time. They took into account three stages of disease: (i) sustainment, where the goal of surveillance is to either detect or maintain disease freedom; (ii) investigation, where the goal is to learn more about an epidemic or endemic disease; and (iii) implementation, where surveillance is used as a source of information for mitigation strategies.

A conceptual framework like this emphasizes the dynamic nature of surveillance programs and makes a compelling case for the necessity of system-based empirical methods to confront them. This paradigm has the advantage of being able to take into account substantial heterogeneity and feedback mechanisms in this socioeconomic overlay, depending on the type of disease at issue and the availability of data. In addition to modeling the evolution of surveillance resources based on their effectiveness over time and accounting for external drivers that may influence uptake, the analysis presented here is inherently dynamic. This results in a set of empirical tools that combine and overlay the framework found in Häsler et al. (2011) and risk factors identified in Gilbert et al. (2013).

Our analysis begins with a summary of the broad ideas that guide this strategy, and then it provides a generic example of how these techniques could be used to manage disease in Scotland.

7.2 Definition

The process of continuously evaluating a population's health and illness status is called *disease monitoring*. The process of selecting people from the public to evaluate their health or disease status may be repeated or continuing. The illness under observation could be a particular infectious disease, a particular production sickness, or just general health issues. It is possible to define the population at the level of a herd, region, or country.

When a system is referred to as "disease surveillance," it means that if data show that a disease's prevalence or incidence is higher than a certain threshold, some sort of targeted action will be implemented. Analogous to illness monitoring, population sampling for the purpose of evaluating health or disease status can be continuous or recurrent, and the population can be characterized at the national, regional, or herd level. Typically, surveillance is focused on a particular illness.

Three elements are necessary for disease surveillance systems: a predetermined illness level threshold (a predetermined critical level at which action will be taken), a preset disease monitoring system, and planned directed actions (interventions).

A disease control program (DCP) is the culmination of an intervention strategy, disease control techniques, and monitoring and surveillance tactics used over an extended period of time to lower the incidence of a particular disease.

An example of a DCP is a disease eradication program (DEP), where the goal of the program is to eradicate a particular disease (the organism causing the condition).

During the French Revolution, the word "surveillance" was originally used to refer to "keeping watch over a group of persons thought to be subversive." Epidemiologists and other professionals involved in animal health have used the word widely when discussing the tracking and management of health-related events in animal populations. Early detection of any shift in an animal population's health status depends on disease surveillance. It is also crucial to establish the extent of a recognized disease or to offer evidence that no diseases are present. In animal health programs, the phrases "surveillance" and "monitoring" are sometimes used interchangeably. Monitoring an animal population for the emergence of a particular illness or a collection of diseases is known as animal disease surveillance. Identifying a disease or set of diseases, tracking changes in prevalence, and figuring out the pace and direction of disease propagation are the main goals of monitoring animal diseases. Thus, by definition, monitoring is insufficient to stop or manage a health issue. On the other hand, prevention or control of the health issue under observation is a part of surveillance. In real-world field scenarios, monitoring typically happens after an early response if surveillance efforts reveal the onset or spread of a disease. Numerous methods for implementing surveillance can also be utilized for monitoring, and vice versa. The lines separating these two concepts in practice frequently become hazy. However, the differences are more related to the goals than the methods used.

An examination or study in which data are methodically gathered for a particular goal or theoretical hypothesis is referred to as a "survey." This kind of study has a set time limit, which is typically quite brief. On the other hand, surveillance and monitoring entail the continuous, methodical gathering of data and information. Surveys are more commonly utilized to provide an answer to a particular study issue with an exploratory and scientific focus.

The methods employed in survey research are comparable to those in monitoring and surveillance. In theory, a sequence of surveys can be thought of as a monitoring system that might change into a surveillance system in the case that steps are taken to stop or manage the illness. Because the terms "surveillance," "monitoring," and "survey" contain a number of common elements, it makes sense to treat them as a single subject for the duration of this chapter.

To encapsulate the ideas and methods, several writers have suggested using the name "monitoring and surveillance system" (MOSS) (Doherr and Audigé 2001). In such sense, the term "monitoring" refers to an ongoing, flexible process of gathering information about illnesses and the factors that contribute to them within a specific community, devoid of any kind of direct control measures. A particular type of monitoring known as surveillance involves the implementation of control or eradication actions in response to the exceeding of predetermined threshold values related to the infection or disease condition. Monitoring is therefore a necessary component of any program aimed at controlling disease (Noordhuizen et al. 1997; Office International des Epizooties (OIE) 2000). In this chapter, the term "MOSS" will be used from now on, and surveys are included in it unless specified differently.

7.3 A Survey of Potential Methods for Examining the Surveillance System's Configuration

A few possible approaches that more accurately represent the intricacy of the issue at hand are as follows. These techniques depart from optimization methods (Cannon 2009), but they can serve as a preliminary approximation of the surveillance problem's complexity without taking feedback effects into account. One way to formulate this kind of challenge is to explicitly represent the system that is being shown as a system dynamics (or SD) problem. In this way, different tactics for disease control itself (Rich 2008) as well as the allocation of resources for mitigation and surveillance might adhere to different decision criteria created within the model (Duintjer Tebbens and Thompson 2009). Homer and Hirsch (2006) looked at the tradeoffs between therapeutic and diagnostic interventions in a general public health model in this way. It will be evident soon enough that a model of animal illness surveillance may readily adopt such an approach.

The capacity to integrate pertinent socioeconomic factors that may affect how resources are allocated is another benefit of a systems approach. For example, Ulli-Beer et al. (2007) tried to optimize government budget resources toward incentives for successful waste management by incorporating socioeconomic behavior and attitudes toward trash and recycling decisions in a model. The cost implications of various tactics from the epidemiological side were not taken into consideration in Rich's (2007) proposal to link economic decisions with biological determinants of disease. Various approaches of modeling economic actors can be used, depending on the production system, regional variety, level of analysis, and availability of data (Figure 7.1).

A straightforward S-I-R (susceptible-infected-recovered) model of disease transmission is created, following the progression of individual animals or herds between various natural disease states. The rectangles in the diagram stand for stocks of animals or herds at any particular time, meaning the quantity of animals or herds in the susceptible, infected, or removed states. The broad arrows represent the movements of herds or animals across several states. These would be the differential equations supporting the actors' transitions between states in the mathematical language of S-I-R models. Stocks and flows (and parameters) are related by the small circles and thin arrows that link them to stocks, flows, or other circles. These can include herd or animal populations, vaccine efficacy rates, and rates of disease transmission, among other things.

The model includes the transitions from susceptible to recovered (by vaccination) and from recovered to susceptible (due to declining immunity). It also allows for the addition of other disease states, such as latency and incubation periods

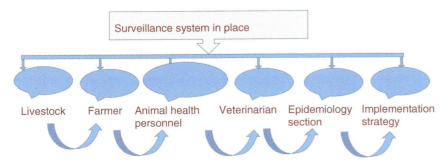

Figure 7.1 Flow of information in surveillance and management.

(Rich 2008). Complex, nonlinear differential equation systems can be graphically represented using iThink modeling, which is a strong benefit. Functional forms that relate stocks, flows, and parameters in accordance with accepted epidemiological theory are, in fact, hidden behind the graphical interface. Two diamond shapes at the top and bottom represent decision-making processes. The types of information needed to make a choice are inputs into these decision processes (linked by thin dotted lines), and the decisions made result in actions that are defined as parameters.

Two major decisions are made in this model: the distribution of resources for monitoring and the implementation of mitigating actions in response to the results of surveillance. The size of the population to be surveyed, budgetary considerations, unit prices for various measurements, and objectives relating current illness incidence to real incidence are taken into account while making decisions about surveillance in this model. As previously mentioned, this model incorporates feedbacks between the decision set for surveillance decisions and the evolving course of the disease.

Similar to how surveillance methods, financial constraints, expenses associated with mitigation, and the effectiveness of detection all affect mitigation options, these factors also have an impact on how the disease progresses (and, subsequently, which surveillance approach is chosen).

What about the socioeconomic factor overlays? The system dynamics model can be applied here in conjunction with a wide range of alternative economic theories. According to Rich (2007), economic decisions that affect entry and exit rates (such as animal births, decisions about slaughter or breeding) and transmission rates (such as risk factors in production, rates of trade between areas, etc.) may link epidemiology and economics. The economics of surveillance activities themselves may be impacted if, for instance, various tactics increase producer costs, which may then change their production patterns and, as previously mentioned, affect the transmission of illness.

Depending on the situation, the socioeconomic side of the model's precise structure will change. Rich (2007) used a livestock population model that divided animals into age cohorts based on the market's desire for livestock products. Given that S-I-R models typically have daily or weekly disease time steps, a population structure method like this would be more suitable for shorter-cycle species like chicken. A more general strategy would be to explicitly express typical farm production decisions as a mathematical programming model, where different resource and other technological restrictions are taken into account while agents of different typologies strive to maximize earnings. These kinds of models have been applied in Scotland to examine how farm- or herd-level decisions are affected by mitigations of animal health (Weldegebriel et al. 2009).

The level of agent aggregation in system dynamics models is sometimes excessively broad, which is a drawback. The system under consideration in an SD model represents a representative system or agent (or average of agents), which might not adequately portray the diversity of farm kinds and system actors. These guidelines may be based on epidemiology (such as responses to disease regimens) or economic phenomena (such as decisions to purchase or hold cattle in response to changes in market pricing). The ability to include several components of the overall model, such as a behavioral feedback model, an on-farm illness model, and a between-farm movement model, with only a few clear interactions between these modules, is one benefit of this technique. This implies that each module's internal workings can then be completely redesigned without affecting the others. The primary drawbacks of this strategy are the computational demands of these numerical techniques, the intricacy of the underlying code, and the ensuing challenges in summarizing and assessing the model. Nonetheless, separating the behavioral feedback, movements, and on-farm disease modules in this manner fits well within an object-oriented programming framework and significantly enhances the readability of the code for each component of the model while maintaining all its potential complexity.

The central component of this model is an object class that represents a population of actors. It has methods that can be used from the outside to create and delete players from the population, and to summarize and return each actor's latent and observable states. This high-level object is a single realization of the system under study, and it has fixed parameters that control its demography: how many and what kinds of actors are there, how these actors behave, the parameters that control test results and the spread of disease, and the economic model to be applied. Several, potentially heterogeneous lower level objects that belong to an actor class are set up using parameters. Each of these objects has methods to interact with other actors, methods to return the observed and latent state of that actor (with internal rules defining the relationship between these states), and a set of internal rules defining how these interactions affect that actor's behavior. While more elaborate farm classes deriving from the parent class of actor will probably incorporate complex on-farm disease dynamic models and diagnostic test representations, in the simplest instance these actors need to contain nothing extra at all. Physical heterogeneity, including herd size, farm type, animal breed, and proximity to water sources, can also be incorporated into the actor class through parameter values taken from a distribution describing all actors at class initialization. Farmers' responses to external stimuli can also be varied.

The regulator class objects in the metapopulation object represent the government and media influences on the system. These entities will receive information about the observed disease state of the actors and will shape the actors' behavior based on how the government and media respond to this observed disease state. Ultimately, an additional regulator class governs the system's economic aspects, and interactions between this entity and each actor further shape the activities of these actors. A specific amount of time is allotted to each metapopulation object to run, during which time the necessary data are taken out of the system and another instance of the class is called and permitted to execute. This yields a whole distribution of possible results for a given parameter set, which represents system variability. The entire procedure can be repeated using multiple draws from probability distributions describing the uncertainty in these parameter estimates to ascertain the sensitivity of the system to the parameter values used, since most of the parameters used to set up the simulation are probably at least partially unknown.

This framework offers a wide range of possible applications in disease monitoring scenarios and other situations where behavioral influences between numerous actors need to be addressed due to the inherent flexibility of our method. Therefore, it is our goal that this framework be applied in a generic and adaptable manner, and that new and updated classes be actively developed to enable the framework to simulate new diseases and populations.

7.4 MOSS Data Collection Method

The gathering of data, which can be categorized as active or passive, is a key element of every MOSS. Unfortunately, some writers have misused these concepts to categorize passive vs aggressive surveillance (Lilienfeld and Stolley 1994). If an action is a component of the definition of a monitoring system, then it cannot be passive. Consequently, the terms "active" and "passive" will only be used in reference to the data-gathering method in this chapter.

The systematic or routine recording of cases of a certain disease or set of diseases with the specific intention of monitoring or surveilling others is known as an active data collection for a MOSS. Typically, a population is specified for a system based on a certain area or time period. This ought to give every member of the specified population a known, frequently equal chance of being chosen. The event of interest, its anticipated prevalence, and the diagnostic tests that are now available determine which population is suitable for identification. Interviews or letters may be used to get information from owners on the health-related incident. Biological samples can be obtained at carcase rendering facilities, abattoirs, or during farm visits. A MOSS's active data gathering may also include screening biological sample banks for certain diseases or lesions or checking animal medical records (either the files or electronic databases) for particular entries.

Examples of such a system include the MOSSes for brucellosis and tuberculosis that are conducted on a regular basis in a number of nations, the sero-surveys for infectious bovine rhinotracheitis (IBR) and enzootic bovine leucosis (EBL) in Switzerland (Stärk 1996), the screening for contagious bovine pleuropneumonia (CBPP) in abattoirs in Switzerland (Stärk 1996), the bovine spongiform encephalopathy (BSE) of fallen stock and emergency slaughtered cattle in Switzerland and Europe (Doherr et al. 1999, 2001), and the screening of "downer cows" in the United States. Additional instances include the United Kingdom's scrapie surveillance (Simmons et al. 2000) and postal scrapie surveys conducted in the Netherlands, Switzerland, and the UK (Baumgarten et al. 2002). Mail or interview surveys and the collection of biological samples for laboratory testing are two examples of national MOSSes (Traub-Dargatz et al. 2000a,b).

When population based, one of the main drawbacks of active data collecting for a MOSS is its high cost in cases where the target disease is not commonly observed. The higher the sample size needed for detection, the lower the illness prevalence. When the prevalence drops to extremely low levels (<0.1%), it is frequently impractical to increase the sample size any further due to financial limitations, issues with diagnostic laboratories' operational capacity, or just issues with the selected test system (e.g., tests not sensitive and specific enough to distinguish between zero and very low prevalence levels). From low prevalence to the likelihood of disease freedom, the situation shifts. The emphasis today is on identifying a health-related event if it happens in the defined population at a frequency over the threshold, rather than on estimating prevalence.

In Europe, mandatory falling stock surveillance for BSE is one instance where all animals within a specific population are subjected to testing. Due to the anticipated extremely low prevalence (<0.1%) of detected cases in this program, all cattle that fall and are older than 24 months must be checked. The average prevalence in this high-risk target population between January 2001 and April 2002 was roughly 0.05%, or one instance for every 2000 samples analyzed. Healthcare providers, at their discretion, submit clinical or subclinical questionable cases to the health authorities as part of the passive data-gathering process (Lilienfeld and Stolley 1994). As a result, the system's validity depends only on these specialists' desire to protect data flow. In the field of veterinary medicine, the awareness and degree of information regarding a specific disease among veterinarians, animal producers, and animal owners might have an impact on the passive data-gathering process. An additional crucial element of this kind of data gathering is the availability of a diagnostic laboratory program to validate and support cases. Inconsistency in data collecting across communities and for different diseases is the primary drawback of passive data gathering. Thus, one should proceed cautiously when comparing different passively acquired MOSS data.

The three main factors influencing the efficacy of the MOSS are illness awareness, the educational background of the data sources (owners/producers, regulatory veterinarians, and practitioners), and the type of disease covered by the MOSS. An illness having a high case-fatality rate, for example, might be reported more frequently than one having a low case-fatality rate. Even when a disease's true prevalence and incidence are lower, one with greater public awareness – due to, say, extensive advertising or educational programs – may be more likely to be reported than one with less awareness. It should be mentioned that early disease identification cannot be guaranteed by using passive data collection methods. Data gathered passively for a MOSS may reveal a shift in a trend that calls for additional research. Then, often, an active approach to data collection might be used.

For diseases that must be reported to the authorities under legal requirements, certain nations have used the phrase "notifiable animal diseases." Specific zoonotic diseases and the majority of OIE List A diseases meet the requirements to be included on the notifiable list. While most governments have adopted passive data collection for MOSSes, these notifiable diseases by definition should necessitate active data gathering. The primary cause of this is the absence of a carefully thought-out study design to actively track and identify cases of these illnesses. Three groups of MOSS activities have been identified by other writers (Doherr and Audigé 2001) based on the data-gathering method: sentinel networks, active networks, and passive networks. Passive data gathering was thought to include baseline data collecting as a subcategory. A surveillance-derived disease trend, from our perspective, differs from baseline data. Since disease trends might vary over time, it could be incorrect to refer to these statistics as "baseline data" in this context. The technique of actively gathering data for a MOSS using a chosen sample to represent the population is referred to as "sentinel networks."

7.5 Targeted Surveillance

The phrase "targeted surveillance" is gaining popularity, and it basically means concentrating the MOSS sampling on high-risk populations – also known as targeted populations – that have particular, well-established risk indicators. Fallen cow stock in Europe is an example of a target population since these high-risk livestock have higher rates of BSE than do normally healthy cattle. Large-scale processed hamburger meat is another target population since it is linked to a higher risk of *Escherichia coli* O157:H7 than raw meat. The major goal of putting this surveillance strategy into practice is to make the system more effective. When the two following circumstances are met, this design is suitable: the disease in question is less common in the general population than in the targeted group, and certain risk factors have been identified or are known. Therefore, before considering this approach, sufficient knowledge of the disease and its epidemiology is necessary. Targeted surveillance is occasionally employed to guarantee that a highly susceptible population is free of a particular disease. For example, the primary goal of the surveillance program for downer cows and cattle suspected of exhibiting neurological indications of BSE in the United States is to demonstrate the absence of BSE.

One useful strategy for deliberately implementing an action that can quickly lessen the impact of a disease is targeted surveillance. A veterinary teaching hospital's nosocomial infection MOSS, which focuses *Salmonella* surveillance on equine colic cases, is an illustration of this strategy in action. This is because, compared to other hospital-admitted individuals, these cases are more vulnerable to this infection (Kim et al. 2001).

7.6 Implications of the Trade Regulation Change on MOSS Planning and Implementation

The Agreement on the Application of Sanitary and Phytosanitary Measures (SPS), which lays out the fundamental guidelines for food safety and standards pertaining to the health of animals and plants, is one of the accords that was included in the treaty that formed the World Trade Organization (WTO).

Trade choices pertaining to agricultural products have undergone a significant transformation as a result of the SPS Agreement. Its primary goal is to prevent SPS measures from being used as unjustified trade barriers. The agreement stipulates that all actions must be supported by science and not unduly restrictive, while acknowledging that nations have the right to protect the health of their citizens and their agricultural sector. The significance of SPS has been emphasized more in the SPS Agreement, specifically calling for enhanced surveillance and monitoring systems, sufficient laboratory diagnosis, risk analysis capabilities, and quality assurance. The agreement requires a nation to use scientifically grounded surveillance efforts to demonstrate the state of animal health. The design, implementation, and results of MOSSes for animal diseases in both animals and animal products are therefore being monitored by a nation's veterinary services, livestock businesses, and international bodies (Zepeda et al. 2001).

The need for MOSS that is backed by science has coincided in a number of nations with a cutback in government veterinary services' budgets and staff. As a result, several nations have made an effort to determine the best ways to meet both domestic and global standards for animal health. Many strategies and tactics for MOSS in animal health programs have been discussed in the past 10 years. When a disease is at or close to zero prevalence, which is the most significant result of this kind of investigation, the disease or its agent is declared eradicated from a nation. This kind of MOSS aims to demonstrate (with known confidence) that a pathogen or disease, if it exists in a region or nation, is present at or below a practically undetectable (acceptably low) prevalence. The phrase "freedom from disease" may be deceptive, despite the fact that it is still often employed. Freedom is synonymous with total absence, a notion that is currently deemed intolerable.

Present methods often entail gathering data from several sources and using them to present a compelling argument regarding the prevalence of a disease in a nation. A systematic survey that is statistically valid is one type of evidence that is frequently requested or employed. Well-established theory and methodologies, along with the capacity to generate a quantified probability estimate for the presence of disease, are the main benefits of using surveys. The level of verification of disease status must increasingly satisfy quantitative standards mandated by international legislation; for instance, the probability of the illness's presence at a prevalence in animals of 0.2% or higher must be less than 1%. Additional forms of evidence that could be employed are data gathered passively, an evaluation of the veterinarian services' quality, livestock movement records, environmental and geographic factors, sentinel herds, abattoir monitoring, and so on.

It has come to light that this strategy has a number of issues. Often, structured surveys are too costly or unworkable to obtain the necessary degree of proof. This is a result of the extremely large sample sizes required in situations when there is very little prevalence and low sensitivity and specificity in the applied tests. Variability in specificity and sensitivity as well as a dearth of trustworthy estimates of these test accuracy characteristics for the group being studied exacerbate this challenge. Because of this, surveys by themselves may not always be sufficient to ascertain a person's genuine disease condition. To determine the overall likelihood that a disease does not exist or is below the threshold prevalence, it is necessary to compile the evidence from all the various sources. However, currently, there are no recognized methods for estimating the strength of the evidence offered by passively gathering data for a MOSS or for aggregating probability estimates from several different sources into a single estimate of the likelihood that the disease will not exist. It is suggested that a variety of analytical techniques could be used to address these issues, such as:

- a standardized method for estimating the power of a complex MOSS through scenario tree analysis and stochastic simulation (A. Cameron, personal communication)
- better use of methods to elicit and combine expert opinion as additional information to data generated by a MOSS (K. Stärk, personal communication)
- strategies to modify the value of data sources for a MOSS based on the amount of time that has passed since their generation (Schlosser and Ebel 2001)
- Bayesian approaches to the combination of data from multiple sources of MOSS (Suess et al. 2002).

Whether one or more of the aforementioned strategies are employed, it is important to make sure that the underlying ideas and the resources needed to put them into practice are solid and widely accessible to those who require them. Utilizing these strategies would necessitate the following tasks.

1) List all potential sources of proof that the illness is not present.
2) Create a scenario tree for each source and analyze it separately to determine the likelihood that the MOSS would detect an infected animal, assuming one is present. Ranges and probability estimates are needed for every branch of the tree. These ought to be obtained from trustworthy data sources, if any, or, in the absence of trustworthy data, from properly structured expert opinion techniques.
3) Using stochastic techniques, ascertain the probability distribution surrounding the point estimate of the likelihood of detecting illness based on a scenario tree and provide measures of confidence for both estimates.

4) Modify each number to reflect the amount of time that has passed since the data were collected.
5) To get a general probability and confidence level, add all the estimations from all the sources of information.
6) In the event that the resulting probability falls short of meeting international standards, fill the probability gap by conducting a (relatively modest) structured survey or using sensitivity analysis to see which approach may be most successful in raising the level of confidence.

While there are few instances of some of these strategies being used, many nations are finding it difficult to adapt to the new global trade landscape. In order to demonstrate the absence of a disease and comply with the SPS Agreement, countries and international organizations must make a major effort. International financing agencies must modify their funding practices and show a willingness to assist in the development of sustainable infrastructure in order to give developing nations access to the global economy.

7.7 Conclusion

This chapter has demonstrated that interoperability and semantic consistency are the most widely used of the four integration strategies. Furthermore, it is clear that the idea of systems integration in health surveillance is still relatively new, though it has gained popularity recently. Integration mechanisms appear to have the ability to enhance surveillance performance, despite the paucity of formal evaluations; further quantitative research is required to validate this. Integration of surveillance systems will be heavily influenced by technological improvement in the future. Large volumes of heterogeneous data must be linked and managed for the integration and successful operation of surveillance systems to require technological innovation and strengthened data management systems. A thorough evaluation of the integrated systems should take sustainability, impact, efficiency, effectiveness, and relevance into account.

References

Baumgarten, L., Heim, D., Fatzer, R. et al. (2002). Assessment of the Swiss approach to scrapie surveillance. *Veterinary Record* 151 (18): 545–547.

Bennett, R., McClement, I., and McFarlane, I. (2010). An economic decision support tool for simulating paratuberculosis control strategies in a UK suckler beef herd. *Preventive Veterinary Medicine* 93 (4): 286–293.

Cannon, R.M. (2009). Inspecting and monitoring on a restricted budget – where best to look? *Preventive Veterinary Medicine* 92: 163–174.

Department for Environment, Food, and Rural Affairs, UK (2011). A review of the implementation of the Veterinary Surveillance Strategy (VSS). https://assets.publishing.service.gov.uk/media/5a78c2a740f0b63247699f54/pb13568-vss-review-110204.pdf (accessed 19 January 2024).

Doherr, M.G. and Audigé, L. (2001). Monitoring and surveillance for rare health-related events: a review from the veterinary perspective. *Philosophical Transactions of the Royal Society B: Biological Sciences* 356: 1097–1106.

Doherr, M.G., Oesch, B., Moser, B. et al. (1999). Targeted surveillance for bovine spongiform encephalopathy (BSE). *Veterinary Record* 145: 672.

Doherr, M.G., Heim, D., Fatzer, R. et al. (2001). Targeted screening of high-risk cattle populations for BSE to augment mandatory reporting of clinical suspects. *Preventive Veterinary Medicine* 51: 3–16.

Duintjer Tebbens, R.J. and Thompson, K.M. (2009). Priority shifting and the dynamics of managing eradicable infectious diseases. *Management Science* 55 (4): 650–663.

Gilbert, W.H., Häsler, B.N., and Rushton, J. (2013). Influences of farmer and veterinarian behaviour on emerging disease surveillance in England and Wales. *Epidemiology and Infection* 142: 1–15.

Hadorn, D.C. and Stärk, K.D.C. (2008). Evaluation and optimization of surveillance systems for rare and emerging infectious diseases. *Veterinary Research* 39: 57.

Häsler, B., Howe, K.S., and Stärk, K.D.C. (2011). Conceptualising the technical relationship of animal disease surveillance to intervention and mitigation as a basis for economic analysis. *BMC Health Services Research* 11 (1): 225.

Häsler, B., Howe, K.S., Di Labio, E. et al. (2012). Economic evaluation of the surveillance and intervention programme for bluetongue virus serotype 8 in Switzerland. *Preventive Veterinary Medicine* 103 (2): 93–111.

Hauser, C.E. and McCarthy, M.A. (2009). Streamlining 'search and destroy': cost-effective surveillance for invasive species management. *Ecology Letters* 12: 683–692.

Hoinville, L.J., Alban, L., Drewe, J.A. et al. (2013). Proposed terms and concepts for describing and evaluating animal health surveillance systems. *Preventive Veterinary Medicine* 112 (1–2): 1–12.

Homer, J.B. and Hirsch, G.B. (2006). System dynamics modeling for public health: background and opportunities. *American Journal of Public Health* 96 (3): 452–458.

Jost, C.C., Mariner, J.C., Roeder, P.L. et al. (2007). Participatory epidemiology in disease surveillance and research. *Revue Scientifique et Technique OIE* 26 (3): 537–549.

Kim, L.M., Morley, P.S., Traub-Dargatz, J.L. et al. (2001). Factors associated with *Salmonella* shedding among equine colic patients at a veterinary teaching hospital. *Journal of the American Veterinary Medical Association* 218 (5): 740–748.

Lilienfeld, D.E. and Stolley, P.D. (ed.) (1994). *Foundations of Epidemiology*, 3e. New York: Oxford University Press.

Millar, H.H. (1995). Planning annual allocation of fisheries surveillance effort. *Fisheries Research* 23: 345–360.

Moran, D. and Fofana, A. (2008). An economic evaluation of the control of three notifiable fish diseases in the United Kingdom. *Preventive Veterinary Medicine* 80: 193–208.

Noordhuizen, J.P.T.M., Frankena, K., van der Hoofd, C.M., and Graat, E.A.M. (ed.) (1997). *Application of Quantitative Methods in Veterinary Epidemiology*. Wageningen, The Netherlands: Wageningen Press.

Office International des Epizooties (OIE) (2000). *Recommended Standard for Epidemiological Surveillance Systems for Rinderpest*International Animal Health Code Part 3, Section 3.8, Appendix 3.8.1. Amsterdam: Office International des Epizooties.

Prattley, D.J., Morris, R.S., Stevenson, M.A., and Thornton, R. (2007). Application of portfolio theory to risk-based surveillance resources in animal populations. *Preventive Veterinary Medicine* 81: 56–69.

Rich, K.M. (2007). New methods for integrated models of animal disease control. American Association of Agricultural Economics Annual Meeting, Portland.

Rich, K.M. (2008). An interregional system dynamics model of animal disease control: applications to foot-and-mouth disease in the Southern Cone of South America. *System Dynamics Review* 24 (1): 67–96.

Schlosser, W. and Ebel, E.D. (2001). Use of a Markov-chain Monte Carlo model to evaluate the time value of historical testing information in animal populations. *Preventive Veterinary Medicine* 48: 167–175.

Simmons, M.M., Ryder, S.J., Chaplin, M.C. et al. (2000). Scrapie surveillance in Great Britain: results of an abattoir survey, 1997/98. *Veterinary Record* 146 (14): 391–395.

Stärk, K.D. (1996). Animal health monitoring and surveillance in Switzerland. *Australian Veterinary Journal* 73 (3): 96–97.

Stärk, K.D.C., Regula, G., Hernandez, J. et al. (2006). Concepts for risk-based surveillance in the field of veterinary medicine and veterinary public health: Review of current approaches. *BMC Health Service Research* 6: 20.

Suess, E.A., Gardner, I.A., and Johnson, W.O. (2002). Hierarchical Bayesian model for prevalence inferences and determination of a country's status for an animal disease. *Preventive Veterinary Medicine* 55: 155–171.

Traub-Dargatz, J.L., Garber, L.P., Hill, G.W. et al. (2000a). Overview of the initial phase of the National Animal Health Monitoring Systems (NAHMS) Equine '98 Study. Ninth Meeting of the International Society of Veterinary Epidemiology and Economics, Breckenridge.

Traub-Dargatz, J.L., Garber, L.P., Fedorka-Cray, P.J. et al. (2000b). Fecal shedding of *Salmonella* spp. by horses in the United States during 1998 and 1999 and detection of *Salmonella* spp. in grain and concentrate sources on equine operations. *Journal of the American Veterinary Medical Association* 217 (2): 226–230.

Ulli-Beer, S., Andersen, D.F., and Richardson, G.P. (2007). Financing a competitive recycling initiative in Switzerland. *Ecological Economics* 62: 727–739.

Weldegebriel, H.T., Gunn, G.J., and Stott, A.W. (2009). Evaluation of producer and consumer benefits resulting from eradication of bovine viral diarrhoea (BVD) in Scotland, United Kingdom. *Preventive Veterinary Medicine* 88 (1): 49–56.

Zepeda, C., Salman, M.D., and Ruppanner, R. (2001). International trade, animal health, and veterinary epidemiology: challenge and opportunities. *Preventive Veterinary Medicine* 48: 261–272.

8

Epidemiological Studies, Measures of Disease Frequency, and Mortality

Samuel U. Felix[1,2], Samuel C. Maureen[3], Simpson Monya[2], Mariam Yakubu[2], and Njideka Adeniyi[2]

[1] *Faculty of Veterinary Medicine, National Animal Production Research Institute, Ahmadu Bello University, Zaria, Nigeria*
[2] *Department of Food and Animal Science, Alabama A&M University, Normal, AL, USA*
[3] *JayCare Medical Centre, Crestwood Medica Center, Huntsville, AL, Kaduna, Nigeria*

8.1 Introduction

Epidemiology is essential for understanding the patterns and causes of health-related events within populations, guiding public health policies and interventions. It involves a variety of research designs, including both observational and experimental studies, each suited to address particular research questions. Observational studies, like cohort and case-control studies, investigate the relationships between exposures and outcomes, while experimental studies, such as randomized controlled trials, determine causality through controlled interventions. The selection of a study design is influenced by the research goals, practicality, and ethical considerations. Key measures in epidemiology, such as disease frequency, offer insights into the disease burden within populations. Prevalence indicates the proportion of individuals with a particular condition at a specific time or over a defined period. Incidence reflects the rate at which new cases of a disease emerge, providing critical information about the risk of developing the condition. Mortality, which refers to the occurrence of death in a population, is a vital outcome in epidemiological studies. Mortality rates are crucial indicators of population health, enabling comparisons across different regions, demographics, and timeframes. Age-specific and age-standardized mortality rates offer a deeper understanding of how diseases affect various age groups and help adjust for differences in population age distributions (Forbes et al. 2023).

8.1.1 Epidemiological Studies

Epidemiology is the scientific field dedicated to examining the distribution and determinants of health-related occurrences, primarily diseases, within populations. It employs diverse research methodologies to uncover patterns, causative factors, and risk elements associated with health outcomes (Sapkota 2023). Epidemiological studies are of central importance in public health and systematically explore and explain the distribution and determinants of events related to health, with particular attention to diseases, in populations. These studies offer vital insights into the occurrence, patterns, and factors influencing the development and disease transmission (Zeeb et al. 2023). Epidemiological studies fall into two main categories: observational and experimental (Morabia 2023). Table 8.1 outlines the most prevalent types of studies, providing their alternate names and units of study.

8.1.1.1 Observational Studies
Observational studies permit the natural progression of events without any interference from the investigator, who merely observes and measures. These studies encompass both descriptive and analytical categories:

1) Descriptive studies focus on presenting a straightforward account of disease occurrence within a population. Typically, they serve as the initial phase in epidemiological investigations.
2) Analytical studies delve deeper into the exploration of connections between health status and various variables.

Epidemiology and Environmental Hygiene in Veterinary Public Health, First Edition. Edited by Tanmoy Rana.
© 2025 John Wiley & Sons, Inc. Published 2025 by John Wiley & Sons, Inc.

8 Epidemiological Studies, Measures of Disease Frequency, and Mortality

Table 8.1 Classification of epidemiological study.

Study types	Other names	Unit of study
Observational studies		
Descriptive studies		
Analytical studies		
Ecological	Correlational	Populations
Cross-sectional	Prevalence	Individuals
Case-control	Case-reference	Individuals
Cohort	Follow-up	Individuals
Experimental studies or Intervention studies		Individuals
Randomized controlled trials		
Cluster randomized controlled trials	Clinical trials	
Field trials	Community intervention studies	
Community trials		Healthy people Communities

While genuinely descriptive studies are uncommon, most epidemiological studies possess an analytical nature. Although basic descriptive studies are infrequent, the information they offer in health statistics reports serves as a valuable resource for generating ideas for epidemiological research. Even a small amount of descriptive data, such as may be involved in case series outlining the characteristics of persons with a specific illness, without comparison to a reference population, often provides a stimulus for more complete epidemiological investigations. An illustrative instance is the 1981 report detailing four young men with an unusual form of pneumonia, which spurred an extensive array of epidemiological studies on the subsequently identified condition, known as acquired immunodeficiency syndrome (Rosenbaum and Rubin 2023).

8.1.1.2 Experimental Studies

Experimental or intervention studies are designed to actively modify a factor related to disease, such as an exposure or behavior, or to influence the course of a disease through treatment. These studies are similar in design to experiments in other scientific fields but are subject to additional constraints due to their potential impact on participants' health (Baker et al. 2023). Key experimental study designs include:

1) Randomized controlled trials (RCTs), often referred to as clinical trials, where patients are the subjects.
2) Field trials, which involve healthy individuals as participants.
3) Community trials, where entire communities are the units of study.

In all epidemiological research, it is essential to clearly define what constitutes a case of the disease under investigation. This involves specifying the symptoms, signs, or other criteria that indicate an individual has the disease. Similarly, it is crucial to have a precise definition of what it means for a person to be exposed to the factor under study. This definition should include all relevant characteristics that identify someone as having been exposed. Without clear and consistent definitions for both disease and exposure, interpreting the results of epidemiological studies becomes highly problematic (Baker et al. 2023).

8.1.2 Observational Epidemiological Study

8.1.2.1 Descriptive Studies

An initial phase in epidemiological inquiries often involves providing a straightforward depiction of a community's health status. This portrayal relies on readily accessible data or data garnered from specific surveys. Typically, national health statistics centers in many countries conduct such studies. These purely descriptive investigations refrain from delving into the analysis of connections between exposure and outcomes. They commonly hinge on mortality statistics, examining death patterns across specified time frames or in various nations, differentiating by age, sex, or ethnicity (Ge et al. 2023).

8.1.2.2 Ecological Studies

Ecological (or correlational) studies are valuable for generating hypotheses, with the primary units of analysis being groups rather than individuals. For example, an association was identified between the average sales of an anti-asthma medication and an unusually high number of asthma-related deaths across various provinces in New Zealand. To confirm such observations, it is crucial to thoroughly test these findings, controlling for potential confounding variables to rule out the possibility that other factors, such as differences in disease severity among populations, might explain the observed relationship (Spake et al. 2023).

Ecological studies can be conducted by comparing populations in different locations simultaneously or by analyzing the same population in a single location over different time periods (time series). Time series studies can reduce some of the socioeconomic confounding often encountered in ecological studies. In daily time series studies, confounding is virtually eliminated, as individuals serve as their own controls over a short time frame. Although ecological studies are relatively simple to conduct and thus appealing, they often pose challenges in interpretation. It is rarely feasible to directly examine the various potential explanations for the findings. Ecological studies generally rely on data collected for other purposes, and information on different exposures and socioeconomic factors may be incomplete or unavailable. Additionally, because the analysis is conducted at the group level, it is not possible to establish a direct link between exposure and effect at the individual level (Zhou et al. 2023).

Despite these challenges, ecological studies have the advantage of utilizing data from populations with diverse characteristics or from different sources. For example, the increase in mortality during the 2003 heatwave in France (Figure 8.1) was correlated with rising temperatures, although increased daily air pollution also played a role. The elevated death rate mainly affected the elderly, with immediate causes often linked to heart or lung disease (Zhou et al. 2023).

8.1.2.3 Ecological Fallacy

The ecological fallacy is a logical error that occurs when conclusions about individuals are incorrectly drawn from data that is aggregated at the group level. This fallacy happens when one assumes that a relationship observed in a group applies equally to individuals within that group. The error lies in inferring individual characteristics based solely on patterns observed in larger groups, which can lead to inaccurate conclusions. It is important to recognize that correlations at the group level do not necessarily translate to the same correlations at the individual level (Lundh 2023).

An ecological fallacy, or bias, arises when inappropriate conclusions are drawn based on ecological data. This bias occurs because the association seen between variables at the group level does not necessarily reflect the association that exists at the individual level. For instance, assuming that all individuals from an ethnic group with a higher average income in a particular region must also have a high income exemplifies the ecological fallacy. Another example would be concluding that because regions with higher education levels tend to vote for a specific political party, every educated individual in those regions must support that party (Tobias et al. 2023).

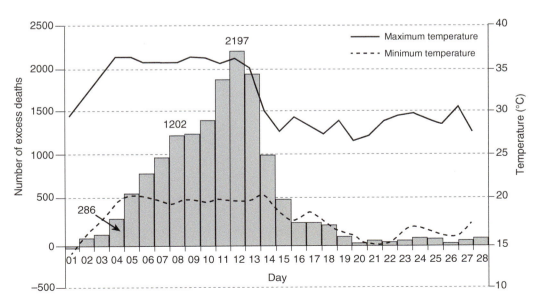

Figure 8.1 Mortality during the 2003 heat wave.

8.1.2.4 Cross-sectional Studies

Cross-sectional studies, often known as prevalence studies, are designed to measure the occurrence of diseases by assessing both exposure and outcome simultaneously. One of the challenges in these studies is understanding the direction of the observed associations, specifically whether the exposure occurred before or after the observed effect. If it can be established that the exposure preceded the effect, the data from a cross-sectional study may be treated similarly to cohort study data. Cross-sectional studies are generally easier and more cost-effective to conduct, making them particularly useful for examining exposures related to inherent characteristics of individuals, such as ethnicity or blood type. In the case of sudden disease outbreaks, cross-sectional studies that measure various exposures can be a convenient first step in identifying potential causes. The information gathered from these studies is also crucial for assessing the healthcare needs of populations (Savitz and Wellenius 2023).

Repeated cross-sectional surveys, which utilize independent random samples and standardized definitions and methods, provide valuable indicators of trends over time. Each survey should have a clearly defined objective, and valid surveys require well-crafted questionnaires, adequately sized and appropriately sampled populations, and a high response rate. Many countries routinely conduct cross-sectional surveys on representative population samples, focusing on personal and demographic characteristics, illnesses, and health-related behaviors. These surveys are essential for examining the frequency of diseases and associated risk factors in relation to variables such as age, sex, and ethnicity (Rindfleisch et al. 2008).

8.1.2.5 Case-control Studies

Case-control studies relatively provide a straightforward technique for investigating the causes of diseases, particularly those that are rare. These studies involve comparing individuals who have a specific disease or outcome (cases) with a suitable control group that does not have the disease or outcome. The comparison focuses on assessing the presence of a potential cause or exposure in both groups. While data on the disease are collected at a specific point in time, the exposure data are evaluated retrospectively, looking back to a prior time (Figure 8.2) (Gupta and Sadhukhan 2023).

The World Health Organization (WHO) Global InfoBase, accessible at http://infobase.who.int, is an online tool and data repository that compiles, stores, and presents information on chronic diseases and their associated risk factors. The InfoBase covers risk factors for chronic diseases such as overweight/obesity, blood pressure, cholesterol levels, alcohol consumption, tobacco use, fruit and vegetable intake, physical inactivity, and diabetes. Launched in 2002, it enhances access to country-reported chronic disease risk factor data for health professionals and researchers, ensuring that sources are traceable and survey methodologies are comprehensive.

It is important to recognize that case-control studies are longitudinal in nature, which sets them apart from cross-sectional studies. The term "retrospective" is often associated with case-control studies because researchers look back from the occurrence of the disease to identify potential causes. However, "retrospective" in this context refers to the direction of inquiry, not the timing of data collection. A case-control study can be retrospective, relying entirely on past data, or prospective, involving the ongoing collection of data over time (Gupta and Sadhukhan 2023).

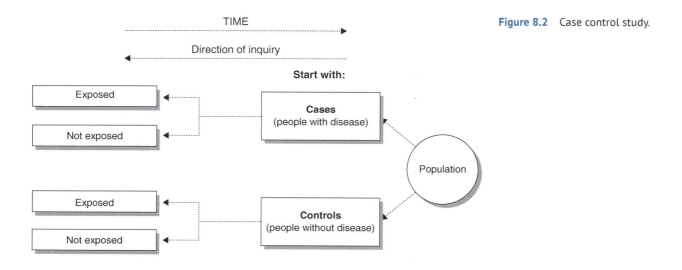

Figure 8.2 Case control study.

8.1.2.6 Selection of Cases and Controls

Exposure

One of the key things to be taken into consideration in any case-control study is the onset of the study itself and the duration of exposure both for cases and controls. In the case-control design, the status of the exposure is almost always required to be ascertained subsequent to the development of the disease, Types of studies 45, that is retrospective data and usually by direct questioning of the affected person or a relative or friend. The informant may be biased by awareness of the hypothesis under study or of the nature of the disease experience. Researchers in Papua New Guinea compared histories of meat consumption by individuals who had enteritis necroticans, with people without the disease. Proportionately more peopleIn the case-control study, the procedure starts with the careful selection of cases, which must be representative of all cases of a defined population group. The cases should be selected based on having the disease and not on the exposure. Controls are persons without the disease. One of the major challenges facing population-based case-control studies is how to efficiently find and recruit control subjects without excessive costs. Critical for this, among other things, will be a need for controls to be selected in such a way as to reflect the population from which cases were drawn, specifically, exposure prevalence. Selection of cases and controls should not depend on their exposure status, and their exposure status should be classified in the same manner for both. Cases and controls do not need to be representative; they can be limited to subgroups: for example, persons aged 65 years and over, men, or women. Controls should ideally include individuals who would have been identified as case subjects if they had developed the disease. Ideally, case-control studies use new (incident) cases to avoid the complexities involved in teasing apart factors related to causation and survival (or recovery). In practice, studies often must be conducted using prevalence data, as has frequently been done in case-control studies of congenital malformations. Although case-control studies can be used to estimate the relative risk of contracting a particular disease, they cannot furnish the absolute incidence of the disease. A much higher percentage of those who had had the disease than those not affected reported consuming meat previously e who had had the disease reported prior meat consumption than those who were not affected. Sometimes, biochemical measurements are made which are supposed to determine the exposure, but such measurements may not represent relevant past exposure, for example, the concentration of lead in blood or cadmium in urine. Exposure markers, for example, even lead in blood at age 6 years, are not good markers of exposure at age 1–2 years–the age of greatest sensitivity to lead. This can be avoided if the exposure can be estimated from an established recording system (for example, stored results of routine blood testing or employment records) or where the case-control study is prospective, such that the exposure data are collected before the disease develops (Virani et al. 2023).

Odds Ratio

The measure of the association in a case-control study is an estimate of the relative risk computed through the calculation of the odds ratio. It represents the comparison of the odds of exposure among cases with the odds of exposure among controls. The following is the calculation of the odds ratio (Table 8.2):

$$OR = (50 / 11) \div (16 / 41) = 50 \times 4111 \times 16 = 11.6$$

The estimates from the odds ratios would indicate that recent consumption of meat in cases was 11.6 times that in the controls. This measure would have a special value in the case of a rare disease and one comparable to the risk ratio. Exposure in cases and controls has to be representative of the general population for odds ratio to be a valid estimate. However, because in case-control studies neither the incidence of the disease in each of the two groups is known, the absolute risk will not be calculated. The odds ratio reported has to go with the confidence interval to give a measure of the precision around

Table 8.2 Odd ratio: Disease and exposure.

		Exposure (recent meat ingestion)		
		Yes	No	Total
Disease (enteritis necroticans)	Yes	50	11	61
	No	16	41	57
	Total	66	52	118

the point estimate. The confidence interval helps one to comprehend the range at which the true value of the odds ratio can fall with some level of significance concerning an association measure. Therefore, cases were 11.6 times more likely than controls to have recently eaten meat. The odds ratio immediately approaches the risk ratio, especially when a disease is rare. But this means a good approximation of the odds ratio can be achieved only if cases and controls represent the general population as far as the exposure is concerned. However, an absolute risk cannot be calculated as the incidence of disease is unknown. Where an odds ratio is reported, the confidence interval observed around the point estimate.

Cohort Studies

Cohort studies, otherwise known as follow-up or incidence studies, start with a cohort that is, at the beginning, disease-free. Further on, the cohort is divided according to possible cause exposure: some persons are exposed, and others are not. Specific variables of interest have to be defined and measured, and the whole cohort is followed forward in time, seeing cases of the disease develop, comparing the group with exposure to that without exposure. In this design, data on exposure and disease are required at different time points; therefore, by definition, cohort studies are longitudinal, just as the case-control study is. Cohort studies are often called prospective studies, but this terminology is ambiguous and best avoided. The "prospective" in this terminology refers to the timing of data collection, not to the exposure-effect relationship. Thus, there are prospective and retrospective cohort studies. Cohort studies give an overview of information concerning the causation of diseases and provide a direct measure of risk for a given disease. Although conceptually simple, cohort studies are actually major enterprises that require follow-up over extended periods, especially when diseases have long induction periods. For instance, the induction period for radiation-induced leukaemia or thyroid cancer is measured in many years, so exposure cohorts must be followed up over long periods of time. Cohort studies usually involve long-term exposures, and the accurate assessment of these exposures generally requires data collection over extended periods. For some exposures, like tobacco use, where habits are relatively stable, information about past and current exposure can be obtained at the time the cohort is defined. Cohort studies can be used to study acute effects as well as chronic effects, even when the cause-effect relationships are not immediately apparent for acute effects. In this regard, one of the important challenges in a cohort study is that measurement or data collection on individual exposure might not be possible. Secondly, in a case where a disease under investigation is very uncommon both in the exposed and in the unexposed, the study may encounter problems in acquiring an adequately large study group.

Cohort studies can also be relatively inexpensive if routine sources of information on mortality or morbidity are incorporated as part of the follow-up. The Framingham study, initiated in 1948, is a classic example of a cohort study in which a wide variety of risk factors are under study in relation to a variety of illnesses, such as cardiovascular and respiratory diseases and musculoskeletal disorders. The study design has contributed knowledge on public health immensely. Similarly, large cohort studies have been initiated in China wherein baseline data collection on demographic characteristics, medical histories, and major cardiovascular risk factors was done from a representative sample of 169 871 men and women aged 40 and older in 1990. This shall be followed up regularly in the cohort over time.

One particular type of cohort study is the investigation of identical twins, in whom one can control for the confounding effect of genetic variation between exposed and non-exposed individuals. Twin studies have produced impressive evidence supporting a number of cause-effect relations for chronic diseases. The Swedish twin registry is one such representative data source that can be exploited to answer a large number of epidemiological questions. The genetically similar pairs of twin studies offer a good opportunity for studying the effects of environmental factors on health outcomes, controlling for genetic variations (Figure 8.3).

Historical Cohort Studies

Costs can sometimes be minimized by adopting a historical cohort approach design that involves the identification of individuals from records of past exposure. In such cases, the associated research design is called a historical cohort study because all relevant information about exposure and disease has already been collected at the initiation of the study itself. For example, the records of the exposure of military personnel to radioactive fallout at nuclear bomb testing sites were used to investigate the question of whether the fallout causes the development of cancer during the past three decades. This design is relatively common in studies examining occupational exposures and cancer. Such historic cohort studies use existing data and records, reducing the degree of active follow-up and the amount of data collection required of participants. This has the added advantage, in the investigation of health outcomes occurring several years after past exposures under study chicas porno (Ben-Shlomo et al. 2023).

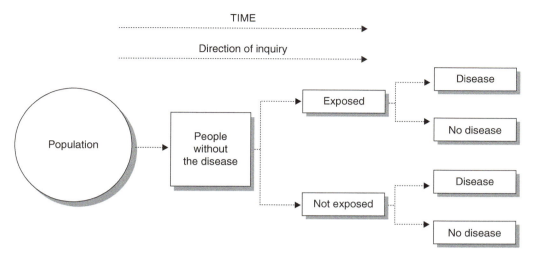

Figure 8.3 Epidemiological cohort study.

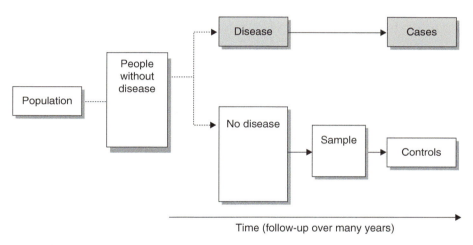

Figure 8.4 Nested case control studies.

Nested Case-control Studies

The nested case-control design makes cohort studies less expensive. Both cases and controls are selected from a defined cohort where already some information with regard to exposures and risk factors has become available. The additional information on new cases and controls specially selected for the study will be collected and analyzed. This design is more useful when the measurement of exposure is expensive. An example of a nested case-control study by Wild et al. is given in, 2023 (Figure 8.4).

8.1.3 Experimental Epidemiology

The experimentation or intervention must include deliberate changes in a variable in one or more groups of subjects. This may pertain to the removal of some dietary factor suspected of causing allergies or the introduction of a new kind of treatment to only a certain group of patients. An intervention is assessed for its effect by comparing the outcomes of the experimental group with a control group. Because the interventions are strictly based on the protocol of the study, such a design has to be bound by critical ethical considerations. For instance, no patient should be deprived of appropriate treatment as a consequence of their participation in an experiment; the kind of treatment being tested must be based upon current knowledge and must be in compliance with the ethical standard. Obtaining informed consent from study participants is generally required in almost all situations. Interventional studies are almost always designed as a randomized controlled trial, field trial, or community trial. These designs reassure the reliability of the results and ethical treatment of participants in the study while adding valuable data about the efficiency of interventions.

8.1.3.1 Randomized Controlled Trials

A randomized controlled trial (RCT) is an epidemiological experiment, really, carefully designed to test the influence of an intervention (a treatment for some disease, often referred to as a clinical trial). The underlying concept behind the RCT involves randomly assigning patients to two groups: one that receives the intervention and another with a control intervention; outcomes are measured by making a comparison between these groups. The greatest strength of randomization in an RCT is to ensure that the groups to be compared at baseline are similar. Random allocation puts all patients in the intervention and control groups by chance. Proper selection and randomization will go a long way in ensuring that any differences observed between groups, once the study design has been put in place, are solely because of chance and not because of any conscious or unconscious biases of the investigators. It is this randomness that controls for any type of potential confounding and hence increases the validity of inter-group comparison, enabling a clearer assessment of the true impact of the intervention under study. Randomized controlled trials are proposed as one of the gold standards in clinical research that help to establish causation and evaluate the efficacy of the interventions (Kandi and Vadakedath 2023) (Figure 8.5).

8.1.3.2 Field Trials

In contrast to clinical trials, field trials involve healthy people who are presumed to be at risk. Data collection occurs "in the field," typically among members of the general population who are not institutionalized. Since subjects are free of disease, and the objectives are to prevent diseases that may occur with fairly low frequency, field trials are usually complex and often expensive undertakings. One well-known example of a large field trial was a test of the Salk vaccine for the prevention of poliomyelitis, which involved more than one million children. Use of field trials is especially good at measuring the interventions aimed at reducing exposure without measurement of the occurrence of health effects. For example, several protective measures against pesticide exposure have been tested by field trials, and the monitoring of children's blood lead levels has been used to quantify the protection afforded by removal of lead paint in the home environment. While the logistic complexity and possible high costs of field trials, involving healthy subjects and prevention of relatively rare diseases, are great, they can indeed provide insight into intervention effectiveness in real-world settings. More importantly, on-field intervention studies can be made more discrete and are therefore less resource-intensive, as they perhaps do not need as long a follow-up or the measurement of disease outcomes (Jutten et al. 2023).

8.1.3.3 Community Trials

In community trials, whole communities are treated in groups. Such an experimental design can be particularly well-suited when there are likely to be social determinants of the disease and if prevention is targeted on a group basis. A classic example is cardiovascular disease. However, large community intervention trials can raise unforeseen methodological problems.

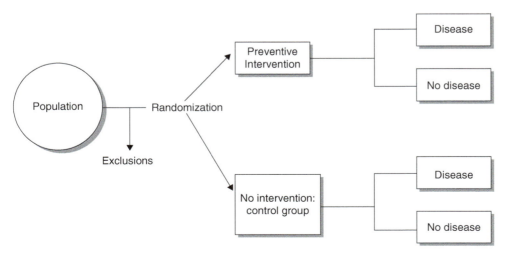

Figure 8.5 Controlled randomized trial.

Community trials involve the implementation of interventions at a community level to test an intervention's effect on a change in health outcome variables with the participation of the entire community. To this effect, combined strategies in the form of public health campaigns, policy changes, or community-wide education programs are employed in the trials. While community trials have this advantage of assessment of the effect of intervention in contrast to community settings and the difficulties of assessing the conundrum of community dynamics and confounding might be challenges in design and interpretation of results, community trials often are important in understanding the effectiveness of interventions in promoting health and preventing diseases within the much larger canvas of social and environmental factors. This type of experiment involves treatment groups as communities, not individuals. This is particularly appropriate in cases of diseases that are influenced by social conditions, and for which group behavior is appropriate in preventing undesirable occurrences. Cardiovascular disease serves as an excellent example of a disease condition appropriate for community trials, though unanticipated methodological problems can arise in large community intervention trials (Volpp et al. 2023).

8.1.3.4 Limitations of Community Trials
Such designs necessarily have limitations because only a few communities can be included in any study, and it is usually impossible to randomly allocate them. Other methods must be used to ensure that any differences observed at the end of the study are due to the intervention and not because of underlying community differences. It is also difficult to isolate the communities receiving intervention from more general social trends. One of the major challenges is overcoming design limitations when there are major positive changes, quite unexpectedly, in the control sites for some risk factors. Thus, it is not at all times that one can draw a definitive conclusion about overall effectiveness of a community-wide effort.

8.1.3.5 Potential Errors in Epidemiological
Epidemiological studies seek to offer precise assessments of disease occurrence or other outcomes, yet the potential for measurement errors introduces challenges. Epidemiologists diligently work to minimize errors and evaluate the impact of those that cannot be eradicated. Errors can stem from random or systematic sources, and addressing these issues is a key focus in the field of epidemiology.

8.1.3.6 Random Error
Random error is what occurs when measurements in a sample differ from the true population value, purely by chance, and thus provide wrong measures of association. The three largest sources of random error include individual biological variation, sampling error, and measurement error. Since we are able to study only a sample of the population, random error can never be completely eliminated. One of the major reasons for sampling error is the small sample size, which is not representative of all variables present within a population. Increasing the size of the study is definitely the best way to reduce this error. Biological variation among individuals is obvious and no measurement can ever be completely accurate. Rigorous protocols and enhanced precision in individual measures reduce measurement error. Investigators should be aware of how measurements have been made in any particular study and to recognize that errors may occur with the techniques. Quality control within laboratories should be systematic to provide a documented record of the accuracy and precision of measurements.

8.1.3.7 Sample Size
The study's sample size must be sufficiently large to provide adequate statistical power for detecting meaningful differences. Calculations for sample size can be performed using standard formulas outlined in Chapter 4, but several pieces of information are necessary for the calculation:

1) The required level of statistical significance for detecting a difference.
2) The acceptable error rate or chance of missing a real effect.
3) The magnitude of the effect under investigation.
4) The prevalence of the disease in the population.
5) The relative sizes of the groups being compared.

In reality, logistic and financial considerations often influence sample size determination, requiring a compromise between sample size and costs. The World Health Organization (WHO) has published a practical guide for determining sample size in health studies. Additionally, improving the precision of a study involves ensuring that the groups being compared are of appropriate relative size.

8.1.3.8 Systematic Error

In epidemiology, systematic error, also known as bias, arises when study outcomes consistently deviate from the actual values. A study characterized by minimal systematic error is considered highly accurate, and accuracy remains independent of sample size. Epidemiological investigations can be influenced by numerous sources of systematic error, encompassing more than 30 distinct types of bias. The primary biases include selection bias and measurement (or classification) bias.

8.1.3.9 Selection Bias

Systematic differences between people selected for a study and those not selected lead to selection bias. One obvious form of selection bias is due to participant volunteerism, either because they are ill or because they have a certain exposure that may be of concern. For example, respondents to a questionnaire on the health effects of smoking may differ in their smoking patterns from nonrespondents, with nonrespondents being heavier smokers. Bias, therefore, may also occur in research into children's health dependent on parental cooperation. For instance, in a cohort study of neonates, there might be varying responses to the 12-month follow-up depending on the socio-economic groups of the parents. Bias arises when those who respond or continue to respond to a study are different from those who are never recruited or who drop out of the study prematurely–information bias in an estimate of the exposure–outcome relationship. An important form of selection bias occurs when the disease or factor being studied itself makes people unavailable for the study. For example, in a factory where workers are exposed to formaldehyde, those who experience a high degree of irritation to the eyes are more likely to resign or quit their jobs. The less affected remaining workers may then lead to a prevalence study being highly misleading with respect to the association of formaldehyde exposure with eye irritation in the workplace. This large selection bias is called the healthy worker effect in occupational epidemiology studies. Workers need to be well enough to work; therefore, in general, the severely ill and disabled are excluded from the workforce. Likewise, if health center examinations are utilized and those not participating are not followed up, such study is bound to lead to biased results given the fact that the unwell patients could be at home or in the hospital. Any epidemiological study design has to deal with and take into consideration possible selection bias.

8.1.3.10 Measurement Bias

Measurement bias is what happens if measurements or disease or exposure classifications of individual subjects are made inaccurately, so that they do not reflect what one wishes to measure. It may derive from many sources, which may be more or less important. The biochemical or physiological measurements themselves are intrinsically imprecise, and different laboratories may obtain quite different results from the same specimen. It is possible to reduce measurement bias if specimens from exposed and control groups are analyzed in a random fashion over different laboratories, rather than all the specimens from the exposed group in one laboratory and those from the control group in another. The important form of measurement bias in retrospective case-control studies is recall bias. It happens when cases and controls remember information differently. Cases may be more likely to recall past exposure, especially if it is widely known to be associated with the studied disease, such as lack of exercise and heart disease. Differential recall may exaggerate an associated effect with the exposure, for instance, if heart cases are more likely to report on past sedentary living, or underestimate it if cases are more likely than controls to deny past exposure. This tends to underestimate the true strength of the relationship and can then lead to apparent discrepancies between different epidemiological study results in situations in which measurement bias occurs equally in both groups being compared. Observer bias may be brought into the measurements by knowledge of the exposure status on the part of the investigator, the laboratory technician, or the participant. To reduce bias, measurements may be made in a blinded or double-blind manner. A blind study indicates that the participant classification is not available to investigators, whereas the double-blind study is one in which neither the investigators nor the participants know about the latter's classification.

8.1.3.11 Confounding

One major problem associated with epidemiological research is confounding. This occurs when there is another exposure in the population being studied, itself being related to the disease and exposure of interest. The potential problem occurs when this is a factor extraneous to the variable of interest, a determinant or risk factor for the end health outcome in its own right, and found differentially distributed among the subgroups so defined. Confounding is said to occur if the effects of two different exposures, or risk factors, have not been distinguished adequately, and then the analysis attributes the observed effect to one variable rather than the other. For a variable to be a confounder, two conditions must be met (Figure 8.6).

Confounding is what happens as a result of the fact that risk factors are not randomly distributed to the source population and the study population and may therefore generate incorrect estimates of effect. Although it sounds somewhat like bias,

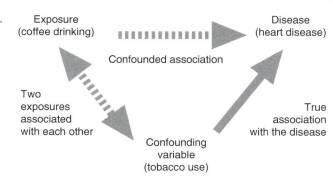

Figure 8.6 Confounding situations.

it is not the same thing. Systematic error in the research design does not cause confounding. Common examples of confounders used in epidemiological studies include age and social class. For example, an association that was seen between high blood pressure and coronary heart disease may simply be due to simultaneous variation of both those variables with increasing age. In that case, it will be important to recognize the opportunity for confounding by age and to take appropriate measures to avoid its effects. When that is done, it will become clear whether or not high blood pressure really does increase the risk of suffering from coronary heart disease.

8.1.3.12 The Control of Confounding

There are several strategies to handle confounding, either at the design phase or during the analysis of research outcomes in epidemiology. Common ways of controlling confounding in the design of an epidemiological study include randomization, restriction, and matching. Confounding at the analysis level may be controlled by stratification and statistical modeling.

8.1.3.13 Randomization

In experimental studies, randomization is the best way to ensure that potential confounding variables are equally distributed among groups that are being compared. The sample sizes need to be of an adequate size to avoid a random maldistribution of such variables. Randomization avoids an association of potentially confounding variables with the exposure under study.

8.1.3.14 Restriction

One way to control confounding is to limit the study to people who have particular characteristics. For example, in a study on the effects of coffee on coronary heart disease, participation in the study could be restricted to nonsmokers, thus removing any potential effect of confounding by cigarette smoking

8.1.3.15 Matching

Matching is a method of selecting study subjects such that some possible confounding variables are equally distributed between the two groups being compared. For example, in a case-control study on exercise and coronary heart disease, each patient with heart disease may be matched for age group and sex so that confounding by age and sex does not occur. Matching has been very broadly used in case-control studies, but it may cause problems with the selection of controls if the matching criteria are too strict or too numerous. This is called overmatching. Matching may be expensive in terms of time and money and is particularly useful when there is a danger that there will be no overlap at all between cases and controls; for example, when the cases are likely to be older than the controls.

8.1.3.16 Stratification and Statistical Modelling

In full-cohort studies, it is usually preferable to deal with confounding in the analysis phase rather than in the design phase. The way that confounding is controlled in this situation is called stratification, in which the strength of associations is measured within well-defined and homogeneous categories, called strata, of the confounding variable. For example, if age is a confounder, the association may be measured within 10-year age groups. Similarly, if sex or ethnicity is a confounder, one assesses the association separately in men and women or in different ethnic groups. There are methods for summarizing the overall association by creating a weighted average of the estimates obtained in each different stratum.

While stratification is conceptually simple and relatively easily done, it is limited by study size in application and may not satisfactorily deal with multiple factors simultaneously. In these cases, multivariate statistical modeling becomes

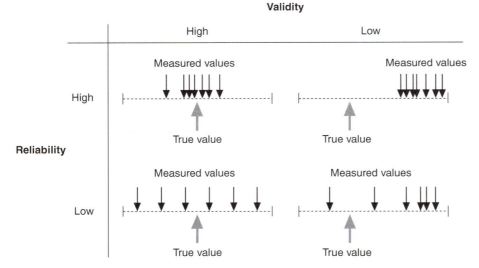

Figure 8.7 Validity and reliability.

necessary to estimate the strength of associations while simultaneously controlling for several confounding variables. There are a number of statistical techniques that help enable such comprehensive analyses.

8.1.3.17 Validity
Validity refers to how close the test comes to measuring what it is supposed to measure. A study is considered valid if its results are accurate and near the true value, free from systematic errors, and at least minimizing random errors. Even in a low-reliability but high-validity setting, measurements taken may be different, although their average will be very close to the real value. Conversely, high reliability (or repeatability) in measurements does not guarantee validity, as all of the measurements could be quite far from the true value. There is again a classification for the term 'validity' into two: internal and external (Figure 8.7).

8.1.3.18 Internal Validity
Internal validity refers to how well the results obtained are correct about what is being studied in that particular group of people. For example, measurements of blood haemoglobin must distinguish accurately participants with anemia as defined in the study. Systematic error introduced by analysis of the blood in a different laboratory might result in different readings, but the evaluation of associations with anemia, measured by a single laboratory, may be internally valid. While it must be at least internally valid, the results of even a perfectly internally valid study are of no consequence if they cannot be compared with those of other studies. Systematic error, all forms of which are sources of internal validity threats, can be improved upon through good design and attention to detail.

8.1.3.19 External Validity
External validity, or generalizability, refers to the degree to which the findings of a study apply to people not in the study (or, for example, to laboratories not involved in it). Internal validity is a prerequisite for, but does not ensure, external validity, and is easier to achieve. External validity requires external quality control of measurements and judgments about the degree to which a study's results can be generalized. This does not require that the study sample be representative of a reference population. For example, evidence that the effect of lowering blood cholesterol in men is also relevant to women requires a judgment about the external validity of studies in men. External validity is assisted by study designs which examine clearly-stated hypotheses in well defined populations. Such results should point toward supporting the external validity of a study if similar findings are replicated in studies with other populations.

8.1.3.20 Measuring Disease Frequency
Several measures of disease frequency are based on the concepts of prevalence and incidence. Epidemiologists, however, have not yet agreed on a set of definitions for terms used in this field. In this text we generally use the terms as defined in Last's Dictionary of Epidemiology.

Table 8.3 Differences between incidence and prevalence.

	Incidence	Prevalence
Numerator	Number of new cases of disease during a specified period of time	Number of existing cases of disease at a given point of time
Denominator	Population at risk	Population at risk
Focus	Whether the event is a new case Time of onset of the disease	Presence or absence of a disease Time period is arbitrary; rather a "snapshot" in time
Uses	Expresses the risk of becoming ill The main measure of acute diseases or conditions, but also used for chronic diseases More useful for studies of causation	Estimates the probability of the population being ill at the period of time being studied. Useful in the study of the burden of chronic diseases and implication for health services

8.1.3.21 Population at Risk

An important factor in the calculation of all measures of disease frequency is a correct estimate of the numbers of people under study. Ideally, these numbers should include only those people who are potentially susceptible to the diseases being studied. For example, men should not be included in the calculation of the frequency of cervical cancer.

The population who are susceptible to a given disease are referred to as the population at risk, and may be defined by demographic, geographic or environmental factors. For example: occupational injuries occur only among working people, so the population at risk is the workforce; in some countries brucellosis occurs only among people handling infected animals so the population at risk comprises those working on farms and in slaughterhouses.

8.1.3.22 Incidence and Prevalence

The distinction must be made: incidence refers to the rate of occurrence of new cases arising in a given period in a specified population, whereas prevalence refers to the frequency of existing cases in a defined population at a particular point in time. These are fundamentally different measures of occurrence (Table 8.3). There may be low incidence and a high prevalence – as for diabetes – or a high incidence and a low prevalence – as for the common cold. Colds occur more frequently than diabetes but last only a short time, whereas diabetes is essentially lifelong

Prevalence and incidence measurements count cases in defined populations at risk. The number of cases can be reported without reference to the population at risk to provide a general indication of the magnitude of a health problem or of short-term trends in a population, such as during an epidemic. Case number information, although crude, is included in WHO's Weekly Epidemiological Record; it gives some indication of how an epidemic of communicable disease is developing. In the context of a narrowly-defined population and short period of time, often during a disease outbreak, the term "attack rate" is used interchangeably with incidence. The attack rate can be most simply calculated as the number of people affected divided by the number exposed. Thus, in the investigation of a food-borne disease outbreak it can be calculated in terms of each type of food eaten and then the rates compared to identify the source of infection. Data on prevalence and incidence become considerably more useful if they are converted into rates. A rate is obtained by dividing the number of cases by the corresponding number of people in the population at risk, usually expressed as cases per 10n people. Some epidemiologists reserve the term "rate" for measurements of disease occurrence per time unit. In this book, the term "disease" is used throughout in its broad sense and includes clinical disease, adverse biochemical and physiological changes, injuries, and mental illness.

8.1.3.23 Prevalence

Prevalence (P) of a disease is calculated as follows:

$$P = \frac{\text{Number of people with the disease or condition at a specified time}}{\text{Number of people in the population at risk at the specified time}} \times 10^{N}$$

Data on the population at risk are not always available and in many studies the total population in the study area is used as an approximation. Prevalence is expressed in many instances as cases per 100, or per 1000 population. In this

Increased by:	**Decreased by:**	**Figure 8.8** Prevalence in epidemiology.

Longer duration of the disease — Shorter duration of the disease

Prolongation of life of patients without cure — High case-fatality rate from disease

Increase in new cases (increase in incidence) — Decrease in new cases (decrease in incidence)

In-migration of cases — In-migration of healthy people

Out-migration of healthy people — Out-migration of cases

In-migration of susceptible people — Improved cure rate of cases

Improved diagnostic facilities (better reporting)

case, P has to be multiplied by the appropriate factor: 10n. If data have been collected for one point in time, P is the "point prevalence rate." Sometimes it is more convenient to use "period prevalence rate," calculated as the total number of cases at any time during a specified period, divided by the population at risk midway through the period. Similarly, a "lifetime prevalence" is the total number of persons known to have had the disease for at least some part of their lives. Apart from age, several factors determine prevalence (Figure 8.8). In particular: • the severity of illness (if many people who develop a disease die within a short time, its prevalence is decreased); • the duration of illness (if a disease lasts a short time its prevalence is lower than if it lasts a long time); • the number of new cases (if many people develop a disease, its prevalence is higher than if few people do so). Since prevalence can be influenced by many factors unrelated to the cause of the disease, prevalence studies do not usually provide strong evidence of causality. However, prevalence measures are useful in estimating the need for preventive action, health care, and health service planning.

8.1.3.24 Incidence

Incidence refers to the rate of occurrence of new events in a population. Variable time periods for which the individuals are free from the disease and thus stand a chance or are "at risk" of developing it are included. In the count of incidence, the numerator is the number of new events happening in a specified period, and the denominator is the population "at-risk" of experiencing this event in that period. The most accurate way of calculating incidence is to calculate what Last calls the "person-time incidence rate."[11] Each person in the study population contributes one person-year to the denominator for each year (or day, week, month) of observation before disease develops, or the person is lost to follow-up. Incidence (I) is calculated as follows:

$$P = \frac{\text{Number of new events in a specified period}}{\text{Number of new events in a specified period}} \times 10^{N}$$

The numerator strictly refers only to first events of disease. The units of incidence rate must always include a unit of time, cases per 10n and per day, week, month, year, etc. For each individual in the population, the time of observation is the period that the person remains disease-free. The denominator to be used in calculating incidence therefore represents the sum of all the disease-free person-time periods during the period of observation of the population at risk.

Since it may not be possible to measure the periods of time when someone was disease-free, the denominator often has to be estimated by multiplying the average size of the study population by the length of time of the study period. This is reasonably accurate if the population size is large and stable, and incidence is low–for example, with stroke.

8.1.3.25 Cumulative Incidence

Cumulative incidence, on the other hand, is a much more simplistic way of expressing the occurrence of a particular disease or health status. Contrasted to incidence, it only measures the denominator at a study's beginning. The following formula may be used to calculate CI:

$$C.I = \frac{\text{Number of people who get a disease during a specified period}}{\text{Number of people free of the disease in the population at risk at the beginning of the period}} \times 10^N$$

Cumulative incidence is usually expressed as cases per 1000 population. As for example, the cumulative incidence for stroke during the eight-year follow-up was 2.3 per 1000 (274 cases of stroke, divided by the 118 539 women who entered the study). From a statistical perspective, the cumulative incidence is the probability that the members of the population contract the disease during the time period of interest. The period may be of any length, but it is usually several years or even the whole lifetime. In this way, the cumulative incidence rate is essentially a "risk of death" concept, as used in actuarial and life-table calculations. One of the strong points about cumulative incidence rates is their simplicity, which makes them useful in health information being communicated to the general public.

8.1.3.26 Case Fatality

Case fatality refers to the severity of a disease, usually defined as the proportion of cases with a given disease or condition that die in a specified period. It is expressed as a percentage.

$$\text{Case fatality} \left(\%\right) \frac{\text{Number of deaths from diagnosed cases in a given period}}{\text{Number of diagnosed cases of the disease in the same period}} \times 100$$

8.1.3.27 Mortality

Epidemiologists often explore the health status of a population in terms of data that are routinely collected: in many high-income countries, for example, the fact and cause of death are recorded on a standard death certificate, to which there is also attached information on age, sex, and place of residence. The International Statistical Classification of Diseases and Related Health Problems (ICD) concerns itself with providing guidelines on the classification of deaths.14 The procedures are revised from time to time to keep up with new diseases and changes in case-definitions, and are used today for coding causes of death. The International Classification of Diseases is now in its 10th revision, so therefore goes by the name ICD-10.

8.1.3.28 Death Rates

The Death rate/crude mortality rate of all deaths or a specific cause of death is calculated as:

$$\text{Death rate} = \frac{\text{Number of deaths during a specified period}}{\text{Number of persons at risk of dying during the same period}} \times 10^N$$

The main limitation of the crude mortality rate is that it does not allow for the fact that the probability of dying is not constant and varies according to age, sex, race, socioeconomic class, and other factors. It is generally inappropriate for comparing different time periods or geographical areas. For example, patterns of death in newly occupied urban developments with many young families are likely to be very different from those in seaside resorts, where retired people may choose to live. Comparisons of mortality rates between groups of diverse age structure are usually based on age-standardized rates.

8.1.3.29 Age-specific Death Rates

The death rates may, however, be expressed not only for a whole population, but also for particular subgroups therein defined either by age, race, sex, occupation, or geographical location, or for specific causes of death. For example, the ageand sex-specific death rate is defined as:

$$= \frac{\text{Total number of deaths occurring in a specific age and sex group of the population in a defined area during a specified period}}{\text{Estimated total population of the same age and sex group of the population in the same area during the same period}} \times 10^{N}$$

8.1.3.30 Proportionate Mortality

Proportionate mortality, actually a ratio, is sometimes used to describe the mortality in a population: the number of deaths from a given cause per 100 or 1000 total deaths in the same period. Proportionate mortality does not convey information about the risk of members of a population contracting or dying from a disease. Comparisons of proportionate rates between groups may show interesting differences. However, unless the crude or age-group-specific mortality rates are Measuring health and disease 25 known, it may not be clear whether a difference between groups relates to variations in the numerators or the denominators. For example, the proportional mortality rates for cancer would be much higher in countries with a large proportion of old people and high per capita incomes than in poor countries with few elderly if actual lifetime risk for the same cancers is about the same.

8.1.3.31 Infant Mortality

Infant mortality rate is one of the common indicators used to capture the level of health in a community. It measures the rate of death among children in the first year of their lives, whose denominator is the number of live births in the same year. The infant mortality rate is calculated as:

$$\text{Infant mortality rate} = \frac{\text{Number of deaths in a year of children less than 1 year of age}}{\text{Number of live births in the same year}} \times 1000$$

The use of the infant mortality rate as an indicator of overall health status in a population is based on the assumption that it is particularly sensitive to socioeconomic changes and to health care interventions. While infant mortality has declined in all world regions, wide differences persist both between and within countries.

Child mortality rate The child mortality rate –under-5 mortality rate – is based on deaths of children aged 1–4 years, and is often used as a general health indicator. Injuries, malnutrition and infectious diseases are common causes of death in this age group. The under-5 mortality rate describes the probability – expressed per 1000 live births – of a child dying before reaching 5 years of age. In parentheses are the areas of uncertainty around the estimates for middle-income and lowincome countries.

8.1.3.32 Maternal Mortality Rate

Maternal mortality is the risk of a mother's death related to pregnancy or childbirth, but unrelated to accidental or incidental causes. The rate varies from about 3 per 100 000 live births in high-income countries to over 1500 per 100 000 live births in low-income countries.3 But even this comparison does not reflect the much greater lifetime risk of dying from pregnancy-related causes in poorer countries.

$$\text{maternal mortality rate} = \frac{\text{Number of maternal deaths in a given geographic area in a given year}}{\text{Number of live births that occurred among the population of the given geographic area during the same year}} \times 10^{n}$$

8.1.3.33 Adult Mortality Rate

The adult mortality rate is the probability of dying between 15 and 60 years of age per 1000 population. Adult mortality rate is an indicator that assesses health inequalities among principal working age groups across countries. In nearly all countries, the probability of dying in adulthood is higher for men than for women; however, this variation across countries is very huge.

References

Baker, M.G., Masterson, M.Y., Shung-King, M. et al. (2023). Research priorities for the primordial prevention of acute rheumatic fever and rheumatic heart disease by modifying the social determinants of health. *BMJ Global Health 8* (Suppl 9): e012467.

Ben-Shlomo, Y., Mishra, G.D., and Kuh, D. (2023). Life course epidemiology. In: *Handbook of Epidemiology* (ed. W. Ahrens and I. Pigeot), 1–31. New York, NY: Springer New York.

Forbes, H.J., Travers, J.C., and Johnson, J.V. (2023). Supporting the replication of your research. In: *Research Ethics in Behavior Analysis* (ed. D.J. Cox, J.J. Finney, and M.A. Barnes), 237–262. Academic Press.

Ge, Y., Zhang, G., Meqdad, M.N., and Chen, S. (2023). A systematic and comprehensive review and investigation of intelligent IoT-based healthcare systems in rural societies and governments. *Artificial Intelligence in Medicine* 146: 102702.

Gupta, R.D. and Sadhukhan, S.K. (2023). Epidemic investigation and control. In: *Statistical Approaches for Epidemiology: From Concept to Application* (ed. R. Mukhopadhyay and R. Bhattacharya), 183–201. Cham: Springer International Publishing.

Jutten, R.J., Papp, K.V., Hendrix, S. et al. (2023). Why a clinical trial is as good as its outcome measure: a framework for the selection and use of cognitive outcome measures for clinical trials of Alzheimer's disease. *Alzheimer's & Dementia 19* (2): 708–720.

Kandi, V. and Vadakedath, S. (2023). Clinical trials and clinical research: a comprehensive review. *Cureus 15* (2): e35077.

Lundh, L.G. (2023). Person, population, mechanism. Three main branches of psychological science. *Journal for Person-Oriented Research 9* (2): 75.

Morabia, A. (2023). History of epidemiological methods and concepts. In: *Handbook of Epidemiology* (ed. W. Ahrens and I. Pigeot), 1–33. New York, NY: Springer New York.

Rindfleisch, A., Malter, A.J., Ganesan, S., and Moorman, C. (2008). Cross-sectional versus longitudinal survey research: concepts, findings, and guidelines. *Journal of Marketing Research 45* (3): 261–279.

Rosenbaum, P.R. and Rubin, D.B. (2023). Propensity scores in the design of observational studies for causal effects. *Biometrika 110* (1): 1–13.

Sapkota, K. (2023). Descriptive and analytical epidemiology. In: *Statistical Approaches for Epidemiology: From Concept to Application* (ed. R. Mukhopadhyay and R. Bhattacharya), 1–18. Cham: Springer International Publishing.

Savitz, D.A. and Wellenius, G.A. (2023). Can cross-sectional studies contribute to causal inference? It depends. *American Journal of Epidemiology 192* (4): 514–516.

Spake, R., Bowler, D.E., Callaghan, C.T. et al. (2023). Understanding 'it depends' in ecology: a guide to hypothesising, visualising and interpreting statistical interactions. *Biological Reviews* 98: 983–1002.

Tobias, D.K., Papatheodorou, S., Yamamoto, J.M., and Hu, F.B. (2023). A primer on systematic review and meta-analysis in diabetes research. *Diabetes Care 46* (11): 1882–1893.

Virani, S.S., Newby, L.K., Arnold, S.V. et al. (2023). 2023 AHA/ACC/ACCP/ASPC/NLA/PCNA guideline for the management of patients with chronic coronary disease: a report of the American Heart Association/American College of Cardiology Joint Committee on Clinical Practice Guidelines. *Circulation 148* (9): e9–e119.

Volpp, K.G., Berkowitz, S.A., Sharma, S.V. et al. (2023). Food is medicine: a presidential advisory from the American Heart Association. *Circulation 148* (18): 1417–1439.

Wild, P., Miller, A.B., Goff, D.C. Jr., and Bammann, K. (2023). Cohort studies. In: *Handbook of Epidemiology* (ed. W. Ahrens and I. Pigeot), 1–37. New York, NY: Springer New York.

Zeeb, H., Stronks, K., Agyemang, C., and Spallek, J. (2023). Epidemiological studies on migrant health. In: *Handbook of Epidemiology* (ed. W. Ahrens and I. Pigeot), 1–27. New York, NY: Springer New York.

Zhou, X., Lu, Y., Hu, S. et al. (2023). New perspectives on temporal changes in occupancy characteristics of residential buildings. *Journal of Building Engineering 64*: 105590.

9

Animal Disease Alerts and Forecasting

Amitava Roy[1] and Tanmoy Rana[2]

[1] *Department of Livestock Farm Complex, West Bengal University of Animal & Fishery Sciences, Kolkata, West Bengal, India*
[2] *Department of Veterinary Clinical Complex, West Bengal University of Animal & Fishery Sciences, Kolkata, West Bengal, India*

9.1 Introduction

Early outbreak detection is crucial for minimizing morbidity and death by implementing disease prevention and control measures on time. A lot of public health authorities have been inspired to create early disease outbreak detection systems using non-diagnostic information, which is frequently derived from electronic data collected for other purposes, by the World Trade Centre and Anthrax terrorist attacks of 2001 (Ackelsberg et al. 2002), as well as the recent West Nile virus and SARS outbreaks (Kulldorff et al. 2005). The threat of newly emerging infectious diseases to the human population is increasing. Climate changes that result in increased burdens of vector-borne diseases and the subsequent introduction of zoonotic diseases include greater temperatures and changed patterns of rainfall. It is well known that many global epidemics are extremely susceptible to short-term variations in the weather and alterations in the environment (Mills et al. 2010). "Forecasting" is the process of keeping an eye on particular risk factors in order to anticipate circumstances that may give rise to a particular disease's onset and subsequent spread. According to Myers et al. (2000), disease forecasting assists in predicting the course of illness, alerting medical professionals, and implementing control measures to stop disease outbreaks. People who are sick enough to visit a treatment centre voluntarily report diseases to authorities; as a result, these facilities are only useful for early diagnosis and treatment of infections (Linthicum et al., 1999). Alternatively, active disease surveillance could help avert an outbreak or limit the pace of transmission at an early stage of an epidemic. This entails "searching" for evidence of disease proactively through routine and ongoing monitoring in endemic areas (Ogden et al. 2010). A number of weather satellites are operated by the National Oceanic and Atmospheric Administration (NOAA) to gather operational data for climate prediction and weather forecasting. In addition to NOAA and NASA, a number of nations in the European Union, Japan, Canada, and India have remote sensing satellites that offer worldwide observations to forecast the onset of disease (Hargrove et al. 2009). Over the past 20 years, there has been a significant evolution in the use of geographic information system (GIS) to map the distribution of vector species and disease risks (Beck et al. 2000). This chapter's goals are to provide an overview of the advancements made in the use of disease surveillance systems to investigate the biology of pathogens that cause zoonotic and animal diseases, as well as to suggest areas for future research on disease forecasting (Table 9.1).

9.2 The Purpose of Forecasting

The following goals are used in the disease forecasting process (Myers et al. 2000):

1) Investigate the modes of transmission and learn how to stop the spread of epidemic diseases;
2) To assess how well disease control initiatives are working;

Epidemiology and Environmental Hygiene in Veterinary Public Health, First Edition. Edited by Tanmoy Rana.
© 2025 John Wiley & Sons, Inc. Published 2025 by John Wiley & Sons, Inc.

Table 9.1 The list of diseases of common interest provided (Adapted from GLEWS (2013)).

Nonzoonotic diseases	Zoonotic diseases
Black quarter	Q fever
Classical swine fever (CSF)	Bovine spongiform encephalopathy (BSE)
Contagious bovine pleuropneumonia (CBPP)	West Nile virus
Foot and mouth disease (FMD)	Anthrax
Peste des petits ruminants (PPR)	Tularemia
African swine fever (ASF)	Brucellosis (*Brucella melitensis*)
Haemorrhagic septicemia	Venezuelan equine encephalomyelitis
	Crimean congo hemorrhagic fever
	Japanese encephalitis
	Nipah virus
	Food borne diseases
	Rift valley fever (RVF)
	Marburg hemorrhagic fever
	Rabies
	Sheep pox/goat pox
	Ebola virus
	Highly pathogenic avian influenza (HPAI)

3) Strategies for illness control and emergency readiness;
4) To exhibit an understanding of illness epidemiology;
5) To examine the significance of diseases from the perspective of public health;

Early warning systems are expected to be not only practical but also essential weapons in the fight against the resurgence and spread of infectious diseases, thanks to developments in disease monitoring systems, epidemiological modeling, and information technology (Myers et al. 2000).

9.3 Early Warning: What Is It?

Early warning refers to the prompt and efficient response provided by accredited organizations, enabling people who are at risk of harm to take preventative or mitigation measures and get ready for a successful reaction (Grasso and Singh 2011). The idea behind Early Warning and Response (EWS) is to address a disease epidemic in its early phases. Early detection of epidemics with a recognized zoonotic potential for illness may facilitate management measures that can lower rates of morbidity and mortality in humans, from the standpoint of public health. According to Farnswortha et al. (2010), one of the primary applications of early warning systems is education as a tool for comprehending the essential components of early environmental hazard detection and response.

9.4 Initiatives for Early Warning

In the area of early warning, numerous initiatives have already been launched at the national and regional levels. Internationally, EWS systems have been built by Food and Agriculture Organization (FAO), Office International Des Epizooties (OIE), and World Health Organization (WHO). These systems methodically gather, check, evaluate, and act upon information from a range of sources, including unofficial media reports and informal networks (WHO 2006).

9.5 Role of International Organizations in Taking the Lead in Early Warning System Development

9.5.1 The Early Warning System of the Office International Des Epizooties (OIE)

On January 25, 1924, OIE was founded in Paris. The Office retained its previous acronym, OIE, but changed its name to the World Organization for Animal Health in May 2003. This organization has established a search and verification mechanism for animal health information in order to notify the OIE of newly discovered or reemerging diseases that have not yet been formally reported. The framework's goal is to strengthen regional alliances and national governments' ability to combat transboundary animal diseases (TADs). Emergency funding is quickly raised to send OIE Reference Laboratories experts to a nation to evaluate its epidemiological condition and determine what steps need to be taken (FAO 2011).

Access to all data stored in OIE's new World Animal Health Information System (WAHIS) is possible through the World Animal Health Information Database (WAHID) Interface. The previous web interface, known as the Handistatus II System, is replaced, and it is greatly expanded. Instant notifications and follow-up reports from Country/jurisdiction Members informing of extraordinary epidemiological events occurring in their jurisdiction currently provide a wide range of information. An assessment by each member nation every six months regarding the occurrence, progression, and absence of diseases on the OIE list as well as data of epidemiological importance to other nations (OIE 2013).

9.5.2 Food and Agriculture Organization

After FAO was founded in 16th October, 1945, Canada moved its headquarters to Rome, Italy. The primary objective of FAO is to provide food security for everybody. FAO created an EWS system through its 1994-established special EMPRES priority initiative (FAO 2011). The web-based EMPRES worldwide Animal illness Information System (EMPRES-i) was created to facilitate both regional and worldwide illness information in order to enhance veterinary services. Accurate and up-to-date disease information facilitates progressive control and eradication of TADs, such as emergent zoonoses, by improving early warning and reaction. The goal of EMPRES-i is to provide clarification on disease incidents that are reported to FAO from various sources, including government Ministries of Agriculture and Health, field mission reports, partner NGOs, and country or regional project reports. EMPRES employs both official and unauthorized sources of information for verification (FAO 2002). The creation of software programmes like the Transboundary Animal Disease Information System (TAD info), Transboundary Animal Diseases Simulator (TAD simulator), and Good Emergency Management Practise (GEMP) has been a key component of the EMPRES initiative for early warning and early response (FAO 2011).

9.5.3 World Health Organization

WHO was founded on April 7, 1948, and is based in Geneva, Switzerland. Its mission is to promote global public health. WHO provides aid to impacted nations through the coordination of international investigations, provision of supplies, and technical guidance (Formenty 2009). In order to address the global threat of emerging and epidemic-prone diseases in humans, as well as to get ready for the swift deployment and coordination of international resources in the event of a collaborative outbreak of international significance, the Global Outbreak Alert and Response Network (GOARN) is expanding on both new and existing partnerships of national and international institutions and networks (Ridder and Formenty 2011). According to Jebara (2004), GOARN seeks to enhance national outbreak preparation by assessing risks of rapidly emerging epidemic disease threats, providing affected human populations with timely access to appropriate technical support, and maintaining containment and control of outbreaks. In order to manage vital information about outbreaks and guarantee precise and prompt communications between important international public health professionals, such as WHO Regional Offices, Country Offices, cooperating centres, and partners in the GOARN, WHO has created a comprehensive "Event Management System." In order to help WHO and the GOARN prepare more effectively, respond more quickly, and manage resources more efficiently, this system creates a dynamic picture of Alert and Response Operations and offers information for action in a methodical manner. In order to support the operational aspects of alert and response of the new International Health Regulations (WHO 2013a), the WHO event management system is being further strengthened.

9.6 Global Early Warning and Response System (GLEWS)

The OIE, FAO, and WHO created alert and response mechanisms, on which Global Early Warning System (GLEWS) is a collaborative system, adds significant value (WHO 2010). When necessary, the GLEWS collaborates on cooperative field missions to assess and contain outbreaks, exchanges information, and performs epidemiological analyses to help predict, prevent, and control hazards to animal health, including zoonoses. Representatives from FAO, OIE, and WHO voluntarily joined the GLEWS effort from its inception since they all had the same goal of improving EWS capabilities for the benefit of the global community. Throughout the EWS phase, mutual benefits have been found through partnership (FAO-OIE-WHO 2010). For highly pathogenic avian influenza (HPAI), Rift Valley fever (RVF), and other vector-borne illnesses, well defined GLEWS are available; GLEWS is being developed for the remaining illnesses (Ahmed et al. 2009). The GLEWS Management Committee (GMC) oversees general GLEWS operations and is in charge of monitoring the strategic plan and the execution of the GLEWS agreement. The GLEWS Task Force, co-chaired by FAO, OIE, and WHO, is tasked with carrying out various responsibilities, with guidance and decisions coming from the GLEWS Management Committee (WHO 2010). The information gathered through the various tracking and verification channels of each organization will be fed into a GLEWS electronic platform where it will be further analyzed, monitored, and/or sent out as Early Warning Messages upon notification of a rumor, suspicion, or forecast regarding a disease outbreak.

9.6.1 Aims of GLEWS

Selected OIE and FAO cooperating centres, OIE and FAO laboratories, and WHO collaborating centres will be used for the specific study and modeling of trends. Only in the event when a joint onsite assessment or intervention mission is clearly indicated, will a GLEWS Emergency Response be required (FAO-OIE-WHO 2010; Formenty 2009).

1) Improved containment and worldwide readiness;
2) Enhanced nation-level identification of extraordinary epidemiological occurrences;
3) Enhanced alert timeliness and sensitivity, as well as enhanced national surveillance and monitoring systems;
4) Increase international openness and adherence to OIE reporting requirements;
5) Enhance the quality of field animal health information and offer technical assistance;
6) Strengthening the connection between veterinary and medical laboratories;
7) Offer the impacted nations prompt, effective, and coordinated support.

9.6.2 GLEWS Combined Risk Assessment for Zoonotic Diseases

In order to evaluate and offer solutions to reduce the risks connected to the appearance or spread of animal infections at the animal/human/ecosystem interface, risk analysis is crucial. One of the key areas that has lately received significant attention for enhanced cooperation between FAO, OIE, and WHO to manage the introduction of pathogens – particularly emergent zoonotic pathogens – is risk analysis (WHO 2013b). As intended, joint risk assessments for priority zoonotic illnesses as CCHF, RVF, H5N1 HPAI, rabies, and Brucellosis will first be carried out in certain locations. Using data on reported outbreaks, surveillance operations conducted by nations, and combining this information with other datasets including land use, trade, livestock population, animal movement, etc., risk analysis and mapping methodologies will be developed and validated within this framework. Tools for risk mapping are crucial for improving the sensitivity and accuracy of early warning systems. The global community will have access to early warning messages for efficient response and to support disease surveillance and control efforts at the interface of the animal-human-ecosystem (FAO 2011).

9.6.3 The Following National and Regional Networks Support GLEWS (Angot 2009)

i) National authorities	ii) WHO (194 member states)	iii) Regional organizations: EC, SADC, ASEAN, CAN
iv) Laboratory and epidemiological networks	v) FAO (191 member nations)	vi) FAO (191 member nations)
vii) Unofficial surveillance programs (PROMED, GPHIN)	viii) OIE (178 member countries)	ix) International reference laboratories
	x) Other partners	

9.6.4 The GLEWS Method for Treating Highly Pathogenic Avian Influenza (HPAI)

Following the emergence of the highly pathogenic avian influenza H5N1 (HPAI H5N1), which caused the avian influenza (AI) crisis, nations have been on high alert to stop the disease's spread and reduce the possibility of a human pandemic (Martin et al. 2007a,b). The FAO Early Warning System for Global Avian Influenza Monitoring emphasizes the possibility of improved information sharing and integration among important stakeholders, as well as improved comprehension of the illness (Martin et al. 2006). One example of generating disease information is the EMPRES I disease tracking list (DTL). The list includes all verified outbreaks in domestic poultry and wild birds, as well as ongoing and completed studies globally. For a one-year period, the DTL also shows the daily incidence's temporal progression. The unverified occurrences on this list are shared with national and regional field personnel, as well as important partner institutions, who are asked to confirm and authenticate them, follow up, and look for trustworthy sources of information.

Risk maps are created that display the locations of proven outbreaks in wild birds and poultry. To visualize disease outbreaks and comprehend the epidemiological processes causing TADs to originate and spread, EMPRES I was connected to a GIS (Gilbert et al. 2007). These illustrations highlight how crucial GIS is for locating spatial or spatiotemporal patterns that can be utilized to create more exacting tests of causality. To sum up, the ultimate objective of early warning systems is to enable timely response in the most economical way while making information and risk-assessment results available to all pertinent stakeholders (Martin et al. 2007a,b).

9.6.5 Vector-Borne Diseases: Rift Valley Fever (RVF) and the GLEWS Approach

Remotely sensed data of vegetation and rainfall have been included into regional and GLEWSs to predict RVF before it reaches epidemic proportions in sections of East Africa that are known to be susceptible to RVF epidemics. Protecting sustainable livestock production and enabling developing nations to lawfully engage in domestic, regional, and global trade are the ultimate goals of such systems (Davies and Martin 2003), throughout irregular periods, epidemics of RVF have occurred throughout eastern and southern Africa. Above-average rainfall following a drought and the existence of exotic animal breeds that are sensitive have been linked to these epidemics (Martin et al. 2006). These forecasts make use of data sets such as the satellite vegetation index and cold cloud duration (CCD), which are connected with variations in the climate (Davies and Martin 2003). The normalized difference vegetation index (NDVI) is produced using measurements from the Advanced Very High Resolution Radiometer sensor (AVHRR) onboard polar-orbiting satellite series managed by the NOAA (Davies and Martin 2003). In order to monitor vector populations and RVF virus activity in East Africa, vegetation index maps have been utilized in conjunction with ground data to establish a correlation between these two factors. In fact, NDVI statistics for the research area and viral isolation data spanning a 25-year period were used in a thorough analysis. The NDVI ratio reaches 0.43–0.45 as the water table rises to the point where floods may happen (Linthicum et al. 1987). The primary benefit of employing remote sensing to forecast the presence of RVF in East Africa is the system's comparatively low cost, which makes it possible to implement preventive actions like immunizing vulnerable animals and controlling mosquito larvae (Linthicum et al. 1987). The FAO has made considerable use of this technology in order to alert nations that are at a higher risk of contracting the disease (Paweska et al. 2008).

9.6.6 Early Warning System (EWS) Components Include

According to Myers et al. (2000), there are three parts to EWS: modeling the current environmental data, conducting routine surveillance of the disease of interest, and using predictive models to anticipate future risk in conjunction with ongoing environmental and epidemiological surveillance.

a) *Disease surveillance:*
An interactive disease surveillance system, or sentinel network, is a system in which health care providers routinely gather health data over a large geographic region (often at the national level) (CDC 2010). The majority of developed countries have laws requiring the reporting of several infectious illnesses. According to Childs and Gordon (2009), prompt data collection and evaluation of regional and national statistics facilitate the early identification of shifts in the prevalence of illnesses. Additionally, the database offers details for organizing and carrying out interventions (Childs and Gordon 2009). Health information systems that may predict sickness are in high demand as a result of the sentinel systems' expansion from autonomous national networks to coordinated worldwide information systems (Flahault

et al. 1998). According to current knowledge, a facility-based sentinel surveillance system can be a valuable tool for tracking infectious diseases, directing future research, assessing preventative measures, and forecasting epidemics (Shalala 1998).

b) ***Developing a model:***

Modeling is a key component of disease forecasting, and it can be based on two approaches: the statistical method, which establishes statistical correlations between historical case numbers and environmental variables, and the biological approach, which aims to capture the biology of the transmission mechanisms (Myers et al. 2000). In summary, samples from as wide a range of environmental conditions as possible are needed for the statistical approach. Predictions derived from this approach make the assumption that the future will look like the past, i.e. that the relationships between case numbers and environmental variables that have already been established will continue to exist (Frisen 1992). The biological approach necessitates information on every parameter and variable thought to be crucial to transmission. Theoretically, predictions derived from this method can take into account the effects of environmental modifications or interventions, provided that the effects of each on the important transmission parameters are determined. It should be evident from the foregoing that only the statistical technique is feasible in the absence of complete information of all the transmission paths for any given disease. This explains why the statistical approach was taken in a large portion of the early epidemiology of diseases like cancer that were poorly understood. Although statistical models can be quite effective, biological process-based models should always be used first because their development reveals our complete ignorance of the systems we research. Real progress will only be made by tackling this ignorance (Frisen 1992).

c) ***Prognosticating and forecasting diseases:***

A fundamental trade-off between the advance times that predictions may offer and their specificity lies at the core of early warning systems. Long-range forecasts typically offer the fewest specific cautions, but they have the benefit of giving planners a fair amount of advance time. Conversely, systems that rely on early case detection offer very detailed information on the exact time and location of outbreaks, but they also leave little time for corrective action to be taken. A dependability estimate ought to be included in any risk forecast (Livestock and Dairy Development Department 2012). Activities aimed at preventing and controlling epidemics typically entail a series of steps, and it's critical to acknowledge the potential value of a variety of indicators that can be used to form an integrated prediction strategy. Recently, a hierarchical tracking system for malaria outbreaks in Africa's highlands has been developed (Cox et al. 1999).

9.7 Geographical Information System (GIS)

An automated system called GIS is used to input, store, analyze, and output spatial data. These data were used to predict diseases in conjunction with population data and historical disease records (Connor et al. 1995).

Applications of GIS (Khan 1999):
  i) Research disease variation and geographic distribution
 ii) Map populations at risk and stratify risk factors
iii) Forecast epidemics
iv) Monitor diseases and interventions over time
  v) Locate nearest Health facility
vi) Keep an eye on health facilities, regular medical personnel, equipment, and supplies delivered to service areas.

9.8 Disease Prognosis in India

In order to create a system of disease monitoring and surveillance of economically significant livestock illnesses and to develop strategic control strategies, the ICAR established the Project Directorate on Animal Disease Monitoring and Surveillance (PD_ADMAS) in India in 1987. Even though the country's health care infrastructure has expanded significantly over the years, the disease surveillance system has not received the attention it deserves because of the outbreaks of swine flu (2009), bird flu (2006), and Crimean-Congo hemorrhagic fever (2011), which brought to light the system's shortcomings (PD_ADMS 2011).

9.8.1 Network for Surveillance of Animal Diseases

Currently, our nation's animal illness monitoring network gathers data from sick animals and provides it to a veterinarian at a government hospital or pharmacy for clinical diagnosis. The information is subsequently forwarded to the State Veterinary authority at the district, taluka, and block levels. At the district, state, or regional levels, diagnostic laboratories share illness information. The Department of Animal Husbandry, Dairying and Fisheries (DADF), Ministry of Agriculture, Government of India, is the primary channel via which the State Governments exchange this information at the national level (Hemadri and Kumar 2013).

9.8.2 Centre for Animal Disease Research and Diagnosis (CADRAD)

Since 2001–2002, the Department of Animal Husbandry & Dairying, Ministry of Agriculture (Govt. of India) has recognized it as the Central Disease Diagnostic Laboratory (CDDL), providing it with a particular mandate, a technical plan, and financial assistance. Nonetheless, there are five regional illness diagnosis laboratories: one each in Guwahati (Northeastern), Jallandhar (Northern), Bangalore (Southern), Kolkata (Eastern), and Pune (Western). Delhi, Mumbai, Chennai, Kolkata, Bangalore, Hyderabad are the six quarantine stations (Hemadri and Kumar 2013).

Disease surveillance and ICAR (*Hemadri and Kumar 2013*):
  I) Foot and Mouth Disease Project Directorate (PDFMD);
 II) Animal Disease Monitoring and Surveillance Project Directorate (PD_ADMAS);
III) Laboratory for Animal Disease with High Security (HSADL, IVRI);

9.8.3 PDADMAS (Project Directorate on Animal Disease Monitoring and Surveillance) Bangalore

This organization is in charge of monitoring serious, commercially significant animal illnesses, such as zoonoses. Information technology advancements have made it possible to establish a National Livestock Disease Information System, which is currently desperately needed.

1) "Epi- InfoTM (Analysis Project On Forecasting/Forewarning Livestock Disease)"
2) "National Animal Disease Referral Expert System (NADRES)" is the second.

9.8.4 Epi- InfoTM (Analysis Project on Livestock Disease Forecasting/Forewarning)

With the help of GIS, PD_ADMAS has created the novel India.admas-Epitrak epidemiology software, a dynamic and interactive database pertaining to cattle diseases. This software is helpful to field veterinarians, administrators, technocrats, students, veterinarian colleges, and administrators because it meets the needs of data retrieval, analysis, and essential reporting of disease events as and when they occur (Hemadri and Kumar 2013).

9.8.5 NADRES (National Animal Disease Referral Expert System)

Part of a mission mode sub project supported by the National Agricultural Technology Programme, this one focuses on weather-based animal disease forecasting and building an animal health information system through disease monitoring and surveillance (NADRES 2011).

9.9 Conclusion

A stronger ability to manage and contain disease outbreaks is made possible by early diagnosis and prompt action. The improvement of disease analysis, early detection, and the stoppage of disease transmission depend on animal disease surveillance. For the benefit of the global community, GLEWS uses the most modern developments in communication and information technologies to enhance the early warning systems of the OIE, FAO, and WHO. Veterinary public health research can benefit greatly from the use of GIS, particularly when it comes to ecological analysis, mapping, and surveillance of newly emerging zoonoses. For certain vector-borne diseases, RVF, HPAI, and other conditions, well-defined

GLEWS are available; GLEWS is currently being developed for the remaining diseases. In India, the PD_ADMAS and other surveillance and information networks are independent, so a thorough evaluation of the animal disease surveillance system is required as it could influence significant policy choices. The effectiveness of the national disease monitoring programme and the level of knowledge among farmers, technicians, field veterinarians, and extension professionals regarding the clinical and epidemiological characteristics of illnesses are key factors in the successful implementation of EWS.

References

Ackelsberg, J., Balter, S., Bornschelgel, K. et al. (2002). Syndromic surveillance for bioterrorism following the attacks on the World Trade Center-New York City, 2001. *MMWR. Morbidity and Mortality Weekly Report* 51: 13–15.

Ahmed, J., Bouloy, M., Ergonul, O. et al. (2009). International network for capacity building for the control of emerging viral vector borne zoonotic diseases: ARBO-ZOONET. *Euro Surveillance* 14 (12): 1–4.

Angot, J.L. (2009). The governance of veterinary services and their role in the control of avian influenza. *Revue Scientifique et Technique (Office International des Épizooties)* 28: 397–400.

Beck, L.R., Lobitz, B.M., and Wood, B.L. (2000). Remote sensing and human health: new sensors and new opportunities. *Emerging Infectious Diseases* 6: 217–226.

CDC (Centers for Disease Control and Prevention). (2010) Climate Change and Public Health. Available: http://www.cdc.gov/nceh/climatechange Accessed on 16 June 2013.

Childs, J.E. and Gordon, E.R. (2009). Surveillance and control of zoonotic agents prior to disease detection in humans. *Mount Sinai Journal of Medicine* 76: 421–428.

Connor, S.J., Thomson, M.C., Flasse, S.P., and Williams, J.B. (1995). The use of low-cost remote sensing and GIS for identifying and monitoring the environmental factors associated with vector borne disease transmission. *GIS for Health and the Environment* 1: 75–87.

Cox, J.S., Craig, M.H., Le Sueur D, Sharp, B. (1999) Mapping Malaria Risk in the Highlands of Africa. MARA/HIMAL Technical Report; Durban.

Davies, G. and Martin, V. (2003) Recognizing Rift Valley fever. FAO Animal Health Manual 17.

FAO (2002). Towards a global early warning system for animal diseases. *EMPRES (Transboundary Animal Diseases Bulletin)* 20: 1.

FAO-OIE-WHO (2010) The FAO-OIE-WHO Collaboration Sharing responsibilities and coordinating global activities to address health risks at the animal-human-ecosystems interfaces A Tripartite Concept Note. http://www.glews.net/wpcontent/uploads/2011/04/html Accessed on 15th July 2013.

Farnswortha, M.L., Westb, C.H., Fitchett, S. et al. (2010). Comparing national and global data collection systems for reporting, outbreaks of H5N1 HPAI. *Preventive Veterinary Medicine* 95: 175–185.

Flahault, A., Dias-Ferrao, V., Chaberty, P. et al. (1998). Flunet as a tool for global monitoring of influenza on the web. *Journal of the American Medical Association* 280: 1330–1332.

Food and Agriculture Organization (FAO) (2011) Challenges of animal health information systems and surveillance for animal diseases and zoonoses. Proceedings of the international workshop organized by FAO, 23-26 November 2010, Rome, Italy.

Formenty, P. (2009) When animal disease strikes to human an integrated approach in time and space. Epidemic and Pandemic alert & Response, International meeting on emerging diseases 2009, Vienna, Austria.

Frisen, M. (1992). Evaluation of methods for statistical surveillance. *Statistics in Medicine* 11: 1489–1502.

Gilbert, M., Xiao, X., Chaitaweesub, P. et al. (2007). Avian influenza, domestic ducks and rice agriculture in Thailand. *Agriculture, Ecosystems & Environment* 119: 409–415.

GLEWS Global Early warning system for major animal diseases including zoonoses (2013) GLEWS disease priority list Available at http: www.glews.net Accessed on 10th May 2013.

Grasso, V. and Singh, A. (2011) Early Warning Systems: of-Art Analysis and Future Directions. Draft report United Nations Environment Programme (UNEP) 1–10.

Hargrove, W.W., Spruce, J.P., Gasser, G.E., and Hoffman, F.M. (2009). Toward a national early warning system for forest disturbances using remotely sensed canopy phenolog. *Photogrammetric Engineering & Remote Sensing* 75: 1150–1156.

Hemadri, D. and Kumar, G.B. (2013) Vision 2050. Project Directorate on Animal Disease Monitoring & Surveillance, Hebbal, Bengaluru available at http: http://www.pdadmas.ernet.in Accessed on 18th July 2013.

Jebara, K.B. (2004). Surveillance, detection and response: managing emerging diseases at national and international levels. *Revue Scientifique et Technique (Office International des Épizooties)* 23 (2): 709–715.

Khan, O.A. (1999). The first international health NICD- geographics conference. *American Journal of Public Health* 1 (2): 55–65.

Kulldorff, M., Heffernan, R., Hartman, J., and Assunc R., Mostashari, F. (2005). A space-time permutation scan statistic for disease outbreak detection. *PLoS Medicine* 2 (3): 216–224.

Linthicum, K.J., Bailey, C.L., Davies, F.G., and Tucker, C.J. (1987). Detection of Rift Valley fever viral activity in Kenya by satellite remote sensing imagery. *Science* 235: 1656–1659.

Linthicum, K.J., Anyamba, A., Tucker, C.J. et al. (1999). Climate and satellite indicators to forecast Rift Valley fever epidemics in Kenya. *Science* 285: 397–400.

Livestock and Dairy Development Department (2012) Animal Disease Management -Assessment and Way Forward Punjab Government Efficiency Improvement Programme *Crown agents*: 7-9.

Martin, V., Sims, J., Lubroth, D. et al. (2006). Epidemiology and ecology of highly pathogenic avian influenza with particular emphasis on South East Asia. *Developments in Biologicals* 124: 23–36.

Martin, V., Dobschuetz, S., Lemenach, A. et al. (2007a). Early warning, database, and information systems for avian influenza surveillance. *Journal of Wildlife Diseases* 43 (3): S71–S76.

Martin, V., Simone, L., Lubroth, J. et al. (2007b). Perspectives on using remotely-sensed imagery in predictive veterinary epidemiology and global early warning systems. *Geospatial Health* 2 (1): 3–14.

Mills, J., Kenneth, N., Gage, L., and Khan, A. (2010). Potential influence of climate change on vector-borne and zoonotic diseases: a review and proposed research plan. *Environmental Health Perspectives* 118 (11): 1507–1513.

Myers, M.F., Rogers, D.J., Cox, J. et al. (2000). Forecasting disease risk for increased epidemic preparedness in public health. *Advances in Parasitology* 47: 309–330.

National Animal Disease Referral Expert System (NADRES) 4:362– (2011) PDADMAS News January-June 2011. 1(1): Available at http: http://www.nadres.res.in Accessed on 18th July 2013.

Ogden, N.H., Bouchard, C., Kurtenbach, K. et al. (2010). Active and passive surveillance and phylogenetic analysis of *Borrelia burgdorferi* elucidate the process of Lyme disease risk emergence in Canada. *Environmental Health Perspectives* 118: 909–914.

OIE (World Organization for Animal Health) (2013) World Animal Health Information System (WAHIS) Available on http://www.oie.int/wahis2/public/index.php. Accessed on 3rd September 2013.

Paweska, J., Blumberg, L., Weyer, J. et al. (2008). Rift Valley fever outbreak in South Africa. *NHLS Communicable Diseases Surveillance Bulletin* 6 (2): 1–2.

Project Directorate on Animal Disease Monitoring and Surveillance PD_ADMS. (2011) PDADMAS News January-June 2011 1(1): Available on http: http://www.pdadmas.ernet. Accessed on 18th July 2013.

Ridder, B.A. and Formenty, P. (2011) From Forecasting to Control of Zoonotic Diseases: Linking Animal and Human Systems. Available at http:outbreak@who.int/outbreak network Accessed on 1st June 2012.

Shalala, D.E. (1998). Collaboration in the fight against infectious diseases. *Emerging Infectious Diseases* 4: 15–18.

WHO (World Health Organization) (2006) Global Early Warning and Response System for Major Animal Diseases, including Zoonoses (GLEWS). Final version adopted by the three organizations tripartite 2006:1-26

WHO (World Health Organization) (2010) Global Early Warning System for Major Animal Diseases, Including Zoonoses (GLEWS). At http://www.who.int/zoonoses/outbreaks/glews Accessed on 15th July 2013.

WHO (World Health Organization) (2013a) Outbreak surveillance and response in humanitarian emergencies: WHO guidelines for EWARN implementation. Geneva, Switzerland: Available http://www.who.int/disease control emergencies/publications html Accessed 30th March, 2013.

WHO (World Health Organization) (2013b) Zoonoses and Veterinary public health Available at http://www.who.int/zoonoses/outbreaks/glews/en Accessed on 10th May, 2013.

10

Strategies of Disease Management: Prevention, Control, and On-farm Biosecurity

Harshit Saxena[1], Akhilesh Kumar[1], Varun Kumar Sarkar[1], Manav Kansal[2], and Kartikey Verma[3]

[1] Division of Medicine, ICAR-IVRI, Izatnagar, Bareilly, India
[2] ICAR-IVRI, Izatnagar, Bareilly, India
[3] CoVSc & AH, SVPUAT, Mathura, India

Health is a state of complete physical, mental, and social well-being and not merely the absence of disease and infirmity. Disease is any harmful deviation from the normal structural or functional state of an organism, generally associated with certain signs and symptoms and differing in nature from physical injury (Encyclopaedia Britannica).

Infectious diseases are caused by agents such as virus, bacteria, fungi, rickettsia, etc., while noninfectious diseases are caused by any metabolic disturbances, poisoning, drug toxicity, etc. (Table 10.1).

10.1 Strategies of Disease Management: Prevention

Prevention refers to all those measures that are applied before the disease sets in or while the infection is in its early stage. Prevention of disease can be divided into three levels: primary prevention, secondary prevention, and tertiary prevention (Table 10.2).

10.1.1 Disease Prevention Strategies

10.1.1.1 Vaccination Programs

Vaccination is a process of building active immunity in the targeted animal. Vaccination refers to administration of an antigen consisting of live, attenuated or dead bacterium, virus or fungi into the body of susceptible animals. Vaccination works on the principle of memory formation by helper T cells which on subsequent encounter with the same antigen in future results in its destruction by the immune cells of the body. There are multiple strategies used to vaccinate animals (Tables 10.3, 10.4, 10.5, 10.6).

- *Emergency vaccination*: A specific type of vaccination program that is implemented in response to an outbreak or potential outbreak of a specific disease. It is used when there is urgent need to quickly control and contain the spread of a disease within a population of farm animals.
- *Ring vaccination*: Involves vaccinating animals in a defined geographical area surrounding an outbreak or infected premises, creating a ring of vaccinated animals to prevent the spread of the disease. Generally animals within a 5 km radius of the outbreak are vaccinated.
- *Systematic vaccination*: Immunization in affected nations that strives to lessen a disease's incidence, prevalence, or effect in order to prevent, control, and maybe eradicate it. The goal of routine immunization in free nations or zones is to either stop the spread of a disease from an infected adjacent country or zone or to lessen its effects in the event that it does spread.
- *Blanket vaccination*: Involves immunizing all vulnerable animals in a region, nation, or zone.
- *Targeted vaccination*: Entails immunizing a portion of the vulnerable animal population.

Epidemiology and Environmental Hygiene in Veterinary Public Health, First Edition. Edited by Tanmoy Rana.
© 2025 John Wiley & Sons, Inc. Published 2025 by John Wiley & Sons, Inc.

Table 10.1 Disease, common name, etiology, transmission, common symptoms, and treatment.

Disease	Species affected	Common name	Etiology	Transmission	Signs and symptoms	Prevention and control
Anthrax	Cattle, buffalo, sheep, goat, pig, human	Gorhi, gilt, goli	*Bacillus anthracis*	Contaminated blood	Swellings over body, especially around neck	Annual vaccination
Brucellosis	Cattle, buffalo, sheep, goat, horse, human	Bang disease	*Brucella* spp.	Food and water contaminated with discharge	Abortion storm during 9th month of pregnancy	Vaccination in female calves at 4–8 months of age
Hemorrhagic septicemia	Cattle, sheep, buffalo, swine	Shipping fever, galghotu	*Pasturella* spp.	Contaminated food, water, pastures; contact with infected animal	Swellings on neck, dewlap, and throat	Premonsoon vaccination
Black quarter	Cattle and buffalo	Sujaa	*Clostridium chauvoei*	Blood-contaminated food and water	Lameness in leg and crepitating sound when pressed	Annual vaccination
Foot and mouth disease	All cloven-footed animals	Muh khur	Aphthovirus	Aerosol, contact with infected animals	Sores on feet, mouth and tongue; lameness	Polyvalent vaccination seasonally
Hog cholera	Porcine	Swine fever	Pestivirus	Contaminated food and water; contact with infected animal	Sudden rise of fever	Vaccination at 6–8 months of age
Babesiosis piroplasmosis	Cattle, buffalo, sheep	Cattle tick fever, Texas fever	*Babesia bigemina*	Blood-sucking ticks (*Rhipicephalus*)	High temperature, red to dark brown urine	Dipping during tick season
Bloat	Cattle, buffalo, sheep, goat	Aphara	Accumulation of gas/foam in rumen	Greedy feeding; excessive feeding	Greatly distended abdomen	Reduce concentrate feeding
Milk fever	Cattle and buffalo at early lactation period	Zilchighi-ka bukhar	Acute fall in blood calcium	Occurs generally in first month of lactation	Head prostration, loss of appetite	IV administration of calcium gluconate

Table 10.2 Comparison of primary prevention, secondary prevention, and tertiary prevention.

Parameters	Primary prevention	Secondary prevention	Tertiary prevention
Targeted population	Healthy population	Diseased population	Diseased population
Primary initiative	Preventing exposure to casual factors of disease	Activities including early diagnosis of disease	Therapeutic activity is applied on a symptomatic population
Aim for the reduction of diseases	Incidence of disease	Prevalence of disease	Complications of the disease
Action	Quarantine, vaccination	Tuberculin test, rose Bengal plate test (RBPT) for brucellosis	Therapy or rehabilitation

Table 10.3 Routine prophylactic schedule for cattle and buffalo.

Disease	Vaccine	Dose and method	Age and time of vaccination
Foot and mouth disease	A polyvalent inactivated aqueous aluminum hydroxide and saponin adjuvanted vaccine comprising serotypes O, A22, C and Asia 1	2 ml deep intramuscular route	First at the age of four months then twice in a year
Anthrax	Anthrax spore vaccine prepared from *Bacillus anthracis* Sterne strain suspended in glycerine	Dose should be not less than 10 million spores/dose given via intramuscular route	First vaccine is given at the age of six months then repeated annually before monsoon
Black quarter	Formalin-inactivated *Clostridium chauvoei* culture, adjuvanted with aluminum hydroxide gel or alum precipitated vaccine	5 ml subcutaneous route	First vaccination is done at the age of six months and is then repeated annually
Hemorrhagic septicemia	Formaldehyde inactivated culture of *Pasteurella multocida* with aluminum hydroxide gel adjuvant or oil adjuvant or alum precipitated vaccine	3 ml intramuscular or subcutaneous route	First vaccination is done at 4–6 months of age and then repeated annually at least 15–20 days prior to monsoon
Brucellosis	Live *Brucella abortus* strain 19 vaccine	Dose should be not less than 4×10^{10} viable organisms and given subcutaneously	Female calves between 4–8 months of age are vaccinated once for life
Buffalopox	A live attenuated vaccine (BPXV Vij/96 strain)	The recommended dose is 0.5 ml (containing a minimum of 3.0 $\log^{10}$ TCID50) to be inoculated intradermally on the abaxial surface of the tail	Animals older than four months of age can be vaccinated with this vaccine
Infectious bovine rhinotracheitis	Modified live virus vaccines (MLV strain of the IBR virus)	2 ml subcutaneously or intramuscularly	Calves vaccinated before the age of six months should be revaccinated after six months of age
Theileriosis	Live schizonts are cultured in lymphoblast cell culture and attenuated through extended *in vitro* passage	The recommended dose is 3 ml given subcutaneously	Three months of age and above

Table 10.4 Vaccination schedule for sheep and goats.

Disease	Vaccine	Dose and method	Age and time of vaccination
Sheep pox	Live attenuated freeze-dried vaccine prepared from Roumanian (RF) strain of sheep pox virus Live attenuated sheep pox vaccine (Srinagar strain)	The dose of vaccine is 0.1 ml for all age groups and is given intradermally in the caudal fold or tip of the ear	First dose at three months of age. Booster repeated every year
Enterotoxemia vaccine	Formalin-inactivated culture of *Clostridium perfringens* type D and epsilon toxoid adjuvanted with aluminum hydroxide gel	3–5 ml subcutaneous route	In lambs, first vaccination is done at the age of four months if dam is vaccinated or at one week if dam is unvaccinated, then repeated annually before the monsoon
Peste des petits ruminants	Live attenuated indigenous PPR vaccine (PPRV/Sungri/96 strain)	The recommended dose is 1.0 ml (containing a minimum of 2.5 $\log^{10}$ TCID50) to be inoculated by subcutaneous route in the neck region	First dose at four months of age; revaccinate once in three years. Avoid vaccination in advanced pregnancy
Goat pox	Live attenuated vaccine (Uttarkashi strain)	The dose of vaccine is 0.1 ml for all age groups and is given intradermally in the caudal fold or tip of the ear	First dose at three months of age. Booster repeated every year
Bluetongue	Multivalent inactivated pentavalent bluetongue vaccine containing most prevalent serotypes 1, 2, 10, 16, and 23	Dose: 2 ml subcutaneously	First at the age of four months and booster 28 days after first vaccination
Sore mouth, scabby mouth, orf or contagious ecthyma	A live attenuated vaccine (ORFV Muk 59/05 strain)	The recommended dose is 0.20 ml (containing a minimum of 3.0 $\log^{10}$ TCID50 vaccine virus) to be inoculated by intradermal route with scarification on the inner aspect of thigh	Animals older than four months of age can be vaccinated

10 Strategies of Disease Management: Prevention, Control, and On-farm Biosecurity

Table 10.5 Vaccination schedules for pig.

Disease	Vaccine	Dose and method	Age and time of vaccination
Classic swine fever	Live attenuated lapinized CSF virus	1 ml intramuscular route	First dose at the age of 25–30 days, booster after one month and thereafter every six months
Hemorrhagic septicemia (HS)	HS oil adjuvant vaccine	2 ml intramuscular or subcutaneous route	First dose at 4–6 months of age. Booster repeated every year, preferably before the rainy season (May–June)
Anthrax	Anthrax live spore vaccine	0.5 ml intramuscular route	First dose at six months of age. Booster repeated every year, preferably in May to June
Foot and mouth disease (FMD)	FMD inactivated polyvalent vaccine	1 ml intramuscular route	First dose at four months of age. Booster at six months of age. Repeated every six months

Table 10.6 Vaccination schedule for equines.

Disease	Vaccine	Dose and method	Age and time of vaccination
Equine herpesvirus 1	Formalin inactivated vaccine prepared from an indigenous EHV 1 (strain Hisar-90-7)	2 ml intramuscular route	Six months of age or older At five months of pregnancy followed by two boosters at 7th and 9th months of pregnancy
Equine influenza	Inactivated vaccine A/eq/Katra (Jammu)/06/08 (H3N8) EIV isolate adjuvant with aluminum hydroxide	1 ml intramuscular route	First vaccination in animals above six months of age followed by a booster vaccine after 4–5 weeks and then repeated annually
Equine abortion	*Salmonella abortus equi* vaccine	First two doses 10 ml and third dose 20 ml to be repeated at 10 days interval and given by intramuscular route	Booster every year

Source: ICAR (2020).

- *Barrier vaccination*: Involves vaccinating animals over a certain line to prevent the spread of disease across that line, for example two areas that are divided by water bodies/oceans.
- *Dampening down vaccination*: Vaccination typically used in areas where it is not feasible or practical to vaccinate the entire population; it is often employed during disease outbreaks or in high-risk areas to provide immediate protection to vulnerable animals.

10.1.1.2 Quarantine

Quarantine refers to separation of healthy animals from infected/suspected animals. There are some protocols for the introduction of new animals in the farm, some key components are given below:

- *Isolation*: New animals should be kept in separate housing from the existing population.
- *Duration*: The duration of quarantine varies depending on disease risk and requirements, but normally it should be around 30 days.
- *Veterinary examination*: The new animal should undergo a thorough veterinary examination upon arrival.
- *Monitoring*: During the period of quarantine, the animal should be carefully watched and monitored for any signs of illness.
- *Gradual integration*: After the quarantine period is completed, introduce the new animal gradually to the existing population.

10.1.1.3 Early Disease Diagnosis

Early diagnosis of disease relies on finding a causative organism without much clinical manifestation of the disease. General tests used for early disease diagnosis in farm animals include the following.

- *Blood tests*: Blood can be taken for analyzing various parameters such as complete blood count, total leukocyte count, differential leukocyte count, serum biochemistry, serological tests, etc. Thin and thick blood smears are also made for the detection of haemoprotozoans.

- *Fecal examination*: Fecal samples can be examined for the presence of parasites such as flat or round worms, coccidia, and protozoa. Techniques such as fecal sedimentation or flotation were found more useful in detection parasitic eggs as compared to direct fecal examination.
- *Polymerase chain reaction (PCR)*: PCR is a molecular technique applied most widely to detect the presence of specific pathogens by amplifying their genetic material several times. It is one of the most sensitive tests used for the detection of even small number of pathogens.
- *Milk testing*: Some pathogens have the ability to spread via milk in dairy animals. Milk samples can be analyzed for the detecting the presence of mastitis-causing bacteria, *Brucella* spp., somatic cell counts and milk composition (e.g., fat, protein, SNF [solids not fat] content).
- *Enzyme-linked immunosorbent assay (ELISA)*: It is a commonly used serological test that detects the presence of or antigens in blood or other body fluids. It can be used to detect the presence of specific antibodies or pathogens.

10.1.1.4 Host Movement

Movement of hosts from an area with high risk of disease to a low-risk area is an effective measure for disease prevention. Seasonal migration of livestock from an area where vectors are very active to an area where vectors are low is an example.

10.1.1.5 Improvement in Environment, Husbandry, and Feeding

There are fewer chances of disease occurrence in animals that are reared with balanced feeding, proper housing facilities, and good environmental conditions than in those reared under poor conditions.

10.1.1.6 Animal Comfort

By keeping the animal in open, curtain-sided free stall barns, the incidence of respiratory infections can be reduced as compared to animal housed in overcrowded places. Confined to small congested areas.

10.1.1.7 Calf Health

Nowadays, disease prevention is linked to gut health. There is a major shift toward seeking improved calf health through timely and adequate colostrum feeding because colostrum contains various preformed antibodies which provide passive immunity to the calves against various harmful pathogens.

10.1.1.8 Udder Health

Udder health is very important in prevention of any disease. Pre and post milking teat disinfection is vital and blanket application of antibiotic therapy at drying off is commonly adopted strategy for mastitis control at dairy farms.

10.1.1.9 Tools of Epidemiology

Epidemiological tools play a crucial role in preventing disease spread by forecasting the disease transmission trend. Examples of the contributions of epidemiology include calculation of adequate sample size, understanding the effects of factors among animals in a study, and prediction of epidemics in advance.

10.1.1.10 Disposal of Carcase

Massive mortality events can result from disease outbreaks or natural disasters. When faced with a disease outbreak, animals in the affected region need to be culled and disposed of safely, requiring practical and economically sensible measures (Kim and Pramanik 2016). There are various methods for carcase disposal, such as burial, incineration, rendering, composting, anaerobic digestion, and alkaline hydrolysis.

- *Burial*: carcases are disposed of in cemeteries, ditches, or open-bottomed receptacles called "mortality pits." Due to the introduction of infectious pathogens into the human food chain and environmental contamination, this approach has been outlawed in the majority of developed nations. Large-scale burial in various calamities and disasters may cause infections and chemical byproducts of decomposition will contaminate ground and surface water. The survival of pathogens has been significantly decreased by the use of hydrated lime $Ca(OH)_2$ in burial. Even though there is a very minimal likelihood that burying carcases may contaminate drinking water, certain infectious material, including anthrax spores or prions, can be found in the soil after the carcase has decomposed. Burial sites should be placed far from livestock areas and be deep enough to minimize the possibility of infectious pathogens being transferred back to the surface (Baba et al. 2017).

- *Burning*: in many nations, especially developing ones, it is customary practice to burn carcases on pyres within farms. In outbreaks of diseases like foot and mouth disease (FMD) and anthrax, the burning of carcases has been documented. Transmissible spongiform encephalopathy-related biosecurity issues still exist since open-air combustion seldom reaches high enough incineration temperatures (Scudamore et al. 2002).
- *Incineration*: animal byproducts or carcases are burned at high temperatures ($850\,°C$) to create an inorganic ash during the incineration process. The procedure is anticipated to eliminate all infectious pathogens. With the exception of alkaline hydrolysis, it is widely agreed that incineration kills prion proteins more efficiently than the alternatives (NABC 2004). In terms of zoonotic and animal pathogens, particularly tough spore-forming bacteria like *Bacillus anthracis*, the high temperature of cremation also totally eliminates them (DEFRA 2008).
- *Composting*: composting is a straightforward procedure that may be used in specialized facilities, on-farm utilizing enclosed windrows or in-vessel approaches, or both (NABC 2004; DEFRA 2008). Usually, the procedure entails stacking carcases between strata of carbon-rich substrate like straw, sawdust, or rice hulls, with a final coating of carbon-rich substrate applied to the entire pile. Larger carcsses are usually laid down in single layers, whereas poultry might be piled many times. The compost piles are then aerated or flipped (NABC 2004). The process fundamentally consists of two phases: a primary thermophilic phase, which lasts for a few weeks and generates temperatures as high as $70\,°C$, and a secondary mesophilic phase, which lasts for many months and normally ranges from 30 to $40\,°C$. It has been demonstrated that the temperatures produced during the thermophilic phase of carcase or meat waste composting significantly lower bacterial, viral, protozoal, and helminth populations (Gwyther et al. 2011).
- *Anaerobic digestion*: in order to create methane (biogas), which may be used as a fuel source, anaerobic digestion entails the decomposition of organic material under anaerobic circumstances (Ward et al. 2008).
- *Alkaline hydrolysis*: alkaline hydrolysis is a relatively recent technique that was created in the 1990s. It catalyzes the hydrolysis of biological material using sodium hydroxide or potassium hydroxide to produce a sterile aqueous solution that is composed of peptides, amino acids, sugars, and soaps (NABC 2004). The concentration of the alkali is added to the carcases in either solid or solution form, depending on the weight of the carcase material, in a steel alloy container. To considerably speed up the process, the container is then sealed and heated to $150\,°C$ for up to six hours while under high pressure (Kalambura et al. 2008).

10.2 Strategies of Disease Management: Control

The term *control* refers the strategies that are applied post infection to minimize the further spread of disease by decreasing its spreading intensity. Control is an ongoing process and requires continuous monitoring backed by financial support. Strategies that are applied to control disease spread in farm animals include the following.

10.2.1 Chemoprophylaxis

Chemoprophylaxis refers to the use of chemical agents such as drugs or medications to prevent the development or spread of infectious diseases. It involves the administration of specific drugs to individuals which are at risk of contracting a particular disease in order to reduce the likelihood of infection or to minimize the severity of the disease if infection occurs.

10.2.2 Chemotherapy

Proper treatment of the diseased animal under supervision of a veterinarian with chemical agents that inhibit or destroy the disease-causing agents without much affecting the body of the host.

10.2.3 Slaughter

Slaughter techniques play a crucial role in controlling infections in farm animals. Key aspects of the slaughter process that help minimize the risk of infection include the following.

- *Preslaughter management*: good management practices before animals are brought to the slaughterhouse can help reduce the prevalence of infections. These include maintaining proper hygiene, providing appropriate housing and nutrition, and implementing vaccination programs.

- *Biosecurity measures*: strict biosecurity protocols should be in place to prevent the introduction of infectious agents to the slaughterhouse. This involves controlling access to the facility, proper cleaning and disinfection procedures, and ensuring that personnel follow hygiene practices, such as wearing protective clothing and sanitizing equipment.

There are different techniques of slaughtering.

- *Preemptive slaughter*: this technique is employed as an emergency response strategy during disease outbreaks, particularly when dealing with highly contagious diseases. It includes culling of infected animals and those animals that have been exposed to the causative factor of the disease.
- *Blanket culling*: a drastic control measure that is applied typically in situations where there is a severe disease outbreak, a high risk of disease transmission, or a need for rapid disease containment. The primary objective of blanket culling is to control the spread of infectious diseases by removing the entire population of animals at risk.
- *Stamping out*: the stamping out method of slaughter is aimed at complete elimination of carriers of infection from the infected premises. It refers to culling of all susceptible/infected/vaccinated/unvaccinated animals in the infected premises and thereafter disposal of carcases by burial or burning. The policy is accompanied by complete disinfection procedures.

10.2.4 Control of Internal Parasites by Deworming

Deworming refers to administration of chemical drugs into the body of the animal to prevent any parasitic infestations. Parasitic worms infect all types of animals. Parasite infestation not only causes nuisance to the animal but also leads to huge economic losses, as in case of *Ostertagi* spp. Some worms have modified mouth parts to suck blood from the host, as in case of *Fasciola* which tends to suck 0.5 ml blood per day inside the host. The worms generally thrive in hot and humid areas so it is imperative in these areas to deworm the livestock regularly (Table 10.7).

Specific deworming methods and medications vary depending on the type of animal involved, the parasite, and local guidelines. Some common deworming methods include the following.

- *Oral medications*: provide broad-spectrum coverage rather than working on specific parasites. Available in the form of tablets, liquids, and pastes.
- *Pour on*: some dewormers come in the form of spot-on treatments that are applied to the skin, typically between the shoulder blades of the animal. These are commonly used for removal of ectoparasites such as fleas and ticks but also have efficacy for internal parasites.
- *Injectible dewormers*: generally subcutaneous injections are given as deworming drugs into the body of the animal when oral administration is not feasible. Examples include ivermectin.

Table 10.7 Deworming schedule recommended for buffalo calves by National Dairy Research Institute scientists.

Age of the calf	Deworming as per doses recommended by manufacturers of the drug
Days 3, 4, and 5	Sulmet® full dose on 3rd day and ½ dose on 4th and 5th days
Day 7	Piperazine
30 days	Sulmet
1½ months	Piperazine
2½ months	Piperazine
3½ months	Phenovis®
Four months	Sulmet
Five months	Piperazine
Six months	Phenovis
Seven months	Piperazine
Nine months	Phenovis
Twelve months	Phenovis

The frequency of deworming depends on several factors like age of the animal, health status of the animal, lifestyle, environmental conditions, parasite load in the feces, etc. Young animals should preferably be dewormed every month while older livestock stock should be dewormed every 4–6 months. Pregnant females should be dewormed after parturition.

- *Deworming schedule for pigs*: the recommended time to deworm pregnant sows is 7–10 days before the anticipated due date. Piglets should receive the same treatment when they are a month old. Later, the veterinarian can choose the frequency based on the physical condition and the level of worm infestation in a particular location.
- *Deworming schedule for sheep and goats*: deworming should start at about three months old. Deworming should be performed in May or June each year, before the start of the monsoon season. Deworming should be performed twice a year, premonsoon and postmonsoon, in areas where water logging is an issue (IVRI 2021).

10.2.5 Disinfection

Disinfection is a crucial control measure for disease management, particularly in preventing the transmission of infectious diseases. It involves the process of eliminating or reducing the number of microbes, such as bacteria, viruses, and fungi, on surfaces, objects, or in the environment. Commonly used disinfectants include the following.

- *Alcohol-based disinfectants*: alcohol-based disinfectants, such as isopropyl alcohol (rubbing alcohol) and ethanol, are effective against a broad range of bacteria and viruses. They are commonly used for disinfecting skin, medical instruments, and small surfaces.
- *Chlorine-based disinfectants*: chlorine-based disinfectants, like sodium hypochlorite (bleach), are highly effective against bacteria, viruses, and fungi. They are commonly used for disinfecting surfaces, countertops, and washing areas. Diluted bleach solutions are also used for sanitizing drinking water and treating contaminated surfaces.
- *Quaternary ammonium compounds (quats)*: quats, such as benzalkonium chloride, are commonly used disinfectants, surface cleaners, and disinfectant wipes. They are effective against a wide range of microorganisms and are often used in healthcare facilities, food service areas, and public spaces.
- *Hydrogen peroxide*: hydrogen peroxide is a versatile disinfectant that is effective against bacteria, viruses, and fungi. It is commonly used for disinfecting wounds, sterilizing medical equipment, and cleaning surfaces. Hydrogen peroxide can be found in various concentrations and is often used as a diluted solution for disinfection purposes.
- *Phenolic compounds*: phenolic compounds, such as ortho-phenylphenol (OPP) and triclosan, are commonly found in household disinfectants and some hand sanitizers. They have broad-spectrum antimicrobial properties and are effective against many bacteria and viruses.
- *Quaternary ammonium hydrogen peroxide (QAC-HP)*: QAC-HP is a combination disinfectant that blends quaternary ammonium compounds with hydrogen peroxide. It provides a synergistic effect, enhancing the antimicrobial activity. QAC-HP disinfectants are often used in healthcare facilities, laboratories, and high-risk environments.
- *Iodine-based disinfectants*: iodine-based disinfectants, such as povidone-iodine, are effective against a wide range of bacteria, viruses, and fungi. They are commonly used for presurgical skin preparation, wound cleansing, and disinfecting medical instruments.

10.3 Strategies of Disease Management: Biosecurity Measures

Biosecurity refers to a set of management practices which reduce the potential for the introduction and spread of disease-causing organisms onto and between sites. Biosecurity includes all the procedures that are used to prevent the introduction of disease (Figure 10.1).

The measures aim to protect human, animal and plant health, as well as the environment. Types of biosecurity measures include the following.

10.3.1 Locational Biosecurity

Locational biosecurity, also known as spatial biosecurity, refers to the implementation of biosecurity measures based on specific location or premises. It involves designing and implementing strategies to prevent the introduction or spread of

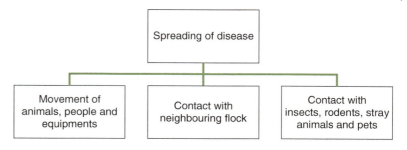

Figure 10.1 Flow diagram showing factors responsible for spreading disease.

diseases or harmful biological agents within a particular area, such as livestock farm. Some key aspects of locational biosecurity are listed below.

- The farm should be located at an elevated and well-ventilated place.
- The farm should be at least 1 km away from any farm
- The farm should be set away from water ways/water pools.
- The farm should be set away from any nearby village poultry/backyard poultry to reduce the chances of disease spread.
- In poultry farms, broiler and layer units should not be established in close vicinity to avoid transmission of diseases.

10.3.2 Structural Biosecurity

Structural biosecurity refers to the physical infrastructure and design features implemented to prevent the entry or spread of diseases, pathogens, or harmful biological agents within a facility, building, or premises. Some key aspects of structural biosecurity are as follows.

- *Orientation of farm*: the long axis of the farm should be in an east–west direction while windows and open areas should be in north–south direction in tropical countries.
- *The farm should be single storey*; multistorey farm should be discouraged.
- *Fencing and barriers*: appropriate fencing to restrict the movement of animals on the farm.
- *Cleaning and disinfection facilities*: foot baths of appropriate dimensions filled with disinfectant should be provided at the farm entrance. The cleaning facilities should have proper drainage systems and be equipped with adequate supplies of cleaning equipment.
- *Waste management*: proper waste disposal facilities should be available near the farm. The waste should be disposed of after suitable treatment and away from any human dwellings and agricultural establishments.

10.3.3 Operational Biosecurity

Operational biosecurity includes day-to-day practices and procedures implemented on a farm to prevent the introduction and spread of diseases and pathogens among livestock. It includes behavioral aspects of working personnel to minimize the risk of disease transmission. Key aspects of operational biosecurity are listed below.

- *Protective clothing and equipment*: provision of protective clothing to the working personnel inside the farm such as boots, gloves, sleeves, facemasks, head masks, or other personal protective equipment.
- *Vaccination and disease prevention*: periodic vaccination of farm animals against common diseases to enhance their immunity and reduce the chances of getting infection.
- *Training and education for farm personnel*: it is very important that the staff working on the farm should know the significance of biosecurity practices and protocols. Regularly update staff on emerging diseases and practices to combat spread.

10.3.4 Continuous Biosecurity

Continuous biosecurity is an ongoing and comprehensive approach to protecting and maintaining the security of biological materials, facilities, and systems. It involves measures and practices aimed at preventing the accidental or intentional release of harmful biological agents, as well as mitigating the risks associated with biological threats.

References

Baba, I.A., Banday, M.T., Khan, A.A. et al. (2017). Traditional methods of carcass disposal: a review. *Journal of Dairy, Veterinary & Animal Research* 5 (1): 21–27.

DEFRA (2008). *Sector Guidance Note IPPC SG8: Integrated Pollution Prevention and Control (IPPC), Secretary of State's Guidance for the A2 Rendering Sector*. London: DEFRA Publications.

Gwyther, C.L., Williams, A.P., Golyshin, P.N. et al. (2011). The environmental and biosecurity characteristics of livestock carcass disposal methods: a review. *Waste Management* 31 (4): 767–778.

ICAR (2020). Vaccine for livestock and poultry. https://icar.org.in/sites/default/files/2022-06/Vaccines-for-Livestock-and-Poultry.pdf (accessed 6 February 2024).

IVRI (2021). Vaccination and Annual Health Calendar for Sheep and Goat. www.ivri.nic.in/Extension/Download/IVRI-FFL-8-2021.pdf (accessed 30 July 2023).

Kalambura, S., Krička, T., Jurišić, V., and Janječić, Z. (2008). Alkaline hydrolysis of animal waste as pre-treatment in production of fermented fertilizers. *Cereal Research Communications* 36: 179–182.

Kim, G.H. and Pramanik, S. (2016). Biosecurity procedures for the environmental management of carcasses burial sites in Korea. *Environmental Geochemistry and Health* 38: 1229–1240.

NABC (2004). Carcass Disposal: A Comprehensive Review. Report Written for the USDA Animal and Plant Health Inspection Service, National Agricultural Biosecurity Centre, Kansas State University.

Scudamore, J.M., Trevelyan, G.M., Tas, M.V. et al. (2002). Carcass disposal: lessons from Great Britain following the foot and mouth disease outbreaks of 2001. *Revue Scientifique et Technique* 21 (3): 775–787.

Ward, A.J., Hobbs, P.J., Holliman, P.J., and Jones, D.L. (2008). Optimisation of the anaerobic digestion of agricultural resources. *Bioresource Technology* 99 (17): 7928–7940.

11

Economic Impact on Animal Diseases

Justin Davis K[1], Athira K[1], and Javed Jameel A[2]

[1] *Department of Veterinary Epidemiology and Preventive Medicine, College of Veterinary and Animal Sciences, Kerala Veterinary and Animal Sciences University, Pookode, India*
[2] *Department of Veterinary Clinical Medicine, Ethics and Jurisprudence, College of Veterinary and Animal Sciences, Kerala Veterinary and Animal Sciences University, Pookode, India*

> *"Man is an animal that makes bargains: no other animal does this – no dog exchanges bones with another."*
>
> Adam Smith

11.1 Introduction

Economics is the science that primarily deals with decision making and simply measures things in monetary units (International Federation for Animal Health 2013; Dijkhuizen et al. 1995; Dijkhuizen and Morris 1996). It is also defined as the study of utilizing scarce resources with competing demands (Rushton 2017). The economics of animal health is continuously evolving and a subject area with wide scope and importance (Rushton 2009; Rushton and Gilbert 2016). *Animal health economics* can be described as the discipline that offers a broad framework of concepts, procedures, and data to support the decision-making process in optimizing animal health management programs (Dijkhuizen et al. 1996; Ramsay et al. 1999).

> Economics or "the allocation of scarce resources" is vital to the development of veterinary medicine and services. Food safety and food security are the large returns to relatively limited investments.
>
> *Dr Faouzi Kechrid, recipient of WASAVA award for global meritorious service,*
> *International Federation for Animal Health (2013)*

Livestock disease outbreaks affect both microeconomics and macroeconomics. The impact of animal disease outbreaks is complex and heterogeneous and varies from region to region across the world (Kappes et al. 2023). The difference in approach of an animal health specialist and an economist to an outbreak of disease is depicted in Figure 11.1. The animal health specialist defines the disease list and the process of managing the diseases without reference to economic context or impact, whereas the focus of the economist is to determine the cost of the animal disease or to assess the economic viability of a prevention and control strategy.

> Every country in the world deals with the burden of animal disease, and for many, that burden is, unfortunately, quite large. But there's a huge gap in our knowledge of the real costs of animal disease — to our livestock economy, global trade and to human health and prosperity. We're trying to fill that gap.
>
> *Thomas L. Marsh, Professor, School of Economic Sciences/Paul G. Allen School of Global Animal Health*

Globalization in the agricultural sector and international trade have increased the chances for new animal disease introductions and spread across borders. Outbreak of an economically important animal disease would have serious impacts on producers, trade of animal products, marketing chains, and the gross agricultural income. Approximately

---

Epidemiology and Environmental Hygiene in Veterinary Public Health, First Edition. Edited by Tanmoy Rana.
© 2025 John Wiley & Sons, Inc. Published 2025 by John Wiley & Sons, Inc.

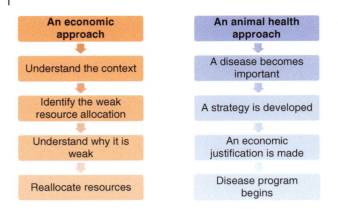

Figure 11.1 Differences between an economic and an animal health approach. *Source:* Rushton (2017); Huntington et al. (2021).

one-half of agricultural income comes from the animal product sector. Understanding how animal disease affects productivity from the livestock sector and the food chain is a complex, multidisciplinary problem (Armbruster 2005). The costs of animal diseases can vary as societies and economies evolve, making monitoring and surveillance programs important (International Federation for Animal Health 2012). Intergovernmental organizations with a mission relevant to animal health and production include the World Organisation for Animal Health (WOAH), the World Health Organization (WHO), and the Food and Agriculture Organization (FAO). They recognize the need for improving the use and application of epidemiology and social sciences tools (diagnostics, data analysis and risk assessments, and communication) for managing zoonotic and high-impact diseases of animals and humans (Perry et al. 2023).

11.2 Economics of Animal Disease

Evans in 2003 categorized the economic impacts of animal diseases into six areas: production effects, market and price effects, trade effects, impacts on food security and nutrition, human health and the environment, and financial costs (Pritchett et al. 2005). They pose threats to public health, economy, environment, animal production and welfare. The WOAH estimates that 60% of human infectious diseases are zoonotic and three out of the five (75%) emerging infectious diseases in humans are of animal origin (World Trade Organisation 2020; Dharmarajan et al. 2022; World Organisation for Animal Health 2023a).

Livestock disease outbreaks affect the economy through increased mortality, reduced productivity, loss of trade, decreased market value, food insecurity, and control costs (Krishnamoorthy et al. 2019). With advances in livestock production in the mid to late nineteenth century, there was a rise in economic diseases such as rinderpest (RP), foot and mouth disease (FMD), classic swine fever, contagious bovine pleuropneumonia (CBPP), and highly pathogenic avian influenza, leading to more investments in veterinary services, education, and research (International Federation for Animal Health 2012).

The economic impact of a zoonotic pathogen or animal disease is the function of infection intensity, disease frequency, the effect of the disease on human health, productivity in animals, and response to treatment (Rushton 2009). Both zoonotic and livestock diseases cause a multitude of disease-specific impacts on an economy. For example, highly pathogenic influenza and FMD have severe impacts on domestic and international trade markets. The international markets for beef are segmented on the basis of FMD status, where they fetch higher premium prices for supplying countries that are both FMD free and which do not vaccinate their herds (Perry and Sones 2007). Countries with both epidemic and endemic FMD had significant impacts extending from the farm-level to the national-level economy. Economic loss of over 12 million US$ was reported from the FMD outbreak in the United States in 2001, of which 50% loss was in trade and tourism (McLeod and Rushton 2007). Moreover, the presence of endemic FMD in most of sub-Saharan Africa closes most high-value export markets for beef such as the European Union, United States, Japan, and Korea. McLeod and Rushton (2007) noted that zoonotic diseases like brucellosis have relatively limited market impacts compared to diseases such as FMD, which only affect animals (Rich and Perry 2011).

The economic and social impacts of livestock disease have been globally recognized in both developed and developing countries. For improved animal health, quantifying the economic impact of an animal disease outbreak is important for formulating prevention and control strategies (Barratt et al. 2019). The scientific foundation for the discipline of animal health economics was laid in Australia by Morris in 1969 and in England by Ellis in 1972. These two authors successfully introduced a simple but essential economic principle, called the "equimarginal principle" in making veterinary decisions. In essence, the principle focuses on increasing disease control input to the level where the cost of an additional input balances with the return from the additional output. Since then, increasing effort has been made to apply this principle in the various areas of animal health economics (Dijkhuizen et al. 1995).

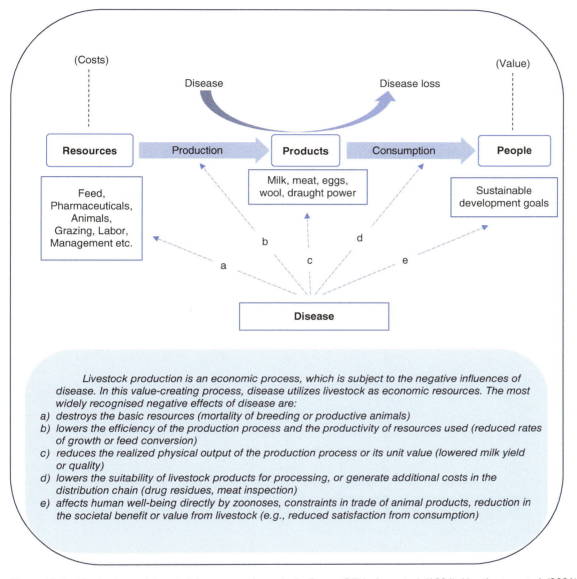

Figure 11.2 The basic model underlying economic analysis. *Source:* Dijkhuizen et al. (1996); Huntington et al. (2021); McInerney (2003).

11.2.1 Basic Economic Model

The basic economic model primarily comprises three major components: people, products, and resources. *People*, who want things and make decisions, act as the driving force for economic activity. *Products* are goods and services that satisfy people's needs and are considered as the outcome of economic activity. *Resources* are the physical factors and services that form the basis for generating the products, for starting an economic activity (Dijkhuizen et al. 1996). These three components can be put together to explain the basic conceptual model that underlies economic analysis (Figure 11.2).

The economic costs of animal disease can be categorized as either direct or indirect costs (Figure 11.3). *Direct costs*

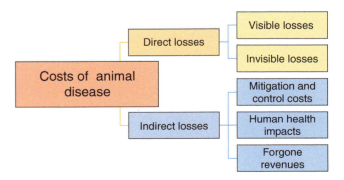

Figure 11.3 Costs of animal disease. *Source:* Adapted from International Federation for Animal Health (2012).

have an immediate impact on livestock populations and agriculture, whereas *indirect costs* are the mitigation or control efforts, losses in trade and other revenues, and impacts on human health. Estimating the costs of animal disease globally is a difficult task due to the variation in costs of resources, livestock product prices, and productivity. But we are able to gain a meaningful sense of the social and economic costs from disease outbreaks (International Federation for Animal Health 2012). In 2006, animal health monitoring systems budgeted around 150 million US$ per year for monitoring and surveillance programs of livestock diseases (Paarlberg et al. 2008).

11.2.1.1 Direct Losses

As a country's animal disease status changes over time, we assume direct costs as the sum of losses from the first confirmation of a notifiable disease outbreak to the disease freedom status.

Direct losses include visible losses and invisible losses.

- *Visible losses* include animal deaths and illness or stunting from disease or subsequent control methods.
- *Invisible losses* include reduced fertility or changes in herd.

11.2.1.2 Indirect Losses

Economic losses incurred in markets after the declaration of disease freedom are defined as indirect costs. To avoid double counting, using disease status as a marker, we could say that when direct costs end, indirect costs begin. Indirect costs include the shocks in markets (revenue foregone) as a result of changes in prices of commodities for producers and consumers, after disease freedom is declared (Barratt et al. 2019).

Indirect losses include the following.

- *Mitigation and control costs* include the costs of drugs, vaccines, surveillance, and labor needed to carry out control measures.
- *Human health impacts* include the costs that arise when animal diseases affect human populations, such as treatment costs and losses in productivity due to illness or death.
- *Foregone revenues* include the indirect economic impacts of animal diseases resulting from curtailed market access, losses in consumer confidence, and knock-on effects on other sectors of the economy.

Disease outbreaks often have broader, longer-term multiplier effects that extend beyond principal markets (Pritchett et al. 2005). Indirect costs are an important aspect of an animal disease outbreak and larger in magnitude than direct costs. It is usually underestimated or not considered when estimating the true costs of an outbreak. In zoonotic diseases, the direct costs can be more than 20 billion US$ and indirect losses over 200 billion US$. Indirect costs are also of concern because the costs of disease do not stop at the farm gate, within the agricultural sector, or after disease freedom is declared and should be included in the prevention and control strategies and policies. This will be particularly important if alternative policy options led to significantly different indirect cost outcomes and hence different decision choices are indicated (Barratt et al. 2019).

11.2.2 Common Modeling Techniques in Animal Health Economics

Models, especially mathematical models (defined set of equations), are essential tools for understanding animal health economics (Dijkhuizen et al. 1996). Basically, there are two different modeling approaches to be considered: a *positive approach* and a *normative approach*. The positive approach (empirical modeling) includes description of relevant processes and uses statistical or epidemiological data for analysis. In animal health economics, the normative approach, which includes computer simulation techniques (mechanistic modeling), is more important (Dijkhuizen et al. 1996). The major functions of mathematical models are included in Figure 11.4.

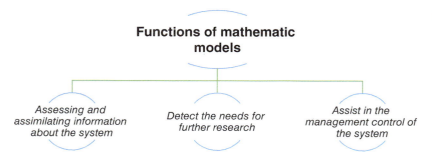

Figure 11.4 Functions of mathematic models. *Source:* Adapted from Dijkhuizen et al. (1996).

To perform an economic analysis of animal diseases and their control, a wide range of modeling techniques are available. The choice of modeling technique will depend on a number of factors, such as the nature of the problem, the resources available, and the availability of data on the problem. The classification of livestock models is shown in Figure 11.5.

A *static model* does not contain time as a variable and cannot analyze or simulate the effect over time, compared to a *dynamic model*. A model that makes definite predictions for quantities like milk production and liveweight is called *deterministic*. A *stochastic model* contains probability distributions or random elements to deal with uncertainty in prices and performances. With random elements, repeated runs of the model ("replicates") are necessary to provide insight into the variation in outcome. An *optimization model* determines the optimum solution given the objective function and restrictions, whereas a *simulation model* calculates the outcome of predefined sets of input variables like disease control strategies (Dijkhuizen et al. 1995).

For the conceptual framework of disease control programs and policies, economic analysis is inevitable. The most common economic modeling approaches (Figure 11.6) used in veterinary medicine are partial budgeting, cost–benefit analysis, and decision analysis (Smith 2006). The common modeling techniques and their indications are described in Table 11.1. Cost–benefit analyses (CBAs) focus on the direct costs of animal disease, including animal mortality, morbidity, and associated response costs (Barratt et al. 2019).

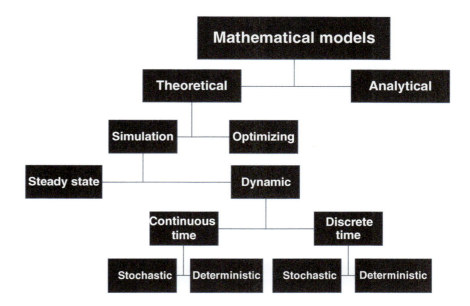

Figure 11.5 Classification of livestock models. *Source:* Rushton (2009)/CAB International.

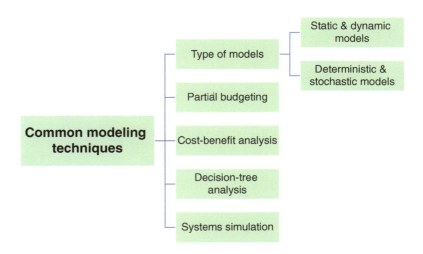

Figure 11.6 Common modeling techniques in animal health economics. *Source:* Adapted from Dijkhuizen et al. (1995).

Table 11.1 Common modeling techniques, definitions, and indications.

Common modeling techniques	Definition	Indication
Partial budgeting	Quantification of the economic consequences of a specific change in farm procedure; requires the simplest data collection of all the methods	If the proposed analysis concerns a simple economic comparison of disease control measures on a farm, e.g., the effect of dry cow therapy to control mastitis
Cost–benefit analysis	Procedure for determining the profitability of proposed courses of action over an extended period of time	If the subject of research deals with more long-term disease control programs at regional or national levels
Decision tree analysis	Graphical method of expressing, in chronological order, the alternative actions available to the decision maker and the choices determined by chance	If there are multiple possible outcomes of the proposed courses of action and chance is an important factor in determining which outcome occurs
Systems simulation	Creating a mathematical model of the system under consideration (e.g., animal, farm, population), which can then be manipulated by input modification	If there are complex feedback loops whereby the effect of one decision about the control of the disease flows through to influence some aspect of animal production, which in turn flows back to influence a variable further back in the production system

Source: Smith (2006)/CRC Press.

11.3 Economic Impact of Transboundary Animal Diseases

Transboundary animal diseases (TADs) are those animal diseases which can easily spread to other countries in epidemic proportion and whose control or management requires cooperation between several countries (Food and Agriculture Organization 1997; Otte et al. 2004). One of the critical distinguishing features of these diseases is their ability to spread rapidly across borders (Food and Agriculture Organization 1997). The prevention and control of TADs require regional or international initiatives to achieve the millennium development goals and food security. Some of the most important TADs of livestock and poultry (Figure 11.7) are FMD, RP, contagious bovine pleuropneumonia (CBPP), RVF, peste des petits

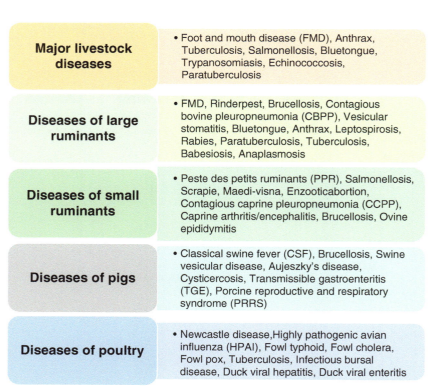

Figure 11.7 Major diseases of livestock (large ruminants, small ruminants, pigs and poultry). *Source:* Adapted from Rushton (2009).

ruminants (PPR), bovine spongiform encephalopathy (BSE), classic swine fever (CSF), African swine fever (ASF), avian influenza (AI), and Newcastle disease (ND) (Otte et al. 2004).

Transboundary animal diseases (Otte et al. 2004) are defined as:

> Those that are of significant economic, trade and/or food security importance for a considerable number of countries; which can easily spread to other countries and reach epidemic proportions; and where control/management, including exclusion, requires cooperation between several countries.

The economic impact of a TAD can be assessed at global or national level and from the perspectives of different stakeholders. The impact could be a threat to national income, a potential drain on budget, and an impediment to international trade. The major economic impacts of TADs on different stakeholders and methods for estimating them are tabulated in Tables 11.2 and 11.3 respectively.

In developed countries, the main economic impact of TADs arises from market disruption and costs of disease control, whereas in developing countries, losses from disease infection or the costs of control applied by farmers should be

Table 11.2 Economic impacts of TADs.

Stakeholders	Major impacts
Livestock producers, traders, and processors and retailers of livestock products	TAD may represent a threat to livelihood, a need to invest in prevention measures, and a source of friction with state veterinary services
Animal health providers and suppliers of vaccines and drugs	TAD as a source of revenue from drug and vaccine sales
Consumers	TAD as a threat to health (if the disease is zoonotic), and may be disadvantaged if a severe disease outbreak affects food prices or disrupts the food supply
National level	TAD can reduce revenue from tourism if it restricts access to rural areas or discourages people from visiting an infected country

Source: Mcleod et al. (2016)/Food and Agriculture Organization of the United Nations.

Table 11.3 Methods for estimating the economic impact of a TAD.

Level	Reasons	Possible methods
Global/ regional	• Explain or justify the focus on a particular disease on the part of the international community. • Determine future policy directions of governments and intergovernmental organizations with regard to "emerging" TADs, or those that are spreading or have changed location	• Spreadsheet modeling • Macroeconomic modeling • May be supported by epidemiological studies/modeling
National/ sector ± stakeholder[a]	• Explain or justify the focus on a particular disease on the part of a government. Demonstrate to government the savings that may be gained by financing TAD prevention measures. Estimate the costs incurred in controlling an outbreak as a matter of public accountability. Estimate impacts on food supply or consumption	• Comparison of national statistics before and after outbreak • Macroeconomic modeling • Simulation modeling • Choice models and related methods • May be supported by epidemiological studies/modeling
Stakeholder	• Assess where control efforts should be directed or who might contribute to funding them	• Choice models and related methods • Simulation modeling • Sustainable livelihoods analysis • Value chain analysis • May be supported by epidemiological studies/modeling.

[a] An analysis at national level will often include impacts for specific stakeholder groups as well as the national impact.
Source: Mcleod et al. (2016)/Food and Agriculture Organization of the United Nations.

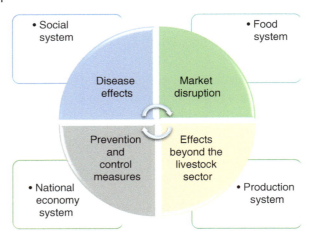

Figure 11.8 Context and sources of the impact TADs. *Source:* Mcleod et al. (2016)/Food and Agriculture Organization of the United Nations.

considered. The economic impacts of TADs are classified based on the context (production system, food system, national economy, social system) and their source (Mcleod et al. 2016). Figure 11.8 depicts the context and sources of the impact of TADs. Among the four main sources of impact, the first three (disease effects, market disruption, control measures) are experienced within the livestock sector and the fourth one has effects beyond the livestock sector.

- *Disease effects* include mortality and loss of production caused by clinical or subclinical disease, affecting the social system.
- *Market disruption* caused by consumer fears, supply shortage causing market shocks, restrictions on international trade in livestock and livestock products. Disease spread and the effectiveness of prevention and control measures are affected by the way in which production and marketing of food are organized and regulated.
- *Control measures* include the costs and benefits of measures applied by farmers, governments, and industry to prevent or control disease outbreaks.
- *Effects beyond the livestock sector* include impacts on human health, the public health system, tourism, and wildlife. Scale and intensity of production affect the way in which livestock owners experience the impact of TADs. Each type of producer has a perception of TADs that relates to their own experience, and this affects the way they react to and deal with TADs.

11.3.1 Economic Viability of an Intervention to Prevent or Control a TAD

An intervention to prevent or control a TAD could be anything from a large government program to the measures applied by an individual farmer. An intervention is considered economically viable when the benefits it generates are at least as high as the costs it incurs (Figure 11.9). The WOAH global animal disease control and eradication strategies for FMD, PPR, dog-mediated rabies, African swine fever (ASF), and their goals are depicted in Table 11.4.

The costs and benefits of TAD prevention and control interventions are classified within and beyond the livestock sector (Table 11.5, Figure 11.9). The costs of TAD prevention and control are mostly incurred within the livestock sector, but there may also be costs beyond the sector (public health). There may be new costs incurred in order to implement the intervention, as well as opportunity costs which include the output value that is lost as a result of implementing the intervention. The potential benefits within and beyond the livestock sector are of two types: additional output and reduced costs. Prevention and outbreak control appear as both benefits and costs. This reflects the fact that early investment and more stringent outbreak control measures and policies are required to create savings from reduced disease incidence.

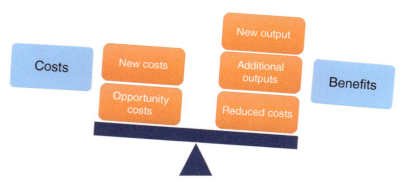

Figure 11.9 Costs and benefits of TAD prevention and control interventions: an intervention is economically viable when the benefits it generates are higher than the costs it incurs. *Source:* Adapted from Mcleod et al. (2016)/Food and Agriculture Organization of the United Nations.

11.3 Economic Impact of Transboundary Animal Diseases | 163

Table 11.4 WOAH global animal disease control and/or eradication strategies.

Disease	Global strategy	WOAH partners	Duration	Goal
Foot and mouth disease (FMD)	Global FMD control strategy	FAO	2012–2027	To reduce the global burden of FMD and the risk of reintroduction of the disease into free areas
Peste des petits ruminants (PPR)	Global strategy for the control and eradication of PPR	FAO	2015–2030	PPR eradication by 2030
Dog-mediated rabies	Zero by 30: the global strategic plan to end human deaths from dog-mediated rabies by 2030	WHO, FAO, Global Alliance for Rabies Control	2018–2030	To end human deaths from dog-mediated rabies by 2030
ASF	Global control of African swine fever, a GF-TADs initiative	FAO	2020–2025	Global control of ASF

Source: Adapted from Awada et al. (2023).

Table 11.5 Classification of costs and benefits of TAD prevention and control interventions.

Classification of costs and benefits		Within the livestock sector	Beyond the livestock sector
Costs	New costs	Prevention and preparedness costs	Public health investment
		Outbreak control costs	Higher food prices for consumers
	Opportunity costs	Costs of changes to management or production systems	Costs to tourism or wildlife
Benefits	New outputs	Increased asset and output value	Human lives saved or quality-adjusted life-years increased
		Reduced prevention and treatment costs	Public health treatment costs reduced
	Reduced costs	Reduced costs of outbreak control	Tourist sector outbreak control costs reduced

Source: Mcleod et al. (2016)/Food and Agriculture Organization of the United Nations.

Table 11.6 Average annual cost of disease control programs by type of disease.

Disease	Average annual cost per program (million USD)
Foot and mouth disease (FMD)	35.9
Bovine tuberculosis	20.9
Brucellosis	3
Bovine viral diarrhea	2.6
Transmissible spongiform encephalopathy (TSE)	2.3
Rabies	1.2
Bluetongue	1.2
Classic swine fever (CSF)	1.2

Source: Adapted from Rushton and Gilbert (2016).

According to the survey on national veterinary services among the member countries of the World Organisation for Animal Health (OIE), the majority of the countries have their own disease specific control programs. The most expensive disease specific control programs were for FMD (35.9 million USD) and bovine brucellosis (20.9 million USD) (Table 11.6 and Figure 11.10).

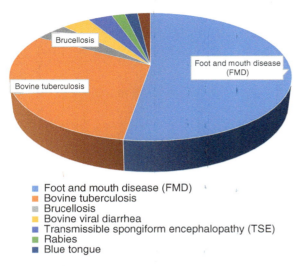

Figure 11.10 Average annual cost of major disease control programs. *Source:* Adapted from Rushton and Gilbert (2016).

11.4 Global Burden of Animal Diseases Program

The Global Burden of Disease (GBD) study for human health has created a comprehensive dataset of diseases, injuries, and risk factors that is used to measure epidemiological levels, disease emergence, and trends worldwide. But for animal diseases, we lack these dataset equivalents. Globally, around 1.3 billion people depend on farm animals for their living and each year, 300 billion US$ is lost due to animal diseases in livestock. The impact of animal diseases on the economy is irreparable considering its ripple effects on trade, food supply, and human health and we lack the ability to bring economic science and veterinary science under one umbrella (World Organisation for Animal Health 2023b).

The Global Burden of Animal Diseases (GBADs) hosted by the WOAH is a multiinstitutional collaborative program aiming at data collection, analysis, and generation of information for evidence-based investment plans, to facilitate the allocation of resources and support high-quality evaluation of existing animal health investments (Rasmussen et al. 2022). In 2021, the WOAH and its partners (Bill and Melinda Gates Foundation) secured more than 7 million US$ to roll out the GBADs (World Organisation for Animal Health 2023b). The six key components of a GBADs program (Figure 11.11) identified were disease classification, data collection, disease losses, animal health expenditure, sustainability, and equitability (Rushton et al. 2018).

- *Disease classification*: involves key areas of case definition, applicability in the field and with existing data, and engagement with animal owners and healthcare advisers.
- *Data collection*: there was agreement on the importance of clarity on the types of data to be collected from the public and private sectors and that ownership and commercial sensitivities are thought through and treated with transparency.
- *Disease losses*: covers the need for a framework that captures what losses will be included, how they will be measured, and how they will be reported.
- *Animal health expenditure*: public and private costs need to be separated and costs for different disease issues need to be attributed.

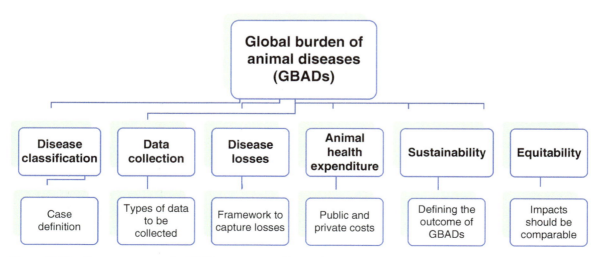

Figure 11.11 Key components of a GBADs programme. *Source:* Adapted from Rushton et al. (2018).

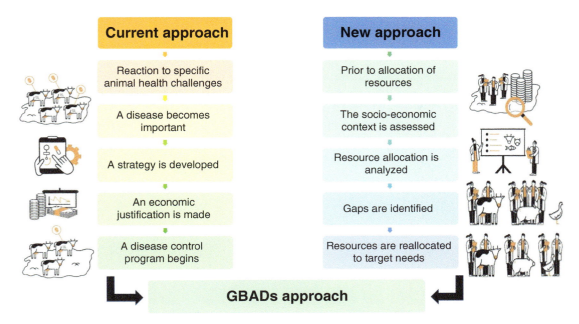

Figure 11.12 GBADs approach to evaluating the burden of animal diseases. *Source:* World Organisation for Animal Health (2023b).

- *Sustainability*: identified the need for a mapping exercise to determine who should be linked to a process of defining the outcomes of GBADs in a structured and timely way.
- *Equitability*: impacts in low-income countries must be presented in a way that is comparable to impacts in high-income countries.

The new approach proposed by the GBADs program will capture the wider social and environmental impacts when evaluating the burden of animal diseases (Figure 11.12). The GBADs program will help quantify the positive and negative impacts of animal production systems on society and the environment, and will offer solutions to support smallholders, businesses, and society as a whole (Rushton 2017; World Organisation for Animal Health 2023b).

11.5 Estimation of Economic Losses Due to Animal Diseases

Animal diseases such as FMD, hemorrhagic septicemia (HS), mastitis, PPR, and surra in cloven-footed domestic animals occupy the top position among livestock diseases due to their wide host range, short duration of immunity, and economic impact on livestock production (Singh et al. 2014). A study by the World Bank found that, over the last couple of decades, zoonotic emerging diseases have created global costs of 6 billion US$ (Grace et al. 2015). Moreover, each year there is a 1 in 100 chance of the world experiencing a 1 trillion US$ pandemic. In low-income countries, zoonoses and diseases which recently emerged from animals make up 26% of the infectious disease burden and 10% of the total disease burden (Grace et al. 2015).

The total economic loss due to diseases in bovines was worked out as the sum of (A) mortality loss, (B) loss in milk yield, and (C) cost of treatment of affected animals (Singh et al. 2014).

The total economic loss is expressed as $T = A + B + C$.

11.5.1 Loss from Mortality

This was worked out as the product of the number of dead animals (D) due to the disease and probable market value (P) of the animal: $A = D \times P$.

11.5.2 Loss in Milk Yield

$$B = B_1 + B_2 + B_3$$

$B_1 = value\ of\ direct\ loss\ due\ to\ reduction\ in\ milk\ yield$: for the proportion of cows in milk in the herd, the losses were expressed in terms of reduction in milk yield, which through the price of milk could be directly converted into monetary terms. When a cow died as a result of the disease, the adopted market value was assumed to reflect its production worth. Double counting or costing was avoided. The immediate fall in milk production in lactating cows is never regained later and therefore constituted a significant loss.

The loss due to direct decline in milk production was estimated using the formula:

$$B = (I - D)P_1 L Z M$$

where:

I = number of infected animals
D = number of animals that died
P = proportion of animals in milk
Z = annual average milk yield per milch animal
L = proportion of lactation lost
M = price of milk.

$B_2 = loss\ of\ milk\ due\ to\ increased\ abortion$: abortion can occur due to specific disease, particularly in late pregnancy, and leads to increased calving index, besides loss of calves. Assuming the time for abortion as eight months from conception, and a delay of six months in the next conception, the calving index is increased by 13.5 months in aborting cases, and the milk loss due to increased abortions can be estimated from the equation:

$$B_2 \left[(12 / C_1) - \left\{ 12 / (C_1 + 13.5 A) \right\} \right] (I - D)P_1\ Y M$$

where:

C_1 = calving index
A = increased abortion rate
Y = average lactation yield per milch animal.

$B_3 = milk\ loss\ due\ to\ increased\ intercalving\ period$: the problem of nonconception caused by a disease increases the intercalving period and thus lower numbers of animals will be in milk at any given time. As a result of nonconception or delayed conception, milk output is reduced. An average delay of three months in the next conception was assumed for all the animals affected by the disease. The loss of milk was calculated by the reduction in proportion of lactating animals in any year multiplied by the average milk yield per in-milk bovine per year and by the price M.

$$B_3 \left[(12/C_1) - \left\{ 12/(C_1 + 3) \right\} \right] (I - D)P_1\ Y\ M$$

11.5.3 Treatment Costs

$$C = I\ T_c$$

where T_c = average treatment cost of an infected animal.

11.5.4 Transboundary Animal Diseases

11.5.4.1 Foot and Mouth Disease

Foot and mouth disease is a rapidly spreading, highly contagious disease of cloven-footed animals like cattle, buffalo, goats, sheep, and pigs, and is endemic in India. These endemic countries contain three-quarters of the world's FMD-susceptible livestock and most of the world's poorest livestock keepers (Grace et al. 2012). Economic losses caused by the disease are mainly due to loss in milk production, reduction in draught power, and loss of body weight leading to reduced yield of meat (Figure 11.13, Table 11.7).

11.5 Estimation of Economic Losses Due to Animal Diseases

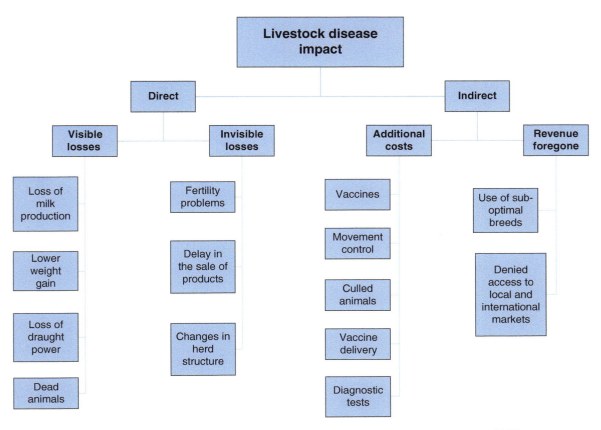

Figure 11.13 The impacts of foot and mouth disease. *Source:* Rushton (2009); Knight-Jones et al. (2017).

Table 11.7 Components of losses due to FMD in different species.

	Species			
Livestock disease impact	Cattle and buffalo	Goat	Sheep	Pig
Direct visible losses	Mortality	Mortality	Mortality	Mortality
	Direct milk loss	Direct milk loss	Wool loss	—
Direct invisible losses	Reproductive failure • Increased abortions • Increased calving interval	Reproductive failure • Increased abortions • Increased calving interval	Reproductive failure • Increased abortions • Increased calving interval	Reproductive failure • Increased abortions • Increased calving interval
Direct visible losses	Draught power loss	Body weight loss	Body weight loss	Body weight loss
Direct visible losses	Reduction in growth of calves	—	—	—
Indirect additional costs	Treatment cost	Treatment cost	Treatment cost	Treatment cost
Indirect losses (revenue foregone)	Opportunity cost[a]	Opportunity cost[a]	Opportunity cost[a]	Opportunity cost[a]

[a] Includes the cost of higher feeding and rearing inputs in surviving infected animals, loss due to extra human labor on longer rearing times in young stock, cost of permanent disability, extra human labor for nursing of animals and disinfection of housing, transportation of sick animals for treatment.
Source: Adapted from Knight-Jones and Rushton (2013).

Table 11.8 Global FMD impact due to vaccination costs and direct, visible production losses in affected stock by region.

	Impact US$			
	Production losses	Vaccination	Total	
Region	Median	Median	90% range	Median
China	1.9 billion	2.2 billion	2.5–7 billion	4 billion
India	1.9 billion	0.2 billion	1–4 billion	2.1 billion
Rest of Asia	1.2 billion	70 million	0.7–3 billion	1.3 billion
Africa	2.3 billion	20 million	1–5 billion	2 billion
Europe and Turkey	35 million	20 million	0.03–0.1 billion	0.06 billion
Middle East	0.2 billion	30 million	0.1–0.5 billion	0.22 billion
South America	0.1 billion	0.7 billion	0.5–1.4 billion	0.8 billion
Total	7.6 billion	2.5 billion	6.5–21 billion	11 billion

Source: Adapted from Knight-Jones et al. (2017).

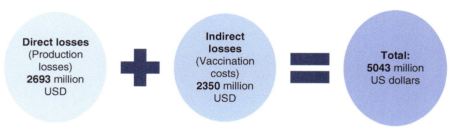

Figure 11.14 Global economic impact of FMD in China, India, Asia, Africa, Europe, the Middle East, and South Africa. *Source:* Adapted from Singh et al. (2013).

The global economic impact of FMD under current control conditions was calculated using spreadsheet models in seven regions of the world (China, India, the rest of Asia, Africa, Europe, the Middle East, and South Africa). The impacts were categorized as direct (production losses) and indirect (vaccination) costs (Table 11.8, Figure 11.14). According to the researchers, around 20 million cattle, 11 million pigs, 11 million goats, and 9 million sheep are affected by FMD in a year (Singh et al. 2013). The total losses per infected animal due to FMD in cattle, buffalo, sheep, goats, and pigs were ₹12 532, ₹21 682, ₹2023, ₹3046, and ₹2830 respectively (Knight-Jones and Rushton 2013).

11.5.4.2 Rabies

Dog-mediated rabies remains a global zoonosis of major public health, agricultural, and economic significance. It causes a loss of over 1.8 million disability-adjusted life-years (DALYs) every year, with direct and indirect economic costs (postexposure prophylaxis, animal tests, dog vaccination, and livestock losses) totaling 5.5 billion US$ per year. The global cost of canine rabies due to human mortality is estimated as 120 billion US$ (Rushton and Knight-Jones 2015; Anderson et al. 2014; Hampson et al. 2015).

11.5.4.3 Brucellosis

Bovine brucellosis is one of the most common neglected zoonotic diseases in the world, causing huge losses to the dairy industry (Gemechu 2017). Economic impact can include direct (e.g., reduced milk yield, increased mortality) and indirect (e.g., vaccination, culling) costs. Direct impacts may further be classified as visible (e.g., abortion, repeat breeding), invisible (e.g., lower fertility), additional costs (e.g,. treatment, vaccination), and revenue forgone (e.g., distress selling). Loss may comprise only those parameters that reduce benefits (e.g., reduced milk yield, reduced weight gain, reduced fertility, increased replacement cost, increased mortality, etc.) while cost would comprise amounts spent for treatment and control of the disease (e.g., biosecurity, vaccination, movement control, disease surveillance, research, etc.) (World Organisation for Animal Health 2016).

11.5.4.4 Lumpy Skin Disease

Lumpy skin disease (LSD) is a recently emerged devastating viral disease of cattle and water buffalo causing significant economic losses. It is a vector-borne disease, endemic in most African countries, which has spread to 35 new countries and territories in the Middle East, Southeast Europe, Western, Central, and Southeast Asia in the past 10 years (Awada et al. 2023). The economic losses in LSD are higher due to decreased feed intake, milk production, weight conversion, damage to hides, abortion and infertility, and ban on international trade. The annual financial cost of clinical LSD included the average production losses, due to morbidity and mortality arising from milk loss, beef loss, traction power loss, and treatment and vaccination costs at the herd level (Deka et al. 2018).

11.5.5 Climate-sensitive Diseases

Climate change may affect animal health by increasing the frequency and severity of climate events and associated diseases like heat stress, adaptation of livestock systems to new environments, promoting the emergence of novel pathogens, and creating environmental conditions that increase contact among pathogens, vectors, and hosts (Kappes et al. 2023).

The three important climate-sensitive diseases for which economic losses are estimated are trypanosomosis, tick-borne diseases (TBDs), and RVF. Trypanosomosis in cattle causes an annual loss of 5 billion US$ and over the long run the agricultural income of Africa had gone down to 4.5 billion US$ in a year (Tuppurainen et al. 2017). Among the TBDs, East Coast fever is one of the most economically important diseases of cattle as it causes high mortality, morbidity, and other production losses (Shaw et al. 2014). Associated losses with the disease include the high cost of chemical acaricides to manage the disease and its negative environmental impacts (Olwoch et al. 2008). RVF epidemics in Kenya during 2006 caused losses of over 32 million US$, apart from the devastating socioeconomic impacts arising from mortality in young stock, abortions, closure of markets, and enforcement of export restrictions (Perry 2009). Estimates of the economic impact of various TADs are shown in Table 11.9.

> Good governance of public and private components of veterinary services, appropriate surveillance, early detection and rapid response mechanisms are the best actions for animal disease prevention and control, with positive impacts on animal production, health and welfare, as well as humankind.
>
> *Dr Bernard Vallat, Director General (2000–2015), World Organisation for Animal Health,*
> *International Federation for Animal Health (2013)*

11.6 Advances in Estimating the Cost of Animal Disease Outbreaks

The traditional cost–benefit assessment (CBA) methods frequently face pitfalls in estimating the direct costs of disease due to more dynamic markets. But the current assessment methods are mainly targeting the evaluation of indirect costs that helps to improve the decision-making process and assessment of the economic expenses of animal disease epidemics.

11.6.1 Vector Error Correction Model

Time series analysis is the econometric technique that correlates data statistically and provides information about alterations in market dynamics at the beginning of a disease outbreak. Indirect costs are defined as the economic losses faced in markets following the declaration of disease independence. The multivariate vector error correction model (VECM) is an epidemiological tool and a time series model that helps to capture market dynamics after a disease freedom or outbreak is

11 Economic Impact on Animal Diseases

Table 11.9 Estimate of economic impact of animal diseases.

Disease	Value of impact	Scale/period	References
Foot and mouth disease (FMD)	2.1 million US$ per month	Average monthly cost of disease outbreak	Rushton and Gilbert (2016)
	6.5 to US$ 21 billion	Global annual impact taking into account only production losses and vaccination costs in endemic areas	Knight-Jones et al. (2017)
	>1.5 billion US$ a year	Outbreaks in FMD-free countries and zones	Knight-Jones et al. (2017)
	8 billion GBP	Cost of controlling the 2001 UK outbreak (3 billion public sector and more than 5 billion private sector)	Rich and Wanyoike (2010)
	481 million GBP	Direct cost to agriculture (231) and gross cost to tourism (250) of the 2001 FMD outbreak in Scotland	National Audit Office of the UK Government (2002)
	2700 million US$	South Korean livestock sector 2010–2011	Mcleod et al. (n.d.)
	1600 million US$	Taiwan, direct costs and loss of exports, 1997	Royal Society of Edinburgh (2002)
	230 million US$	Cost to Kenyan farmers in the early 1980s	Yang et al. (1999)
	7–9 million US$ per year	Cost to the Uruguayan economy through lost export opportunities prior to eradication in 1997	Ellis and Putt (1981)
Rabies	8.6 billion US$ per year	Economic burden of dog-mediated rabies	Anderson et al. (2014)
	37.5 million US$ per month	Average monthly cost of disease outbreak	Rushton and Gilbert (2016)
	5.5 billion US$ per year	Global burden of endemic canine rabies	Anderson et al. (2014)
	120 billion US$	Global cost for canine rabies	Rushton and Knight-Jones (2015)
Brucellosis	58.8 million US$ per year	Economic loss due to brucellosis in India based on active surveillance program	Leslie et al. (1997)
	3.4 billion US$	Median loss to livestock sector, mainly to dairy sector	Kollannur et al. (2007)
Classic swine fever (CSF)	2.34 billion US$	Cost of controlling the 1997–1998 outbreak in The Netherlands	Singh et al. (2015)
	2.7 million US$ per year	Cost to smallholders in Haiti	Meuwissen et al. (1999)
	2.5 million US$	Direct costs of reported outbreaks in Chile	Otte (1997)
	50 million US$	Annual losses in Mexico, Brazil, and Dominican Republic from 1997 to 2001	Pinto (2000)
Contagious bovine pleuropneumonia (CBPP)	2 billion US$ per year	Annual cost to African famers	Otte et al. (2004)
	44.8 million Euro per year	Annual cost in Africa	Pinto (2003)
H7N9 High-pathogenicity avian influenza (HPAI)	6.5 billion US$	Chinese livestock sector 2012–2013	Mcleod et al. (n.d.)
H5N1 HPAI	5–10 billion US$	Cost to Asian economy	Tambi et al. (2006)
	214 million US$ at 2005 prices	Vietnamese poultry sector 2003–2010	Bio-Era (2005)
	124.7 million US$	Direct costs to Vietnamese farmers	McLeod et al. (2013)
	107–120 million US$	Direct costs of 2003–2004 outbreaks	World Organisation for Animal Health (2007)

Table 11.9 (Continued)

Disease	Value of impact	Scale/period	References
HPAI	2.65 million US$	Cost of an outbreak in the USA in 1983–1984	World Bank (2004)
	8.3 million US$	Average monthly cost of disease outbreak	Rushton and Gilbert (2016)
Peste des petits ruminants (PPR)	12 million US$ per year	Annual value of disease losses and control costs	United States Department of Agriculture (2005)
	34.08 million US$ per year	Goat mortality from PPR in Bangladesh	Government of Kenya (2008)
Lumpy skin disease (LSD)	2217.26 million US$	Net economic loss due to LSD in India	Honhold and Sil (2001)
	141, 1000, 1176 US$	Median losses per affected lactating cow, for dead cow and total economic loss of LSD outbreak at herd level in Ethiopia	Singh et al. (2023)
	2093.99 GBP	Turkey, total economic loss of GBP 2093.99 per herd was reported	Molla et al. (2017)
	8.6 million, 6.7 million, 5.3 million EUR	Net economic losses due to LSD in Bulgaria, Former Yugoslav Republic of Macedonia and in Albania	Sevik and Dogan (2017)
	1.45 billion US$	Net loss due to LSD in South, East and Southeast Asian countries	Casal et al. (2018)
Equine influenza	2.1 million US$ per month	Average monthly cost of disease outbreak	Rushton and Gilbert (2016)
Newcastle disease	2.1 million US$ per month	Average monthly cost of disease outbreak	Rushton and Gilbert (2016)
Transmissible spongiform encephalopathy (TSE)	10.3 million US$ per month	Average monthly cost of disease outbreak	Rushton and Gilbert (2016)

declared (Roche et al. 2020). The indirect costs of different vaccine stock strategies due to FMD were first predicted using this epidemiological model. According to Corbyn (Roche et al. 2020), indirect costs are more predictable when vaccination is utilized as opposed to culling in the FMD control strategies.

11.6.2 OutCosT

OutCosT (OUTbreak COSting Tool) is a spreadsheet-based tool jointly developed by the FAO and researchers at the Autonomous University of Barcelona (Spain), that enables countries to assess the financial burden of animal disease outbreaks and their control measures (FAO 2022). It helps to estimate the direct costs of disease outbreaks and their control with good precision. It can simulate and calculate the costs of alternative management strategies and disease outbreaks in past and future scenarios. Estimating the economic burden of livestock diseases emphasizes the need for early detection and cost-effective prevention and control strategies. The tool has been validated with data from four countries in three continents for ASF and will be soon available for cattle, sheep, and goat diseases (Corbyn 2022). It calculates the costs of disease prevention and control policies, and surveillance activities, as well as awareness and training campaigns.

11.7 Conclusion

The concept of animal health economics and estimating the cost of animal diseases in monetary units is a continuously evolving research area. Zoonotic diseases pose a challenge to both human and animal health. A wide range of strategies have to be employed to mitigate the impact of animal diseases, considering climate change, the diverse nature of disease pathogens, and their interrelationships with animal hosts. Most countries have very rudimentary disease reporting and mitigation strategies. However, advances in vaccinology, disease monitoring, and surveillance programs will help to tackle this problem. Merging economics with epidemiology is one of the strategies adopted to ensure sustainability in food security and human health. A systematic, multidisciplinary approach in assessing the GBADs will be helpful to study the economic impact of animal diseases.

References

Anderson, A., Shwiff, S., Gebhardt, K. et al. (2014). Economic evaluation of vampire bat (*Desmodus rotundus*) rabies prevention in Mexico. *Transboundary and Emerging Diseases* 61: 140–146.

Armbruster, W.J. (2005). Economic impacts of animal disease management and policy. *International Food and Agribusiness Management Review* 8: 20–22.

Awada, L., Gregory, K., Hutchison, J. et al. (2023). Current animal health situation worldwide in regard to selected global strategies and infection with lumpy skin disease virus: analysis of events and trends. In: *Proceedings of 90th General Session, World Assembly of OIE Delegates*. Paris: World Organisation for Animal Health.

Barratt, A.S., Rich, K.M., Eze, J.I. et al. (2019). Framework for estimating indirect costs in animal health using time series analysis. *Frontiers in Veterinary Science* 6: 190.

Bio-Era (2005). Economic risks associated with an influenza pandemic. In: *Prepared testimony of James Newcomb, Managing Director for Research, Bio Economic Research Associates, before the United States Senate Committee on Foreign Relations*.

Casal, J., Allepuz, A., Miteva, A. et al. (2018). Economic cost of lumpy skin disease outbreaks in three Balkan countries: Albania, Bulgaria and the former Yugoslav Republic of Macedonia (2016–2017). *Transboundary and Emerging Diseases* 65: 1680–1688.

Corbyn, A. (2022). An analysis of the indirect costs of animal health over time. *Health Economics Outcome Research* 8: 5.

Deka, R.P., Magnusson, U., Grace, D., and Lindahl, J. (2018). Bovine brucellosis: prevalence, risk factors, economic cost and control options with particular reference to India – a review. *Infection Ecology & Epidemiology* 8: 1555448.

Dharmarajan, G., Li, R., Chanda, E. et al. (2022). The animal origin of major human infectious diseases: what can past epidemics teach us about preventing the next pandemic? *Zoonoses* 2: 1–13. http://dx.doi.org/10.15212/zoonoses-2021-0028.

Dijkhuizen, A.A. and Morris, R.S. (1996). *Animal Health Economics: Principles and Applications*, 1e. Sydney: Post Graduate Foundation in Veterinary Science.

Dijkhuizen, A.A., Huirne, R.B.M., and Jalvingh, A.W. (1995). Economic analysis of animal diseases and their control. *Preventive Veterinary Medicine* 25: 135–149.

Dijkhuizen, A.A., Huirne, R.B.M., and Morris, R.S. (1996). Economic decision making in animal health management. In: *Animal Health Economics: Principles and Applications* (ed. A.A. Dijkhuizen and R.S. Morris), 13–23. Sydney: Post Graduate Foundation in Veterinary Science.

Ellis, P.R. and Putt, S.N. (1981). The Epidemiological and Economic Implications of a Foot-and mouth Disease Vaccination Programme in Kenya.

Food and Agriculture Organization (1997). *Prevention and Control of Transboundary Animal Diseases*. Rome: FAO.

Food and Agriculture Organization (2022). New tool helps estimate the costs of animal disease outbreaks. www.fao.org/europe/news/detail/New-tool-helps-estimate-the-costs-of-animal-disease-outbreaks/en (accessed 18 January 2024).

Gemechu, R. (2017). Review on economic importance's of rabies in developing countries and its controls. *Archives of Preventive Medicine* 2: 15–21.

Government of Kenya. (2008). Emergency project for the control of peste des petits ruminants (PPR) in Kenya: situation analysis and concept note.

Grace, D., Gilbert, J., Randolph, T., and Kang'ethe, E. (2012). The multiple burdens of zoonotic disease and an eco-health approach to their assessment. *Tropical Animal Health and Production* 44: 67–73.

Grace, D., Bett, B., Lindahl, J., and Robinson, T. (2015). *Climate and Livestock Disease: Assessing the Vulnerability of Agricultural Systems to Livestock Pests under Climate Change Scenarios*. Copenhagen, Denmark: CGIAR Research Program on Climate Change, Agriculture and Food Security.

Hampson, K., Coudeville, L., Lembo, T. et al. (2015). Estimating the global burden of endemic canine rabies. *PLoS Neglected Tropical Diseases* 9: e0003709.

Honhold, N. and Sil, B.K. (2001). Epidemiology, Economic Impact and Control of PPR in Bangladesh. Internal Report of the ARMP Project.

Huntington, B., Bernardo, T.M., Bondad-Reantaso, M. et al. (2021). Global Burden of Animal Diseases: a novel approach to understanding and managing disease in livestock and aquaculture. *Revue Scientifique et Technique* 40: 567–584.

International Federation for Animal Health. (2012). The costs of animal disease. www.bft-online.de/fileadmin/bft/publikationen/IFAH_Oxford-Analytica_The-Costs-of-Animal-Disease_October2012.pdf (accessed 18 January 2024).

International Federation for Animal Health (2013). The Costs of Animal Diseases and Societal Benefits from Healthy Animals. International Federation for Animal Health Annual Report 2012. www.vetanco.com/en/wp-content/uploads/sites/5/2016/02/The-costs-of-anial-diseases-and-societal-benefits-from-healthy-animals.pdf (accessed 18 January 2024).

Kappes, A., Tozooneyi, T., Shakil, G. et al. (2023). Livestock health and disease economics: a scoping review of selected literature. *Frontiers in Veterinary Science* 10: 1168649.

Knight-Jones, T.J.D. and Rushton, J. (2013). The economic impacts of foot and mouth disease – what are they, how big are they and where do they occur? *Preventive Veterinary Medicine* 112: 161–173.

Knight-Jones, T.J.D., McLaws, M., and Rushton, J. (2017). Foot-and-mouth disease impact on smallholders – what do we know, what don't we know and how can we find out more? *Transboundary and Emerging Diseases* 64: 1079–1094.

Kollannur, J., Rathore, R., and Chauhan, R. (2007). Epidemiology and economics of brucellosis in animals and its zoonotic significance. *ISAH Tartu Estonia* 83: 466–468.

Krishnamoorthy, P., Kurli, R., Patil, S.S. et al. (2019). Trends and future prediction of livestock diseases outbreaks by periodic regression analysis. *Indian Journal of Animal Sciences* 89: 369–376.

Leslie, J., Barozzi, J., and Otte, M.J. (1997). The economic implications of a change in FMD policy: a case study in Uruguay. *Epidemiologie et Sante Animale* 31/32: 10.21.1–10.21.3.

McInerney, J.P. (2003). Economics in the veterinary domain: further dimensions. In: *Application of Quantitative Methods in Veterinary Epidemiology* (ed. J.P.T.M. Noordhuizen, K. Franken, M.V. Thrusfield, and E.A.M. Graat), 321–333. Wageningen: Wageningen Academic Publishers.

McLeod, A. and Rushton, J. (2007). The economics of animal vaccination. *Revue Scientifique et Technique* 26: 313–326.

McLeod, A., Trung, H.X., and Long, N.V. (2013). Estimating the economic impacts of emerging infectious diseases (EIDs) in animals in Vietnam. In: *Report to project 'Support to Knowledge Management and Policy Dialogue through the Partnership on Avian and Pandemic Influenza (KMP-API)' for the Ministry of Agriculture and Rural Development*. Vietnam.

Mcleod, A., Pinto, A., Lubroth, J. et al. (2016). *Economic Analysis of Animal Diseases*. Rome: FAO.

Meuwissen, M.P.M., Horst, S.H., Huirne, R.B.M., and Dijkhuizen, A.A. (1999). A model to estimate the financial consequences of classical swine fever outbreaks: principles and outcomes. *Preventive Veterinary Medicine* 42: 249–270.

Molla, W., de Jong, M.C., Gari, G., and Frankena, K. (2017). Economic impact of lumpy skin disease and cost effectiveness of vaccination for the control of outbreaks in Ethiopia. *Preventive Veterinary Medicine* 147: 100–107.

National Audit Office of the UK Government (2002). *The 2001 Outbreak of Foot and Mouth Disease Report by the Comptroller and Auditor General*. London: HMSO.

Olwoch, J.M., Reyers, B., Engelbrecht, F.A., and Erasmus, B.F.N. (2008). Climate change and the tick-borne disease, theileriosis (East Coast fever) in sub-Saharan Africa. *Journal of Arid Environments* 72: 108–120.

Otte, M.J. (1997). *Consultancy Report on Cost-Benefit of Different Vaccination Strategies for the Control of Classical Swine Fever in Haiti*. Rome: FAO.

Otte, J., Nugent, R., and McLeod, A. (2004). Transboundary animal diseases: assessment of socio-economic impacts and institutional responses. In: *Livestock Policy Discussion Paper*. Agal: FAO.

Paarlberg, P.L., Seitzinger, A.H., Lee, J.G., and Mathews, K.H. Jr. (2008). *Economic Impacts of Foreign Animal Disease*. Washington, DC: United States Department of Agriculture http://www.ers.usda.gov/webdocs/publications/45980/12171_err57_1_.pdf.

Perry, B.D. (2009). Economic impact of tick-borne diseases in Africa. *Onderstepoort Journal of Veterinary Research* 76: 49.

Perry, B.D. and Sones, K.R. (2007). *Global Roadmap for Improving the Tools to Control Foot-and-Mouth Disease in Endemic Settings. Report of a workshop held at Agra, November 29–December 1*. Nairobi: International Livestock Research Institute.

Perry, B.D., Rich, K.M., and Perez, A.M. (2023). Editorial: Challenging standards and paradigms to support animal disease prevention and control. *Frontiers in Veterinary Science* 10: 1208023.

Pinto, J. (2000). Hazard analysis on farm and at national level to maintain classical swine fever disease free status in Chile. PhD thesis, University of Reading.

Pinto, J. (2003). *Estimacion del Impacto de la Peste Porcina Clasica en Sistemas Productivas Porcinos en America Latina: Estudios de Casos en Tres Paises*. Santiago de Chile: FAO.

Pritchett, J., Thilmany, D., and Johnson, K. (2005). Animal disease economic impacts: a survey of literature and typology of research approaches. *International Food and Agribusiness Management Review* 8: 23–45.

Ramsay, G.C., Philip, P., and Riethmuller, P. (1999). The economic implications of animal diseases and disease control at the national level. *Revue Scientifique et Technique* 18: 343–356.

Rasmussen, P., Shaw, A.P.M., Munoz, V. et al. (2022). Estimating the burden of multiple endemic diseases and health conditions using Bayes' Theorem: a conditional probability model applied to UK dairy cattle. *Preventive Veterinary Medicine* 203: 105617.

Rich, K.M. and Perry, B.D. (2011). The economic and poverty impacts of animal diseases in developing countries: new roles, new demands for economics and epidemiology. *Preventive Veterinary Medicine* 101: 133–147.

Rich, K.M. and Wanyoike, F. (2010). An assessment of the regional and national socio-economic impacts of the 2007 Rift Valley fever outbreak in Kenya. *American Journal of Tropical Medicine and Hygiene* 83: 52–57.

Roche, X., Rozstalnyy, A., Tago Pacheco, D. et al. (2020). *Introduction and Spread of Lumpy Skin Disease in South, East and Southeast Asia: Qualitative Risk Assessment and Management*. Rome: FAO.

Royal Society of Edinburgh. (2002). Inquiry into Foot and Mouth Disease in Scotland, July 2002. https://www.scribd.com/document/61435188/Foot-and-Mouth-Disease-in-Scotland (accessed 24 January 2024).

Rushton, J. (2009). *The Economics of Animal Health and Production*, 1e. Oxford: CAB International.

Rushton, J. (2017). Improving the use of economics in animal health – challenges in research, policy and education. *Preventive Veterinary Medicine* 137: 130–139.

Rushton, J. and Gilbert, W. (2016). The economics of animal health: direct and indirect costs of animal disease outbreaks. *Revue Scientifique et Technique* 33: 710–735.

Rushton, J. and Knight-Jones, T. (2015). The impact of foot and mouth disease. In: *Proceedings of the FAO/OIE Global Conference on Foot and Mouth Disease Control*, 205–209. Rome: FAO and OIE.

Rushton, J., Bruce, M., Bellet, C. et al. (2018). Initiation of global burden of animal diseases programme. *Lancet* 392: 538–540.

Sevik, M. and Dogan, M. (2017). Epidemiological and molecular studies on lumpy skin disease outbreaks in Turkey during 2014–2015. *Transboundary and Emerging Diseases* 64: 1268–1279.

Shaw, A.P.M., Wint, G.R.W., Cecchi, G. et al. (2014). Mapping the economic benefits to livestock keepers from intervening against bovine trypanosomosis in Eastern Africa. *Preventive Veterinary Medicine* 113: 197–210.

Singh, B., Prasad, S., Sinha, D.K., and Verma, M.R. (2013). Estimation of economic losses due to foot and mouth disease in India. *Indian Journal of Animal Sciences* 83: 964–970.

Singh, D., Kumar, S., Singh, B., and Bardhan, D. (2014). Economic losses due to important diseases of bovines in Central India. *Veterinary World* 7: 579–585.

Singh, B.B., Dhand, N.K., and Gill, J.P.S. (2015). Economic losses occurring due to brucellosis in Indian livestock populations. *Preventive Veterinary Medicine* 119: 211–215.

Singh, A., Kour, G., Dhillon, S.S. and Brar, P.S. (2023). Impact of lumpy skin disease in India: socio-behavioural analysis, epidemiology and economics. https://doi.org/10.21203/rs.3.rs-2478979/v1 (accessed 24 January 2024).

Smith, R.D. (2006). The cost of disease. In: *Veterinary Clinical Epidemiology*, 217–222. New York: Taylor and Francis.

Tambi, N.E., Maina, W.O., and Ndi, C. (2006). An estimation of the economic impact of contagious bovine pleuropneumonia in Africa. *Revue Scientifique et Technique* 25: 999–1012.

Tuppurainen, E., Alexandrov, T., and Beltran-Alcrudo, D. (2017). *Lumpy Skin Disease – A Field Manual for Veterinarians*. Rome: FAO.

United States Department of Agriculture (2005). *High-Pathogenicity Avian Influenza: A Threat to U.S. Poultry*. Riverdale, MD: Animal and Plant Health Inspection Service.

World Bank. (2004). Technical Annex for a Proposed Credit of SDR 3.5 million (US$5 Million Equivalent) to the Socialist Republic of Viet Nam for an Avian Influenza Emergency Recovery Project. World Bank Rural Development and Natural Resources Sector Unit East Asia and Pacific Region.

World Organisation for Animal Health. (2007). Cost of national prevention systems for animal diseases and zoonoses in developing and transition countries. https://www.woah.org/app/uploads/2021/03/oie-costs-of-national-prevention-systems-finalreport—exec-sum.pdf (accessed 24 January 2024).

World Organisation for Animal Health (2016). *Infection with Brucella abortus, Brucella melitensis and Brucella suis*. Rome: World Organisation for Animal Health.

World Organisation for Animal Health. (2023a). One Health. https://www.woah.org/en/what-we-do/global-initiatives/one-health/ (accessed 24 January 2024).

World Organisation for Animal Health. (2023b). The Global Burden of Animal Diseases (GBADs). https://gbads.woah.org (accessed 24 January 2024).

World Trade Organisation. (2020). Future resilience to diseases of animal origin: the role of trade. www.wto.org/english/tratop_e/covid19_e/resilience_report_e.pdf (accessed 24 January 2024).

Yang, P.C., Chu, R.M., Chung, W.B., and Sung, H.T. (1999). Epidemiological characteristics and financial costs of the 1997 foot-and-mouth disease epidemic in Taiwan. *Veterinary Record* 145: 731–734.

12

International Laws and Regulations on Controlling Livestock Diseases

Bhavanam Sudhakara Reddy, Sirigireddy Sivajothi, and Kambala Swetha

College of Veterinary Science, Sri Venkateswara Veterinary University, Proddatur, Andhra Pradesh, India

12.1 Introduction

The overall aim of the livestock health and disease control scheme in India is to improve the animal health sector by implementing prophylactic vaccination programs against various diseases of livestock and poultry, capacity building, disease surveillance, and strengthening of the veterinary infrastructure. It is envisaged that implementation of the scheme will ultimately lead to prevention and control, subsequently eradicating disease, increasing access to veterinary services, promoting higher productivity from animals, boosting trade in livestock and poultry and their products, and improving the socioeconomic status of livestock and poultry farmers.

Some of the laws and regulations at international level are mentioned below.

The Prevention and Control of Infectious and Contagious Diseases in Animals Act 2009: An Act to provide for the prevention, control, and eradication of infectious and contagious diseases affecting animals, for prevention of outbreak or spreading of such diseases from one state to another, and to meet the international obligations of India for facilitating import and export of animals and animal products and for matters connected therewith or incidental thereto.

Control and Diseases of Animals Act – Malawi: An Act to consolidate and amend the law relating to the control and diseases of animals. This Act makes provision for measures to prevent the spreading of diseases affecting animals in Malawi. The Minister may declare any creature to be an animal and any animal disease is a disease for purposes of this Act. The Minister, the Chief Veterinary Officer or any other authorized person may declare any area within Malawi to be an infected area and specified provisions of this Act shall apply to such area. The Minister may also place restrictions on the importation or exportation of animals, establish quarantine stations and make rules for purposes of this Act. Other provisions of this Act concern, among other things, slaughter of animals ordered by a veterinary officer, examination of animals and other inspections, seizure of stray animals and measures regarding dangerous dogs. Implemented in Control and Diseases of Animals Act 1967 [1].

Diseases of Animals Rules 1923: These Rules carry into effect provisions of the Control and Diseases of Animals Act concerning a wide variety of matters including: measures regarding stray animals, disinfection, use of private land for the quarantine of straying animals, prohibition of removal of grass or herbage from infected land, powers of inspectors, precautionary measures, testing and branding of animals, quarantine and restrictions on exhibition and sale of animals [2].

Compulsory Reporting of Cattle Deaths Notice 1925: This Notice of the Chief Veterinary Officer stipulates that in specified districts the notification of death occurring among cattle must be notified by the owner of cattle or a person in charge of cattle to the nearest veterinary officer [3].

Prohibition of Treatment except by Veterinary Officers 1928: This Notice prohibits the treatment of trypanosomiasis except by a veterinary officer or persons acting under his or her direction. Owners of animals suspected to suffer from the disease are required to contact a veterinary officer [4].

Diseases of Animals (Cattle) Rules 1942: These Rules specify duties of all owners or persons in charge of cattle in an area prescribed by the Chief Veterinary Officer. Owners or persons in charge of cattle shall furnish information concerning the state of health of animals owned or in charge and shall take all measures in respect of the cattle as a veterinary officer may

---

Epidemiology and Environmental Hygiene in Veterinary Public Health, First Edition. Edited by Tanmoy Rana.
© 2025 John Wiley & Sons, Inc. Published 2025 by John Wiley & Sons, Inc.

direct. Any person who fails to comply with any requirement made under these Rules shall be punished as specified. Implemented in Control and Diseases of Animals Act 1967 [5].

Diseases of Animals (Stock Route) Rules 1958: These Rules stipulate that no movement of cattle may take place on the stock route approved by the Chief Veterinary Officer unless the fee payable under these Rules has been paid and that all cattle using the stock route shall be branded or otherwise marked in a manner approved by the Chief Veterinary Officer. Implemented in Control and Diseases of Animals Act 1967 [6].

Movement of Farm Animals Rules 1968: These Rules place restrictions on the movement of farm animals, i.e., cattle, sheep, goats, poultry, and swine. Movement of an animal from one district to another without a permit from a veterinary inspector or other authorized persons is prohibited. Movement of diseased animals requires a permit from a veterinary officer. Owners of land may detain trespassing farm animals for which no permit was obtained. Diseases among animals from which a permit was obtained shall be notified [7].

Control and Diseases of Farm Animals Rules 1968: These Rules make provision for measures to prevent the spreading of diseases among farm animals, i.e., cattle, sheep, goats, and swine. Measures include the record keeping and notification of death or disease of animals by owners or persons in charge of a farm, examination by veterinary inspectors, isolation of animals, disinfecting of stables and vehicles and removal of grass, etc. from infected areas [8].

Animals Quarantine Rules 1968: These Rules concern the quarantine of animals imported into Malawi and stray animals suffering from disease. They also require owners of land on which carcases of stray animals are found to bury or burn such carcases and to inform the police and prohibit the removal of grass, dung, etc. from areas where animals are quarantined or isolated. The Chief Veterinary Officer shall have the powers to sell unclaimed animals and may erect fences on (private) land for the purpose of isolation or quarantine of animals [9].

Prevention of Trypanosomiasis Rules 1968: These Rules concern the prevention of spreading of trypanosomiasis. Measures that may adopted include the disinfecting of animals in decontamination sheds or tsetse fly barriers and the issuance of directions regarding traveling in infected areas [10].

Swine Fever Rules 1968: These Rules concern permits for the removal of pigs from areas declared to be infected with swine fever under Section 4 of the Control and Diseases of Animals Act. A permit shall be issued by an inspector in the form as set out in the Schedule to these Rules. The Rules concern also the confinement of pigs and their detention and destruction [11].

Animals (Import) Rules 1968: These Rules place restrictions on the importation of animals, including importation of semen, eggs and animal by-products including vaccines. No person shall import animals or animal by-products except under a permit from the Chief Veterinary Officer [12].

Control of Dogs Rules 1969: These Rules make provision for the control of dogs for purposes of the Control and Diseases of Animals Act. Dogs shall be registered with the registering authority in each district in accordance with these Rules. Failure to register a dog in accordance with these Rules is declared to be an offence [13].

Eradication of East Coast Fever Rules 1969: These Rules make provision with respect to the prevention of East Coast fever. Measures to control the spreading of this disease affecting animals include declaration of eradication areas and infected areas by the Chief Veterinary Officer and restrictions on movement of animals from and to eradication areas and infected areas, disinfecting of animals [14].

Declaration of Diseases of Animals 1969: This Notice declares the disease denominated "Rift Valley fever" to be a disease for purposes of the Control and Diseases of Animals Act [15].

Prevention of Rabies Rules 1969: These Rules make provision with respect to the prevention of rabies. Measures to control the spreading of rabies include notification, inspection, restrictions on movement of animals, vaccination, marking of dogs, and destruction and disposal of diseased animals [16].

Control and Diseases of Animals (Veterinary Services Fees) Rules 1973: These Rules prescribe fees for specified services provided by the government in connection with the prevention of the spreading of diseases affecting animals. A part of the fees collected shall be paid by the government to the district council or chief of the area where the fees were collected [17].

Control and Diseases of Animals (Prohibition of Importation of Animals) Order 1990: This Order in general prohibits the importation of animals of a kind specified in the First Column of the Schedule from the country specified in relation to such animals as specified in the Second Column of the Schedule prohibited on account of the presence in that country of the disease specified in the Third Column of the Schedule. The Schedule specifies livestock and by-products thereof from Zimbabwe due to foot and mouth disease in that country [18].

12.2 Some Diseases of Animals Acts in Botswana

Diseases of Animals Act Botswana: An Act to provide for the prevention and control of diseases of animals; to regulate the import, export, and movement of animals; to provide for the quarantine of animals in certain circumstances; and to provide for matters incidental to and connected with the foregoing.

In this Act, "disease" is defined as the diseases listed in Section 2 and other diseases which the Minister, by notice in the Gazette, may declare to be diseases for the purposes of this Act. Every owner of an animal affected by any disease shall notify the disease to the authorities and keep the animal(s) affected separate from healthy animals (Section 3). The Director of Veterinary Services may by notice published in the Gazette: (i) declare any area to be an infected area as regards any disease named in such notice; (ii) alter the limits of an area; (iii) declare an area free from disease; (iv) prohibit movement into or out of the area of any animal, carcase, litter, dung, or fodder, except under a permit issued by a veterinary officer (Section 4). In the absence of any other provision made by Regulations under this Act, the provisions of Section 5 shall apply to any infected area. Section 6 provides for the import and export of animals and animal products and the declaration of infective agents. The Minister may be announced or notified the, establish quarantine stations. The Minister may also declare stock-free zones (Section 8). Section 10 deals with stock in transit. Other sections provide for slaughter of infected animals and compensation, powers to order seizure of stock, manufacture and sale of any vaccine serum, serum, virus, biological product, therapeutic substance or other similar products used for treatment of diseases, evidence of certificates, and regulation-making powers of the Minister (20 sections) [19].

Disease of Stock Regulations 1926: These Regulations make provision with respect to the prevention of animal diseases. They introduce various measures to control movement and hygiene of stock, such as import control (regulations 4 and 5), inoculation (6); examination (7); slaughter (12); stock-free zones (14); inspection (15); destruction of stock (24); isolation of stock (28); impounding of stray stock (45); branding of cattle (50); etc. Regulations 75–102 contain special measures for specific diseases. Regulation 3 specifies diseases for the purpose of these Regulations. Importation of stock shall be imported only after having obtained a permit from the Director of Veterinary services (reg. 5). The Minister may, by Notice in the Official Gazette, declare any area to be a diseased area (reg. 84) [20].

These Regulations provide for the compensation of healthy cattle which come into contact with infected animals. All animals driven under supervision to a quarantine camp shall become property of the government at the moment they first enter the gate (reg. 6). Owners will be paid the amount for which the government is able to sell such animals, in cash (reg. 8). Animals will be listed and valued by an expert on entry into the camp (reg. 9). Regulation 18 provides for the importation of butter and cheese from Zimbabwe (20 regulations) [21].

Diseases of Stock (Poultry) Regulations 1941: No person shall introduce into Botswana, except from the Republic of South Africa, any poultry unless such poultry is accompanied by: (i) a written permit by the Principal Veterinary Officer authorizing the introduction of such poultry; (ii) a certificate, issued by a veterinarian authorized thereto by the government of the country of origin, showing: (i) that poultry examined was found healthy and free from diseases specified in this provision; (ii) in the case of domestic fowl, the tuberculin test was carried out; (iii) in the case of turkeys, geese, and ducks, that the premises where the poultry came from was free from tuberculosis; (iv) agglutination tests in respect of specified fowl and turkeys were carried out and found negative. Regulation 4 deals with the introduction of birds (5 regulations) [22].

Diseases of Animals (Inoculation) Order 1952: This Order, made under regulation 22 of the Diseases of Stock Regulations, requires all bovines in Botswana to be inoculated annually against anthrax [23].

Diseases of Animals (Muzzling) Order 1954: This Order, made under regulation 83 of the Diseases of Stock Regulations, provides that the Director of Veterinary Services, veterinary officers, livestock officers, and stock inspectors may order any dog or other species of carnivora or monkey in Botswana to be isolated, muzzled, or destroyed [24].

Movement of Stock (Restriction) Order 1960: Movement of all stock is prohibited in Botswana, except under permit issued for each removal by a person authorized by the Director to issue such a permit (2 sections) [25].

Foot-and-Mouth Disease (Conveyance of Products) Order 1960: The vegetable and animal products specified in the Schedule are declared to be vegetable and animal products likely to convey or spread foot-and-mouth disease. (Schedule: "Any of the following products: hay, manure, bedding, fodder, hides, skins, milk or cream, bones, meat, whether dried or fresh, riems, horns or hoofs, game trophies or skins, blood, hair, meat offals, hide and skin pieces and trimmings") [26].

Stock Diseases (Semen) Regulations 1968: No person shall introduce, or cause to be introduced any semen unless accompanied by a permit of the Director. The Director grants permit to such conditions as may appear necessary or expedient for the prevention of spreading of animal diseases. Also sale, disposal, collection of semen or artificial insemination requires a permit of the Director. Contravention of the above rules shall be fined [27].

Diseases of Animals (Declaration of Stock-Free Zones) Order 1982: This Order declares any area specified in the Schedule to the Order to be a stock-free zone for the purposes of control of disease. Any stock in an area declared to be a stock-free zone shall be removed immediately by the owner or the person having possession or custody of such stock from such area. Not doing so is declared to be an offence [28].

Diseases of Animals (Prohibition of Use of Anabolic Hormones and Thyrostatic Substances) Regulations 1987: These Regulations prohibit the manufacture, importation, use, handling, storage, transportation, distribution, and sale of anabolic hormones and thyrostatic substances for use in animals. The Regulations also define certain exemptions from this rule. The Director of Animal Health and Production shall decide on sampling and testing of animals and animal produce for residues of the anabolic hormonal or thyrostatic substances. The Regulations define measures and offences in relation to the presence of prohibited residues in animals or food [29].

Prohibition of Sale of Imported Cattle to the Botswana Meat Commission for Export to the European Union Regulations 1998: These Regulations provide that the Botswana Meat Commission shall not buy or slaughter for export to the European Union any cattle branded in accordance with these Regulations. These Regulations require any cattle imported in Botswana, i.e., cattle not born and bred in Botswana, to be branded within seven days of importation with a sign "No EU." Penalties are prescribed [30].

Declaration of Foot and Mouth Disease (Infected Area) Order (S.I. No. 3 of 2003). 2003: This Order declares a specified area to be an infected area for the purposes of Section 4 of the Diseases of Animals Act and prohibits the movement of cloven hoofed animals and their products into or out of the area, except under and in accordance with a permit issued by a veterinary officer [31].

Diseases of Animals (Stock Feed) Regulations 2004: These Regulations control the production, placing on the market and use of feed for any animal that has been prescribed to be stock for the purposes of these Regulations and the use of substances of animal origin in fertilizer and disposal of animal waste. The restrictions aim to reduce the danger of spreading animal diseases through substances of animal origin. No poultry excreta, meat and bonemeal, or any other protein of animal origin shall be used as animal feed or in animal feed or used as fertilizer on any pasture land or any land to which stock has uncontrolled access. Feed intended for retail shall be labeled in accordance with these Regulations [32].

Diseases of Animals (BSE Control [Removal of Specified Risk Material]) Regulations 2004: These Regulations require that specified risk material of every animal that is slaughtered by an abattoir or export slaughterhouse shall be removed immediately after the slaughtering of that animal, and shall be burned or buried. The Minister may, by Statutory Instrument, specify the parts of a bovine animal that are likely to be contaminated with the agent that causes BSE [33].

Diseases of Animals (Livestock Identification and Trace-back) Regulations 2005: These Regulations provide for inspection of export slaughterhouses and introduce a system of identification of cattle for the purposes of the Diseases of Animals Act. The Director of Animal Health and Production or any veterinary officer may inspect export slaughterhouses so as to ensure that meat hygiene at the slaughter house conforms to best practice and to control livestock identification and trace-back records. No person shall submit any animal to export slaughter house unless such person has obtained a permit from the Director in accordance with Regulation 57 of the Diseases of Stock Regulations. The Director shall maintain aq trace-back register and slaughterhouses shall keep records of trace-back data. Importation of animal identification devices shall be approved by the Director [34].

Diseases of Animals (Animal Information and Traceability System) Regulations (S.I. No. 7 of 2018) 2018: These Regulations consist of seven parts divided into 22 articles: Part I Preliminary, Part II Stock traceability manager and other support personnel, Part III Stock traceability manager and other support personnel, Part IV Identification of animals, animal identification devices and manner of tagging animals, Part V Control of movement of imported animals, Part VI Management of animals for slaughter and inspection of export slaughter houses and abattoirs, Part VII General provisions. The aims of this Regulation are to appoint a stock traceability manager and other personnel able to register the animals, the owners of the animals and of the holdings. Moreover, the Regulations outline the management of animals for slaughter and inspection of export slaughterhouses and abattoirs. The last part of the Regulations covers general provisions with a focus on product traceability, information security, disclosure of official information, and an article on offences and penalties [35].

12.3 Regulations in Victoria

The Livestock Disease Control Regulations (the Regulations) operate under the Livestock Disease Control Act 1994 (the Act) in Victoria to: provide requirements to protect Victorian livestock from disease, maintain and enhance domestic and international market access. The legislation also aims to protect public health by preventing diseases that are transmissible to humans, by providing compensation for certain livestock losses, and by supporting the operation of livestock traceability systems for the purposes of market access and disease and residue control. The Regulations provide requirements, infringement offences and penalties that relate to the testing, notification, and prevention of livestock diseases, the identification and movement of livestock, the import of livestock, livestock products, fodder and fittings into Victoria, the seizure and disposal of certain livestock, fodder and fittings, and livestock-related compensation claims.

Livestock Disease Control Regulations 2017 S.R. No. 57/2017 Authorized Version incorporating amendments as at 1 February 2020: Part 1 Preliminary. 1 Objectives – the objectives of these Regulations are (i) to provide for the timing and manner of the notification of livestock diseases; (ii) to provide for the manner in which certain livestock are identified; (iii) to provide for the manner of certification of, and restrictions relating to, livestock, livestock products, fodder or fittings introduced into Victoria; (iv) to set out the standards and record-keeping requirements relating to testing for livestock diseases; (v) to set out requirements for the prevention of livestock diseases; (vi) to provide for the recording or forwarding of information relating to the movement of identified livestock; (vii) to provide for matters relating to claims for compensation for losses incurred due to livestock disease; (viii) to provide for other matters required to be prescribed under the Livestock Disease Control Act 1994.

These Regulations are made under Section 139 of the Livestock Disease Control Act 1994. 3 Commencement – these Regulations come into operation on 1 July 2017. 4 Revocation – the Regulations listed in Schedule 1 are revoked.

Livestock Disease Control Act 1994 No. 115 of 1994 Authorized Version incorporating amendments as at 5 April 2023: The Parliament of Victoria enacts as follows: Part 1 Preliminary. 1 Purposes – the main purposes of this Act are to provide for the prevention, monitoring, and control of livestock diseases and to provide compensation for losses caused by certain livestock diseases. 2 Commencement – (1) Section 1 and this section come into operation on the day on which this Act receives the Royal Assent. (2) Subject to subsection (3), the remaining provisions of this Act come into operation on a day or days to be proclaimed. (3) If a provision referred to in subsection (2), other than section 92(2), does not come into operation within the period of 12 months beginning on, and including, the day on which this Act receives the Royal Assent, it comes into operation on the first day after the end of that period [36–38].

Australia (Victoria) – Livestock Disease Control Regulations 2017: These Regulations, consisting of 112 sections divided into 13 Parts and six Schedules, establish the requirements for livestock disease controls. The objectives of these Regulations are: (i) to provide for the timing and manner of the notification of livestock diseases; (ii) to provide for the manner in which certain livestock are identified; (iii) to provide for the manner of certification of, and restrictions relating to, livestock, livestock products, fodder, or fittings introduced into Victoria; (iv) to set out the standards and record keeping requirements relating to the testing for livestock diseases; (v) to set out requirements for the prevention of livestock diseases; (vi) to provide for the recording or forwarding of information relating to the movement of identified livestock; (vii) to provide for matters relating to claims for compensation for losses incurred due to livestock disease; and (viii) to provide for other matters required to be prescribed under the Livestock Disease Control Act 1994 [39].

Livestock Disease Control Act 1994: This Act provides for the prevention, monitoring, and control of livestock diseases and for the compensation for losses caused by certain livestock diseases. Livestock means any nonhuman animal, and any fish or bird, whether wild or domesticated, egg intended for hatching or bee. The objectives of the Act include: protect public health by preventing, monitoring, and controlling diseases transmissible from livestock to humans; to protect domestic and export markets for livestock and livestock products by preventing, monitoring, and controlling livestock diseases; to provide for the preventing, monitoring, and eradication of exotic livestock diseases and to facilitate the operation of livestock identification and tracking programs for disease and residue control and market access (Section 4). The Act consists of 149 sections and is divided into the following parts: Preliminary (i); Provisions applying to diseases generally (ii); Exotic diseases (iii); Provisions for particular livestock (iv); Compensation (v); Duty and records (vi); Administration (vii); Enforcement (viii); Regulations (ix); and Repeals, amendments and transitional provisions (x).

The Act contains several principles and provisions that contribute to the food safety and quality legislation; one of the Act's objectives is to protect public health by preventing, monitoring, and controlling diseases transmissible from livestock to humans. Firstly, the Act empowers the Governor in Council to make orders that prohibit importing, transporting, selling, or handling livestock products that have been declared infected; the Act also recognizes responsibilities of owners and others for diseases affecting livestock products, establishing duties and penalties (e.g., notification, separation of livestock products). Section 45, for instance, establishes a prohibition of use of cow, goat, sheep, or buffalo for dairying if an inspector is of the opinion that it would be deleterious to the health of human beings or unfit for human consumption [40].

Livestock Disease Control Regulations 1995: The objectives of these Regulations are to provide for the eradication, prevention, monitoring, and control of diseases in livestock and generally prescribe forms, penalties, and other matters authorized by the Livestock Disease Control Act 1994. The Regulations cover notification of livestock diseases (Part 2), identification of livestock (Part 3), introduction of livestock into Victoria (Part 4), testing for diseases (Part 5) and prevention of spread of diseases (Part 6). They also cover compensation (Part 7), record of sales (Part 7A), licences and enforcement [41].

Livestock Disease Control Regulations 2006: These Regulations implement the Livestock Disease Control Act 1994 by providing for the timing and manner of the notification of livestock diseases; the manner in which certain livestock are identified; the manner of certification of, and restrictions relating to, livestock, livestock products, fodder, or fittings introduced into Victoria; standards and record keeping requirements relating to the testing for livestock diseases; requirements for the prevention of livestock diseases; the recording or forwarding of information relating to the movement of identified livestock; and for matters relating to claims for compensation for losses incurred due to livestock disease [42].

Livestock Disease Control Regulations 2017: These Regulations, consisting of 112 sections divided into 13 Parts and six Schedules, establish the requirements for livestock disease controls. The objectives of these Regulations are: (i) to provide for the timing and manner of the notification of livestock diseases; (ii) to provide for the manner in which certain livestock are identified; (iii) to provide for the manner of certification of, and restrictions relating to, livestock, livestock products, fodder, or fittings introduced into Victoria; (iv) to set out the standards and record keeping requirements relating to the testing for livestock diseases; (v) to set out requirements for the prevention of livestock diseases; (vi) to provide for the recording or forwarding of information relating to the movement of identified livestock; (vii) to provide for matters relating to claims for compensation for losses incurred due to livestock disease; and (viii) to provide for other matters required to be prescribed under the Livestock Disease Control Act 1994 [39].

12.4 Regulations in India

In India, a scheme was initiated to reduce the risk to animal and human health and to increase livestock productivity by reducing disease burden and with certain other objectives.

- To implement a critical animal disease control program to eradicate PPR by 2030 by vaccinating all sheep and goats and to control CSF by vaccinating the entire pig population.
- To provide veterinary services on farm through MVUs.
- To assist states with control of animal disease by prevention and control of important livestock and poultry diseases as per the state's priorities.

Some of the livestock disease control measures adopted in India are listed below.

12.4.1 Assistance to States for Control of Animal Diseases (ASCAD)

This covers activities for vaccination against economically important diseases of livestock and backyard poultry duly prioritized by the state as per the disease(s) prevalence and losses to the farmers. Due emphasis shall also be given to vaccination against zoonotic diseases like anthrax and rabies for which assistance shall be given to the states as per proposals received from them. Another activity that has been prioritized is control of emergent and exotic diseases. This includes surveillance and related activities to check ingress of exotic diseases as well as emergent/reemergent livestock/poultry diseases. Assistance shall also be given for ring vaccination to inhibit spread of disease (in cases of disease outbreaks) as well as payment of compensation to farmers for culling of poultry, elimination of infected animals, and destruction of poultry feed/eggs, including operational costs. A third activity under the ASCAD component is research and innovation, publicity and awareness, training, and allied activities. Publicity and awareness and training are existing activities under the extant ASCAD but research and innovation is a newly proposed activity. Under this activity it is envisaged that funds may be released to recognized private/public institutions, other ministries/departments, etc. toward collaboration in research and innovation/trainings/capacity building/crisis management mock drills, etc. The funding pattern is 60:40 center:state except the north-east states and Himalayan region where it is 90:10 center:state; 100% central assistance to states, for training and control of emergent exotic diseases and conducting training/holding workshops. Grants are also provided as compensation to farmers for culling of birds, elimination of infected animals, and destruction of feed/eggs including operational costs (50:50 center:state).

12.4.2 Peste des Petits Ruminants Eradication Program (PPR-EP)

Peste des petits ruminants, also known as sheep and goat plague, is a highly contagious animal disease affecting domestic and wild small ruminants. It is caused by a virus belonging to the genus *Morbillivirus*, family Paramyxoviridae. Once introduced, the virus can infect up to 90% of an animal herd, and the disease kills anywhere up to 70% of infected animals. This component will cover the entire sheep and goat population in the country under carpet vaccination against PPR, for 100% effective coverage of the entire eligible small ruminant population. Funding pattern – 100% central assistance to states.

12.4.3 Establishment and Strengthening of Existing Veterinary Hospitals and Dispensaries (ESVHD)

In order to help states establish new veterinary hospitals and dispensaries as well as strengthen/equip existing ones, including running mobile veterinary ambulances, the Department provides financial assistance under this component.

12.4.4 Mobile Veterinary Units

To increase on-farm accessibility of veterinary services, funds for MVUs will be provided to states under this scheme, with one MVU approximately for one lakh livestock population. These MVUs will be customized fabricated vehicles for veterinary healthcare with equipment for diagnosis, treatment, and minor surgery, audiovisual aids and other basic requirements. The MVUs need to be positioned at strategic locations in order to minimize travel time and to provide services within targeted time.

12.4.5 Call Centers

A state-level call center would also be set up/aligned with the existing call center in each state. The call center would function as the pivot whilst supporting mobile veterinary services. It would receive calls from livestock rearers/animal owners and transmit them to the veterinary doctor at the call center. The decision on directing the MVU would be based on the emergent nature of the veterinary case as decided by the veterinarian at the call center. The call center would also be responsible for monitoring the movement and use of the MVUs. The call center should also confirm actual services through the mobile number of the animal owner and share the data with the state concerned.

12.4.6 Classic Swine Fever Control Program (CSF-CP)

Swine fever is a highly contagious and economically significant viral disease of pigs. The severity of the illness varies with the strain of the virus, the age of the pig, and the immune status of the herd. Acute infections, which are caused by highly virulent isolates and have a high mortality rate in naive herds, are more likely to be diagnosed rapidly. CSF-CP will be implemented in the whole country with the target being 100% eligible pig population; funding pattern 100% central assistance to states [43].

12.5 Animal Health Law

The European Parliament and the Council adopted Regulation (EU) 2016/429 on transmissible animal diseases ("Animal Health Law") in March 2016. It has been applicable since 21 April 2021.

Overall, the single, comprehensive new Animal Health Law supports the EU livestock sector in its quest for competitiveness and creating a safe and smooth EU market of animals and their products, leading to growth and jobs in this important sector. The huge number of legal acts are streamlined into a single law. Simpler and clearer rules enable authorities and those having to follow the rules to focus on key priorities: preventing and eradicating disease. Responsibilities are clarified for farmers, vets, and others dealing with animals. The rules allow greater use of new technologies for animal health activities – surveillance of pathogens, electronic identification and registration of animals. Better early detection and control of animal diseases, including emerging diseases linked to climate change, will help to reduce the occurrence and effects of animal epidemics. It offers more flexibility to adjust rules to local circumstances, and on emerging issues such as climate and social change. It sets out a better legal basis for monitoring animal pathogens resistant to antimicrobial agents, supplementing existing rules and Regulations on veterinary medicines and on medicated feed.

References

1 www.fao.org/faolex/results/details/en/c/LEX-FAOC092011 (Laws of Malawi, Cap. 66:02, pp. 1–8) LEX-FAOC092011

2 www.fao.org/faolex/results/details/en/c/LEX-FAOC092013 (Laws of Malawi, Cap. 66:02, pp. 13–22) LEX-FAOC092013

3 www.fao.org/faolex/results/details/en/c/LEX-FAOC092015 (Laws of Malawi, p. 23) LEX-FAOC092015

4 www.fao.org/faolex/results/details/en/c/LEX-FAOC092014 (Laws of Malawi, Cap. 66:02, p. 23) LEX-FAOC092014

5 www.fao.org/faolex/results/details/en/c/LEX-FAOC092020 LEX-FAOC092020

6 www.fao.org/faolex/results/details/en/c/LEX-FAOC092022 LEX-FAOC092022

7 www.fao.org/faolex/results/details/en/c/LEX-FAOC092060 LEX-FAOC092060

8 www.fao.org/faolex/results/details/en/c/LEX-FAOC092059 LEX-FAOC092059

9 www.fao.org/faolex/results/details/en/c/LEX-FAOC092028 (Laws of Malawi, Cap. 66:02, pp. 38–40) LEX-FAOC092028

10 www.fao.org/faolex/results/details/en/c/LEX-FAOC092027 (Laws of Malawi, Cap. 66:02, p. 37) LEX-FAOC092027

11 www.fao.org/faolex/results/details/en/c/LEX-FAOC092024 (Laws of Malawi, Cap. 66:02, pp. 35–36) LEX-FAOC092024

12 www.fao.org/faolex/results/details/en/c/LEX-FAOC092012 (Laws of Malawi, Cap. 66:02, pp. 9–10) LEX-FAOC092012

13 www.fao.org/faolex/results/details/en/c/LEX-FAOC092066 (Laws of Malawi, Cap. 66:02, pp. 59–64) LEX-FAOC092066

14 www.fao.org/faolex/results/details/en/c/LEX-FAOC092065 (Laws of Malawi, Cap. 66:02, pp. 54a–56) LEX-FAOC092065

15 www.fao.org/faolex/results/details/en/c/LEX-FAOC092063 (Laws of Malawi, Cap. 66:02, p. 49) LEX-FAOC092063

16 www.fao.org/faolex/results/details/en/c/LEX-FAOC092061 (Laws of Malawi, Cap. 66:02, pp. 43–48) LEX-FAOC092061

17 www.fao.org/faolex/results/details/en/c/LEX-FAOC092018 (Laws of Malawi, Cap. 66:02, pp. 25–26) LEX-FAOC092018

18 www.fao.org/faolex/results/details/en/c/LEX-FAOC117755 LEX-FAOC117755

19 www.fao.org/faolex/results/details/en/c/LEX-FAOC006474 www.laws.gov.bw. LEX-FAOC006474

20 www.fao.org/faolex/results/details/en/c/LEX-FAOC016942 www.laws.gov.bw Diseases of Stock (Quarantine and Compensation) Regulations 1930.

21 www.fao.org/faolex/results/details/en/c/LEX-FAOC006486

22 www.fao.org/faolex/results/details/en/c/LEX-FAOC006487

23 www.fao.org/faolex/results/details/en/c/LEX-FAOC091455

24 www.fao.org/faolex/results/details/en/c/LEX-FAOC066206

25 www.fao.org/faolex/results/details/en/c/LEX-FAOC006497

26 www.fao.org/faolex/results/details/en/c/LEX-FAOC006498

27 www.fao.org/faolex/results/details/en/c/LEX-FAOC019064

28 www.fao.org/faolex/results/details/en/c/LEX-FAOC065991

29 www.fao.org/faolex/results/details/en/c/LEX-FAOC065989

30 www.fao.org/faolex/results/details/en/c/LEX-FAOC066253

31 www.fao.org/faolex/results/details/en/c/LEX-FAOC065802

32 www.fao.org/faolex/results/details/en/c/LEX-FAOC066207

33 www.fao.org/faolex/results/details/en/c/LEX-FAOC065990

34 www.fao.org/faolex/results/details/en/c/LEX-FAOC065988

35 www.fao.org/faolex/results/details/en/c/LEX-FAOC196347

36 www.legislation.vic.gov.au/in-force/statutory-rules/livestock-disease-control-regulations-2017/005

37 https://agriculture.vic.gov.au/biosecurity/protecting-victoria/livestock-disease-control-regulations-2017#h2-0

38 https://agriculture.vic.gov.au/biosecurity/protecting-victoria/livestock-disease-control-regulations-2017

39 www.fao.org/faolex/results/details/en/c/LEX-FAOC175442

40 www.fao.org/faolex/results/details/en/c/LEX-FAOC046193

41 www.fao.org/faolex/results/details/en/c/LEX-FAOC046504

42 www.fao.org/faolex/results/details/en/c/LEX-FAOC105637

43 https://dahd.nic.in/schemes-programmes/lh-dc#:~:text=Assistance%20to%20States%20for%20Control,and%20losses%20to%20the%20farmers

13

Role of OIE in Global Trade in Animals and Animal Products

Somu Yogeshpriya[1] and Tanmoy Rana[2]

[1] *Department of Veterinary Medicine, Veterinary College and Research Institute, Tamil Nadu Veterinary and Animal Sciences University, Orathanadu, India*
[2] *Department of Veterinary Clinical Complex, West Bengal University of Animal & Fishery Sciences, Kolkata, India*

13.1 Introduction

The international community was given a completely novel and critically needed international decision-making forum to prevent the regional and global spread of contagious and trade-sensitive animal diseases and zoonoses with the establishment of the Office International des Epizooties (OIE) as an independent intergovernmental international organization in 1924 (OIE 2008). Membership has since increased to 172 nations and territories from the original 28. The original goals of the OIE, now known as the World Organization for Animal Health, are still relevant today. Through the years, these goals have been expanded to include the overarching goal of advancing animal health worldwide.

Foreign animal ailments have the potential to have a large negative influence on animal health, production, and trade, making them a serious concern to nations all over the world. Imported animal disease must be quickly controlled and eradicated in order to safeguard the long-term prosperity of a nation's animal agricultural industry. Global market growth, intensification of animal production methods, and the ongoing evolution of infectious pathogens have all had a significant impact on how we design and implement national animal health systems, including risk-based legislation, to prevent the spread of animal diseases.

The study by Zepeda et al. (2001) confirmed that diseases have been known to spread across borders in a number of instances. A cattle epidemic was once again introduced to Europe in 1920 when rinderpest spread to Belgium from cattle coming from India and headed for Brazil while passing via the port of Antwerp (OIE, 1999). The introduction of foot and-mouth disease (FMD) from Brazil to Mexico in the 1950s resulted in the death of 1 million sheep, calves, and goats as well as a significant socioeconomic disaster. Hispaniola saw an epidemic of African swine disease in 1978, which could only be contained by wiping out the whole island's swine population. Particularly in Haiti, this had a profound impact on the rural population's already insecure way of life.

13.2 Benefits and Barriers of International Trade

With the above considerations, the validity of the zero-risk approach to trade concerns might be questioned.

- Risk can be decreased in every aspect of safety, but it is scientifically impossible to reduce it to zero. Scientific evidence provides some clarity regarding the possibility of risk absence but cannot confirm risk absence.
- Political lines are not respected by nature. As a result, a disease can spread across a political border undetected, whether there is international trade or not.
- International travel and trade are facts of our current global community, and risk will always exist (no matter how small). Unwarranted technical obstacles to trade can lead to trafficking as a means of getting around such barriers, which can seriously threaten agricultural security and have the opposite effect to what is intended.

Epidemiology and Environmental Hygiene in Veterinary Public Health, First Edition. Edited by Tanmoy Rana.
© 2025 John Wiley & Sons, Inc. Published 2025 by John Wiley & Sons, Inc.

13.3 OIE Internal Standards, Guidelines, and Recommendations for Animal and Aquatic Health

13.3.1 Establishment of the World Trade Organization (WTO) and the Sanitary and Phytosanitary Measures (SPS) Agreement

The WTO was founded in 1995 to handle the demands and difficulties of modern-day global commerce and market liberalization. The group's first task was to deal with agricultural trade and nontariff trade restrictions. Its joint efforts led to the creation of the SPS Agreement, which establishes fundamental guidelines for actions meant to safeguard the health of people, animals, and plants. These actions should be technically sound, based on a risk assessment, and on internationally accepted standards and recommendations. In a nutshell, the SPS Agreement permits nations to defend themselves against unwelcome pests and disease agents that could endanger the health of people, plants, and animals, but not in a way that unfairly restricts trade. When trade policies are created in accordance with international norms to make sure that trade flows as smoothly, reliably, and freely as possible, trade ties are more stable. As a result, when nations uphold the WTO and SPS Agreement, the global agriculture trade community benefits.

13.3.1.1 Role of WTO
3) International organization dealing with the rules of trade between nations.
4) WTO agreements are negotiated and signed by Members and ratified in their parliaments.
   - Require good reasons for restricting trade.
   - Aim to make trade stable, predictable, and transparent.
   - Provide a "court" for legal disputes.
   - Reduce conflict.
5) WTO accords, like the SPS Agreement, give states the tools to set up a framework to enable trade based on generally accepted norms for food safety and animal health.

13.3.1.1.1 Role of WTO in Codex and OIE
1) WTO SPS Agreement works in tandem with international standard-setting bodies.
2) FAO/WHO Codex Alimentarius:
   - Codex establishes science-based food standards.
   - Codex standards are recognized by the SPS Agreement in the area of food safety.
3) World Organization for Animal Health (OIE):
   - OIE establishes science-based standards for animal health.
   - OIE recognized by the SPS Agreement as the international standard-setting body for animal health and zoonoses.

13.3.1.2 Agreement on the Application of Sanitary and Phytosanitary Measures (SPS Agreement)
- Basic rules for food safety, animal, and plant health measures in trade.
- Measures do not act as unnecessary barriers to trade.
- Regulations must be based on science.
- Multilateral framework of rules/disciplines to guide development, adoption, and enforcement of SPS measures.
- SPS measures which may, directly or indirectly, affect international trade.

13.3.1.2.1 Core Principles of SPS Agreement
- Nondiscrimination
- Scientific justification
- Equivalence
- Regionalization
- Transparency
- Technical assistance; special and differential treatment
- Control, inspection, and approval procedures

13.3.1.2.2 Scientific Justification
- Ensure that any animal health or food safety-related measure is based on scientific principles.
- Ensure that any animal health or food safety-related measure is applied only to the extent necessary to protect human or animal life or health, not maintained without sufficient scientific evidence and the least trade restrictive and consistent.
- Risk assessment exception includes insufficient scientific evidence; provisional measure and seek to obtain additional information; review measure within a reasonable period of time.

13.3.1.2.3 Importance of Transparency
- Regulatory changes affects market access.
- Enhanced clarity and predictability.
- Advance warnings.
- Improve accountability and responsiveness of regulatory system.

13.3.1.2.4 Obligations in the SPS Agreement
- Notification of draft SPS regulations.
- Designation of National Notification Authority.
- Establishment of National Enquiry Point.
- Publication of SPS regulations.

13.3.1.2.5 Specific Trade Concerns of SPS Agreement
- Highly pathogenic avian influenza (HPAI)
- Bovine spongiform encephalopathy (mad cow disease).
- Veterinary drug maximum residue limits (MRLs).
- Foot and mouth disease.
- African swine fever.
- Delays in approval procedures for meat and dairy products.
- COVID-19 related restrictions.

13.3.1.3 Codex Alimentarius Commission Mandate
- To protect the health of consumers.
- To ensure fair practices in international food trade.
- To coordinate all food standardization work done by international organizations.

13.3.1.4 Codex Committee on Residues of Veterinary Drugs in Foods
- To determine priorities for the consideration of residues of veterinary drugs in foods.
- To recommend maximum levels of such substances.
- To develop codes of practice.
- To consider methods of sampling and analysis for the determination of veterinary drug residues in foods.

13.4 Epidemiology and Risk Analysis

Risk analysis and regionalization are crucial to the interaction between epidemiology and international trade. Animal health risk analysis depends on epidemiological information; without it, the process would just be a random, biologically incoherent game of chance (Zepeda et al., 2001).

Hazard identification, risk assessment, risk management, and risk communication constitute the various steps in the process of animal health risk analysis. Its goals are to determine any potential risks related to a commodity, evaluate the likelihood of its introduction, establishment, and spread within the importing nation, and calculate any potential repercussions from that introduction (OIE, 1999). Risk analysis has been used formally and informally for many years in veterinary services, despite the fact that it is a relatively new analytical approach (Figure 13.1).

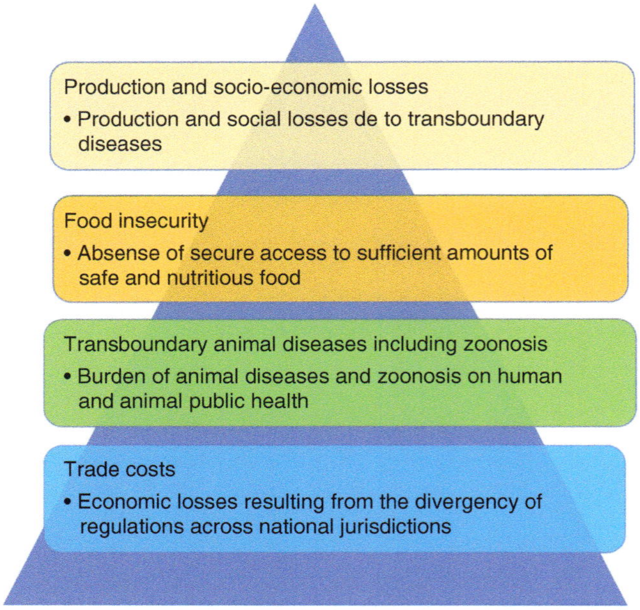
Production and socio-economic losses
• Production and social losses de to transboundary diseases
Food insecurity
• Absense of secure access to sufficient amounts of safe and nutritious food
Transboundary animal diseases including zoonosis
• Burden of animal diseases and zoonosis on human and animal public health
Trade costs
• Economic losses resulting from the divergency of regulations across national jurisdictions

Figure 13.1 Unsafe and unfair trade.

In accordance with the SPS Agreement, the International Plant Protection Convention (IPPC) for plant health issues and the Codex Alimentarius Commission (Codex) for food safety both received comparable mandates. One of the basic tenets of the SPS Agreement is that the OIE's standards should be founded on research and have as their primary goal the protection of human and animal health without placing unrealizable restrictions on trade. This crucial provision must be respected in trade negotiations by nations who have signed the SPS Agreement and are also OIE members (Bruckner, 2004).

Therefore, countries are encouraged to implement the minimal requirements, recommendations, and guidelines established by the OIE and, whenever possible, incorporate them into their national legislation. Should an importing nation require a level that is higher than the OIE requirements advised for trade purposes, it must be supported by science and be based on an analysis of the risks associated with the import (World Trade Organisation, 1995). OIE standards are already the result of a risk assessment by default, therefore they typically do not need to go through the process again for trade-related purposes.

The Terrestrial Animal Health Code and the Aquatic Animal Health Code of the OIE contain the standards to be applied in the international trade in terrestrial and aquatic animals and their products. These standards are democratically adopted by members of the OIE after debate by specialist ad hoc groups under the guidance of the OIE Specialist Commissions: the Scientific Commission for Animal Diseases, the Biological Standards Commission, the Aquatic Animal Health Standards Commission, and the Terrestrial Animal Health Standards Commission.

Standards are revised and updated on a continuous basis. The companion complementary volumes, the OIE Manual of Diagnostic Tests and Vaccines for Terrestrial Animals (OIE, 2008) and a similar manual for aquatic animals, specify reference techniques for diagnosing animal diseases, tests that are prescribed and recommended for trade purposes, and export certification and quality requirements for vaccines for specific animal diseases. While the focus of this chapter will mainly be on animal health issues related to terrestrial animals, the same principles apply to aquatic animals.

The OIE standards reflect a horizontal and a vertical dimension. The horizontal standards are described in Volume I and vertical standards in Volume II of the 2008 edition of the Code. Horizontal standards are those describing generic aspects, such as ethics in international trade or the quality of national veterinary services, a *sine qua non* condition for importing countries to trust the reliability of health certificates accompanying consignments of animals and products in cross-border trade. These certificates must be issued exclusively by the veterinary services under the full responsibility of the government of the exporting country.

Other guidelines and recommendations to facilitate trade are also described in the Code, such as procedures for pathogen inactivation; disposal of carcases and dead animals; recommendations for disinfection and transport of animals by land, air or sea; identification and traceability of animals and products; requirements for border control and quarantine stations; import risk analysis; equivalence; obligations and ethics in international trade; zoning and compartmentalization; transfer of biological material and other animal welfare considerations such as slaughter of animals.

13.5 Concepts of Disease as Trade-facilitating Measures

As a consequence of the above, the idea of safe commodity trade has been incorporated into the Code, which includes provisions allowing for the unrestricted trade of items like milk and milk products, semen, hides and skins, gelatin and collagen from hides and skins, and deboned skeletal muscle from cattle younger than 30 months from countries with BSE (OIE, 2008).

The same theory holds true for matured, deboned bovine meat that has had its pH lowered to below 6 in order to protect it against the FMD virus. Expanding on this idea as a trade-facilitating approach for other OIE-listed diseases would require more study.

However, adopting a strategy that relies entirely on the systematic inactivation of viruses in the products would be foolish and irresponsible and would lead to Members reducing their animal disease surveillance efforts and their policies for the prevention and management of possible biological disasters. The benefits of animal health policies for reducing poverty and improving public health provide an adequate reason for funding and sustaining surveillance networks and quick response systems to deal with threats and risks to animal health.

It is a nonnegotiable requirement that all Members adhere to OIE criteria for the quality and evaluation of veterinary services in order to ensure the efficacy of surveillance at national, regional, and global levels. The trustworthiness of the veterinary certificates they issue is another duty of the veterinary services in addition to their surveillance role. These certifications are included with every shipment of animals or animal products shipped around the world.

In order to ensure that granting everyone access to regional and global markets will not jeopardize the security of international trade, compliance with OIE standards for a country's quality of veterinary services ensures that these certificates are issued under circumstances that guarantee their dependability.

13.6 Conclusion

In order to compete in the global market for trade in animals and animal products, developing nations are under increasing pressure to enhance the quality of their veterinary services. The demands made on developing nations by mostly developed nations to adhere to international disease prevention standards have also led to an increase in the demands made on these developing nations' human, financial, and technological resources.

The OIE is committed to facilitating and promoting the international trade in animals and animal products for all its Members as much as is possible within the limits of its resources, in accordance with the mandate set forth in the Agreement on the Application of SPSs of the WTO and the mandate given to the OIE by its International Committee. This goal cannot be accomplished quickly; it requires patience and a logical, scientific approach to decision making in the future.

References

Brückner, G.K. (2004). Working towards compliance with international standards. *Revue Scientifique et Technique* 23: 95–107.

OIE (1999). *75 Years 1924 ± 1999*. Paris: Office International des Epizooties.

OIE (2008). *Terrestrial Animal Health Code*, 17e. Paris: Office International des Epizooties.

World Trade Organization (1995). *The Results of the Uruguay Round of Multilateral Trade Negotiations: The Legal Texts: Agreement on the Application of Disease Control and Phytosanitary Measures*. Geneva: World Trade Organization.

Zepeda, C., Salmana, M., and Ruppanner, R. (2001). International trade, animal health and veterinary epidemiology: challenges and opportunities. *Preventive Veterinary Medicine* 48: 261–271.

14

Comparative Epidemiological Studies

Maninder Singh and Jay P. Yadav

Department of Veterinary Public Health and Epidemiology, College of Veterinary Science, Guru Angad Dev Veterinary and Animal Sciences University, Rampura Phul, India

14.1 Introduction

In populations, diseases do not occur randomly. There are exposures/factors/determinants which are responsible for the occurrence of disease. Therefore, the study and identification of exposures responsible for disease/outcome are at the core of epidemiology. The determination and establishment of exposures responsible for occurrence of disease help in establishment of causality of disease/outcome.

Every epidemiological study aiming to identify the factors of disease and its control and prevention starts with the descriptive epidemiology, in which the data are collected on the "who," "when," and "where" of the disease. This information and other collected data help in identification of exposures/factors which are further evaluated for causality or association between exposure and disease (even if causality is not confirmed). This step is called analytical epidemiology and involves comparison of the exposure and outcome in different groups of participants to determine the relative occurrence and association.

This chapter describes the various studies used in analytical epidemiology. Before proceeding further, it must be understood that in these studies, "comparison" is the core component, i.e., the study compares the exposure and outcome in different groups. Based upon the differences in occurrences of exposure and outcome in the groups, the association between exposure and outcome or causality is established.

In epidemiology, studies are basically categorized into two types: observational study and experimental study. Observational studies are further divided as indicated in Figure 14.1.

14.2 Observational Studies

Observational studies have gained their name as the exposure and outcome are observed in study participants under natural conditions. The investigator does not have control over exposure and thus cannot alter it but rather collects the data from the study participants in field conditions.

Observational studies are further categorized into cohort studies, case–control studies, and cross-sectional studies.

14.2.1 Cohort Study

A cohort study begins with the selection of participants based on exposure. At the initiation of the study, some participants will have exposure and others will not; both types are followed over a period of time to evaluate for the occurrence of the outcome of interest (Setia 2016a). The outcome may occur only once (e.g., death) or multiple times (e.g., diarrhea). This type is called a "prospective cohort study" (Figure 14.2).

Another type of cohort study is called a "retrospective cohort study" in which the outcome has already occurred in the past. But essentially the study design of a retrospective cohort study is the same as that of the prospective cohort study. Therefore, the investigators start with the exposure at the baseline in the past and follow up to collect the data on the

---

Epidemiology and Environmental Hygiene in Veterinary Public Health, First Edition. Edited by Tanmoy Rana.
© 2025 John Wiley & Sons, Inc. Published 2025 by John Wiley & Sons, Inc.

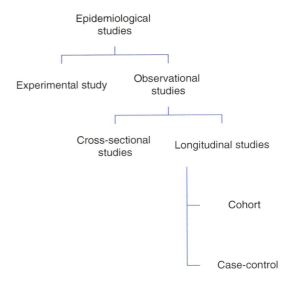

Figure 14.1 Classification of epidemiological studies.

outcome. As the information is retrieved from the past, the retrospective study is useful only if past records are available. As a cohort study involves a time period, it is a type of longitudinal study. In general terms, the study answers the question "what will happen?"

The prospective cohort design is most suitable for studying rare exposures while the retrospective cohort design is useful in studying rare outcomes. Further, the prospective design is time-consuming and expensive while retrospective studies, as the outcome has already occurred, are relatively quick and inexpensive. Another advantage of the retrospective cohort study is that multiple exposures can be studied simultaneously. However, the retrospective design has one major limitation of "recall bias," i.e., there is every possibility that the participants will not be able to recall the exposures being studied. Also, the composition of study participants may not be representative of the population and thus the retrospective design may not be suitable to establish causality. In the prospective cohort study, the temporality associated with exposure and disease gives a better indication of the causality. Further, the prospective cohort study is most suitable in multiple outcomes to a given exposure.

Cohort studies are helpful in determination of cumulative incidence (incidence risk) and incidence rate for the outcome in the population. The data obtained by the exposure followed by the outcome are analyzed for their association by relative risk (also called "risk ratio"). Relative risk is the comparison of risk of outcome in the exposed group with the risk of outcome in the unexposed group. The calculation of relative risk is shown in Figure 14.3.

In Figure 14.3, $(a/a+b)$ is the risk of disease in the exposed group, also called the incidence of disease in the exposed group. $(c/c+d)$ is the risk of disease in the unexposed group, also called the incidence of disease in the unexposed group.

- Relative risk is >1 when the risk of disease in exposed individuals, i.e. $(a/a+b)$, is higher than the risk of disease in unexposed individuals, i.e. $(c/c+d)$. This means that the exposure actually increases the occurrence of disease. If relative risk is 2, this means that the risk of disease in the exposed group is twice the risk of disease in the unexposed group.
- Relative risk is <1 when the risk of disease in the exposed individuals, i.e. $(a/a+b)$, is lower than the risk of disease in unexposed individuals, i.e. $(c/c+d)$. This means that the exposure actually prevents the occurrence of disease and therefore is beneficial.
- Relative risk = 1 when the risk of disease in exposed individuals, i.e. $(a/a+b)$, is equal to the risk of disease in unexposed individuals, i.e. $(c/c+d)$. This means that the exposure does not have any impact on disease.

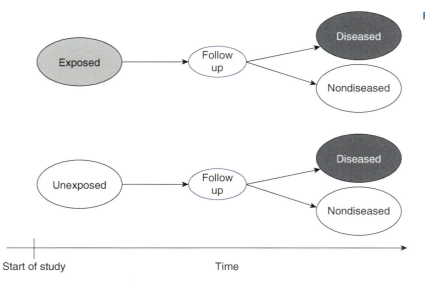

Figure 14.2 Cohort study design.

Some examples of cohort studies from research articles in the veterinary field are given below.

14.2.1.1 Prospective Cohort Study

Van Cleef et al. (2015) identified the transmission of livestock-associated MRSA from pigs to pig farmers using a prospective cohort design in The Netherlands; 171 household members on 49 farrowing pig farms were study participants. The study confirmed the transmission and carriage of livestock-associated MRSA in pig farmers in the study period.

	Disease +	Disease –
Exposure +	a	b
Exposure –	c	d

Relative Risk = Risk of disease in the exposed group/Risk of disease in the unexposed group

Relative Risk = {(a/a+b)/(c/c+d)}

Figure 14.3 Calculation of relative risk in cohort study.

14.2.1.2 Retrospective Cohort Study

In a study by Chaters et al. (2018) in Kenya, the investigators analyzed the impact of foot and mouth disease (FMD) on the fertility of the cattle. The herd in which the FMD outbreak (i.e., exposure) had occurred in the past was selected. The data on fertility in the FMD-infected animals and noninfected animals were collected and analyzed. It was found that the age at first calving was 2.7 months higher in the FMD-infected group than the noninfected group, reducing the production lifespan in the former. Also, conception rates were poorer in the former than the latter. The study expected the losses to be lower in the vaccinated group than the nonvaccinated group.

14.2.2 Case–control Study

A case–control study is a type of longitudinal study which starts with the participants being selected based on the outcome. The participants with outcome (called cases) and without outcome (called controls) are selected and assessed for exposure in the past (Setia 2016b) (Figure 14.4). Therefore, the study is inherently retrospective in nature. In general language, the study answers the question "what happened?" To identify the cases, case definition should be as specific as possible. The participants in the control group should be from the same study population. To make sure that cases and controls are similar in certain characteristics and to control confounders, matching in respect of certain criteria, e.g., genetics, farm management, is often used in case–control studies.

The advantages of the case–control study are that as it is inherently retrospective in nature, it is relatively fast and inexpensive. It is appropriate for rare diseases and diseases with long latent periods. Further, multiple exposures can be examined at the same time. The case–control study is very commonly used in outbreak settings involving shorter incubation periods. The disadvantage of this type of study is that it is not a good design for rare exposures and multiple outcomes. The study design is prone to selection bias, recall bias, and observation bias. Moreover, it is difficult to determine the prevalence of disease as the population being exposed is not available as the participants have been selected on the basis of outcome.

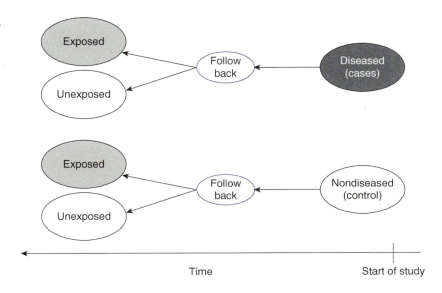

Figure 14.4 Case–control study design.

14 Comparative Epidemiological Studies

Odds Ratio = Odds of disease in the exposed group/Odds of disease in the unexposed group

Odds Ratio = (a/c)/(b/d) = ad/bc

Figure 14.5 Calculation of odds ratio in a case–control study.

For the same reason, relative risk to determine the association between the exposure and the outcome cannot be calculated; instead, the odds ratio is calculated as indicated in Figure 14.5.

The interpretation of the odds ratio is same as that of relative risk.

- Odds ratio is >1 when the odds of disease occurrence in exposed individuals is higher than the odds of occurrence of disease in unexposed individuals.
- Odds ratio is <1 when the odds of disease occurrence in exposed individuals is lower than the odds of disease occurrence in unexposed individuals.
- Odds ratio = 1 when the odds of disease occurrence in exposed individuals is equal to the odds of disease occurrence in unexposed individuals.

For example, Chimera et al. (2022) studied FMD outbreaks which occurred in Malawi and Tanzania from 1957 to 2019 using a matched case–control study. The study was conducted to determine the spatiotemporal pattern and risk factors associated with FMD in the region. A higher density of cattle, goats, and pigs was positively associated with risk of FMD in the region and had an odds ratio ˃1.

In case of outbreak settings, whenever multiple exposures are investigated, the attributable fraction for each exposure is calculated to identify the exposure responsible for the outbreak. The exposure for which the attributable fraction is close to 100% has the greater chance for being the main exposure factor for the outbreak. Attributable fraction is calculated as below:

$$\text{Attributable fraction}: \left\{\left(a \,/\, a+b\right)-\left(c \,/\, c+d\right)\right\} / \left(a \,/\, a+b\right)$$

In hospital settings, frequently a case–case study is adopted instead of a case–control study. For example, if we want to study diarrhea caused by enterohemorrhagic *Escherichia coli* in dogs, diarrhea caused by other infectious agents in the dogs in the same hospital will be selected as a control in place of healthy dogs. Further, a case–control–case study design may also be conducted in such settings.

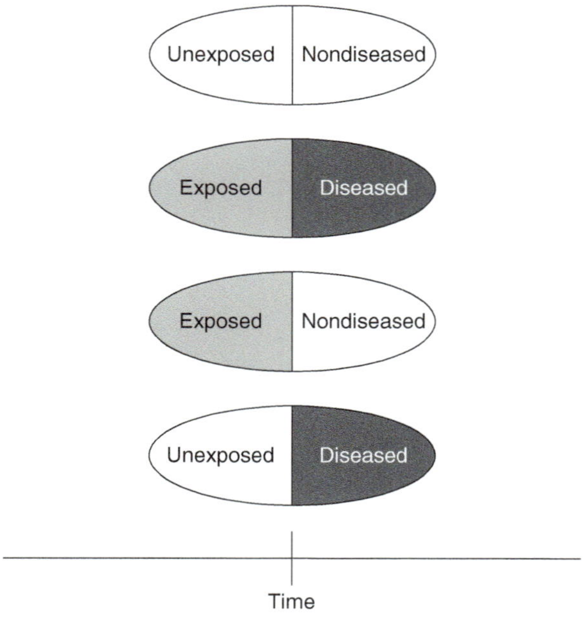

14.2.3 Cross-sectional Study

In the cross-sectional study, the investigator measures the outcome and exposures in the study participants at the same time. Participants are selected based on certain inclusion and exclusion criteria (Setia 2016c). The selected participants are investigated further for exposure and disease at the same time (Figure 14.6). This study design is most suitable for population-based surveys and therefore is helpful in determination of prevalence of exposures and diseases in populations. The information collected from this study may help in designing future cohort studies to confirm causality. In general language, the study answers the question "what is happening?" In a cross-sectional study, the prevalence odds ratio is calculated to determine the association between exposure and outcome. Mathematically, the prevalence odds ratio is the same as the odds ratio.

Figure 14.6 Cross-sectional study design.

For example, Fonseca et al. (2023) did a cross-sectional study in Canadian dairy herds to investigate the impact of use of intramammary and systemic antimicrobials on the *Escherichia coli* isolated from fecal samples, The study found that the *E. coli* isolates from animals with antimicrobial exposure had 18% higher odds of being resistant to any antimicrobial than those not receiving antimicrobials.

A cross-sectional study is useful for public health planning, monitoring, and evaluation of control programs as it is relatively fast and inexpensive. However, cross-sectional study design is poor in establishing causal relationships and cannot calculate the incidence of a disease.

14.3 Experimental Study

In epidemiology, this would be better called an "interventional study" as vaccines, drugs, or medical devices are frequently used exposures in experimental settings to calculate their intervention attributes. In an experimental study, unlike observational studies, the investigator has the discretion to change the exposures between groups and follow for the differences in outcome between groups. Experimental studies are helpful in proving causality or evaluating different interventions.

One of the most commonly used experimental studies is the clinical trial. Clinical trials are generally randomized and are called randomized controlled clinical trials in which the investigator randomly distributes the exposure to the study participants. To prevent the biases associated with allotment of exposures and selection bias, single-blind (participants are unaware of the type of intervention assigned) and double-blind (both investigator and participants are unaware of the type of intervention assigned and to whom assigned) methods are adopted. Nonrandomized community trials are adopted for mass interventions such as impact of vaccination on disease prevalence.

14.4 Biases Associated with Epidemiological Studies

Bias is the "systematic deviation of results or inferences from truth or the processes that lead to such deviation" (Merck Veterinary Manual). There are multiple sources in a study which can introduce bias and thus false results. As it is difficult to completely avoid bias in a study, investigators try to minimize their effects.

The different sources of bias in a study are explained below.

- *Selection bias*: occurs in a case–control study when the selected controls are not truly representative of the population from which cases are selected.
- *Recall bias*: occurs when the study participants do not remember the exposure correctly. It is significant in case–control and retrospective cohort studies in which the information on exposures is collected from previous times. Frequently, cases remember exposures better than the controls.
- *Observation bias*: associated with the investigator as the investigator does not correctly record exposures and/or outcomes in the study participants.
- *Confounding*: a very important reason for bias in epidemiological studies, confounding occurs when a variable different from the exposure and outcome leads to an association between the exposure being studied and disease. Such a variable is called a "confounder" and is statistically associated with both exposure and disease, due to which it leads to a spurious association between the exposure and disease, even when in fact such an association does not exist. For example, parity of cattle can be a confounder for locomotor disorders, which can make a spurious association between other variables such as high milk yield and locomotor disorders.

14.5 Conclusion

The choice of epidemiological study is based on the aim of the study, time period, and resources available. Retrospective designs are relatively fast and inexpensive but prospective designs are better for studying rare exposures. Cross-sectional designs are good for population-based surveys. Relative risk and odds ratio are the measures used to determine association between exposure and disease.

References

Chaters, G., Rushton, J., Dulu, T.D., and Lyons, N.A. (2018). Impact of foot-and-mouth disease on fertility performance in a large dairy herd in Kenya. *Preventive Veterinary Medicine* 159: 57–64.

Chimera, E.T., Fosgate, G.T., Etter, E.M.C. et al. (2022). Spatio-temporal patterns and risk factors of foot-and-mouth disease in Malawi between 1957 and 2019. *Preventive Veterinary Medicine* 204: 105639.

van Cleef, B.A., van Benthem, B.H., Verkade, E.J. et al. (2015). Livestock-associated MRSA in household members of pig farmers: transmission and dynamics of carriage, a prospective cohort study. *PLoS One* 10 (5): e0127190.

Fonseca, M., Heider, L.C., Stryhn, H. et al. (2023). Intramammary and systemic use of antimicrobials and their association with resistance in generic Escherichia coli recovered from fecal samples from Canadian dairy herds: a cross-sectional study. *Preventive Veterinary Medicine* 216: 105948.

Setia, M.S. (2016a). Methodology series module 1: cohort studies. *Indian Journal of Dermatology* 61 (1): 21–25.

Setia, M.S. (2016b). Methodology series module 2: case–control studies. *Indian Journal of Dermatology* 61 (2): 146–151.

Setia, M.S. (2016c). Methodology series module 3: cross-sectional studies. *Indian Journal of Dermatology* 61 (3): 261–264.

15

Clinical Trials, Diagnostic Testing, and Risk Analysis

Negin Esfandiari[1] and Mohammadreza Najafi[2]

[1] *Department of Food Hygiene and Quality Control, Division of Epidemiology, Faculty of Veterinary Medicine, University of Tehran, Tehran, Iran*
[2] *Department of Pathobiology, Faculty of Veterinary Medicine, Urmia University, Urmia, Iran*

15.1 Clinical Trials

A planned experiment conducted on volunteers in their regular setting is known as a controlled trial. These studies must be carefully planned and carried out because they frequently involve client-owned animals and because of their size and scope, it would be exceedingly challenging to reproduce them in order to confirm the results.

The evaluation of easily manipulable interventions, such as therapeutic or preventive items, diagnostic techniques, and animal health programs, benefits particularly from controlled trials. The majority of trials are designed to evaluate a single intervention, and this is actually where they excel (Figure 15.1).

The result could be a measure of productivity, performance, or lifespan, or it could be a specific health characteristic (such a clinical condition, for example). The research groups are made up of individuals, herds, or other groupings and are created by randomly assigning the intervention(s) under evaluation. Controlled trials are frequently referred to as clinical trials. However, some authors limit its application to clinical trials and/or tests of therapeutic products.

There are two measures of validity for clinical trials: internal and external. The degree to which conclusions from a study are applicable to the sample of patients being studied is referred to as *internal validity*. The extent to which research findings can be extrapolated to the entire population from which the sample was chosen, such as the target group, is known as *external validity* (also known as generalizability).

Internal validity is the primary prerequisite for external validity; for example, incorrect conclusions from a clinical experiment will also be incorrect when applied to a larger group of patients. However, if study participants are not representative of the general patient community, a study may yield valid results but still lack external validity.

Comparison of two "treatment arms" – a group receiving the treatment and a control group not receiving it – is a crucial component of a clinical trial with good design. A concurrent control group is chosen at the same time as the group getting treatment, whereas a historical control group is created using data from the past. Typically, concurrent control groups are recommended.

The control group may be given a different (standard) treatment to which the first treatment under trial is being compared (a "positive" control group), no treatment (occasionally referred to as a "negative" control group), or a placebo (a substance with no therapeutic effect that is visually similar to the treatment under trial so that those administering and receiving the treatment and placebo cannot distinguish one from the other).

15.1.1 Case Definition

The selection of patients who fit the case definition is the first step in a clinical trial. It is not as simple as it might seem at first. A set of clinical symptoms that includes all actual cases of a disease while excluding associated but unrelated disorders may be challenging to describe. Few patients would exhibit the whole spectrum of disease signs and symptoms; as a

---

Epidemiology and Environmental Hygiene in Veterinary Public Health, First Edition. Edited by Tanmoy Rana.
© 2025 John Wiley & Sons, Inc. Published 2025 by John Wiley & Sons, Inc.

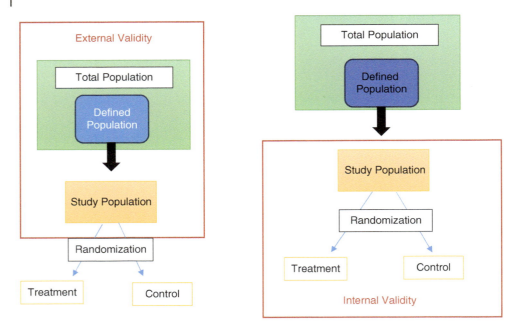

Figure 15.1 External and internal validity of a clinical trial.

result, minimal diagnostic criteria must frequently be defined. The case definition grows increasingly more stringent and encompasses a decreasing number of instances as the number of signs and symptoms needed to meet it rises. Additionally, when several clinics are involved, the case definition criteria should be applied consistently.

When subjects are incorrectly assigned to categories (such as cases or controls, or exposure status), misclassification bias – a type of information bias – occurs. This might be caused, for instance, by a diagnostic test's insufficient sensitivity and/or specificity or by inadequate data gathered from medical or other records.

15.1.2 Selecting the Controls

15.1.2.1 Historical Controls

We might make use of historical controls, a comparison group from the past. We currently have a therapy that we think would be quite beneficial, and we would like to test it in a group of patients; however, we are aware that a comparison group is necessary. We will thus go to the records of patients with the same condition who received treatment prior to the release of the new medicine in order to compare.

This kind of design seems basic and appealing by nature. There are, however, several issues with using historical controls (Figure 15.2). First, if we start the trial now, we can collect patient data extremely carefully. However, we cannot accomplish that for past patients whose medical records we must abstract. Clinical, not research, records were created. Thus, if at the end of the study we find a difference in outcome between patients treated in the early period (historical controls) and patients treated in the later period (current), we will not know if the difference was due to a difference in data quality or a true difference in outcome. In historical control studies, study group data are typically not comparable.

The second issue is that ancillary supportive therapy, living conditions, nutrition, and lifestyles change over time, so we cannot be sure that a difference in outcome between the early and later groups is due to the therapy. Thus, if we see a difference and rule out data quality differences, we will not know if the difference is due to the intervention we are studying or to changes in numerous other things throughout calendar time.

This design can be useful, though. When a disease is always fatal and a new medicine becomes available, a drop in case fatality that parallels drug use strongly suggests that the drug is working. However, it is still possible that environmental factors caused the fall.

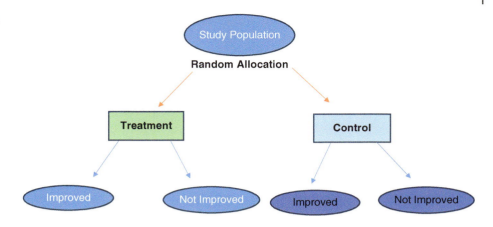

Figure 15.2 Designing of a clinical trial.

15.1.2.2 Simultaneous Nonrandomized Controls

There are various methods that could be used to choose controls in a nonrandomized manner. One method is to group patients according to the day of the month on which they were admitted to the hospital. The assignment system in this case is predictable, and doctors may be able to forecast what the following patient's assignment will be. As such knowledge raises the possibility of bias on the part of the researcher regarding the treatment group to which each participant will be assigned, the goal of randomization is to eliminate the possibility that the researcher will know what the assignment of the next patient will be.

15.1.2.3 Random Allocation

Randomized controlled trials, in which patients are assigned at random to treatment and control groups, are the most effective technique to evaluate the particular effects of a clinical intervention. Randomization is used to ensure that all prognostic factors are distributed equally among the treatment and control groups. If there are few patients, the researcher can determine whether randomization has been achieved by comparing the distribution of a few patient characteristics between the groups.

15.1.2.4 Stratified Randomization

Patients may be randomized separately within each stratum if specific patient features are known to be associated with prognosis. Patients may then be divided into groups (called strata) with comparable prognoses.

The likelihood of unequal cohorts during the randomization process is decreased by prior stratification, even though it is possible to stratify after the data have been collected analytically.

15.1.3 Specifying the Intervention

The intervention's nature must be made crystal clear. For evaluating new items, a fixed intervention (one without flexibility) is appropriate. For products that have been in use for some time and for which there is a body of knowledge that has been utilized in clinical settings, a more lenient methodology may be suitable.

When possible, the initial treatment assignment should be kept a secret to prevent clinical judgments from being impacted by group assignment.

If participants are going to be in charge of some or all of the interventions, it is imperative that they have clear instructions on how to administer or implement the intervention. Additionally, a means of monitoring the intervention administration process should be established, and the system for ensuring that the right therapy is administered to the right animal must be kept as straightforward as feasible.

15.1.4 Inclusion and Exclusion Criteria

There must be established eligibility and admittance requirements for the use of animals in trials. These should be included in the protocol and contain a clear description of the disease for which the treatment is being evaluated and the standards for determining the condition's diagnosis. The opposite of inclusion criteria is exclusion criteria. Avoid using too many exclusion criteria or you will risk compromising external validity. It might be wise to account for some aspects either during the analysis or in the trial design through stratification.

15.1.5 Cross-over Design

Each person in a cross-over trial receives both therapies (in sequence). The initial intervention, however, is still chosen at random. This method is only appropriate for therapy evaluations if the subject's condition is stable and the duration of the intervention effect is minimal. Between procedures, there might need to be a "wash-out" phase. Since the same individual receives both levels of the intervention, it has the advantage of increasing the study's power.

15.1.6 Factorial Designs

Trials examining two or more interventions are especially well suited to this design, especially if there is a chance that the therapies will work in concert or in opposition to one another. The study patients are given access to every potential combination of treatments (e.g., neither treatment, treatment 1 only, treatment 2 only, and both treatments). The treatment effects are typically not confounded (i.e., they are unrelated to or orthogonal to the intervention) and the analyses are simple because the designs are typically balanced. Normally, one should not try to evaluate more than two or three therapies because it becomes difficult to interpret any potential relationships.

15.1.7 Cluster Randomized Trials

In a cluster (group) randomized trial, the experimental unit is a group of people, and the groups themselves – rather than the people who make up those groups – are assigned at random.

15.1.8 Community Trials

In a community trial, the entire community serves as the experimental unit. Human medicine has conducted many community experiments, such as fluoridating the public water supply to reduce tooth cavities.

15.1.9 Multicenter Trials

A multicenter trial may need to be planned if there are insufficient subjects at one location. The necessity to take into consideration within- and between-center differences is a crucial component. Although a multicenter trial complicates the protocol and execution of the trial, it can improve the generalizability of the results (because the trial typically covers a larger geographic area) and also increases the opportunity to identify interaction effects (such as different responses by center). A strategy for statistical efficiency in multicenter trials is to keep the number of individuals per center roughly constant.

15.1.10 Superiority, Equivalence, and Noninferiority Trials

Trials of superiority are intended to identify differences between treated and untreated groups. In these trials, efficacy is firmly established but sometimes, comparisons of two therapies are made without trying to show which is superior. Equivalence studies may be used to show that, within specified bounds, the effects of each treatment are equivalent.

The noninferiority trial, a special case of an equivalence trial, aims to show that a therapy is not worse than an established one. This is typical in early therapeutic effect trials, where it is frequently desired to show that a new treatment is not inferior to (i.e., equal to) a known preparation, while it may also be equivalent to or superior.

15.1.11 Follow-up and Compliance

Making sure that all groups are followed strictly and equally is a crucial step. While a brief observation period after the intervention makes this procedure easier, it must be lengthy enough to guarantee that all relevant outcomes have been observed and recorded. No matter how much time and effort is put into follow-up, some participants will inevitably leave the research due to drop-out or noncompliance. Therefore, especially for studies with lengthy follow-up periods, it is important to periodically check in on the progress of all research participants.

Regular communication with all participants is crucial for limiting study losses. There may be incentives to continue participating in the study. It is important to make an attempt to ascertain whether study participants are adhering to the protocol in addition to optimizing retention in the study.

Participants must follow the trial designers' instructions, or adhere to therapy, in order for a trial to be successful; this is called *compliance*. Poor compliance will limit the trial's statistical power.

15.1.12   Masking or Blinding

The use of masking (or blinding) is essential in the fight against bias in controlled trials. The phrases single, double, and triple blindness are not consistently used, which is unfortunate.

In a single-blind study, the participant is not aware of the nature of the intervention used on specific study participants. This feature should ensure that subjects in the various intervention levels receive equal follow-up and supervision. A double-blind study is one in which the intervention assignment is kept a secret from the participant as well as a few members of the study team (i.e., those in charge of delivering the interventions and evaluating the results). This characteristic aids in ensuring that subjects receiving various levels of intervention are evaluated equally. In a triple-blinded trial, those analyzing the data are likewise blinded to the treatment that each group underwent. This feature is intended to guarantee that the analysis is carried out objectively.

It is frequently necessary to utilize a placebo to make sure that the important people continue to be blind. A placebo is a substance that is given to animals in the groups assigned to receive the comparative treatment and is identical to the substance being tested. In many drug trials, the placebo simply serves as the drug's delivery system but contains no active substance.

15.1.13   Assessment of Outcome

The number of primary outcomes in a controlled trial should be no more than one or two, and the number of secondary outcomes should be no more than three. The objectively measurable outcomes are preferred when choosing the outcomes to be measured, while the latter cannot always be avoided.

Per-protocol or intent-to-treat analysis is possible. An intent-to-treat analysis includes data from all subjects assigned to a certain intervention, regardless of whether they completed the trial or followed the protocol. As indicated, such an analysis will yield a cautious assessment of the intervention's effect, but it may reflect the expected response when employed in a similar group. Per-protocol analyses contain only patients who followed the procedure and completed the study. This approach may measure response if the intervention is implemented as planned, but it will likely bias future intervention effect estimates for two reasons. First, noncompliance is unlikely to be random, and noncompliers may not be representative of all intervention participants, hence the estimate of effect may be biased. Second, future intervention use will never be 100% compliant, so evaluating an effect under this assumption is unwise.

15.1.14   Informed Consent and Other Ethical Considerations

Owners of animals enrolled in a trial should be informed of the trial's goals and overall plan, and their willingness to participate should be recorded before the research actually starts. This is a case of informed consent. In previous veterinary studies, this has been poorly reported.

Although veterinary schools and research institutes frequently include ethical review committees that can evaluate informed consent, veterinary professionals and other potential clinical trial participants might not have access to these reviews. However, a number of official veterinary organizations have proposed ethical criteria for the conduct of research in regular veterinary practice, including clinical trials.

The ethical criteria for controlled trials of pharmaceuticals and medical treatments on animals have two main parts. The first is an ethics review conducted by a board that is concerned with the participants' ethical treatment, and the second is a review conducted by an animal welfare committee that is concerned with the welfare of the animal subjects. Each country will have its own specific rules and laws.

15.1.15   Limitations of Clinical Trials

The primary constraint is financial; clinical trials are typically expensive to conduct because it may be necessary to screen several animals in order to find one that meets all inclusion criteria and none of the exclusion criteria, and it typically becomes expensive to maintain animals in particular conditions in order to control exposure. To control all potential risk factors and scenarios that could affect the outcome, they typically need solid records. However, they are the best option to prove a causal relationship between a potential risk factor and an outcome.

15.1.16 In Practice

The best method currently available for evaluating the efficacy of treatment is randomized controlled clinical trials. The bulk of therapeutic questions are, however, resolved through alternative methods, particularly uncontrolled and nonrandomized trials, due to several practical constraints. The majority of case reports and uncontrolled clinical studies are primarily driven by the urge to deliver some type of treatment.

15.2 Diagnostic Testing

The Greek words *dia* (apart) and *gignoskein* (to recognize or know) are where the word "diagnosis" originates. In its simplest form, diagnosis refers to the capacity for differentiation or discrimination. Therefore, a diagnostic test is any tool or process that can distinguish between a diseased person and a person who does not have a disease.

15.2.1 The Quality of a Test

The capacity of a test to deliver precise and accurate results while avoiding measurement errors is referred to as its quality. Many diagnostic tests have important measurement error limitations which could be brought on by the measurement tool, the operator, or both.

15.2.1.1 Accuracy
A test's accuracy is its capacity to recognize the actual (true) value. By calibrating the tool or the user, accuracy can be increased.

15.2.1.2 Precision
The ability of a test to function consistently while using the same sample multiple times is known as precision. By measuring the same sample more than once and using the average of those measurements as the outcome, precision can be increased (Figure 15.3).

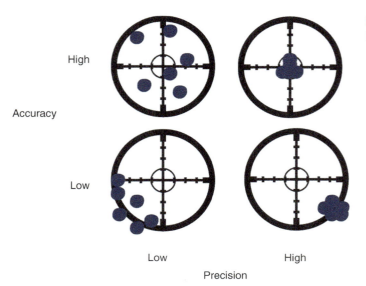

Figure 15.3 Graphical representation of accuracy and precision of a diagnostic test.

15.2.1.3 Sensitivity

Sensitivity is a test's capacity to identify truly positive animals, or the capacity to accurately diagnose affected animals. The percentage of people with an illness (denominator) who respond positively to the diagnostic test (numerator) is the formula use to determine a test's sensitivity.

$$Sensitivity = \frac{True\ positive}{True\ positive + False\ negative}$$

15.2.1.4 Specificity

The ability of a test to accurately identify unaffected animals, or the capacity to identify truly negative animals, is known as specificity. The percentage of unaffected animals (denominator) that respond negatively to the diagnostic test (numerator) is the formula used to determine a test's specificity.

$$Specificity = \frac{True\ negative}{True\ negative + False\ positive}$$

The accuracy of the positive outcomes is referred to as sensitivity, and the accuracy of the negative results is referred to as specificity. As a result, both are markers of how well a test performs in terms of correctly classifying a patient as affected or unaffected. The better the test, the higher the sensitivity and specificity. Over 90% sensitivity and specificity are regarded as high and relevant test results.

When testing an animal, professionals want to know how certain they can be of the outcome. How likely is it, in other words, that an animal with a positive test genuinely has the illness or that an animal with a negative test is actually unaffected? The positive predictive value (PPV) and negative predictive value (NPV), respectively, provide this information.

15.2.1.5 Positive Predictive Value

Positive predictive value determines the likelihood of an animal to truly be affected if it has a positive test. To put it another way, it examines the percentage of test-positive animals (denominator) that are actually affected (numerator).

$$PPV = \frac{TP}{TP + FP}$$

15.2.1.6 Negative Predictive Value

The NPV expresses the probability that an animal that tests negative is actually unaffected. In other words, the percentage of test-negative animals (denominator) that are actually unaffected (numerator) is examined.

$$NPV = \frac{TN}{TN + FN}$$

Clinicians may choose to run several tests simultaneously or sequentially to prevent potential issues caused by the use of unreliable tests.

15.2.1.7 Parallel Testing

Parallel testing refers to the simultaneous administration of two or more tests to detect the same condition. In this case, if any test yields a positive result, the animal is deemed to be affected. Because more genuine positive animals will be found using this method, the testing process will be more sensitive. The high percentage of false-positive animals, which rises with repeated tests, is a drawback of this testing methodology. Additionally, the method of testing is expensive because all animals go through all diagnostic procedures.

15.2.1.8 Serial Testing

When testing in series, an initial test is carried out first, and a follow-up confirmatory test is only carried out if the initial test yields the desired result (positive or negative). As only some animals are subjected to many tests, this lowers overall expenses while simultaneously improving the overall testing's specificity. Screening is a specific kind of serial testing in which a first diagnostic test is carried out to separate affected and unaffected people as much as feasible.

15.2.2 Reliability of Tests

The issue of a test's repeatability or reliability is another consideration when evaluating diagnostic and screening procedures. No matter how sensitive and specific a test is, if the results cannot be replicated, the test's value and use are obviously poor. The factors that affect test result variability are intrasubject variation (variation within a single subject), intraobserver variation (variation within a single reader's interpretation of test results), and interobserver variation (variation between different readers' interpretations of test results).

15.2.2.1 Intrasubject Variation

Many times, even over a short period of time, the numbers acquired when measuring certain attributes change. It is obvious that this, along with the circumstances in which some tests are performed, may cause varied outcomes in the same person. As a result, while analyzing any test results, it is crucial to take into account the testing environment, including the time of day.

15.2.2.2 Intraobserver Variation

Readings of the same test findings provided by the same observer can often differ from one another. The extent to which subjective elements influence the observer's judgments varies between tests and examinations, and the bigger the subjective component in the reading, the more likely it is that there will be intraobserver variation in the readings.

15.2.2.3 Interobserver Variation

Variation between observers is another crucial factor. Often, two examiners do not arrive at the same conclusion. An essential consideration is the degree to which observers concur or disagree.

15.2.3 In Practice

No matter how sensitive and specific a test may be, if the results cannot be repeated, the test is not very useful. Therefore, when assessing such tests, it is important to take into account all these factors mentioned as well as the intended use of the test.

Animal populations with certain diseases are subjected to diagnostic tests (most notably herds and flocks). Therefore, before a testing plan is created or the results can be properly interpreted, it is important to understand the features of each disease.

15.3 Risk Analysis

Risk analysis is a formal process for determining the probability and consequences of unfavorable outcomes in a particular group, while taking into account exposure to probable hazards and the nature of their impacts. This includes the control (typically reduction) of exposure likelihood.

15.3.1 Definition of Risk

Risk is the likelihood of an event happening and how damaging it would be for the environment and human (and animal) health.The possibility that an event will take place and the severity (i.e., the impact, magnitude, or seriousness) of the consequences of that occurrence are the two components that make up risk. The latter can range from being somewhat harmless to being disastrous.

"Very low," "low," "medium," and "high" are popular classifications for risk in qualitative descriptions. Additionally, risk can be classified as "negligible" or "nonnegligible" (usually understood to be "below very low"). It is also possible to utilize descriptions that blend elements from each of these levels.

A quantitative explanation frequently concentrates on likelihood, which is the possibility that an event (exposure to a hazard) will occur during a predetermined period of time.

Risk does not indicate an existing issue or a determined conclusion. It is the potential of future harm. Consequently, it cannot be measured, only estimated.

Today, risk analysis is used to address a variety of veterinary difficulties. Import risk analysis is a significant area. The possibility of importing diseases from other nations exists even though they may exist in low numbers and be effectively controlled (or eradicated).

Food safety risk analysis is the second important branch of veterinary risk analysis. Most food safety risk analyses, as opposed to import risk analyses, relate to domestic issues, with an emphasis on the processes used in food production and risk reduction or mitigation measures. In import risk assessments, risk is typically expressed in terms of likelihood while severity is not considered. This frequently occurs because it may be challenging to assess severity.

Nowadays, rather than solely depending on the rather subjective assessments of individual scientists or parties, veterinary risk analysis has emerged to analyze the hazards associated with certain diseases as objectively as possible.

15.3.2 Components of Risk Analysis

Following the OIE (2013) guidelines, there are four main components of import risk analysis: hazard identification, risk assessment, risk management, and risk communication. For food safety risk analysis, the recognized guidelines were published by the Codex Alimentarius Commission (CAC) (1999) which will be explained below.

15.3.2.1 Hazard Identification

The definition of hazards (such as a pathogen) is known as hazard identification. Sometimes published information may help with this, but more often it involves careful reading of the literature and discussions with experts and those who could be affected by the risks. In food safety risk analysis, hazard identification is part of risk assessment (Figure 15.4).

15.3.2.2 Risk Assessment

The steps in the OIE framework are:

- *entry assessment*: determination of the likelihood of a commodity (e.g., an imported animal) being contaminated or infected with hazards, and a description of the pathways by which the hazards can be introduced into the environment
- *exposure assessment*: the estimation (qualitatively or quantitatively) of the magnitude, frequency, duration, and route of exposure of humans or animals to hazards
- *consequence assessment*: similar to hazard characterization. However, it also can include indirect effects
- *risk estimation*: descriptions of the nature and magnitude of risk, either to health or to the environment.

The steps in the CAC framework are:

- *hazard identification*
- *hazard characterization*: qualitative or quantitative evaluation of the nature of the adverse health effects associated with hazards
- *exposure assessment*: the estimation (qualitatively or quantitatively) of the magnitude, frequency, duration, and route of exposure of humans or animals to hazards
- *risk characterization*: descriptions of the nature and magnitude of risk, either to health or to the environment.

In both situations, thorough examination of the pertinent literature is required, and formal metaanalysis may be conducted in addition to expert opinion gathering.

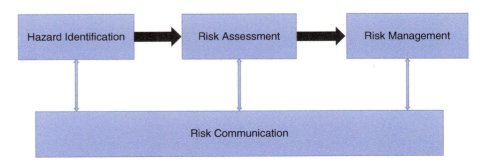

Figure 15.4 Components of risk analysis.

15.3.2.3 Risk Management

Risk management is the process of choosing risk control strategies while taking into account social norms, legal obligations, and cost considerations. It is not about decisions that will be made in the future but rather about decisions that must be made now, specifically about speculative or unclear aspects of decision outcomes.

Construction of a risk matrix (probability impact matrix), which evaluates risks according to their two components – likelihood and severity of consequences – can be used to prioritize management.

15.3.2.4 Risk Communication

The goal of risk communication is to inform and facilitate discussion among all interested parties (such as legislators, the general public, and livestock owners) about the hazards and risks. Given that risk analysts' perceptions of risk frequently differ from those of the general public, risk communication is crucial.

Risk communication should not come last. When establishing the hazard and the risk question as well as developing the strategy for the entire risk analysis, it is crucial to take into account how the results of the risk assessment will be communicated. If not, the activity might be pointless.

15.3.2.5 Qualitative or Quantitative Assessment?

In today's society, when a degree of intellectual superiority is frequently associated with numerical outputs, there may be a temptation to believe that a quantitative assessment is "better" than a qualitative one. However, the majority of risk assessments are suited for qualitative evaluation, which is also the most popular type of assessment to support everyday decisions.

Quantification could be necessary to examine a problem more thoroughly and evaluate different control strategies. This requires building a mathematical model, which comes with challenges related to data quality and availability, selection of suitable statistical distributions, assumptions, and validation.

15.3.2.6 Acceptable Level of Risk

In order to implement effective risk management methods, the outcomes of risk assessments must be meaningfully interpreted. The latter implicitly depend on the accepted level of risk (or, more precisely, on the options that involve a particular amount of risk).

As a result, determining acceptable levels of risk is complicated, and should take into account psychological and economic considerations. This demonstrates that social, economic, and political factors, rather than scientific ones, are typically taken into account when deciding the acceptable amount of risk.

15.3.3 In Practice

The limitations of risk analysis, which could raise more problems than answers, should be understood by veterinarians. Risk analyses may produce inaccurate conclusions, and the dangers and processes that are the subject of the analysis typically involve some degree of uncertainty.

However, risk analysis can be a useful tool for identifying and managing risk in many veterinary medicine areas rather than trying to implement a "zero-risk" strategy that is not adaptable to new information, changing economic conditions, and changing political demands.

References

Codex Alimentarius Commission (CAC) (1999). *Principles and Guidelines for the Conduct of Microbiological Risk Assessment.* Rome: FAO.

OIE (2013). *Chapter 2.1. Risk analysis. In: Terrestrial Animal Health Code*, 12e. Paris: World Animal Health Organisation.

Further Reading

Dohoo, I.R., Martin, S.W., and Stryhn, H. (2009). *Veterinary Epidemiologic Research.* VER, Inc.

Gordis, L. (2013). *Epidemiology E-Book.* St Louis: Elsevier Health Sciences.

Smith, R.D. (2020). *Veterinary Clinical Epidemiology: From Patient to Population.* Boca Raton: CRC Press.

Thrusfield, M. and Christley, R. (2018). *Veterinary Epidemiology.* Hoboken: Wiley.

Villarroel, A. (2015). *Practical Clinical Epidemiology for the Veterinarian.* Hoboken: Wiley.

16

Observational Studies

Ashemi Yusuf[1], Amitava Roy[2], and Tanmoy Rana[3]

[1] *World Bank Regional Disease Surveillance System Enhancement Project, Abuja, Nigeria*
[2] *Department of Livestock Farm Complex, West Bengal University of Animal & Fishery Sciences, Kolkata, India*
[3] *Department of Veterinary Clinical Complex, West Bengal University of Animal & Fishery Sciences, Kolkata, India*

16.1 Introduction

Veterinarians, epidemiologists, and academics are very interested in learning what factors contribute to diseases and how we may prevent or lessen their negative impacts. To accomplish this, we must determine the most effective research strategy. The type of study selected will depend on the objectives of the study and the context in which it will be conducted. Our goal is to compile as much relevant data as we can to help us make wise choices. Avoiding reliance on inaccurate, outdated, or biased information is important. But not all studies are equally trustworthy.

A hierarchy of research evidence can be used to decide which evidence to include when answering a particular question. The evidence in the lower levels of this hierarchy is based on the opinions of a small number of people, whereas the evidence in the upper levels is derived from carefully designed studies that are less likely to be affected by biases. As a result, the designs near the top of the pyramid offer the most convincing evidence, while they are frequently rarer than those at lower levels. Observational studies seem to fall somewhere in the middle of the hierarchy but it is crucial to remember that a study's conception, execution, and analysis determine its level of quality. For making precise and reliable judgments about causes or relationships, these criteria are essential. Even though every study design presents its own set of difficulties, without proper planning and reporting, studies could inadvertently suggest erroneous relationships.

Based on a straightforward enquiry: "Did the researcher deliberately change population parameters or randomly allocate factors (disease or hypothesized risk factors) to animals and assess the effect on disease occurrence?," epidemiological study designs can be broadly divided into two categories. If the response is "Yes," the design will be experimental. If the response is "No," the design is observational, and this chapter will center on that.

Therefore, studies in the experimental category involve an intervention, such as the manipulation of a study factor (treatment, exposure) with or without control and randomization of participants to the factor (treatment, exposure) groups, while studies in the observational category include those that do not involve any intervention or experiment.

16.2 Objectives and Application of the Strengthening the Reporting of Observational Studies in Epidemiology (STROBE) Statement

A paper reporting on one of the three primary study designs used in analytical epidemiology – cohort, case–control, or cross-sectional – should follow the guidelines of the STROBE Statement. These suggestions are not guidelines for planning or carrying out studies; rather, they serve as direction on how to describe observational research effectively. Additionally, even though clear reporting is a requirement for evaluation, the checklist is not a tool to assess the caliber of observational research.

The STROBE Statement is presented here along with an explanation of its creation. We provide justification for the inclusion of the many checklist items, methodological background, and published instances of what we consider transparent

---

Epidemiology and Environmental Hygiene in Veterinary Public Health, First Edition. Edited by Tanmoy Rana.
© 2025 John Wiley & Sons, Inc. Published 2025 by John Wiley & Sons, Inc.

reporting in a thorough companion study, the Explanation and Elaboration piece (Vandenbroucke et al., 2007). We strongly advise using the STROBE checklist in conjunction with the explanation piece, which is freely available on the websites of PLoS Medicine, Annals of Internal Medicine, and Epidemiology (www.epidem.com).

16.2.1 STROBE Components

A list of 22 factors known as the STROBE Statement is thought to be necessary for accurate reporting of observational research (Table 16.1). These refer to the title and abstract of the article (item 1), the methods (items 2 and 3), the results (items 13–17), and the discussion sections (items 18–21), as well as extra information (item 22 on funding). While four items (6, 12, 14, and 15) are design specific and have various variations for all or part of the item, there are 18 items that are shared by all three designs. Information should be provided separately for exposed and unexposed groups in cohort and cross-sectional studies, or for cases and controls in case–control studies, for specific items (marked by asterisks). Despite being offered here as a single checklist, the STROBE website also offers separate checklists for each of the three study designs.

16.2.2 Observational Study Design

The objective of an observational study design is to carefully examine the distribution of an exposure (the factor being studied) and/or an outcome of interest (the disease or effects or results being observed) without purposefully influencing or interfering with the natural course of events.

Unlike experimental studies, which are simple and involve the researcher deliberately controlling how the study subjects are assigned to different groups, they may expose some to a particular risk factor while keeping others from it, or they may assign some to receive a new treatment while keeping others from receiving it. Things are typically more complicated in observational studies than they are in experiments, particularly when it comes to researching animals. The researcher makes a thorough plan before setting out to determine how frequently an illness or medical condition occurs. To find potential risk factors for an illness, they may also examine patterns of exposure (such as being exposed to specific substances) with the occurrence of diseases. Studying how environmental elements like air pollution affect horses' respiratory issues is one instance. The researcher would study several herds of horses, gauge their exposure to air pollution, and gauge the frequency of respiratory illnesses. They can ascertain if there is a connection between air pollution and respiratory issues in horses by evaluating the data. In this instance, the researcher takes the role of an observer, gathering data without actively getting involved or changing the variables. To comprehend the link between exposure and disease consequences, they rely on data collection and observation of natural events.

Observational studies have the advantage of allowing us to acquire data or explore a variety of variables that may affect results. Furthermore, whether or not the study is done, the subjects are frequently already unavoidably exposed to the risk factor under investigation. This means that instead of deliberately exposing a certain group of study participants to the risk factor, researchers can look into the impact of these naturally occurring exposures.

An investigator may perform an observational study for one of three general purposes: to discover relationships, to forecast an outcome, or to identify possibly causative associations. Cross-sectional, cohort, and case–control observational designs are the three most popular types.

The various kinds of observational studies that can be used by researchers studying animal health will be given a general overview in this chapter. It is crucial to remember that each of the several observational study designs we will be discussing has its own advantages and disadvantages. You should briefly mention these restrictions as you investigate them.

16.2.3 Cross-sectional Study

One significant category of observational study design that is frequently confused with surveys is cross-sectional studies. Cross-sectional studies go beyond surveys, which typically concentrate on the distribution and prevalence of diseases over time and space, and among individuals. These studies assess the presence or absence of disease and potential risk factors in a random sample of animals drawn from a larger population at one particular period. This method enables the simultaneous measurement of outcomes and risk factors. The study begins with no knowledge of the animals' exposure to particular risk factors or the existence of a specific disease. As the investigation develops and the animals are examined or evaluated, these specifics are identified. Cross-sectional studies therefore assess prevalence.

16.2 Objectives and Application of the Strengthening the Reporting of Observational Studies in Epidemiology (STROBE) Statement

Table 16.1 The STROBE statement: checklist of matters to be covered in observational study reports.

	Item number	Recommendation
Title and abstract	1	a) In the title or abstract, mention the study's design using a popular phrase.
		b) Give an informed, balanced account of what was done and what was discovered in the abstract.
Introduction		
Background/ rationale	2	Describe the scientific context and justification for the reported study.
Objectives	3	Describe your precise goals and any established hypothesis.
Methods		
Study design	4	Early in the text, highlight the important study design components.
Setting	5	Describe the context, the places, and the pertinent times, such as the recruiting, exposure, follow-up, and data collecting periods.
Participants	6	a) Cohort study – explain the eligibility requirements, as well as the sources and procedures used to choose participants. Describe the follow-up procedures. Give the eligibility requirements, sources, and procedures used to determine the case and choose the control in a case–control study. Explain why you chose the cases and controls you did.
		Give the eligibility requirements, as well as the sources and procedures used to choose participants, for a cross-sectional study.
		b) Cohort study – provide matching criteria and the number of exposed and unexposed subjects for matched studies.
		Give matching criteria and the number of controls per case for matched case–control studies.
Variables	7	All outcomes, exposures, predictors, potential confounders, and effect modifiers should be precisely defined. Describe the diagnostic standards, if any.
Data sources/ measurement	8^a	Provide information on data sources and evaluation (measurement) procedures for each variable of interest.
		If there are multiple groups, explain how assessment methods are comparable.
Bias	9	Describe any initiatives made to address potential bias sources.
Study size	10	Describe how the study size was determined.
Quantitative variables	11	Describe the methods used to handle quantitative variables in the analyses. Describe the classifications that were chosen, if relevant, and why.
Statistical methods	12	a) Describe all statistical techniques, including confounding correction techniques.
		b) Outline any techniques applied to study subgroups and interactions.
		c) Describe how any missing data were accounted for.
		d) If appropriate, describe how loss to follow-up was handled in the cohort trial.
		Describe how the matching of cases and controls was handled in a case–control study, if relevant.
		Cross-sectional study – if appropriate, describe analytical procedures, taking sampling technique into consideration.
		e) Provide any sensitivity analysis descriptions.
Results		
Participants	13^a	a) Describe the numbers of participants at each step of the trial, including those who were possibly eligible, were eligible, and were not eligible.
		Determined to be eligible, included in the study, followed up with, and analyzed.
		b) State the grounds for your absence at each stage.
		c) Take into account using a flowchart.

(Continued)

Table 16.1 (Continued)

	Item number	Recommendation
Descriptive data	14[a]	a) Describe the study participants' characteristics (e.g., demographic, clinical, and social) and provide details on exposures and potential risks.
		b) List the number of individuals for whom each relevant variable has missing data.
		c) Cohort study: compile follow-up time information (such as the average and overall amount).
Outcome data	15[a]	Report the number of outcome events or summary measures over time for a cohort study.
		Reporting statistics for each exposure category or exposure summary measures in a case–control study
		Cross-sectional study: indicate the number of outcome instances or summary metrics.
Main results	16	a) Provide unadjusted estimates, confounder-adjusted estimates, if necessary, and their accuracy (for example, a 95% confidence range). Report category boundaries when continuous variables were categorized.
		b) Clearly state which confounders were adjusted for and why they were included.
		c) If applicable, take into account converting estimates of relative risk into absolute risk for a significant time period.
Other analyses	17	Report any further analyses that were performed, such as sensitivity analyses, analyses of subgroups and interactions.
Discussion		
Key results	18	Summarize the main findings in relation to the study's goals.
Limitations	19	Talk about the study's limitations while considering any possible bias or imprecision sources. Discuss any potential bias's magnitude and direction.
Interpretation	20	Give a cautious general interpretation of the data taking into account the aims, constraints, variety of analysis, and results from comparable studies. Deaths and other pertinent information.
Generalizability	21	Discuss how broadly (externally valid) the study's findings can be applied.
Other information		
Funding	22	Give the funding source and the sponsors' roles for the current study and, if applicable, the initial research on which this article is based.

Note: The STROBE checklist is best used in conjunction with this article.

[a] Give such information separately for cases and controls in case–control studies, and, if applicable, for exposed and unexposed groups in cohort and cross-sectional studies.

Cross-sectional studies allow researchers to actively investigate a number of risk factors at once, which is useful for comprehending complicated phenomena that are influenced by a number of factors. To ascertain the relevance of each element, however, it may be necessary to carry out intricate statistical analysis. It is common practice to employ cross-sectional study designs as a starting point for a preliminary analysis of suspected health-related factors. They act as a foundational step or starting point for performing subsequent study designs in the greater hierarchy of evidence. For example, if a link between a certain disease and an exposure is found in a cross-sectional study, this knowledge can be used to build cohort or case–control studies to further explore and determine if the link is causal or not.

16.2.4 Randomized Controlled Trials

The criteria for inclusion in the study sample must be stated at the beginning of a randomized controlled trial (e.g., in terms of age, sex, diagnosis, etc.). Similar to other epidemiological studies, the subjects chosen for this one should be an accurate representation of the population to which the findings will be applied. A reliable guidance to managing the less severe forms of the illness encountered in general practice may not be provided by a comparison of two treatments for rheumatoid arthritis in a group of hospital patients. Subjects who meet the entrance requirements are prompted to provide their permission to participate. How much the remaining volunteers may be said to represent the target population must be determined when the refusal rates are high. For instance, they might be generally younger than the refusers. Is this significant in light of the research question?

The comparator therapies are then randomly assigned to the participants who agree to participate. You can accomplish this by using published random number tables or computer-generated random numbers. Randomization is frequently done in blocks when patients enter the study sequentially (for example, as they are admitted to the hospital). Therefore, patients may be randomly assigned in blocks of six in a trial that compares two therapies, A and B. Three of the initial six participants in the trial would be randomly assigned to undergo treatment A and three to receive treatment B. In each subsequent batch of six patients, treatments would be distributed using a similar method. The benefit of this approach is that it avoids significant imbalances in patient numbers receiving various therapies, which might occasionally happen by accident. Additionally, it makes sure that the proportion of each treatment stays generally consistent throughout the trial, minimizing the possibility of confounding by external variables that fluctuate over time.

Major outcome factors can occasionally be discovered when people first enroll in a study. For instance, the presence of specific dysrhythmias at the time of hospital admission may be a significant indicator of outcome in a trial of treatment for acute myocardial infarction. Because of the randomization method, these prognostic indicators will typically be distributed equally among the various treatment groups. However, there is the option to stratify subjects at entrance according to the prognostic variable (for example, differentiating patients with and without dysrhythmias), and then randomly assign individuals individually within each stratum in blocks as an additional measure of protection against unintentional confounding.

It may be preferable for those in charge of management to be "blinded" to which treatment has been assigned when the result is influenced by other facets of a patient's management in addition to the therapies being compared. However, preparations must be made to enable quick deblinding if treatment-related issues arise. The criteria for removing a patient from therapy should, to the extent practicable, be laid out in advance. However, the clinical team responsible for the patient must have the final say. Even if a patient withdraws from an experimental treatment, follow-up care and outcome evaluation should continue. Trial endpoints range from more subjective sensations and physical indications to more objective outcomes like hemoglobin concentration or birth weight.

By keeping the assessor unaware of the course of therapy, bias in the evaluation of subjective outcomes can be avoided. For instance, using a pharmacologically inactive placebo as a comparison may be useful when evaluating a new migraine analgesic based on reported levels of symptoms. Otherwise, there is a chance that patients will think they are getting something better just because it is new. Similarly, it is advisable to keep the examiner in the dark regarding which patient received which treatment if the end goal is a subjective bodily indicator (such as the severity of a skin rash). It is critical to monitor both potential negative effects and the results that treatment is meant to improve. While the treated group in a trial of the cholesterol-lowering medication clofibrate exhibited a lower incidence of nonfatal myocardial infarction, their overall mortality was higher than that of the untreated controls. This higher than average mortality could not be traced to a single cause of death, but may have been caused by unanticipated therapeutic side-effects. Readers interested in learning more about the techniques employed should consult a more in-depth work because the statistical analysis of randomized controlled trials is too complex to be covered in a book of this length.

Regardless of the analytical method used, it is crucial to compare participants in accordance with the therapy to which they were randomly assigned, even if this treatment was not finished. It might not even have been started in other circumstances. Otherwise, the negative effects of selective therapy cessation might go unnoticed. In one trial, for instance, participants were removed from medication if they experienced severe heart failure, a potential side-effect of beta-blockers, in an effort to lower mortality following myocardial infarction. Patients with more serious infarcts and consequently worse prognoses were more likely to get cardiac failure as a result of the experimental medication. It would be anticipated that fewer of these people will get cardiac failure while taking a placebo. Any benefits from the beta-blocker would have tended to be falsely inflated if the withdrawals had been left out of the analysis. Examining results in light of the actual treatments used at the same time is also beneficial. If only those who chose not to receive the treatment were to profit from randomization, that would raise suspicions.

On the basis of calculated statistical power, the size of a randomized controlled trial may be selected in advance. These calculations, which work best when done in partnership with a medical statistician, call for specification of the expected distribution of outcome measures as well as the difference in outcomes between treatments that is worth finding. This strategy has a drawback in that the trial may go on after enough information has accumulated to demonstrate that one treatment is unmistakably superior. As a result, some patients would unnecessarily receive inadequate care. Monitoring the trial's findings at regular intervals with predetermined criteria for calling a halt if one treatment seems obviously superior is one way to get around this problem.

16 Observational Studies

The requirement to seek participants' agreement after being given adequate notice presents another issue with randomized controlled trials. Some patients find it difficult to comprehend why a doctor would choose to treat patients at random as opposed to using their best judgment. Due to this challenge, a different design has been developed that might be used to compare a novel treatment to traditional care. All patients who meet the entrance requirements are randomized, and those who are assigned to conventional treatment are given normal care. Those assigned to the new treatment are asked to agree to this but, if they decline, they will receive standard care. Thus, the requirement for randomization explanation is removed. However, two vulnerabilities must be set up in opposition to this. First, the prime analysis follows randomization, just like in any experiment that uses randomization. Differentials in outcomes might be hidden if a sizable minority of patients reject the new therapy. Second, neither the patient nor the clinical team may be made ignorant of the course of treatment. The nature of the study and the endpoints being measured will determine how important this constraint is.

16.2.5 Experimental Population Research

However, it is also possible to conduct experimental interventions at the level of populations. Individual participants are typically divided into treatment groups in experimental research, and these groups are then compared.

Interventions can be distributed randomly in populations, just like in studies of people. Randomization might not be very useful if there are only a few populations being compared. In order to achieve the greatest possible comparability between various intervention groups, it could be preferable to assign interventions in a purposeful and planned manner. Comparing the study and control populations before and after the intervention can help to increase the control of residual confounding.

Experimental research is typically time-consuming and expensive, much like longitudinal studies. Consequently, it should not be started without a valid reason. It does offer the most convincing proof of cause and effect, however, if well planned and executed.

16.3 Limitations and Consequences of STROBE

The STROBE Statement was created to support writers when they write up analytical observational studies, editors and reviewers when they contemplate publishing such papers, and readers when they critically evaluate published articles. Through an open approach, the checklist was created while taking into consideration the knowledge gathered from other efforts, particularly CONSORT. Researchers examined the pertinent methodological studies and empirical research, and thoroughly iteratively consulted on each subsequent draft. Thus, the checklist provided here is the result of input from numerous people with various backgrounds and viewpoints. This consultation process had a significant positive impact on the explanatory piece (Vandenbroucke et al., 2007), which is meant to be used in conjunction with the checklist.

According to Vandenbroucke et al. (2007), observational studies have a variety of uses, ranging from the discovery of novel results to the support or denial of earlier findings. Some research is purely exploratory and generates intriguing theories. Others look for evidence to support clearly defined hypotheses. Another sort of study meticulously plans the collecting of fresh data on the basis of an existing premise. Since readers always need to know what was planned (and what was not), what was done, what was discovered, and what the results signify, the current checklist can be helpful for all of these research types. The CONSORT statement currently has four extensions (Gagnier et al., 2006). The STROBE Extension to Genetic Association research (STREGA) effort (Ioannidis et al., 2006) is the first extension to STROBE for gene–disease association research. To prevent effort duplication, anyone looking to expand on the STROBE Statement should get in touch with the coordinating committee first.

The STROBE Statement should not be taken as an attempt to impose a fixed framework on the reporting of observational research. The checklist items should be covered somewhere in the article in sufficient length and with clarity, although the sequence and format in which they are presented rely on the author's preferences, the journal's style, and the customs of the research field. Consider discussing the reporting of findings under a number of different headings, while keeping in mind that authors may discuss a number of headings in a single section of text or in a table. Additionally, item 22, which deals with the source of funding and the function of funders, could be covered in an appendix or in the article's section on methodologies. Avoid attempting to standardize reporting. An editor of a specialized medical publication requested that authors of randomized clinical trials "CONSORT" their articles before submitting them (Ormerod, 2001). We do not think manuscripts should be "STROBEd," in the sense of dictating vocabulary or style. Encourage writers to incorporate narrative aspects into their works, such as the description of illustrative situations, to enhance the key details of their research and to make the articles more engaging to read (Schriger, 2005).

It should be made clear that the STROBE Statement was not created as a tool for evaluating the caliber of published observational research. Other organizations have created these tools, which were the focus of a systematic review (Sanderson et al., 2007). The Explanation and Elaboration study included a number of examples of good reporting from studies whose findings were not supported by more research; the key aspect was the effective reporting, not the caliber of the research. But if authors and journals use STROBE, problems like confounding, bias, and generalizability might become more transparent. This could help temper the overzealous reporting of new findings in the scientific community and popular media (Bartlett et al., 2002), and enhance the methodology of studies over time. Improved reporting may also make it easier to decide when and what topics should be the focus of future investigations.

STROBE and other recommendations for reporting research are to be viewed as dynamic texts that demand ongoing evaluation, improvement, and, if necessary, modification. One idea for expanding the reach of STROBE is to republish this article in specialized publications and journals that are published in other languages. The coordinating group should be consulted in advance by any organizations or individuals who want to translate the checklist into other languages. In the future, the checklist will be revised in light of feedback, criticism, fresh data, and practical experience. We encourage readers to leave feedback on the STROBE website (www.strobe-statement.org).

References

Bartlett, C., Sterne, J., and Egger, M. (2002). What is newsworthy? Longitudinal study of the reporting of medical research in two British newspapers. *BMJ* 325: 81–84.

Gagnier, J.J., Boon, H., Rochon, P. et al. (2006). Reporting randomized, controlled trials of herbal interventions: an elaborated CONSORT statement. *Annals of Internal Medicine* 144: 364–367.

Ioannidis, J.P., Gwinn, M., Little, J. et al. (2006). A road map for efficient and reliable human genome epidemiology. *Nature Genetics* 38: 3–5.

Ormerod, A.D. (2001). CONSORT your submissions: an update for authors. *British Journal of Dermatology* 145: 378–379.

Sanderson, S., Tatt, I.D., and Higgins, J.P. (2007). Tools for assessing quality and susceptibility to bias in observational studies in epidemiology: a systematic review and annotated bibliography. *International Journal of Epidemiology* 36: 666–676.

Schriger, D.L. (2005). Suggestions for improving the reporting of clinical research: the role of narrative. *Annals of Emergency Medicine* 45: 437–443.

Vandenbroucke, J.P., von Elm, E., and Altman, D.G. for the STROBE Initiative(2007). Strengthening the reporting of observational studies in epidemiology (STROBE): explanation and elaboration. *PLoS Medicine* 4: e297.

17

Nature of Data, Data Collection, and Management

Abbas Rabiu Ishaq

Paws and Claws Specialist Veterinary Clinic, Riyadh, KSA

17.1 Meaning of Data

According to the Cambridge English dictionary, data is a collection of information commonly in the form of numbers or facts that are gathered to be examined/processed. These, when processed, form the basis of making decisions. Data may be an electronic form of information that is stored and processed by a computer. The singular form is *datum*, though the form "data" is commonly seen as an uncountable singular form that requires a singular verb when used in a sentence. Data is a collection of qualitative and quantitative variables (Ajayi 2017). Data is information that is coded into a suitable format for ease of processing (Ajayi 2017).

17.2 Data Curation

This is the continuous process of data management throughout its cycle in order to make it suitable for the primary purpose (Pennock 2007). This comprises content creation, selection, classification, transformation, validation, and preservation (Curry et al. 2010).

17.3 Data Collection

17.3.1 Focus Group

This is a method of data collection whereby the moderator/facilitator discusses with a group of 6–12 persons termed the focus group questions relating to the research topic (Plummer 2017).

17.3.1.1 Advantages of Focus Group Data Collection

Individuals forming the focus group have liberty to deliberate on ideas, making it possible to generate new ideas (Onwuegbuzie et al. 2009). It provides an easy way of gathering information about a topic of interest (Lin et al. 2017) in a relaxed environment, avoiding the tension of person-to-person interviews (Onwuegbuzie et al. 2009). It produces abundant data which can be easily analyzed (Onwuegbuzie et al. 2009)

17.3.1.2 Disadvantages of Focus Group Data Collection

There is the possibility of one individual dominating the discussion, making the information biased. There is need for high skills from moderators which may not always be obtainable (Onwuegbuzie et al. 2009).

Epidemiology and Environmental Hygiene in Veterinary Public Health, First Edition. Edited by Tanmoy Rana.
© 2025 John Wiley & Sons, Inc. Published 2025 by John Wiley & Sons, Inc.

17.3.2 Observation

This is an important data collection tool that uses relatively unstructured approaches (Aktinson and Hammersley 1998) to produce unique insight and introspection. This method fall into three categories: direct observation, participant observation, and unobtrusive observation (Twycross and Shorten 2016).

17.3.2.1 Advantages of Observation

Observation data collection allows collection of many varieties of information such as actions and speech. It gives first-hand information about events (Twycross and Shorten 2016) and captures numerous data to be analyzed (Meriläinen et al. 2010). Collection of digital data format is easy through observation, and this can be subjected to repeated views (Meriläinen et al. 2010). Field notes are easily jotted down (Emerson et al. 2011).

17.3.2.2 Disadvantages

Researchers may face serious ethical challenges (Emerson et al. 2011).

Participant observation is a mode of observation data collection in which the researcher is the subject of the research (Young and Barrett 2001). Its major advantage is that more accurate information is achieved. The drawback arises from the inability of the researcher to be unbiased (Burawoy 1991).

17.3.3 Interviews (In-Depth/Unstructured Interviews)

This is a form of conversation (Lofland and Lofland 1995) to provide knowledge about a specific topic of interest (Rorty et al. 1980). It mimics natural conversations in many aspects, though maintaining the differences between the researcher and participants in terms of roles (Rubin and Rubin 2011).

17.4 Nature of Data

Data can be based on nature/origin/collection methods and classified into primary and secondary. Data can be qualitative or quantitative (Hammersley 2007), small or big (Miller 2010). Small data are usually generated to answer specific research questions by limited volumes, short time intervals, narrowed varieties, and noncontinuity (Kitchin and Lauriault 2015).

17.4.1 Small Data

Small data comes from experiments and is characterized by precision, such as the scores of students in a class for a specific subject (Faraway and Augustin 2018). After acquisition of data, there comes the need to make it easily handled by graphical presentation or frequency tabulation, known as frequency distribution (Gravetter and Wallnau 2000). Frequency tables are organized ways of displaying various observations and the number of times they occur (Gravetter and Wallnau 2000) using arbitrary measures called class intervals (Dawson 2004). The difference between the lower and higher value of the class (class width) is meant to be constant across a given table and should not overlap (Gravetter and Wallnau 2000). These relatively small data can be managed using descriptive statistics or elementary data analysis by any measures of central tendencies and dispersion (Tukey 1977).

17.4.2 Big Data

Big data is a form of information that exhibits massive complexity and variations and presents difficulties in storage, visualization, analysis, and result deductions (Sagiroglu and Sinanc 2013). Big data is seen as an explosion or expansion of information that is readily available for proper coverage (Fan et al. 2018). Stonebraker (2012) defines big data as information having big volume, big velocity, or big variety. It has also been described as data that has a size that makes it part of the problem and outruns traditional analytical techniques.

17.4.2.1 Acquiring Big Data

Lyko et al. (2016) describe the method of acquiring big data in terms of velocity, volume, variety, and value (4Vs). For instance, "velocity" uses a connector layer to gather, convert, and add paralleled data to an index (Asur and Huberman 2010).

Another method is the Oracle, which uses three steps to process data prior to storage in a Hadoop distributed file system (HDFS) or "not only SQL" (NoSQL). The steps are data retrieval and storage in scalable storage (such as HDFS), data reorganization and secondary storage and lastly analysis using analytical algorithms (McAfee et al. 2012).

17.4.2.2 Goals of Analyzing Big Data
- To allow for accurate prediction of future observations.
- To get an idea of the relationship that exists between its characteristics and responses in scientific research (Bickel et al. 2008).
- To allow for exploration of hidden information about subgroups, thus limiting the chances of having outliers.
- Extraction of the most important features shared across substudy groups (Strohbach et al. 2016).

17.4.2.3 Challenges/Constraints of Big Data
Big data poses challenges that are mostly encountered during analysis.

- Because it originates from different sources, statistical bias, heterogeneity, and experimental variations may arise.
- High dimensional approach creates room for unnecessary information/noise and spurious relativities.
- Instability of algorithm and huge computing costs (Strohbach et al. 2016).

17.4.2.4 Uses/Applications of Big Data
17.4.2.4.1 Neurological Sciences
Neuroimaging techniques such as fMRI, electrophysiology, and positron emission tomography offer detailed information about the complex neuronal networks in the brain. This aids in the diagnosis of conditions such as anxiety, attention deficit hyperactive disorder(ADHD), depression, Alzheimer disease, and schizophrenia (Jonides et al. 2006). fMRI is a noninvasive way of producing hundreds of scanned 3D brain images (Visscher and Weissman 2011). These images are shared with databases such as ADHD-200 (HD-200 Consortium 2012) and autism brain imaging data exchange (ABIDE) (Di Martino et al. 2014).

17.4.2.4.2 Economics and Finance
Corporate organizations/businesses use data-oriented mechanisms to provide forecasted information of targeted clients, associated risks, and business efficiency (Cai and Liu 2011a,b; Agarwal et al. 2012). This includes business variants such as transaction records, consumer confidence, stock prices, high-frequency trades, derivative trades, and currency rates (Fan et al. 2018).

One example is trying to analyze the financial and economic panel of a large incorporation with robust variables using the commonly known vector autoregressive (VAR) (Bai 2003; Forni et al. 2005). The analyzer is expected to encounter numerous errors that may make the final output less significant or potentially insignificant (Song and Bickel 2011). Venturing into spatial assumption, which deploys numerous analytical approaches, makes it easier and offers a more reliable output (Han and Liu 2013).

Another instance where a big data approach should be applied is business risk management and optimization of portfolio (Cochrane 2009; Dempster and Thompson 2002). Only 1000 stocks may contain as much as 500 500 co-variance estimates (Fan et al. 2008; Bickel and Levina 2008). Employment of direct and inverse co-variance matrices may limit the chances of error (Stock and Watson 2002; Bai and Ng 2002).

17.4.2.4.3 Genomics
The application of a big data approach in genomics helps biologists to study biological functions, instead of capitalization on the sequences. This helps in unveiling masked rare genetic disorders (Worthey et al. 2011; Chen et al. 2012) and determining the relationship between certain gene sequences and diseases (Cohen et al. 2004; Han and Pan 2010). Another reason for using big data in biomedical imaging is that it allows concurrent monitoring for genes and proteins. This gives first-hand information for the interaction that exists between regulatory proteins and neurological activities (Bickel et al. 2009). Big data in genomics helps in reducing biases (such as batch effect and block effect) that may arise from experimental variations (demographic and environmental) (Leek and Storey 2007).

Public gene data banks such as Gene Expression Omnibus (GEO) and National Center For Biotechnology Information (NCBI) have a stock of over 500 000 gene expression profiles in the form of exon arrays (Liu et al. 2012a), ribonucleic acid sequencing (RNA-seq) and microarrays (Fan et al. 2013, 2018). This makes the formerly cumbersome gene sequencing analysis a bit easier and more comprehensive (Edgar et al. 2002).

17.4.2.4.4 Other Applications of Big Data

This includes social media (Asur and Huberman 2010), internet security, digital books/archives, and personalized medicine (Fan et al. 2018).

17.4.2.4.5 Hidden Characteristics of Big Data

Noise Accumulation   Noise accumulation is the numerous errors encountered during big data collection. This arises because big data takes a wider topic coverage with numerous variables (Donoho 2000; Hastie et al. 2009; Bühlmann and Van De Geer 2011). One way to minimize this noise is by selection of subsets that have the best signal-to-noise ratios, known as sparse modeling (Bühlmann and Van De Geer 2011). Noise accumulation can be caused by spurious correlation, measurement errors, incidental endogeneity, or the heterogeneous nature of big data (Hastie et al. 2009).

Incidental Endogeneity   This is when a predictive variable shows some level of correlation with anticipated residual noise (Engle et al. 1983). This salient feature is encountered when relating certain gene sequences with inheritable disorders (Valiathan et al. 2012). One implication of endogeneity is that it causes inconsistency in selection of models (Fan and Liao 2014).

Spurious Correlation   This happens when random variables that are not correlated turn out to show some sample correlations upon subjection to a high dimension approach (Fan and Lv 2008).

Heterogeneous Nature   The fact that big data originates from various subgroups will give rise to contrasting information for the attached variables (Fan et al. 2018). A better understanding of these co-variations that exist within and between subgroups, such as the beneficial and adverse effects of chemotherapeutic agents, relationship between genes and certain diseases and so on, can only be achieved using big data approaches (Hastie et al. 2009).

17.4.2.4.6 Approaches to Overcome Errors in Handling of Big Data

Independence Screening of Variables   This is employed in extremely high dimension data with high anticipated computational errors that cannot be handled by quasi-likelihood (Fan and Lv 2008). This technique has more comprehensive computational accuracy and theoretical advantages (Genovese et al. 2012; Fan and Song 2010). The idea behind independent variable screening is to use marginal contribution of co-variate to ascertain its importance and remove the least important variables (Fan and Lv 2008; Fan and Song 2010). The limitation of this technique is that it does not use co-variance of matrix of a variable and cannot measure multivariate effects of variables on the response variable (Ke et al. 2014). Independence variable screening can be in the form of nonparametric screening (Fan et al. 2011), principled sure independence screening (Zhao and Li 2012), correlation screening (Hall and Miller 2009), distance correlation (Li et al. 2012a), rank correlation (Li et al. 2012b), and iterative screening (Fan et al. 2009).

Eliminating Incidental Endogeneity   This feature means the commonly used data analysis methods are full of flaws. Dealing with this employs other techniques such as high dimensional linear regression model (Fan et al. 2011), least-square methods (Example Lasso), and focused generalized methods of moments (FGMMs) (Fan et al. 2011).

Using Sparest Solution in Independence Set   This is a more straightforward way of overcoming big data errors compared to penalized quasi-likelihood. It has approaches such as loss of function, likelihood, or quasi-likelihood (Fan 2013). Loss of function is the use of an estimation equation, from which a high confidence set can be derived directly (Liang and Zeger 1986). Another way of estimating sparsity is by recruiting a weighed variable to attain the value of another (Fan 2013) via linear programming discriminant rule and Gaussian graphic model (Cai and Liu 2011a,b; Liu et al. 2012b). The overall aim of this technique is to cope with measurement errors and even endogeneity (Gautier and Rose 2011).

Penalized Quasi-Likelihood   This technique minimizes the chances of recording too much noise while dealing with big data by assigning a target variable through which the anticipated noise can be traced (Akaike 1974). Data analysts employ penalty functions such as soft thresholding penalty (Tibshirani 1996; Donoho and Johnstone 1994), minimax concavity penalty (Zhang 2010), hard thresholding penalty (Antoniadis 1997; Antoniadis and Fan 2001), and smoothly clipped absolution deviation (Fan and Li 2001).

Impacts of Big Data   The impacts (undesirable) seen in big data fall into one of the two categories: infrastructural needs such as hardware specifications or computation (Fan et al. 2014).

Impacts on Infrastructure Demands   The impacts of big data on the infrastructures needed for optimal processing can be overcome by employing Hadoop (also core Hadoop). This comprises HDFS and MapReduce (Shvachko et al. 2010). MapReduce is a programming model, while HDFS is a tool for analyzing, processing and storage of big unstructured data (Dwivedi and Dubey 2014).

MapReduce   This is an easy-to-program and reliable means of handling data sizes of petabytes developed by Google (Dean and Ghemawat 2004). It uses parallel computing to handle up to 10 petabytes in 24 hours (Feldman et al. 2010). A major advantage of MapReduce over other parallel computing methods is that it merges parallel and sequential computation (Kang et al. 2008).

A proper MapReduce class (MRC) will consider the available memory's ability to accommodate the data at hand, number of machines available, and time-frame to completion (Feldman et al. 2010).

Hadoop/Core Hadoop   Hadoop is a Java program for handling clusters of hardware similar to the Google file system. It has the ability to process large data from different computers by enabling parallel processing, thus consuming minimal time and hardware (Honnutagi 2014). HDFS splits big data into smaller portions known as nodes, which are individually processed by different machines, thus limiting encountered errors to a definite one (Honnutagi 2014).

17.4.2.4.7   Architecture of HDFS

A cluster of HDFS consists of a single NameNode for metadata storage, a master server and many DataNodes, known as slaves, for application data storage (Hadoop 2014). Reading data files from HDFS involves six simple steps. This starts with a client clicking the open file system, which triggers the distribution file system to locate blocks of NameNodes. This allows the client to read the input data file stream, second data stream reading, locating best DataNodes, and final closure (Honnutagi 2014).

17.4.2.4.8   Impacts on Computation

Big Data Dimension Reduction and Random Projection   This is a big data preprocessing technique that produces compressed information as it maintains the vital information. This includes principal component analysis (PCA) (Golub and Van Loan 2012), random projection (RP) (Johnson 1984), discrete cosine transform (DCT) (Rao and Yip 2014), and latent semantic indexing (LSI) (Deerwester et al. 1990).

Small Data Storage   This is achieved using magnetic random-access memory (MRAM) (Comstock 2002), floppy disk (Amankwah-Amoah 2016), hard disk drives (Masood and Shyen 2016), compact disks (CD), and magnetooptical (MO) disks (Kawata and Kawata 2000).

Big Data Storage Techniques   This involves the use of highly sophisticated storage databases that use in-memory and columnar storage techniques such as "not only SQL" (NoSQL), MapReduce (MapR), Hortonworks (Andersen and Culler 2016), cloud storage (Yamato et al. 2014), high-density data storage (HDDS) (Li et al. 2010), and Cloudera (Rouse 2014).

17.5   Data Analysis

17.5.1   Measures of Central Tendency

Central tendency helps in recognizing the centrality/central value of sets of data (Bhattacharyya 2017). It is a statistical way of achieving a single value that is a suitable representative of a whole (Manikandan 2011a). The most common methods of measurement of central tendencies are mean (arithmetic mean, harmonic mean, geometric mean), mean deviation, median (Anilkumar and Samiyya 2013), and mode (Bhattacharyya 2017).

17.5.1.1 Mean (Arithmetic Mean)

This is the middle estimation of the various observations in each set of data. It can be reached by adding individual figures $(X_1 + X2 + X3 + X4 + \cdots + X_n)$ and dividing by the number of observations (N). Thus, mean $C = (\Sigma Xn/N)$ for ungrouped/raw data while group data is the summation of the product of observations and their various frequencies, divided by summation of all frequencies/cumulative frequency (Bhattacharyya 2017). Grouped data mean can be calculated using the formula Mean $(\dot{X}) = \Sigma f\chi / \Sigma n$ (where Σ is summation, f is the frequency, n is number of observations, and χ is the mid-point of class interval) (Kaliyadan and Kulkarni 2019).

17.5.1.2 Median

The median is the middle observation when all observations in a data set are arranged in ascending/descending order of magnitude. In other words, it is the 50th percentile (Gravetter and Wallnau 2000) or positional average (Manikandan 2011b). To find the median observation in a set of information, you use the formula $(n + 1)/2$ th for odd numbers of observations and $(n/2 + 1)$ th for even-numbered observations (Gravetter and Wallnau 2000). For example, for a set consisting of five items, the median is the third figure while for a set of six items, the mean is the average of the third and fourth items.

17.5.1.3 Mode

Mode is the observation/value that appears the most in a given data set. It is the value with the highest frequency (Norman and Streiner 2008). A single data set can have more than a single mode in several instances (Kaliyadan and Kulkarni 2019).

Measures of dispersion are statistical tools used to describe the extent of variability. This consists of range, interquartile range, and standard deviation (Manikandan 2011c).

17.5.1.4 Standard Deviation

Standard deviation is a measure of dispersion used to ascertain the spread of data toward the mean. It is calculated using $SD = \sqrt{(\chi - \dot{X})^2} / n - 1$ (Lee et al. 2015).

17.5.1.5 Interquartile Range

Interquartile range is the difference between the first and third quartiles or the difference between the 25 and 75 percentiles (Gravetter and Wallnau 2000).

17.5.1.6 Range

Range of given data is the difference between the smallest and largest observation. It is characterized by ease of calculation and high sensitivity to outliers (Swinscow and Campbell 2002).

17.6 Sample Questions

1 A survey was conducted at the Paws and Claws Specialist Veterinary Clinic, Riyadh, KSA on the types of feeds given to indoor cats. Owners were asked about the feed types they offer due to increased rates of urinary stones seen on radiographs of various cats. A total of 50 cats were targeted; 27 were given only dry feed, 16 were fed a combination of wet and dry, while the rest were maintained on strictly wet food.
   a) Create a table that will make the information condensed and comprehensive.
   b) From the table, deduce the modal feed type used.
   c) Create a pie chart for the information.

2 A survey was conducted to determine the amount of feed taken by cats under hospitalization (irrespective of age and disease condition). A total of 100 cats were considered for a duration of 24 hours and the feed amounts taken by individual cats in grams are as follows.

72	16	51	80	0	42	5
17	23	74	81	35	59	88
19	11	32	18	39	19	66
93	0	15	34	61	28	16
18	36	27	83	15	42	9
47	94	13	46	19	61	53
16	32	68	19	79	32	43
73	0	21	88	43	8	88
33	5	16	71	82	51	15
60	56	24	29	40	93	23

a) Create a standard frequency distribution table with fix class width.
b) Use the table to calculate:
   i) mean
   ii) median
   iii) mode
   iv) first quartile
   v) third quartile
   vi) interquartile range
   vii) standard deviation.
c) Create a histogram.
d) Create a frequency polygon.

17.6.1 Solutions

1 a)

Feed type	Frequency	Sector (degrees)
Dry	27	194.4
Combination	16	115.2
Wet	7	50.4
Total	50	360

b) Dry feed has the highest number of subjects as shown in the table, by definition; dry feed is the mode.
c)

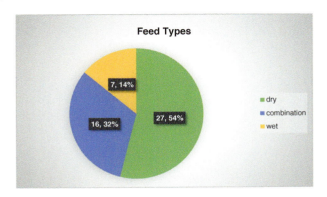

222 | *17 Nature of Data, Data Collection, and Management*

2 a) Class width is the difference between the higher class limit and the lower class limit.
Therefore to find class width $= 9 - 0 = 9$, $29 - 20 = 9$, $99 - 90 = 9$, so 9 is the class width.

Class	F	X	FX	CF	CB	$(X-\bar{X})$	$(X-\bar{X})^2$	$F(X-\bar{X})^2$
0–9	8	4.5	36	8	0–9.5	−37.5	1406.25	11 250
10–19	23	14.5	333.5	31	9.5–19.5	−27.5	756.25	17 393.75
20–29	8	16.5	130	39	19.5–29.5	−25.7	660.49	5283.92
30–39	12	34.5	414	51	29.5–39.5	−9.5	90.25	1083
40–49	9	44.5	400.5	60	39.5–49.5	2.5	6.25	56.25
50–59	11	54.5	599.5	71	49.5–59.5	12.5	156.25	1718.75
60–69	9	64.5	580.5	80	59.5–69.5	22.5	506.25	4556.25
70–79	6	74.5	447	86	69.5–79.5	32.5	1056.25	6337.5
80–89	9	84.5	760.5	95	79.5–89.5	42.5	1806.25	16 256.25
90–99	5	94.5	472.5	100	89.5–99.5	52.5	2756.25	13 781.25
Total	$\sum F = 100$		$\sum FX = 4176$					$\sum 77\,716.92$

b) i) Mean $\left(\bar{X}\right) = \dfrac{\sum FX}{\sum F}$

$$= \dfrac{4174}{100}$$

$$= 41.74$$

$$\bar{X} = 42$$

ii) Median $= \underbrace{L + \left(\sum f\right)/(2-\mathrm{fa})\mathrm{c}}_{f}$

$$= 29.5 + \underbrace{(100/2 - 39)10}_{12}$$

$$= 29.5 + \left(\dfrac{11}{12}\right)10$$

$$= 29.5 + \left(1.22\right)10$$

$$= 29.5 + 12.2$$

$$= 42.1$$

iii) Mode $= L + \left(\dfrac{D1}{D1 + D2}\right)\mathrm{c}$

$$= 10 + \left(\dfrac{15}{15 + 15}\right)10$$

$$= 10 + \left(\dfrac{15}{30}\right)10$$

$$= 10 + \left(0.5\right)10$$

$$= 10 + 5$$

$$= 15$$

iv) First Quartile $Q_1 = L + \left(\dfrac{KN}{4} - CF \right) i$

$$Q_1 = 9.5 + \left(\frac{20 - 8}{23} \right) 10$$

$$Q_1 = 9.5 + \left(\frac{12}{23} \right) 10$$

$$Q_1 = 9.5 + (0.5)10$$

$$Q_1 = 9.5 + 5$$

$$Q_1 = 14.7$$

v) Third Quartile $Q_3 = L + \left(\dfrac{(3)KN}{4} - CF \right) i$

$$Q_3 = 59.5 + \frac{(3)100}{4} = \frac{300}{4} = 75$$

$$Q_3 = 59.5 + \left(\frac{75 - 71}{9} \right) 10$$

$$Q_3 = 59.5 + \left(\frac{4}{9} \right) 10$$

$$Q_3 = 59.5 + (0.44)10$$

$$Q_3 = 59.5 + 4.44$$

$$Q_3 = 62.9$$

vi) Interquartile $(Q3 - Q1)$

$$Q_3 = L + \left(\frac{(3)KN}{4} - CF \right) i - Q_1 = L + \left(\frac{KN}{4} - CF \right) i$$

$$= 59.5 + \left(\frac{75 - 71}{9} \right) 10 - 9.5 + \left(\frac{20 - 8}{23} \right) 10$$

$$= 59.5 + \left(\frac{4}{9} \right) 10 - 9.5 + \left(\frac{12}{23} \right) 10$$

$$= 59.5 + (0.44)10 - 9.5 + (0.5)10$$

$$= 59.5 + 4.44 - 9.5 + 5$$

$$= 62.9 - 14.7$$

$$= 48.2$$

vii) Standard Deviation (SD)

$$\text{Formula} = \sqrt{\frac{\Sigma F \left(X - \bar{X} \right) 2}{\Sigma F}}$$

$$SD = \sqrt{\frac{77716.92}{100}}$$

$$SD = \sqrt{777.1692}$$

$$SD = 27.87$$

c)

Class Interval	Frequency
0–9	8
10–19	23
20–29	8
30–39	12
40–49	9
50–59	11
60–69	9
70–79	6
80–89	9
90–99	5
Total	100

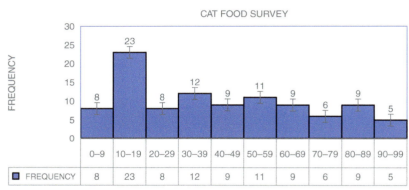

d)

Class Mark	Frequency
4.5	8
14.5	23
24.5	8
34.5	12
44.5	9
54.5	11
64.5	9
74.5	6
84.5	9
94.5	5

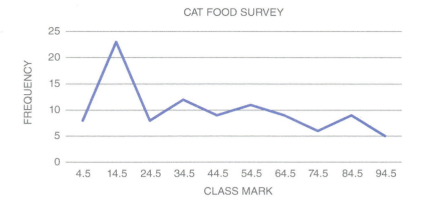

References

Agarwal, A., Negahban, S., and Wainwright, M.J. (2012). Noisy matrix decomposition via convex relaxation: optimal rates in high dimensions. *Annals of Statistics* 40: 1171–1197.

Ajayi, V.O. (2017). Primary sources of data and secondary sources of data. Benue State University. 1 (1): 1–6.

Akaike, H. (1974). A new look at the statistical model identification. *IEEE Transactions on Automatic Control* 19 (6): 716–723.

Aktinson, P. and Hammersley, M. (1998). Ethnography and participant observation. In: *Strategies of Qualitative Inquiry*, 248–261. Thousand Oaks: Sage.

Amankwah-Amoah, J. (2016). Competing technologies, competing forces: the rise and fall of the floppy disk, 1971–2010. *Technological Forecasting and Social Change* 107: 121–129.

Andersen, M. P. and Culler, D. E. (2016). {BTrDB}: optimizing storage system design for timeseries processing. *14th USENIX Conference on File and Storage Technologies (FAST 16)*.

Anilkumar, D.R.P. and Samiyya, N.V. (2013). Refining measure of central tendency and dispersion. *IOSR Journal of Mathematics* 6: 1–4.

Antoniadis, A. (1997). Wavelets in statistics: a review. *Journal of the Italian Statistical Society* 6: 97–130.

Antoniadis, A. and Fan, J. (2001). Regularization of wavelet approximations. *Journal of the American Statistical Association* 96 (455): 939–967.

Asur, S. and Huberman, B. A. (2010). Predicting the future with social media. *2010 IEEE/WIC/ACM International Conference on Web Intelligence and Intelligent Agent Technology*.

Bai, J. (2003). Inferential theory for factor models of large dimensions. *Econometrica* 71 (1): 135–171.

Bai, J. and Ng, S. (2002). Determining the number of factors in approximate factor models. *Econometrica* 70 (1): 191–221.

Bhattacharyya, S. (2017). Measures of central tendency and measures of dispersion in graphical demonstration. *International Multidisciplinary Research Journal* 4.

Bickel, P.J. and Levina, E. (2008). Covariance regularization by thresholding. *Annals of Statistics* 36: 2577–2604.

Bickel, P., Buehlmann, P., Yao, Q. et al. (2008). Sure independence screening for ultrahigh dimensional feature space Discussion. *Journal of the Royal Statistical Society, Series B (Statistical Methodology)* 70 (5): 883–911.

Bickel, P.J., Brown, J.B., Huang, H., and Li, Q. (2009). An overview of recent developments in genomics and associated statistical methods. *Philosophical Transactions of the Royal Society A: Mathematical, Physical and Engineering Sciences* 367 (1906): 4313–4337.

Bühlmann, P. and Van De Geer, S. (2011). *Statistics for High-Dimensional Data: Methods, Theory and Applications*. New York: Springer Science and Business Media.

Burawoy, M. (1991). Teaching participant observation. In: *Ethnography Unbound: Power and Resistance in the Modern Metropolis* (ed. M. Burawoy, A. Burton, A. Ferguson, et al.), 291–300. Oakland: University of California Press.

Cai, T. and Liu, W. (2011a). A direct estimation approach to sparse linear discriminant analysis. *Journal of the American Statistical Association* 106 (496): 1566–1577.

Cai, T. and Liu, W. (2011b). Adaptive thresholding for sparse covariance matrix estimation. *Journal of the American Statistical Association* 106 (494): 672–684.

Chen, R., Mias, G.I., Li-Pook-Than, J. et al. (2012). Personal omics profiling reveals dynamic molecular and medical phenotypes. *Cell* 148 (6): 1293–1307.

Cochrane, J. (2009). *Asset Pricing*. Princeton: Princeton University Press.

Cohen, J.C., Kiss, R.S., Pertsemlidis, A. et al. (2004). Multiple rare alleles contribute to low plasma levels of HDL cholesterol. *Science* 305 (5685): 869–872.

Comstock, R.L. (2002). Review modern magnetic materials in data storage. *Journal of Materials Science: Materials in Electronics* 13: 509–523.

Curry, E., Freitas, A., and O'Riáin, S. (2010). The role of community-driven data curation for enterprises. In: *Linking Enterprise Data*, 25–47.

Dawson, B. (2004). Methods of evidence-based medicine and decision analysis. In: *Basic and Clinical Biostatistics*, vol. 326 (ed. S. White). New York: McGraw Hill/Lange.

Dean, J. and Ghemawat, S. (2004). MapReduce: simplified data processing on large clusters. https://static.googleusercontent.com/media/research.google.com/en//archive/mapreduce-osdi04.pdf (accessed 24 January 2024).

Deerwester, S., Dumais, S.T., Furnas, G.W. et al. (1990). Indexing by latent semantic analysis. *Journal of the American Society for Information Science* 41 (6): 391–407.

Dempster, M.A.H. and Thompson, G.W.P. (2002). Dynamic portfolio replication using stochastic programming. www.jbs.cam.ac.uk/wp-content/uploads/2020/08/wp0025-1.pdf (accessed 24 January 2024).

Di Martino, A., Yan, C.G., Li, Q. et al. (2014). The autism brain imaging data exchange: towards a large-scale evaluation of the intrinsic brain architecture in autism. *Molecular Psychiatry* 19 (6): 659–667.

Donoho, D. L. (2000). High-dimensional data analysis: the curses and blessings of dimensionality. https://dl.icdst.org/pdfs/files/236e636d7629c1a53e6ed4cce1019b6e.pdf (accessed 24 January 2024).

Donoho, D.L. and Johnstone, I.M. (1994). Ideal spatial adaptation by wavelet shrinkage. *Biometrika* 81 (3): 425–455.

Dwivedi, K. and Dubey, S. K. (2014). Analytical review on Hadoop distributed file system. 5th International Conference – Confluence the Next Generation Information Technology Summit.

Edgar, R., Domrachev, M., and Lash, A.E. (2002). Gene expression omnibus: NCBI gene expression and hybridization array data repository. *Nucleic Acids Research* 30 (1): 207–210.

Emerson, R.M., Fretz, R.I., and Shaw, L.L. (2011). *Writing Ethnographic Fieldnotes*. Chicago: University of Chicago Press.

Engle, R.F., Hendry, D.F., and Richard, J.F. (1983). Exogeneity. *Econometrica: Journal of the Econometric Society* 51: 277–304.

Fan, J. (2013). Features of big data and sparsest solution in high confidence set. In: *Past, Present, and Future of Statistical Science* (ed. X. Lin, C. Genest, D. Banks, et al.), 531–548. London: Routledge.

Fan, J. and Li, R. (2001). Variable selection via nonconcave penalized likelihood and its oracle properties. *Journal of the American Statistical Association* 96 (456): 1348–1360.

Fan, J. and Liao, Y. (2014). Endogeneity in high dimensions. *Annals of Statistics* 42 (3): 872.

Fan, J. and Lv, J. (2008). Sure independence screening for ultrahigh dimensional feature space. *Journal of the Royal Statistical Society, Series B (Statistical Methodology)* 70 (5): 849–911.

Fan, J. and Song, R. (2010). Sure independence screening in generalized linear models with NP-dimensionality. *Annals of Statistics* 38: 3567–3604.

Fan, J., Fan, Y., and Lv, J. (2008). High dimensional covariance matrix estimation using a factor model. *Journal of Econometrics* 147 (1): 186–197.

Fan, J., Samworth, R., and Wu, Y. (2009). Ultrahigh dimensional feature selection: beyond the linear model. *Journal of Machine Learning Research* 10: 2013–2038.

Fan, J., Feng, Y., and Song, R. (2011). Nonparametric independence screening in sparse ultra-high-dimensional additive models. *Journal of the American Statistical Association* 106 (494): 544–557.

Fan, J., Liao, Y., and Mincheva, M. (2013). Large covariance estimation by thresholding principal orthogonal complements. *Journal of the Royal Statistical Society, Series B (Statistical Methodology)* 75 (4): 603–680.

Fan, J., Han, F., and Liu, H. (2014). Challenges of big data analysis. *National Science Review* 1 (2): 293–314.

Fan, J., Sun, Q., Zhou, W. X., and Zhu, Z. (2018). Principal component analysis for big data. https://arxiv.org/abs/1801.01602

Faraway, J.J. and Augustin, N.H. (2018). When small data beats big data. *Statistics and Probability Letters* 136: 142–145.

Feldman, J., Muthukrishnan, S., Sidiropoulos, A. et al. (2010). On distributing symmetric streaming computations. *ACM Transactions on Algorithms (TALG)* 6 (4): 1–19.

Forni, M., Hallin, M., Lippi, M., and Reichlin, L. (2005). The generalized dynamic factor model: one-sided estimation and forecasting. *Journal of the American Statistical Association* 100 (471): 830–840.

Gautier, E. and Rose, C. (2011). High-dimensional instrumental variables regression and confidence sets. https://arxiv.org/abs/1105.2454 (accessed 24 January 2024).

Genovese, C.R., Jin, J., Wasserman, L., and Yao, Z. (2012). A comparison of the lasso and marginal regression. *Journal of Machine Learning Research* 13 (1): 2107–2143.

Golub, G.H. and Van Loan, C.F. (2012). *Matrix Computations*. Baltimore: Johns Hopkins University Press.

Gravetter, F.J. and Wallnau, L.B. (2000). Hypothesis tests with two independent samples. In: *Statistics for the Behavioral Sciences*, 5e (ed. V. Knight, F. Stoddard, and R. Bruckman). Belmont: Wadsworth/Thomson Learning.

Hadoop, A. (2014). https://hadoop.apache.org/ (accessed 24 January 2024).

Hall, P. and Miller, H. (2009). Using generalized correlation to effect variable selection in very high dimensional problems. *Journal of Computational and Graphical Statistics* 18 (3): 533–550.

Hammersley, M. (2007). The issue of quality in qualitative research. *International Journal of Research and Method in Education* 30 (3): 287–305.

Han, F. and Liu, H. (2013). Transition matrix estimation in high dimensional time series. Presented at International Conference on Machine Learning, 172–180.

Han, F. and Pan, W. (2010). A data-adaptive sum test for disease association with multiple common or rare variants. *Human Heredity* 70 (1): 42–54.

Hastie, T., Tibshirani, R., Friedman, J.H., and Friedman, J.H. (2009). *The Elements of Statistical Learning: Data Mining, Inference, and Prediction*, vol. 2. New York: Springer.

HD-200 Consortium (2012). The ADHD-200 consortium: a model to advance the translational potential of neuroimaging in clinical neuroscience. *Frontiers in Systems Neuroscience* 6: 62.

Honnutagi, P.S. (2014). The Hadoop distributed file system. *International Journal of Computer Science and Information Technologies (IJCSIT)* 5 (5): 6238–6243.

Johnson, W. B. (1984). Extensions of Lipshitz mapping into Hilbert space. Conference on Modern Analysis and Probability.

Jonides, J., Nee, D.E., and Berman, M.G. (2006). What has functional neuroimaging told us about the mind? So many examples, so little space. *Cortex* 42 (3): 414–417.

Kaliyadan, F. and Kulkarni, V. (2019). Types of variables, descriptive statistics, and sample size. *Indian Dermatology Online Journal* 10: 82–86.

Kang, U., Tsourakakis, C., Appel, A. P., Faloutsos, C., and Leskovec, J. (2008). Hadi: Fast Diameter Estimation and Mining in Massive Graphs with Hadoop. Technical Report CMU-ML-08-117. School of Computer Science, Carnegie Mellon University, Pittsburgh.

Kawata, S. and Kawata, Y. (2000). Three-dimensional optical data storage using photochromic materials. *Chemical Reviews* 100 (5): 1777–1788.

Ke, T., Jin, J., and Fan, J. (2014). Covariance assisted screening and estimation. *Annals of Statistics* 42 (6): 2202.

Kitchin, R. and Lauriault, T.P. (2015). Small data in the era of big data. *GeoJournal* 80: 463–475.

Lee, D.K., In, J., and Lee, S. (2015). Standard deviation and standard error of the mean. *Korean Journal of Anesthesiology* 68 (3): 220–223.

Leek, J.T. and Storey, J.D. (2007). Capturing heterogeneity in gene expression studies by surrogate variable analysis. *PLoS Genetics* 3 (9): e161.

Li, H., Xu, Q., Li, N. et al. (2010). A small-molecule-based ternary data-storage device. *Journal of the American Chemical Society* 132 (16): 5542–5543.

Li, G., Peng, H., Zhang, J., and Zhu, L. (2012a). Robust rank correlation based screening. *Annals of Statistics* 40: 1846–1877.

Li, R., Zhong, W., and Zhu, L. (2012b). Feature screening via distance correlation learning. *Journal of the American Statistical Association* 107 (499): 1129–1139.

Liang, K.Y. and Zeger, S.L. (1986). Longitudinal data analysis using generalized linear models. *Biometrika* 73 (1): 13–22.

Lin, M.F., Hsu, W.S., Huang, M.C. et al. (2017). "I couldn't even talk to the patient": barriers to communicating with cancer patients as perceived by nursing students. *European Journal of Cancer Care* 26 (4): e12648.

Liu, H., Han, F., Yuan, M. et al. (2012a). High-dimensional semiparametric Gaussian copula graphical models. *Annals of Statistics* 40: 2293–2326.

Liu, H., Han, F., and Zhang, C.H. (2012b). Transelliptical graphical models. *Advances in Neural Information Processing Systems* 25.

Lofland, J. and Lofland, L.H. (1995). Developing analysis. In: *Analyzing Social Setting*, 3ee, 183–203. Belmont: Wadsworth.

Lyko, K., Nitzschke, M., and Ngonga Ngomo, A.C. (2016). Big data acquisition. In: *New Horizons for a Data-Driven Economy: A Roadmap for Usage and Exploitation of Big Data in Europe* (ed. J.M. Cavanillas, E. Curry, and W. Wahlster), 39–61. New York: Springer.

Manikandan, S. (2011a). Frequency distribution. *Journal of Pharmacology and Pharmacotherapeutics* 2 (1): 54–56.

Manikandan, S. (2011b). Measures of central tendency: the mean. *Journal of Pharmacology and Pharmacotherapeutics* 2 (2): 140.

Manikandan, S. (2011c). Measures of dispersion. *Journal of Pharmacology and Pharmacotherapeutics* 2 (4): 315.

Masood, I. and Shyen, V.B.E. (2016). Quality control in hard disc drive manufacturing using pattern recognition technique. In: *IOP Conference Series: Materials Science and Engineering*, 012008. Bristol: IOP Publishing.

McAfee, A., Brynjolfsson, E., Davenport, T.H. et al. (2012). Big data: the management revolution. *Harvard Business Review* 90 (10): 60–68.

Meriläinen, M., Kyngäs, H., and Ala-Kokko, T. (2010). 24-hour intensive care: an observational study of an environment and events. *Intensive and Critical Care Nursing* 26 (5): 246–253.

Miller, H.J. (2010). The data avalanche is here. Shouldn't we be digging? *Journal of Regional Science* 50 (1): 181–201.

Norman, G.R. and Streiner, D.L. (2008). *Biostatistics: The Bare Essentials*. New Haven: PMPH USA.

Onwuegbuzie, A.J., Dickinson, W.B., Leech, N.L., and Zoran, A.G. (2009). A qualitative framework for collecting and analyzing data in focus group research. *International Journal of Qualitative Methods* 8 (3): 1–21.

Pennock, M. (2007). Digital curation: a life-cycle approach to managing and preserving usable digital information. *Library and Archives* 1 (1): 1–3.

Plummer, P. (2017). Focus group methodology. Part 1: design considerations. *International Journal of Therapy and Rehabilitation* 24 (7): 297–301.

Rao, K.R. and Yip, P. (2014). *Discrete Cosine Transform: Algorithms, Advantages, Applications*. New York: Academic Press.

Rorty, R., Taylor, C., and Dreyfus, H.L. (1980). A discussion. *Review of Metaphysics* 34 (1): 47–55.

Rouse, M. (2014). Internet of Things (IOT). http://whatis.techtarget.com/definition

Rubin, H.J. and Rubin, I.S. (2011). *Qualitative Interviewing: The Art of Hearing Data*. London: Sage.

Sagiroglu, S. and Sinanc, D. (2013). Big data: a review. 2013 IEEE International Conference on Collaboration Technologies and Systems (CTS).

Shvachko, K., Kuang, H., Radia, S., and Chansler, R. (2010). The hadoop distributed file system. 2010 IEEE 26th Symposium on Mass Storage Systems and Technologies (MSST).

Song, S. and Bickel, P. J. (2011). Large vector auto regressions. https://arxiv.org/abs/1106.3915 (accessed 24 January 2024).

Stock, J.H. and Watson, M.W. (2002). Forecasting using principal components from a large number of predictors. *Journal of the American Statistical Association* 97 (460): 1167–1179.

Stonebraker, M. (2012). What does 'big data' mean? https://cacm.acm.org/blogs/blog-cacm/155468-what-does-big-data-mean/fulltext (accessed 24 January 2024).

Strohbach, M., Daubert, J., Ravkin, H., and Lischka, M. (2016). Big data storage. In: Cavanillas, J. M., Curry, E., and Wahlster, W. (eds) New Horizons for a Data-Driven Economy: A Roadmap for Usage and Exploitation of Big Data in Europe. New York: Springer, pp. 119–141.

Swinscow, T.D.V. and Campbell, M.J. (2002). *Statistics at Square One*, 111–125. London: BMJ.

Tibshirani, R. (1996). Regression shrinkage and selection via the lasso. *Journal of the Royal Statistical Society, Series B (Statistical Methodology)* 58 (1): 267–288.

Tukey, J.W. (1977). *Exploratory Data Analysis*. Reading: Addision-Wesley.

Twycross, A. and Shorten, A. (2016). Using observational research to obtain a picture of nursing practice. *Evidence-Based Nursing* 19 (3): 66–67.

Valiathan, R.R., Marco, M., Leitinger, B. et al. (2012). Discoidin domain receptor tyrosine kinases: new players in cancer progression. *Cancer and Metastasis Reviews* 31: 295–321.

Visscher, K.M. and Weissman, D.H. (2011). Would the field of cognitive neuroscience be advanced by sharing functional MRI data? *BMC Medicine* 9 (1): 1–6.

Worthey, E.A., Mayer, A.N., Syverson, G.D. et al. (2011). Making a definitive diagnosis: successful clinical application of whole exome sequencing in a child with intractable inflammatory bowel disease. *Genetics in Medicine* 13 (3): 255–262.

Yamato, Y., Muroi, M., Tanaka, K., and Uchimura, M. (2014). Development of template management technology for easy deployment of virtual resources on OpenStack. *Journal of Cloud Computing* 3: 1–12.

Young, L. and Barrett, H. (2001). Adapting visual methods: action research with Kampala street children. *Area* 33 (2): 141–152.

Zhang, C.H. (2010). Nearly unbiased variable selection under minimax concave penalty. *Annals of Statistics* 38: 894–942.

Zhao, S.D. and Li, Y. (2012). Principled sure independence screening for cox models with ultra-high-dimensional covariates. *Journal of Multivariate Analysis* 105 (1): 397–411.

18

Systematic Reviews in Epidemiological Studies

Pratistha Shrivastava[1] and Raghvendra Mishra[2]

[1] Department of Veterinary Parasitology, Institute of Veterinary Sciences and Animal Health, SOADU, Bhubaneswar, India
[2] Department of Veterinary Public Health, M.B. Veterinary College, Dungarpur, India

18.1 Introduction

A systematic review serves as a potent research instrument designed to locate and consolidate all pertinent evidence related to a specific research query (Denison et al. 2013). It represents an advancement over a conventional literature review as it applies systematic techniques to meticulously search for, evaluate, and integrate the available evidence. The process it follows closely resembles that of a scientific experiment, placing utmost importance on transparency (and reproducibility) of the methods employed, and ensuring consistent treatment of all the gathered evidence (Figure 18.1).

The primary goal of systematic reviews is to encompass all relevant literature related to the review question, without bias toward the direction or significance of the results. This comprehensive approach leads to reduced bias and increased confidence in the conclusions drawn. A well-conducted systematic review plays a pivotal role in the scientific community by presenting a concise summary of existing evidence while also highlighting areas where knowledge gaps exist. This makes systematic reviews a crucial catalyst for further research.

Moreover, systematic reviews serve decision makers by providing them with consolidated and reliable information, which can be instrumental in shaping policies. For instance, the Cochrane Collaboration is renowned for producing and maintaining systematic reviews that assess the effectiveness of healthcare interventions primarily through randomized trials.

Furthermore, systematic reviews can also amalgamate the findings from observational studies, offering a comprehensive view of the evidence on a particular topic. This integration of diverse sources of information contributes to a more robust and informed understanding of the subject matter.

Systematic reviews offer valuable insights that can shape future interventions and research. They may identify potential interventions worthy of inclusion in randomized trials or delve into underlying causative factors, exploring the association between risk factors and the outcome of interest.

The utility of systematic reviews spans beyond medicine and extends to a wide array of scientific disciplines. Researchers at all levels, including early career researchers (ECRs), may opt to undertake systematic reviews, with such reviews even forming a part or the entirety of a PhD thesis.

While conducting a systematic review can be a substantial undertaking requiring considerable time, the potential benefits are significant as they provide a comprehensive summary of all the available evidence pertaining to a specific question. One advantage is the avoidance of primary data collection, which can be expensive and time-consuming. Additionally, engaging in review work provides researchers with a broad exposure to a particular topic and epidemiological research in general, which can be invaluable for their academic and professional growth .

It is strongly recommended that systematic reviews involve a minimum of two reviewers working independently throughout the process, including screening abstracts, data extraction, and assessing the risk of bias. This approach helps reduce the possibility of reviewer bias and enhances the reliability of the review findings. Conducting a systematic review can be challenging, especially for those without prior experience, and therefore additional support and direction may be necessary to embark on such a project.

Epidemiology and Environmental Hygiene in Veterinary Public Health, First Edition. Edited by Tanmoy Rana.
© 2025 John Wiley & Sons, Inc. Published 2025 by John Wiley & Sons, Inc.

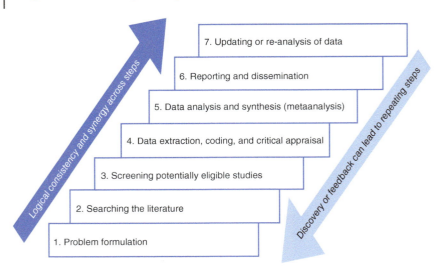

Figure 18.1 Diagrammatic representation of a systematic review.

To address this need, we have developed a guidance article specifically aimed at ECRs, providing a straightforward outline of how to initiate a systematic review. While the article serves as a helpful starting point, it is not a comprehensive guide and instead directs readers to other resources for further information. It emphasizes that the systematic review process is applicable to various study types, encompassing both observational and trial designs, and works with data collected using quantitative or qualitative approaches.

However, for this particular chapter, the focus will be on reviewing observational studies that have utilized quantitative methods. If ECRs are interested in conducting reviews of qualitative research, they are encouraged to seek alternative resources for guidance. One such resource is the Cochrane Qualitative and Implementation Methods Group website (https://methods.cochrane.org/qi/), which can serve as a valuable starting point for exploring this topic further.

Identifying the necessity for a systematic review is a crucial step before initiating the process. To avoid duplicating existing research efforts, it is essential to conduct a thorough literature search. This search should specifically target systematic reviews that have already been conducted on your topic. Additionally, it is beneficial to check databases that record prospective systematic reviews, such as PROSPERO. In the event that you discover an existing systematic review on your topic, you should carefully consider whether another review is warranted at this time. Factors to ponder include whether relevant research has been published since the existing review, or if there are any gaps or limitations in the existing review that justify the need for a new one. By critically assessing the current state of research and identifying areas that can benefit from further investigation, you can determine whether proceeding with a systematic review is appropriate and valuable. This process ensures that the effort put into the review will lead to meaningful contributions to the existing body of knowledge.

Developing a protocol is a crucial step that should be undertaken before commencing your systematic review, and it is essential to ensure that all reviewers are in agreement with it. There are several reasons why this is important.

- *Focus and purpose*: creating a protocol helps to clearly define the purpose and objectives of the systematic review. It ensures that all reviewers have a shared understanding of the review's scope, research questions, and goals, which helps maintain consistency and avoids potential disagreements during the process.
- *Methodological consistency*: the protocol sets out a predefined plan for how the review will be conducted. It outlines the search strategy, inclusion and exclusion criteria for studies, data extraction methods, and assessment of risk of bias, among other aspects. This consistency in methodology is crucial for producing reliable and reproducible results.
- *Reference and guidance*: the protocol serves as a reference document throughout the review process. For instance, during the screening phase, having clear details of the inclusion criteria readily available in the protocol can facilitate efficient and accurate article screening.

By having a well-structured and agreed-upon protocol in place, the systematic review process becomes more systematic and transparent, and ultimately enhances the quality and credibility of the review's findings. Indeed, a well-structured protocol is essential for ensuring consistency among all reviewers involved in the systematic review.

To create an effective protocol, the initial step is to accurately define the primary objectives of the review, along with providing relevant background information. The review question should be stated clearly, and it can be a broad question or broken down into specific, focused objectives. Taking sufficient time to carefully craft the review question is crucial, as it will directly impact the design of the search strategy.

When dealing with etiological questions (questions related to causes or factors contributing to an outcome), the search strategy should concentrate on gathering information related to both the exposure and the outcome. This approach looks for an overlap between the two distinct subjects. For instance, when exploring the relationship between peripheral neuropathy and subsequent falls as a consequence, searching for articles that address this specific relationship will yield fewer results compared to searching for articles about either peripheral neuropathy or falls alone. This method, known as an exposure/outcome model, allows for a more targeted and relevant search, ultimately aiding in the comprehensive retrieval of pertinent literature for the systematic review. By carefully defining the review question and adopting appropriate search strategies, the protocol ensures that all reviewers are well equipped to conduct the review in a consistent and systematic manner.

The methods section of the protocol is a critical component that outlines the entire process of the systematic review. It provides comprehensive details about how the review will be conducted. The key elements to include in the methods section are as follows.

- *Search strategy*: describe the databases to be searched (e.g., PubMed, Scopus, Web of Science) and the specific years of publication that will be covered. Explain the search terms and keywords that will be used to identify relevant studies. Mention any filters or limitations applied to the search, such as language restrictions.
- *Screening process*: explain how the screening of studies will be carried out. This typically involves two stages: screening of titles and abstracts to identify potentially relevant studies, followed by full-text screening to determine final inclusion. Specify the criteria that will be used for each screening stage.
- *Data retrieval*: describe additional methods for obtaining data, such as screening the reference lists of included studies and contacting authors for unpublished or additional information.
- *Inclusion criteria*: clearly outline the inclusion criteria that studies must meet to be considered for the review. These criteria should directly relate to the review question and research objectives. Be specific and provide sufficient detail to enable other researchers to apply the same criteria.

By including these crucial details in the methods section of the protocol, the systematic review becomes transparent, reproducible, and comparable. It ensures that the review process is conducted in a rigorous and standardized manner, allowing for accurate and reliable findings that can contribute meaningfully to the research field (Figure 18.2).

By combining the use of MeSH terms and free-text terms in the search strategy, researchers can ensure a comprehensive and targeted search for relevant articles in databases (Table 18.1). MeSH terms provide a standardized and systematic way to identify articles related to specific subject headings, while free-text terms offer flexibility in capturing variations in language and concepts that may not yet be indexed with MeSH terms.

Spending sufficient time developing and clearly defining the inclusion criteria is crucial for the success of the systematic review. Well-defined inclusion criteria ensure that the correct papers are selected to answer the review question and save valuable time during the later stages of the review process. When formulating the inclusion criteria, researchers should consider the following factors.

- *Sample/population of interest*: specify the characteristics of the study population that are relevant to the research question. This could include demographic details (e.g., age, gender, health condition) or other specific traits.
- *Independent variable*: identify the main exposure or intervention being investigated in the included studies.

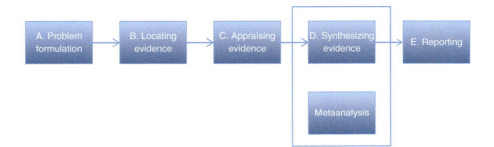

Figure 18.2 A methods section protocol.

18 Systematic Reviews in Epidemiological Studies

Table 18.1 Two main approaches to searching databases for articles.

Approach	Description
MeSH (Medical Subject Headings) terms	Denoted by a trailing slash, e.g. Accidental Falls/
	The complete set of MeSH terms can be searched at www.nlm.nih.gov/mesh
	It is customary to use the explode operator beforehand, indicating to the database that you want articles with the given term and relevant subcategories, e.g., exp Accidental Falls
	For the EMBASE database, MeSH terms are represented as "EMTREE" terms and include the complete MeSH vocabulary
	Check for terms assigned to relevant articles you already have as they can guide your MeSH term selection
Free-text terms	Useful when there are no applicable MeSH terms for your area of interest, or for newer articles that may not have been indexed with MeSH terms yet
	Denoted by double-quotation marks, followed by a full stop and then the fields of interest. For example, "falls."ti,ab searches for the word "falls" in the title and abstract of all articles
	It is beneficial to brainstorm synonyms (e.g., "peripheral neuropathy," "peripheral sensory loss") and include alternative spellings (e.g., "haemoglobin" and "hemoglobin") to capture all relevant variations of terms that authors might use in the literature

- *Outcomes*: clearly state the outcomes of interest that the included studies should have examined and reported.
- *Study design and setting*: define the types of study designs (e.g., randomized controlled trials [RCTs], observational studies) that will be included, and consider any specific settings that are relevant to the research question.
- *Language*: decide whether studies published in languages other than the language(s) understood by the reviewers will be included.
- *Publication type*: specify any criteria related to the publication status (e.g., peer-reviewed articles, conference abstracts) that will be considered.

The methods section of the protocol should also outline the following details.

- *Data extraction*: explain how data will be extracted from the selected studies. Define the specific data points that will be collected and the format in which the data will be recorded.
- *Risk of bias assessment*: describe how the risk of bias in each included article will be evaluated. This may involve using standardized tools or criteria to assess the quality of the studies.
- *Data synthesis*: explain the methods that will be employed to synthesize the data from the included studies. This could include narrative synthesis, metaanalysis, or other statistical approaches.

By meticulously defining these aspects in the methods section, researchers ensure a systematic and transparent review process. Additionally, it helps other researchers understand and replicate the review, enhancing the credibility and reliability of the findings.

The protocol for a systematic review does not need to be rigid and unchangeable. It is acceptable and sometimes necessary to make edits and adaptations during the course of the review to improve its clarity, functionality, and effectiveness. However, any modifications should be agreed upon by all reviewers involved in the process, and consistency in the selection of articles should be maintained.

Sometimes, the initial inclusion criteria may not yield sufficient evidence to answer the review question conclusively. In such cases, it is perfectly valid to revisit and revise the inclusion criteria to ensure that all relevant evidence is captured.

It is crucial to keep a detailed record of any changes made to the protocol and the reasons behind those changes. This log serves as valuable documentation for other researchers who may wish to replicate the review and arrive at the same conclusions. Transparency in documenting protocol changes enhances the credibility and reproducibility of the review process.

Additionally, it is highly beneficial to consult established systematic review guidelines during the protocol development stage. These guidelines provide valuable frameworks and checklists that help in designing a robust and comprehensive protocol. Many journals also require authors to adhere to these guidelines when submitting their systematic review articles for publication.

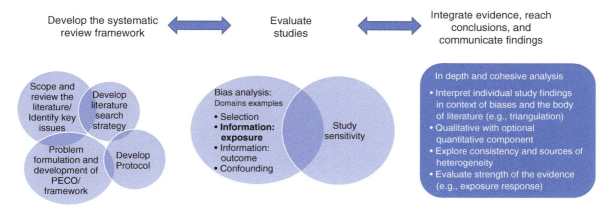

Figure 18.3 Components of a systematic review.

Two commonly used systematic review guidelines are:

- *PRISMA (Preferred Reporting Items for Systematic Reviews and Meta-Analyses)*: a comprehensive guideline for reporting systematic reviews and meta-analyses
- *MOOSE (Meta-analysis Of Observational Studies in Epidemiology)*: a guideline specifically tailored for conducting metaanalyses of observational studies.

Adhering to these guidelines ensures that the systematic review is conducted with high standards of transparency and rigor, which ultimately strengthens the impact and credibility of the review's findings (Figure 18.3).

18.2 Searching

18.2.1 Searching Databases

The search strategy for a systematic review involves searching relevant databases that contain published peer-reviewed literature. MEDLINE and EMBASE are considered primary sources and it is highly recommended to search them simultaneously to ensure comprehensive coverage of the literature. However, it is important to note that other databases might also be relevant to your review question, and it is beneficial to explore additional databases to ensure thoroughness.

The Centre for Reviews and Dissemination (CRD) provides a valuable resource to identify relevant databases for your topic. By referring to its list, you can find additional databases that may contain pertinent literature.

Once you have selected the databases to use, you need to choose a search system to run your searches. Many institutions' libraries subscribe to specific search systems such as OVID or ATHENS. It is often convenient to use the system to which your institution has access.

To design an effective search strategy, it is advisable to seek the guidance of an information specialist, often available through your institution's library. Information specialists are skilled in conducting systematic literature searches and can assist you in constructing a comprehensive and precise search strategy.

Collaborating with an information specialist ensures that your search strategy is optimized to retrieve all relevant articles while minimizing the risk of missing essential studies. Their expertise contributes to the overall quality and reliability of your systematic review.

MeSH terms assigned to articles in the MEDLINE database are a powerful tool for locating articles related to a particular topic. MeSH terms provide a standardized way of categorizing and indexing articles, making it easier to find relevant literature.

To begin the search process, it is beneficial to browse through the different MeSH terms on the US National Library of Medicine website. This helps researchers gain a better understanding of the available terms and how they can be used to construct an effective search strategy.

However, since MeSH terms may not cover all relevant aspects of a topic, it is essential to supplement them with free-text terms. These are specific words or expressions that may be found in different sections of the article, such as the title or abstract. By incorporating free-text terms, the search strategy becomes more comprehensive, capturing additional relevant articles that might not be explicitly indexed with MeSH terms.

To conduct the search effectively, the MeSH terms and free-text terms for each factor under investigation should be combined using the "OR" operator. This produces a broader set of articles that contain any of the specified terms related to the factor.

Once the initial search retrieves a large number of articles, the next step is to refine the results to focus on the research question. This is achieved by using the "AND" operator to combine the MeSH and free-text terms for each factor, along with the other relevant inclusion criteria defined in the protocol. The "AND" operator ensures that only articles that meet all the specified criteria are included in the final selection.

By employing a combination of MeSH terms and free-text terms, and strategically using "OR" and "AND" operators, the search strategy becomes powerful and targeted, capturing all relevant articles while maintaining precision to answer the research question accurately.

An important consideration in designing is the search strategy for a systematic review. While it is essential to aim for comprehensive coverage of relevant literature, the screening process must be manageable and practical. Some searches have the potential to yield an overwhelming number of results, making it challenging to review all articles in a reasonable time-frame.

To address this issue, researchers can employ additional criteria to limit the number of articles returned. For example, they may choose to include only articles published after a certain date or to exclude certain types of studies, such as animal studies.

However, this process involves a balance. On one hand, researchers must ensure the search is sensitive enough to capture all relevant studies that meet the inclusion criteria. On the other hand, they must consider the time and resource burden of screening a large number of articles.

Restrictions placed on the search should be carefully considered during the review's assessment of potential biases. Generally, the fewer restrictions placed on the search, the better, as this approach minimizes the risk of inadvertently excluding important studies.

It is worth noting that in some cases, researchers may conduct an initial scoping search to assess the volume of potentially relevant articles. This scoping search can help researchers make informed decisions about additional search restrictions based on the feasibility of screening the identified articles.

Ultimately, the goal is to strike a balance between a comprehensive search and a manageable screening process, ensuring that the systematic review remains rigorous and unbiased while also being practical to conduct within the available resources and time constraints.

Gray literature refers to sources of information that are not indexed in traditional publication databases. These sources can include conference abstracts, government reports, theses, and other unpublished or noncommercially published materials. Including gray literature in a systematic review can be valuable, as it may provide access to research findings and data that are not available through conventional databases. To identify relevant conference abstracts, researchers can manually screen conference proceedings or use databases like Zetoc from the British Library, which provides access to conference information. Additionally, the libraries of relevant institutions or centers may be helpful in identifying relevant PhD dissertations that could be valuable for the review.

For reviews related to healthcare, the Health Technology Assessments (HTA) database, available on the CRD website, is a valuable resource for identifying gray literature. However, it is essential to bear in mind that searching for gray literature can be time-consuming. Researchers must weigh the potential benefits of including gray literature against the time burden it may impose on the review process. Including gray literature can enhance the comprehensiveness and validity of the review, but it is essential to strike a balance between the effort spent on searching for it and the potential value it may add to the review's findings. Researchers should carefully assess the relevance and impact of including gray literature in their specific review context and make informed decisions based on the available resources and time constraints.

18.3 Handling and Screening Search Result

18.3.1 Handling Search Results

After conducting the searches, the results will typically be in the form of a list of articles, conference abstracts, or other types of gray literature (if included in the search). Depending on the scope of the search, the number of results to be processed can be substantial, potentially resulting in multiple lists if searches were conducted across various sources. To handle and screen these data carefully and consistently, researchers need to adopt an appropriate method for organizing the results. It is essential to use a structured and systematic approach to manage the screening process efficiently. Storing the results in an appropriate program or format for screening is highly recommended. Some common methods include the following.

- *Microsoft Word document*: researchers can create a table or a structured document to list the article titles, abstracts, and other relevant details. This approach provides a straightforward way to review and evaluate each item.
- *PDF files*: if the search results are in PDF format, researchers can use annotation tools to mark the articles as relevant or irrelevant during the screening process.
- *Reference management software*: reference management tools like Reference Manager or Endnote offer more advanced features for organizing and screening search results. These software programs allow researchers to create libraries of references, tag articles as relevant or irrelevant, and add notes or comments.

Using reference management software can be particularly advantageous for larger-scale systematic reviews, as it facilitates collaboration among reviewers and streamlines the screening process. Regardless of the method chosen, it is essential to document the screening process thoroughly, including the reasons for including or excluding each article. This documentation ensures transparency and reproducibility, as well as enabling verification of the review's results.

By adopting an appropriate and structured approach to handling and screening the search results, researchers can efficiently manage the review process and maintain consistency in their evaluations, resulting in more reliable and accurate findings.

Using reference management software offers the advantage of easily identifying and removing duplicate articles from the search results. Duplicate articles may arise when researchers use multiple sources for their search, and managing them manually could be time-consuming and prone to errors. Reference management software streamlines this process, improving efficiency and accuracy in identifying and eliminating duplicates.

In the end, the choice of how to manage search results may come down to personal preference and the specific needs of the review. Different researchers may have their preferred methods or workflows. What matters most is consistency and meticulous documentation of the methods used.

In a systematic review, maintaining consistency throughout the entire process is crucial to ensure the validity and reliability of the results. By adhering to a well-defined protocol, using standardized data management approaches, and recording all decisions and methods, researchers can enhance the transparency and reproducibility of the review.

Keeping a comprehensive record of the methods employed in the review is essential for several reasons.

- *Facilitates transparency*: detailed documentation enables other researchers to understand and replicate the review's process, contributing to the review's credibility.
- *Ensures accuracy*: recording methods and decisions helps to prevent errors and provides a clear trail for validation and verification.
- *Facilitates updating*: if the review is to be updated or revised in the future, well-documented methods help streamline the process.
- *Allows peer review*: transparent methods allow for constructive feedback during the peer review process, leading to potential improvements in the review.

By being consistent, transparent, and thorough in all aspects of the systematic review, researchers can produce a robust and reliable synthesis of evidence that contributes meaningfully to the field of study.

18.3.2 Screening Search Result

The primary purpose of screening is to identify sources of information that are relevant to the review question and meet the specified inclusion criteria. To achieve this, it is crucial for the reviewers to refer back to the protocol regularly and consistently throughout the screening process. The inclusion and exclusion criteria outlined in the protocol serve as the foundation for the screening process. Reviewers use these criteria to determine whether each article or source of information aligns with the research question and meets the predefined requirements for inclusion in the review. For maximum reliability and to minimize potential bias, screening should be conducted by at least two reviewers working independently. Each reviewer assesses the eligibility of the articles or sources without influence from others. This independent screening process helps ensure that a comprehensive evaluation is performed and that diverse perspectives are considered.

In cases where there are disagreements between the two independent reviewers, it is essential to resolve these differences through consensus. A third reviewer, often referred to as an arbitrator or mediator, can be involved to help reconcile conflicting assessments. The third reviewer's role is to objectively evaluate the disputed articles and facilitate an agreement between the two initial reviewers. Maintaining a collaborative and transparent process during screening is crucial to ensure the reliability and validity of the systematic review's results. Adherence to the agreed-upon protocol, independent screening, and resolution of disagreements through consensus contribute to a rigorous and credible review that offers meaningful insights into the research question.

The screening of published articles in a systematic review generally involves two main phases.

1) *First phase – title and abstract screening*: in the initial phase, researchers look at the exported references from their search results. During this stage, they review the titles and abstracts of the articles to identify potentially relevant papers. The goal is to narrow down the initial set of search results to a smaller subset that appears to be relevant to the review question and meets the inclusion criteria.
2) *Second phase – full-text screening*: in the second phase, researchers obtain a copy of the potentially relevant papers identified during the title and abstract screening phase. They read the full text of these articles carefully and thoroughly to make a final decision on whether they meet all the specified inclusion criteria for the systematic review. Articles that meet the criteria are included in the review, while those that do not are excluded.

It is important to emphasize that both phases of screening involve an assessment of the relevance of the articles based on the predefined inclusion criteria outlined in the protocol. The screening process aims to identify articles that are most suitable for answering the review question and meet the specific requirements of the research.

Conducting both title and abstract screening and full-text screening ensures a thorough and comprehensive evaluation of the articles, leading to a high-quality and reliable systematic review. The process involves collaboration between reviewers and adhering to the review protocol to maintain consistency and minimize bias.

Screening can indeed be a time-consuming process, especially during the initial stages. However, with practice and familiarity with the review question and inclusion criteria, it generally becomes more efficient and quicker.

To manage the screening process effectively, it is advisable to follow these practices.

1) *Record progress*: after each screening session, make a note of how far you have progressed in the list of articles. This record helps ensure that you start from the correct point in the next session, avoiding duplication and maintaining continuity.
2) *Start with titles*: begin the screening process by looking at the titles of the articles. Often, titles provide sufficient information to make quick decisions about their relevance to the review question. If the title clearly indicates that the article is not relevant, it can be excluded at this stage, saving time on further evaluation.
3) *Use abstracts for further evaluation*: if the relevance of an article is not immediately apparent from the title, review the abstract for additional information. Abstracts usually provide a summary of the article's content and research findings. This can help make a more informed decision about whether the article meets the inclusion criteria.
4) *Create a list of potentially relevant papers*: if you are unsure about the relevance of an article after reviewing the abstract, add it to a list of potentially relevant papers. These are articles that require a full-text review to determine if they meet the inclusion criteria.
5) *Assess full-text for final decision*: once you have the full text of the potentially relevant papers, read them thoroughly to make a final decision on their inclusion in the review. Having the complete article in front of you provides a comprehensive view of the study's details and allows for a more accurate evaluation.

By following these practices and maintaining a systematic approach, researchers can streamline the screening process, making it more manageable and efficient. Consistent and careful screening is essential to ensure that only relevant and high-quality studies are included in the systematic review, leading to reliable and meaningful results.

It is crucial to keep a detailed and organized record of the papers identified during the screening process. This record serves several essential purposes.

- *Identification and tracking*: the record, often in the form of a list, should contain sufficient information about each potentially relevant paper, such as the title, first author, year of publication, and unique identifiers like PubMed IDs. This information allows researchers to easily identify and locate the papers again, especially when reporting the methods and results in the systematic review.

- *Flow diagram*: the number of papers included and excluded at each stage of the screening process is a critical component of the flow diagram. The flow diagram visually represents the screening process, indicating the flow of papers from the initial search results to the final inclusion in the review. Transparently reporting this information enhances the review's reproducibility and facilitates readers' understanding of the study selection process.
- *Reasons for exclusion*: for the papers obtained in full but subsequently excluded from the review, it is essential to record the specific reasons for their exclusion. These reasons are also reported in the flow diagram and provide valuable context and transparency to readers. Common reasons for exclusion might include not meeting the inclusion criteria, inadequate study design, or insufficient data.

By maintaining a well-documented and comprehensive record throughout the screening process, researchers can ensure the accuracy and transparency of their systematic review. This documentation is valuable during the reporting phase and when presenting the review's methodology and results to the scientific community. It enhances the credibility and reproducibility of the review and allows other researchers to follow the study selection process accurately. Screening conference abstracts can be a quicker process compared to screening full papers because there is no need for a second phase of obtaining the full version. However, it is essential to be aware that the information provided in conference abstracts is often more limited compared to full papers. This limitation can make it more challenging to determine whether the abstracts meet the inclusion criteria for the systematic review. While conference abstracts can offer valuable insights and preliminary findings, they may not provide enough detail to fully assess the study's relevance and methodology. Therefore, it becomes even more crucial to rigorously apply the inclusion criteria when screening conference abstracts.

In some cases, due to the limited information in the abstracts, researchers might need to contact the study authors for additional details to determine if the abstract meets the inclusion criteria. This could involve requesting the full paper or any supplementary information that clarifies the study design, methodology, or results. Contacting the study authors for further information is a valuable practice when necessary. Authors are usually willing to provide additional details about their research, and this can help ensure that the review's conclusions are based on accurate and complete information. However, it is important to document all communications with study authors during the review process, as this information should be reported transparently in the systematic review. Researchers should include the details of any correspondence with authors in the review's documentation and potential publication. By applying a rigorous and systematic approach to screening conference abstracts and, when needed, seeking additional information from study authors, researchers can enhance the quality and reliability of their systematic review findings. This approach ensures that the review's conclusions are based on a comprehensive understanding of the available evidence.

18.4 Identification of Additional Sources Following Screening

18.4.1 Citation Searching

Citation searching is a valuable method for discovering relevant literature that may have been overlooked during the initial search process. There are two main components to citation searching.

- *Checking bibliographies*: in this component, researchers review the bibliographies of papers that have already been identified and included in the systematic review. By examining the reference lists of these papers, researchers can identify earlier articles that have been cited by the included papers. This process is known as backward citation searching. It allows researchers to uncover older literature that might not have appeared in the initial search results but could be highly relevant to the review question.
- *Checking citation indexes*: in this component, researchers use citation indexes like the ISI citation index through Web of Science to identify later articles that have cited the papers included in the review. This process is known as forward citation searching. By identifying more recent articles that cite the included papers, researchers can access up-to-date literature that may not have been available at the time of the initial search.

Both backward and forward citation searching are relatively simple and quick methods to discover relevant literature. They offer an opportunity to find additional studies that might have been published before or after the initial search date. These methods can be especially valuable in systematic reviews as they help ensure the review is as comprehensive and up to date as possible. By incorporating citation searching into the systematic review process, researchers can reduce the

18.4.2 Contacting Authors

Contacting experts in the field is a crucial aspect of a comprehensive search strategy for a systematic review. These experts, often the authors of relevant studies, possess valuable knowledge and expertise in the specific area of interest, making them an excellent resource for identifying any articles or studies that might have been missed during the initial database search. When contacting authors, it is essential to be respectful and professional. Researchers can reach out to authors to share their current list of included articles and ask if there are any additional relevant studies they might be aware of. If new articles are suggested by the authors, it is important to contact the corresponding author(s) of these articles as well.

During this communication with authors, researchers may also seek clarity on specific details or finer points of the published articles. However, it is critical to maintain consistency throughout the process. All authors should be asked the same questions and provided with the same opportunity to contribute to the review. This ensures that no bias is introduced into the review.

In some cases, researchers may request authors to conduct further analyses on their data to facilitate the inclusion of these analyses in a metaanalysis, if applicable. Specific and well-defined requests with clear instructions, such as providing a table for authors to fill out, can make it easier for authors to respond and contribute valuable information. Throughout the review process, it is essential to acknowledge and properly credit the help received from authors in the write-up of the systematic review. Proper attribution of contributions is crucial for maintaining scientific integrity and acknowledging the expertise and assistance provided by authors.

By engaging with experts and authors in a respectful and consistent manner, researchers can enhance the quality and comprehensiveness of their systematic review, leading to more robust, and informative findings.

18.4.3 Data Extraction

Data extraction is a critical step in a systematic review that involves locating and synthesizing relevant information from the included papers. Using a standardized data extraction form offers several advantages, including providing consistency and structure to the extraction process. When designing the data extraction form, it should be tailored specifically to the research question and objectives of the systematic review. The form should capture the necessary information required to answer the review question effectively and perform any planned analyses. Researchers should consider what descriptive information and data they wish to present in the final review paper, as this will help guide the selection of data to extract.

Key considerations when designing the data extraction form include the following.

- *Relevance to research question*: ensure that the data to be extracted are directly relevant to the research question and contribute to the review's objectives. Avoid including extraneous information that does not directly relate to the study's purpose.
- *Clarity and structure*: organize the data extraction form in a clear and structured manner. Use headings and subheadings to categorize the information to be extracted. This clarity aids both the data extraction process and subsequent data synthesis.
- *Guidance notes*: provide a set of guidance notes to accompany the data extraction form. These notes should explain the meaning and context of each data field, clarify any potential areas of ambiguity, and offer instructions for consistent data extraction.
- *Consistency between reviewers*: the guidance notes are particularly important in ensuring consistency between different reviewers involved in the data extraction process. All reviewers should have a shared understanding of the data extraction requirements to avoid discrepancies in extracted data.
- *Pilot testing*: before starting the full data extraction, consider pilot testing the data extraction form with a small subset of included papers. This pilot phase allows reviewers to identify any potential issues or ambiguities in the form and make necessary adjustments before proceeding with the full extraction.

By using a well-designed and tailored data extraction form with clear guidance notes, researchers can systematically and accurately extract the relevant information from the included papers. This process ensures that the review's findings are based on reliable and comprehensive data, contributing to the review's overall rigor and credibility. Piloting the data extraction form on a couple of studies that meet the review's inclusion criteria is a crucial step in the systematic review process. This pilot testing allows researchers to assess the appropriateness and effectiveness of the form in capturing the relevant data while excluding unnecessary information. It helps ensure that the form is well designed and tailored to the specific needs of the review.

When creating the data extraction form, it is essential to include key information that allows for proper identification and reference of each study. This information typically includes the aspects listed below.

1) *Paper title*: the title of the paper is essential for identifying and referencing each study accurately.
2) *Authors*: including the names of the authors allows for proper attribution and acknowledgment of the study's contributors.
3) *Type of publication*: indicating the type of publication (e.g., original research article, review, metaanalysis, etc.) helps categorize the studies appropriately.
4) *Year of publication*: the publication year is necessary for tracking the temporal distribution of the included studies and assessing the currency of the evidence.
5) *Citation information*: other citation details, such as the journal name, volume, page numbers, and DOI (Digital Object Identifier), provide comprehensive referencing information for the review.
6) *Source of the paper*: it is useful to include where the paper was found, such as the database from which it was retrieved (e.g., MEDLINE) or any other sources, such as reference lists of other papers or conference proceedings.
7) *Study type and data*: the specific data to be extracted will depend on the review question and the types of studies available. For example, in clinical trials, data may include details about the study design, participants, interventions, outcomes, and results. In qualitative studies, data may include information on the research methodology, participants, data collection methods, and themes.

By piloting the data extraction form and including the necessary information, researchers can ensure that the form captures all relevant data while maintaining consistency and efficiency throughout the review process. This comprehensive approach enhances the accuracy and validity of the systematic review's findings. The content of the form can indeed vary based on the specific research question being addressed and the types of studies included in the review. Here is a summary of the key information to consider including in the data extraction form.

18.4.3.1 Study Description
- Aims and objectives of the study.
- Study setting, including geographical location and time period.
- Study design, such as cohort, case–control, RCT, etc.
- Recruitment procedures used to select participants.
- Inclusion and exclusion criteria used to define the study population.
- Length of follow-up for longitudinal studies.

18.4.3.2 Participant Description
- Baseline characteristics of study participants, including age, gender, and relevant demographics.
- Follow-up characteristics, if applicable.
- The target population and the final number of subjects studied for the outcome.

18.4.3.3 Description of Exposure (or Intervention) and Outcome Measurements
- Detailed description of the measurement of exposure and outcome, including the instruments or tools used, protocols, and reliability measures.
- For intervention studies (RCTs), a description of the intervention, randomization, and blinding procedures.

18.4.3.4 Statistical Data/Results
- Statistical techniques used in the study, such as regression, t-tests, etc.
- Confounding factors that were adjusted for in the analysis.
- Results of the study analysis, including the direction and magnitude of associations and the precision of estimates.
- Conclusions drawn from the study based on the results.

18.4.4 Risk of Bias Assessment

Conducting a risk of bias assessment, also known as a quality assessment, is a crucial step in a systematic review. The purpose of this assessment is to evaluate the potential for bias in individual studies included in the review. Bias, in this context, refers to flaws in the design or conduct of the study that could affect the validity and reliability of its findings in relation to the review question. It is important to clarify that when assessing the risk of bias, the focus is not on critiquing the authors themselves but rather on identifying any potential methodological limitations that may impact the study's results. The risk of bias assessment is valuable during the synthesis process because it helps differentiate between studies that provide reliable estimates in relation to the review question and those that may have introduced bias and therefore need to be interpreted with caution.

There are several approaches to conducting a risk of bias assessment, and there is no one-size-fits-all method suitable for all systematic reviews. Some common options include the following.

- *Standard assessment tools*: researchers may use standardized assessment tools, such as those provided in the Cochrane Handbook or the RTI item bank, to evaluate the risk of bias in included studies. These tools offer a systematic and structured approach to assess various aspects of study quality.
- *Customized assessment*: alternatively, researchers may choose to develop their own risk of bias assessment tool tailored to the specific needs of the review. Customized tools allow for greater flexibility in addressing the unique aspects of the research question and the included study designs.

Whichever approach is chosen, it is important to be transparent and explicit about the risk of bias assessment process in the systematic review report. This includes detailing the criteria used for assessment and how the assessments were conducted. Additionally, the findings of the risk of bias assessment should be taken into account during the data synthesis and interpretation stages to appropriately weigh the evidence from different studies. By conducting a rigorous risk of bias assessment, researchers can enhance the credibility and reliability of their systematic review findings, providing a more robust basis for drawing conclusions and making recommendations.

18.5 Results Synthesis

18.5.1 Narrative Synthesis

Writing a narrative synthesis of the results is a crucial step in a systematic review. It involves summarizing the information from the included studies, highlighting their characteristics, and presenting the key findings without interpretation. Here is an outline of the process.

1) *Characteristics of included studies*: start by providing a concise summary of the characteristics of the included studies. This may include details such as the study setting (geographical location, time period), study design (cohort, case–control, RCT, etc.), exposure and outcome measures used, and any co-variates that were measured.
2) *Summarize key findings*: present a clear and succinct summary of the key findings from each study. Focus on the main results related to the review question, avoiding interpretation at this stage. Consider grouping studies based on similarities in design, population, or exposure to facilitate clarity.
3) *Addressing consistency and variability*: discuss the overall direction of effect observed across the included studies. Identify any results that are not consistent with an apparent trend. Examine variations in findings among studies and consider potential reasons for discrepancies, such as differences in study design, population characteristics, or measurement methods.
4) *Accounting for risk of bias*: discuss the impact of the risk of bias assessment on the interpretation of the results. Analyze how the findings from studies with low, moderate, or high risk of bias differ in relation to the review question. Be transparent about the implications of bias on the overall conclusions.

5) *Consideration of Metaanalysis*: if appropriate, explore the potential for conducting a metaanalysis to synthesize the results quantitatively. Determine if the included studies are similar enough in terms of design and outcomes to warrant statistical pooling of data. If a metaanalysis is not feasible, provide a clear rationale for the decision.

6) *Tables and graphics*: complement the narrative synthesis with tables and graphics to present the summarized data visually. Tables can be used to display study characteristics, key results, and risk of bias assessments. Graphics, such as forest plots or funnel plots (if applicable), can aid in visualizing the results of metaanalyses.

7) *Limitations and strengths*: acknowledge the limitations and strengths of the included studies and the review process itself. Be transparent about any uncertainties or potential sources of bias that may impact the conclusions.

8) *Implications and future research*: conclude the narrative synthesis by discussing the implications of the findings for practice, policy, or future research. Identify areas where further investigation is needed to address gaps in knowledge.

By following these steps, researchers can present a comprehensive and unbiased narrative synthesis of the results in their systematic review, providing valuable insights to readers and contributing to evidence-based decision making.

18.5.2 Metaanalysis

Metaanalysis is a powerful statistical technique used to combine the results of multiple independent studies to obtain a more precise and comprehensive estimate of the measure of association. It can enhance the statistical power of the analysis and provide a more robust and reliable conclusion. However, before conducting a metaanalysis, it is essential to carefully assess whether it is appropriate to combine the results of the included studies. There are several considerations to take into account.

- *Homogeneity of studies*: the studies included in the metaanalysis should be reasonably homogeneous in terms of study design, participant characteristics, exposure or intervention, and outcome measurements. If the studies are too dissimilar, the results may not be meaningful when combined, and the metaanalysis may be inappropriate.

- *Clinical heterogeneity*: even if the studies are similar in design, there may still be clinical heterogeneity due to differences in patient populations, treatment protocols, or other factors. If there is substantial clinical heterogeneity, the results may not be generalizable or appropriate for statistical pooling.

- *Statistical heterogeneity*: statistical heterogeneity refers to variations in effect sizes among the included studies beyond what would be expected due to chance alone. If significant statistical heterogeneity is present, it may indicate underlying differences between studies that could affect the validity of the combined estimate.

- *Outcome measures*: the outcome measures reported in the included studies should be conceptually similar and measured in a comparable way. If the outcome measures are too diverse, combining them in a metaanalysis may not provide meaningful results.

- *Publication bias*: publication bias occurs when studies with positive or significant results are more likely to be published, leading to an overestimation of the overall effect size. It is crucial to assess and address publication bias in a metaanalysis to avoid biased conclusions.

If the studies are sufficiently homogeneous, both clinically and statistically, and their outcome measures are conceptually comparable, then a metaanalysis can be conducted. However, if heterogeneity is present or the studies are too diverse, a narrative synthesis or a qualitative systematic review may be more appropriate.

It is important for researchers to conduct sensitivity analyses and explore potential sources of heterogeneity before proceeding with a metaanalysis. This way, the robustness and generalizability of the combined estimate can be thoroughly assessed and reported. Additionally, transparency in the reporting of the metaanalysis methods and findings is essential for readers to understand the validity and limitations of the results.

Metaanalysis requires having numerical estimates of the effect of the exposure or intervention in question in a consistent and comparable form across studies. This typically involves having effect sizes such as risk ratios, odds ratios, hazard ratios, or mean differences that quantify the association between the exposure and the outcome of interest. These effect sizes should ideally measure the same outcome variable (or a comparable outcome) and should be expressed in a consistent metric, such as per unit change in exposure or a common reference category for categorical exposures. Having effect sizes in a similar form allows for meaningful statistical pooling and synthesis of the results across studies.

When conducting a metaanalysis, researchers have two main sources for obtaining effect size estimates.

- *Published results*: many studies report effect size estimates and associated measures of uncertainty (e.g., confidence intervals) in their published articles. Researchers can extract these estimates directly from the publications and use them in the metaanalysis. It is essential to use the effect sizes that are most relevant to the research question and outcome of interest.
- *Contacting authors*: in some cases, the published results may not provide the necessary effect size estimates in a compatible form for metaanalysis. In such situations, researchers may consider contacting the authors of the original studies to request additional information or data needed for the metaanalysis. This may involve asking authors to provide effect size estimates that were not initially reported or to reanalyze their data to obtain the required effect measures.

When contacting authors, it is essential to be clear about the specific information or data needed and to provide a rationale for the request. Researchers should also be prepared to explain the purpose and significance of the metaanalysis and how their study fits into the broader context of the research question. Obtaining effect size estimates from authors can enhance the completeness and accuracy of the metaanalysis. However, researchers should be aware that not all authors may be able or willing to provide the requested information, and it is essential to account for potential nonresponse or missing data in the analysis.

In summary, metaanalysis relies on having consistent and comparable effect size estimates. Researchers can use published results or, if necessary, contact authors to obtain the required effect measures to ensure a meaningful and informative metaanalysis.

While traditional metaanalysis is a widely used statistical technique for combining the results of multiple studies, newer and more sophisticated methods, such as network metaanalysis (NMA), are being developed to address specific challenges and questions in evidence synthesis. Network metaanalysis is an extension of traditional metaanalysis that allows for the simultaneous comparison of multiple interventions (including both direct and indirect comparisons) within a network of RCTs. It is particularly useful when there are multiple treatment options for a specific condition or disease, and head-to-head comparisons between all treatments may not be available in individual studies. In NMA, both direct evidence (from studies directly comparing two interventions) and indirect evidence (derived from comparing interventions indirectly via a common comparator) are combined to estimate the relative effectiveness of different interventions.

This approach can provide valuable insights into the comparative effectiveness of various treatments and can help inform decision making in clinical practice and healthcare policy. However, these newer metaanalysis techniques come with their own methodological challenges.

- *Assumptions*: NMA relies on certain assumptions, and violations of these assumptions can impact the validity of the results. For example, the transitivity assumption assumes that the distribution of effect modifiers is consistent across the different treatment comparisons.
- *Data availability*: NMA requires a sufficient number of studies comparing various interventions to ensure reliable and robust estimates. If there are limited or sparse data for certain comparisons, the precision of the results may be compromised.
- *Complexity*: NMA can be more complex than traditional pairwise metaanalysis, in terms of both conducting the analysis and interpreting the results. This complexity may require specialized statistical expertise to perform appropriately.
- *Reporting and interpretation*: proper reporting and interpretation of NMA results require careful attention to detail, including transparency in methods and assumptions, as well as the communication of findings in a clear and understandable manner.

Given the complexity and potential pitfalls of these advanced metaanalysis techniques, it is crucial to consult with a statistician or methodologist with relevant expertise when planning and conducting such analyses. This can help ensure that the chosen method is appropriate for the research question and that the analysis is conducted and interpreted correctly.

In conclusion, while newer metaanalysis techniques like NMA offer valuable advancements in evidence synthesis, it is essential to approach their implementation with caution and seek expert guidance to ensure methodological rigor and validity.

There are several options for conducting a metaanalysis using different software packages, each with its advantages and limitations.

- *General-purpose statistical packages (SPSS®, SAS, R, Stata)*: these widely used statistical packages offer various functionalities, including the ability to perform metaanalyses. They are powerful and flexible, allowing for complex statistical analyses. R, in particular, is free and has a vast user community that develops and shares various metaanalysis packages. However, commercial packages like SPSS, SAS, and Stata may require the purchase of licenses, which can be expensive.

- *Software specifically designed for metaanalysis (RevMan, Metawin, CMA)*: There are software packages explicitly developed for metaanalysis, such as RevMan (Review Manager), Metawin, and Comprehensive Metaanalysis (CMA). These tools are designed to streamline the process of conducting metaanalyses and often provide specialized features for effect size calculations, forest plots, and other metaanalysis-related tasks. However, they may have limitations in terms of data formats and graphical customization compared to general-purpose statistical packages.
- *Microsoft Excel*: Microsoft Excel, although not specifically designed for metaanalysis, can still be used to perform basic metaanalyses and produce forest plots. It is more accessible and may already be available to many researchers as part of Microsoft Office. There are guides available that provide step-by-step instructions for conducting metaanalyses in Excel. However, Excel may lack some of the advanced features available in dedicated metaanalysis software.

Regardless of the software used, it is essential to ensure data accuracy and consistency. As mentioned, having two reviewers independently enter the data for the metaanalysis helps minimize errors and ensures the reliability of the results. Each option has its pros and cons, and the choice of software may depend on the specific needs, budget constraints, and familiarity of the researchers with the tools. It is always good practice to seek advice from experts or consult methodological resources when conducting metaanalyses to ensure the appropriate selection and proper execution of the chosen software.

18.5.3 Sensitivity Analysis and Assessing Bias

These are important aspects of conducting a metaanalysis and help researchers gain a deeper understanding of the results and the potential sources of variability across studies.

1) *Sensitivity analysis*: sensitivity analysis is a crucial step in metaanalysis, where researchers explore the robustness of the overall effect size by examining whether the effect differs across subgroups or by investigating the impact of excluding certain studies from the analysis. By categorizing studies based on relevant characteristics (e.g., age group, study design, intervention type), researchers can perform separate metaanalyses for each subgroup to see if the effect varies between them. This process allows for a more nuanced understanding of the overall effect and provides insights into potential effect modifiers.
2) *Heterogeneity assessment*: heterogeneity refers to the variability in effect sizes observed across different studies. It can arise due to genuine differences in study populations, interventions, or other factors that affect the outcome. The Q-statistic and I2 value are commonly used to assess heterogeneity. The Q-statistic tests whether the observed variation is beyond what would be expected by chance alone, while the I2 value quantifies the percentage of total variation attributable to heterogeneity.
   - If heterogeneity is low and not statistically significant, a fixed-effects model is appropriate, assuming a common true effect size across all studies.
   - If heterogeneity is high and statistically significant, a random-effects model is more appropriate, taking into account the variation between studies due to both random sampling error and systematic differences.

The presence of heterogeneity does not necessarily invalidate the metaanalysis but it should be thoroughly investigated to understand its potential sources and implications. Subgroup analyses and metaregression can help explore the sources of heterogeneity and identify possible effect modifiers.

Conducting sensitivity analysis and assessing heterogeneity are essential steps in the metaanalysis process, as they enhance the reliability and interpretability of the results. Researchers should carefully interpret the findings and consider the implications of potential effect modifiers and sources of heterogeneity when drawing conclusions from the metaanalysis. Even though a metaanalysis combines data from multiple studies to provide a more comprehensive estimate of the effect size, the presence of bias in the original studies can still influence the metaanalysis result. It is crucial to be aware of potential sources of bias and to take them into consideration during the interpretation of the findings.

Here are some important points to consider when interpreting the results of a metaanalysis.

- *Assessing bias*: conducting a sensitivity analysis to examine the effect estimates of studies with low and high risk of bias is one way to assess the possibility of bias in the metaanalysis. Additionally, researchers can use tools such as the Cochrane Risk of Bias tool to assess the methodological quality of individual studies included in the metaanalysis.
- *Publication bias*: publication bias occurs when studies with positive or statistically significant results are more likely to be published than those with negative or nonsignificant results. This bias can lead to an overestimation of the effect size in the metaanalysis. Researchers can use methods like funnel plots or statistical tests (e.g., Egger's test) to explore the

presence of publication bias. Moreover, searching for unpublished data, such as gray literature or contacting experts in the field, can help mitigate the impact of publication bias.

- *Heterogeneity and subgroup analyses*: high heterogeneity among the studies can be an indicator of potential sources of bias or effect modification. By conducting subgroup analyses based on study characteristics, researchers can explore whether the effect size varies between different subgroups. This can provide insights into possible reasons for the observed heterogeneity.
- *Confidence intervals*: paying attention to the width and precision of the confidence intervals around the effect estimate is important. A wide confidence interval indicates greater uncertainty in the results and should be taken into account when interpreting the findings.
- *External validity*: consider the generalizability of the results to the broader population or specific subgroups of interest. The included studies might have certain limitations or characteristics that affect the applicability of the results to other settings or populations.

In conclusion, being cautious and critical when interpreting the results of a metaanalysis is essential. Researchers should carefully assess the potential sources of bias and heterogeneity, consider the confidence intervals, and evaluate the external validity of the findings to draw reliable and meaningful conclusions from the metaanalysis.

Reference

Denison, H.J., Dodds, R.M., Ntani, G. et al. (2013). How to get started with a systematic review in epidemiology: an introductory guide for early career researchers. *Archives of Public Health* 71 (1): 21.

19

Statistical and Mathematical Modeling

Ashish C. Patel

Veterinary College, Kamdhenu University, Anand, India

Epidemiology is a discipline which deals with the study of infectious diseases in a population. It is concerned with all aspects of epidemic, e.g., spread, control, vaccination strategy, etc.

Statistical and mathematical modeling have a significant role in epidemiology for the prediction method as well as to understand how and why infections are spread. Models also cover the current status of infection, to what extent it may be spread, how much of the community will be infected within a particular time interval, how to mitigate outbreaks, how to prevent or restrict infection among individuals within and between populations. Infectious diseases caused by a known etiological agent are easier to control but infectious diseases caused by multiple etiological agents are difficult to control. When a new infectious disease emerges or there is an outbreak of a known infectious disease, epidemiologists collect, analyze, and interpret information to indicate interventions to mitigate further spreading.

Many infectious diseases cross regional, national, and international boundaries, and not limited to particular castes or communities. Infectious agents initially affecting only one region of the world can spread to other regions and ultimately may become a pandemic. The best example of this is COVID-19. Such diseases may have several types based on their extent of spread.

Infectious diseases are basically of two types: acute infectious diseases which remain for a short period (days/weeks), e.g., influenza, chickenpox, etc., and chronic infectious diseases which remain for longer periods (month/year), e.g., hepatitis. In general the spread of an infectious disease depends upon various factors such as a susceptible population, infective population, immune class, and mode of transmission of infection. To understand and control infectious diseases, it is necessary to understand statistical and mathematical models to control further spread (Brauer and Castillo-Chavez, 2000).

19.1 Importance of Statistical and Mathematical Modeling in Epidemiology

In epidemiology, the question may arise, what is the relationship of epidemiology and statistical/mathematical models? Why are these models important in epidemiology? Can we control/mitigate infectious diseases without any knowledge of models? The aim of epidemic modeling is to understand and if possible control the spread of disease. In this context the following questions may arise.

- What is the rate of spread of infectious disease?
- How much of the total population are infected or will be infected?
- What control measures could be used?
- What will be the effects of migration/environment?
- To what extent will the disease persist?

Statistical and mathematical analysis allows us to take information from individuals and classify them into certain groups according to age, caste, time point, weather, etc. This may help us to understand from where the infection has originated, how it might be spreading and thereby to understand the use of potential resources for prevention and containment in restricted

Epidemiology and Environmental Hygiene in Veterinary Public Health, First Edition. Edited by Tanmoy Rana.
© 2025 John Wiley & Sons, Inc. Published 2025 by John Wiley & Sons, Inc.

zones. This kind of data analysis from the field may be useful for the generation of hypotheses. In order to test hypotheses about disease prevalence, we need more sophisticated approaches/designs/models to minimize bias and quantify the role of chance.

The aims of such analysis may be:

- to understand the magnitude of infectious diseases in a population in terms of transmission, new cases, and existing cases
- to analyze the prognosis of infections, complications of infections, and posttreatment infections; for example, there was an outbreak of fungal infection mucormycosis due to continuous steroid treatment for COVID-19.
- to determine risk factors of infection, including the frequency of infection acquisition and progression from infection to disease, sequelae, different clinical outcomes, etc.
- to evaluate the efficacy and effectiveness of preventive measures (vaccines) and curative measures (treatments)
- to guide policymakers regarding prevention, control, and eventual elimination of the infectious disease.

19.2   Assumptions for Statistical and Mathematical Models

Some general assumptions are common to all statistical and mathematical models.

- The mode of transmission of an infection is either by direct or indirect contact between an infected individual and a susceptible individual.
- There is no latent period for the infection once a susceptible individual comes into contact with an infected individual. The infection is transmitted rapidly when the contact takes place.
- All susceptible individuals are equally susceptible and all infected ones are equally infectious.
- It is assumed that the population in which the infection spreads is large enough to take care of fluctuations in the spread of the disease. So a deterministic model is considered. A deterministic model allows you to calculate a future event exactly, without the involvement of randomness.
- The population size is fixed and considered as closed.

    If X (t)- population of susceptible,

    Y (t)- population of infected while,

    If B is the average contact number with susceptible which leads to new infection per unit time per infective,

    Then

$$Y\left(t+\Delta t\right) = Y\left(t\right) + BY\left(t\right)\Delta t$$

which in the limit $\Delta t \rightarrow 0$ gives $dY/dt = BY$ (t) which represents the rate of change of y with respect to t.

19.3   Differences between Statistical and Mathematical Models

- There is a basic difference between a mathematical model and a statistical model. In the mathematical model, there is no random error term in the equation, whereas the statistical model includes the random error term.
- The simplest example of a regression model as $Y = a + bx$ represents a mathematical model as $Y = a + bx + e$ represent a statistical model, where a is an intercept, b is the slope of the straight line (for a given population) and e is the random error component.
- The statistical model expresses relationship between a dependent variable (Y) and an independent variable (X) when both X and Y are continuous variables.
- Statistical models can be used for prediction of dependent variables per unit change in independent variables. Also for prediction of a mean value of Y for a given value of X (my/x) in the population.
- A regression line that fits well indicated by small error or deviations between observed values and predicted values by model. The main objective of epidemiological studies is to evaluate the association between exposure of individuals to infection/disease and the occurrence of a specific disease.
- In epidemiological investigation, it is essential to determine the status of disease from the effects of certain risk factors/ causative agents or co-variates. This can be handled by using a multiple regression model which gives the relationship between a dependent variable and a set of independent predictors.
- The effect of other factors that explain or produce confounding can be controlled at either the design stage or analysis stage of the research exercise.

Table 19.1 Classification and description of time series models.

Time series model	Model description	Type of model: stationary/nonstationary
Autoregressive model (AR)	Present values explained linearly based on previous values and present residuals	Stationary
Moving average (MA)	Present values of time series explained linearly for previous values and time series residuals	Stationary
Autoregressive moving average (ARMA)	As a combination of AR and MA, present values of time series are explained linearly for current values but also previous and present residuals	Stationary
Autoregressive integrated moving average (ARIMA)	Based on the ARMA model, but a differencing procedure transforming nonstationary data to stationary data	Nonstationary
Seasonal autoregressive integrated moving average (SARIMA)	Based on the ARIMA model, but also includes seasonal differencing, in case of data with periodic patterns	Nonstationary

19.4 Time Series Regression (TSR) Model

- Time series regression models for forecasting of infectious diseases are of prime importance for determining the behavior of the disease spread and to create better policies to overcome the problem.
- This model gathers past information on a scale of time. Then the constructed model is applied for forecasting the future values of the series. Many researchers have developed time series models to enhance the prediction precision of the disease.
- The main time series models used for forecasting the infectious diseases are autoregressive time series models such as AR (Auto Regressive), MA (Moving Average), ARMA (Auto Regressive Moving Average), ARIMA (Auto Regressive Integrated Moving Average), and SARIMA (Seasonal Auto Regressive Integrated Moving Average).
- These time series models help forecast the forthcoming propensity of the phenomenon, risks, and distribution or dilation trend of different diseases.
- Autoregressive models are classified into two categories: stationary and nonstationary time series models. The model is termed stationary if it mean, variance, autocorrelation, and other parameters are stationary over time. A model is termed strictly stationary when the mean, variance, and co-variances are fixed over fixed time intervals, i.e., weekly, monthly, fortnightly, etc.

There are several stationary and nonstationary TSR models used in epidemiology as shown in Table 19.1.

19.5 SI (Susceptible to Infected) Model

As it is observed that B depends upon the susceptible population, so β = average number of contacts between susceptible and infected which leads to new infection per unit time per susceptible per infective (Figure 19.1), then:

$$B = \beta X(t), \text{ which gives, } dy/dt \left(\text{the rate of change of } y \text{ with respect to } t\right)$$
$$= \beta X(t) Y(t)$$
$$= \beta (N - Y) Y$$

where $N = X + Y$ is the total population, which is fixed as per assumption.

19.6 SIS Model (No Immunity Model)

Pathogen causes illness for a period of time followed by immunity as:

S (Susceptible) $\rightarrow$ I (Infected)
S: Previously unexposed to the pathogen.

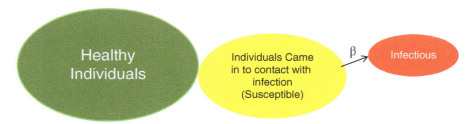

Figure 19.1 Susceptible to Infected (SI) Model. As shown in the figure, the larger circle indicates the larger number of individuals who are healthy, a few of whom come into contact with infection, resulting in susceptibility which then converts to infectious. β indicates the average number of individuals who come into contact with infection which leads to new infection per unit time per susceptible per infective.

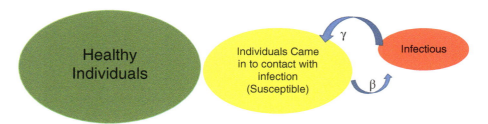

Figure 19.2 In the Susceptible-Infectious-Susceptible (SIS) (No Immunity) Model, infected cases are again susceptible after recovery. This model is applied to diseases which have the common occurrence of reinfection and relapse cases, e.g., cough, throat infection, some cases of COVID-19.

I: Currently colonized by the pathogen.
Proportion of population: $S = X/N$, $I = Y/N$.
We ignore demography of population (death/birth and migration).

- Recovery rate is inversely proportional to infectious period. So it is taken to be constant though infection period (time spent in the infectious class) is distributed about a mean value and can be estimated from the clinical data.
- In this model, it is assumed that the whole population is divided into two classes, susceptible and infective, and that if an individual is infected then it remains in that class. However, this is not always the case, as an infected person may recover from the disease (Figure 19.2).
- If γ is the rate of recovery from infective class to susceptible class, then:

$$dS/dt = \gamma I - \beta SI$$

$$dI/dt = \beta SI - \gamma I$$

$$dI/dt = \beta\left[(1 - 1/R0) - I\right], I, R0 = \beta/\gamma$$

$S^* = 1/R0$ and $I^* = 1 - 1/R0$, feasible if $R0 > 1$

19.7 SIR (Susceptible–Infected–Recovered) Model

Pathogen causes illness for a period of time followed by immunity.

S (Susceptible) → I (Infected) → R (Recovered)
S: Previously unexposed to the pathogen.
I: Currently colonized by the pathogen.
R: Successfully cleared from the infection.
Proportion of population: $S = X/N$, $I = Y/N$, $R = Z/N$.
We ignore demography of population (death/birth and migration) (Hethcote, 2000).

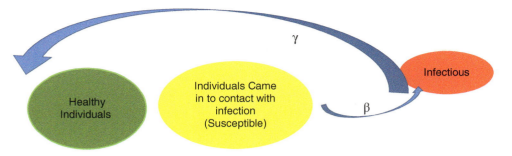

Figure 19.3 The Susceptible–Infected–Recovered (SIR) model computes theoretical infections with a contagious infection in a closed population over time. This model involves the number of susceptible people, infected cases, and recovered individuals.

In view of the above assumption, the SIR model is given by:

$dS/dt = -\beta SI$

$dI/dt = -\beta SI - \gamma I$

$dR/dt = \gamma I$ as with conditions of $S(0) > 0; I(0) > 0$ and $R(0) = 0$

where $1/\gamma$ is average infectious period. If $S(0) < \gamma/\beta$, then initially $dI/dt < 0$ and the infection will be cured. Thus, for an infection to enter, $S(0) > \gamma/\beta$ or if γ/β: removal rate is small enough then the disease will spread (Figure 19.3).

- SIR models are very general in nature as these models follow a black box approach and do not consider the mechanism of transmission of a disease.
- In fact, the structure of a disease plays an important role in the modeling. It may be noted that a disease can be transmitted directly or indirectly.
- The direct mode of transmission could be by viral agents (COVID-19, SARS, measles, rubella, chickenpox) or by bacteria (TB, meningitis, gonorrhea). Generally, viral causative agents confer immunity against reinfection while there is no such immunity with a bacterial causative agent. The indirect mode of transmission could be due to vectors or carriers (malaria).
- So, for modeling of most communicable diseases, the factors mentioned below should be considered.
  1) *Age-structured population*: many diseases spread with contact in a group of a given age structure, e.g., measles, chickenpox, and other childhood diseases spread mainly by contact between children of similar age group.
  2) *Incubation period*: it is often assumed that the latent period of disease is very small and that there is no incubation time for the disease to show. This is not true with diseases like typhoid. Such considerations will give rise to time delay models.
  3) *Variable infectivity*: in diseases like HIV/AIDS, infective individuals are highly infective in the initial stages. Thereafter, they have a relatively low infectivity for a long period before again becoming highly infective before developing full-blown AIDS.
  4) *Spatial nonuniformity*: it is well known that bubonic plague was carried from place to place by rats. Thus, spatial spread becomes important in such cases, which will lead to a system of partial differential equations (PDEs).
  5) *Vertical transmission*: in some diseases, the offspring of infected members may be born infective (AIDS). This is called vertical transmission.
  6) *Models with compartments*: in many cases the population can be placed in different compartments, where intercompartmental interaction takes place, e.g., in malaria.
  7) *Stochastic models*: so far we have considered only deterministic models, and random effects have not been taken into account. The random effect is negligible for larger populations but when the population is smaller, stochastic models will be required.

19.8 Recent Statistical Modeling for COVID-19 Pandemic

Scientists have been working on COVID-19 epidemiological modeling to understand the disease outbreak and its spread. For instance, Hoertel et al. (2020) suggested a random agent-based microsimulation (ABM) model for the COVID-19 epidemic in France. They described the effect of nontherapeutic interventions (natural remedies) on the incidence of COVID-19 and mortality. They also discussed the model with different suppressive measures and effect of lockdown during COVID-19. They have calculated R0 for their model to predict the pattern of infection spread. Based on study data, they also described the effect of lockdown, physical distancing, and mask wearing on disease spread and reduction of mortality rates.

Hsiang et al. (2020) studied the different statistical models and epidemiological studies for the transmission dynamics of COVID-19. They collected data on 1700 local, regional, and national nonpharmaceutical interventions assigned during COVID-19 in China, Italy, the United States, France, South Korea, and Iran. Then they applied reduced-form econometric methods, to determine the impact of policies on economic growth and empirically measure the effect that these anticontagion policies had on the growth rate of infections. They found that anticontagion policies definitely slowed this growth and can be helpful in making well-informed decisions regarding whether or when these policies should be applied, intensified, or lifted, and they may support policy making in the more than 180 other countries in which COVID-19 has been reported.

Baggett et al. (2020) described the use of descriptive statistics for characterization of COVID-19 samples as the percentage of PCR positive and the symptom profile of persons with RT PCR-confirmed infections of COVID-19. Initially, numerous symptomatic persons had been considered as COVID negative based on rapid screening tests, prior symptom screening, and self-referrals. Based on RT PCR testing, it was suggested that the rapid screening test may be detected as false negative. These results suggested that the RT PCR test should be advisable for asymptomatic persons who live with symptomatic persons with COVID-19.

Banerjee et al. (2020) used population-based cohort data on the primary and secondary care electronic health records from England. They estimated one-year mortality caused by routine health issues through simple models and excessive mortality caused by COVID-19. They also published an online prototype risk calculator for estimating excess deaths.

Rai et al. (2021) described the impact of social media awareness on the transmission dynamics of COVID-19 in India.

19.9 Conclusion

In this chapter, I have discussed the concept of statistical and mathematical modeling and their importance in epidemiological studies for predicting infectious disease spread. I have covered assumptions and the difference between statistical and mathematical modeling in epidemiological studies. Time series regression models are used for forecasting of infectious diseases and to understand the behavior of the disease spread in order to determine the best health policies to mitigate any outbreak. The main time series models are autoregressive models including AR, MA, ARMA, ARIMA, and SARIMA. The AR models are classified into stationary and nonstationary. I have also covered SI, SIS, and SIR models and discussed which model should be used for specific infectious diseases and why.

References

Baggett, T.P., Keyes, H., Sporn, N., and Gaeta, J.M. (2020). Variation in COVID-19 hospitalizations and deaths across New York City boroughs. *JMMA* 323: 2192–2195.

Banerjee, A., Pasea, L., Harris, S. et al. (2020). Estimating excess 1-year mortality associated with the COVID-19 pandemic according to underlying conditions and age: a population-based cohort study. *Lancet* 395: 1715–1725.

Brauer, F. and Castillo-Chavez, C. (2000). *Mathematical Models in Population Biology and Epidemiology*. New York: Springer.

Hethcote, HW. (2000). The mathematics of infectious diseases. *SIAM Review* 42 (4): 599–653.

Hoertel, N., Blachier, M., Blanco, C. et al. (2020). A stochastic agent-based model of the SARS-CoV-2 epidemic in France. *Nature Medicine* 26: 1–5.

Hsiang, S., Allen, D., Annan-Phan, S. et al. (2020). The effect of large-scale anti-contagion policies on the COVID-19 pandemic. *Nature* 584: 262–267.

Rai, R.K., Khajanchi, S., Tiwari, P.K. et al. (2021). Impact of social media advertisements on the transmission dynamics of COVID-19 pandemic in India. *Journal of Computational and Applied Mathematics* 2021 (27): 1–6.

20

Health Schemes and Its Importance

Sabhyata Sharma[1], Abhishek Pathak[1], Abhinav Meena[1], and Sandeep Kumar[2]

[1] *Department of Veterinary Parasitology, Apollo College of Veterinary Medicine, Jaipur, Rajasthan, 302031, India*
[2] *Cluster University of Jammu, 180001, Jammu and Kashmir, India*

20.1 Introduction

Numerous variables, such as disease, starvation, bad management, and improper use of the best genetic material, limit the number of livestock that may be produced. The main goals of animal health initiatives are to protect human health by battling zoonoses, to ensure a steady supply of food for a growing human population, and to promote domestic and international trade in animals and animal products (Temple, 1970). The required interventions must be both economically sensible and technically sound. One of the industries with the quickest rate of growth is the livestock industry, particularly in low- and middle-income nations due to the rising demand for meals derived from animals. More than a billion people depend on the livestock industry for their livelihoods, a major number of whom are small-scale livestock farmers and pastoralists. Many of the Sustainable Development Goals (SDGs) are supported by livestock systems, which significantly reduce poverty and improve nutrition and health. In addition to benefits, the rapid expansion of livestock production to meet the demands of a growing population also carries risks if livestock systems are not adequately managed. Concerns regarding the security of food and nutrition, as well as the health of people, animals, and the environment, are raised by these threats (WHO, 2005). Some of the most important dangers to animal health and welfare include developing illnesses, zoonotic diseases, and transboundary animal diseases. Both the trade in livestock and its byproducts as well as human wellbeing are hampered by these diseases.

It is important to acknowledge that the occurrence and spread of these diseases, whether they are zoonotic or not, invariably have significant negative effects on the economy and society. Both the trade in livestock and its byproducts as well as human well-being are hampered by these diseases. It is important to acknowledge that the occurrence and spread of these diseases, whether they are zoonotic or not, invariably have significant negative effects on the economy and society. Human-wildlife interface livestock systems, as well as large scale commercial systems with densely populated, homogeneous populations, each have their own distinct ecological characteristics. These systems operate in a more globalized context characterized by population expansion, economic growth, fast urbanization and land use expansion, unsustainable resource exploitation, increased human and animal movement, and climate change. It is a continuing challenge for regulatory and technical authorities, as well as livestock producers, to stay current with these developments and make the appropriate corrections. With more opportunities for interspecies interactions and pathogen spillover due to all of these factors, the environment is becoming more conducive to the emergence and rapid spread of diseases, necessitating integrated solutions as part of a comprehensive all-systems approach to disease prevention and control. The Emergency Prevention System for Animal Health (EMPRES-AH), which is intended to "control epidemic animal diseases as well as emerging diseases on a regional and global basis, through international cooperation involving early warning, rapid reaction, enabling research, and coordination," is at the core of FAO's animal health programme. It is also crucial to the health and well-being programme. The EMPRESAH Strategic Plan for 2023–2026 is described in this chapter, and it offers a fresh method for fusing biosecurity and One Health to aid Members in managing threats to animal health through improved early warning and progressive biosecurity management pathways. In order to advance towards the SDGs, the Plan also supports the FAO Strategic Framework (2022–2031) and sustainable livestock transformation.

Epidemiology and Environmental Hygiene in Veterinary Public Health, First Edition. Edited by Tanmoy Rana.
© 2025 John Wiley & Sons, Inc. Published 2025 by John Wiley & Sons, Inc.

20.2 One Health Programme

A sustainable balance and optimization of the health of people, animals, and ecosystems are the goals of the integrated, unifying approach known as "One Health." It acknowledges how interconnected and dependent the health of people, domestic and wild animals, plants, and the larger environment (including ecosystems) is. The COVID-19 pandemic, a human health emergency brought on by an animal-transmitted virus, and the global impact and reaction to it underscore the necessity for coordinated action across sectors to safeguard health and prevent disruption of food systems. As part of the transformation of the agri-food system for the health of humans, animals, plants, and the environment, FAO recommends a One Health approach. The work on sustainable agriculture, the health of animals, plants, forests, and aquaculture, food safety, antimicrobial resistance (AMR), food security, nutrition, and livelihoods are involved. A One Health strategy is crucial for advancement in order to anticipate, prevent, detect, and control diseases that transfer from animals to humans, address AMR, assure food safety, stop dangers to human and animal health resulting from the environment, as well as combat many other issues. In order to accomplish the Sustainable Development Goals (SDGs), a One Health approach is also essential. In particular, the Quadripartite, which consists of FAO, the United Nations Environment Programme (UNEP), the World Health Organisation (WHO), and the World Organisation for Animal Health (WOAH), works with partners to promote systemic health. In order to protect farmers' livelihoods from the effects of plant and animal diseases, the FAO focuses on eradicating hunger, promoting food security, food safety, and healthy diets, preventing and controlling transboundary diseases, zoonoses, and AMR, and enhancing the sustainability and resilience of agri-food systems with benefits for One Health. Working together for one health, we are one globe.

20.3 FAO's Role

In order to simultaneously address the health of humans, animals, plants, and the environment, FAO helps members in developing and implementing effective joint One Health strategies and capacities. To secure health security from communities to the national and international level, a One Health approach is utilized to create and implement programmes, biosecurity initiatives, enabling policies, and, where applicable, regulatory frameworks. One Health in the transformation of agri-food systems is a crucial Priority Programme Area and a component of the FAO's Strategic Framework (2022–2031). As a centre of technical knowledge, FAO supports One Health in preserving the wellbeing of people, animals, plants, and the environment. It also supports the management and conservation of natural resources, ensures food security, makes it easier for people to access safe and nourishing food, combats AMR, advances efforts to adapt to and mitigate climate change, and encourages sustainable fisheries and agricultural production. The FAO promotes the sharing of epidemiological data and laboratory information across sectors and borders in order to anticipate, prevent, identify, and respond to plant, animal, and zoonotic disease outbreaks and AMR, which can lead to more effective early warning, coordinated planning, and response. One Health is coordinated across various FAO divisions by the Joint Centre for Zoonotic Diseases and Antimicrobial Resistance in order to integrate One Health into FAO activities.

In order to address health hazards at the interface of humans, animals, plants, and the environment, and to advance health and sustainable development, FAO engages externally with UNEP, WHO, and WOAH as the Quadripartite. The Tripartite (FAO, OIE, WHO) cooperation, which was enlarged in March 2022 with the signing of the Memorandum of Understanding (MoU), served as the foundation for the Quadripartite partnership.

20.4 Epidemic Diseases: Eradication Versus Control

By definition, the control of epidemic livestock illnesses has a geographic focus (country, region, continent), whereas programmes for improving farmer and/or local community health and production are more common. When performed consistently across a designated area, veterinarian interventions in the first scenario are most effective. In the latter, depending on the clinical circumstances and farming practices, interventions can differ from farm to farm.

The urge to evaluate current disease control initiatives and, if possible, transition from the control phase to an eradication phase is developing among veterinary services. The International Office of Epizootics (OIE) is developing new rules based on a three-stage process that a nation must undertake before being recognized internationally as being free of an epizootic disease in order to assist this.

Regional, subregional, and national eradication will undoubtedly be advantageous for the affected areas. However, doing so might not be economical because maintaining a high degree of emergency readiness is expensive and necessary to guarantee the state of freedom. Therefore, it may be stated that total eradication offers the best long-term economic return.

The following criteria have been identified as crucial elements for effective disease eradication based on the experience of the FAO European Commission for the Control of Foot-and-Mouth Disease and current efforts of the FAO-coordinated Global Rinderpest Eradication Programme (GREP):

1) The use of high-quality, internationally recognized vaccinations that have been independently verified for efficacy and safety.
2) Organized mass immunization efforts that result in the verifiable elimination of chronic endemicity.
3) Establishing and maintaining national veterinary services that are competent to plan a thorough and ongoing control and monitoring programme.
4) Adherence to the applicable OIE recommendations and deadline for the declaration of freedom from infection and disease.
5) The availability of a national laboratory service that can offer or develop quick and efficient differential diagnosis services.
6) Formulation of a successful plan to stop the etiological agent's reintroduction.
7) Creation of successful regional and national emergency plans, including a practiced action plan in case of an outbreak. A stamping-out policy should be put into place as part of this.

The following legal authority granted to national veterinary agencies must be used to support these measures:

1) The right to collect samples for laboratory testing; the requirement that the owner and/or pertinent municipal authorities notify them of any suspicious cases.
2) The ability to compel mandatory quarantines of sick locations, preferably with animal slaughter and ring vaccination, as well as the authority to seize pertinent materials.
3) The provision of recompense.
4) Sanitation precautions and other suitable practices on contaminated sites.
5) The ability to impose restrictions on the movement of livestock and to halt vehicles and herds in order to check the animals.
6) The ability to establish protection and monitoring zones in order to put additional, intense control measures into place; the ability to carry out emergency vaccination drives.

Although eradicating epidemic diseases globally or regionally would be the ultimate goal, control remains the only realistic objective in the majority of cases. This is due either to the epidemiological complexity of the disease, as in the case of vector-transmitted illnesses like African horse sickness, African swine fever, and Rift Valley fever, or to the lack of adequate tools to achieve eradication, such as effective and safe vaccines and systems for accurate diagnosis and surveillance.

20.5 A Strategy for Disease Eradication at the Global Level

Without a coordinated international effort in obtaining disease intelligence and implementing control measures, eradication at the global or regional level cannot be achieved. Due to their mandates, international organizations like the FAO, OIE, and the World Health Organization (WHO) have a significant role to play in this.

A successful preventative campaign is a key component in the elimination of any major epidemic disease. A new priority programme dubbed Emergency Prevention System (EMPRES) for Transboundary Animal and Plant Pests and Diseases has been launched by FAO as a result of this realization. Through FAO assistance, including technical coordination of control/eradication actions, the animal-illnesses component of EMPRES seeks to boost the response of member countries in prevention and/or their prompt response to emergencies caused by significant transboundary pests and diseases. The Global Rinderpest Eradication Programme (GREP), run by the FAO, aims to completely eradicate rinderpest by the year 2010. The GREP Secretariat was established by the Animal Production and Health Division of FAO with the following responsibilities to help with the execution of this programme:

1) Coordinating meetings are organized.
2) The world reference laboratory is encouraged to support targeted investigations, applied research, and global virus surveillance.

20 Health Schemes and Its Importance

3) Forming advisory scientific committees to help the project.
4) Coordination of risk analysis research and campaigns.
5) Backing for worldwide surveillance.
6) The creation of technical guidelines and the distribution of information and data.

The Pan-African Rinderpest Campaign (PARC), the Western Asia Rinderpest Eradication Campaign (WAREC), and the South Asia Rinderpest Eradication Campaign (SAREC) are the three regional campaigns in Africa, West Asia, and South Asia, respectively (WHO 2005). The GREP Secretariat within FAO will therefore provide the technical linkage between these campaigns. The efficiency of national operations, including the veterinary services, local infrastructures, and the availability of sufficient funding, ultimately determines the success of regional initiatives (Welte and Terán 2004). In each of the regional campaigns, FAO is providing technical support in the areas of epidemiology, such as surveillance and sero-monitoring, vaccination quality control, and the development of communication initiatives to encourage community engagement, in order to assure national success (WHO 2005).

20.6 A Strategy for Disease Eradication at the Continental Level

The primary animal disease that restricts international trade is foot-and-mouth disease (FMD). Additionally, it adversely affects weight increase, milk yield, and draught power, which consequently reduces agricultural production. The current distribution of FMD around the world in some ways reflects the current state of the global economy: all OECD nations are free of the illness and have a programme that aims to completely eradicate the virus. In order to maintain their ability to engage in international trade, middle-income nations like many South American nations conduct extensive FMD control campaigns. In contrast, low-income nations with minimal involvement in the international trade of animals and animal products, such as Sub-Saharan Africa and some regions of Asia, have few examples of successful control programmes (WHO 2005). The national veterinary services, the coordinating function of the South American Commission for the Control of Foot-and-Mouth Disease (COSALFA), as well as the technical support of the World Health Organization all contributed to the success of the ongoing continental plan for the eradication of FMD from the Americas, the Hemispheric Programme for Eradication of Food and Mouth Disease, which has already led to several countries in the region attaining disease-free status (WHO 2005). This demonstrates the value of global cooperation and ought to serve as an example for other developing nations working to eradicate or control regional illness. The first Joint FAO/OIE/Pan-American Health Organization (PAHO) Conference on the Perspective for the Eradication of Foot and Mouth Disease in the Next Millennium and the Impact on Food Security and World Trade was held in 1996, most likely in Brazil (WHO 2005). It is appropriate that an extensive long-range review of FMD eradication strategies in the next millennium will take place in South America (Robinson and Production 2003).

20.7 Control of Endemic Diseases

20.7.1 Brucellosis

The most significant zoonotic disease in the Near East, brucellosis is still an issue in many nations. In accordance with standards developed in partnership with the countries of the region, the FAO, WHO, and OIE are putting together project documents for a regional brucellosis control programme. The program's strategy is centered on immunizing the entire herd or flock of cattle, buffalo, sheep, goats, and camels, regardless of their age or gender. The incidence of the disease is anticipated to be reduced to a point where the idea of eradicating the disease is feasible after a period of 15–20 years of widespread immunization. A more effective vaccination and/or serological tests that can distinguish between infected and vaccinated animals will have been developed in the meantime to match the revised objective.

20.7.2 Tick- and Tick-borne Diseases

The goal of the FAO initiative on ticks and tick-borne diseases is to raise awareness of the emergence of tick acaricide resistance and to promote integrated techniques for controlling ticks and tick-borne diseases, including immunization when appropriate. The Coordinated Programme for the Control of Ticks and Tick-Borne Diseases in Central, East, and Southern

Africa, now in its third phase, has been guided by this idea. The program's goal is to control ticks and tick-borne diseases in cattle using strategic tick control and cost-effective immunization against theileriosis, heart-water, anaplasmosis, and babesiosis. Together with the World Acaricide Resistance Reference Centre in Berlin, Germany, and through the organization of workshops like those held in Zimbabwe, Malawi, and Brazil in 1994, FAO supports work on the assessment of acaricide resistance on a global scale.

When specific conditions support the idea, as they did with the Caribbean's *Amblyomma variegatum* infestation, tick removal is taken into consideration. The Programme for the Eradication of *A. variegatum* and its associated diseases, Heartwater and Dermatophilosis, from the Caribbean has been certified operational after more than seven years of investigations and talks. This came after agreements between the FAO and the Caribbean Community Secretariat (CARICOM) and the Inter-American Institute for Cooperation on Agriculture (IICA).

Through carefully planned surveys, the campaign has now officially started, and work is being done to map the tick's distribution. In order to get rid of this dangerous insect from the area before the year 2000, a pilot eradication programme with the most community involvement has already been started in Anguilla. A large-scale eradication programme will then be planned and carried out. The launch of the campaign comes at an ideal moment given the recent reports of additional *A. variegatum* infection foci in Dominica and new locations in Barbados.

20.7.3   Insect Borne Diseases

The most significant animal health issue in sub-Saharan Africa, according to many experts, is African animal trypanosomiasis (AAT), which is spread by Tsetse flies. The coordination necessary for a concerted effort to address this intricate, multifaceted issue is provided by FAO through its Programme for the Control of African Animal Trypanosomiasis and Related Development. A Geographical Information System (GIS) has been developed by the FAO team that deals with insect-borne diseases to measure the economic and agricultural effects of AAT and to pinpoint the regions where its management is most likely to result in higher agricultural productivity. In the semi-arid and subhumid regions, the disease is gradually taking greater significance. Control initiatives are particularly effective where agriculture is developing.

The *Trypanosoma evansi*, or Surra, *Trypanosomiasis equiperdum*, or Dourine, and the non-cyclically transmitted *Trypanosoma vivax* are the three types of non-tsetse-transmitted animal trypanosomiasis (NTTAT), which has a much wider geographic distribution. Additionally dynamic is the *T. evansi* distribution scenario. Recent Surra flare-ups in cattle in Indonesia and in carabaos, the swamp buffalo, in the Philippines are thought to be related to transboundary movement of people and animals. The FAO Field Programme is looking into the latter outbreaks.

FAO has turned its focus to the prevention of new outbreaks of both New World Screw worm (NWS) and Old-World Screw worm (OWS), as well as of other exotic diseases, following the successful conclusion of the screw worm eradication campaign in the Libyan Arab Jamahiriya supported by the Screw worm Emergency Centre for North Africa (SECNA), which involved the active participation and collaboration of the Mexico/United States Commission on Screw worm (WHO 2005). The majority of training initiatives to far have been focused on North Africa. A request for funds from donors has been made for a plan to eradicate NWS in Jamaica. This strategy is expected to result in a widespread eradication effort in the Caribbean. Improvements are still being made to the methods for NWS surveillance, control, and eradication using the Sterile Insect Technique (SIT), with the hope that the outcomes will be highly advantageous for all affected nations (WHO 2005). The FAO is very concerned about the rapidly spreading issue of anthelmintic resistance in sheep parasites, and money have been dedicated to initiatives aiming to map the scope of the issue in developing nations (Lubroth 2012). The southern region of Latin America has been assessed by a recent survey funded by the FAO Technical Cooperation Programme (TCP). The findings are alarming: more than 75% of farms exhibit issues with resistance to two of the three primary anthelmintic groups currently available for chemical management, and an increasing number exhibit resistance to all three. Similar issues exist in eastern and southern Africa, according to a consultant that was hired to assess the situation in a few African nations (WHO 2005).

Hydatidosis, cysticercosis, and trichinellosis are three parasitic zoonotic illnesses that continue to be a big issue, resulting in human misery and large losses from discarded meat and organs. TCP has enabled the evaluation of current activities in various South American nations. FAO is developing control methods in partnership with the Veterinary Public Health Units of WHO and PAHO (Leforban et al. 2002).

FAO has turned its focus to the prevention of new outbreaks of both New World Screw worm (NWS) and Old-World Screw worm (OWS), as well as of other exotic diseases, following the successful conclusion of the screw worm eradication campaign in the Libyan Arab Jamahiriya supported by the Screw worm Emergency Centre for North Africa (SECNA), which involved the active participation and collaboration of the Mexico/United States Commission on Screw worm (WHO 2005). The majority of training initiatives to far have been focused on North Africa. A request for funds from donors has been made for a plan to eradicate NWS in Jamaica (Lubroth 2012)

20.7.4   Non-Infectious and Production Diseases

In many parts of the world, the significant effort to control the major infectious and parasitic diseases has been largely effective. However, it hasn't always led to the anticipated rise in productivity and livestock output. Numerous significant production-related diseases, such as helminth infections, as well as reproductive problems, dietary issues, and other untreated non-infectious conditions are among the many and various causes of this. These are only a small portion of a complicated collection of situations that hinder output. Additional issues may include a lack of government incentives, incorrect price policies, and a failure to provide animal health services.

The FAO has focused more on creating programmes to control helminths and non-infectious diseases over the past few years. Governments have been made more aware of the economic impact of these illnesses and disorders as well as the obstacles they impose on efforts to increase livestock productivity through a variety of initiatives. Publication of educational materials and the creation of production data through pilot projects are examples of activities.

The FAO is very concerned about the rapidly spreading issue of anthelmintic resistance in sheep parasites, and money have been dedicated to initiatives aiming to map the scope of the issue in developing nations. The southern region of Latin America has been assessed by a recent survey funded by the FAO Technical Cooperation Programme (TCP). The findings are alarming: more than 75% of farms exhibit issues with resistance to two of the three primary anthelmintic groups currently available for chemical management, and an increasing number exhibit resistance to all three. Similar issues exist in eastern and southern Africa, according to a consultant that was hired to assess the situation in a few African nations.

Hydatidosis, cysticercosis, and trichinellosis are three parasitic zoonotic illnesses that continue to be a big issue, resulting in human misery and large losses from discarded meat and organs. TCP has enabled the evaluation of current activities in various South American nations. FAO is developing control methods in partnership with the Veterinary Public Health Units of WHO and PAHO.

Animals can suffer from micromineral deficits (P, Cu, Co, Zn, Cu-Mo-S interactions), which are well known in many parts of the world. They might significantly lower food security and animal output for both consumers and livestock owners. However, even though the knowledge for control is accessible, control cannot always be attained due to the lack of mineral supplements or fertilizers.

20.7.5   Animal Health Delivery at Herd Level

FAO's livestock programme is increasingly emphasizing an integrated approach to livestock production and enhancement of food security (WHO 2005). This strategy aims at focusing much technical and social expertise on priority livestock systems. Two such systems are mixed farming (crop and livestock) in high potential areas and peri-urban dairy production.

One arm of this integrated approach is a Herd Health and Production Programme (HH&PP) protocol, which includes the following interactive steps for delivering animal health within farming systems (WHO 2005):

1) Agree with farm management on proposed production and acceptable risk targets.
2) Define and develop the tools and technologies required to collect the necessary data.
3) Interpret the data gathered from all sources.
4) Develop and agree upon a plan of action that includes concrete steps to reach the production and acceptable risk targets set in step one.
5) Monitor and evaluate progress and begin again at step one.

Through the use of pilot programmes that follow the HH&PP protocol and close results monitoring, this approach enables private veterinary practices to provide clinical and HH&PP services and defines areas of responsibility in a way that fosters close collaboration between the private sector and public services (Lubroth 2012). Additionally, it is possible to form national consultation committees of interested parties for HH&PPs to further define the idea and how it will be delivered, to adapt the strategy to local circumstances, and to publicize the findings (Leforban et al. 2002). These consultation groups would include of service providers from the public and private sectors, as well as livestock input producers, educators, and other interested parties.

20.7.6 Enabling Domains

The key tools for the international control of animal diseases are the availability of adequate information, proper services for the diagnosis of disease conditions, vaccines of appropriate quality and a functional veterinary service. Emerging trends in all four areas will affect future strategies for the control of animal diseases (Lubroth 2012).

20.7.7 Information

The international exchange of information concerning animal diseases is coordinated by OIE, which classifies infectious diseases into List A and List B, reflecting the contagiousness of the disease and its relative economic importance for international trade in animals and animal products (Domenech et al. 2006). It is the responsibility of the Chief Veterinary Officer of each country to notify the international community, through the OIE, whenever an outbreak of an epizootic disease is encountered and periodically to update OIE on the disease situation in the country. Every year FAO publishes the FAO/OIE/WHO *Animal Health Yearbook*, which details the disease status of each member country of OIE, WHO and FAO (WHO 2005).

It is widely acknowledged that the official information provided in the yearbook frequently represents the bare minimum known about the disease situation in many developing countries. The three international organizations have recently evaluated the quality and impact of the information contained in the yearbook. It is now well acknowledged that veterinary services must create reliable information systems in order to expand their offerings and increase the accuracy of data on disease incidence and the outcomes of diagnostic tests or surveillance (Sota, 1995). Additionally, this would provide governments the ability to create community-level plans for improving the health and production of livestock. This computer programme, HANDISTATUS, was developed at the request of OIE, FAO, the Inter-American Institute for Cooperation on Agriculture (IICA), and other organizations (Domenech et al. 2006).

In order to enable each national veterinary service to easily be informed of the disease status of every member country of OIE and/or FAO, FAO and OIE want to establish a system that would substantially improve such an interchange of disease information. Making sure poor nations can access and efficiently utilize the system will be a global challenge. PANAFTOSA, which is actively creating numerous information systems with IICA and others, has built a comparable complete disease-notification system for vesicular illnesses for South America. The PROPEXAN initiative, which aims to prevent the most common animal diseases in Latin America and the Caribbean, plays an essential supporting role in this regard. The majority of the countries where this project has been active are in Central America, the Caribbean, and the Andean area. Its headquarters are in Panama, and it provides officials from the neighboring nations with formal and practical in-service training on topics including animal health inspection, animal quarantine, and the epidemiology, prevention, identification, and eradication of exotic animal diseases.

20.7.8 Diagnosis

Current trends in animal disease diagnostic technology are moving towards an improved flow of samples and data from herd level to the veterinary clinic, national laboratories, regional reference laboratories and world reference laboratories (Domenech et al. 2006). While conventional techniques in veterinary diagnosis should not be overlooked, the use of modern diagnostic technology based on molecular biotechnology is dramatically gaining ground, and polymerase chain reaction (PCR), monoclonal antibody probes, enzyme-linked immunosorbent assays are now becoming standard, primary diagnostic tools in industrialized countries. There is a need for technology transfer, however, in order to establish these technologies in developing countries (WHO 2005).

FAO has been addressing this issue from four aspects (WHO 2005):

1) Educating and making decision-makers aware. Senior scientists in underdeveloped nations have been the target of a series of awareness workshops designed to help them understand the possibilities that the new technology in animal health provide. When a specialized role has been identified, FAO has called for special expert consultations to provide advice, either by itself or in collaboration with other organizations like the International Atomic Energy Agency (IAEA).

2) Laboratory scientists and workers receive hands-on training. This has taken the shape of practicing specific methods at the bench for particular goals. The Joint FAO/IAEA Division's training of employees from poor nations in the enzyme-linked immunosorbent test (ELISA) technology has been the most comprehensive initiative. Through this project,

surveillance programmes like the rinderpest sero-monitoring network for GREP and the FMD sero-monitoring network that is being created in South America in partnership with PANAFTOSA have been made possible.

3) Biotechnology networks at FAO. These are now being created in South America, India, and Eastern Europe. The main goal of the operations in South America is to improve the ability of the region to diagnose diseases that are not yet included in the great PAHO programme. In order to facilitate the exchange of knowledge, information, and reagents through a system of TCDC (Technical Cooperation among Developing Countries), the FAO Regional Office in Latin America and the Caribbean has been creating a network of top laboratories known as REDLAB.

4) The tracking of key disease pathogens on a global scale. This is done by using a network of reference laboratories that have been chosen for their proven proficiency in delivering referral diagnoses for the disease(s) for which they have been assigned. For instance, the FAO has designated PANAFTOSA as the FAO Regional Reference Laboratory for the Americas and the Pirbright Laboratory of the Institute for Animal Health of the United Kingdom as the FAO World Reference Laboratory for FMD. Similar to this, in order to assist GREP (WHO 2005), FAO has just named the Pirbright Laboratory as the FAO World Reference Laboratory for Rinderpest. The information produced by the network of reference laboratories is proving to be of utmost significance in molecular epidemiology and the monitoring of global disease. The FAO, OIE, and WHO networks all complement one another.

20.7.9 Vaccines

Three main challenges have been the focus of recent trends in vaccine development: vaccine technology, vaccine quality, and vaccination monitoring. While subunit genetically engineered or synthetic peptide vaccines have not yet produced outstanding results, recent advancements in vaccine technology have been linked to the consolidation of cell culture and fermentation technologies, gene deletion, gene manipulation of vaccine viruses, and viral-vector recombinant vaccines. The FAO has produced a thorough analysis and set of recommendations for veterinary vaccinations.

Vaccine quality perceptions and attitudes have also changed throughout time. Most developing nations now generally agree that vaccinations should be produced in accordance with good manufacturing practices (GMP) (WHO 2005). The idea that FAO is currently promoting was first offered by the UK Veterinary Medicines Directorate and was supported at the FAO Expert Consultation on Quality Control of Veterinary Vaccines in Developing Countries held in 1991, specifically.

The ingredients must be of appropriate purity, in the right proportions, and processed correctly; the containers must be robust with a secure closure; and the labelling must be accurate and enlightening. "Medicines (vaccines) must be manufactured with appropriate quality control procedures in premises that are licensed, and inspected (Lubroth 2012)."

The Pan African Veterinary Vaccine Centre (PANVAC), an initiative of the Organization of African Unity/Interafrican Bureau for Animal Resources (OAU/IBAR), has led the way in advancing these ideas of vaccine quality in Africa with technical support from the FAO. The majority of PANVAC's effects have been seen in the enhancement of rinderpest vaccine quality, as shown by the fact that from 33% in 1985 to around 80% in 1992, more vaccine batches produced in Africa have met international quality requirements. Additionally, as seen by the variety of reasons why vaccines are rejected, testing quality has reached international standards.

With the development of ELISA technology, sero-monitoring for vaccine monitoring has become a reality (WHO 2005). The largest sero-monitoring network in the world is the Pan-African Rinderpest Campaign (PARC) sero-monitoring network, which is overseen by the Joint FAO/IAEA Division (Lubroth 2012). The use of the ELISA technique with standardized and highly specific reagents, standardized hardware, and standardized computer software, supported by a well-controlled quality-assurance programme for the reagents and techniques, and consistent technical advice from FAO/IAEA staff members and the scientist responsible for developing and standardizing the technique, are the key components of this network (Lubroth 2012). All those in charge of the national testing programme will also receive a uniform training package. Now, it is FAO policy to apply the strategy to other GREP-affiliated regions of the world.

20.7.10 Veterinary Sciences

Effective control of animal diseases requires a competent veterinary service with a clearly defined chain of management and reporting command. Additionally, the veterinary service has to have sufficient laboratory support for disease surveillance and diagnosis. The laboratory shall report directly to the national Chief Veterinary Officer (or Director of Veterinary Services) regarding responsiveness to priority infectious illnesses and areas of their control needing laboratory support.

Government intervention in all veterinary concerns is not required for an efficient veterinary service. National veterinary associations and international organizations must provide substantial support for initiatives aimed at establishing a thriving private veterinary programme (Otte and Chilonda, 2000). It is important to keep in mind from the perspective of controlling animal diseases that a disease outbreak is first noticed by the farmer, herder, or pastoralist, or by those in charge of routine on-farm animal health activities, typically private veterinary staff and/or community-based extension workers. It is necessary to build structures that incentivize private vets with licenses to carry out tasks like routine vaccines, farm testing, and even clinical inspections. However, such licensed veterinary inspectors should be permitted to charge reasonable fees for services provided and should be fairly compensated by the government for tasks delegated to them.

National veterinary services must function both within a regional and an international environment in order to control animal illnesses. Major epizootic disease outbreaks should be reported to OIE, FAO, and, in the case of zoonotic illnesses, WHO as well, as they are of acute concern to adjacent nations. Each nation within a region needs to have a robust national veterinary service that openly shares disease information with other nations in order to effectively control epizootic illnesses.

Developing nations, in particular, will need to enhance and modernize their veterinary services and stop viewing them as merely an element of an agricultural extension service, as is obvious from trends in the global control of epizootic illnesses.

20.7.11 Contribution of Isotopic and Nuclear Techniques

Immunological and molecular technologies produced from and connected to nuclear energy have significant and frequently novel roles in the control of animal health. They can provide substantial advantages over alternative approaches since they are simple to use, quick, sensitive, precise, and sturdy. This involves the use of point-of-care products, which helps farmers, extension agencies, and veterinary authorities control and remove diseases that have a detrimental impact on animal productivity and health.

A more accurate evaluation of the risks of disease transmission is made possible by the use of stable isotope ratios, which allow for the tracking of animal movements. It is now possible to create attenuated vaccines that contain metabolically active but non-replicating pathogens that are able to elicit a potent immune response and memory, particularly in cases of parasitic diseases that result in significant production losses across the globe.

20.8 Conclusions

The control of infectious and epizootic diseases is a requirement for the development of economically viable cattle. The international objective for major epidemic diseases (OIE List A) is to eradicate the disease rather than only contain it. In addition to a properly established chain of management command in member countries, this asks for the purposeful enhancement of all facets of veterinary services. In surrounding nations, diverse strategies are frequently utilized to control endemic diseases, whether they are brought on by bacteria, viruses, or parasites. Control strategy standardization and harmonization are goals.

It is also being discussed how to control production disorders that are chronic or non-infectious and necessitate the provision of strategic clinical veterinary services at the farm level. Government services must accommodate the private sector in its efforts to provide continuous veterinary services to livestock owners in order to recognize the size of losses brought on by non-infectious and productivity disorders. Private veterinary practices and the production or import of necessary supplies should be allowed by law. The objectives of all these services must be raised food productivity, raised food security, and raised producer profitability. Through its many different interventions, the FAO's Animal Health Service works tirelessly to advance the idea of a comprehensive veterinary system that depends on a strong public service and a thriving commercial sector.

References

Domenech, J., Lubroth, J., Eddi, C. et al. (2006). Regional and international approaches on prevention and control of animal transboundary and emerging diseases. *Annals of the New York Academy of Sciences* 1081 (1): 90–107.

Leforban, Y., Gerbier, G., and Rweyemamu, M. (2002). Action of FAO in the control of foot and mouth disease. *Comparative Immunology, Microbiology and Infectious Diseases* 25 (5–6): 373–382.

Lubroth, J. (2012). FAO and the one health approach. In: *One Health: The Human-Animal-Environment Interfaces in Emerging Infectious Diseases: Food Safety and Security, and International and National Plans for Implementation of One Health Activities* (ed. J.S. Mackenzie, M. Jeggo, P. Daszak, and J.A. Richt), 65–72. Berlin, Heidelberg: Springer Berlin Heidelberg.

Otte, M.J. and Chilonda, P. (2000). *Animal Health Economics: An Introduction*, 12. Rome, Italy: Animal Production and Healthy Division (AGA), FAO.

Robinson, A. and Production, A. (2003). *Guidelines for Coordinated Human and Animal Brucellosis Surveillance*. Rome, Italy: FAO.

Sota, C.A. (1995). International collaborative research: role of FAO and other international organizations on animal health programs in Latin America and the Caribbean. *Veterinary Parasitology* 57 (1–3): 11–17.

Temple, R.S. (1970). Animal production programs of FAO. *Journal of Animal Science* 30 (4): 643–649.

Welte, V.R. and Terán, M.V. (2004). Emergency prevention system (empres) for transboundary animal and plant pests and diseases. the empres-livestock: an FAO initiative. *Annals of the New York Academy of Sciences* 1026 (1): 19–31.

World Health Organization (2005). *WHO/FAO/OIE Guidelines for the Surveillance, Prevention and Control of Taeniosis/Cysticercosis*. World Organisation for Animal Health.

21

Animal Health, Management, and Nutritional Epidemiology

Amitava Roy[1], Tanmoy Rana[2], and Arkaprabha Shee[3]

[1] *Department of Livestock Farm Complex, West Bengal University of Animal & Fishery Sciences, Kolkata, India*
[2] *Department of Veterinary Clinical Complex, West Bengal University of Animal & Fishery Sciences, Kolkata, India*
[3] *Subject Matter Specialist (Animal Sc.), Dhaanyaganga Krishi Vigyan Kendra, Sargachi, Murshidabad, India*

21.1 Introduction

According to the FAO (2009), livestock products account for about half of global agricultural production. Consumer demand for animal-sourced foods, nonfood products (like hides), production inputs (like fertilizer for crops), as well as for other, nonmarket objectives (like culture) is met through the production of livestock.

Global demand for meat and dairy products is predicted to rise by 63% and 30%, respectively, by 2050 (Revell 2015), as a result of rising population and rising incomes fueled by economic expansion in rural regions (Beegle and Christiaensen 2019). By 2050, the average demand for all animal source foods will rise from 1.4 billion to 2.0 billion tonnes, assuming no changes in per capita consumption (Henchion et al. 2021). Over the period 1973–2013, animal milk and meat output in developing nations increased from 31% and 22% of worldwide meat and milk production, respectively, to 63% and 53% of the same global production. Because of the ongoing development in demand for food items derived from animals brought on by real income and population growth, the value of livestock product share in agriculture will continue to rise (Cohen 2006).

Due to internal and foreign market shocks, livestock disease externalities have a detrimental influence on productivity and distort values, creating market inefficiencies. Due to domestic and international market shocks that cause market inefficiencies, livestock illness externalities have a detrimental influence on productivity and skew values (FAO 2016). Livestock disease outbreaks and occurrences in production are a threat to the herd's health and the viability of commercialized livestock product markets, as well as their expansion to meet demand and smallholder farming methods (FAO 2009). Additionally, livestock diseases may promote harmful and unsustainable practices. When used excessively, antibiotics can have negative effects, including antimicrobial resistance. For instance, antibiotics designed to promote growth may be utilized to enhance animal size or treat persistent diseases. Episodic or unforeseen illness outbreaks diminish animal output in a similar way, but they can also unintentionally affect the supply and demand for other market items.

Consumer demand in retail markets may be distorted by unfavorable news and publicity related to a disease outbreak, but shortages or surpluses may result from distortions in unrelated markets (Hennessy and Marsh 2021). The health of human and wildlife populations, as well as the environment and climate change, can all be directly impacted by livestock disease and/or its externalities. This may happen as a result of effects on the neighborhood's local environments around livestock production systems (Kock 2005). For instance, disease vector feedback loops between cattle and wildlife may exist (Horan et al. 2008). There are more opportunities for zoonotic contact between wildlife and livestock vectors as a result of human encroachment into wildlife regions for urban development and/or livestock production. As a result of climatic changes, zoonotic pathogens have been encouraged to reemerge (Cutler et al. 2010) and production environments with higher burdens of livestock disease have been created (Ahmed et al. 2019), drawing attention to the interaction between livestock, wildlife, and the climate as well as the pathways by which disease spreads. While we appreciate the complexity and significance of the livestock–wildlife connection, we do not fully address it in this review and leave it for future work.

The necessity and application of government response and eradication programs, trade bans, and trade restrictions show the significance of animal disease in production and its impact on the health of populations and markets. The cost–benefit

Epidemiology and Environmental Hygiene in Veterinary Public Health, First Edition. Edited by Tanmoy Rana.
© 2025 John Wiley & Sons, Inc. Published 2025 by John Wiley & Sons, Inc.

21.2 Production

A discussion of the expenditures associated with a few cattle diseases opens this section. The effects of climate change on production environments and disease transmission within these environments are next explored, followed by the spread of cattle disease to humans and the environment.

The loss of production or a decline in production efficiency are two direct economic effects of clinical and subclinical livestock illness situations. Lack of productivity has an impact on income, wealth, and food access. Production conditions and market conditions will have an impact on how much of a financial burden there will be. A local farm economy that is diversified with different sources of revenue could be more resilient and bear less weight. In contrast, the local economy may be less resilient, the burden may be greater, and local food security may be compromised if it depends heavily on one or a small number of sensitive commodities. Diseases and lower animal productivity can have long-lasting effects on livestock output in a number of "hidden" ways (such as longer reproductive cycles that result in fewer offspring), which frequently outweigh the losses brought on by obvious illness (Otte et al. 2004). Examples of livestock health issues include lameness in the feet, ketosis, mastitis, and infertility. These issues may also be related to transboundary illnesses with significant worldwide impact, such as lumpy skin disease, sheeppox, goatpox, and foot and mouth disease (FMD).

Due to their widespread occurrence and severe and protracted nature, foot diseases are a persistent issue in dairy cattle. Costs in milk production, extended calving intervals, excessive culling, additional veterinary visits and treatments, as well as labor costs for the farmer and trimmer are some ways in which foot problems have an economic impact. A Dutch farm with 65 cows reported total foot diseases expenditure of $4899 per year ($75 per cow), ranging from $3217 to $7001. The severity of claw diseases and production, fertility, and performance were found to have phenotypic correlations in one study on Spanish dairy cows (Charfeddine and Pérez-Cabal 2017). The presence of sole ulcer or white line disease was linked to reduced milk production, particularly in cows in their second or later lactations, according to the authors' analysis of three prevalent claw disorders: dermatitis, sole ulcer, and white line disease. Furthermore, when compared to a mild condition, severe sole ulcer or white line disease caused milk losses to quadruple (Charfeddine and Pérez-Cabal 2017). According to Charfeddine and Pérez-Cabal (2017), each affected cow resulted in annual costs of $10.8, $50.9, and $43.2 for dermatitis, sole ulcers, and white line disease. More than half of the increased costs were caused by milk losses, longer calving intervals, and premature culling (Charfeddine and Pérez-Cabal 2017).

In the dairy business, lameness is a significant problem (Dolecheck and Bewley 2018). In contrast to earlier research, which indicated that the prevalence of lameness in north-eastern United States herds in 2008 reached as high as 55% (von Keyserlingk et al. 2012), Cutler et al. (2010) assessed the prevalence of lameness in United States herds to be 10% in 2014. The top three primary health issues in dairy farmers' herds in the United Kingdom are lameness, mastitis, and fertility (Leach et al. 2010). Lowered milk supply and reproductive performance, increased cow culling, and other diseases are some of the clinical and subclinical consequences of ketosis (Raboisson et al. 2014). Steeneveld et al. (2020) observed differences in annual net cash flows of farms in the no ketosis scenario (i.e., no risk) and the base scenario (i.e., 1% probability of clinical ketosis and 11% probability of subclinical ketosis) in a study conducted in a typical Dutch dairy context. According to them, the average herd level costs of ketosis were €3613 for the basic scenario and €7371 for the high-risk scenario, or two times the probability of developing clinical and subclinical ketosis (Steeneveld et al. 2020). Poxvirus infections, including lumpy skin disease, sheeppox, and goatpox, can potentially result in large losses for livestock producers through morbidity, mortality, control efforts, and reduced trade (Limon et al. 2020).

Livestock that has been infected may exhibit symptoms including weight loss, decreased milk production, depression, lethargy, fever, and in extreme circumstances death. Additionally, sheeppox and goatpox can impair the production of cashmere and wool, while lumpy skin disease lowers the quality of hide. In a study of backyard and transhumance farmers in north-east Nigeria, farmers reported that they sold cattle, sheep, and goats for 47%, 58%, and 57% less than they would have for a healthy animal. Additionally, Limon et al. (2020) observed that the milk output of cows that were clinically affected fell by 65% and by 35% when they recovered. The median live weight loss for cattle, sheep, and goats was 10%, 15%, and 17%, respectively. Economic losses at the farm level range from US$10 to US$6340 depending on the afflicted species and production method (Limon et al. 2020).

The effects of FMD have been thoroughly investigated after outbreaks or anecdotally, but they have been poorly characterized in places where it is endemic (Lyons et al. 2015). In a study to determine the effect on milk output in 218 lactating cattle during a 29-day FMD outbreak, at the herd level, yields declined from an average of 20 to 13 kg (a 35% decrease) per cow per day, with recovery occurring about two months after the outbreak's termination (Lyons et al. 2015). A 2008–2018 retrospective examination of FMD exposure in cattle in endemic areas in East Africa demonstrated decreased milk production and reproductive performance (Reagan 2020). Calving intervals and lameness are additional factors to take into account when comparing endemic illness and long-term animal productivity.

Through morbidity, mortality, and the expenses of prevention and control, livestock illnesses result in losses to production systems. While diseases typically present as apparent ailments, they can have a hidden impact on productivity in a variety of ways, such as longer production cycles and slower population growth.

21.3 Impact of Climate Change on Animal Diseases

Climate change is closely related to production conditions and subsequent implications, and it may have a significant impact on the epidemiology of infectious animal diseases (Bett et al. 2017). Although there may be some good effects of climate change on animal health, this review is most interested in the negative effects that result in higher costs for raising cattle. The occurrence of infectious diseases that are highly dependent on environmental and climatic conditions, such as an increase in heat-related illnesses and stress, extreme weather events, the adaptation of animal production systems to new environments, and the emergence or reemergence of infectious diseases are just a few of the ways in which these may occur (Forman et al. 2008). These activities have an impact on the biology of the hosts, diseases, and vectors, as well as on the environment by enhancing their growth and contact (Bett et al. 2017). Finally, livestock value chains are directly and indirectly impacted by climate change-induced effects on animal health and well-being, which have repercussions for society as a whole.

The host's physiology is impacted by the temperature outside, which in turn affects how well the host can fight against infection (Bett et al. 2017). The ideal temperature range for most farm animals is between 10 °C and 30 °C, and temperatures above this range negatively impact animal health and well-being, feed intake, milk production, reproductive performance, and wool production (Das et al. 2016). According to the National Research Council (National Research Council US 1981), for every unit increase in temperature above ideal temperatures, feed intake for goats, pigs, and chickens decreases by 3–5%. When exposed to extremely high temperatures, pigs in particular are vulnerable to heat stress (Forman et al. 2008). Heat stress in the dairy industry is seen as a serious issue in Chinese Taipei. According to Bett et al. (2017), heat stress lengthens the cycle, decreases the symptoms of estrus, and increases the risk of fetal death.

The pace of development, geographic distribution, and geographic persistence of infections and vectors, as well as the dynamics of vector-borne disease transmission, are all substantially influenced by temperature and moisture (Bett et al. 2017). Arthropods typically exhibit greater metabolic rates at high temperatures, which promotes increased eating, reproduction, and maturation (Ahumada et al. 2004). Key epidemiological characteristics including infection rates and the distribution of infections in the vector are significantly influenced by temperature. By speeding up the reproduction of diseases in vectors, higher temperatures decrease the incubation period of pathogens. Pathogens that spend a portion of their life cycle outside the host can also be affected by temperature and humidity (Madeira et al. 1998). Climate has an impact on the developmental phases of the vectors that spread diseases to sheep, goats, cattle, and horses (Forman et al. 2008), including nematodes, mosquitoes, ticks, and flies.

Climate change has an impact on the geographic distribution of infections, hosts, and vectors. Evidence for this has been discovered, for instance, on the bluetongue virus-transmitting *Culicoides imicola* (Wilson and Mellor 2009). The geographic range and dispersion of parasites and vectors are usually constrained by temperature and moisture (Kimaro and Chibinga 2013). For instance, in east and southern Africa, the range of vectors is frequently constrained by high wintertime mortality rates and poor summertime population recovery rates. Warmer places may see increases in populations of some vectors that were previously uninhabitable whereas warmer regions may continue to be favorable for vectors if there is also an increase in precipitation or humidity. The rate at which parasites develop may shift as a result of climate change, increasing the number of parasite generations in some cases and subsequently extending the parasites' range in both time and space. One example of a disease whose geographic and temporal spread could be altered is the New World screwworm

(*Cochliomyia hominivorax*), which already impacts animals in South America. In Brazil, it has been demonstrated that the amount of precipitation and temperature are closely connected with the spread of screwworm (Pinto et al. 2008). The prevalence of animals harboring screwworm larvae varies significantly from season to season in some parts of Brazil, with summer witnessing the highest incidence followed by spring, winter, and autumn (Pinto et al. 2008).

The temporal and geographic distribution of infectious diseases in South America's endemic regions and their spread to disease-free areas are projected to shift as a result of climate change. This includes diseases spread by vectors like New World screwworm, West Nile fever, vesicular stomatitis, and bluetongue (Pinto et al. 2008). Although bluetongue outbreaks have been documented in Europe in the past, the frequency of its importation after 1998 has been shocking. Bluetongue virus has been identified in six strains in 12 nations, and it has been discovered that it can be found roughly 800 km farther north than previously thought (Wilson and Mellor 2009). According to Pinto et al. (2008), the main cause of the expansion of tick-borne diseases like bluetongue, *Culicoides imicola* (a native European midge), screwworm, and tick-borne diseases throughout Europe, South America, and Africa is climate change. El Niño/Southern Oscillation (ENSO) in Africa has been connected to diseases spread by biting midges and mosquitoes (Anyamba et al. 2002). According to predictions, some regions of Africa will likely experience a change in the geographic range of some ticks, such as *Rhipicephalus appendiculatus* (Olwoch et al. 2008). Typhoon occurrences were reported to be associated with outbreaks of bovine ephemeral disease (1996) and dengue fever (2001) in Chinese Taipei (Forman et al. 2008). According to Forman et al. (2008), climate-induced bird migration may change the geographic distribution of viruses including West Nile virus and highly pathogenic avian influenza (HPAI).

21.4 Zoonoses and Other Negative Effects

Zoonoses are a crucial factor to take into account in production settings. Dairy cattle are susceptible to diseases caused by microorganisms that can be transferred from cows to people. Such dairy diseases as brucellosis, TB, and Q fever were almost completely under control thanks to eradication campaigns and the advent of pasteurization. Due to the illegal drinking of raw milk, there have only been a few occurrences of food-borne illnesses in recent years. Numerous significant public health concerns, including antibiotic use and the resulting microbial resistance in humans, bovine spongiform encephalopathy (including variant Creutzfeldt–Jakob disease), and other challenges are currently being faced by the cow sector. Additional indirect connections exist between animals and people due to environmental or ecosystem health (Taylor et al. 2001). The use of antimicrobial medications places bacteria under a selection pressure that may cause some bacterial strains to acquire antibiotic resistance. The possibility that zoonotic germs could spread microbial resistance from animals to humans is a source of concern. Consuming nonpathogenic bacteria is more likely to result in the transmission of resistance to human diseases (LeBlanc et al. 2006). Concern over this spillover effect for the environment, animal health, and human health is rising.

Disease spillover is an intricate and concerning public health issue. While the development of pasteurization assisted in the elimination of the majority of zoonotic worries, concerns about the connection between animal and human diseases and the potential transmission of microbial resistance from animals to people are becoming more and more pressing.

21.5 Prevention and Treatment of Animal Diseases

Beyond a primary focus on productivity, the rising emphasis on animal production for promoting food security has brought food safety issues to the forefront. While foods derived from animals provide vital micro- and macronutrients for the growth of body and brain (Grantham-McGregor et al. 2007), eating tainted food increases the risk of contracting a disease (Vipham et al. 2020). With children under five bearing 40% of this burden in low-income areas and the total burden being calculated at 33 million disability-adjusted life-years (Havelaar et al. 2013), evaluation of the impact of food-borne disease has found that it is comparable to the burden of the "big three" diseases, namely HIV/AIDS, malaria, and tuberculosis. Risks of zoonosis rise in places where food is produced, both commercially and at home (Headey and Hirvonen 2016). Urbanization and production intensification both contribute to the geographic concentration of human and cattle populations, which increases the risk of zoonotic transmission (Hassell et al. 2017). According to Vipham et al. (2020), underdeveloped communities frequently lack the infrastructure and resources necessary to handle livestock in a sanitary and hygienic manner during production, adding to the difficulty of achieving the sanitary requirements for trade market access.

A key production practice for reducing adverse effects on both production and human health is the prevention and treatment of livestock disease. Producers must pay to prevent and treat livestock diseases. Profit-maximizing or expenditure-loss frontier frameworks or more generally, cost and benefit frameworks that include profits as part of benefits are frequently used to analyze investments in disease mitigation (Kaniyamattam et al. 2020). The decision-making process for producer-level disease control, however, might not take into account more important considerations relating to external effects on human health and other production systems. Profit-maximizing circumstances show that producers are not expected to eradicate all sickness and will only do so when individual private gains surpass individual costs in the absence of any disease control regulations (Havelaar et al. 2015).

Public policy is used to handle disease preventive and treatment issues that producers do not feel are best served by their involvement but that may have detrimental effects on parties not directly involved in production (Salmon et al. 2018). These topics, which in general focus on preventive and service delivery, include systematic vaccination and disease vector control, surveillance, diagnostics, and animal quarantine measures, drug quality control, food and hygiene inspection, and veterinary research and extension (Umali et al. 1994); all these topics are related to prevention and service providing. Regulation mandating veterinary control for administration also addresses difficulties related to drug misuse that have production-enhancing advantages but pose risks to public health and the environment (Lhermie et al. 2020). Public spending on illness prevention and treatment, which has been successful in reducing disease incidence, has contributed to growing fiscal deficits, necessitating a review of policy design and the creation of incentives for greater private engagement (Bicknell et al. 1999). In order to promote effective policy outcomes, particularly in Africa and Asia, it is also necessary to address the researcher–government connection and the sharing of information between the two parties (Serra et al. 2020).

21.6 What Function Does Nutritional Epidemiology Play in the Determination of Causality?

The fact that nutritional epidemiology mostly uses observational data – which is thought to be less reliable than experimental data in establishing causality – is one of the main objections leveled against it. The typical hierarchy of evidence from diverse study designs is shown in Figure 21.1. Although they are at the top of the hierarchy, randomized trials with strict endpoints are typically not the best or most practical study design to address nutritional epidemiological queries about the long-term effects of particular foods or nutrients (unless they can be put into a pill).

Nutritional epidemiologists often rely on prospective cohort studies, the strongest observational study design for reducing bias and determining causality, when there is a lack of data from big randomized control trials (RCTs) on hard endpoints. Since they are prospective in nature, they are less susceptible to a number of flaws that frequently afflict retrospective or cross-sectional study designs, such as reverse causation, recall bias, and selection bias. When the outcome affects the exposure rather than the other way around, this is known as reverse causality. Because cross-sectional research and retrospective case–control studies evaluate exposure and result simultaneously, this is a typical worry. Because participants are followed throughout time, prospective cohort studies can reduce the probability of reverse causation by visible disease.

These studies can also investigate the level of reverse causation from subclinical disease through lag analyses. Because prospective cohort studies start with a disease-free population at baseline and are followed up to determine incident cases

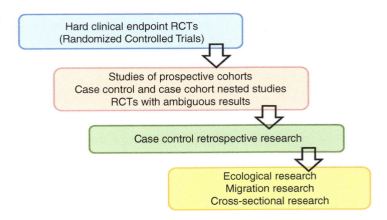

Figure 21.1 Research plan hierarchy in nutritional epidemiology. Randomized controlled trial (RCT).

that develop over time, they are superior to retrospective case–control studies in that the issues of selection bias (controls not being representative of the underlying population that gave rise to cases) and recall bias (knowledge of disease status affecting recall of diet) can be largely minimized. This is demonstrated by the lack of replication of erroneous associations between total calorie intake and colon cancer (Giovannucci and Goldin 1997) and lipids and breast cancer (Giovannucci et al. 1993) in large prospective cohort studies.

Confounding is a significant issue when dealing with any form of observational data. An unaccounted-for confounder introduces bias into the relationship between exposure and disease since it is linked with both the exposure and the outcome but is not caused by either. Randomly allocating individuals to treatment groups eliminates all forms of measurable and unmeasured confounding, which is the major reason why randomized trials are preferred for determining causation, assuming the sample size is large enough. Researchers must rely on their subject matter expertise to recognize and account for all pertinent confounders in observational study designs like prospective cohort studies in order to account for this kind of bias. Once information on these variables has been gathered, the researcher can statistically account for confounders in a regression model or limit the data to a particular subset to reduce residual confounding. When the most important confounders are taken into account, a well-conducted cohort study can replicate the results of a randomized trial (Hernán and Robins 2006).

Sensitivity analysis defines the amount of unmeasured confounding required to totally cancel out an impact, which further reinforces the conclusions. Furthermore, a prospective design permits ongoing tracking of confounders and lessens the risk of residual confounding because updated information may minimize measurement error in confounder evaluation, and further confounder information can be gathered as necessary.

21.7 What Function Do Nutritional Epidemiological Studies Play in the Development of Policy?

National organizations like the American Diabetes Association, American Heart Association, American College of Cardiology, US Preventive Services Task Force, and Food and Drug Administration have used well-defined grading systems to assign the weight of evidence in different study types when rating the quality of the strength of the evidence (US FDA 2014). In most scales, properly conducted RCTs with illness endpoints are the highest level of evidence, and prospective cohort studies are one level below RCTs. Evidence from prospective cohort studies in conjunction with smaller RCTs with intermediate endpoints is frequently taken into account for substantiating dietary claims or developing policy in the absence of major RCTs with disease endpoints.

For instance, the US Department of Agriculture (USDA)/US Department of Health and Human Services Dietary Guidelines Advisory Committee has heavily relied on evidence from prospective cohort studies, in addition to evidence from RCTs, to assess the relationships between particular dietary factors and chronic disease risk (Spahn et al. 2011), which forms one of the pillars for making dietary recommendations for the US population. The following discussion examines three instances of epidemiological data influencing policy change. Based on observational data from the United Kingdom from the 1970s, folate was originally recognized as a crucial nutrient in preventing neural tube abnormalities (NTDs), including anencephaly and spina bifida (Smithells et al. 1980). In the 1980s, case–control studies revealed that women who took prenatal folate supplements had a lower chance of giving birth to children with NTDs than those who did not (Bower and Stanley 1989). At the time, there was only one prospective cohort trial, but the findings indicated that periconceptual folate supplementation had a potent protective effect (Milunsky et al. 1989). This link was supported by observational studies looking at blood folate levels (Wald et al. 1996) and randomized trials of folate supplementation (Czeizel and Dudas 1992).

Trans fatty acids (TFAs) are a highly effective example of nutritional epidemiology influencing policy. In the early twentieth century, TFAs were initially created to stabilize vegetable fat at room temperature, and they quickly gained use in the production of food. In the 1950s, Ancel Keys hypothesized that TFAs might be linked to heart disease (Keys et al. 1957), but it was not until the 1990s that experimental data revealed that TFAs might both raise LDL cholesterol and lower HDL cholesterol (Mensink and Katan 1990). This connection was confirmed by later epidemiological data from the Nurses' Health Study (Willett et al. 1993). Scientists argued for a decrease in TFAs in foods as more evidence accumulated (Willett and Ascherio 1994), and the FDA authorized a proposal for manufacturers to disclose TFAs in the nutrition facts label of foods in 2003. TFAs are a highly effective example of nutritional epidemiology influencing policy.

21.8 Conclusion

Animal health issues have a complex global influence on markets and livelihoods that varies from place to region. Selected, recent information regarding the effects of and attention to animal disease throughout production, disease prevention and treatment, animal welfare, trade and regulation has been discussed in this analysis.

The effects of animal sickness on human health and food security have drawn attention to the need to combine economics and epidemiology. Impacts on supply, market pricing, and trade are just a few of the factors that influence policy; there are also implications on human health. There is a knowledge vacuum on the distribution of animal disease burden within value chains and its impact on the overall economy due to the varied structure of livestock and livestock product value chains in both developed and undeveloped countries. In order to evaluate the effects of the animal disease burden segregated among all actors and economies that make up value chains, precise and suitable data as well as institutional information must be obtained. A multidisciplinary approach involving information, population and production systems, economic and epidemiological analysis, animal health ontology, and human health implications is necessary to evaluate the worldwide burden of animal disease. It would be easier to obtain information on the immediate and long-term effects of animal disease on industries and economies if work could be done to reduce the burden of animal disease. Evaluating how animal disease burden is distributed across the value chain and its impact on the value chain and economy better informs policy and allows targeted investment from private and public organizations (Marsh et al. 2017).

References

Ahmed, H., Yoder, J., de Glanville, W.A. et al. (2019). Economic burden of livestock disease and drought in Northern Tanzania. *Journal of Development and Agricultural Economics* 11: 140–151.

Ahumada, J.A., Laoointe, D., and Samuel, M.D. (2004). Modeling the population dynamics of *Culex quinquefasciatus* (Diptera: Culicidae), along an elevational gradient in Hawaii. *Journal of Medical Entomology* 41: 1157–1170.

Anyamba, A., Linthicum, K.J., Mahoney, R. et al. (2002). Mapping potential risk of Rift Valley fever outbreaks in African savannas using vegetation index time series data. *Photogrammetric Engineering and Remote Sensing* 68: 137–145.

Beegle, K. and Christiaensen, L. (2019). *Accelerating Poverty Reduction in Africa*. Washington, DC: World Bank.

Bennett, R. (2003). The 'direct costs' of livestock disease: the development of a system of models for the analysis of 30 endemic livestock diseases in Great Britain. *Journal of Agricultural Economics* 54: 55–71.

Bett, B., Kiunga, P., Gachohi, J. et al. (2017). Effects of climate change on the occurrence and distribution of livestock diseases. *Preventive Veterinary Medicine* 137: 119–129.

Bicknell, K.B., Wilen, J.E., and Howitt, R.E. (1999). Public policy and private incentives for livestock disease control. *Australian Journal of Agricultural and Resource Economics* 43: 501–521.

Bower, C. and Stanley, F.J. (1989). Dietary folate as a risk factor for neural-tube defects: evidence from a case-control study in Western Australia. *Medical Journal of Australia* 150: 613–619.

Charfeddine, N. and Pérez-Cabal, M.A. (2017). Effect of claw disorders on milk production, fertility, and longevity, and their economic impact in Spanish Holstein cows. *Journal of Dairy Science* 100: 653–665.

Cohen, B. (2006). Urbanization in developing countries: current trends, future projections, and key challenges for sustainability. *Technology in Society* 28: 63–80.

Cutler, S.J., Fooks, A.R., and Van der Poel, W.H.M. (2010). Public health threat of new, reemerging, and neglected zoonoses in the industrialized world. *Emerging Infectious Diseases* 16: 1–7.

Czeizel, A.E. and Dudas, I. (1992). Prevention of the first occurrence of neural-tube defects by periconceptional vitamin supplementation. *New England Journal of Medicine* 327: 1832–1825.

Das, R., Sailo, L., Verma, N. et al. (2016). Impact of heat stress on health and performance of dairy animals: a review. *Veterinary World* 9: 260–268.

Dolecheck, K. and Bewley, J. (2018). Animal board invited review: dairy cow lameness expenditures, losses and total cost. *Animal* 12: 1462–1474.

Ekboir, J., Jarvis, L.S., Sumner, D.A. et al. (2002). Changes in foot and mouth disease status and evolving world beef markets. *Agribusiness* 18: 213–229.

FAO (2009). *The State of Food and Agriculture: Livestock in the Balance*. Rome: Food and Agriculture Organization of the United Nations.

FAO (2013). *World Livestock 2013 – Changing Diseases Landscapes*. Rome: Food and Agriculture Organization of the United Nations.

FAO (2016). *Economic Analysis of Animal Diseases. FAO Animal Production; Health Guidelines, No. 18*. Rome: Food and Agriculture Organization of the United Nations.

Forman, S., Hungerford, N., Yamakawa, M. et al. (2008). Climate change impacts and risks for animal health in Asia. *Revue Scientifique et Technique* 27: 581–597.

Giovannucci, E. and Goldin, B. (1997). The role of fat, fatty acids, and total energy intake in the etiology of human colon cancer. *American Journal of Clinical Nutrition* 66 (Suppl 6): 1564S–1571S.

Giovannucci, E., Stampfer, M.J., Colditz, G.A. et al. (1993). A comparison of prospective and retrospective assessments of diet in the study of breast cancer. *American Journal of Epidemiology* 137: 502–511.

Grantham-McGregor, S., Cheung, Y.B., Cueto, S. et al. (2007). Developmental potential in the first 5 years for children in developing countries. *Lancet* 369: 60–70.

Hassell, J.M., Begon, M., Ward, M.J., and Fèvre, E.M. (2017). Urbanization and disease emergence: dynamics at the wildlife–livestock–human interface. *Trends in Ecology & Evolution* 32: 55–367.

Havelaar AH, Cawthorne A, AnguloF,Bellinger D, Corrigan T, Cravioto A, et al. WHOInitiative to Estimatethe Global Burdenof Foodborne Diseases. Lancet.2013; 381: S59.

Havelaar, A.H., Kirk, M.D., Torgerson, P. et al. (2015). World Health Organization global estimates and regional comparisons of the burden of foodborne disease in 2010. *PLoS Medicine* 12: 1923.

Headey, D. and Hirvonen, K. (2016). Is exposure to poultry harmful to child nutrition? An observational analysis for rural Ethiopia. *PLoS One* 11: 590.

Henchion, M., Moloney, A., Hyland, J. et al. (2021). Trends for meat, milk and egg consumption for the next decades and the role played by livestock systems in the global production of proteins. *Animal* 15: 100287.

Hennessy, D.A. and Marsh, T.L. (2021). Economics of animal health and livestock disease. *Handbook of Agricultural Economics* 5: 4233–4330.

Hernán, M.A. and Robins, J.M. (2006). Estimating causal effects from epidemiological data. *Journal of Epidemiology and Community Health* 60: 578–586.

Horan, R.D., Wolf, C.A., Fenichel, E.P., and Mathews, K.H. (2008). Joint management of wildlife and livestock disease. *Environmental and Resource Economics* 41: 47–70.

Kaniyamattam, K., Hertl, J., Lhermie, G. et al. (2020). Cost benefit analysis of automatic lameness detection systems in dairy herds: a dynamic programming approach. *Preventive Veterinary Medicine* 178: 104993.

Keys, A., Anderson, J.T., and Grande, F. (1957). Prediction of serum-cholesterol responses of man to changes in fats in the diet. *Lancet* 273: 959–966.

Kimaro, E.G. and Chibinga, O.C. (2013). Potential impact of climate change on livestock production and health in East Africa: a review. *Livestock Research for Rural Development* 25: 1–11.

Kock, R.A. (2005). What is this infamous 'wildlife/livestock disease interface'? A review of current knowledge for the African continent. Conservation and Development Interventions at the Wildlife/Livestock Interface: Implications for Wildlife, Livestock and Human Health, No. 30, 1–13.

Leach, K.A., Whay, H.R., Maggs, C.M. et al. (2010). Working towards a reduction in cattle lameness: 1. Understanding barriers to lameness control on dairy farms. *Research in Veterinary Science* 89: 311–317.

LeBlanc, S.J., Lissemore, K.D., Kelton, D.F. et al. (2006). Major advances in disease prevention in dairy cattle. *Journal of Dairy Science* 89: 1267–1279.

Lhermie, G., Sauvage, P., Tauer, L.W. et al. (2020). Economic effects of policy options restricting antimicrobial use for high risk cattle placed in US feedlots. *PLoS One* 15: 239135.

Limon, G., Gamawa, A.A., Ahmed, A.I. et al. (2020). Epidemiological characteristics and economic impact of lumpy skin disease, sheeppox and goatpox among subsistence farmers in Northeast Nigeria. *Frontiers in Veterinary Science* 7: 8.

Lyons, N.A., Alexander, N., Stärk, K.D.C. et al. (2015). Impact of foot-and-mouth disease on milk production on a large-scale dairy farm in Kenya. *Preventive Veterinary Medicine* 120: 177–186.

Madeira, N.G., Amarante, A.F.T., and Padovani, C.R. (1998). Effect of management practices on screw-worm among sheep in São Paulo state, Brazil. *Tropical Animal Health and Production* 30: 149–157.

Marsh, T.L., Pendell, D.L., and Knippenberg, R. (2017). Animal health economics: an aid to decision making on animal health interventions – case studies in the United States of America. *Revue Scientifique et Technique* 32: 137–145.

Mensink, R.P. and Katan, M.B. (1990). Effect of dietary trans fatty acids on highdensity and low-density lipoprotein cholesterol levels in healthy subjects. *New England Journal of Medicine* 323: 439–445.

Milunsky, A., Jick, H., Jick, S.S. et al. (1989). Multivitamin/folic acid supplementation in early pregnancy reduces the prevalence of neural tube defects. *JAMA* 262: 2847–2852.

National Research Council (US) Subcommittee on Environmental Stress (1981). *Effect of Environment on Nutrient Requirements of Domestic Animals*. Washington, DC: National Academies Press.

Olwoch, J.M., Reyers, B., Engelbrecht, F.A., and Erasmus, B.F.N. (2008). Climate change and the tick-borne disease, theileriosis (East Coast fever) in sub-Saharan Africa. *Journal of Arid Environments* 72: 108–120.

Otte, M.J., Nugent, R., and McLeod, A. (2004). *Transboundary Animal Diseases: Assessment of Socio-Economic Impacts and Institutional Responses*. Rome: Food and Agriculture Organization.

Pinto, J., Bonacic, C., Hamilton-West, C. et al. (2008). Climate change and animal diseases in South America. *Revue Scientifique et Technique* 27: 599–613.

Raboisson, D., Mounié, M., and Maigne, E. (2014). Diseases, reproductive performance, and changes in milk production associated with subclinical ketosis in dairy cows: a meta-analysis and review. *Journal of Dairy Science* 97: 7547–7563.

Reagan, A.B.L. (2020).Quantifying production losses associated with foot and mouth disease outbreaks on large scale dairy farms in Nakuru County, Kenya. PhD thesis, Egerton University.

Revell, B. (2015). Meat and milk consumption 2050: the potential for demand-side solutions to greenhouse gas emissions reduction. *EuroChoices* 14: 4–11.

Salmon, G., Teufel, N., Baltenweck, I. et al. (2018). Trade-offs in livestock development at farm level: different actors with different objectives. *Global Food Security* 17: 103–112.

Serra, R., Kiker, G.A., Minten, B. et al. (2020). Filling knowledge gaps to strengthen livestock policies in low-income countries. *Global Food Security* 26: 100428.

Smithells, R.W., Sheppard, S., Schorah, C.J. et al. (1980). Possible prevention of neural-tube defects by periconceptional vitamin supplementation. *Lancet* 1: 339–340.

Spahn, J.M., Lyon, J.M., Altman, J.M. et al. (2011). The systematic review methodology used to support the 2010 Dietary Guidelines Advisory Committee. *Journal of the American Dietetic Association* 111: 520–523.

Steeneveld, W., Amuta, P., van Soest, F.J.S. et al. (2020). Estimating the combined costs of clinical and subclinical ketosis in dairy cows. *PLoS One* 15: 230448.

Taylor, L.H., Latham, S.M., and Woolhouse, M.E.J. (2001). Risk factors for human disease emergence. *Philosophical Transactions of the Royal Society of London. Series B, Biological Sciences* 356: 983–989.

Tisdell, C. (1995). Assessing the approach to cost-benefit analysis of controlling livestock diseases of McInerney and others. https://ideas.repec.org/p/ags/uqseah/164427.html (accessed 24 January 2024).

Umali, D.L., Feder, G., and de Haan, C. (1994). Animal health services: finding the balance between public and private delivery. *World Bank Research Observer* 9: 71–96.

US FDA (2014). Guidance for industry: evidence-based review system for the scientific evaluation of health claims – final. www.fda.gov/Food/GuidanceRegulation/GuidanceDocumentsRegulatoryInformation/ucm073332.htm#system (accessed 24 January 2024).

Vipham, J.L., Amenu, K., Alonso, S. et al. (2020). No food security without food safety: lessons from livestock related research. *Global Food Security* 26: 100382.

Von Keyserlingk, M.A.G., Barrientos, A., Ito, K. et al. (2012). Benchmarking cow comfort on North American freestall dairies: lameness, leg injuries, lying time, facility design, and management for high-producing Holstein dairy cows. *Journal of Dairy Science* 95: 7399–7408.

Wald, N.J., Hackshaw, A.D., Stone, R., and Sourial, N.A. (1996). Blood folic acid and vitamin B12 in relation to neural tube defects. *British Journal of Obstetrics and Gynaecology* 103: 19–24.

Willett, W.C. and Ascherio, A. (1994). Trans fatty acids: are the effects only marginal? *American Journal of Public Health* 84: 722–724.

Willett, W.C., Stampfer, M.J., Manson, J.E. et al. (1993). Intake of trans fatty acids and risk of coronary heart disease among women. *Lancet* 341: 581–585.

Wilson, A.J. and Mellor, P.S. (2009). Bluetongue in Europe: past, present and future. *Philosophical Transactions of the Royal Society B: Biological Sciences* 364: 2669–2681.

22

Vaccines and Vaccination

J. Jyothi[1] and M. Bhavya Sree[2]

[1] *Department of Veterinary Medicine, P.V. Narasimha Rao Telangana Veterinary University, Hyderabad, India*
[2] *Student, P.V. Narasimha Rao Telangana Veterinary University, Hyderabad, India*

Animal vaccination is the immunization of a domestic, livestock or wild animal (National Office of Animal Health 2020). The first animal vaccine was for chicken cholera in 1879, invented by Louis Pasteur (National Museum of American History 2020). The production of such vaccines encounters issues in relation to the economic difficulties of individuals, governments, and companies (Donadeu et al. 2019). Regulation of animal vaccinations is much lower compared to regulation of human vaccinations. Vaccines are categorized into conventional and next-generation vaccines (Thomas 2016). Animal vaccines are the most cost-effective and sustainable method of controlling infectious veterinary diseases (Jorge and Dellagostin 2017).

The Global Rinderpest Eradication Program is a large-scale international collaboration involving vaccination, local and international trade restrictions, and surveillance. This effort may be one of veterinary medicine's greatest achievements and rinderpest may soon become only the second disease (after smallpox) to be globally eradicated.

The rabies vaccine is another example of the impact of a successful animal vaccination program.

22.1 Objectives of Vaccination

- To vaccinate the largest possible number of individuals in the population at risk.
- To vaccinate each individual no more frequently than necessary.
- To vaccinate only against agents to which the animal has a realistic risk of exposure and subsequent development of serious disease.
- Veterinary vaccines have had, and continue to have, a major role in protecting animal health and public health, reducing animal suffering, enabling efficient production of food animals to feed the burgeoning human population, and greatly reducing the need for antibiotics to treat food and companion animals.
- Vaccinating animals helps by stimulating an immune response without causing the disease itself. This creates early exposure to disease-causing organisms, so that the animal's immune system is able to recall the infectious agent to which the animal is vaccinated.
- Vaccination helps provide sustainable and economic stability for farmers and the communities they serve.
- When animals are not well cared for, it leads to reduced resistance to diseases and the development of clinical diseases.
- Animals in poor health, poor body condition or stressed should not be vaccinated because the vaccine will not be effective.

22.2 Nonliving Vaccines for Animals

Vaccines may contain either living or killed organisms or purified antigens from these organisms. Vaccines containing living organisms tend to trigger the best protective responses. Killed organisms or purified antigens may be less immunogenic than living ones because they are unable to grow and spread in the host. Thus, they are less likely to stimulate the immune system

Epidemiology and Environmental Hygiene in Veterinary Public Health, First Edition. Edited by Tanmoy Rana.
© 2025 John Wiley & Sons, Inc. Published 2025 by John Wiley & Sons, Inc.

in an optimal fashion. On the other hand, they are often less expensive and may be safer. Living viruses from vaccines infect host cells and grow briefly. The infected cells then process the viral antigens, triggering a response dominated by cytotoxic T cells, a type 1 response. Killed organisms and purified antigens, in contrast, commonly stimulate responses dominated by antibodies, a type 2 response. This type of response may not generate optimal protection against some organisms.

As a result, vaccines that contain killed organisms or purified antigens usually require the use of adjuvants to maximize their effectiveness. Adjuvants may, however, cause local inflammation and multiple doses or high doses of antigen increase the risks of producing hypersensitivity reactions. Killed vaccines should resemble the living organisms as closely as possible. Chemical inactivation should cause minimal change to their antigens. Compounds used in this way include formaldehyde, ethylene oxide, ethyleneimine, acetyl ethyleneimine, and beta-propiolactone.

22.2.1 Subunit Vaccines

Although vaccines containing whole killed organisms are economical to produce, they contain many components that do not contribute to protective immunity. They may also contain toxic components such as endotoxins. Thus, depending upon costs, it may be advantageous to identify, isolate, and purify the critical protective antigens. These can then be used in a vaccine by themselves. For example, purified tetanus toxin, inactivated by treatment with formalin (tetanus toxoid), is used for active immunization against tetanus. Likewise, the attachment pili of enteropathogenic *Escherichia coli* can be purified and incorporated into vaccines. The antipilus antibodies protect animals by preventing bacterial attachment to the intestinal wall.

22.2.2 Antigens Generated by Gene Cloning

The DNA encoding the desired antigens may be inserted into its vector, which then expresses the protective antigen. The recombinant vector is grown and the antigens encoded by the inserted genes are harvested, purified, and administered as a vaccine. An example of such a vaccine is one directed against the cloned subunit of *E. coli* enterotoxin. The cloned subunits are antigenic and function as effective toxoids.

A purified subunit antigen, called OspA, encoded by a gene from *Borrelia burgdorferi*, effectively protects dogs against Lyme disease. A similar type of vaccine may be developed through the use of bacterial "ghosts," which are bacteria that have been emptied of their contents, especially their DNA.

22.2.3 DNA Plasmid Vaccines

Animals may also be immunized by injection of DNA encoding viral antigens. This DNA is inserted into a bacterial plasmid, a piece of circular DNA that acts as a vector. When the genetically engineered plasmid is injected, it is taken up by host cells. The DNA is then transcribed, and mRNAs are translated to produce the vaccine protein. The transfected host cells thus express the vaccine protein in association with major histocompatibility complex class I molecules. This results in the development of not only neutralizing antibodies but also cytotoxic T cells.

22.3 Modified Live Vaccines for Animals

22.3.1 Attenuated Vaccines

The use of live organisms in vaccines presents many advantages. For example, they are usually more effective than inactivated vaccines in triggering cell-mediated immune responses. However, their use also presents potential hazards. Thus, the virulence of a live organism used for vaccination must be attenuated so that it is able to replicate but is no longer pathogenic.

The level of attenuation is critical to vaccine success. Underattenuation will result in residual virulence and disease (reversion to virulence); overattenuation will result in an ineffective vaccine. Attenuated vaccines should not be used to vaccinate species for which they have not been tested or approved. Pathogens attenuated for one species may be over- or underattenuated in others. Thus, they may either cause disease or fail to provide adequate protection.

Traditional methods of attenuating organisms have been by prolonged tissue culture or culture in eggs. These have relied on random mutations, an unpredictable process.

Although few bacterial vaccines have been attenuated in this way (the most obvious examples are *Brucella* strain 19 and the Sterne strain of anthrax), the bacterial genome is usually too large to generate effectively and irreversibly attenuated mutants. It has proven much easier to attenuate viruses with their relatively small genomes. Many of the currently available viral vaccine strains were attenuated in this way.

22.3.2 Gene-deleted Vaccines

Molecular genetic techniques now make it possible to modify the genes of an organism so that it becomes irreversibly attenuated. Deliberate deletion of the genes that code for proteins associated with virulence is an increasingly attractive procedure.

For example, gene-deleted vaccines were first used against the Aujeszky disease herpesvirus in swine. In this case, the thymidine kinase gene was removed from the virus. Herpesvirus requires thymidine kinase to return from latency. Viruses from which this gene has been removed can infect neurons but cannot replicate and cause disease.

Similar genetic manipulation can also be used to restrict the ability of bacteria to grow *in vivo*. For example, a modified live vaccine is available that contains streptomycin-dependent *Mannheimia haemolytica* and *Pasteurella multocida*.

These mutants depend on the presence of streptomycin for growth. When used in a vaccine, the absence of streptomycin will eventually result in the death of the bacteria but not before they have stimulated a protective immune response.

22.3.3 Virus-vectored Vaccines

Another way to produce a highly effective living vaccine is to insert the genes that encode protective antigens into an avirulent "vector" organism. The most widely used vaccine viral vectors are large DNA viruses such as poxviruses (fowlpox, canarypox), vaccinia virus, adenoviruses, and some herpesvirus. These viruses have a large genome that facilitates insertion of new genes. They also express relatively high levels of the recombinant antigen. In at least some cases, vectored vaccines appear able to induce immunity even when high levels of maternal antibody are present.

Canarypox-vectored vaccines incorporating genes from canine distemper virus are now used to immunize dogs, and a similar vaccinia vector containing the gene encoding rabies glycoprotein is effective in protecting dogs and cats against rabies virus.

Fowlpox virus and herpesvirus recombinant vaccines are widely used in the poultry industry. For example, one vector is fowlpox virus, into which Newcastle disease virus HA and F genes are incorporated. It has the benefit of conferring immunity against fowlpox virus as well.

22.4 Route of Administration of Vaccination in Animals

The most common method of vaccine administration is by subcutaneous (SC) or intramuscular (IM) injection. This approach is excellent for relatively small numbers of animals and for diseases in which systemic immunity is important.

In addition, the veterinarian can be sure an animal has received the appropriate dose of vaccine. However, local immunity is sometimes more important than systemic immunity, and in these cases it is more appropriate to administer the vaccine at the site of microbial invasion. For example, intranasal vaccines protect:

- cattle against infectious bovine rhinotracheitis
- cats against feline rhinotracheitis and calicivirus infections
- poultry against infectious bronchitis and Newcastle disease.

Unfortunately, these techniques require handling each individual animal. Spraying of vaccines enables the vaccines to be inhaled by all the animals in a herd, group, or flock – an obvious advantage when the unit is large. This method is commonly used in the poultry industry.

22.5 Combination Vaccines for Animals

Because of the complexity of many disease syndromes or to avoid giving animals multiple injections, it is common to use mixtures of organisms in single vaccines.

For example, for bovine respiratory disease complex, combined vaccines are available for bovine respiratory syncytial virus, infectious bovine rhinotracheitis virus, bovine viral diarrhea virus, parainfluenza 3 virus, and *Mannheimia haemolytica*. Combination vaccines that save considerable time and effort are also commonly used in dogs and cats.

When a mixture of antigens is given to an animal simultaneously, they may compete with one another. However, manufacturers have recognized this and modified vaccines accordingly. Vaccines should never be mixed indiscriminately because one component may dominate and interfere with responses to the other components.

The simultaneous administration of multiple vaccines to an animal does not present difficulties to the immune system of normal, healthy animals.

22.6 Vaccination Schedules for Animals

Although it is not possible to devise precise schedules for each vaccine, certain principles are common to all methods of active immunization. Newborn animals are passively protected by maternal antibodies and, in general, cannot be vaccinated until maternal immunity has waned. If stimulation of immunity is deemed necessary at this stage, the mother may be vaccinated during late pregnancy, timing the doses so that peak antibody levels are reached at the time of colostrum formation.

It is important to note that modified live vaccines against viruses that cause abortion should not be used in pregnant animals, because the vaccine itself may cause abortion. Neonatal animals are protected against disease caused by that specific pathogen while sufficient maternal antibodies are present. However, passive antibody titers decrease exponentially. These maternal antibodies may drop below protective levels while at the same time preventing successful immunization. Inactivated vaccines are not very effective in conferring protective immunity in the face of maternal antibodies.

Modified live vaccines, however, may induce a protective primary immune response and some immunological memory. Because the precise time of loss of maternal immunity cannot be predicted, young animals must usually be vaccinated multiple times to ensure successful immunization, and appropriate biosecurity measures should be used until immunity develops.

The interval between vaccine doses depends on an animal's immunological memory. The duration of this memory depends on multiple factors, such as the nature of the antigen, the use of live or dead organisms, the adjuvants used, and the route of administration.

Some vaccines may induce immunity that persists for an animal's lifetime. Other vaccines may require boosting only once every 2–3 years. Even killed viral vaccines may protect some animals against disease for many years. Unfortunately, the minimal duration of immunity has rarely been reliably measured.

22.7 Risk Factors for Vaccination

Risk factors to be considered include host factors specific to that animal, environmental factors, and agent factors specific to that vaccine. Animals that are malnourished, are ill with another disease or condition, or are stressed are unlikely to respond well to vaccination.

Young animals (for example, puppies and kittens less than 16 weeks of age) may still have significant levels of antibodies from their mother, taken in when they nursed in their first day of life. These antibodies may inactivate the vaccine, rendering it useless. Environmental factors look at the population as a whole.

The more animals there are in the population, the greater the likelihood that any one animal will be exposed to a given virus. Those animals that are exposed to new animals, for example by introduction of a new pet, or by boarding or grooming, are at greater risk.

22.8 Importance of Veterinary Vaccines

22.8.1 Safe and Efficient Food Production

Veterinary vaccines are used in livestock and poultry to maintain animal health and to improve overall production. More efficient animal production and better access to high-quality protein are essential to feed the growing population. Vaccines that preserve animal health and improve production are important components in meeting this need.

Recently, vaccines have been developed to reduce the shedding of organisms that cause food-borne diseases in people. Vaccines for *E. coli* O157:H7 in cattle and *Salmonella enteritidis* in chickens are available. These vaccines typically do not improve the health of the vaccinated animal, but they reduce the shedding of pathogens that may contaminate animal products for human consumption. The severity of the *S. enteritidis* outbreak in people in the United States in 2010 due to consumption of contaminated eggs could have been reduced or prevented if the chickens had received the *S. enteritidis* vaccine.

22.8.2 Control of Zoonotic Diseases

Vaccines to control zoonotic diseases in food animals, companion animals, and even wildlife have had a major impact on reducing the incidence of zoonotic diseases in people. Without rabies vaccines, it is unlikely that families would be willing to keep cats and dogs as pets.

Recombinant vaccinia-vectored rabies vaccines have also been used successfully in baits for oral vaccination campaigns to reduce the incidence of rabies in wild animals (Pastoret and Brochier 1996). Vaccines for brucellosis were instrumental in the *Brucella abortus* eradication program in the United States.

Many countries have severe problems with brucellosis in cattle, small ruminants, and people due to a lack of available *Brucella* vaccines for animals (FAO 2010).

22.8.3 Control of Emerging and Exotic Diseases of Animals and People

Emerging and exotic animal diseases are a growing threat to human and animal health and jeopardize food security. Increases in human and animal populations, with accompanying environmental degradation and globalized trade and travel, enhance opportunities for transfer of pathogens within and between species. The resulting diseases pose enormous challenges now and for the future. Both types of production present unique challenges for disease emergence and control. Emerging zoonotic diseases of both food and companion animals are a major threat to public health. It is inevitable that the world will continue to experience emerging disease outbreaks in the coming decades. Rapid development of animal vaccines can play a key role in controlling such diseases.

22.8.4 Reduction in the Need for Antibiotics

Veterinary vaccines reduce the need for antibiotics to treat infections in food-producing and companion animals. There are increasing concerns related to antibiotic resistance associated with the extensive use of antibiotics in veterinary and human medicine (Singer et al. 2003).

If regulatory requirements for a biologics company to obtain and maintain a license to produce the vaccine were to increase, then the cost of the vaccine would increase and producers would opt to use less vaccine and more antibiotics. Affordable and available vaccines reduce reliance on antibiotics for animal health.

22.9 Advances in Vaccinology

Much progress has been made in vaccine development in recent years but significant challenges remain. Animal and human infectious disease experts need to work together to prepare for new and emerging diseases. Veterinary vaccines must be pure, safe, potent, and effective and they must be economical or they will not be widely used.

Proper standards and production controls in the manufacture of veterinary vaccines are essential for ensuring quality products for animal disease control. The regulatory process for evaluation of vaccines must ensure adequate evaluation of biologics but be efficient for both the regulatory agencies and the biologics manufacturers.

Keeping the costs of animal vaccines low will encourage more use of vaccines and less use of antibiotics. It will also enable the use of food safety vaccines that do not have an economic advantage for the producer or health advantage to the animal, but have important public health benefits.

22.10 Conclusion

The fact that so many people depend on livestock and poultry for their livelihoods and as a source of food limits policy options, complicates local and global trade decisions, and raises political sensitivities. It is inevitable that the world will continue to experience the emergence of new human and animal diseases in the coming decades. The challenge mandates the need for the medical, veterinary, and public health communities to work together locally and internationally. Veterinary vaccines will continue to be an important tool to protect human health, animal health, food safety, and food security and must be accessible and economical.

References

Donadeu, M., Nwankpa, N., Abela-Ridder, B. et al. (2019). Strategies to increase adoption of animal vaccines by smallholder farmers with focus on neglected diseases and marginalized populations. *PLOS Neglected Tropical Diseases* 13: e0006989.

Food and Agriculture Organization of the United Nations (FAO). *Brucella melitensis* in Eurasia and the Middle East. FAO Animal Production and Health Proceedings No. 10. (2010). Rome: FAO.

Jorge, S. and Dellagostin, O.A. (2017). The development of veterinary vaccines: a review of traditional methods and modern biotechnology approaches. *Biotechnology Research and Innovation* 1: 6–13.

National Museum of American History (2020). *The Antibody Initiative – Veterinary Vaccines and Serums*. Washington, DC: National Museum of American History.

National Office of Animal Health (2020). *Vaccination for Animal Health: An Overview*. Stevenage, UK: National Office of Animal Health.

Pastoret, P.-P. and Brochier, B. (1996). The development and use of a vaccinia-rabies recombinant oral vaccine for the control of wildlife rabies; a link between Jenner and Pasteur. *Epidemiology and Infection* 116: 235–240.

Singer, R.S., Finch, R., Wegener, H.C. et al. (2003). Antibiotic resistance – the interplay between antibiotic use in animals and human beings. *Lancet Infectious Diseases* 3: 47–51.

Thomas, S. (2016). *Vaccine Design: Methods and Protocols. Vaccines for Veterinary Diseases*, vol. 2. Champaign: Humana Press.

Section 2

Impact of Environmental Hygiene in Veterinary and Public Health

23

Aims, Scope, Administration, and Importance of Veterinary Public Health

Chandra Shekhar

Department of Veterinary Public Health & Epidemiology, College of Veterinary Science & Animal Husbandry, Acharya Narendra Deva University of Agriculture & Technology, Ayodhya, India

23.1 Introduction

Health is a state of complete physical, mental, and social well-being and not merely the absence of disease or infirmity. Medical and veterinary professionals have traditionally focused respectively on the improvement of human health and livestock health and production as their primary objectives, respectively. Public health may be defined as "the science of preventing disease, prolonging life and promoting health and efficiency through organized community efforts." Veterinary public health (VPH) is an essential component of public health which includes various types of cooperation between the disciplines that link the health triad that is people–animals–environment, and all of its interactions. Examples related to this triad include zoonoses, chemical residues, animal production systems, nature conservation, wildlife, and water pollution. VPH impacts on human health by reducing exposure to hazards arising from animals, animal products, and their environment. Examples of these hazards include zoonoses, vector-borne and other communicable diseases, chemicals and drugs used in animals, envenomations, and injuries from exposure to animals (WHO 2002).

The concept of VPH originated in ancient Egypt, when healer priests drew no distinctions between caring for human patients and animals. They gained much knowledge from the anatomy and diseases of animals, which they applied to the healing of humans (Schwabe 1978). The "One Medicine" approach prevailed until the nineteenth century. Since then, the gulf between human and animal physicians has been increasing, mainly because of changes in political and cultural rules rather than scientific logic (Schwabe 1978). The term "veterinary public health," according to Schwabe (1984) was introduced after World War II by public health administrators in the US Public Health Service to designate those areas of public health in which veterinary medicine shares particular interests. Newly emerging and reemerging infections are recognized as a global problem, and 75% of these are potentially zoonotic (Taylor et al. 2001). The reemerging zoonoses together with other issues such as bioterrorism, antimicrobial resistance, pollution incidents, xenotransplantation, and the socioeconomic importance of food production make a collaborative interprofessional approach to VPH more urgent.

In 1975, VPH was defined by a Joint FAO/WHO Expert Committee on VPH as "a component of public health activities devoted to the application of professional veterinary skills, knowledge and resources to the protection and improvement of human health" (WHO 1975). The World Health Organization (WHO) defined VPH as "the sum of all contributions to the physical, mental and social well-being of humans through an understanding and application of veterinary science" (Figure 23.1) (WHO 2002). VPH is a major part of public health in which human health and well-being are the central tasks. In recent years the VPH has gained increasing importance because immense changes have occurred in animal production processes and agricultural structures (Khatun et al. 2019).

Many significant developments have occurred in VPH. The predominant concern of VPH during the 1970s and for most of the 1980s related to risks of chemical pollution of the environment and the food chain (e.g., from pesticides, natural toxins, and drug residues in food, and groundwater pollution from animal waste). However, in recent years emerging and reemerging zoonotic diseases have acquired global significance for VPH. These include *Salmonella enteritidis* in poultry, the most frequently reported zoonotic disease in many countries, multidrug-resistant *Salmonella typhimurium*, Rift Valley fever in East Africa, Marburg and Ebola viral hemorrhagic fevers in Africa, the Arabian Peninsula, and Egypt, the New

---

Epidemiology and Environmental Hygiene in Veterinary Public Health, First Edition. Edited by Tanmoy Rana.
© 2025 John Wiley & Sons, Inc. Published 2025 by John Wiley & Sons, Inc.

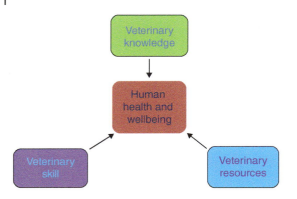

Figure 23.1 Role of veterinary public health.

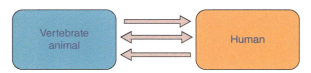

Figure 23.2 Transmission of zoonotic disease.

World screw worm (*Cochliomyia hominivorax*) in north Africa and new rabies-like viruses in bats in Australia and Europe. Zoonoses may be defined as "those diseases and infections that are naturally transmitted between vertebrate animals and humans" (Figure 23.2). About one infectious disease has been experienced every year during recent past and scientists have reported that out of a total 1415 known infectious diseases of humans, 868 (61%) are of zoonotic importance (Pal and Siddiky 2011). Over 70% of new diseases of humans have an animal origin, with the potential of becoming local and major public health threats (FAO 2017).

23.2 Aims of Veterinary Public Health

The main aim of VPH is the contribution of veterinary science to public health; that is, protection and improvement of human health. An additional aim of VPH is to protect the health of animals and the environment. In the past, VPH evolved to deal with three different issues: combating animal diseases, performing meat inspection, and control of zoonoses (Pal and Siddiky 2011).

23.3 Scope of Veterinary Public Health

The concept of "One World, One Health" was coined in view of the rapid emergence and reemergence of zoonotic pathogens and their rapid spread through foods, international travel and trade, which has created new challenges and opportunities for veterinary services. Thus, the role of veterinarians has been realized in safeguarding animal and human health. In the nineteenth century, Robert Virchow, a German physician, stated that there is no dividing line between animal and human medicine, nor should there be. Later on, William Osler, a Canadian physician, used the term "One Medicine." In 1984, Calvin W. Schwabe, an epidemiologist, supported the integration of human and veterinary medicine and encouraged the veterinary and medical professions to coordinate with each other to prevent zoonotic diseases (Krishna 2011).

The scope of VPH is multidisciplinary; besides dealing with animal disease, it is concerned with zoonoses, food-borne disease, and environmental health (Kouba 1992), involving veterinarians, health professionals, and scientists as well as paraprofessionals who treat, control or prevent zoonotic diseases (Ortega et al. 2004). VPH concerns all areas of food production and safety, zoonosis control, environmental protection, and animal welfare (Khatun et al. 2019).

Veterinary public health involves not only veterinarians in governmental, nongovernmental and private sectors, but also other professionals such as physicians, nurses, microbiologists, food technologists, sanitarians, environmental specialists, agricultural scientists, paraveterinary staff, and auxiliaries who contribute to the treatment, control, and prevention of diseases of animal origin. VPH directly improves human health by reducing exposure to hazards arising from animals and animal products, for example hazards due to zoonoses and other communicable diseases, vector-borne diseases, chemicals and veterinary drugs used in animals, envenomations, and injuries from occupational and recreational exposure to animals.

23.4 Domains of Veterinary Public Health

The important domains of VPH include the following.

23.4.1 The Core Domains of Veterinary Public Health

The core domains of VPH include epidemiology, diagnosis, control, prevention and elimination of zoonoses; biomedical research; food protection; management of health aspects of laboratory animal facilities and diagnostic laboratories; health education and extension; and production and control of biological products and medical devices. Other VPH domains may include management of public health emergencies, management of domestic and wild animal populations, and protection of drinking water and the environment.

23.4.2 Emerging Domains in Veterinary Public Health

The specific emerging domains in VPH that significantly contribute to public health include the following.

- Investigation, epidemiology, and control of nonzoonotic and communicable diseases.
- Epidemiology and prevention of noninfectious diseases (including the promotion of healthy lifestyles).
- Risk analysis, cost–analysis, effectiveness analysis, cost–benefit, health economics, and other methods of evaluating health service delivery and public health programs.
- Administration, leadership, and management of public health and environmental agencies, including government institutions, nongovernmental organizations (NGOs), and academic institutions.
- Social, mental, and behavioral aspects of human–animal relationships (including animal-facilitated therapy and development of animal welfare standards).
- The social context of delivery of VPH services, especially to rural women who have traditionally been underserved by the veterinary services, yet who have great potential for preventing zoonotic diseases and diseases of animal origin.

23.4.3 Other Contributions of Veterinary Public Health

Veterinary public health contributes to many areas of public health that are not related to animals, including the design and analysis of public health programs. The efficiency of such programs, particularly in developing countries, can be improved by ensuring that VPH skills are fully integrated at both local and national levels. Moreover, there may be widespread changes within the immediate scope of VPH itself that may involve the following issues.

23.4.3.1 Farming Methods

These include changes in the intensity of livestock production; aquaculture and game farming; the need to adopt environmentally friendly approaches; genetic engineering and transgenesis; the use of additives and antimicrobials in feedstuffs, and safe sourcing of feedstuffs; the use of antimicrobial agents for growth promotion and disease prophylaxis; waste disposal; advancement of women's rights in rural areas; ruralization of urban areas (as people move to cities, bringing their livestock and culture from rural areas with them).

23.4.3.2 Food Production Chain

This includes a change in focus from individual animals to herds and populations, and systems-based controls, e.g., hazard analysis critical control point (HACCP); increased responsibility of personnel at all points in the food production chain to certify the quality of all phases of production and the final products; development and implementation of new technologies for food and feed production, preservation and commercialization, and related problems of toxic residues and improved standards of hygiene; and new social needs, in particular greater attention to consumers' requirements.

23.4.3.3 Trade, Travel, and Movement

These include continuing expansion of international travel and trade in animals and animal products; changes in food habits associated with travel or migration; implementing and ensuring compliance with the requirements of international agreements and conventions (e.g., the World Trade Organization [WTO] Agreement on the application of Sanitary and Phytosanitary [SPS] measures) and national regulations, both to allow access to international markets and to guarantee the internal market by certification of products; changes in consumer expectations, including export and tourist markets, and increased consumer awareness.

23.4.3.4 Interactions Between Humans and Animals

These include changing incidence of animal-related hazards associated with tourism; role of companion animals and human well-being; new requirements connected with increasing urban and periurban animal populations; and biomedical applications, e.g., xenotransplantation.

23.4.3.5 Natural and Man-made Disasters

These include increasing demand for VPH services to respond to nonepidemic emergencies such as weather-related problems, earthquakes, industrial and nuclear accidents, and to man-made epidemics.

23.4.3.6 Emerging and Reemerging Zoonotic Diseases

These include expansion and increasing importance of zoonoses.

23.4.3.7 Reduced Resources

These include reduced governmental funding and a trend toward privatization of services; maintaining sustainability of traditional VPH services; developing alternative mechanisms for delivery of VPH services; commitments and priorities of national governments; poor perception and understanding of VPH within the public health sector.

23.4.3.8 Pace of Change

These include reliance on new disciplines and improved evidence-based decision making within VPH, e.g., risk analysis, social and gender analysis; information overload, media attention and the need for rapid and accurate communication; the need for flexibility and innovation.

23.5 Administration of Veterinary Public Health

In 1995, the 48th World Health Assembly adopted resolution WHA48.13 (WHO 1995), in which efforts were made to strengthen national and global surveillance of infectious diseases, and diseases due to antimicrobial-resistant microorganisms. As a result, a new department that included a team of VPH officers with expertise in the areas of zoonoses, foodborne disease surveillance and control, and other related subjects (WHO 1997) was established at WHO Headquarters in Geneva. The WHO subsequently further strengthened its commitment to surveillance and control of infectious diseases (WHO 1999).

The functions, activities, and resources of VPH are dispersed throughout various agencies and sectors such as agriculture, health, and the environment. A VPH program may act as a focal point with liaison functions, or it may have extensive operational responsibilities for providing technical cooperation to national programs. Organizational requirements of VPH at the international level include global and regional coordination units, country and intercountry advisers, and specialized reference centers. The important role of a VPH program is to serve as a catalyst for intersectoral action, especially between agriculture and the health sectors, where functions and resources related to food production and the control of zoonotic diseases exist. An effective institutional program should be established to coordinate and oversee intersectoral collaboration. An example of such a program is the Inter-American Meeting, at the Ministerial Level, on Animal Health (RIMSA), which is convened by the Pan American Health Organization (PAHO) with the participation of representatives from the Ministries of Health and Agriculture of the countries in the WHO Region of the Americas. The WHO, FAO, and OIE routinely collaborate on VPH subjects of common interest. However, stronger political commitment by Member States can make this collaboration more effective.

The unexpected link between bovine spongiform encephalopathy (BSE) and variant Creutzfeldt–Jakob disease (vCJD) called for close intersectoral cooperation to elucidate this connection. Hantaviruses, and West Nile virus (WNV) in the Americas, are examples of zoonotic agents causing human illness and death that require rapid responses from, and teamwork between, physicians, veterinarians, and biologists. Resistance to antimicrobial agents among zoonotic bacteria has also become an issue of increasing concern for animal production and human health.

The aim of VPH is to protect human health, animals, and the environment from risks that are rapidly evolving as a result of dramatic changes, which requires strong intersectoral cooperation, resource mobilization, and community participation. To ensure food quality and safety, VPH must focus on integrating health professions and food chain and environmental partners in a single system. Within VPH, close liaison must exist between veterinarians, medical and other health professionals, including epidemiologists, food technologists, occupational health workers, environmental specialists, and laboratory personnel. The role of VPH is important in developing an integrated "farm-to-table" approach to ensure food safety (Figure 23.3). Animal production, animal health and welfare, and food safety are closely linked so the role of VPH is essential to achieve the necessary integration. VPH professionals need strong scientific and technical competence in the prevention and control of zoonotic and food-borne diseases, and skills in disaster management.

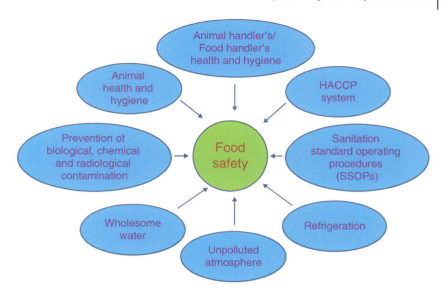

Figure 23.3 Methods of ensuring food safety.

To serve VPH and address relevant problems, the collaborating and reference centers should focus on appropriate goals. In recent decades, decreasing attention paid by governments and development agencies to infectious diseases has led to the closure of some collaborating and reference centers, or a drastic reduction in their functions, through lack of funding. Therefore, there is need for ongoing financial support to collaborating and reference centers to sustain their activities. Support from the WHO, FAO, OIE, and other international or national agencies can help collaborating and reference centers to attract funding. Alternatively, they can form consortia or partnerships with other centers to develop a problem-orientated approach. Centers should also team up with other health and science professionals, including professionals associated with the health of domestic and wild animals.

23.6 Importance of Veterinary Public Health

The primary challenge for effective implementation of VPH is to establish an effective VPH system, with staff well trained in the broad areas of public health and preventive medicine and well integrated in the public health team. Unfortunately, in many countries veterinarians focus mainly on clinical or meat inspection work. In order to achieve VPH objectives, WHO experts stressed the need for the establishment of a VPH unit staffed with public health veterinarians to deal with major issues such as zoonoses control and protection of foods of animal origin, and for close collaboration between the different professional groups, especially veterinarians, public health workers, and environmental professionals, which can contribute to VPH goals (Kakkar et al. 2013). The major importance of VPH includes the following factors.

23.6.1 Prevention, Control, and Eradication of Zoonoses

Human health is inextricably linked to animal health and this link between human and animal populations, and with the surrounding environment, is particularly close in developing regions where animals provide transportation, draught power, and clothing as well as proteins such as milk, meat, and eggs (Malinda 2011). In recent years, the occurrence of zoonotic diseases has increased due to alteration of the environment, establishment of human settlements in formerly uninhabited areas, a greater demand for animal protein, intensification of animal production, and increased trade in animals, animal products, and other foodstuffs.

Veterinary public health expertise is an essential component of the public health response to emerging and reemerging infectious diseases. Veterinarians and other VPH professionals, however, have more to offer to the public health response than expertise in traditional surveillance and control of zoonotic diseases. VPH professionals are essential partners, together with other public health officials, and agricultural and diagnostic laboratory staff. VPH staff are needed to develop and enhance surveillance of outbreaks of emerging and reemerging diseases, and to monitor changes in the incidence and epidemiology of these diseases. Prevention and control of emerging infectious diseases is a multidisciplinary and multifaceted endeavor which requires the skill and expertise of many healthcare providers, including VPH professionals. VPH leadership is particularly needed to develop and implement guidelines for the diagnosis, prevention, and control of zoonotic diseases.

23.6.2 Protection of Food

Veterinary public health service has the responsibility to conduct antemortem inspection of animals and postmortem inspection of carcases to ensure wholesome meat for human consumption (Buntain 2004). Globalization of trade has facilitated the spread of food-borne diseases, such as BSE in cattle. Therefore, food and livestock feed need to be closely monitored during production, processing, handling, and distribution.

The emergence and reemergence of zoonotic diseases might be the consequence of new patterns in food trade. Enterohemorrhagic *Escherichia coli* (EHEC) was initially confined to North America until the mid-1990s, but at present it occurs throughout the world. *Salmonella enteritidis* and the multidrug-resistant *Salmonella typhimurium* (DT 104) via eggs have likewise spread widely since they were first detected in the United Kingdom. BSE has also spread rapidly from the United Kingdom to many countries since the 1980s and now threatens to become endemic in certain European countries.

Each year, millions of people are affected by food-borne and water-borne diseases and thousands die, especially children in developing countries. Improper methods of food production, storage, handling, and preparation have resulted in many widespread outbreaks. Food animals are the reservoir for many emerging and important food-borne pathogens such as *E. coli* O157:H7, nontyphoidal *Salmonella* spp., *Campylobacter* spp., and *Yersinia* spp. Therefore, VPH leadership is essential to respond to the threat posed by these pathogens, particularly in the development of sustainable, integrated safety measures for the reduction of health risks along the entire food chain, from the point of primary production to the consumer (the "farm-to-table" approach).

Antimicrobials have undoubtedly saved the lives of millions of people. However, the widespread use of antimicrobials in hospitals, health centers, the community, and agriculture has led to the emergence of resistance among bacteria (WHO 2000). Antimicrobials are commonly used in food-producing animals for growth promotion, prophylaxis, and treatment. However, such use can also lead to the development of antimicrobial-resistant pathogens, which may be transmitted to humans through the food supply. Therefore, VPH leadership is essential to evaluate and respond to the human health consequences of using antimicrobials in food-producing animals. HACCP is a preventive risk management approach that has been extensively used by food industries to increase product safety (Kaba et al. 2017).

23.6.3 Protection and Preservation of Environment

A core function of the VPH service is to protect the environment (Cifuentes 1992). The steadily increasing global population is responsible for a range of complex social and environmental changes causing a rise in global temperature. Towns and cities across the globe are expanding as rural populations move into urban areas in search of work, education, health, and basic services. Moreover, as some urban industries have developed, others have collapsed, changing the urban structure and cohesion. The consequent movements of people and animals form new settlements and ecological niches with unprecedented features. In developing countries, subsistence farming and animal husbandry have evolved in cities as a result of these changes. Large-volume, high-density livestock-rearing systems also generate huge quantities of wastes and pollutants. These represent short- and long-term risks to animal and human health, as well as to the environment. Such risks can be extreme in poor countries. The climatic changes also increase the risks of vector-borne and other diseases in humans and animals, such as malaria, cold-water vibriosis in fish, etc.

An inextricable link between humans, pets, livestock, wildlife, and their ecological environment is evident which requires integrated approaches to human and animal health along with their respective social and environmental contexts (Figure 23.4). Because veterinarians work at the interface of human, animal, and environmental health, they are uniquely positioned to view this dynamic through the lens of public health impact. Significant changes in land use, expansion of large and intensified animal production units, and microbial contamination and chemical pollution of land and water sources have created new threats to animal and human health (Allard 2002).

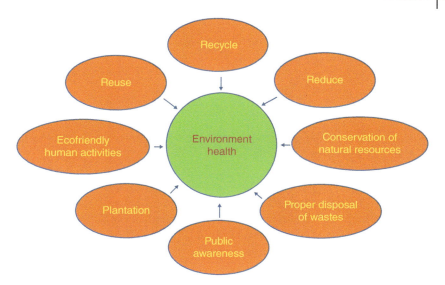

Figure 23.4 Methods of protection of the environment.

23.7 Challenges to Veterinary Public Health and Its Future Trends

Significant changes in land use, expansion of large and intensified animal production units, and microbial contamination and chemical pollution of land and water sources have created new threats to animal and human health (Allard 2002). Outbreaks of severe acute respiratory syndrome (SARS), West Nile virus (WNV), avian influenza (H5N1), swine flu, Nipah virus, and anthrax have proved a strong association between human and livestock, including wildlife. This increased human–animals interface has put livestock producers, consumers, and traders and processors of livestock products at higher risk of contracting zoonotic diseases. Hence the importance of collaborative research and effective veterinary and health services for the prevention and control of zoonotic diseases has increased many-fold (Pal and Siddiky 2011). This situation necessitates the establishment of effective partnerships between human health and veterinary administration and services with the aim of improving human health and well-being in the context of "One World, One Health" (Figure 23.5). Zoonotic and emerging infectious disease events have given rise to increasing calls for efforts to build global VPH capacities (Kakkar et al. 2013).

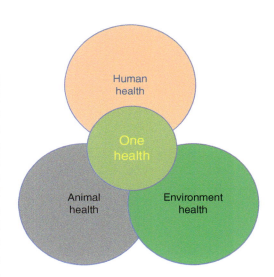

Figure 23.5 One Health approach.

23.8 Conclusion

In recent years, problems due to widespread emerging and reemerging zoonotic diseases, including food-borne diseases, and environmental problems have increased significantly. Therefore, public health veterinarians, physicians, other health professionals, and environmental health specialists need to work in close collaboration to achieve the One Health goal. New information and new approaches for the efficient and cost-effective delivery of reliable and accurate information to VPH users in both developing and developed countries are required. International organizations such as the WHO, FAO, and OIE can assist in harmonizing surveillance systems, facilitating agreement on the types of data that should be shared internationally, and assuring quality control for surveillance data. These agencies should also be encouraged to facilitate the timely summarization and dissemination of VPH information to their Member States. Moreover, the Global Surveillance and Early Warning System (GLEWS) is important for global surveillance and intelligence of health threats and to help regions and countries to enhance their capacities in surveillance, risk assessment, prevention, and risk management of animal diseases, including zoonoses, and to support rapid response mechanisms in partnership with the WHO and OIE.

References

Allard, D.G. (2002). The 'farm to plate' approach to food safety – everyone's business. *Canadian Journal of Infectious Diseases & Medical Microbiology* 13 (3): 185–190.

Buntain, B.J. (2004). Emerging challenges in public health protection, food safety and security: veterinary needs in the USDA's Food Safety and Inspection Service. *Journal of Veterinary Medical Education* 31 (4): 334–340.

Cifuentes, E.E. (1992). Protección del medio ambiente y actividades de salud pública veterinaria [Protection of the environment and veterinary public health activities]. *Revue Scientifique et Technique* 11 (1): 191–203.

Food and Agriculture Organization of the United Nations (FAO). (2017). FAO'S global animal diseases surveillance and early warning system. www.fao.org/documents/card/en?details=a84b70f3-51a2-4731-b49d-dd6f809f24a2/ (accessed 2 February 2024).

Kaba, T., Zerihun, T., Abera, B., and Kassa, T. (2017). A review on the role of veterinary public health and its current challenges. *Archives on Veterinary Science and Technology* 2017 (4): 1–6.

Kakkar, M., Abbas, S.S., Kumar, A. et al. (2013). Veterinary public health capacity-building in India: a grim reflection of the developing world's under preparedness to address zoonotic risks. *WHO South-East Asia Journal of Public Health* 2 (3): 187–191.

Khatun, M.M., Islam, M.A., and Rahman, M.M. (2019). Current status of veterinary public health activities in Bangladesh and its future plans. *BMC Veterinary Research* 15 (1): 164.

Kouba, V. (1992). Veterinary public health in world-wide animal health and production. *Revue Scientifique et Technique* 11 (1): 241–254.

Krishna, L. (2011). Veterinary public health and zoonotic disease control in India. In: *Veterinary Public Health and Zoonotic Disease Control in SAARC Countries* (ed. S.K. Pal and M.N.A. Siddiky). Bangladesh: SAARC Agriculture Centre.

Malinda, L. (2011). Veterinary profession has long protected animal and public health. Symposium underscores achievements over the year. *Journal of the American Veterinary Medical Association* 15: 3–5.

Ortega, C., de Meneghi, D., de Balogh, K. et al. (2004). Importancia de la salud pública veterinaria en ia actualidad: el proyecto SAPUVET [The current importance of veterinary public health: the SAPUVET project]. *Revue Scientifique et Technique* 23 (3): 841–849.

Pal, S.K. and Siddiky, M.N.A. (ed.) (2011). *Veterinary Public Health and Zoonotic Disease Control in SAARC Countries*. Bangladesh: SAARC Agriculture Centre.

Schwabe, C.W. (1978). *Cattle, Priests, and Progress in Medicine*. Minnesota: University of Minnesota Press.

Schwabe, C.W. (1984). *Veterinary Medicine and Human Health*, 3e. Baltimore/London: Williams and Wilkins Press.

Taylor, L.H., Latham, S.M., and Woolhouse, M.E. (2001). Risk factors for human disease emergence. *Philosophical Transactions of the Royal Society of London. Series B, Biological Sciences* 356 (1411): 983–989.

World Health Organization (WHO) (2000). *Overcoming Antimicrobial Resistance. World Health Organization Report on Infectious Diseases*. Geneva, World Health Organization.

World Health Organization (WHO) The Veterinary Contribution to Public Health Practice. World Health Organization Technical Report Series. (1975).

World Health Organization (WHO) (1995). *Communicable Diseases Prevention and Control: New, Emerging and Reemerging Infectious Diseases*. Geneva, World Health Organization.

World Health Organization (WHO) (1997). *EMC Annual Report 1996*. Geneva, World Health Organization.

World Health Organization (WHO) (1999). *Removing Obstacles to Healthy Development: Report on Infectious Diseases*. Geneva, World Health Organization.

World Health Organization (WHO) (2002). Future Trends in Veterinary Public Health. World Health Organization Technical Report Series.

24

Role of Veterinarians in Public Health

Pratistha Shrivastava[1], Simant Kumar Sahoo[2], and K.M. Venkatesh[3]

[1] *Department of Veterinary Parasitology, Institute of Veterinary Science and Animal Husbandry, SOADU, Bhubaneswar, India*
[2] *Veterinary Officer, Odisha State Government, Gajapati, India*
[3] *Veterinary Practitioner, Tamil Nadu, India*

24.1 Introduction

Many veterinarians, whether directly or indirectly, play a crucial role in achieving public health objectives. Veterinary public health efforts encompass many domains, including diagnosis, surveillance, epidemiology, and control, prevention, and elimination of zoonotic diseases. In routine practice, most private veterinary practitioners actively contribute to public health. They develop expertise in diagnosing acute and chronic diseases in animals, including those with zoonotic potential, which can affect not only the animal owners and their families but also the broader communities in which they live. Both small and large animal veterinarians contribute to this important aspect of public health (Figure 24.1).

Examples of public health activities carried out by veterinarians include the following.

- *Performing routine health examinations*: veterinarians conduct regular health check-ups for animals, ensuring early detection of any potential health issues and preventing the spread of diseases.
- *Maintaining immunization regimens*: vaccinations are a crucial aspect of preventing infectious diseases in animals. Veterinarians administer vaccinations according to recommended schedules to safeguard the health of pets and livestock.
- *Implementing parasite control programs*: controlling parasites in animals is vital to prevent the transmission of diseases to humans and other animals. Veterinarians devise and implement effective parasite control strategies.
- *Advising on risks for immunocompromised individuals*: veterinarians offer guidance to individuals with weakened immune systems about the potential risks associated with animal contact, helping them take necessary precautions to stay safe.
- *Facilitating the use of guide and service dogs*: veterinarians play a role in training and certifying guide and service dogs, assisting people with disabilities in their daily activities, thus enhancing their independence and overall well-being.
- *Promoting the human–animal bond*: veterinarians advocate for the benefits of the human–animal bond, especially for vulnerable groups like the disabled, elderly, war veterans, and those with posttraumatic stress disorder (PTSD). This bond can have therapeutic effects, improving mental and emotional health.

These activities demonstrate how veterinarians actively contribute to public health by safeguarding both animal and human populations.

The well-being of communities is optimized when veterinarians adopt a "herd health" perspective, addressing health issues collectively and utilizing relevant epidemiological principles. Alongside their direct services, veterinary practitioners play a vital role by promptly reporting disease events and trends to state public health and regulatory agencies. Moreover, they actively collaborate with human medical professionals to combat zoonotic diseases, which have the potential to affect both animals and humans.

Additionally, veterinarians offer their expertise and guidance to local health boards and commissions, contributing valuable insights to public health discussions. These meaningful relationships and partnerships between veterinarians and various health organizations are only possible due to the inseparable connection between animal and human health.

Epidemiology and Environmental Hygiene in Veterinary Public Health, First Edition. Edited by Tanmoy Rana.
© 2025 John Wiley & Sons, Inc. Published 2025 by John Wiley & Sons, Inc.

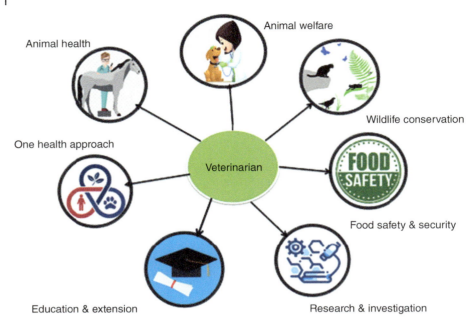

Figure 24.1 The multifaceted roles of veterinarians.

Recognizing this interdependence and working collaboratively helps to ensure effective disease monitoring, control, prevention, and overall enhancement of community health for both animals and humans. By acknowledging the mutual impact of animal and human health, veterinarians play a crucial role in safeguarding the well-being of entire communities.

Veterinarians play a crucial role not only in managing direct zoonotic diseases in animals but also in diagnosing, investigating, and controlling indirect zoonoses and nonzoonotic communicable diseases that have an impact on human health. Examples of these diseases include the following.

- *West Nile disease*: veterinarians may encounter cases of West Nile disease in pet animals. This mosquito-borne viral infection can pose a risk to both animals and humans.
- *Coccidioidomycosis (valley fever)*: this fungal infection, also known as valley fever, can affect animals and may have implications for human health as well.
- *Bovine leukosis*: veterinarians are involved in diagnosing and managing bovine leukosis, a viral disease affecting cattle.
- *Foot and mouth disease (FMD)*: FMD is a highly contagious viral disease that can impact cloven-hoofed animals. It can have significant consequences for the food supply, national economy, and the livelihood of farmers.
- *Fowlpox*: veterinarians may encounter cases of fowlpox, a viral disease affecting birds, including poultry. It can impact the poultry industry and pose challenges to food production.

These examples highlight the critical role veterinarians play in safeguarding public health by addressing diseases that can affect animals, humans, and even the nation's economy and food supply. Their expertise in diagnosing, investigating, and controlling these diseases is vital in maintaining a healthy and resilient society. By managing both direct and indirect health threats, veterinarians contribute significantly to the overall well-being of communities and the nation as a whole.

The rising vulnerability of livestock to infectious diseases can be attributed to several contributing factors.

- *Increasing intensity and concentration of production agriculture*: as agricultural operations intensify and concentrate, there is a higher density of livestock in specific areas. This close proximity can facilitate the rapid spread of infectious diseases within the population.
- *Genetic convergence of food-producing species*: the genetic similarity among food-producing species makes them susceptible to common diseases, increasing the risk of widespread outbreaks.

- *Accessibility of livestock to external contact*: despite rigorous biosecurity measures, livestock can still come into contact with external sources of infection, such as wildlife, other livestock, or contaminated equipment, which can introduce and spread diseases.
- *Scale and frequency of animal transport*: domestic and international transportation of animals can facilitate the rapid dissemination of infectious agents across regions and even countries.
- *Increasing size of feedlots*: the larger the feedlot, the greater the number of animals living in close quarters, which creates an environment conducive to disease transmission.
- *Lack of immunity to foreign animal diseases*: when livestock are exposed to pathogens they have not encountered before, they may lack immunity, making them highly susceptible to foreign animal diseases.
- *Relatively porous nature of national borders*: the ease of movement across national borders allows diseases to spread across regions and countries more rapidly.
- *Shortage of trained foreign animal disease diagnosticians and epidemiologists*: a lack of professionals with expertise in diagnosing and controlling foreign animal diseases can hinder timely and effective response efforts.

These factors collectively contribute to the vulnerability of livestock to infectious diseases, emphasizing the importance of robust biosecurity measures, surveillance, and cooperation between veterinary authorities to mitigate disease outbreaks and protect animal and human health.

While some significant diseases transmitted by food-producing animals, such as brucellosis, tuberculosis, and coxiellosis/Q fever, have been successfully eradicated or controlled in North America and Europe through measures like pasteurization and inspections at slaughter, there are many other food-borne diseases that remain widespread. Examples include listeriosis, salmonellosis, and staphylococcosis, among others. These illnesses contribute significantly to the national burden of food-borne morbidity and mortality.

Despite various safety measures, food-borne diseases of animal origin continue to pose a substantial public health concern. In the USA alone, there are approximately 20 000 reported cases of food-borne illnesses each year, leading to around 4200 hospitalizations and 80 deaths. It is evident that pathogens transmitted by food-producing animals are responsible for the majority of these cases.

To address this ongoing challenge, it is essential for authorities and stakeholders to continue implementing rigorous food safety protocols, surveillance, and monitoring throughout the entire food production and supply chain. Proper handling, processing, and preparation of food products of animal origin remain critical in minimizing the risk of food-borne illnesses and ensuring public health protection. Additionally, ongoing research and collaboration between public health agencies, veterinary authorities, and the food industry play a crucial role in identifying and controlling emerging food-borne pathogens effectively.

The management of health aspects in laboratory animal facilities and diagnostic laboratories has become increasingly critical due to the challenges posed by resurgent infectious diseases and the need to develop novel therapeutics. Maintaining healthy laboratory animal colonies is essential for conducting effective research and diagnostic efforts. Veterinarians play a key role in ensuring the success of these services while upholding principles of humane treatment.

As the demand for specialized veterinary services in these fields grows, international collaboration and reference centers are gaining importance. These centers often focus on zoonotic diseases (infectious diseases that can be transmitted from animals to humans) and comparative medicine, which involves studying diseases and treatments across different species (Figure 24.2).

Given the complexity and specialization required, only a few countries possess the capacity to provide comprehensive services in this domain. Hence, there is an increasing emphasis on international collaboration, where countries and institutions work together to pool resources, knowledge, and expertise. These collaborations not only improve the capacity to address health challenges but also facilitate sharing of information and best practices.

The role of international collaboration and reference centers is particularly crucial in regions with limited local surveillance, diagnostic capabilities, and response capacity, especially tropical areas where zoonotic diseases often emerge. These centers aid in detecting and managing disease outbreaks, helping to prevent potential pandemics and safeguard global health. As the importance of these centers continues to grow, there will be a rising need for trained and experienced veterinary personnel. The expertise of these professionals is essential in tackling complex health issues, advancing research, and ensuring effective disease control measures.

The management and maintenance of laboratory animal facilities and diagnostic laboratories are of the utmost importance in addressing emerging infectious diseases. Collaborative efforts on an international scale, coupled with a skilled veterinary workforce, will play a vital role in successfully managing health challenges, particularly zoonotic diseases, and advancing medical research.

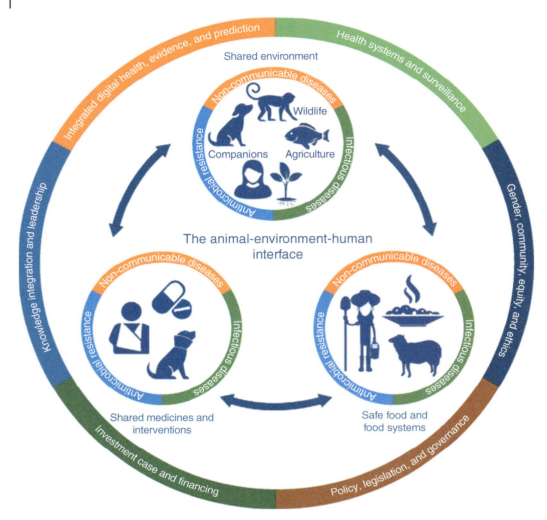

Figure 24.2 Navigating the convergence of animals, environments, and humans: a holistic approach to public health.

In biomedical research, it is essential to build on the information gathered from public health surveillance to develop a comprehensive understanding of the complex interactions between hosts, parasites, vectors, pathogens, and the environment. Establishing a clear causal link between human and animal diseases relies heavily on research efforts that often involve a combination of molecular studies, mathematical modeling, and experimental epidemiology, which can be carried out in both field and laboratory settings.

One of the primary challenges faced in research on endemic and resurgent zoonoses is the lack of fundamental knowledge regarding host–parasite interactions. Understanding how these interactions occur is crucial for effectively controlling and managing such diseases. Unfortunately, for many zoonotic species, the specific route of transmission to humans remains uncertain, making it challenging to design targeted prevention strategies.

Additionally, in some cases, the molecular biology of the infectious agents in human and animal hosts may differ significantly. For instance, research efforts are focused on identifying virulence factors for *E. coli* O157:H7, a strain associated with severe food-borne illness in humans. Understanding why these virulence factors exhibit different expressions in people and cattle is crucial to gaining insights into the mechanisms of infection and potential interventions.

To bridge these knowledge gaps, researchers need to employ a multidisciplinary approach that integrates various scientific methods and collaboration between human and veterinary health professionals. By studying the genetics, behavior, and ecological factors of pathogens and their hosts, researchers can gain a deeper understanding of zoonotic diseases and develop strategies for disease prevention and control.

The World Health Organization (WHO) emphasizes the importance of continued research in this field to improve our ability to combat zoonotic diseases effectively. Advances in biomedical research will contribute to better surveillance, diagnosis, and treatment of zoonoses, ultimately enhancing global health and safeguarding against potential outbreaks.

Health education and extension efforts play a vital role in promoting public awareness of both infectious and noninfectious diseases. While academic institutions, particularly land-grant universities, take the lead in training new veterinary practitioners and providing continuous education to those already in practice, all veterinarians actively participate in educating the public about health-related risks.

Veterinarians act as important conduits of health information to the public, helping individuals and communities understand the potential threats posed by diseases and how to prevent or manage them effectively. Their role goes beyond treating individual animals; they also serve as advocates for public health and well-being. Figure 24.3 describes the interaction between different components of public health.

As the field of health education evolves, there is a growing need for multidisciplinary collaborations between various academic disciplines. At the collegiate level, this means fostering relationships between schools of medicine, veterinary medicine, sociology, and basic sciences. This interdisciplinary approach allows for a broader understanding of health issues, including their societal, environmental, and biological aspects.

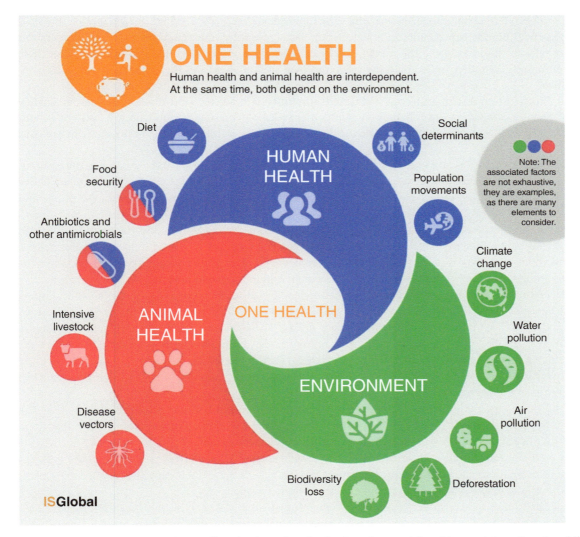

Figure 24.3 Intersecting worlds: unveiling the dynamics of animal, environmental, and human interactions in public health. *Source:* Lancet One Health Commission.

By collaborating with professionals from diverse fields, veterinarians can gain a more holistic perspective on health challenges, which is critical for developing comprehensive solutions. This approach also enables them to address complex issues, such as zoonotic diseases and their impact on both animal and human populations.

Health education and extension efforts empower communities to make informed decisions about their health and the health of their animals. By working together with the public, veterinarians can foster a culture of prevention and responsible care, ultimately contributing to improved public health outcomes.

Veterinarians not only provide medical care to animals but also serve as educators, raising awareness about infectious and noninfectious diseases. Collaborating with other disciplines enriches their knowledge and ensures a more integrated and effective approach to health education and extension. This concerted effort contributes to healthier communities and a better understanding of the complex interplay between human, animal, and environmental health.

Enabling appropriate knowledge and awareness among the public about disease risks requires a delicate balance of risk perception and risk awareness. Community stakeholders play a crucial role in resolving risks, making it essential to communicate effectively with them. However, it is important to note that most epidemiologists are typically employed by governmental or industrial stakeholders, which might not always be perceived as representing the public's interests directly.

In this context, veterinary practitioners have a unique opportunity and, some might argue, a responsibility to bridge the gap between expert knowledge and public awareness. Veterinarians, being trusted members of the community, can serve as credible sources of information about disease threats and their management.

By staying informed about disease threats and up to date on the latest scientific research, veterinary practitioners can provide accurate and relevant information to the public. They can translate complex scientific concepts into accessible language, helping community members understand the risks they face and the measures they can take to protect themselves and their animals.

In addition to their clinical roles, veterinarians can engage in community outreach and education initiatives. By actively participating in public health campaigns and collaborating with other stakeholders, such as public health authorities, animal welfare organizations, and local government agencies, they can strengthen collective efforts to manage disease risks effectively.

Furthermore, veterinarians can act as advocates for the public, ensuring that the interests and concerns of the community are taken into account when formulating disease control strategies and policies. By being knowledgeable and proactive in disseminating credible information, veterinary practitioners can foster trust and cooperation between the public and relevant stakeholders.

Overall, veterinary practitioners have a significant role to play in promoting risk awareness and risk resolution within their communities. By leveraging their expertise and credibility, they can empower the public with the knowledge needed to make informed decisions regarding disease prevention and management. This proactive approach not only benefits public health but also strengthens ties between veterinary professionals and the communities they serve.

The production and control of biological products and medical devices for animals involve a shared responsibility among various government agencies, primarily the Food and Drug Administration (FDA), the United States Department of Agriculture (USDA), and the Environmental Protection Agency (EPA). The FDA, specifically its Center for Veterinary Medicine, is primarily responsible for regulating animal drugs, animal feeds, and most veterinary devices. It oversees the approval process, ensuring that these products are safe and effective for their intended use in animals.

The USDA regulates animal vaccines and biologics. It evaluates and approves vaccines and biologics intended for animal use, ensuring that they meet the necessary safety and efficacy standards.

When it comes to pesticides used on animals, the regulatory responsibility is split between the FDA and the EPA. The FDA oversees certain flea and tick products for animals while the EPA regulates others. This division ensures that these products are safe for animals and do not pose risks to human health or the environment.

Veterinarians play a crucial role within each of these governmental agencies. They actively contribute to the development and evaluation of novel products, such as drugs, vaccines, and medical devices. Their expertise in veterinary medicine and animal health is vital in assessing the safety and efficacy of these products.

Simultaneously, veterinarians act as consumer protectors, safeguarding the public from false or misleading claims related to these products. They ensure that accurate information is provided to consumers, enabling them to make informed decisions about the use of biological products and medical devices for their animals.

Overall, veterinarians play a central role in the regulatory process, ensuring that animal drugs, vaccines, and medical devices meet the necessary quality standards and contribute to the overall health and well-being of animals while also safeguarding consumers and the environment. Their expertise and commitment are essential in balancing innovation and safety in the veterinary products industry.

The regulation of storage, use, and transfer of biological agents is a crucial aspect of biosecurity and public safety. Due to their inherent virulence and potential for transmission, access to certain disease pathogens, known as select agents, has been restricted to authorized facilities and legitimate purposes. The Federal Select Agent Program (FSAP) plays a central role in overseeing the possession, use, and transfer of these select agents and toxins. It is a collaborative effort jointly administered by two federal agencies: the Centers for Disease Control and Prevention (CDC) and the USDA's Animal and Plant Health Inspection Service (APHIS). The FSAP aims to prevent the misuse or accidental release of these dangerous agents, which have the potential to cause severe threats to public health, animal health, or plant health, as well as the products derived from animals or plants. The program sets strict regulatory guidelines for entities handling and conducting research involving select agents to ensure compliance with safety protocols and prevent any risks to human, animal, or environmental well-being.

Laboratories and facilities that work with select agents are subject to rigorous inspections, security measures, and reporting requirements to maintain the highest level of biosecurity and safety. By monitoring and regulating the possession and transfer of these biological agents, the FSAP helps minimize the potential for intentional or accidental harm associated with these dangerous pathogens. Stringent oversight and regulation of select agents are critical in safeguarding public health and preventing the deliberate or unintentional release of harmful agents that could have devastating consequences. The collaborative efforts between the CDC and APHIS in the FSAP ensure that the storage, use, and transfer of biological agents are closely monitored and controlled, protecting both human and animal populations as well as agriculture and environment.

Government and legislative activity involve the active engagement of veterinarians at various levels of state and federal agencies. Many veterinarians are employed in the government sector, contributing their expertise to a range of important roles and responsibilities.

At the federal level, over 3000 veterinarians hold positions in various agencies. The USDA employs a significant portion of these veterinarians. Within the USDA, veterinarians are involved in activities related to animal health, food safety, and agricultural research and development. Other federal agencies that employ a considerable number of veterinarians include the Department of Defense (DoD), specifically the Army and Air Force, and the Department of Health and Human Services (DHHS), which includes the CDC, the FDA, and the National Institutes of Health (NIH). Within these agencies, veterinarians contribute to public health programs, research, and regulatory initiatives.

While some veterinarians are engaged in direct animal care within the government sector, the vast majority of opportunities lie in public health programs. Veterinarians in these roles are often involved in disease surveillance, outbreak investigations, food safety assessments, and research projects focused on understanding zoonotic diseases.

The expertise of veterinarians is valuable in addressing public health challenges, safeguarding food safety, and protecting both animal and human health. Their contributions to government and legislative activities play a critical role in shaping policies and strategies that have far-reaching impacts on public health and well-being. By utilizing their knowledge and skills, veterinarians in the government sector contribute to the overall health and safety of communities and the nation as a whole.

Veterinarians in government and legislative roles have a wide range of responsibilities that encompass various aspects of public health, animal health, and food safety. Examples of their contributions include the following.

- *Food safety inspection programs*: veterinarians play a crucial role in overseeing food safety inspection programs, ensuring that the food supply is safe for consumption. They assess food-processing facilities, inspect meat and poultry products, and monitor the implementation of proper sanitation practices to prevent food-borne illnesses.
- *Disease surveillance and outbreak investigation*: veterinarians are involved in disease surveillance programs, monitoring the health of animals and detecting potential outbreaks. They investigate outbreaks of infectious diseases, both in animals and humans, to identify the source, assess the risk, and implement control measures.
- *Laboratory animal care*: veterinarians in government agencies are responsible for overseeing the welfare and health of laboratory animals used in research. They ensure that animals are treated ethically and follow appropriate guidelines for their care and use.
- *Biomedical research*: veterinarians contribute to biomedical research by providing expertise in animal models and ensuring that research involving animals is conducted ethically and adheres to animal welfare standards.
- *Public health program management and leadership*: veterinarians take on leadership roles in managing public health programs. They develop and implement strategies for disease control, conduct risk assessments, and design preventive measures to protect both animal and human populations.

- *Zoonotic disease management*: as zoonotic disease experts, veterinarians actively participate in monitoring and controlling diseases that can spread between animals and humans. Their knowledge is invaluable in preventing and managing potential outbreaks.
- *Policy development*: veterinarians contribute to the development of public health policies related to animal health, food safety, and disease control. Their input helps shape regulations and guidelines that ensure the well-being of both animals and humans.

Overall, veterinarians in government and legislative positions play pivotal roles in promoting public health, ensuring food safety, and safeguarding animal welfare. Their diverse expertise and dedication contribute significantly to protecting the health of communities and the nation as a whole.

At the state level, each department of agriculture typically appoints a state veterinarian who plays a crucial role in safeguarding the livestock, poultry, and aquaculture industries, which, in turn, indirectly protects public health. The state veterinarian's primary responsibilities revolve around preventing, detecting early, containing, and eradicating economically significant livestock, poultry, and fish diseases, some of which may be transmissible to humans. The state veterinarian takes charge of regulating the importation, transportation, and processing of animals within the state. This ensures that disease risks are minimized and controlled when animals are moved across borders. Additionally, they are responsible for controlling and eradicating contagious diseases that affect poultry and livestock, aiming to protect the state's agricultural interests.

The regulation of fish farming is also under the purview of the state veterinarian, ensuring that aquaculture practices are managed to prevent disease outbreaks and protect the state's fish population.

In times of emergencies, such as disease outbreaks or natural disasters affecting animals, the state veterinarian coordinates and implements emergency response programs to mitigate the impact on the agriculture industry.

Furthermore, the welfare of farm animals is closely monitored by the Office of the State Veterinarian. When cases of animal cruelty arise, the office conducts investigations and, when necessary, initiates prosecutions to ensure the humane treatment of animals within the state's jurisdiction.

In summary, the state veterinarian plays a pivotal role in protecting the economic interests of the livestock, poultry, and aquaculture industries while also safeguarding public health by preventing the spread of diseases that can impact both animals and humans. Their oversight and regulatory efforts ensure that agricultural practices are conducted responsibly and in compliance with animal welfare standards, contributing to the well-being of both animals and the general public.

The role of veterinarians in government and legislative activities is crucial in protecting public health and advancing policies that serve national interests. In this context, state public health veterinarians (SPHVS) play a significant role in zoonotic disease control and prevention, with a primary focus on safeguarding public health. They are employed in every state in different nations, primarily within health department divisions of epidemiology, toxicology, or environmental health.

State public health veterinarians work directly on identifying, monitoring, and controlling zoonotic diseases. By collaborating with various public health departments and agencies, they contribute to preventing disease outbreaks, ensuring early detection and implementing appropriate measures to protect public health.

Another aspect of governmental activity involving veterinarians is legislative engagement. While the number of veterinarians serving in legislative roles is relatively small, their impact is significant. They play key roles in formulating laws, rules, and regulations aimed at protecting public health, domestic preparedness, and national defense. Veterinarians serve in various capacities, including as representatives in the United States House of Representatives and in senior leadership positions within several United States Cabinet-level departments, such as the USDA, DHHS, DoD, and Department of Homeland Security (DHS). They also serve as legislative liaisons for professional associations like the American Veterinary Medical Association (AVMA).

Practicing veterinarians actively support these legislative efforts, contributing to the communicative action that transmits ideas and issues effectively to legislators. By engaging with policymakers and sharing their expertise, practicing veterinarians help shape improved legal and policy outcomes related to public health, animal welfare, and national defense.

Through this collaborative pathway of veterinarians in government roles, ideas are translated into effective policies, ultimately benefiting the health and well-being of both animals and humans. Their contributions in zoonotic disease control, public health, and legislative arenas highlight the vital role of veterinarians in protecting society's health and advancing national interests. Figure 24.4 describes how a veterinarian deals with different components of the environment in order to safeguard the health of human and animals.

Figure 24.4 Veterinarians: safeguarding health across species and beyond.

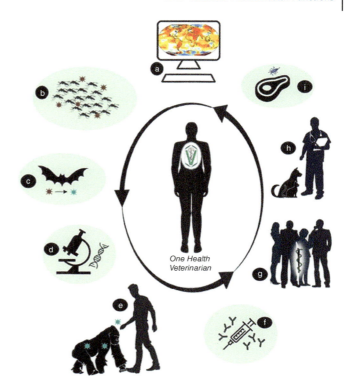

24.2 Essential Public Health Functions

The United States Public Health Service (USPHS), under the DHHS, developed and adopted 10 essential public health functions in 1994. These functions serve as a framework to guide state and local health agencies in achieving their mission of promoting physical and mental health while preventing disease, injury, and disability. The 10 essential public health functions are as follows.

- *Monitor health status*: regularly collect, analyze, and interpret data on the health of populations to identify health trends and potential health hazards.
- *Diagnose and investigate health problems and hazards*: conduct investigations and research to understand the causes of health problems, including infectious diseases, environmental hazards, and other public health threats.
- *Inform, educate, and empower people about health issues*: provide accurate and timely health information to the public to empower individuals to make informed decisions about their health and well-being.
- *Mobilize community partnerships to solve health problems*: collaborate with community organizations, agencies, and stakeholders to address public health challenges and implement effective solutions.
- *Develop policies and plans that support individual and community health efforts*: formulate evidence-based policies and plans to promote health and improve the well-being of the community.
- *Enforce laws and regulations that protect health and ensure safety*: implement and enforce laws and regulations to safeguard public health and ensure safety in various settings, including food safety, environmental health, and disease control.
- *Link people to needed personal health services and assure the provision of healthcare when otherwise unavailable*: facilitate access to healthcare services, especially for underserved and vulnerable populations, to ensure equitable health outcomes.
- *Assure a competent public and personal healthcare workforce*: foster a skilled and well-prepared public health workforce to meet the diverse needs of the community.
- *Evaluate the effectiveness, accessibility, and quality of personal and population-based health services*: continuously assess the performance and impact of health services and programs to improve their effectiveness and quality.
- *Research for new insights and innovative solutions to health problems*: engage in scientific research to advance understanding and find innovative solutions to public health challenges.

These essential public health functions serve as a comprehensive framework for guiding public health efforts at the state and local levels. By addressing these functions, health agencies can effectively promote and protect the health and well-being of their communities.

24.2.1 Monitor Health Status to Identify Community Health Problems

Monitoring health status is a crucial function of public health agencies, as it involves the continuous and systematic collection, analysis, interpretation, and dissemination of specific data related to health outcomes within a community. This process is known as public health surveillance. By implementing surveillance systems, agencies can track and monitor the health of populations over time, allowing them to identify and analyze adverse events, health trends, and disease patterns.

Public health surveillance provides essential baseline data that serve as a foundation for planning, implementing, and evaluating public health practices and interventions. By gathering data on various health indicators, such as disease incidence, mortality rates, behavioral risk factors, and environmental exposures, public health agencies can assess the health needs and priorities of the community.

24.2.2 Diagnose and Investigate Health Problems and Health Hazards in the Community

In addition to surveillance, public health agencies conduct targeted screening programs or surveys to detect specific health problems and hazards within the community. These activities are designed to identify health conditions, risks, or exposures that may be of particular concern.

When health problems or hazards are detected through screening or surveys, public health professionals conduct in-depth investigations to determine their magnitude and impact on the population. This process involves assessing the extent of the issue, identifying risk factors, understanding transmission patterns, and evaluating the effectiveness of existing prevention and control measures.

The findings from these investigations are critical for informing public education and prevention efforts. By understanding the root causes and risk factors associated with specific health problems, public health agencies can design and implement targeted interventions to address the identified issues effectively.

In summary, monitoring health status through public health surveillance and conducting in-depth investigations of health problems and hazards play vital roles in identifying and understanding the health needs and challenges within a community. These activities serve as the basis for evidence-based public health actions aimed at promoting health, preventing diseases, and improving the overall well-being of the population.

24.2.3 Inform, Educate, and Empower People about Health Issues

Once public health priorities have been established through surveillance, detection, and investigation, it is essential to engage in educational activities to disseminate information about health issues. Public health agencies play a vital role in informing and educating the public about health risks, preventive measures, and healthy behaviors. By providing accurate and accessible health information, agencies empower individuals to make informed decisions about their health and well-being.

Educational initiatives may include public health campaigns, workshops, seminars, and community outreach programs. These efforts aim to raise awareness, promote health literacy, and encourage behavior change that can lead to improved health outcomes.

24.2.4 Mobilize Community Partnerships to Identify and Solve Health Problems

Public health agencies can effectively address health problems by collaborating with community partners. Building strong community partnerships is crucial for identifying health challenges and developing comprehensive solutions.

Identifying potential stakeholders who have a vested interest in public health interventions is essential. Community organizations, schools, healthcare providers, local businesses, and other entities can contribute resources, expertise, and support to public health efforts.

Through collaboration and shared responsibility, public health agencies can leverage community strengths and resources to implement effective programs and initiatives that address the specific health needs of the community.

24.2.5 Develop Policies and Plans that Support Individual and Community Health Efforts

Policies and laws are powerful tools in shaping individual behaviors and improving population health outcomes. Public health agencies play a significant role in advocating for and developing evidence-based policies and plans that promote health and prevent diseases. Examples of such policies include regulations on food marketing to children, restrictions on tobacco sales, and promoting safe environments for physical activity. These policy interventions can positively influence behaviors and create supportive environments that encourage healthier choices.

By engaging with policymakers and advocating for health-promoting policies, public health agencies can contribute to creating lasting and sustainable changes that support individual and community health efforts.

In summary, public health agencies play a critical role in informing and empowering the public about health issues, mobilizing community partnerships to address health challenges, and advocating for policies that promote individual and community well-being. These activities are fundamental to achieving public health goals and creating healthier, thriving communities.

24.2.6 Enforce Laws and Regulations That Protect Health and Ensure Safety

To ensure the overall safety and health of the community, public health agencies play a crucial role in enforcing laws and regulations. Simply having policies and laws in place is not sufficient; enforcement is essential to ensure compliance and adherence to health and safety standards.

Public health agencies, working in collaboration with law enforcement and other relevant authorities, monitor and oversee compliance with health-related laws. This includes regulations related to food safety, environmental health, disease control, vaccination requirements, and other public health measures.

Ongoing assessment and education efforts are also undertaken to keep the public informed about existing laws and regulations. By raising awareness and promoting understanding of these rules, agencies encourage community cooperation and support for health protection measures.

24.2.7 Link People to Needed Personal Health Services and Assure the Provision of Healthcare When Otherwise Unavailable

Access to timely and appropriate healthcare services is critical for individuals to prevent and avoid adverse health outcomes and medical costs. Public health agencies work at various levels, from local to federal, to establish and maintain a coordinated system of health care. These agencies help ensure that individuals can access necessary health services, particularly for underserved and vulnerable populations. They collaborate with healthcare providers, community organizations, and social service agencies to address barriers to care, such as geographic location, affordability, and cultural considerations.

Efforts to link people to needed health services include public health outreach programs, health insurance enrollment assistance, community health clinics, and telehealth initiatives. By ensuring access to care, public health agencies contribute to improving health outcomes and reducing disparities.

24.2.8 Assure a Competent Public Health and Personal Healthcare Workforce

A competent and well-trained healthcare workforce is essential for providing effective and efficient care to the community. Public health agencies play a role in assuring the competence of the workforce through various strategies.

Licensing and credentialing processes ensure that healthcare professionals meet established standards and qualifications. Additionally, public health agencies incorporate core public health competencies into personnel systems to ensure that their staff possess the necessary knowledge and skills to carry out their roles effectively.

Continual quality improvement opportunities are provided to members of the public health workforce, fostering ongoing professional development and learning. By investing in the competence of the workforce, public health agencies enhance the overall quality of health services and public health interventions.

In summary, public health agencies enforce laws and regulations, link individuals to necessary health services, and work to ensure a competent and skilled healthcare workforce. These efforts are fundamental to protecting and improving the health and well-being of communities and individuals.

24.2.9 Evaluate Effectiveness, Accessibility, and Quality of Personal and Population-based Health Services

Evaluating the effectiveness, accessibility, and quality of health services is essential for optimizing resource allocation and ensuring that programs and policies achieve their intended outcomes. Public health agencies conduct rigorous evaluations to assess the impact and efficiency of interventions and services.

Through evaluations, agencies determine whether specific public health programs and policies are achieving their desired results in improving health outcomes and addressing health disparities. These assessments provide valuable information on the success of interventions and inform decisions on resource allocation, program continuation, or modification.

Evaluations also examine the accessibility of health services, ensuring that they reach all segments of the population, including vulnerable and underserved groups. By identifying barriers to access and understanding the factors that influence health service utilization, public health agencies can work to improve healthcare equity.

Additionally, evaluations assess the quality of health services, focusing on patient satisfaction, adherence to best practices, and adherence to established standards of care. Improving service quality enhances overall health outcomes and patient experiences.

Cost-effectiveness analyses are also employed to inform policymakers on how to efficiently allocate healthcare resources. By comparing the costs and outcomes of different interventions, public health agencies can identify cost-effective strategies that maximize health benefits within budget constraints.

24.2.10 Support/Sponsor Research for New Insights and Innovative Solutions to Health Problems

Public health agencies play a critical role in supporting and sponsoring research efforts to address emerging health challenges and find innovative solutions. By funding and collaborating on research projects, agencies generate evidence-based insights that guide policy development and program implementation.

Through coordinated research programs, public health agencies gain a deeper understanding of health issues, risk factors, and effective interventions. The evidence obtained from research studies informs the development of evidence-based practices and interventions that improve health and well-being over time.

Research efforts also drive advances in medical and public health knowledge, leading to the development of new interventions, treatments, and preventive measures. By investing in research, public health agencies contribute to the advancement of science and the continuous improvement of public health practices.

Furthermore, research plays a vital role in addressing health disparities and understanding the social determinants of health. Findings from research studies help identify root causes and inform strategies for promoting health equity and reducing health disparities among different population groups.

In summary, public health agencies actively engage in evaluating the effectiveness and quality of health services while ensuring their accessibility to all communities. Additionally, they support and sponsor research efforts to generate new insights and innovative solutions to health problems, leading to continuous improvement and better health outcomes for the population.

25

One Health Concept and Initiatives in Veterinary Public Health

Naveen Kumar[1], Amit Kumar[2], Dinesh Mittal[1], and Manesh Kumar[1]

[1] *Department of Veterinary Public Health and Epidemiology, Lala Lajpat Rai University of Veterinary and Animal Sciences, Hisar, India*
[2] *Department of Veterinary Surgery and Radiology, Lala Lajpat Rai University of Veterinary and Animal Sciences, Hisar, India*

25.1 Introduction

Veterinary medicine is defined as the branch of medicine which deals with diagnosis, treatment, prevention and control of diseases, injuries or disorders in animals. Veterinarians have various significant roles including breeding, production, reproduction, and management of health of high-producing dairy animals, and treatment, prevention, and control of diseases in pets and wild animals. There are high chances of transmission of disease-causing agents between humans, animals, and the environment which are very difficult to control individually by personnel working for the betterment of these components of the ecosystem.

Veterinary science serves human health through the monitoring, prevention, and control of zoonotic disease (infectious disease transmitted from nonhuman animals to humans and vice versa), food safety, and through human applications via medical research using animal species. The first extant record of veterinary medicine is the Egyptian Papyrus of Kahun (Twelfth Dynasty of Egypt) (Thrusfield 2007). Although humans have been associated with animals since prehistoric times, the development of scientific veterinary medicine is comparatively recent. A milestone was the establishment of the first permanent veterinary school at Lyons, France, by Claude Bourgelat in the year 1762, established after observing the devastation caused by cattle plague in French herds. Bourgelat founded the veterinary school to educate students to combat the disease (Thrusfield 2007).

Veterinary medicine has diverse responsibilities spanning biomedical research, ecosystem management, public health, food and agricultural systems, and the care of companion animals, wildlife, exotic animals, and food animals. Veterinarians have expertise in preventive medicine, population health, parasitology, zoonoses, and epidemiology, making them valuable contributors to public health initiatives. The historical background of this profession has consistently centered around safeguarding and enhancing both animal and human health.

25.2 What is Public Health?

Public health, traditionally defined, pertains to a system organized by the public and health professionals working collectively to reduce morbidity and mortality within human communities. The World Health Organization's Expert Committee on Public Health Administration (1952) defined public health as "the science and art of preventing disease, prolonging life, and promoting health and efficiency through organized community efforts." Various ancient civilizations practiced cleanliness and personal hygiene, often for religious reasons. Historical measures for public health included the quarantine of individuals affected by leprosy during the Middle Ages and sanitation improvements following the plague epidemics in the fourteenth century. Internationally, the World Health Organization (WHO) plays a pivotal role, particularly in supporting the implementation of organizational and administrative methods to address health and disease-related challenges in less developed countries. In these nations, health concerns, resource limitations, health personnel education, and other factors must be considered when designing health service systems.

Epidemiology and Environmental Hygiene in Veterinary Public Health, First Edition. Edited by Tanmoy Rana.
© 2025 John Wiley & Sons, Inc. Published 2025 by John Wiley & Sons, Inc.

While human medicine predominantly addresses the diseases of individual patients through clinical and laboratory examinations and the prescription of medications to alleviate symptoms, public health differs significantly. Public health addresses health-related challenges that demand the collective efforts of communities or groups of people, rather than relying solely on individual care. Public health endeavors to manage health-related issues of groups, which may comprise families, tribes, or individuals residing within specific geographical boundaries, such as colonies, villages, tehsils, or towns. Public health's unit of concern encompasses groups bound by such factors as age, such as senior citizens, or lifestyle habits, such as individuals addicted to smoking or alcohol. Modern public health programs are characterized by their reliance on scientifically collected data pertaining to the health of a defined population. They prioritize improvements in health status and the determinants of health, focusing on outcomes rather than processes. Additionally, these programs embody the principle that community members share both individual and collective responsibility for the well-being of all individuals in the community and for the broader well-being of humanity. Furthermore, the various disciplines and activities operating within public health share a foundational common science – epidemiology.

25.3 What is Veterinary Public Health?

Veterinary public health (VPH) services have grown over the last 50 years. Initially, veterinarians were primarily responsible for disease intelligence within the broader field of medical epidemiology. According to the WHO, VPH constitutes a domain dedicated to applying professional veterinary expertise, knowledge, and resources to enhance and protect human health and well-being. This facet of public health centers on veterinarians' efforts, services, and contributions in resolving human health issues originating from animals.

Veterinary and human medicines intersect through their comparative aspects in clinical medicine, physiology, pathology, and population medicine. Notably, veterinarians have advanced VPH through vital roles in epidemiology, environmental hygiene, disease prevention, control, and eradication, health education, public health administration, and zoonoses management. For instance, rabies in humans primarily results from bites by rabid dogs in India. This issue cannot be managed unless it is controlled or eliminated in dogs, wildlife, and other domestic animals in the affected region. Similarly, the consumption of contaminated food may induce various health-related issues in humans, which necessitate the expertise of qualified veterinarians. As a result, activities related to zoonoses and the supply of disease-free livestock products, including poultry and aquatic animal-derived foods, to the human community fall under the purview of VPH activities.

Beyond zoonoses, epidemiology, and food hygiene, VPH encompasses studies relating to environmental health, ecology, pathobiology, toxicology, and animal welfare. In a broader context, it encompasses aspects of veterinary activities as they relate to human health, including comparative medicine, general medicine, and experimental medicine. Consequently, VPH aligns more with public health than veterinary medicine, as public health veterinarians primarily focus on human health influenced by animals. In contrast, veterinary medicine centers on animal health and welfare.

25.4 The Role of Veterinarians in Human Health

Veterinarians and public health practitioners have shared knowledge and insights, often collaborating to address various health challenges. Numerous diseases can affect multiple species, and the insights gained from one species can enhance the understanding of disease in other hosts. Edward Jenner's experiment with cowpox eventually led to the development of the smallpox vaccine. Renowned veterinarians, including Bernhard Bang and Daniel Salmon, played pivotal roles in shaping modern public health policies related to disease control and food hygiene. Veterinarians, with their extensive studies encompassing monogastrics, ruminants, wildlife, and aquatic animals, have effectively become comparative biologists. For veterinarians, human beings are merely another species. Their research, therefore, frequently draws analogies between health-related issues in animals to advance human health.

In ancient times, there was little distinction between human and animal medicines, and individuals often practiced both professions. During the Middle Ages, the services provided by "animal doctors" and "human doctors" began to diverge, although animal doctors continued to contribute to medical practice, particularly in obstetrics and orthopedics. In 1500, the first successful human cesarean operation was performed by a veterinarian, Jacob Nufer. Schools of veterinary medicine established in the eighteenth century offered courses in midwifery, fracture and trauma management, and ocular diseases. Veterinarians were also employed for certifying human deaths. Their contributions to zoonoses research, disease prevention and control, comparative medicine, herd medicine, and experimental medicine are widely acknowledged.

The contributions of veterinarians to microbiology are significant, with Loeffler and Frosch discovering the first animal virus, and Nocard and Roux elucidating the etiology of bovine pleuropneumonia. The discovery of the diphtheria bacillus by Gasten and Ramon underscored the shared objectives of human and veterinary medicine. Furthermore, contributions by Elerman and Bang, who first identified cancer viruses in chickens, and Salmon and Smith, who were pioneers in experimental immunology, are highly regarded.

In 1975, a joint Food and Agriculture Organization (FAO)/WHO Expert Committee on Veterinary Public Health categorized the principal public health functions of veterinarians into three main areas:

- animal-related functions
- biomedical functions, and
- generalist functions.

Animal-related functions encompass human health aspects related to the production, processing, and marketing of animal-derived foods, health-related concerns in other animal industries, zoonoses, technical consultations on human health matters related to animals and their diseases, investigation of risks to humans posed by biting, toxic, venomous, and other dangerous or objectionable animals, supervision of experimental animal colonies maintained by public health laboratories, comparative studies on the epidemiology of noninfectious diseases in animals and humans influenced by environmental or other factors, and the exchange of research information between veterinary scientists and human health experts to enhance community health.

Biomedical functions of veterinarians encompass epidemiology, health laboratory services, general environmental health, which includes radiological health and environmental physiology, food protection, the production and control of biological products, drug evaluation and control, and most aspects of public health research, including research in reproductive physiology and fertility control. In addition to these areas of responsibility in public health, public health veterinarians can also serve in general public health roles as administrators, planners, and coordinators.

25.5 What is One Health?

One Health, as described by the One Health High-Level Expert Panel (OHHLEP), is:

> an integrated, unifying approach that aims to sustainably balance and optimize the health of people, animals, and ecosystems. It recognizes the health of humans, domestic and wild animals, plants, and the wider environment (including ecosystems) are closely linked and interdependent. The approach mobilizes multiple sectors, disciplines, and communities at varying levels of society to work together to foster well-being and tackle threats to health and ecosystems while addressing the collective need for clean water, energy, and air, safe and nutritious food, taking action on climate change, and contributing to sustainable development. (UNEP 2021)

Although One Health is not a recent concept, its importance has increased in recent times due to changes in interactions between people, animals, plants, and the environment. The human population is proliferating and entering into new geographical territories, resulting in closer coexistence with wild and domestic animals, encompassing livestock and pets. Animals have a significant role in human lives, providing food, clothing, livelihoods, travel, recreation, education, and companionship. Proximity to animals and their surroundings has increased the opportunities for diseases to spread between animals and humans. Furthermore, changes in climate and changes in land use, such as deforestation and intensive agricultural practices, have brought about disruptions in environmental conditions and habitats, thus giving diseases new opportunities to move between animals and humans. The movement of people, animals, and animal products has increased due to international travel and trade, thereby permitting diseases to spread rapidly across borders and throughout the world.

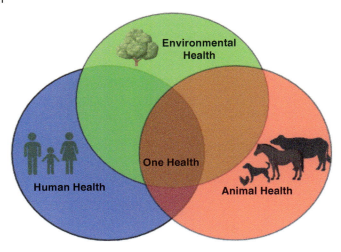

Figure 25.1 One Health triad.

25.6 History of One Health

The idea of "One Health" is not new. Aristotle, around 380 BCE, wrote about animals and their connections to human health. He explored the natural history of diseases that spread between animals and people. Even earlier, Hippocrates, in 490 BCE, talked about how things like the environment could affect human health. In the seventeenth century, an Italian doctor named Lancini also discussed how the environment could spread diseases in both animals and humans. He was one of the first to suggest using mosquito nets to prevent malaria in humans and played a big role in controlling rinderpest in cattle.

Human medicine has a long history but veterinary medicine started as a separate field in China during the Zhou dynasty, between the eleventh and thirteenth centuries. Rudolf Virchow, a renowned physician and pathologist of the nineteenth century, delved into the associations between human and veterinary medicine while studying a roundworm known as *Trichinella spiralis* in swine. He coined the term "zoonosis" to describe an infectious disease that is transmitted between humans and animals. In addition to his medical career, Virchow held various parliamentary positions and underscored the importance of enhancing veterinary education. He emphasized that there should be no dividing lines between animal and human medicine since the knowledge derived from both realms serves as the foundation of all medicine.

In the United States, Dr James H Steele, set up the VPH section at the Centers for Disease Control in 1947, so, he is now known as the father of VPH. The concept of "One Medicine" was coined and advocated by veterinary epidemiologist and parasitologist C.W. Schwabe in 1984. The pioneering efforts of Steele and Schwabe started to have an impact on the education in veterinary medical and medical schools and influenced public policy. Eventually, this approach was further enriched by an ecosystem health perspective that recognized the close connections between environmental factors and the outcomes of animal and human health (Figure 25.1).

The One Health concept arose in September 2004 when a group of global health experts of the Wildlife Conservation Society established it using the "Manhattan Principles" at Rockefeller University in New York. These principles laid out 12 recommendations to encourage greater cooperation among those working on human, animal, and environmental health. The ultimate aim is to improve prevention and response to epidemic diseases that affect both humans and animals, all while maintaining the balance of ecosystems. Over time, these principles were updated to include more aspects, such as pathogen spillover, climate change, and antimicrobial resistance (AMR), which are known as the "Berlin Principles" (Gruetzmacher et al. 2021).

25.6.1 International Collaboration in One Health

While collaboration on various common working streams was already in progress, the formal alliance of the WHO, FAO, and World Organisation for Animal Health (WOAH) was solidified with the publication of the FAO/OIE/WHO Tripartite Concept Note in 2010. The advent of the COVID-19 pandemic further propelled the momentum of One Health, when the heads of the FAO, UNEP, WHO, and WOAH met in November 2020 at the Paris Peace Forum and decided to enhance their cross-sectoral collaboration by creating a multidisciplinary One Health High-Level Expert Panel (OHHLEP) (Figure 25.2), following the United Nations Environment Programme (UNEP).

The One Health Quadripartite Alliance's activities are detailed in the One Health Joint Plan of Action, which was crafted in 2022. This plan serves as a blueprint for a set of actions and initiatives aimed at reinforcing cooperation, communication, capacity development, and coordination. It revolves around six interconnected Action Tracks, all of which work together to promote sustainable health and food systems, reduce global health risks, and enhance ecosystem management by:

- strengthening countries' ability to enhance health systems using a One Health approach
- minimizing the threats arising from emerging or recurring zoonotic epidemics and pandemics

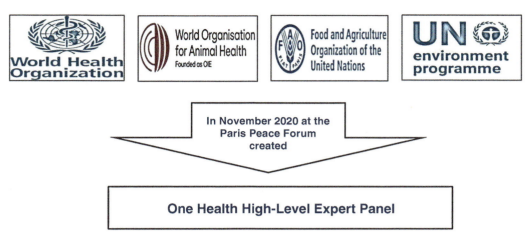

Figure 25.2 Creation of One Health High-Level Expert Panel by the WHO, WOAH, FAO, and UNEP in the year 2020.

- managing and eradicating persistent zoonotic, neglected tropical, or vector-borne diseases
- enhancing the evaluation, control, and communication of risks related to food safety
- combating the concealed epidemic of AMR
- more effectively integrating environmental considerations into the One Health approach.

In May 2021, the OHHLEP appointed 26 international experts from 24 countries to serve as its members. The panel consists of experts with diverse technical knowledge, skills, and experience relevant to One Health, and they collectively represent a broad geographic range. The OHHLEP offers advice to the Quadripartite and performs two main functions.

- Offer policy-relevant scientific evaluations concerning the emergence of health crises linked to human–animal–environment interaction and identify research gaps.
- Direct the creation of a long-term strategic plan to mitigate the risk of zoonotic pandemics like H5N1 avian influenza, MERS, Ebola, and Zika. This includes a monitoring and early warning system, as well as the necessary coordination to integrate and execute the One Health approach, particularly in areas contributing to pandemic risk.

25.7 International Agencies in Veterinary Public Health

The globalization of trade and the dismantling of barriers between countries and continents have led to the global spread of VPH challenges. It is imperative to address these challenges effectively at appropriate international levels. Several international agencies are already engaged in these endeavors, and their mandates evolve according to the changing perceptions of problems in time and place.

25.7.1 World Organisation for Animal Health

The WOAH was initially established as the Office International des Epizooties (OIE) in 1924 as a response to a global cattle plague (rinderpest disease) that devastated livestock and people's livelihoods. Situated in Paris, the WOAH collects information and statistical data on zoonotic infections and publishes this information in its official bulletins.

25.7.2 Food and Agriculture Organization

The FAO of the United Nations, founded in 1945 and headquartered in Rome, is a specialized UN agency leading international efforts to combat hunger and enhance nutrition and food security. The Animal Production and Health Division of the FAO focuses on animal productivity systems, diseases of animals, wildlife, and fish. It is a consultative body to numerous national governments and offers consultation services in the domain of animal diseases with international importance.

25.7.3 World Health Organization

The WHO, an international body under the United Nations headquartered in Geneva, plays a crucial role in epidemiology and the control of zoonoses, food-borne infections and intoxications, and comparative medicine. The WHO's VPH section, a distinct division within the Division of Communicable Diseases, concentrates on zoonoses, food hygiene, and comparative medicine. The VPH section serves as a liaison between the WHO, public health, and the worldwide veterinary profession, creating an organized platform to leverage personnel, information, and general resources to support human health. The WHO is organized into six global regions, each with a regional headquarters. These regions, namely Brazzaville for Africa, New Delhi for Southeast Asia, Alexandria for Eastern Mediterranean, Manila for Western Pacific, Copenhagen for Europe, and Washington for the Americas, collaborate to address global health challenges.

25.8 Initiatives in Veterinary Public Health

Various initiatives have been taken by the WOAH, FAO, WHO, and UNEP to strengthen the health systems by prevention and control of zoonotic diseases, ensuring food safety, biological threat reduction, fighting AMR, etc. Some of the initiatives are as follows.

25.8.1 World Organisation for Animal Health Initiatives

Various global initiatives undertaken by the WOAH, individually or in collaboration with other organizations, are as follows.

25.8.1.1 Global Initiatives for Food Safety

Food containing pathogenic bacteria, viruses, parasites, or harmful chemical substances is responsible for causing over 200 different diseases. Among these illnesses, diarrheal diseases are the most common outcome of consuming contaminated food, affecting approximately 550 million individuals and leading to 230 000 deaths annually. The WHO reports that nearly 600 million people, or roughly 1 in 10 individuals worldwide, experience food-related illnesses each year, with over 400 000 deaths annually attributed to food-borne diseases.

Food-borne illnesses typically result from infections or toxins introduced into the body through contaminated food or water. Food sources that can lead to food-borne illnesses include products of animal origin, fresh fruits and vegetables, and drinking water. Common food-borne pathogens such as *Salmonella*, *Campylobacter*, and *Escherichia coli* affect millions of people each year, sometimes with severe or fatal consequences. For example, salmonellosis outbreaks are often associated with foods like eggs, poultry, and other animal products. *Campylobacter* infections frequently result from consuming raw milk, undercooked poultry, or contaminated drinking water. *Escherichia coli* is associated with unpasteurized milk, undercooked meat, and fresh fruits and vegetables. However, food-borne diseases may also be caused by parasites (e.g., tapeworms like *Echinococcus* spp. or *Taenia solium*), viruses (e.g. *Norovirus* infections), and chemical hazards like veterinary drug residues, chemicals (e.g., dioxins), or environmental pollutants (heavy metals).

The WOAH and the Codex Alimentarius are the global organizations responsible for establishing standards according to the World Trade Organization (WTO) Agreement on Sanitary and Phytosanitary Measures (SPS Agreement). The connection between the WOAH and the Codex is of special significance due to the potential risks to both human health and food safety that can originate at the farm level and subsequent stages throughout the food production process. Therefore, it is essential to customize risk management efforts to identify and manage these risks effectively at the appropriate stages. The WOAH and the Codex work closely together in shaping their individual standards that pertain to the entire food production process. They take deliberate measures to ensure that there are no inconsistencies or gaps between these standards to maintain a harmonious approach (WOAH 2023a).

25.8.1.2 Global Initiatives for Disease Eradication

In order to promote the well-being of both animals and humans, the WOAH has identified the control of animal diseases as one of its primary objectives. Moreover, it has additional objectives, such as preserving the livelihoods of specific communities, alleviating poverty, bolstering the economy, and safeguarding international trade.

25.8.1.2.1 Global Strategies for the Control and/or Eradication of Animal Diseases

The successful eradication of rinderpest in 2011, marking the first ever eradication of an animal disease worldwide, serves as an example that has influenced the strategies currently implemented by the WOAH. According to this strategy, animal diseases with an eradication strategy include African swine fever, bovine tuberculosis, foot and mouth disease, peste des petits ruminants, and rabies, of which bovine tuberculosis and rabies are of public health significance.

25.8.1.3 Global Initiatives to Fight Antimicrobial Resistance

Addressing the global issue of AMR cannot be effectively undertaken by any single organization in isolation. This complex challenge can only be met by a One Health approach that recognizes the interconnectedness and interdependence of animal, human, plant, and environmental health. This is why the WOAH has forged collaborations with other key entities, including the FAO, WHO, and more recently, UNEP. Together, they have established the Quadripartite, an exceptional partnership dedicated to combatting AMR and various other health threats that emerge at the intersection of animal, human, and environmental health. The Quadripartite initiative offers a strategic framework, as well as guidelines and recommendations, to all parties involved in the production, distribution, and administration of antimicrobials (WOAH 2023b).

Actions include enhancing the abilities of member countries to monitor antimicrobial usage and tackle AMR, maintaining uniformity in the standards established by the organizations, assessing and mitigating AMR-related risks on a global scale, and collectively raising awareness, especially during World Antimicrobial Awareness Week (WAAW) from 18 to 24 November every year.

25.8.1.3.1 Building a Global Governance on Antimicrobial Resistance

Due to the multifaceted nature of AMR, effective measures need to be implemented on a global scale. In 2019, the urgent call for coordinated international efforts, the report "No Time to Wait: Securing the Future from Drug-Resistant Infections," was submitted to the Secretary-General of the United Nations. This pivotal report was prepared by the Interagency Coordination Group on Antimicrobial Resistance (IACG), a special group tasked with offering practical recommendations to ensure sustained and impactful actions against AMR. Collaboratively developed with inputs from the Tripartite (FAO, WHO, WOAH) and building upon the WHO's 2015 Global Action Plan on Antimicrobial Resistance (GAP-AMR), which involved the WOAH, this document signifies a crucial milestone. Currently, global, regional, and national efforts in advocacy, collaboration, funding, and action plan execution are all guided by the overarching principles laid out in the strategic framework for collaboration on AMR. Published by the Quadripartite in 2022, this framework is aligned with the objectives of the GAP, aiming to conserve the efficacy of antimicrobials and ensure fair and sustainable access to these essential drugs (WOAH 2023b).

25.8.1.4 Global Initiatives for Biological Threat Reduction

Infectious agents and toxins in animals and animal-derived products pose a persistent and significant threat to various aspects, including animal health, agricultural economies, food security (involving both crops and livestock), food safety, and public health. So, animal pathogens have the potential to be exploited as bioweapons or in acts of bioterrorism due to their substantial impact, cost-effectiveness, ease of acquisition and propagation, and the potential to be surreptitiously transported across borders without detection. Ongoing advancements in biotechnology constantly increase the possibilities for engineering animal pathogens, while the associated costs are decreasing. The WOAH maintains a comprehensive list of all animal pathogens that have been developed for use as bioweapons or possess the potential for such application.

In fulfilling its mission of enhancing animal health, veterinary public health, and animal welfare on a global scale, the WOAH treats the threat posed from accidental or intentional release of animal pathogens with the utmost seriousness. Its strategy for reducing the risk of biothreats revolves around reinforcing, improving, and establishing connections between existing healthcare systems. This strategy aligns with and is reinforced by the WOAH's Fifth Strategic Plan (2011–2015) and included in all its objectives. The biothreat reduction strategy includes five primary areas.

- Policy development, advocacy, and effective communication.
- Maintenance of expertise and the establishment of standards, guidelines, and recommendations.
- Promotion of international collaboration and cooperation.
- Global disease surveillance and intelligence.
- Capacity building and fostering solidarity.

25.8.1.5 Global Initiatives in One Health

These initiatives of the WOAH are designed to aid countries in establishing efficient national health systems characterized by strong organization and adherence to the principles of good governance and One Health. These initiatives primarily focus on the following key areas.

25.8.1.5.1 Enhancing One Health Collaboration in the Field

To effectively address common health risks, it is imperative to have robust and resilient health governance systems at the national level that facilitate multisectoral coordination. However, some countries lack mechanisms for consultation and collaboration among their diverse health sectors.

25.8.1.5.2 Training Health Professionals in One Health

In collaboration with the WHO, the WOAH has developed joint One Health training programs. These initiatives involve conducting multisectoral national seminars in countries to strengthen collaboration between their human and animal health sectors. A dedicated working group comprising WHO and WOAH experts has been established to foster networking and create a global One Health learning community with shared values.

25.8.1.5.3 Building Capacity to Manage Zoonotic Disease Risks

Effective collaboration among all sectors responsible for health is crucial in addressing the challenges posed by zoonoses. The WOAH, in partnership with the FAO and WHO, has jointly produced a guide entitled "Taking a Multisectoral, One Health Approach: A Tripartite Guide to Addressing Zoonotic Diseases in Countries." This guide is adaptable for addressing various health threats at the human–animal–environment interface beyond zoonoses, such as food safety and AMR. It offers principles, best practices, and options to support countries in preventing, preparing for, detecting, and responding to zoonotic threats.

25.8.1.5.4 Strengthening Surveillance Systems

Surveillance protocols play a critical role in the early detection of health risks. Sharing this information enables timely decision making to mitigate the spread of diseases between animals and humans.the WOAH has been implementing the EBO-SURSY Project in West and Central Africa, in partnership with the French Agricultural Research Centre for International Development (CIRAD), the French National Research Institute for Sustainable Development (IRD), and the Pasteur Institute, to bolster early detection systems for the Ebola virus and other viral hemorrhagic fevers. The project, funded by the European Union, involves training professionals from various sectors, including conservationists, forestry services, national veterinary services, epidemiologists, and data managers. This training enables rapid responses after detecting dead or sick wild animals. The project also sheds light on how migrating bats can transmit pathogens over long distances, offering insights into predicting future outbreaks.

25.8.2 World Health Organization Initiatives

The WHO has started numerous initiatives to serve human health, some of them related to VPH as follows.

25.8.2.1 WHO 1+1 Initiative

The WHO 1+1 Initiative was launched in 2019 on World Tuberculosis Day. This initiative is part of a worldwide youth movement aimed at eradicating tuberculosis (TB) by involving and amplifying the voices of young people. The goal is to amplify the power of youth to accelerate progress toward meeting the ambitious 2022 targets set during the UN high-level meeting on ending TB and ultimately achieving the broader objective of ending TB by 2030. The 1+1 Initiative is built on the idea that small actions taken by young individuals can have a significant impact. By tapping into the potential of the younger generation, we can create a social multiplier effect. The concept is simple: if each young person reaches out to another, it can lead to reaching the millions of people needed to put an end to the TB epidemic (WHO 2023a).

The key goals and objectives of the 1+1 Initiative include:

- empowering and mobilizing young people to actively participate in the fight against TB, harnessing their ability to create a multiplier effect through the 1+1 campaign
- acknowledging the valuable contribution of young people and recognizing them as essential stakeholders in the battle to end TB
- embracing the diversity among young people and engaging them across the entire spectrum of activities related to ending TB.

25.8.2.2 Eliminate Yellow Fever Epidemics (EYE) Strategy 2017–2026

The Global Yellow Fever Elimination Strategy (GYFES) is a collaborative effort involving key partners such as Gavi, UNICEF, and the WHO, aimed at addressing the evolving epidemiology of yellow fever, the resurgence of mosquitoes, and the increased risk of urban outbreaks and international transmission (WHO 2023b).

Yellow fever outbreaks continue to pose a threat to countries in Africa and the Americas. Despite progress in immunization efforts, challenges persist in eradicating yellow fever outbreaks, as demonstrated by unprecedented urban outbreaks in 2016. The objectives of the GYFES are designed to confront these challenges.

This strategy strives to establish a worldwide alliance of countries and partners, working in a coordinated manner, to mitigate the escalated risk of yellow fever outbreaks. Moreover, it presents an opportunity to showcase novel approaches to managing the intricate landscape of resurging infectious diseases. The activities supported through this strategy align with the Thirteenth General Programme of Work of the WHO (GPW13), contributing to the overarching goal of preventing epidemics on a large scale. The GYFES gained approval from all African member states during the 67th session of the WHO Regional Committee for Africa and was endorsed by the PAHO Regional Immunization Technical Advisory Group (RITAG) in 2017. It embodies a comprehensive and enduring approach, drawing on past experiences, with the ultimate objective of eradicating yellow fever epidemics by 2026. The strategy is built around three key objectives: safeguarding vulnerable populations, curbing international dissemination, and swiftly managing outbreaks (WHO 2023b).

25.8.2.3 Global Antimicrobial Resistance and Use Surveillance System

In 2015, the GAP-AMR received unanimous approval from WHO member states. The primary objective of GAP-AMR is "to ensure the continued efficacy of effective and safe medicines in treating and preventing infectious diseases, maintaining their quality, promoting responsible use, and ensuring access for all those in need for as long as possible" (WHO 2023c).

Surveillance plays a crucial role in informing policies and responses for infection prevention and control. It is the fundamental tool for assessing the proliferation of AMR and monitoring the effectiveness of local, national, and global strategies. On October 22, 2015, the WHO introduced the Global Antimicrobial Resistance and Use Surveillance System (GLASS), marking the world's inaugural collaborative endeavor to standardize AMR surveillance. The GLASS was formally endorsed by the 68th World Health Assembly through resolution WHA68.7. It was established to support the second objective of the GAP-AMR initiative, which is to "enhance knowledge through surveillance and research" and address knowledge gaps to inform strategies across all levels (WHO 2023c).

The GLASS establishes a uniform method for countries to collect, analyze, interpret, and share data. It also actively facilitates capacity building and monitors the status of both existing and emerging national surveillance systems. Additionally, it promotes a shift from surveillance methods solely relying on laboratory data to a comprehensive system that encompasses epidemiological, clinical, and population-based data. The system is designed to gradually incorporate data from AMR surveillance in humans, which includes monitoring drug resistance and antimicrobial drug use, as well as AMR in the context of the food supply chain and the environment (WHO 2023c).

The GLASS operates across all three tiers of the WHO: its headquarters, regional offices, and country offices. It is bolstered by the WHO AMR Surveillance and Quality Assessment Collaborating Centres Network. The initiative enjoys strong commitment from participating countries and maintains close cooperation with regional AMR networks, such as the Central Asian and European Surveillance of Antimicrobial Resistance (CAESAR), the European Antimicrobial Resistance Surveillance Network (EARS-Net), the Latin American Network for Antimicrobial Resistance Surveillance (Rede Latinoamericana de Vigilancia de la Resistencia a los Antimicrobianos [ReLAVRA]), and the Western Pacific Regional Antimicrobial Consumption Surveillance System (WPRACSS).

25.8.2.4 Global Influenza Surveillance and Response System

Since 1952, global surveillance of influenza has been conducted by the WHO through its Global Influenza Surveillance and Response System (GISRS). This system has successfully built international confidence and cooperation by promoting effective collaboration and the sharing of viruses, data, and benefits. It relies on the commitment of WHO member states to a global public health model (WHO 2023d). The primary mission of GISRS is to safeguard individuals from the threat of influenza by serving as a:

- worldwide mechanism for monitoring, preparedness, and response to seasonal, pandemic, and zoonotic influenza
- global platform for tracking influenza's epidemiology and its associated diseases
- global early warning system for emerging influenza viruses and other respiratory pathogens.

25.8.2.5 Gonococcal Antimicrobial Surveillance Program

Obtaining high-quality and representative data on gonococcal AMR is crucial for monitoring trends in AMR, identifying emerging resistance, and guiding updates to clinical guidelines and public health policies at the global, international, and national levels. Since 1992, the WHO Global Gonococcal Antimicrobial Surveillance Program (GASP) has played a pivotal role in documenting the emergence and spread of AMR in gonorrhea on a global scale. GASP is a worldwide network of laboratories overseen by focal points and regional coordinating centers. In each designated region, the focal point collaborates with its respective WHO regional office to collect data on patterns of antimicrobial susceptibility in gonorrhea from participating countries (WHO 2023e). The primary objectives of the WHO GASP are as follows.

- Ensure that there is effective sentinel surveillance of AMR to inform treatment guidelines in all countries.
- Establish a strategy to rapidly identify patients with gonococcal infections who do not respond to recommended cephalosporin therapy either clinically or microbiologically.
- Ensure the successful clinical management of infected patients and their sexual partners.

To achieve globally accurate and comparable data and to promptly identify emerging resistance, it is essential to standardize gonococcal culture-based AMR monitoring and integrate it with clinical and epidemiological data. In response to these needs, the Enhanced Gonococcal Antimicrobial Surveillance Program (EGASP) was introduced. EGASP is a focused sentinel surveillance program that identifies men with urethral discharge in sentinel sites and clinics in a consecutive manner. During routine clinical activities, demographic, clinical, and behavioral data are collected, and urethral specimens are processed in selected reference laboratories using quality-assured culture techniques and minimum inhibitory concentration (MIC) determination. Laboratory and epidemiological data are combined, verified, analyzed, and shared with the WHO through a dedicated EGASP module in the GLASS-IT platform. Various resources and tools, including the generic EGASP protocol, are available to support the implementation and expansion of EGASP (WHO 2023e).

References

Gruetzmacher, K., Karesh, W.B., Amuasi, J.H. et al. (2021). The Berlin principles on one health-bridging global health and conservation. *Science of the Total Environment* 764: 142919.

Thrusfield, M. (2007). The development of veterinary medicine. In: *Veterinary Epidemiology*, 1–21. Ames: Blackwell.

United Nations Environment Programme (UNEP) (2021). Joint tripartite and UNEP statement on definition of "One Health". www.https://www.unep.org/news-andstories/statements/joint-tripartite-and-unep-statement-definition-one-health (accessed 3 February 2024).

WHO Expert Committee on Public Health Administration & World Health Organization. (1952). Expert Committee on Public-Health Administration : first report [of a meeting held in Geneva from 3 to 7 December 1951]. World Health Organization. https://iris.who.int/handle/10665/40192.

World Health Organization (WHO) (2023a). WHO 1+1 Initiative. www.who.int/initiatives/who-1-1-initiative (accessed 10 October 2023).

World Health Organization (WHO) (2023b). Eliminate Yellow Fever Epidemics (EYE) Strategy 2017–2026. www.who.int/initiatives/eye-strategy (accessed 10 October 2023).

World Health Organization (WHO) (2023c). Global Antimicrobial Resistance and Use Surveillance System (GLASS). www.who.int/initiatives/glass (accessed 10 October 2023).

World Health Organization (WHO) (2023d). Global Influenza Surveillance and Response System (GISRS). www.who.int/initiatives/global-influenza-surveillance-and-response-system (accessed 11 October 2023).

World Health Organization (WHO) (2023e). The Gonococcal Antimicrobial Surveillance Programme (GASP). www.who.int/initiatives/gonococcal-antimicrobial-surveillance-programme (accessed 11 October 2023).

World Organisation for Animal Health (WOAH) (2023b). Antimicrobial resistance. www.woah.org/en/what-we-do/global-initiatives/antimicrobial-resistance/#ui-id-3 (accessed 2 October 2023).

World Organisation for Animal Health (WOAH) (2023a). Food safety. www.woah.org/en/what-we-do/global-initiatives/food-safety/#ui-id-4 (accessed 2 October 2023).

26

Sources and Hazardous Effects of Environmental Contaminants

Atul Kumar[1] and Anil Patyal[2]

[1] *Department of Veterinary Public Health and Epidemiology, CSK HP Agricultural University, Palampur, India*
[2] *Department of Veterinary Public Health and Epidemiology, Dau Shri Vasudev Chandrakar Kamdhenu Vishwavidyalaya, Durg, India*

26.1 Introduction

Environmental contaminants are substances or agents that are present in the environment above the recommended/permissible limits and have the potential to cause harm to human, animal, and plant health, e.g., pesticides, heavy metals, polyaromatic hydrocarbons, organic/inorganic solvents, microplastics (MPs), gases (carbon monoxide, sulfur dioxide, nitrogen oxides), pharmaceuticals, hazardous wastes, endocrine disruptors, electromagnetic radiations, etc. (Singh et al. 2019). Even excessive exposure to light and noise is considered as an environmental pollution and health hazard. These contaminants can be natural or human-made and can come from various sources such as industrial activities, agriculture, transportation, waste disposal, etc.

The presence of contaminants in different compartments of the environment like air, water, and soil can subsequently cause their pollution which adversely affects human health. Air pollutants include gases (such as carbon monoxide, sulfur dioxide, nitrogen oxides), particulate matter (such as PM2.5 and PM10), and chemicals released into the air from industrial processes, vehicle emissions, and burning of fossil fuel. Water contaminants include chemicals (such as heavy metals, pesticides, pharmaceuticals), pathogens (bacteria, viruses), and organic pollutants (such as oil spills) that can contaminate water bodies like rivers, lakes, and groundwater. The major sources of such water contaminants are industrial discharges, agricultural runoff, sewage treatment plants, and waste disposal facilities.

Soil contamination occurs due to the deposition of various pollutants such as heavy metals, pesticides, industrial chemicals, and hazardous waste. These contaminants in soil can have adverse effects on plant growth and soil fertility, and can also enter the food chain (Kumar et al. 2018a). Among organic compounds, persistent organic pollutants (POPs) are resistant to degradation and can persist in the environment for long periods, e.g., polychlorinated biphenyls (PCBs), dioxins, and certain pesticides. They can bioaccumulate in the food chain, posing a risk to human health and wildlife.

Excessive or disturbing noise from industrial activities, transportation (traffic, aircraft), construction, urbanization, and recreational activities can also cause health problems, including hearing loss, stress, and sleep disturbances in humans and wildlife. Excessive or misdirected artificial light can interfere with natural darkness in the environment, leading to disruption of ecosystems and human sleep patterns, and interference with animal behavior. Exposure to high levels of radiation from nuclear power plants, radioactive waste, medical facilities, power lines, electrical appliances, wireless communication devices, and certain industrial processes can probably have detrimental effects on human health and the environment.

Some common sources of environmental contaminants include the following.

- *Industrial activities*: industrial processes can release a wide range of contaminants into the environment. These include air pollutants from factories and power plants, such as emissions of greenhouse gases, sulfur dioxide, nitrogen oxides, and particulate matter. Industrial activities can also produce hazardous waste, chemical spills, and discharges of pollutants into water bodies.
- *Transportation*: vehicles, especially those powered by fossil fuels, emit air pollutants like carbon monoxide, nitrogen oxides, sulfur dioxide, and particulate matter. These exhaust emissions from cars, trucks, ships, airplanes, and trains

Epidemiology and Environmental Hygiene in Veterinary Public Health, First Edition. Edited by Tanmoy Rana.
© 2025 John Wiley & Sons, Inc. Published 2025 by John Wiley & Sons, Inc.

contribute to air pollution, particularly in urban areas with high traffic volumes. Additionally, oil spills from transportation accidents can contaminate water bodies and coastal areas.

- *Agricultural practices*: agricultural activities can contribute to environmental contamination through the use of pesticides, fertilizers, and animal waste. Pesticides and fertilizers can leach into soil and groundwater, polluting water sources. Livestock operations generate large amounts of manure which, if not managed properly, can contaminate waterways with excess nutrients and pathogens.
- *Household and consumer products*: common household products like cleaning agents, paints, solvents, and personal care items may contain chemicals that can be released into the environment. Improper disposal or leakage of these products can contribute to water and soil contamination.
- *Waste disposal and landfills*: improper disposal of solid waste, hazardous waste, and electronic waste can lead to environmental contamination. Landfills can release methane gas and leachates, which can contaminate groundwater and soil. Incineration of waste can release air pollutants and toxic ash.
- *Mining and extraction*: mining operations for minerals, metals, and fossil fuels can result in environmental contamination. Chemicals used in mining processes, such as cyanide and sulfuric acid, can contaminate water sources. Additionally, mining activities can disrupt ecosystems and lead to habitat destruction.
- *Construction and demolition*: construction activities generate dust, noise, and waste materials that can impact the environment. Construction sites can release pollutants into the air and nearby water bodies, especially if proper erosion control and waste management practices are not implemented.
- *Accidental spills and disasters*: accidental spills of oil and chemicals during transportation, storage, or extraction can have severe environmental consequences. Oil spills in oceans, rivers, or coastal areas can harm marine life, while chemical spills can contaminate soil and water. These incidents can have severe and long-lasting effects on ecosystems, water sources, and human health.
- *Natural processes*: natural sources of environmental contaminants include volcanic eruptions, forest fires, and the release of naturally occurring toxic substances like arsenic and mercury from geological formations. While these sources are naturally occurring, they can still have significant impacts on the environment and human health.

It is important to note that efforts are being made to mitigate and regulate these sources of contamination through environmental laws, regulations, and sustainable practices to minimize the release of contaminants into the environment and their subsequent impact.

26.2 Environmental Contaminants and Their Impacts

Contaminants can have various effects on human body systems, depending on the specific type of contaminant and the level of exposure. Pesticides, heavy metals, POPs, solvents, pharmaceuticals, and microplastics are the major environmental contaminants. Therefore, their sources and hazardous impacts have been discussed here in detail (Table 26.1).

26.2.1 Pesticides

Pesticides are chemicals or biological agents used to control pests, including insects, weeds, fungi, and rodents. They are commonly used in agriculture but they can also be found in other settings such as residential areas, public spaces, and industrial sites.

- *Agricultural use*: owing to its agricultural green revolution, India has established its position as a progressive agrarian country. However, at the same time, pesticides have been applied massively to enhance crop production and improve health by destroying pests of food crops (Sharma et al. 2022b). Common agricultural pesticides include herbicides, insecticides, fungicides, and rodenticides. India occupies the fourth position in the world after the USA, Japan, and China in terms of total pesticide production, and the average per hectare usage of pesticides in India has gradually increased from 1.2 g/ha in 1953–1954 to 600 g/ha in 2014–2015. Pesticides have been instrumental in the country's green revolution as they have contributed to the near doubling of food production during the last century (Kumar et al. 2019a). They are also essential in modern agricultural practices because the need to increase food production to feed a rapidly growing human population maintains pressure on modern agricultural practices with judicious use of pesticides and fertilizers. However, th widespread application and indiscriminate use of pesticides can contaminate various environmental compartments

26.2 Environmental Contaminants and Their Impacts | 311

Table 26.1 Environmental contaminants, their sources and effects.

Contaminants	Sources	Impacts		Reference
		Human health	Environment	
Pesticides (OCs, OPs, SP) and POPs (PCBs, pesticides, dioxins)	Electrical transformers and large capacitors, as hydraulic and heat exchange fluids, and as additives to paints and lubricants, agricultural chemicals, municipal and medical waste incineration and backyard burning of trash	Skin lesions, impairment of the immune, endocrine, and nervous systems, kidney damage, congenital disabilities, leukemia, reproductive problems, and carcinogenicity	Water, air, and soil pollution, ecotoxicity, loss of biodiversity	Akhtar et al. (2021)
Heavy metals (Pb, As, Hg, Cd, Cr)	Weathering of rocks, volcanic activity, mining and smelting, metal processing industries, tanneries, lead-based paints, electronic wastes	Skin, bladder, and prostate cancers, hepatotoxicity, renal failure, reduced fertility, Alzheimer and peripheral neuropathy, reproductive, cardiovascular, and immunological toxicities	Water, air, and soil pollution	Sethi et al. (2023)
Organic solvents (toluene, benzene, ethylbenzene, and xylene)	Industries, cleansing agents, paints, adhesives, pharmaceuticals, personal care products, laboratories	Irritation of eyes, nose, throat, and mucosal membranes, thyroid dysfunction, cancers	Water and air pollution, production of ground-level ozone and smog, poor air quality	Uzma et al. (2008)
Biomedical and pharmaceutical wastes	Healthcare facilities, research laboratories, industries	Infectious diseases, antimicrobial resistance, carcinogenicity	Water, air, and soil pollution	Wei et al. (2021)
Air-borne pollutants (hydrocarbons, CO, CO_2, NO, NO_2, SO_3, particulate matter, ozone)	Power stations, refineries, petrochemicals, chemical and fertilizer industries, metallurgical and other industrial plants, municipal incineration, dry cleaners, printing shops, petrol stations, automobiles, forest fires, volcanic erosion, dust storms, and agricultural burning	Acute nasopharyngitis, asthma, pneumonia, diabetes, DNA damage and impaired cellular function, skin redness, damage to the eyes, respiratory and cardiovascular diseases, immunotoxicity	Acid rain, haze, reduction in photosynthesis, climate change, eutrophication	Manisalidis et al. (2020)

(air, water, soil) which can directly or indirectly pose serious risks to the health of humans by causing various effects like partial or complete suppression of the immune response, cancers, endocrine disruptions, neurological disorders, problems with reproduction and birth defects, etc. (Kumar et al. 2018b).

- *Residential and garden use*: pesticides are often used in residential settings for controlling pests in gardens and homes. Homeowners and gardeners use pesticides to eliminate insects, weeds, and other unwanted organisms. Products like insect sprays, weedkillers, and termite treatments are commonly used.
- *Public spaces*: pesticides are used in public areas such as parks, playgrounds, golf courses, and sports fields to maintain esthetics and control pests. Municipalities and landscaping companies may use pesticides to manage weeds, control insects, and prevent diseases in these areas.
- *Structural pest control*: pesticides are employed in the control of pests in and around homes, offices, and warehouses. Professional pest control services use pesticides to manage infestations of insects, termites, rodents, and other pests.
- *Industrial and commercial applications*: pesticides are used in various industrial and commercial sectors. For example, food storage facilities and processing plants may use pesticides to protect stored products from pests. Pesticides may also be used in manufacturing processes to control pests that can damage machinery or products.
- *Public health*: pesticides are used in public health programs to control disease-carrying vectors such as mosquitoes, ticks, and fleas. This includes the use of insecticides for mosquito control, especially in regions where mosquito-borne diseases like malaria, dengue fever, and encephalitis are prevalent.
- *Veterinary applications*: pesticides, known as veterinary pesticides or veterinary medicines, are used to control parasites, ticks, fleas, and other pests that can affect livestock, pets, and animals in zoos and shelters.

The indiscriminate and nonjudicious use of pesticides in different settings can have both positive and negative impacts on the environment, human health, and ecosystems (Rajmohan et al. 2020). Pesticides can enter water bodies through runoff and leaching, contaminating surface water and groundwater. This can disrupt aquatic ecosystems, leading to the decline of fish populations and other aquatic organisms due to a reduction in the resilience of aquatic communities. Their presence in soil impacts soil fertility, beneficial organisms like earthworms, and microbial activity. Long-term use of certain pesticides can lead to the persistence of toxic residues in soil. Pesticides may harm nontarget organisms, like pollinators (bees, butterflies) and natural predators (ladybugs, spiders) that help control pest populations. This can disrupt the ecological balance and have cascading effects on food webs and biodiversity (e.g., ecotoxicity due to usage of dichlorodiphenyl-trichloroethane (DDT) resulted in the decline of bald eagles, snowy egrets, and peregrine falcons in USA and Eurasian sparrow hawks in the UK). Overuse or improper use of pesticides can contribute to the development of pesticide resistance in target pests, making it more challenging to control them effectively.

Exposure to pesticides in humans can cause both acute toxicity and chronic health effects. Exposure to high doses of pesticides, through occupational handling or accidental ingestion, can lead to acute poisoning. Symptoms of acute toxicity may include nausea, dizziness, headaches, respiratory problems, and in severe cases organ damage or even death. Long-term exposure to low levels of pesticides has been associated with various health issues such as cancer, reproductive disorders, neurological effects, endocrine disruption, and developmental abnormalities. It has been observed that farm workers and pesticide applicators face occupational risks due to direct exposure to pesticides during handling, mixing, and application. Without proper safety precautions, they may experience acute or chronic health effects. Sometimes, residues of pesticides can remain on food crops even after application. Consuming these residues, particularly in high concentrations or over a prolonged period, can contribute to dietary exposure and potential health risks.

To minimize these impacts, integrated pest management (IPM) strategies are promoted, which aim to reduce pesticide use through a combination of cultural practices, biological control methods, crop rotation, and targeted pesticide application when necessary. Additionally, stricter regulations, improved pesticide formulations, and public education can contribute to safer and more sustainable pesticide use.

26.2.2 Heavy Metals

Among various contaminants, heavy metal exposure is a growing concern among researchers and environmental scientists (Sethi et al. 2023). Heavy metals are naturally occurring elements with high atomic weights and densities. They can be found in the Earth's crust and can also be released into the environment through various human activities. Metals with recognized toxic effects include lead, mercury, arsenic, cadmium, and manganese.

- *Weathering of rocks*: natural erosion and weathering processes release heavy metals from rocks and minerals into soil and water. This contributes to the presence of heavy metals in the environment.
- *Volcanic activity*: volcanic eruptions can release heavy metals into the atmosphere and deposit them in surrounding areas.
- *Mining and smelting*: mining operations extract metals from the Earth, and smelting processes refine ores to obtain pure metals. These activities can release heavy metals such as lead, mercury, cadmium, arsenic, and nickel into the environment.
- *Metal processing*: industries involved in metal processing, including metal fabrication, plating, and surface treatment, can release heavy metals into the air and water through the use of chemicals and waste disposal.
- *Coal combustion*: burning coal for energy production can release heavy metals such as mercury, lead, and cadmium into the air. These metals are often present in coal as trace elements and are emitted as air pollutants when coal is burned.
- *Waste incineration*: incineration of waste, including electronic waste and medical waste, can release heavy metals present in the waste materials into the air and ash residue.
- *Fertilizers application*: phosphate fertilizers used in agriculture can contain heavy metals as impurities. When these fertilizers are applied to soil, heavy metals like cadmium and lead can accumulate over time.
- *Animal manure*: livestock waste, such as manure and slurry, can contain heavy metals that originate from animal feed, which may include contaminated plants or minerals. Improper management of animal waste can lead to heavy metal contamination of soil and water.
- *Contaminated sites*: former industrial sites, landfills, and areas with improper waste disposal practices can become contaminated with heavy metals. These contaminants can leach into surrounding soil and groundwater.
- *Sewage sludge*: sewage treatment plants produce sludge, which can contain heavy metals from industrial and household wastewater. The application of sewage sludge as fertilizer or its disposal in landfills can introduce heavy metals into the environment.

- *Lead-based paint*: older buildings and homes painted with lead-based paint can deteriorate over time, releasing lead dust or flakes into the environment. This can pose a risk, particularly for children who may ingest or inhale lead-containing particles.
- *Electronics*: electronic devices, such as batteries, circuit boards, and displays, may contain heavy metals. Improper disposal or recycling of electronic waste can result in the release of these metals into the environment.
- *Atmospheric deposition*: heavy metals can be present in air pollution, particularly in areas with high industrial activity or vehicular emissions. These metals can be deposited onto soil, water bodies, and vegetation through rainfall or dry deposition.

High concentrations of heavy metals in the environment can have serious consequences for both water/soil quality and human health. When heavy metals enter the water supply, they can negatively impact the taste, smell, and appearance of the water, making it less appealing for drinking and other uses. In addition, short-term exposure to high levels of heavy metals like cadmium (Cd), lead (Pb), and chromium (Cr) can cause serious health problems characterized by abdominal pain, nausea, vomiting, respiratory distress, neurological disorders, organ damage, and even death. Long-term exposure to lower levels of heavy metals can lead to chronic health effects.

Different heavy metals have different toxicological profiles, but common health concerns include kidney damage, liver dysfunction, respiratory issues, neurotoxicity, developmental disorders, reproductive problems, and increased cancer risk (Mitra et al. 2022). Children and pregnant women are particularly vulnerable to the effects of heavy metal exposure (WHO 2006). The specific health effects of heavy metal exposure depend on a number of factors, including the type of metal, the dose, and the duration of exposure. Some heavy metals, such as mercury and methyl mercury, can bioaccumulate and biomagnify in the food chain. Predatory fish can accumulate high levels of mercury, posing a risk to those who consume them regularly, particularly pregnant women and young children, as evidenced in Minamata disease (Japan). In addition, heavy metal contamination in water bodies can lead to fishery closures, restrictions on fishing, and economic losses for fishing communities. It can also affect aquaculture operations if the cultured species are exposed to contaminated water.

While heavy metals can be toxic in large quantities, some heavy metals, such as iron (Fe), zinc (Zn), and copper (Cu), are essential for the normal growth and development of living beings. However, even essential heavy metals can become toxic if they are present in high concentrations. For example, high levels of iron can cause a metallic taste in the water and can stain clothing and plumbing fixtures. High levels of zinc can interfere with the uptake of other essential elements, such as copper, and can harm aquatic life. High levels of copper can cause digestive problems and liver and kidney damage in humans. Workers in industries like mining, smelting, metal processing, and battery manufacturing may face occupational exposure to heavy metals. They are at higher risk of heavy metal poisoning and associated health effects if proper safety measures are not in place.

Clean-up and remediation of heavy metal-contaminated sites can be expensive, requiring extensive efforts to remove or mitigate the contamination. Therefore, it is important to routinely monitor the levels of all heavy metals in the environment, including essential heavy metals, to ensure that they are within safe levels for human consumption and the environment.

26.2.3 Persistent Organic Pollutants

Persistent organic pollutants (POPs) are chemical substances characterized by their persistence, bioaccumulation, long-range transport, and toxicity. The Stockholm Convention on Persistent Organic Pollutants identifies 29 specific chemicals as POPs. These include pesticides such as DDT, chlordane, hexachlorobenzene (HCB), dieldrin, and others; industrial chemicals like PCBs used in electrical equipment, hexachlorocyclohexane (HCH), and pentachlorobenzene (PeCB); and numerous unintentional byproducts of pulp and paper, pesticide, and plastic manufacturing, including dioxins and furans. POPs are highly resistant to degradation through natural processes, resulting in their persistence in the environment for extended periods ranging from years to decades. Some have half-lives of many centuries (e.g., chloroform 1850 years; and hexachlorethane and trichlorethylene 1.8 billion and 1.3 million years, respectively) (Jeffers et al. 1989).

Persistent organic pollutants can accumulate in the tissues of living organisms, including animals and humans, through the food chain. This means that even at low environmental concentrations, POPs can reach higher levels in organisms, particularly in higher trophic levels. POPs accumulate in adipose tissue and are mobilized during lactation; the concentration of PCBs in a study of breast milk from Nunavik mothers was fourfold that of southern Quebec mothers (Dewailly et al. 1989). POPs can also travel long distances through air and water currents, making them capable of moving far from their original sources of emission. This leads to their global distribution, and they can be found in regions far from their production or use.

Due to their nature, POPs have been associated with various health effects, including developmental abnormalities, reproductive disorders, disruption of hormonal systems, immune system impairments, and increased risk of certain cancers, and they contribute to declines in biodiversity (Akhtar et al. 2021). Although the production and use of some POPs, for example DDT, have ceased in the developed world, their withdrawal from use has been selective. For example, although no longer manufactured, PCBs are still widely found in transformers. Dioxins and furans continue to be released; one often unrecognized source is the burning of vinyl plastics in municipal, hospital, and industrial incinerators.

Because of their acknowledged toxicity, 12 POPs, including organochlorine pesticides, industrial HCB, PCBs, dioxins and furans, were the subject of the Stockholm Convention on Persistent Organic Pollutants under the United Nations Environment Programme, adopted in 2001. This is an international treaty designed to eliminate or restrict the production, use, and release of POPs. It aims to protect human health and the environment from the adverse effects of these pollutants. The treaty includes provisions for the identification, reduction, and elimination of specific POPs, as well as measures for their environmentally sound management and disposal (UNEP 2001).

26.2.4 Solvents

Organic solvents are chemical substances that are widely used in various industries (rubber, plastics) and applications (cleansing agents) due to their ability to dissolve other substances. Organic solvents are commonly used as thinners, diluents, and carriers in paints, coatings, and adhesives to facilitate application and drying. They are used for cleaning and degreasing surfaces, machinery, and equipment in various industries such as automotive, metalworking, electronics, and manufacturing. Organic solvents play a crucial role in the production of pharmaceuticals, chemicals, and synthetic materials, where they are used as solvents, reaction media, or extraction agents. Many personal care products, such as nail polish removers, hair sprays, and perfumes, contain organic solvents. Household cleaning products, including solvents used in carpet cleaners, spot removers, and degreasers, often contain organic solvents. They are also commonly used in laboratories for various applications such as sample preparation, extraction, chromatography, and synthesis.

While they have many useful properties, organic solvents can also have negative impacts on human health and the environment. Many solvents, such as benzene, toluene, xylene, and trichloroethylene, are highly volatile (the so-called volatile organic compounds [VOCs]), and most are lipophilic. The majority are neurodepressants. Studies indicate that toluene and xylene are also neurotoxic to animal fetuses, and result in neuromotor and behavioral effects (Hass et al. 1995; Hougaard et al. 1999). Additionally, some are carcinogens, for example benzene, which is used in the rubber industry, present in paints, vehicle emissions, and tobacco smoke (Clapp 2000). If organic solvents are inhaled as vapors or mists, this can lead to respiratory irritation, dizziness, headaches, nausea, and in some cases long-term health effects like damage to the central nervous system, liver, kidneys, thyroid, and other organs. Prolonged or repeated contact with organic solvents can cause skin irritation, dryness, and dermatitis.

They also affects environmental health, as volatile organic solvents can contribute to the formation of ground-level ozone and smog when they react with nitrogen oxides and sunlight. This can lead to poor air quality and respiratory problems. Improper disposal or release of organic solvents can contaminate water bodies. They can be toxic to aquatic life and may persist in the environment, posing long-term risks to ecosystems.

It is important to handle organic solvents safely, following proper ventilation, personal protective equipment (PPE), and disposal guidelines to minimize exposure and reduce environmental impact. Additionally, industries are encouraged to explore and adopt alternative solvents with lower toxicity and environmental impact to promote safer practices.

26.2.5 Biomedical Wastes and Pharmaceuticals

Biomedical waste, also known as medical or healthcare waste, refers to any waste generated during healthcare activities that may pose a threat to human health or the environment. This waste includes materials such as used needles, syringes, bandages, surgical gloves, cultures, blood-soaked items, pathological wastes, pharmaceuticals, and other potentially infectious or hazardous materials. The improper management of biomedical waste can have several adverse effects on the health of medical staff, outpatients, waste handlers, and people in the nearby community. Biomedical waste may contain pathogenic microorganisms such as bacteria, viruses, and parasites. If not handled and disposed of properly, these infectious agents can spread diseases such as HIV/AIDS, hepatitis A, B, and C, tuberculosis, and other infections (Kumar et al. 2019b).

Biomedical waste, when not managed appropriately, can contaminate soil, water bodies, and air. The open-air storage of biomedical waste can cause the release of a number of harmful gases such as methane and sulfide, which seriously pollute the atmosphere (Hossain et al. 2011; Wei et al. 2021). Additionally, during incineration of biomedical waste, carcinogens such as PCBs and dioxins are released (Windfeld and Brooks 2015). The release of hazardous substances, pharmaceuticals, and chemicals from biomedical waste can pollute water sources and disrupt ecosystems. This can have long-term effects on the environment, including degradation of natural resources and disruption of ecological balance. Due to open-space waste disposal practices, animals and scavengers might be infected, leading to the scattering of waste and the spreading of infections (Bansod and Deshmukh 2023).

Pharmaceuticals include prescription drugs, over-the-counter medications, and veterinary drugs. Different classes of pharmaceuticals such as antibiotics, antiepileptics, anticoagulants, analgesics, antiinflammatories, lipid regulators, steroids, diuretics, contrast media, and antidepressants can have serious impacts on human health and ecosystems (Nassiri and Abdollahi 2017; Sharma et al. 2022a).

The presence of pharmaceuticals in the environment can cause water contamination, ecotoxicity, bioaccumulation and biomagnification, and the emergence of antibiotic resistance among microorganisms. It is important to note that conventional wastewater treatment systems are not designed to remove pharmaceuticals completely, leading to their presence in surface water and groundwater. This results in toxic effects on aquatic organisms and can disrupt aquatic ecosystems, affecting reproduction, growth, behavior, and biodiversity. Certain pharmaceuticals can bioaccumulate in the tissues of organisms and biomagnify through the food chain, potentially leading to higher concentrations in predators and organisms at higher trophic levels. Discharge of pharmaceutical residues, particularly antibiotics, into the environment can contribute to the development and spread of antibiotic resistance in bacteria and other microorganisms.

Therefore, to mitigate the environmental and human health impacts of biomedical wastes and pharmaceuticals, proper disposal and management strategies are essential. Appropriate waste management practices include segregation of waste at the point of generation, using leak-proof and puncture-resistant containers for disposal, proper labeling and color-coding of waste, and following guidelines for treatment and disposal. For pharmaceuticals, drug take-back programs may prove beneficial, wherein unused medications can be safely collected and disposed of by authorized entities. Educating the public about the importance of responsible medication disposal can help prevent environmental contamination.

Regulatory agencies, pharmaceutical companies, and research institutions are actively studying the impacts of biomedical wastes and pharmaceuticals on human health and the environment. Efforts are being made to develop more environmentally friendly waste disposal techniques and drug formulations, improve wastewater treatment technologies, and promote responsible medication use, disposal, and management to minimize their overall impact.

26.2.6 Microplastics

Due to rapid urbanization and industrialization, the presence of microplastics (MPs) in the environment is an emerging area of food safety concern worldwide. MPs are small plastic particles of size range 5 mm to 0.01 mm formed by weathering of larger plastic waste or deliberately made, which have become a major concern. These particles are becoming increasingly ubiquitous in nature and thus are affecting various natural cycles and have been reported in food items and other consumable products. The effects of these particles are a major topic of study all over the world but currently not much is known about the full extent of their effects.

Due to the diverse nature of plastic, its use has increased hugely in the last century. Annual plastic production increased from 1.5 million tonnes in the 1950s to about 245 million tonnes in the 21st century, which means that plastic production has increased 99% since the early 1950s (Law 2017; Zhao et al. 2017). This is due to the ever growing demand for plastic because of the constantly increasing global population and its dependency on this material (Geyer et al. 2017). Disposable single-use plastics, especially packaging made of plastic, are a major contributor to global contamination (Law 2017). And the evidence suggests that this will increase in parallel with population growth by 2050 (Geyer et al. 2017).

It has been reported that approximately 8300 million tonnes of manufactured plastics yielded around 6300 million tons of waste in the world in the year 2015, out of which 12% was incinerated, 79% left unattended in landfills and natural ecosystems, and only 9% has been recycled (Shukla et al. 2022). Poor plastic waste management, rapid urbanization, higher anthropogenic activities, municipal waste dumping, disposal of domestic sewage effluents into water bodies, and lack of strict plastic pollution control legislation are among the reasons for the higher occurrence of MPs in the environment (Shukla et al. 2022).

The durability of plastic, the thing which makes it such a useful material, is the reason for its resistance to degradation, resulting in persistence in the environment (Lebreton et al. 2017). Fragmentation of large plastics by physical, biological, and chemical processes results in loss of structural integrity, resulting in the formation of MPs (Auta et al. 2017). MPs can be further categorized into primary and secondary MPs. Primary MPs are those which are deliberately manufactured in size ranges for use in various industries such as cosmetics and paints. Secondary MPs are formed as a result of degradation of larger plastic wastes in the environment (Shukla et al. 2022).

The occurrence of MPs is a major concern for the international community because of its effects on health, safety, environment, the fishing industry, and the health status of aquatic and terrestrial organisms (Law 2017), with potential human health consequences. MPs enter terrestrial ecosystems through litter, plastic bags, packaging materials, single-use disposables, etc. They undergo degradation to form MPs which enter the food chain, as seen in regurgitated pellets of vultures in Turkey (Torres-Mura et al. 2015). The terrestrial ecosystem also acts as a source of marine plastic contamination through river and canals. Several studies from the marine environment have reported the mortality of aquatic fauna by ingestion of MPs (Gall and Thompson 2015; Li et al. 2016a; Law 2017). Although ingestion of MPs does not result in mortality every time, it can also cause long-term damage to the organism and habitat (Wright et al. 2013).

There are also some reports suggesting that MPs affect the freshwater environment (Eerkes-Medrano et al. 2015). Due to lack of research studies, it is very difficult to assess the impact of MPs in this environment (Wagner et al. 2014). It is widely believed that the freshwater environment acts as an entry pathway into the marine habitat for MPs. It is estimated that between 1.2 and 2.4 million tonnes of plastic enter the sea via rivers every year (Lebreton et al. 2017). This influx suggests much more impact on the environment than only ingestion by organisms.

There are very limited data on the impact of these MPs on human health although it has been suggested that transfer via the food chain is increasing (Derraik 2002). As MPs have reached nearly all ecosystems in the world, it is obvious that these particles are also entering our food chain. There have been many instances of MPs found in food and drink, including bottled water (Mason et al. 2018), sugar, honey (Liebezeit and Liebezeit 2013), salt (Karami et al. 2017), tap water (Kosuth et al. 2018), and beer (Liebezeit and Liebezeit 2014). These MPs are either products of packaging or directly introduced into the food through the environment and manufacturing processes. The magnitude of MP ingestion greatly increases when all the food and environment sources are taken into account.

In some studies, the binding of MPs with polycyclic aromatic hydrocarbons (PAHs), heavy metals, polybrominated diphenylethers (PBDEs), DDT, and PCBs has been proved (Wright et al. 2013). These are added to the plastic in order to improve its physical properties (Wardrop et al. 2016). MPs can shed these additives constantly into the environment, most of which are carcinogenic, toxic or endocrine inhibitors (Eerkes-Medrano et al. 2015). Plastic pellets associated with heavy metals can accumulate at concentration levels much higher than the surrounding environment (Rochman 2013). These chemicals could migrate to upper strata through the food chain (Li et al. 2016b). MPs can also have physical effects similar to large ingested items, causing abrasion and clogging of the digestive system (Wright et al. 2013).

More importantly, after ingestion, MPs can release toxic chemicals (Wardrop et al. 2016). In some studies, disruption of cellular functions and tissues was found in broken hip joints or knee implants made of plastic (Nuss and von Rechenberg 2008). Biological toxicity analysis has proved the potential of MPs to disrupt energy and lipid metabolism and also oxidative stress (Deng et al. 2017). Constant exposure to different MPs through various routes and their cumulative effect in the human body can pose health risks (Karami et al. 2018). Additionally, the likelihood of leaching of additives (e.g., phthalates, bisphenol A, etc.) and monomers (e.g., vinyl chloride, styrene, etc.) from ingested MPs in human consumers cannot be ruled out, and can cause both acute and chronic health effects in humans such as endocrine disruption, cancer, and neurological effects (Shukla et al. 2022).

26.2.7 Air-borne Pollutants

Air-borne pollutants, also known as air pollutants or air contaminants, are substances or particles present in the air that can have harmful effects on human health, ecosystems, and the environment. Some common air-borne contaminants are listed below.

- *Particulate matter (PM)*: particulate matter consists of tiny solid or liquid particles suspended in the air. They vary in size and chemical composition and can be categorized into different size fractions, such as PM10 (particles with a diameter of 10 μm or less) and PM2.5 (particles with a diameter of 2.5 μm or less). Sources of particulate matter include combustion processes (such as vehicle emissions, furnaces, gas stoves, incinerators, and industrial activities), dust and soil, and natural events like wildfires. Smaller particles like PM2.5 can reach the distal airways and therefore are more damaging than larger PM10 particles. Inhalation of PM2.5 particles results in reduced pulmonary function and distal airway disease (Raizenne et al. 1998).

- *Nitrogen oxides (NOx)*: nitrogen oxides are a group of gases that includes nitrogen dioxide (NO_2) and nitric oxide (NO). They are produced during the combustion of fossil fuels, such as in vehicle engines, power plants, and industrial processes (Manisalidis et al. 2020). Nitrogen oxides contribute to the formation of smog, respiratory issues, and acid rain. They have a particular role in the formation of ground-level ozone in outdoor air.
- *Ground-level ozone (O_3)*: ground-level ozone is a secondary pollutant formed by the reaction of VOCs and nitrogen oxides in the presence of sunlight. It is a key component of smog and can be harmful when inhaled. Ground-level ozone is primarily generated by vehicle emissions, industrial processes, and chemical reactions involving pollutants.
- *Sulfur dioxide (SO_2)*: sulfur dioxide is a gas produced from the burning of fossil fuels, particularly those containing sulfur. Major sources include power plants, industrial processes, and fuel combustion in ships and vehicles. While sulfur dioxide is a direct respiratory irritant, it readily dissolves in water and reacts to form acid aerosol particulates, including sulfuric acid, resulting in the formation of acid rain, leading to respiratory problems and harming of plant life.
- *Carbon monoxide (CO)*: carbon monoxide is a colorless, odorless gas produced by the incomplete combustion of fossil fuels. It is primarily emitted from vehicle exhaust, but can also arise from industrial processes and residential combustion sources. High levels of carbon monoxide can be toxic and pose a risk to human health.
- *Volatile organic compounds (VOCs)*: as discussed earlier, VOCs are organic chemicals that easily evaporate at room temperature and can be found in many common products, including paints, solvents, cleaning agents, and personal care products. They contribute to the formation of ground-level ozone and can have short-term and long-term health effects when inhaled.
- *Hazardous air pollutants (HAPs)*: HAPs are a group of air pollutants known to cause serious health effects, including cancer, birth defects, and respiratory problems. They include toxic metals (e.g., lead, mercury), benzene, formaldehyde, and other chemicals. HAPs are often emitted from industrial processes, waste incineration, and certain manufacturing operations.

Efforts to reduce air-borne pollutants involve implementing regulations, adopting cleaner technologies, promoting energy efficiency, and encouraging sustainable practices. Monitoring air quality, improving emission controls, and raising awareness about the health impacts of air pollution are important steps in mitigating the effects of air-borne pollutants.

26.2.8 E-Waste

Rapid development and advancement in technology together with transboundary movement of electronic goods have benefited human activities. But they also engender an undesirable aspect related to the handling and management of electronic wastes. E-waste includes all wastes generated from goods ranging from electronic toys to large household appliances and medical equipment. Products categorized as e-wastes include "white goods" like freezers, washing machines, dryers, etc. and "brown goods" like televisions, radios, computers, game consoles, digital media players, and home entertainment systems.

There is a wide variety of devices that fall under the umbrella of e-wastes but for statistical purposes, it is categorized based on homology in purpose, constituent materials, and typical heft, and similarity in features typical toward the end of life as per the Waste Electrical and Electronic Equipment (WEEE) European Community Directive 2012/19/EU Annex. III. Category 1 includes temperature exchange equipment, e.g., freezers, air conditioners, etc. Category 2 includes screens and monitors, e.g., TVs, laptops, etc. Category 3 is lamps such as fluorescent lamps, LEDs, etc. Categories 4 and 5 include large and small equipment like washing machines, copying equipment, electronic tools and toys, sports equipment, etc. and Category 6 includes small IT and telecommunication equipment such as mobile phones, GPS, etc.

In 2019, more than 50 million metric tonnes of e-waste were generated and this amount is expected to grow exponentially in the next few years. It is now a swiftly growing and valuable waste category owing to elements/metals which can attract high market values. Due to its unsustainable methods of production, distribution, usage, and disposal, only 1/8th to 1/4th of generated e-waste undergoes formal recycling and even less is being salvaged. The bulk of e-waste is processed informally. Since e-wastes contain elements possessing potential environment contamination attributes, such as dioxins, PCBs, lead, mercury, cadmium, and nickel, their improper disposal through landfills or open ground dumping leads to leaching into water and soil. Eventually, these toxicants find their way into the food chain and influence the life expectancy of consumers in several ways (Rather et al. 2017). Populations in proximity to e-waste dumping/recycling sites are more predisposed to serious health implications, especially children, pregnant women, and older or infirm people (Kumar and Gupta 2021).

Concrete action must be taken to stop the release of these toxic compounds into the environment, decrease resource waste by recovering important metals, and safeguard local people and employees from toxic exposure. Legislative frameworks are needed to enhance waste management techniques. Using these rules in conjunction with locally tailored extended producer responsibility (EPR) frameworks, it is possible to develop waste management strategies that benefit the widest possible range of constituents. This in turn would decrease the effect on ecosystems. Partnerships between the public and commercial sectors are essential to the creation and implementation of effective e-waste management plans. Therefore, global collaborations involving producers, consumers, and policy makers are of the utmost significance in curbing the impact of e-waste on human and environmental health.

26.3 Conclusion

To ensure technical advancements, infrastructural developments, and food security, and also to generate enormous profits, various chemicals are being released into the environment. The economic benefits of such activities may be short term but the detrimental effects on ecosystems, biodiversity, and human health are long term. Since human exposure to such harmful contaminants is inevitable, concerns about environmental hygiene and safety are increasing worldwide. To mitigate their impact, environmental regulations, pollution control measures, technological advancements, and sustainable practices are being implemented to reduce the release and exposure of these contaminants.

References

Akhtar, A.B.T., Naseem, S., Yasar, A. et al. (2021). Persistent organic pollutants (POPs): sources, types, impacts, and their remediation. In: *Environmental Pollution and Remediation. Environmental and Microbial Biotechnology* (ed. R. Prasad), 213–246. Singapore: Springer.

Auta, H.S., Emenike, C.U., and Fauziah, S.H. (2017). Distribution and importance of microplastics in the marine environment: a review of the sources, fate, effects, and potential solutions. *Environment International* 102: 165–176.

Bansod, H.S. and Deshmukh, P. (2023). Biomedical waste management and its importance: a systematic review. *Cureus* 15 (2): e34589.

Clapp, R. (2000). Environment and health. *Cancer* 163: 1009–1012.

Deng, Y., Zhang, Y., Lemos, B. et al. (2017). Tissue accumulation of microplastics in mice and biomarker responses suggest widespread health risks of exposure. *Scientific Reports* 7 (1): 1–10.

Derraik, J.G. (2002). The pollution of the marine environment by plastic debris: a review. *Marine Pollution Bulletin* 44 (9): 842–852.

Dewailly, E., Nantel, A., Weber, J.A.P. et al. (1989). High levels of PCBs in breast milk of Inuit women from Arctic Quebec. *Bulletin of Environmental Contamination and Toxicology* 43: 641–646.

Eerkes-Medrano, D., Thompson, R.C., and Aldridge, D.C. (2015). Microplastics in freshwater systems: a review of the emerging threats, identification of knowledge gaps and prioritisation of research needs. *Water Research* 75: 63–82.

Gall, S.C. and Thompson, R.C. (2015). The impact of debris on marine life. *Marine Pollution Bulletin* 92 (1–2): 170–179.

Geyer, R., Jambeck, J.R., and Law, K.L. (2017). Production, use, and fate of all plastics ever made. *Science Advances* 3 (7): e1700782.

Hass, U., Lund, S.P., Simonsen, L. et al. (1995). Effects of prenatal exposure to xylene on postnatal behavior and development in rats. *Neurotoxicology and Teratology* 17: 341–349.

Hossain, M.S., Santhanam, A., Nik Norulaini, N.A. et al. (2011). Clinical solid waste management practices and its impact on human health and environment – a review. *Waste Management* 31: 754–766.

Hougaard, K.S., Hass, U., Lund, S.P. et al. (1999). Effects of prenatal exposure to toluene on postnatal development and behavior in rats. *Neurotoxicology and Teratology* 21: 241–250.

Jeffers, P., Ward, L., Wogtowich, I. et al. (1989). Homogeneous hydrolysis rate constants for selected chlorinated methanes, ethanes, ethenes and propanes. *Environmental Science and Technology* 23: 965–969.

Karami, A., Golieskardi, A., Choo, C.K. et al. (2017). The presence of microplastics in commercial salts from different countries. *Scientific Reports* 7 (1): 1–11.

Karami, A., Golieskardi, A., Choo, C.K. et al. (2018). Microplastic and mesoplastic contamination in canned sardines and sprats. *Science of the Total Environment* 612: 1380–1386.

Kosuth, M., Mason, S.A., and Wattenberg, E.V. (2018). Anthropogenic contamination of tap water, beer, and sea salt. *PLoS One* 13 (4): e0194970.

Kumar, A. and Gupta, V. (2021). E-waste: an emerging threat to "one health". In: *Environmental Management of Waste Electrical and Electronic Equipment* (ed. C.M. Hussain), 49–61. Amsterdam: Elsevier.

Kumar, A., Gill, J.P.S., and Bedi, J.S. (2018a). Multiresidue determination of pesticides in market honey from northern India using QuEChERS approach and assessment of potential risks to consumers. *Current Science* 115 (2): 283–291.

Kumar, A., Gill, J.P.S., Bedi, J.S. et al. (2018b). Pesticide residues in Indian raw honeys, an indicator of environmental pollution. *Environmental Science and Pollution Research* 25: 34005–34016.

Kumar, A., Thakur, A., Sharma, V. et al. (2019a). Pesticide residues in animal feed: status, safety and scope. *Journal of Animal Feed Science and Technology* 7 (2): 73–80.

Kumar, S.R., Abinaya, N.V.,.a., and Venkatesan, A. (2019b). Bio-medical waste disposal in India: from paper to practice, what has been effected. *Indian Journal of Health Sciences and Biomedical Research* 12: 202–210.

Law, K.L. (2017). Plastics in the marine environment. *Annual Review of Marine Science* 9: 205–229.

Lebreton, L.C., Van Der Zwet, J., Damsteeg, J.W. et al. (2017). River plastic emissions to the world's oceans. *Nature Communications* 8 (1): 1–10.

Li, J., Qu, X., Su, L. et al. (2016a). Microplastics in mussels along the coastal waters of China. *Environmental Pollution* 214: 177–184.

Li, W.C., Tse, H.F., and Fok, L. (2016b). Plastic waste in the marine environment: a review of sources, occurrence and effects. *Science of the Total Environment* 566: 333–349.

Liebezeit, G. and Liebezeit, E. (2013). Non-pollen particulates in honey and sugar. *Food Additives and Contaminants: Part A* 30 (12): 2136–2140.

Liebezeit, G. and Liebezeit, E. (2014). Synthetic particles as contaminants in German beers. *Food Additives and Contaminants: Part A* 31 (9): 1574–1578.

Manisalidis, I., Stavropoulou, E., Stavropoulos, A. et al. (2020). Environmental and health impacts of air pollution: a review. *Frontiers in Public Health* 8: 14.

Mason, S.A., Welch, V.G., and Neratko, J. (2018). Synthetic polymer contamination in bottled water. *Frontiers in Chemistry* 6: 407.

Mitra, S., Chakraborty, A.J., Tareq, A.M. et al. (2022). Impact of heavy metals on the environment and human health: novel therapeutic insights to counter the toxicity. *Journal of King Saud University, Science* 34: 101865.

Nassiri, K.N. and Abdollahi, M. (2017). Health risks associated with the pharmaceuticals in wastewater. *Daru* 25 (1): 9.

Nuss, K.M. and von Rechenberg, B. (2008). Biocompatibility issues with modern implants in bone-a review for clinical orthopedics. *Open Journal of Orthopedics* 2: 66.

Raizenne, M., Dales, R., and Burnett, R. (1998). Air pollution exposures and children's health. *Canadian Journal of Public Health* 89 (Suppl 1): S43–S48.

Rajmohan, K.S., Chandrasekaran, R., and Varjani, S. (2020). A review on occurrence of pesticides in environment and current technologies for their remediation and management. *Indian Journal of Microbiology* 60 (2): 125–138.

Rather, I.A., Koh, W.Y., Paek, W.K. et al. (2017). The sources of chemical contaminants in food and their health implications. *Frontiers in Pharmacology* 8: 830.

Rochman, C.M. (2013). Plastics and priority pollutants: a multiple stressor in aquatic habitats. *Environmental Science and Technology* 47 (6): 2439–2440.

Savita, Chopra, V., and Sharma, A. (2019). Environmental contaminants: sources and effects. In: *Evaluation of Environmental Contaminants and Natural Products: A Human Health Perspective* (ed. A. Sharma and M. Kumar), 1–23. Sharjah: Bentham Science Publisher.

Sethi, V., Kumar, A., and Walia, Y.K. (2023). Contamination of natural water and health risk assessment in Western Himalayan region, India. *Water, Air, and Soil Pollution* 234: 388.

Sharma, A., Kumar, A., and Sharma, N. (2022a). Occurrence of antibiotic residues in milk: detection and public health concerns. *Journal of Animal Feed Science and Technology* 10 (1): 23–29.

Sharma, N., Kumar, A., Singh, S. et al. (2022b). Multi-residue determination of pesticides in vegetables and assessment of human health risks in Western Himalayan region of India. *Environmental Monitoring and Assessment* 194: 332.

Shukla, A., Patyal, A., Shakya, S. et al. (2022). Occurrence of microplastics in riverine fishes sold for human consumption in Chhattisgarh, India. *Water, Air, and Soil Pollution* 233: 501.

Torres-Mura, J.C., Lemus, M.L., and Hertel, F. (2015). Plastic material in the diet of the turkey vulture (*Cathartes aura*) in the Atacama Desert, Chile. *Wilson Journal of Ornithology* 127 (1): 134–138.

UNEP (2001). The Stockholm Convention on Persistent Organic Pollutants. www.pops.int/TheConvention/ThePOPs/AllPOPs/tabid/2509/Default.aspx (accessed 5 February 2024).

Uzma, N., Salar, B.M., Kumar, B.S. et al. (2008). Impact of organic solvents and environmental pollutants on the physiological function in petrol filling workers. *International Journal of Environmental Research and Public Health* 5 (3): 139–146.

Wagner, M., Scherer, C., Alvarez-Muñoz, D. et al. (2014). Microplastics in freshwater ecosystems: what we know and what we need to know. *Environmental Sciences Europe* 26 (1): 1–9.

Wardrop, P., Shimeta, J., Nugegoda, D. et al. (2016). Chemical pollutants sorbed to ingested microbeads from personal care products accumulate in fish. *Environmental Science and Technology* 50 (7): 4037–4044.

Wei, Y., Cui, M., Ye, Z. et al. (2021). Environmental challenges from the increasing medical waste since SARS outbreak. *Journal of Cleaner Production* 291: 125246.

WHO (2006). Principles for evaluating health risks in children associated with exposure to chemicals. www.who.int/publications/i/item/9789241572378 (accessed 5 February 2024).

Windfeld, E.S. and Brooks, M.S. (2015). Medical waste management – a review. *Journal of Environmental Management* 163: 98–108.

Wright, S.L., Thompson, R.C., and Galloway, T.S. (2013). The physical impacts of microplastics on marine organisms: a review. *Environmental Pollution* 178: 483–492.

Zhao, S., Danley, M., Ward, J.E. et al. (2017). An approach for extraction, characterization and quantitation of microplastic in natural marine snow using Raman microscopy. *Analytical Methods* 9 (9): 1470–1478.

27

General Aspects of Environmental Hygiene

Udit Jain[1], Faizan ul Haque Nagrami[2], Vijay Laxmi Tripathi[2], Parul[1], Barkha Sharma[1], Shweta Sharma[2], Parul Singh[2], and Shikhar Karan Verma[1]

[1] College of Veterinary & Animal Sciences, DUVASU, Mathura, India
[2] College of Biotechnology, DUVASU, Mathura, India

27.1 Environment

The word "environment" comes from the French verb *environner*, which means to encircle or surround. Environment refers to the totality of all external factors and conditions that have an impact on the survival and growth of any living thing (Figure 27.1). It is the whole of the relationships between the land, water, and human beings and other living things.

Environmental studies have a broad scope that covers many different topics and facets, some of which are listed here.

- The management and conservation of natural resources.
- Ecosystems and biodiversity.
- Control of environmental contamination.
- Social difficulties in the context of growth and the environment.
- Environment and population.

27.2 Importance

Environmental studies are crucial because they address everyday concerns like safe and clean drinking water, sanitary living conditions, clean and fresh air, fertile land, healthy food, and sustainable development. Investing in pollution control technologies will also lower pollution levels and the cost of effluent treatment.

27.3 Need for Public Awareness

There is a Chinese proverb which says "If you plan for one year, plant rice; if you plan for 10 years, plant trees; and if you plan for 100 years, educate people."

The 1992 Rio de Janeiro Earth Summit was a United Nations summit on environment and development (Figure 27.2). The World Summit on Sustainable Development in Johannesburg in 2002 highlighted important worldwide environmental challenges and brought environmental decline to the public's attention.

27.4 Environmental Hygiene

According to one definition, environmental hygiene is "that branch of public health concerned with the control of all those factors in man's surroundings or physical environment which may have detrimental effects on human health and well-being." As an alternative, "all those aspects of public health that are determined by physical, chemical, biological, social,

Epidemiology and Environmental Hygiene in Veterinary Public Health, First Edition. Edited by Tanmoy Rana.
© 2025 John Wiley & Sons, Inc. Published 2025 by John Wiley & Sons, Inc.

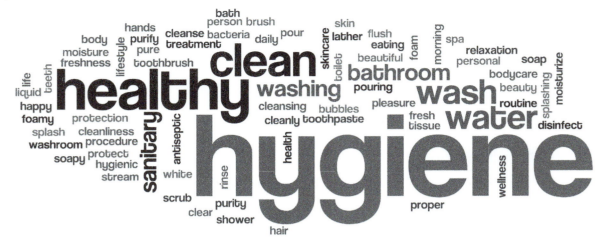

Figure 27.1 Health and hygiene. *Source:* Needy Individuals Support Association. https://nisafoundationngp.org/donations/health-and-hygiene// (accessed December 6 2023).

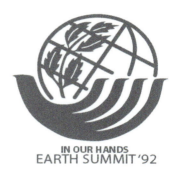

Figure 27.2 Earth Summit 1992, Rio de Janeiro.

and psychological factors in the environment" could be used to describe environmental hygiene. It also comprises theories and methods for identifying, addressing, preventing, and managing environmental variables that may have an impact on the health of current and future generations. Therefore, it includes all the steps required to address the worsening environmental conditions. These steps are intended to monitor the environment and, if necessary, change it to benefit human health.

Historically, air, water, and food contamination by bacteria was a major worry for public health officials. With the start of the industrial period, environmentalists began to pay attention to the issues of chemical contamination. "Normal pollutants" were present in modern industrial and municipal wastes, but they also contained synthetic substances that were foreign to traditional and cutting-edge water treatment methods. In addition, focus is placed on meeting a number of desirable public health requirements. It is important to maintain a high level of environmental hygiene as required by law under the New South Wales Food Act 2003 and Food Regulation 2010.

27.5 Scope of Environmental Hygiene

The areas of concern in environmental hygiene can be summarized as below.

- Water supply, with a focus on giving users access to an adequate supply of safe water.
- Wastewater treatment and water pollution control, including the collection, handling, and disposal of household waste that is water-borne as well as regulation of the quality of surface and ground water.
- Solid waste management, which includes properly handling and discarding waste.
- Vector control.
- Preventing pollutants harmful to human, animal, and plant life from contaminating the soil with human waste.
- Food hygiene, including milk hygiene.
- Air pollution control.
- Radiation pollution control.
- Noise pollution control.
- Occupational health, namely the management of biological, chemical, and physical risks.
- Housing and the area around it, with a focus on the public health elements of private, public, and institutional structures.
- Urban and regional planning.

- Environmental health aspects of air, sea or land transport.
- Accident prevention.
- Public recreation and tourism, particularly environmental health aspects of public beaches, swimming pools, camping sites, etc.
- Sanitation measures during epidemics, emergencies, disastersm and population migration.
- Wildlife and forest conservation.
- Preventive measures to ensure freedom from health risk of the general environment.

27.6 Environmental Hazards

Biological hazards: microbiological, animals (indirect), insects (vectors), food (food-borne infections and intoxications), water (cholera, typhoid), and air (common cold, influenza).
- Chemical hazards: poisons, allergens, irritants, synthetic chemicals.
- Physical hazards: temperature, vibrations/noise, radiation.
- Psychological hazards: stress, anxiety, discomfort, depression.
- Sociological hazards: overcrowding, isolation, traffic, lack of opportunity.

27.7 Objectives of Environmental Hygiene

27.7.1 Prevention and Control of Biological Hazards

The main focus of biological risks is the different infectious diseases that affect humans. Contagious diseases can spread from person to person directly through contact or indirectly through a food source, a body of water (cholera, typhoid), or the air (common cold, influenza). Such diseases may be avoided by altering the environment to block the path of transmission. Humans can be protected from a number of zoonotic illnesses, such as brucellosis, rabies, and tuberculosis, by putting in place the proper environmental control measures.

27.7.2 Prevention and Control of Chemical Hazards

Chemical-related environmental risks to human communities are nothing new. However, in recent years, their magnitude has multiplied greatly. Unprecedented industrial growth has resulted in yearly production of thousands of new chemicals. The associated toxicity and subsequent workplace dangers during production are either not known at all or poorly understood. Many of these pollutants end up in soil, air, surface and ground water. While chemicals from industrial emissions and automotive exhaust are inhaled, residues from agricultural pesticides are consumed with food. Even while the impacts in many circumstances may not be noticeable right away, they may have a long-term (cumulative effect) impact on health.

27.7.3 Prevention and Control of Physical Hazards

Physical environmental risks to health include things like dust, temperature, humidity, machinery, radiation, and sound, among others. These could result in illness, death, or disability. If silica or asbestos dust is inhaled, it can lead to fibrosis, which can occasionally result in physical impairment. Regarding human productivity and performance, temperature and humidity are significant factors. Long-term exposure to radiation, such as that from X-rays, ultrviolet, and infrared rays, can result in skin burns as well as a number of related illnesses and even death. Ionizing radiation overexposure raises the risk of cancer development, genetic mutation, and other biological flaws. Mechanical sounds and vibrations can disrupt the mind and induce hearing loss or impairment. One of the most common environmental risks is noise. Noise levels that are too high have an impact on between 80 and 100 million people. On a daily basis, almost 40 million people suffer negative effects. Visual perception also affects human efficiency and comfort, connected to light type, intensity, color, contrast, and glazing.

27.7.4 Prevention and Control of Sociological and Psychological Hazards

The risks and implications of sociological and psychological factors in relation to the environment must be considered. There is sufficient evidence to conclude that, while genes influence how we react to stimuli, our environments have a greater impact on how we think. Environmental elements like congestion, lack of personal space, limited social contact opportunities, stress from the workplace, traffic, and crowds, among others, are proven to have social and psychological effects on people.

Environmental hygiene thus tries to reduce risks through prevention and control in order to enhance both the quantitative and qualitative aspects of health. This would necessitate a carefully thought-out strategy covering various environmental hygiene components and clearly defined criteria to evaluate its impact on human and animal health. The selection criteria should be supported by scientific research on the short- and long-term impacts of various environmental factors on human and animal health. Along with the socioeconomic position and religious views of the local populace, it should consider both the environmental elements that are present and those that are changing.

27.8 Advances in Environmental Hygiene

Carbon sequestration.
- Bioremediation.
- Rainwater harvesting and artificial discharge.
- Eco-friendly technologies in India.

27.8.1 Carbon Sequestration

This is another name for the geoengineering method of "carbon capture" which is the long-term storage of carbon dioxide (or other forms of carbon) for the purpose of reducing global warming. Worldwide annual carbon emissions are currently almost 33 billion tonnes. The following are some methods for sequestering carbon.

- In plants and soil – terrestrial sequestration ("carbon sinks").
- Underground – geological sequestration.
- Deep in the ocean – ocean sequestration.
- As a solid material (still in development).

27.8.1.1 Terrestrial Carbon Sequestration

This is the process through which atmospheric carbon dioxide is spontaneously taken up by photosynthesis and stored as carbon in biomass and soils (Figure 27.3). Although forests and agricultural lands absorb atmospheric carbon dioxide, 20% of the world's annual carbon dioxide emissions are caused by tropical deforestation. Ways in which to cut greenhouse gas emissions are as follows.

- Preserving the carbon sequestration already present in soils and plants to reduce emissions.
- Increasing carbon storage on agricultural fields by planting trees or switching from conventional to conservation tillage techniques.
- Carbon sequestration rates vary depending on tree species, soil type, regional climate, topography, and management practices.
- After 90 years (1 metric tonne = 1 year), pine plantations in the Southeast United States can accumulate about 100 metric tonnes of carbon per acre.
- When a tree reaches maturity or the organic matter in soils increases to the levels before losses occurred, carbon accumulation eventually reaches a saturation point where further sequestration is no longer possible.
- After this point, the trees or agricultural practices must be maintained to maintain the accumulated carbon and prevent further losses of carbon back to the atmosphere.

27.8.1.2 Geological Sequestration

Storing of carbon dioxide underground in rock formations allows retention o large amounts of carbon dioxide over a long time period held in small pore spaces.

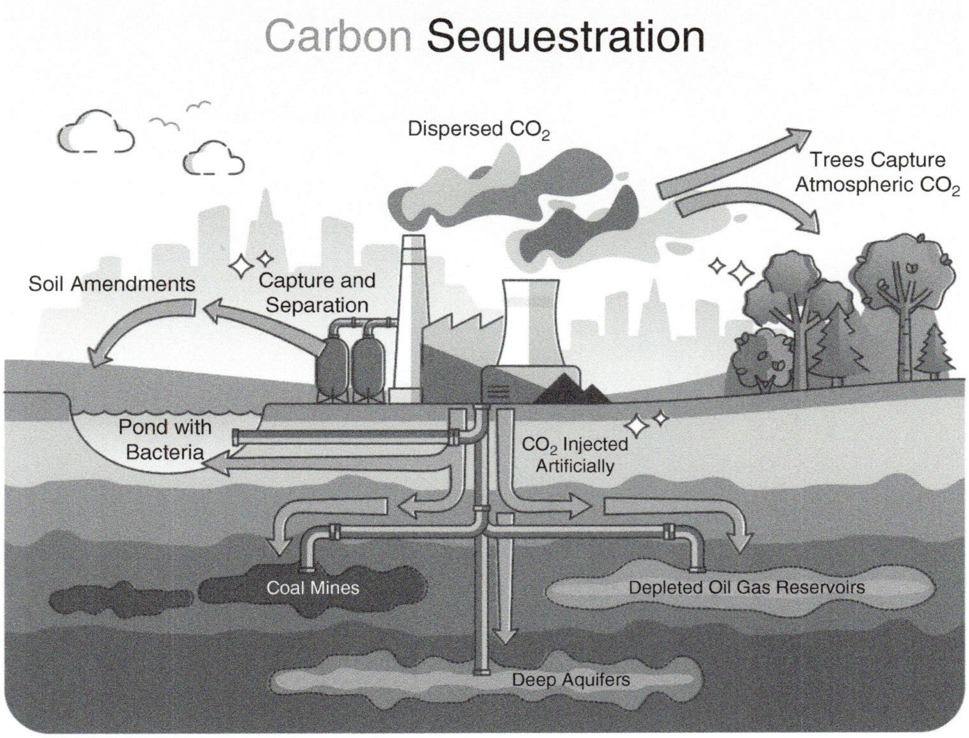

Carbon Sequestration

Figure 27.3 Terrestrial carbon sequestration. *Source:* Amwins, Inc. www.amwins.com/resources-insights/article/carbon-sequestration-101-understanding-the-risks-and-finding-insurance-solutions/ (accessed December 6 2023).

27.8.1.3 Ocean Carbon Sequestration

Carbon is naturally stored in the ocean via two pumps, solubility and biological, and there are analogous human-made methods – direct injection and ocean fertilization. Eventually equilibrium between the ocean and the atmosphere will be reached with or without human intervention and 80% of the carbon will remain in the ocean. Regardless of whether the carbon is introduced into the atmosphere or the ocean, the same equilibrium will be reached. Ocean sequestration's main goal is to accelerate a natural process (Figure 27.4). Capturing, separating, transporting, and injecting CO_2 by direct injection into the deep ocean from land or tankers is required for carbon sequestration. One-third of CO_2 emissions each year already reach the ocean. The ocean contains 50 times as much carbon as the atmosphere.

27.8.2 Bioremediation

This is the process of cleaning up environmental sites contaminated with chemical pollutants by using living organisms to degrade hazardous materials into less toxic substances.

27.8.2.1 Biotechnological Approaches

Biotechnological approaches are essential for

- detecting pollutants
- restoring ecosystems
- understanding the circumstances that can lead to human diseases
- turning waste materials into useful energy.

27.8.2.2 Applying Genetically Engineered Strains to Clean Up the Environment

Escherichia coli to clean up heavy metals.

- Copper, lead, cadmium, chromium, and mercury.
- Biosensors: bacteria capable of detecting a variety of environmental pollutants.

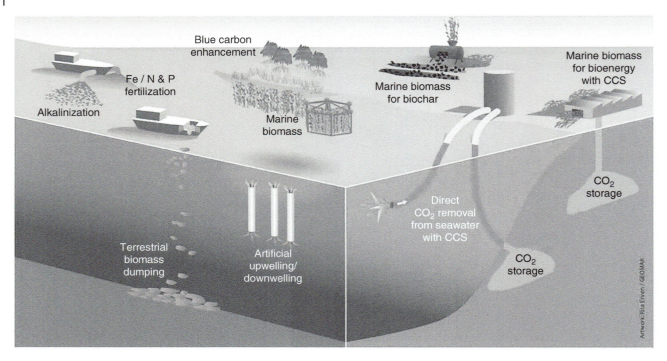

Figure 27.4 Ocean carbon sequestration. *Source:* Rita Erven/GEOMAR. www.iasparliament.com/current-affairs/ocean-carbon-sequestration (accessed December 6 2023).

- Genetically modified plants and phytoremediation.
- Plants that can remove RDX (research department explosive) and TNT (trinitrotoluene).

27.8.2.3 Biodegradation
The use of living organisms such as bacteria, fungi, and plants to degrade chemical compounds.

27.8.2.4 Rain Water Harvesting
Low-lying areas are kept from flooding via rain water gathering. Rain water collection allows dug wells and bore wells to produce consistently by replenishing the groundwater table. It helps in the availability of clean water by reducing salinity and the presence of iron salts.

27.8.2.5 Recharge to Groundwater
This may be undertaken by recharge bore pits, recharge wells, spreading basins, ditches, and hand pumps

27.9 Why is Hygiene Necessary?

Hygiene is defined by the WHO as "the conditions and practices that help maintain health and prevent the spread of diseases." This entails more than just maintaining our cleanliness – it also means abstaining from unhealthy behaviors such as dumping trash on the ground, using the lavatory in public, and many others. By putting such activities into practice, we not only get healthier but also see an improvement in the standard of our lives. Personal hygiene includes maintaining one's physical cleanliness, drinking only hygienic water, washing one's hands after using the restroom, and more. Public hygiene refers to correctly disposing of waste and excrement, which includes waste separation and recycling, routine cleaning, and upkeep of the city's water reservoir. In order to prevent infections, kitchen hygiene is of the utmost importance.

Diseases are transmitted via vectors. As in the cases of typhoid, cholera, and amoebiasis (food poisoning), let's say the vector is polluted with water. We can entirely eliminate our chances of contracting infections by drinking clean water. Pathogens transported by animals and insects can cause several diseases. For instance, roundworms, malaria, and filariasis are carried by flies and mosquitoes. Rats and mosquitoes both thrive in open-air food dumps and stagnant water. We can fully rid our area of mosquitoes by using kerosene or other chemicals to saturate stagnant water bodies. If that isn't possible, we can use mosquito nets to protect ourselves from biting insects while we sleep. Rats enjoy sloppy garbage management. We can avoid leaving food lying around for rats to eat by sorting the rubbish properly.

Another way to catch infections is through close contact with sick people. To meet the medical needs of every citizen, a nation must work to train more doctors. Every citizen should be taught the value of cleanliness, which will manifest itself in how clean our neighborhoods are.

27.10 World Health Organization Scenario on Hygiene

Nearly a quarter of the worldwide burden of disease may be avoided by creating healthier surroundings. The COVID-19 outbreak is yet another reminder of how precarious the balance is between people and the environment. The conditions for good health include clean air, a constant climate, enough water, sanitation, and hygiene, safe chemical use, radiation protection, healthy and safe workplaces, sound agricultural practices, health-supportive towns and built environments, and preserved nature. In 2016, 13.7 million deaths, or 24% of all deaths, may have been prevented by reducing environmental dangers. This indicates that nearly one in four of all deaths worldwide is caused by environmental factors. Numerous disease agents, exposure pathways, and unfavorable environmental circumstances have an impact on the majority of illness and injury categories. The most common disease outcomes are noncommunicable illnesses like cancer, chronic respiratory conditions, and ischemic heart disease. Following closely are injuries, respiratory infections, and stroke.

Activities undertaken by the WHO to advance the global agenda for building healthier environments for healthier populations include:

- giving direction for crucial transitions, such as those in energy and transportation, and encouraging good governance in the areas of health and the environment
- directing research, monitoring changes in health hazards and solution implementation, and guaranteeing information development and dissemination for evidence-based norms and effective remedies
- supportive mechanisms for increasing action in countries and capacity building
- enhancing emergency planning and response capabilities in the event of environmental events and providing pertinent advice on environmental health services and workplace health and safety.

27.11 UNICEF Scenario on Hygiene

In order to stop the spread of infectious diseases and ensure that children enjoy long, healthy lives, good cleanliness is essential. Additionally, it keeps children from skipping class which improves learning results. Maintaining proper hygiene helps families avoid disease and save money on medical expenses. In some circumstances, it can also safeguard a family's social standing and assist people in maintaining their self-confidence. However, without the proper knowledge and skills, enough community support, and the conviction that one's own action can truly make a difference, it can be challenging to practice critical hygiene activities. Inhumane living conditions prevent many youngsters from keeping up with proper hygiene. Maintaining hygiene can be difficult in places with dirty flooring, such as houses, schools, and health centers. It can also be difficult in places without access to water for handwashing. Furthermore, maintaining excellent hygiene is frequently seen as a woman's task, which increases her load of obligation.

The cornerstones of UNICEF's hygiene projects are behavior and societal change. We emphasize handwashing with soap, properly disposing of children's waste, managing and storing drinking water safely, and menstrual hygiene, as these four practices assist children and their families in maintaining good hygiene.

Government disaster preparedness and development initiatives to promote better cleanliness are supported by UNICEF as follows.

- *Encouraging good hygiene practices*: we engage communities through handwashing campaigns, the inclusion of good hygiene practices in school curricula, and the promotion of sanitation.
- *Providing hygiene supplies and services*: we support schools in the construction of handwashing stations and distribute hygiene kits during emergencies to guarantee that everyone has access to the necessary hygiene supplies and services.

- *Assisting girls and women with managing their menstrual hygiene*: we seek to increase girls' and women's self-assurance, knowledge, and abilities so they can safely manage their periods, know what to request when they receive them, and use clean facilities and materials.
- *Working with partners and the business sector*: by collaborating with the private sector to develop innovative hygiene technology and by splitting costs to increase access to hygiene, we help enhance hygiene conditions in communities, workplaces, and other settings.
- *Strengthening the hygiene sector*: we collaborate with governments to improve institutional structures, planning, capacity development, and financing policies – the key tenets of a long-term, sustainable improvement in hygiene.

UNICEF also advocates for increased funding for hygiene activities globally. This includes fostering political leadership for hygiene at all levels and recruiting high-profile champions and political leaders as advocates. Building on local knowledge and promoting positive traditional practices, we continue to develop new strategies and tools to improve key hygiene behaviors, while empowering communities to take their health and well-being into their own hands.

Further Reading

Chu, S.C. and Liaw, C.H. (1998). 1995–1997 study of industrial rainwater catchment systems (I)-(III). Final Report of the Industrial Technology Research Institute, Taiwan.

Liaw, C.H., Chen, H.K, Chang, K.C. and Tsai, Y.L. (2000). Feasibility analysis of rainwater catchment systems in Taiwan. Proceedings of the East Asia 2000 Rainwater Utilization Symposium, Taiwan.

Sengupta, M. and Dalwani, R. (eds). (2008). Ecotechnological Applications for the Control of Lake Pollution. https://sswm.info/sites/default/files/reference_attachments/JOSHI%20and%20JOSHI%202008%20Ecotechnological%20applications.pdf (accessed 5 February 2024).

Sherikar, A.T., Bachhil, V.N., and Thaplyal, D.C. (2001). *Textbook of Elements of Veterinary Public Health*. New Delhi: ICAR.

28

Natural Resources: Definition, Types, Examples, Uses, and Abuses

Udit Jain[1], Faizan ul Haque Nagrami[2], Barkha Sharma[1], Priyambada[2], Parul[1], and Uma Sharma[2]

[1] *College of Veterinary & Animal Sciences, DUVASU, Mathura, India*
[2] *College of Biotechnology, DUVASU, Mathura, India*

28.1 Definition of Natural Resources

Natural resources can be defined as the resources that exist (on the planet) independent of human actions. These are the resources that are created naturally from materials found in the environment. Natural resources include things like air, water, sunlight, soil, rock, plants, animals, and fossil fuels. Natural resources are substances that are found in nature and are useful to humans or may be useful in the future under plausible technological, economic, or social conditions. Examples of such substances include food, materials for construction and clothing, fertilizers, metals, water, and geothermal energy. Natural resources have historically been the purview of the natural sciences.

They serve as the raw material from which other types of capital are created.

28.2 Types of Natural Resources

Depending on their place of origin, natural resources can be grouped as follows (Figure 28.1).

28.2.1 Biotic Resources

Any biological element in the environment is a biotic resource. Examples of biotic resources include forests and their products, crops, birds, animals, fish, and other marine life. Because they replenish and reproduce, these resources are renewable. Coal and mineral oil are biological resources, but they cannot be replenished.

28.2.2 Abiotic Resources

Any environmental elements that are not biological are referred to as abiotic resources. Abiotic resources include things like land, water, air, and minerals like iron, copper, gold, and silver. Since they cannot be produced again or replaced, they are finite and nonrenewable.

There are two categories of natural resources depending on availability (Figure 28.2).

- Renewable natural resources.
- Nonrenewable natural resources.

28.2.3 Renewable

The resources that are consistently available despite their use are those that are renewable. After use, they can be fairly easily recovered or replaced. They are inexhaustive and can be regenerated within a given span of time. For example, water,

---

Epidemiology and Environmental Hygiene in Veterinary Public Health, First Edition. Edited by Tanmoy Rana.
© 2025 John Wiley & Sons, Inc. Published 2025 by John Wiley & Sons, Inc.

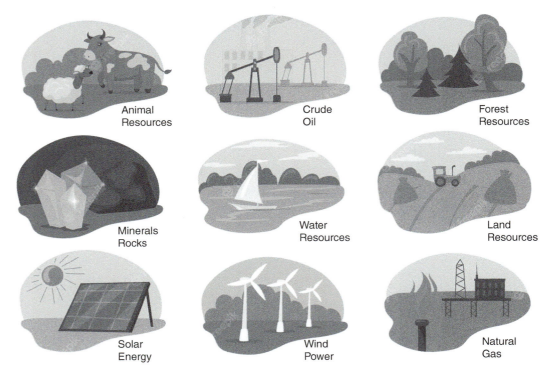

Figure 28.1 Types of natural resources. *Source:* Freepik Company S.L. www.freepik.com/premium-vector/different-types-natural-resources-illustration_16375046.htm (accessed December 6 2023).

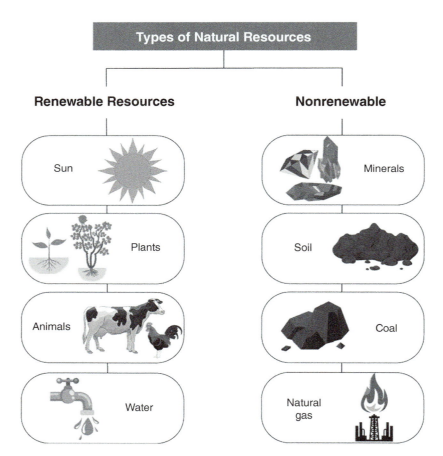

Figure 28.2 Renewable and nonrenewable resources. *Source:* sciencefacts.net. www.sciencefacts.net/what-are-natural-resources.html (accessed December 6 2023).

air, soil fertility, wild plants and animals, human beings and energy resources like wind energy, tidal energy, hydropower, solar energy, and biomass energy are renewable.

Despite the fact that these resources are renewable, it could take decades or centuries to replace them. Organic renewable resources, such as those derived from plants and animals, are distinguished from inorganic renewable resources, which are those derived from nonliving sources like the sun, water, and wind.

28.2.4 Nonrenewable

Once they have been used up or destroyed, nonrenewable resources cannot easily be replaced or recovered. Nonrenewable natural resources are minerals, fossil fuels such as coal and petroleum, and some species of plants and animals. Sometimes, renewable resources become nonrenewable if we exploit them without any control. Some species, if overexploited, become endangered or even extinct. This highlights the numerous reasons why threatened species must be safeguarded at all costs.

Natural resources include:

- forest resources
- mineral resources
- soil resources
- water resources
- food resources
- energy resources.

28.3 Forest Resources

Forests are an important renewable natural resource. The forest ecosystem is dominated by trees, shrubs, and herbs. The world's forests cover 33% of the land area and provide support for insects, birds, and other creatures. Native forests have trees and plants that grow on their own. A man-made forest is one that has been planted with specific tree and shrub species. Boreal coniferous forests can be found between latitudes 55° and 65° north, close to the Arctic Sea. On either side of the planet, between latitudes 30° and 55° north, are temperate forests. Between latitudes 30° north and 30° south and tropical rainforests. Any country's economic development can greatly benefit from the composition and diversity of its forests.

Along with trees, other plants are important for preserving the environment because they cover large areas, produce a variety of goods, and feed living things.

28.3.1 Uses

28.3.1.1 Productive Uses
Forests provide the raw materials required by the paper and pharmaceutical industries, serving a productive purpose. Also available are alkaloids, paints, herbal oils, honey, nuts, wood, turpentine, gum, and food as fuel.

28.3.1.2 Protective Uses
Forests provide a haven for insects, birds, animals, and other creatures, fostering their growth, feeding them, and enabling them to move around freely. During droughts, they halt soil erosion and water loss.

28.3.1.3 Regulative Uses
With the help of forests, the environment's equilibrium can be successfully regulated. A healthy environment, for instance, depends greatly on the regulation of carbon dioxide (CO_2), oxygen (O_2), water (H_2O), and minerals. Forests capture, store, and release solar energy. Starch is created from carbon dioxide and water during the process of photosynthesis in green plants, where it is then stored. Carbon dioxide is taken in during this process, and oxygen is released to help keep the atmosphere in balance and lower the Earth's temperature. The threat posed by an increase in global

temperatures affects people everywhere. One acre of forest can control the carbon cycle, floods, and droughts by absorbing 4 tonnes of carbon dioxide and releasing 8 tonnes of oxygen. The forest also contributes to economic growth and the preservation of land value.

28.3.1.4 Ecological Uses

Wild animals, plants, and millions of species call forests home. Through photosynthesis, they produce oxygen and aid in reducing greenhouse gas emissions that cause global warming. A forest's ability to absorb toxic gases makes it a pollution purifier. In addition to aiding in soil conservation, forests also help control the hydrological cycle.

28.3.1.5 Esthetic Uses

People appreciate the peace and beauty of forests all over the world because forests have the highest esthetic value. Recreational activities and ecosystem research are possible in forests.

28.3.2 Abuses

28.3.2.1 Overexploitation of Forests

A nation's economy benefits greatly from the forest industry. Increased demand for fuel wood due to population growth, as well as an increase in the area covered by industries and urban development, have resulted in overexploitation of forests. On a global scale, we are currently losing forest at a rate of 1.7 million hectares per year. Overgrazing and the conversion of forests into pastures for domestic use are other causes of overexploitation.

28.3.2.2 Deforestation

Deforestation is caused by developing and growing cities, harvesting wood and timber, clearing land for agriculture, and burning or cutting down forests (Figure 28.3). While the long-term effects of deforestation are irreversible, these economic

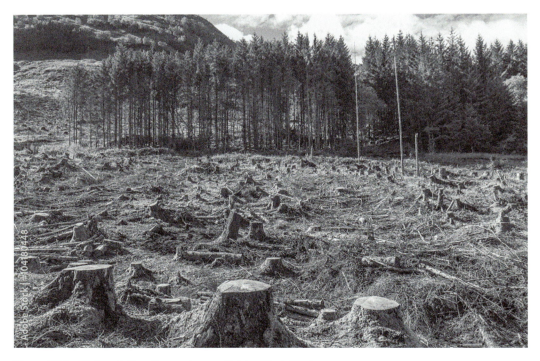

Figure 28.3 Deforestation. *Source:* lowsun/Adobe Stock Photos.

gains are only temporary. Compared to tropical areas, temperate countries have a lower rate of deforestation. If the current rate of deforestation continues, 90% of tropical forests could be lost within the next 60 years. Only 20.6% of India is covered in forests, whereas 33% is needed for ecological balance.

28.3.2.2.1 Causes of Deforestation

Some developed areas have seen an increase in forest area. However, the area covered by forests in developing nations is trending downward, especially in the tropical region. The principal causes of deforestation are:

- shifting cultivation
- commercial logging
- agribusiness expansion
- development projects and increasing food requirements
- wood for fuel
- raw materials for industrial use.

28.3.2.2.2 Major Effects of Deforestation

The environment and other living things are negatively affected and damaged directly by deforestation. The principal reasons for deforestation are:

- soil erosion
- loss of soil fertility
- decrease of rain fall due to effects on the hydrological cycle
- expansion of deserts
- depletion of water table
- loss of biodiversity, flora, and fauna
- environmental changes
- climate change
- disturbance in forest ecosystems.

28.4 Mineral Resources

Minerals are nonrenewable natural resources. They exist naturally as organic, crystalline solids with physical properties. There are thousands of different minerals in the world. The minerals that people use on a daily basis for a variety of purposes heavily influence a nation's economy. About 74 million metric tonnes of iron and steel are extracted worldwide annually. As a result of industrialization and population growth, minerals are exploited. Environmental problems arise when mineral exploitation is pursued by humans in an unscientific manner.

28.4.1 Uses

- Generation of energy using coal, lignite, and uranium.
- Construction, settlements, and housing.
- Ayurvedic medical system.
- Agriculture – fertilizers, seed dressing, and fungicides.
- Weapons and armaments.
- Transportation.
- Development of industrial plants and machinery.
- Communication – telephone wires, cables, and electronic devices.
- Alloys, jewelry (gold, platinum, silver, and diamond).

28.4.2 Abuses

Placer mining, underground mining (for coal seams), and open-cast mining (which removes waste materials from above the mineral-bearing strata before extracting the minerals) have all been used to extract minerals.

28.4.3 Environmental Impact

The mining industry creates the world's largest environmental disaster zones. Each mining stage generates a large amount of waste minerals, which adds to the pollution. Minerals are exploited carelessly, which harms the environment. Water pollution occurs when loose waste from landfills close to water sources is washed. Coal washing operations and mine drainage are additional causes of water pollution. The water surface is contaminated by acid mines. Air pollution is caused by the atmospheric release of toxic gases like carbon monoxide (CO), nitrogen dioxide (NO_2), and sulfur dioxide (SO_2). As soon as they are released into the atmosphere, hydrocarbons, suspended particulate matter, silicon (Si), fluoride (FL), asbestos, and metallic dust damage vegetation and present health risks. Noise pollution is caused by blasting and heavy machinery use. Cutting down trees and soil erosion both occur. Minerals can cause illnesses like silicosis, fluorosis, and asbestosis.

28.4.4 Remedial Measures

Environmentally responsible mining methods are required. Microbes must be utilized in the leaching procedure in order to utilize low-grade ores. Gold-containing iron sulfide ore is extracted using bacteria and *Acidithiobacillus ferrooxidans*. Some bacterial strains can also remove impurities from ore. Growing vegetation in mined areas helps to prevent the release of toxic drainage, which can lessen the adverse effects on the environment.

28.5 Soil Resources

The most limited and priceless resource on which we rely for our daily needs is soil. So we should do everything possible to protect it. India's total area is 328.73 mha, of which 264.5 mha are potential areas for soil resources. Land degradation caused by water scarcity, wind erosion, salinity, alkalinity, and water logging has affected about 187.8 mha. Soil is a thin covering over the land containing organic materials, living organisms, air, and water. Soil is a renewable source but it is regenerated at a very slow rate, i.e., 2.5 cm soil in 200–1000 years. Soil becomes a nonrenewable resource when the rate of erosion is faster than the rate of renewal.

28.5.1 Abuses

Due to rapid population growth, there is an increase in demand for scarce land resources, which are vulnerable to degradation. Natural, human-induced, or anthropogenic activities cause land degradation. Desertification, landslides, volcanoes, earthquakes, floods, and droughts are examples of natural causes. Deforestation, mining, excessive irrigation, building of dams, and increased fertilizer use are all human-made causes. The devastation caused by the floods in Mumbai and Tamil Nadu in November 2005 may have been caused by an increase in greenhouse gases and global temperatures. The average annual rate of land erosion is 20–100 times greater than the rate of renewal. Some of the main reasons for this are human-induced landslides, slopes overirrigated for farming, surface water being directed onto sensitive slopes, forest fires and tree cutting on the slopes, work being done on the slopes, mining, building of roads and railways, the construction of dams and reservoirs, and hydroelectric projects.

28.5.1.1 Soil Erosion

Soil fertility is lost when top soil is moved from one location to another. Asia and Africa account for two-thirds of degraded lands worldwide. Normal soil erosion occurs due to natural processes, and overgrazing, deforestation, and mining can accelerate erosion (Figures 28.4 and 28.5).

Soil erosive forces come in two different varieties. Water and wind are the first climatic agents, while overgrazing damages soil by 35%, mining, and deforestation by 30%, and unscientific farming practices by 28%.

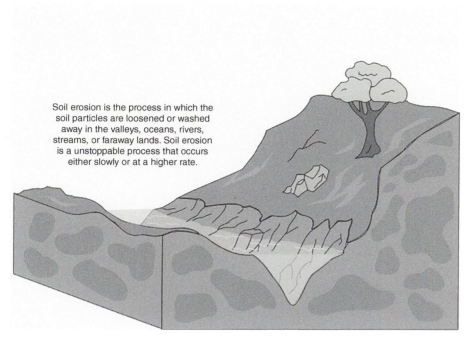

Figure 28.4 What is soil erosion?

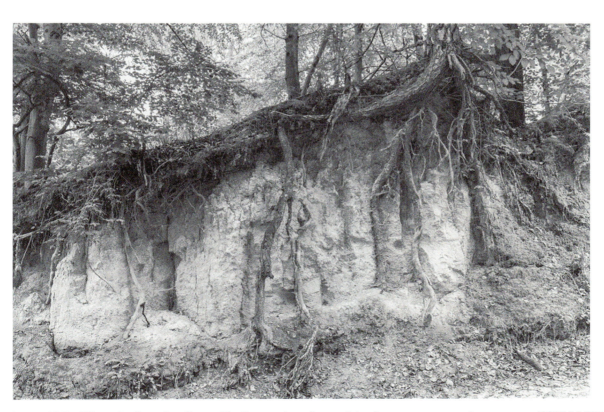

Figure 28.5 Effect of soil erosion. *Source:* The Permaculture Research Institute. www.permaculturenews.org/2017/10/23/soil-erosion-monetary-cost/ (accessed December 28 2023).

28.5.1.2 Desertification

Desertification can range in severity from mild (10–25% productivity drop) to severe (25–50% drop) to extremely severe (more than 50% drop). Overgrazing, deforestation, surface mining, quarrying, unscientific farming, overcultivation, low rainfall, drought, and global warming are the main causes of desertification.

28.6 Water Resources

The essence of life is water. It is a natural resource that is both renewable and necessary. Earth's water is 1.4 billion cubic kilometers in volume, with 93% of that being ocean water, 4.1% being fresh water on land, 0.2% being glaciers, and 0.0001% being air humidity. There are 8 million cubic kilometers of underground water. Water covers 97% of the Earth's surface in total; the Earth would be two feet under water if it were flat. Humans need about 1% of the world's water. The percentage of water in plants and animals' bodies ranges from 60% to 65%. Seventy-seven percent of the total amount of rain falls on the sea, while only 23% falls on land; 84% of water vapor rises from the surface of the sea, compared to 16% from land.

28.6.1 Uses

Nearly all human development activities, including drinking, irrigation, washing, transportation, industrial waste disposal, and coolant for thermal power plants, involve the use of water. The Earth's surface is shaped by water, which also controls the climate. In the entire world, 70% of water is used for agriculture (93% in India and 4% in Kuwait), and 25% is used for industries (70% in Europe and 5% in less developed nations). In the USA, a family of four uses $1000\,\mathrm{m}^3$ of water annually per person, which is significantly more than what is used in developing nations.

28.6.2 Abuses

Due to overpopulation, humans overuse surface water. With very little water, 41% of the world's population (2.4 billion) endures drought. In 2025, this figure will reach 48% (3.5 billion), and by 2050, it will be 9 billion. The amount of groundwater being withdrawn exceeds its level of recharge. As a result, the sediments in aquifers become more compact and the land surface below sinks, causing damage to buildings, pipe fractures, the reversal of sewer canal flows, and tidal flow. Due to groundwater mining, the water table is lowered and seawater intrusion occurs. Brackish water irrigation raises the water table, which can cause salinity and waterlogging issues. Therefore, farming operations will suffer.

28.7 The Importance of Natural Resources

For a variety of reasons, natural resources are very important to human societies. Here are a few main justifications for the significance of natural resources.

28.7.1 Economic Importance

Numerous natural resources are necessary for economic growth. Minerals and fossil fuels, for instance, are essential to industry and transportation, and wood is necessary for the creation of furniture and buildings. Natural resources used to grow crops, like water and fertile soil, are also essential to agriculture. Energy is also produced using natural resources. For example, while fossil fuels are burned to create electricity, clean energy is produced by capturing wind and solar energy.

28.7.2 Environmental Importance

Natural resources play a crucial role in preserving ecosystem balance and supplying habitat for wildlife. For example, forests support a variety of plant and animal species and also help to control the climate and stop soil erosion. Natural resources can be a source of income for a large number of people. For example, forestry and fishing support many communities worldwide through employment and income.

28.7.3 Cultural Importance

For many societies, natural resources also have cultural significance. Indigenous cultures, for example, frequently have a strong bond with the land and depend on natural resources for their way of life. Natural resources play a critical role in sustaining life on Earth, and we must ensure that we safeguard the environment while also allowing it to regenerate itself naturally.

28.8 Threats to Natural Resources

Because natural resources are abundant and unrestricted in the environment, people indiscriminately overuse them, which causes them to become depleted. The following are some serious threats to natural resources.

28.8.1 Overpopulation

More land and forest areas are being cleared, which is destroying the natural vegetation and farms because there are more mouths to feed and people to house. Because of the sharp increase in demand for wood and wood-based goods, forests are being cleared.

28.8.2 Climate Change

Biodiversity and many other abiotic natural resources are being negatively impacted by climate change brought on by excessive human activity. Others will be forced to move to more advantageous environments in order to survive, while species that have become accustomed to their surroundings may perish.

28.8.3 Environmental Pollution

The habitats and health of all living things are directly impacted by air, water, and land pollution. Pollution has an impact on all types of natural phenomena, including soils, rocks, lands, ocean water, fresh water, underground water, and more. It frequently has negative outcomes.

28.9 Conservation of Natural Resources

Natural resources are vital to human survival but not all of them are renewable, making conservation extremely important. Human activity, particularly the use of nonrenewable resources like fossil fuels, is to blame for the dramatic increase in climate change. We can influence our natural environment more favorably if we conserve our natural resources. We can conserve natural resources in our own homes in the following ways.

- *Use less water*: cutting down on the length of showers and turning off the faucets when not in use can help to save water.
- *Turn off the lights*: when not in use, turn off all electronics. LED light bulbs can also be used because they use a very small amount of power.
- *Long-distance vehicle sharing*, biking, and walking all contribute to fuel savings.
- *Use renewable energy*: using solar, wind, and hydroelectric energy can greatly reduce our reliance on fossil fuels and slow the gradual depletion of resources.
- *Use the three Rs* – reduce, reuse, and recycle (Figure 28.6).
- *Compost*: by composting leftover fruit and vegetable scraps, the soil can be enriched. By attracting beneficial organisms, composting reduces the need for pesticides and other dangerous chemicals.
- *Refrain from using plastics* because they are nonbiodegradable waste that pollutes the environment much more quickly.

All these strategies can only be effective if people are aware of them and willing to help protect the environment and natural resources.

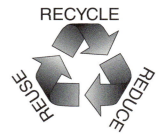

Figure 28.6 Three Rs to conserve natural resources. *Source:* Jemastock/Shutterstock.

Further Reading

Brady, R.L. and Weil, R.R. (1999). *The Nature and Properties of Soils*, 13e. London: Pearson Education.

Gadgil, M. and Guha, R. (1993). *This Fissured Land: An Ecological History of India*. Berkeley: University of California Press.

Kapur, S., Eswaran, H., and Blum, W.E.H. (2011). *Sustainable Land Management*. Singapore: Springer.

Kaushik, A. and Kaushik, C.P. (2018). *Perspectives in Environmental Studies*. New Delhi: New Age International.

Manahan, S. (1999). *Environmental Chemistry*. New York: McGraw Hill.

Odum, E.P. (1959). *Fundamentals of Ecology*. Philadelphia: W.B. Saunders.

O'Riordan, T. and Stoll-Kleemann, S. (2002). *Biodiversity, Sustainability and Human Communities: Protecting beyond the Protected*. Cambridge: Cambridge University Press.

Ramakrishnan, P.S. (2014). *The Cultural Cradle of Biodiversity*. India: National Book Trust.

Schmitz, O.J. (2007). *Ecology and Ecosystem Conservation*. Washington, DC: Island Press.

Sharma, P.D. (2018). *Fundamentals of Ecology*. Meerut: Rastogi Publications.

Singh, J.S., Singh, S.P., and Gupta, S.R. (2017). *Ecology, Environmental Science and Conservation*. New Delhi: S. Chand Publishing.

White, R.E. (2006). *Principles and Practices of Soil Science*. Oxford: Blackwell Publishing.

29

Epidemiology and Environmental Health in Veterinary Medicine

J. Jyothi[1] and M. Bhavya Sree[2]

[1] *Department of Veterinary Medicine, P.V. Narasimha Rao Telangana Veterinary University, Hyderabad, India*
[2] *P.V. Narasimha Rao Telangana Veterinary University, Hyderabad, India*

29.1 Introduction

The primary role of a veterinarian in the arena of epidemiology and environmental health is to provide law enforcement officials, judges, and jury members with the information necessary to make a decision regarding a case associated with offenses against animals.

To prevent the introduction of foreign diseases, veterinarians are employed by state and federal regulatory agencies to quarantine and inspect animals brought into the country. They supervise international and interstate shipments of animals; test for diseases that could threaten animal and human health or the food supply; and manage campaigns to prevent and eradicate diseases, such as tuberculosis and rabies, that pose threats to animal and human health.

Veterinarians serve as epidemiologists in city, county, state, and federal agencies, investigating animal and human disease outbreaks such as food-borne illnesses, influenza, and rabies. They help to ensure the safety of food-processing plants, restaurants, and water supplies.

Urbanization, globalization, and terrorism have brought the need for a stronger, larger, more diverse, and more competent public health workforce to the forefront of public planning (Pappaioanou 2004). A growing number of medical issues are arising from increasing human–wildlife contact, environmental changes, expansion of international travel, antimicrobial misuse, intensification and integration of food production, and growth of the immunocompromised population (World Health Organization 1999). Veterinarians have training that gives them a unique capacity to address public health issues and to help meet public health needs.

On completion of their clinical training, veterinarians take an oath that states: "I solemnly swear to use my scientific knowledge and skills for the benefit of society through . . . the promotion of public health and the advancement of medical knowledge" (American Veterinary Medical Association 1999).

Although veterinary medicine and environmental public health have long had many competencies, practices, and accomplishments in common, it may be useful to reintroduce this important emerging professional partnership.

Veterinary medicine is "real medicine." Schooling consists of a rigorous four-year postbaccalaureate program of medical and surgical training. After successfully passing a national examination, veterinarians in the United States can become licensed to practice on all but human animal species.

Veterinarians are among the few clinicians whose success requires both a solid understanding of the importance of diagnosing and treating the "whole" animal and a thorough application of herd/population health principles and preventive medicine.

Like their physician colleagues, many veterinarians also complete an internship/residency or advanced training that leads to board certification in one or more of the 20 veterinary specialties.

One specialty organization may be of particular interest for the environmental health practice community: the American College of Veterinary Preventive Medicine requires demonstrated proficiency in the public health domains of epidemiology and biostatistics, food safety, infectious and parasitic diseases, environmental health and toxicology, and public administration and health education.

Epidemiology and Environmental Hygiene in Veterinary Public Health, First Edition. Edited by Tanmoy Rana.
© 2025 John Wiley & Sons, Inc. Published 2025 by John Wiley & Sons, Inc.

29 Epidemiology and Environmental Health in Veterinary Medicine

A recent World Health Organization (WHO) technical report defined veterinary public health as "the sum of all contributions to the physical, mental, and social well-being of humans through an understanding and application of veterinary science" (World Health Organization 2002, p. 4). This definition establishes the context – protection and improvement of human health – in which veterinarians make their contribution. It also describes how those who apply the scientific principles of veterinary medicine are part of a core public health practice activity with global impact. There is an explicit understanding that "veterinary public health activities must be carried out in close partnership with other public health efforts to ensure positive health outcomes" (World Health Organization 2002, p. 4).

29.2 Veterinarians in the Current Practice of Public Health

Veterinarians serve many public health roles. Although veterinarians are estimated to make up less than 1% of the public health workforce (Gebbie 2000), recent educational and policy influences have renewed interest in increasing the numbers of veterinary professionals in public health.

Because veterinarians work at the interface of human, animal, and environmental health, they are uniquely positioned to view health through the lens of public health impact. Changes in land use, creation and operation of large terrestrial and marine food production units, and microbial and chemical pollution of land and water sources have created new threats to the health of both animals and humans (Zinsstag et al. 2005).

The intensive responses to the intentional release of anthrax, the periodic contamination of seafood production beds, the spread of West Nile virus, the importation of monkeypox, the widely publicized occurrence of large food-borne disease outbreaks, and the threat of pandemic influenza and COVID-19 all serve as recent models illustrating the impact and burden of disease on the resources of public health infrastructure (Kahn 2006; King 2006).

The need for integrated animal and human health surveillance, diagnostic laboratory systems, and delivery of effective health interventions among animal, human, and public health professions has never been more central (Figure 29.1).

Veterinarians are turning to environmental health scientists and practitioners to develop their understanding that many outbreaks and public health emergencies are failures of veterinary prevention infrastructure. It has been demonstrated that

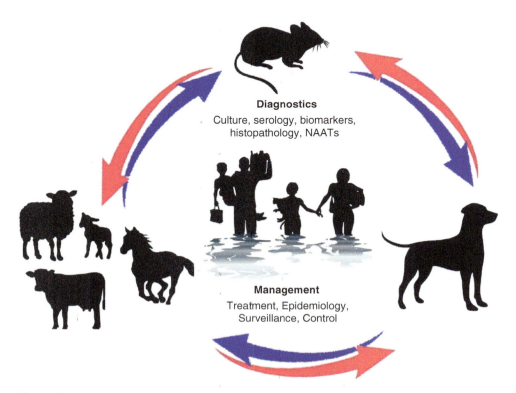

Figure 29.1 Integrated systems for monitoring the health of humans and animals.

the professions can work together to investigate the environmental antecedents that lead to adverse health outcomes (Cassady et al. 2006).

By strengthening epidemiological and laboratory investigations that assess the role of environmental influences, this partnership can help to develop and apply sustainable and effective community health interventions. With their understanding of biological interactions and clinical experience, as well as their roots in preventive medicine, veterinarians are ideal environmental health service partners.

As the profession broadens the perception of what a veterinarian can do, the phrase "one world – one medicine" may signify the acceptance that veterinary medicine is also a human health activity (Figure 29.2). Together with their partners in health protection and promotion, veterinarians can improve public health practice with a renewed focus on the complex interactions that affect environmental, animal, and human health.

Humans live in close association with their pets and other animals (e.g., local wildlife and farm animals). Veterinary epidemiology, like human epidemiology, looks at the association between adverse effects and a selected potential cause of interest, such as exposure to a chemical or a disease agent.

For example, veterinary epidemiology can play a key role in emerging and global disease outbreaks, helping in the understanding and prevention of infections and other emerging diseases, including those transmitted from an animal to other animals, and those possibly transmitted from animals to humans (Figure 29.3).

One example of a veterinary epidemiological study investigated the transmission of *Salmonella typhimurium* from cattle that had received no growth-promoting antibiotics to humans who had direct contact with the sick animals. Other examples are severe acute respiratory syndrome (SARS) and COVID-19. In the investigation of the origins of the SARS outbreak in China, viruses associated with SARS were isolated from Himalayan palm civets found in a live-animal market in Guangdong, China, and evidence of virus infection was also detected in other animals and humans working at the same market. The detection of these viruses in small, live wild mammals in a retail market helped identify at least one means of interspecies transmission: infected animals sold in that market to human customers.

The environment is an important element of the common health of all living organisms, and humans as part of that community benefit from the purity of the soil, water, and air of their habitats. Human communities are also responsible for utilizing natural resources in an environmentally sustainable way.

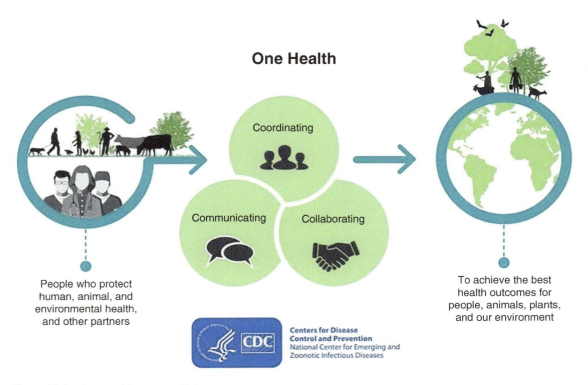

Figure 29.2 One world – one medicine.

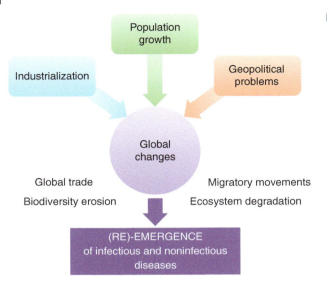

Figure 29.3 Drivers of reemerging diseases.

From among our research themes, the molecular epidemiology and environmental virology of zoonoses, or infectious diseases spread through interaction between different species, explores the traits and routes of transmission of microbes that cause diseases in humans and occur in the environment.

Water is a key route for microbial exposure, and our water-related research is aimed at developing techniques for identifying contamination in water resources and ensuring the quality of water. In terms of antimicrobial resistance, our research focuses on the development of resistance against pharmaceutical agents in microbes and looks into the role of the environment, humans, and animals in the creation and spread of antimicrobial resistance.

Our research in environmental toxicology focuses particularly on the mechanisms of action of dioxins, which supports the risk assessment of dioxins and similar chemicals. Our research is aimed at improving the prevention and control of adverse health effects in humans caused by a range of environmental exposure factors.

Through research, we strive to respond to the topical demand for knowledge pertaining to environmental health, supporting decision making in environmental healthcare. We also investigate control measures employed in environmental healthcare and assess their impact.

The selection of our research topics is guided by the goal of supplementing official activities with the help of research that supports decision making. In order to realize our principle of applying research-based knowledge in decision making, we work closely with various expert and research institutions as well as the authorities.

References

American Veterinary Medical Association (1999). Veterinarian's oath. www.avma.org/resources-tools/avma-policies/veterinarians-oath (accessed 5 February 2024).

Cassady, J., Higgins, C., Mainzer, H. et al. (2006). Beyond compliance: environmental health problem solving, interagency collaboration, and risk assessment to prevent waterborne disease outbreaks. *Journal of Epidemiology and Community Health* 60: 672–674.

Gebbie, K. (2000). *The Public Health Workforce Enumeration 2000*. New York: Center for Health Policy, Columbia School of Nursing.

Kahn, L.H. (2006). Confronting zoonoses, linking human and veterinary medicine. *Emerging Infectious Diseases* 12: 556–561.

King, L. (2006). Veterinary medicine and public health at CDC. *Morbidity and Mortality Weekly Report* 55 (Suppl. 2): 7–9.

Pappaioanou, M. (2004). Veterinary medicine protecting and promoting the public's health and well-being. *Preventive Veterinary Medicine* 62: 153–163.

World Health Organization (1999). Veterinary medicine in public health. *Weekly Epidemiological Record* 19: 154–156.

World Health Organization Study Group on Future Trends in Veterinary Public Health (2002). *Future Trends In Veterinary Public Health: Report of a WHO study group*. Teramo, Italy: World Health Organization.

Zinsstag, J., Schelling, E., Wyss, K., and Mahamat, M.B. (2005). Potential of cooperation between human and animal health to strengthen health systems. *Lancet* 336: 1242–1245.

30

Precision Livestock Farming and Its Advantage to the Environment

Amitava Roy[1] and Tanmoy Rana[2]

[1] *Department of Livestock Farm Complex, West Bengal University of Animal & Fishery Sciences, Kolkata, India*
[2] *Department of Veterinary Clinical Complex, West Bengal University of Animal & Fishery Sciences, Kolkata, India*

30.1 Introduction

Profitable cattle production depends heavily on effective information management (Thysen 2000). Through the use of cutting-edge information and communication technologies (ICT), targeted resource use, and exact control of production process, precision livestock farming (PLF) aims to increase production efficiency while also enhancing animal and human welfare (Cumby and Phillips 2001). In order to allow more efficient technology transfer between scientific and commercial groups, the major goal of this chapter is to briefly cover the state of the art in science today and, more crucially, the commercialization aspects of PLF technologies. By doing this, we hope that PLF will become more than just "the engineers' day-dream" and fulfill earlier writers' predictions that it will be the "animals' friend and the farmers' panacea" (Wathes et al. 2008).

30.2 Scientific Problem

30.2.1 Scientific Theories and PLF Principles

Precision farming has the potential to boost animal and human welfare while increasing production efficiency and cost reduction (Banhazi et al. 2011) through the adoption of electronic data collecting, processing, and application. Livestock managers currently have access to a wealth of knowledge but most of it is not organized in a way that makes it easy to use. For instance, a survey of farmers in southern Australia who were raising cattle on grasslands revealed that over 400 pieces of information might be pertinent for their operations. Numerous sources, including academic institutions, government advisors, producer periodicals, media outlets, technical consultants, and other producers, provide the information. As a result, farm managers frequently ignore many other areas that are as important to boosting productivity and profitability in favor of adopting practices in those areas where they are most interested or where they feel they have the most experience.

Thus, it is important to create a management system that ensures that only the most crucial processes are carried out, that they are all executed accurately and consistently, and that risk is managed. A system like this, based on the Hazard Analysis Critical Control Point (HACCP) method, was created for Australian grazing beef operations and serves as a model for other animal industries (Black and Scott 2002). The following are the guiding principles of the system:

1) Determine which procedures really have a big impact on sustainability, profitability, or productivity. These include procedures that, if not followed correctly, will significantly affect the viability of the business. These procedures ought to include all parts of the firm, from strategic planning for the organizational structure to all facets of production to product sales. It is crucial to limit the number of "essential processes" to just those that, if done incorrectly, will have a significant effect on the organization. All must be administered consistently throughout time, thus the number must be manageable. Only 29 procedures were deemed to be absolutely necessary for maximizing profitability and sustainability across the entire enterprise in the example with grazing beef farms in southern Australia.

Epidemiology and Environmental Hygiene in Veterinary Public Health, First Edition. Edited by Tanmoy Rana.
© 2025 John Wiley & Sons, Inc. Published 2025 by John Wiley & Sons, Inc.

2) Determine the farm or market variables that need to be measured for each critical process in order to make sure it is being done appropriately. Establish the minimum and maximum values for each variable as well as the frequency at which each measurement must be conducted in order to keep the process under control and ensure that it consistently operates within the ideal range.

3) When measurements fall outside specified ranges, take the most advantageous preplanned remedial action. The manager's stress level is significantly reduced by having planned actions when measurement limits are violated because the plan of action, when to implement it, and repercussions are already known. Budgets, whether partial or comprehensive, are a crucial tool for determining the most economically sound course of action.

4) Establish Standard Operating Procedures (SOPs) for each vital process for each particular firm to guarantee that, under typical conditions, the measured values will stay within the predetermined boundaries. Such a procedure means that the manager can "go on leave" confident that all essential business operations will be monitored and accurately carried out by workers. It is important to have both high-level (year calendar and daily actions) and low-level (how to complete a given activity) procedures.

5) Give the workers the tools they need to take the appropriate measures, evaluate the results, and choose the best course of remedial action. These resources must be included in any adoption package. Additionally, staff training using these tools is required.

One of the main causes of the failure of systems like the one described above is the fact that humans have a tendency to grow lax with the implementation of repetitive duties. One strategy for solving this issue is to record measurements and have others check their work. Finding and keeping qualified, motivated employees is a challenge for many rural sectors in industrialized nations. Well-designed adoption programs frequently fail due to a lack of competent workers.

The primary responsibility of PLF is to streamline the data collection, processing, and analysis processes so that the farm manager is presented with solutions rather than issues (Lehr 2011a). The automated measurement, interpretation, and management of these processes will become increasingly important to the application of the described procedure for adopting core enterprise operations. Automation of all measuring systems, interpretation of the readings, detection of important measurement limit breaches, and integrated automatic control systems for each operation to bring it back within allowable limits should all be part of the method.

The global steel business is a prime example of the kind of change required within the animal industries. In contrast to the 1950s, when all tasks were carried out by humans, the entire process is now controlled electronically, and practically all manual job tasks are mechanized and centrally monitored. This is PLF's ideal world, where the use of electronic measurement, interpretation, and control systems achieves the highest levels of animal welfare, environmental sustainability, production, and financial success.

30.2.2 Including Traceability in PLF

Traceability in livestock management has primarily been used for applications that facilitate movement and disease control, such as the European passport system for cattle, the Australian PigPass, and the movement permission across state/provincial borders in Malaysia and Vietnam. Almost no effort has been made to maximize the financial advantages that traceability can provide for cattle operations. The availability of simple, low-cost automated identification systems, the overemphasis on privacy issues related to data collected on-farm, the inconsistent availability of traceability products to farmers, and the overemphasis on specific numbering technologies (simple numbering, barcodes, RFID) are a few of the objective reasons why the integration of traceability and PLF has not advanced further.

The interchange of information along the feed–animal–food cycle is, in our opinion, the most intriguing example of the integration of traceability with PLF. One benefit of this information exchange is that if feed and feed input suppliers have access to slaughterhouse information resulting from the feeding profiles used on the farm, they can significantly enhance the composition of their goods. Additionally, farms can utilize such a system to choose the best feed (or feed supplier). Abattoirs can utilize the system as a foundation for cooperation with farms to produce and source more animals that meet weight and conformation specifications; they can also use the statistics of other farms in the network to optimize their feed consumption/intake. Industry statistics are a crucial instrument for guiding the sector for both governments and the industry itself. Political decision making, benchmarking, lobbying, and business decision making all benefit from the use of reliable statistics.

30.2.3 Technical and Scientific Advancements

The majority of the early PLF developments were started in Europe (EU) or the UK. Researchers at the Silsoe Research Institute in the UK and Leuven University in Belgium were early proponents of the PLF concept. Other EU nations, including Germany, Denmark, the Netherlands, Finland, and the Volcani Research Centre in Israel, saw additional breakthroughs (Halachmi et al. 1998).

Scientists from the UK and Belgium helped Australian PLF projects get off the ground in 2002 (Banhazi et al. 2007). Researchers at the University of Southern Queensland created PLF applications for the beef industry, whereas scientists in South Australia were responsible for the majority of PLF developments relating to the pig industry (Banhazi et al. 2007). Virtual fence methods were thoroughly studied by CSIRO researchers (Umstatter 2011).

Recent advancements in communication technology – including those related to mobile phones, telecommunications, and the internet – offer a significant potential advantage to the creation, use, and worth of PLF. While some clients may prefer independent programs on specific farms, there are several benefits to centralizing data collection, processing, management, and reporting. For processing, storing, and reporting purposes, data gathered by sensors on the farm, for instance, can be transmitted to a central location. This might result in significant time savings for farm managers, which they could use for other, more fruitful responsibilities like those connected to farming and animal husbandry. Only the information necessary for the farm managers' daily needs should be sent to them by the centralized processing, with more in-depth reports made available as needed, such as, for example, the comparative performance of their units through the centralized database.

In summary, an effective PLF system should make its advantages clear to the user and, ideally, should lessen rather than increase the user's management workload (Lehr 2011b).

30.3 Commercial Concerns

30.3.1 Examples of Commercializing PLF Technologies and Their Guiding Principles

There are already a few examples of PLF approaches being commercialized in animal production. Use of robotics in dairying, monitoring water use, egg counting, bird weighing, improved environmental control in poultry houses, computerized feed systems, climate control, automated disease detection, growth measurement, and real-time production site data capture in piggeries are a few examples of commercial applications of PLF techniques (Guarino et al. 2008). Several nations, including Estonia, Denmark, Norway, the UK, Australia, Malaysia, Vietnam, and South Africa, have been investigated for evidence of PLF technologies in laying hens, pigs, dairy animals, and aquaculture fish used in a commercial setting as part of the EU-sponsored BrightAnimal project (Lehr 2011b). Generally speaking, there was little proof that commercial PLF products were being employed on farms. As might be predicted, farmers in technologically advanced nations like Estonia are more likely to embrace technology to improve their lives and lessen their reliance on expensive and difficult-to-find labor. Even so, there is very little technology being used, and important aspects of animal welfare or productivity are not frequently monitored in an automated manner.

The PLF commercialization principles must include the following: (i) verification of the benefits of the PLF technique being proposed; (ii) clear communication to customers of those verified benefits; (iii) identification of the principal beneficiaries (i.e., operator vs owner of the business); (iv) provision of appropriate training and technical support; and (v) proper system specification, installation, commissioning, and monitoring. Unfortunately, academic bodies have up until now mostly led PLF development efforts. In general, commercial companies are not sufficiently involved in the development of PLF technology. Collaboration between smaller specialized companies and bigger generalist corporations is prefered in order to improve the interest of relevant businesses in offering services to farmers. A vital step toward creating commercial PLF tools and products that are desired by customers and sold with confidence is the transfer of PLF technologies to businesses that supply and manage the systems.

30.3.2 Limiting Circumstances for Commercialization

Lack of reliable service options for farmers is the biggest issue with commercialization. Farmers are primarily biologists by nature and only occasionally technologists. A service sector is required to be able to: (i) maintain technological components; (ii) decipher sensor data; (iii) create and routinely transmit straightforward, pertinent advice to farmers; and

(iv) involve users in technological improvements. This service sector would need to employ appropriate business models to prevent farmers from incurring excessive initial investment expenses. Affordable monthly or annual fees, especially those connected to performance enhancements or animal sales, may be compatible with farmers' cash flow. Although farmers frequently invest a portion of their profits in technology, they normally prefer to purchase machinery rather than software or sensors.

For good reason, the food business is generally highly conservative. Despite being one of the biggest global sectors, it has very low profit margins and frequently produces fragile goods. Additionally, the agricultural sector is vulnerable due to its reliance on seasonal demand/supply cycles and meteorological variables. Furthermore, it can be quite challenging to determine the viability of a certain technology and "guesstimate" its advantages, especially for the more daring farmer. In other words, the precise cost–benefit information on PLF that takes into account the complexity of farmers' purchase decisions is a significant missing component. The commercialization process of these technologies depends on proving and demonstrating their economic, welfare, and environmental advantages.

The lack of coordination between researchers, developers, and technology providers is the other major barrier restricting the adoption of PLF technologies on farms. It is exceedingly challenging to improve coordination between PLF tool vendors and developers, yet doing so would lead to the creation of more effective integrated systems. The PLF systems would thereafter become more widely commercialized as integrated systems to better serve the farmers. A lot of PLF "products" were also taken straight from the lab to the farm rather than ever being "productized" (formed into a real "product"). Only a small number of bigger companies with sufficient development budgets have adopted PLF as their driving philosophy.

30.4 Precision Livestock Farming as a Facilitator of Progress: Potential Advantages and Implementation Drivers

It is improbable that PLF would completely transform the cattle industry in the next 10 years. However, sensors will be commonly used around animals in the next 5–10 years, which might allow farmers to efficiently monitor a number of useful indicators for all livestock species. This will make it possible to create and deploy a variety of new services on farms, including individual feeding, heat sensing, health monitoring, and animal localization. Mobile robots will start performing activities like milking outside as well as in sheds. The management of herds and meadows will be improved, and grazing operations' financial results will increase thanks to virtual fencing. In 10 years, the majority of farms in Europe will be computerized and employ software tools to manage their operations.

By adding factual information to the often very subjective (and even emotional) conversation process, PLF can significantly aid in fostering an objective debate on animal welfare. While PLF will not be able to answer every welfare-related enquiry, it will enable interested parties to identify instances of subpar animal care and take appropriate action.

Future GHG emissions will be significant, and PLF can help reduce them by detecting emissions and, if necessary, modifying feeding, temperature, and other factors that affect gas emissions (Frost et al. 2003). Farm businesses involved in the supply chain put a lot of effort into maintaining animals in the best possible conditions, reducing emissions, and offering the greatest livestock product at the most affordable price. PLF can help get these data to other players in the supply chain and, ultimately, to the consumer. It can help consumers make better decisions and serve as the foundation for various business models, such as selling meat according to its protein content, emitted GHG gases, food miles, or other ideas. The sharing of knowledge about the feed–animal–food chain holds enormous promise for increasing livestock productivity. Data on carcase composition could yield highly valuable information for feed producers. Farmers could optimize their feeding practices and select the feed supplier that offers the "best" feed for their livestock. The foundation for such an information exchange is traceability and PLF. If farm profitability in Europe keeps declining, perhaps retailers will start buying farms and demand data exchange along with the supply chain.

In this time, environmental control will significantly improve and most farmers will be aware of their GHG emissions. By capturing gases, modifying their feed, and better managing waste, they are working to cut their emissions, driven by consumers and merchants. PLF will play a part in feeding plans and may have a connection to gas and waste generation.

Precision livestock farming can help prevent the unlawful trade in animals and livestock-related products. Animal trafficking poses serious health and economic issues in nations like Malaysia. Fish banks are severely harmed by the billion dollar industry of illegal and unreported (IUU) fishing. If the information chain could react more quickly, misuse of the fish resource that is currently available may be considerably reduced.

30.5 Observations and Suggestions

- PLF's guiding principles are well known, and frequent PLF technology use could unquestionably help farms to manage their cattle more effectively.
- Traceability integration with PLF would be a good step forward and increase the value of PLF systems.
- Over the past few years, there have been a number of intriguing PLF innovations that have the potential to completely alter livestock management. The PLF/smart farming technologies (if properly implemented) could (i) enhance or at least objectively document the level of animal welfare on farms; (ii) reduce GHG emissions and improve the environmental performance of farms; (iii) lessen illegal product segmentation and facilitate better marketing of livestock products; and (iv) improve rural economy and stabilize rural populations.
- However, when it comes to commercial innovations, there are few instances of PLF technology commercialization, and there are few businesses that are actively engaged in the PLF commercialization process.
- As a result, in order to ensure the proper development and application of PLF products on farms, it is necessary to (i) establish a new service sector to handle the upkeep of hardware tools and the management of collected data; (ii) independently verify the benefits of PLF technologies under real-world farm conditions; and (iii) better coordinate the development and marketing efforts of various industrial and academic partners. It is necessary to enable the commercial sector's participation in the process of professional product development.

A "federation of PLF-focused companies" may also be established with the purpose of creating a "road map" that outlines the actions that must be performed to encourage the commercial adoption of PLF/smart farming technologies. Such a paper could be created as part of a PLF conference or meeting with a commercial focus and should be based on the results of a recently finished worldwide PLF project. Participants in PLF must also work with their local governments to obtain the public funding needed for verification investigations that are unlikely to be covered by private sector funding.

References

Banhazi, T., Dunn, M., and Black, J. (2007). *Development of Precision Livestock Farming (PLF) Technologies for the Australian Pig Industry 3rd European Precision Livestock Farming Conference*. Skiathos: University of Thessaly.

Banhazi, T.M., Tscharke, M., Ferdous, W.M. et al. (2011). Improved image analysis based system to reliably predict the live weight of pigs on farm: preliminary results. *Australian Journal of Multi-disciplinary Engineering* 8 (2): 107–119.

Black, J.L. and Scott, L. (2002). *More Beef from Pastures: Current Knowledge, Adoption and Research Opportunities*. Sydney: Meat and Livestock Australia.

Cumby T R and Phillips V R. (2001). Environmental impacts of livestock production. www.cambridge.org/core/journals/bsap-occasional-publication/article/abs/environmental-impacts-of-livestock-production/5B3AB0867BCCB83DED823435A4833340 (accessed 20 February 2024).

Frost, A.R., Parsons, D.J., Stacey, K.F. et al. (2003). Progress towards the development of an integrated management system for broiler chicken production. *Computers and Electronics in Agriculture* 39 (3): 227–240.

Guarino, M., Guarino, M., Jans, P. et al. (2008). Field test of algorithm for automatic cough detection in pig houses. *Computers and Electronics in Agriculture* 62 (1): 22–28.

Halachmi, I., Edan, Y., Maltz, E. et al. (1998). A real-time control system for individual dairy cow food intake. *Computers and Electronics in Agriculture* 20 (2): 131–144.

Lehr, H. (2011a). Food information management and advanced traceability. In: *Multidisciplinary Approach to Acceptable and Practical Precision Livestock Farming for SMEs in Europe and Worldwide* (ed. I.G. Smith and H. Lehr), 84–111. Halifax: European Commission.

Lehr, H. (2011b). General conclusions and recommendations. In: *Multidisciplinary Approach to Acceptable and Practical Precision Livestock Farming for SMEs in Europe and Worldwide* (ed. I.G. Smith and H. Lehr), 179–188. Halifax: European Commission.

Thysen, I. (2000). Agriculture in the information society. *Journal of Agricultural Engineering Research* 76 (3): 297–303.

Umstatter, C. (2011). The evolution of virtual fences: a review. *Computers and Electronics in Agriculture* 75 (1): 10–22.

Wathes, C.M., Kristensen, H.H., Aerts, J.M., and Berckmans, D. (2008). Is precision livestock farming an engineer's daydream or nightmare, an animal's friend or foe, and a farmer's panacea or pitfall? *Computers and Electronics in Agriculture* 64 (1): 2–10.

31

Biodiversity: Concept, Pattern, Importance, Threats, and Conservation

Jitendrakumar Nayak[1], Varun Asediya[2], Santanu Pal[3], and Pranav Anjaria[1]

[1] *College of Veterinary Science and Animal Husbandry, Kamdhenu University, Anand, India*
[2] *M.B. Veterinary College, Dungarpur, India*
[3] *ICAR – Indian Veterinary Research Institute, Izatnagar, Bareilly, India*

31.1 Introduction

Biodiversity, an intricately woven tapestry of life on our planet, stands as a testament to the grandeur of natural evolution. As the Anthropocene era reshapes the Earth's ecosystems, the symphony of life's diversity faces an unprecedented crescendo of challenges. In this chapter, we embark on an ambitious odyssey to unveil the multifaceted intricacies and ecological significance of biodiversity. We delve into genomics, exploring the nuances of genetic diversity within populations, while tracing the symmetrical patterns of species distributions across varied landscapes. Amidst these revelations, we confront the sobering realities of habitat loss, climatic upheavals, invasive disruptions, and the unsustainable depletion of our natural resources, each note threatening the harmonious composition of life.

However, amidst the profound exploration, glimmers of hope emerge from the horizon of knowledge. Novel frontiers in biodiversity research offer promising avenues for conservation efforts. Advancements in molecular ecology and genomics provide a key to unlock the hidden codes of life's resilience, while the convergence of cutting-edge technologies, including remote sensing and artificial intelligence (AI), opens vistas to comprehend and manage our dynamic ecosystems more adeptly. Equally indispensable is the recognition of the social and political dimensions of conservation, where inclusivity and international collaboration foster a shared responsibility to protect and preserve Earth's priceless heritage.

As this symphony of science and conservation unfolds, we hear a resounding call to action. It implores us, the stewards of our planet, to unite in concert, composing a sustainable future where the melodies of diverse lifeforms persist in eternal harmony. In this transformative symposium of exploration, wisdom, and dedication, we strive to preserve the ethereal beauty of biodiversity, safeguarding the enchanting richness of Earth's ecosystems for posterity.

31.2 Conceptualizing Biodiversity

31.2.1 Genetic Diversity: Unraveling Genomic Insights into Population Dynamics

Genetic diversity underpins the intricate tapestry of biodiversity, governing adaptation and evolutionary processes.

31.2.1.1 Genomic Approaches: From Single Nucleotide Polymorphisms to Metagenomics

Advancements in genomics have revolutionized our understanding of genetic diversity. High-resolution techniques, such as single nucleotide polymorphism (SNP) analysis, enable the detailed exploration of individual genotypes. Metagenomics provides unprecedented insights into the genetic diversity of entire ecosystems, particularly the microbial communities, and their significance in biodiversity dynamics (Exposito-Alonso et al. 2022; Alsammar et al. 2019; Maclot et al. 2020).

Epidemiology and Environmental Hygiene in Veterinary Public Health, First Edition. Edited by Tanmoy Rana.
© 2025 John Wiley & Sons, Inc. Published 2025 by John Wiley & Sons, Inc.

31.2.1.2 Population Genetics: Understanding Genetic Variation and Inbreeding

Population genetics offers powerful tools to study genetic variation within and among populations. Investigating population structure, gene flow, and the influence of genetic drift on the diversity of species deepens our comprehension of biodiversity patterns. Additionally, understanding the implications of inbreeding is crucial for assessing population viability and developing effective conservation strategies (Kardos et al. 2021; Johnston et al. 2019; Teixeira and Huber 2021).

31.2.1.3 Phylogenomics: Illuminating Evolutionary Relationships and Divergence Times

Phylogenomics, an integration of genomics and phylogenetics, provides a wealth of information about the evolutionary history of life. By analyzing entire genomes, we can reconstruct robust phylogenetic trees, uncover ancient species relationships, and estimate divergence times accurately. Phylogenomics offers invaluable insights for biodiversity conservation and sound management decisions (Evangelista et al. 2019; Dembo et al. 2016).

This exploration of genetic diversity enhances our understanding of biodiversity's fundamental mechanisms, guiding us in safeguarding the delicate fabric of life for a sustainable and biodiverse future.

31.2.2 Species Diversity: Integrating Taxonomy, Phylogenetics, and Functional Traits

Species diversity, a cornerstone of biodiversity, necessitates an integrative approach that merges taxonomy, phylogenetics, and functional traits.

31.2.2.1 Species Discovery and Delimitation: Challenges in the Era of Cryptic Diversity

Advancements in genetic and molecular techniques have revolutionized species discovery and delimitation (Rannala 2015; Cicero et al. 2021; Chua et al. 2023; Hillis et al. 2021). However, the existence of cryptic diversity presents challenges, where ostensibly similar species reveal substantial genetic and ecological disparities. The intricacies of detecting and characterizing cryptic species offer insights into biodiversity patterns and conservation implications (Marrone et al. 2023; Cháves-González et al. 2022).

31.2.2.2 Phylogenetic Diversity: Mapping Evolutionary Trees and Biogeographic Patterns

Phylogenetic diversity provides a powerful framework for comprehending species' evolutionary relationships. Robust phylogenetic trees yield insights into historical processes that have influenced contemporary biodiversity. Mapping phylogenetic patterns across geographic regions sheds light on biogeographic mechanisms, including speciation, dispersal, and extinction, revealing the drivers of species distribution and diversity gradients (Figure 31.1) (Hughes et al. 2022; Rosauer et al. 2009; Daru et al. 2020).

31.2.2.3 Functional Traits and Community Ecology: Linking Biodiversity to Ecosystem Functioning

Functional traits, representing the morphological, physiological, and ecological characteristics of species, exert a profound influence on community ecology and ecosystem functioning. The examination of functional diversity's impact on crucial ecological processes, such as nutrient cycling, productivity, and resilience, is essential for comprehending the connection between biodiversity and ecosystem functioning. This understanding plays a pivotal role in devising effective conservation and management strategies in an ever-changing world (de Bello et al. 2021; Carlucci et al. 2020; Hanisch et al. 2020; Sodré and Bozelli 2019).

This integration of taxonomy, phylogenetics, and functional traits empowers researchers to unveil the intricate patterns and processes of species diversity, a crucial endeavor for preserving the remarkable diversity of life on our planet.

31.2.3 Ecosystem Diversity: The Complex Web of Interactions in Diverse Habitats

Ecosystem diversity, encompassing the array of distinct habitats on Earth, provides critical insights into the interwoven relationships within ecological systems (Hoban et al. 2020; Gibb et al. 2020).

31.2.3.1 Ecosystem Typology: From Biomes to Biodiversity Hotspots

Understanding ecosystem diversity begins with classifying habitats into distinct typologies. From broad-scale biomes to localized biodiversity hotspots, unique characteristics and ecological processes define each ecosystem type. The factors that shape these habitats enrich our comprehension of global biodiversity patterns and aid in prioritizing conservation efforts (Mengist et al. 2022; Ntshanga et al. 2021; dos Santos et al. 2019; Grande et al. 2020; Snoeks et al. 2021; Mehring et al. 2020).

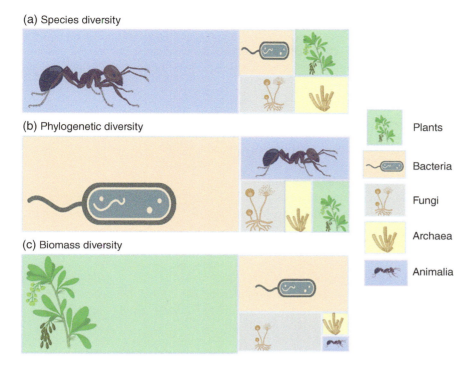

Figure 31.1 Distribution of global biodiversity in the major kingdoms of life through the metrics of (a) species diversity, (b) phylogenetic diversity, and (c) biomass diversity.

31.2.3.2 Trophic Interactions and Food Webs: Biodiversity's Influence on Stability

The dynamic interactions among species within food webs play a central role in shaping ecosystem stability and functioning. The complexity of trophic interactions, from predator–prey relationships to cascading effects on entire ecosystems, is explored. Understanding how biodiversity influences trophic dynamics is pivotal for predicting the consequences of species loss and ecosystem disruptions (Zhao et al. 2023; Rezende et al. 2021; Kohli et al. 2019; Scholl et al. 2023; Danet et al. 2021).

31.2.3.3 Functional Redundancy and Complementarity: Assessing the Importance of Species Roles

Ecosystems often host species that share similar functional traits, known as functional redundancy, or perform unique roles, termed functional complementarity. The significance of both redundancy and complementarity in maintaining ecosystem resilience and stability is explored. Unraveling the intricacies of species roles aids in recognizing key ecological players and informs effective conservation strategies (Streit et al. 2019; Akçakaya et al. 2020; Biggs et al. 2020).

By delving into the complexities of ecosystem diversity, valuable insights into the interconnectedness and functioning of diverse habitats are gained. This knowledge is instrumental in fostering ecological integrity and promoting the conservation of Earth's irreplaceable natural heritage.

31.3 Patterns of Biodiversity

31.3.1 Latitudinal Gradients Revisited: Unraveling Mechanisms Driving Global Patterns

Latitudinal gradients in biodiversity have long fascinated researchers, and this section delves into the underlying mechanisms that shape these global patterns (Zvereva and Kozlov 2021; Nishizawa et al. 2022; Veloy et al. 2022).

31.3.1.1 Historical Biogeography: Disentangling Past Climate and Geological Events

Examination of the historical biogeography of species distribution involves untangling the impacts of past climate fluctuations and geological events. Insights into the evolutionary history of taxa and their dispersal patterns shed light on how historical processes contribute to present-day biodiversity gradients (Wiens and Donoghue 2004; Díaz-Ruiz et al. 2023; Franklin 2023; Nakamura et al. 2023).

31.3.1.2 Contemporary Explanations: Integrating Niche Theory, Evolution, and Climate

Modern theories and frameworks provide complementary explanations for latitudinal biodiversity patterns. The integration of niche theory, evolutionary processes, and climate variables offers a comprehensive understanding of how these contemporary factors interact to influence species diversity along latitudinal gradients (Pau et al. 2011; Wake et al. 2009; Dormann et al. 2010; Carscadden et al. 2020).

31.3.2 Elevational Biodiversity Patterns: Understanding Complexity Across Altitudinal Zones

Elevational gradients offer unique ecological contexts for studying biodiversity patterns.

31.3.2.1 Biodiversity Across Elevational Gradients: Species Richness and Turnover

Species richness varies dramatically with altitude, leading to intriguing patterns of biodiversity across elevational gradients. Understanding the drivers of species turnover within these zones enhances comprehension of elevational biodiversity dynamics and its implications for ecosystem functioning (Albrecht et al. 2021; Fontana et al. 2020; Dzekashu et al. 2022; Cordeiro et al. 2023).

31.3.2.2 Biogeographical Drivers: Climate, Geology, and Topography

The intricate interplay of climate, geology, and topography significantly influences elevational biodiversity patterns (Figure 31.2). Unraveling the biogeographical drivers of species distributions offers valuable insights into the forces shaping diversity across mountainous landscapes (Hanz et al. 2022; Irl et al. 2015).

31.3.3 Temporal Biodiversity Dynamics: Insights from the Fossil Record to Modern Extinctions

31.3.3.1 Paleontological Perspectives: Biodiversity Changes Across Geological Time

Paleontological records provide a unique lens through which historical biodiversity dynamics can be observed. Studying past fluctuations in species diversity enhances the understanding of long-term ecological processes and informs conservation strategies for the future (Kiessling et al. 2023; Pimiento and Antonelli 2022; Rasmussen et al. 2023; López-Antoñanzas et al. 2022; DeMiguel et al. 2021; Saraswati 2022).

31.3.3.2 Historical Context: Lessons from Past Mass Extinctions and Their Relevance Today

Examining past mass extinctions offers essential lessons for addressing contemporary biodiversity crises. Understanding the consequences of past global perturbations can inform the urgency of conservation actions to mitigate ongoing threats to biodiversity (Ceballos et al. 2020; Cowie et al. 2022; Penn and Deutsch 2022).

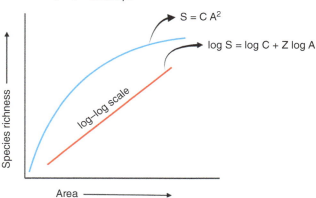

Figure 31.2 Diagram depicting linear species-area relationship on a log scale.

Where, S = Species richness
A = Area
Z = Slope of the line (regression coefficient)
C = Y − intercept

$S = C A^z$

$\log S = \log C + Z \log A$

Exploring the patterns of biodiversity across latitudinal, elevational, and temporal dimensions enhances our appreciation of the intricacies of life's distribution on Earth. This knowledge deepens the commitment to safeguard the incredible diversity of species and ecosystems for future generations.

31.4 The Ecological Significance of Biodiversity

31.4.1 Ecosystem Functioning: Synthesizing the Evidence from Biodiversity-Ecosystem Studies

31.4.1.1 Biodiversity-Ecosystem Functioning Experiments: Patterns and Mechanisms
Analyzing biodiversity-ecosystem functioning experiments provides valuable insights into the patterns and underlying mechanisms that govern the relationship between biodiversity and ecosystem processes. This examination enhances our understanding of how different biodiversity levels impact ecological functions and services (Eisenhauer et al. 2019; Wu et al. 2023a,b; Qiu and Cardinale 2020).

31.4.1.2 Role of Biodiversity in Nutrient Cycling, Productivity, and Resilience
Investigating the role of biodiversity in nutrient cycling, productivity, and ecosystem resilience allows us to appreciate the vital contributions of diverse species to ecosystem stability and functioning. Understanding these processes is pivotal for comprehending the consequences of biodiversity loss and its implications for ecological balance (Nelson et al. 2023; Venkatramanan and Shah 2019; González de Andrés 2019; Leal Filho et al. 2023; Paramesh et al. 2022).

31.4.2 Ecosystem Services and Biodiversity: Assessing Contributions to Human Well-being

31.4.2.1 Quantifying Ecosystem Services: Biodiversity's Role in Supporting Humanity
Quantifying the ecosystem services provided by biodiversity enables us to assess the tangible benefits that nature offers to human societies. This assessment aids in recognizing the significance of preserving biodiversity for the long-term sustenance of human well-being (Hardaker et al. 2022; Liu et al. 2022; Irwin et al. 2022).

31.4.2.2 Cultural Ecosystem Services: Exploring Nonmaterial Benefits of Biodiversity
Beyond tangible benefits, biodiversity enriches human lives through cultural ecosystem services, encompassing spiritual, esthetic, and recreational values. Acknowledging these nonmaterial benefits fosters a holistic understanding of the intricate relationship between biodiversity and human societies (Small et al. 2017; Dou et al. 2021; Anthem et al. 2016; Bieling and Plieninger 2013).

31.4.3 Biodiversity and Trophic Interactions: From Keystone Species to Trophic Cascades

Trophic interactions play a fundamental role in shaping ecosystem dynamics, and this section explores the significance of biodiversity in these ecological processes.

31.4.3.1 Top-down and Bottom-up Regulation: Understanding Trophic Control
Investigating top-down and bottom-up regulation illuminates how trophic interactions influence ecosystem structure and functioning. Understanding the role of key species and trophic cascades enhances our comprehension of the mechanisms by which biodiversity shapes ecological communities (Abdala-Roberts et al. 2019).

31.4.3.2 Impact of Biodiversity Loss on Ecosystem Stability and Resilience
Examining the consequences of biodiversity loss on ecosystem stability and resilience provides critical insights into the vulnerabilities and potential disruptions of ecological systems. Understanding the implications of such losses strengthens the case for conserving biodiversity to maintain ecological integrity. Appreciating the ecological significance of biodiversity through the lens of ecosystem functioning, services, and trophic interactions deepens our understanding of the indispensable role that biodiversity plays in maintaining the delicate balance of our planet's ecosystems (Van Meerbeek et al. 2021; Kéfi et al. 2019; White et al. 2020; Moreno-Mateos et al. 2020; Polazzo et al. 2023; Harvey et al. 2023).

31.5 Anthropogenic Threats to Biodiversity

31.5.1 Habitat Loss and Fragmentation: Evaluating Global and Local Impacts

Anthropogenic activities significantly contribute to habitat loss and fragmentation, posing substantial threats to biodiversity (Figure 31.3).

31.5.1.1 Land Use Change and Habitat Conversion: Identifying Priority Areas for Conservation
Assessing the impact of land use change and habitat conversion on biodiversity allows us to identify priority areas for conservation efforts. Understanding the drivers behind these changes is essential for effective land management and sustainable development practices (Li et al. 2022).

31.5.1.2 Edge Effects and Fragmentation: Implications for Biodiversity Dynamics
Fragmentation alters ecological processes at habitat edges, impacting biodiversity dynamics. Exploring the consequences of edge effects enhances our understanding of how fragmented landscapes influence species interactions and ecosystem functioning (Folharini et al. 2023).

31.5.2 Climate Change and Biodiversity: Assessing Vulnerabilities and Adaptation Strategies

Climate change poses significant challenges to biodiversity, necessitating careful evaluation and proactive responses.

31.5.2.1 Climate-induced Range Shifts: Implications for Species Survival and Biogeography
As climate change drives shifts in species' geographic ranges, understanding the implications for species survival and biogeographic patterns is crucial. Assessing the capacity for species to adapt and migrate informs conservation strategies in a changing climate (Carlson et al. 2022; Beyer et al. 2021; Román-Palacios and Wiens 2020).

31.5.2.2 Ocean Warming and Acidification: Understanding Effects on Marine Biodiversity
Ocean warming and acidification have far-reaching consequences for marine biodiversity. Evaluating the impacts on marine ecosystems and species assists in developing mitigation and adaptation measures for marine conservation (Pörtner 2008; Giddens et al. 2022; Baag and Mandal 2022).

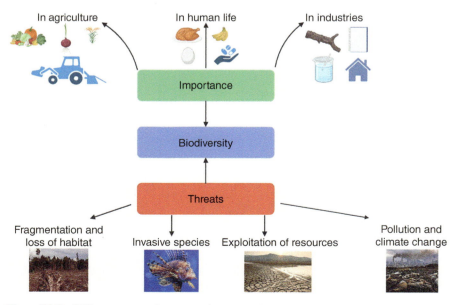

Figure 31.3 Different types of conservation strategies for biodiversity.

31.5.3 Biological Invasions and Global Trade: Managing the Spread of Alien Species

Biological invasions resulting from global trade pose a grave threat to native biodiversity and ecological stability.

31.5.3.1 Invasion Pathways and Hotspots: Preventing New Introductions
Identifying invasion pathways and hotspots helps prevent the introduction of new alien species. Robust biosecurity measures are essential in safeguarding native ecosystems from the harmful effects of invasive species (Meyerson et al. 2022; Nahrung et al. 2023).

31.5.3.2 Impacts of Invasive Species on Native Biodiversity and Ecosystems
Understanding the ecological impacts of invasive species on native biodiversity and ecosystems is critical for implementing effective management strategies and restoration efforts (Hulme 2020).

31.5.4 Overexploitation and Illegal Wildlife Trade: Implications for Fauna and Flora

Unsustainable exploitation and illegal wildlife trade are major contributors to biodiversity loss, requiring urgent attention (Mozer and Prost 2023; Uprety et al. 2021; Wyatt 2021; Hughes et al. 2023).

31.5.4.1 Unsustainable Harvesting: Identifying Threats to Endangered Species
Assessing the extent of unsustainable harvesting practices helps identify and prioritize actions to protect endangered species from overexploitation (Challender et al. 2023; Bolam et al. 2023; Hinsley et al. 2023).

31.5.4.2 Combating Wildlife Trafficking: Strengthening Conservation and Law Enforcement
Combating illegal wildlife trade demands strengthened conservation efforts and law enforcement to curb the illicit activities that threaten the survival of many species (Jiao et al. 2021; Cooney et al. 2017; Kurland et al. 2017).

Addressing these anthropogenic threats to biodiversity is imperative for preserving the rich tapestry of life on Earth. Through proactive measures and collaborative efforts, we can strive to ensure a sustainable future where biodiversity thrives and coexists harmoniously with human society.

31.6 Conservation Strategies: Toward a Sustainable Future

31.6.1 Protected Areas and Beyond: Advancing Conservation Design and Management

Efforts to achieve a sustainable future involve innovative approaches to conservation design and management, extending beyond protected areas (Laffoley et al. 2019; Zhang et al. 2022; Harris et al. 2022). Different types of conservation strategies for biodiversity can be seen in Figure 31.4.

31.6.1.1 Effectiveness of Protected Areas: Assessing Conservation Outcomes and Challenges
Evaluating the effectiveness of existing protected areas is vital in understanding their contribution to biodiversity conservation. Identifying conservation outcomes and addressing challenges will inform strategies to enhance their ecological impact (Gjerde and Rulska-Domino 2012; Sink et al. 2023).

31.6.1.2 Landscape-scale Conservation: Incorporating Connectivity and Multiple Land Uses
Expanding conservation efforts to a landscape-scale framework allows for the incorporation of connectivity and diverse land uses. Integrating conservation with sustainable land management practices fosters ecological resilience and ensures the long-term viability of ecosystems (Pitman et al. 2017; Rodrigues et al. 2022; Costanza and Terando 2019).

31.6.2 Biodiversity Offsets and Compensatory Mitigation: Evaluating Trade-offs and Effectiveness

In pursuit of a sustainable future, biodiversity offsets and compensatory mitigation offer potential solutions to balance conservation and development needs.

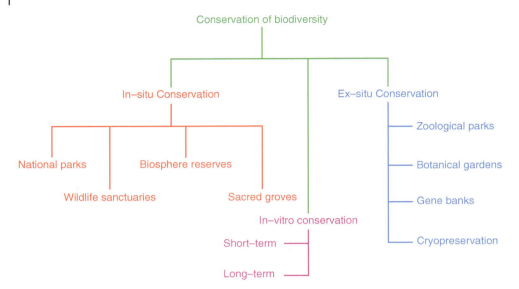

Figure 31.4 Diagram depicting the importance and threats of biodiversity. *Source:* Tired Earth. www.tiredearth.com/articles/what-are-the-main-types-of-habitat-loss (accessed December 28 2023)/dimakig/Shutterstock/piyaset/Adobe Stock Photos/24Novembers/Adobe Stock Photos.

31.6.2.1 Biodiversity Offset Policies: Balancing Conservation and Development Needs

Examining the effectiveness of biodiversity offset policies aids in striking a balance between conservation goals and development imperatives. Understanding trade-offs is essential for devising robust policies that safeguard biodiversity (Moilanen et al. 2020).

31.6.2.2 Improving Mitigation Strategies: Lessons from Successes and Failures

Learning from both successful and unsuccessful mitigation strategies provides valuable insights. Building upon lessons learned empowers us to develop more effective approaches to mitigate the impacts of development on biodiversity (Grimm and Köppel 2019; Bezombes et al. 2017; Accatino et al. 2018).

31.6.3 Integrating Biodiversity into Land Use Planning and Corporate Sustainability

Navigating the complex landscape of biodiversity integration within land use planning and corporate sustainability is akin to charting unexplored territory. Drawing insights from both triumphs and tribulations in mitigation strategies serves as our compass, guiding us towards innovative pathways for harmonizing development with biodiversity conservation. This section embarks on a journey through novel methodologies and real-world examples, unveiling the transformative potential of weaving biodiversity seamlessly into the fabric of land use planning and corporate sustainability frameworks.

31.6.3.1 Spatial Planning for Biodiversity: Incorporating Conservation Goals into Development

Incorporating conservation goals into spatial planning ensures that land development aligns with biodiversity conservation objectives. By integrating ecological principles into development processes, we can minimize the negative impacts on natural habitats (Harlio et al. 2019).

31.6.3.2 Corporate Biodiversity Stewardship: Fostering Sustainable Business Practices

Encouraging corporate biodiversity stewardship involves promoting sustainable business practices that prioritize biodiversity conservation. Embracing corporate responsibility toward biodiversity contributes to a more resilient and sustainable global economy (Fowler and Hope 2007; Konietzko et al. 2023; Vieira Nunhes et al. 2021; Chausson et al. 2023).

31.7 Emerging Frontiers in Biodiversity Research and Conservation

As biodiversity research and conservation continue to evolve, this section explores the cutting-edge frontiers that hold great promise for advancing our understanding and protection of Earth's diverse ecosystems.

31.7.1 Advancements in Molecular Ecology and Genomics: Revolutionizing Biodiversity Studies

Recent breakthroughs in molecular ecology and genomics are transforming the way we study and conserve biodiversity.

31.7.1.1 Environmental DNA and Metabarcoding: Transforming Biodiversity Monitoring

The application of environmental DNA (eDNA) and metabarcoding techniques is revolutionizing biodiversity monitoring. Noninvasive eDNA analysis allows for the detection of species presence and distribution in various ecosystems, offering new insights into biodiversity patterns (Akoijam and Joshi 2022; Van der Jeugt et al. 2022; Rodríguez-Ezpeleta et al. 2021; Banerjee et al. 2022; Xiong et al. 2022; Miya 2022; Bautista et al. 2023; Aucone et al. 2023).

31.7.1.2 Genomics and Conservation: Integrating Genotype-phenotype Studies

The integration of genomics with conservation biology has opened new avenues for understanding the genotype-phenotype relationships in species. Genomic studies provide valuable information on species' adaptive capacities and their responses to environmental changes, enhancing conservation strategies (Henry et al. 2023; Kafkas et al. 2023; Hongo et al. 2023; van den Brandt et al. 2023; Nelson et al. 2019; Mighell et al. 2020).

31.7.2 Technology for Conservation: Remote Sensing, Artificial Intelligence, and Citizen Science

Leveraging technology is a game-changer in biodiversity conservation, with remote sensing, AI, and citizen science playing pivotal roles.

31.7.2.1 Remote Sensing Applications in Biodiversity Research and Monitoring

Remote sensing technologies, such as satellite imagery and LiDAR, enable the assessment of large-scale biodiversity patterns and ecosystem dynamics. They offer a comprehensive view of habitats and facilitate data-driven decision making for conservation efforts (Kerry et al. 2022; Cavender-Bares et al. 2022; Kacic and Kuenzer 2022; Davies et al. 2023; Griffith et al. 2023).

31.7.2.2 Artificial Intelligence and Machine Learning: Harnessing Big Data for Conservation

Artificial Intelligence and machine learning algorithms are instrumental in analyzing vast volumes of ecological data. They aid in species identification, habitat mapping, and predicting biodiversity trends, supporting evidence-based conservation strategies (Shivaprakash et al. 2022; Silvestro et al. 2022; Santangeli et al. 2020; Kwok 2019; Rezapouraghdam et al. 2021).

31.7.3 Social and Political Dimensions of Biodiversity Conservation

Recognizing the social and political dimensions of biodiversity conservation is essential for achieving effective and inclusive conservation outcomes (de Oliveira Caetano et al. 2023; Dayer et al. 2020; de Freitas et al. 2023).

31.7.3.1 Biodiversity and Social Equity: Promoting Justice and Inclusivity

Addressing the connections between biodiversity conservation and social equity is crucial for ensuring fair and equitable outcomes for local communities. Empowering marginalized groups to participate in conservation efforts fosters more sustainable and socially just outcomes (Friedman et al. 2018).

31.7.3.2 Global Governance and Conservation: Strengthening International Collaboration

The protection of global biodiversity demands strengthened international collaboration and governance. Collaborative efforts are necessary to address cross-border conservation challenges, such as transboundary species and habitats, and to promote sustainable practices on a global scale (Gallo-Cajiao et al. 2023; Rogers Van Katwyk et al. 2023; Bai and Zhu 2023; Piskulova 2023; Pyć 2023; Elnaiem et al. 2023).

31.8 Conclusion

In this chapter, we embarked on a thrilling expedition through the boundless realms of biodiversity, unearthing the enigmatic intricacies that animate our planet's web of life. From the microscopic wonders of genetic diversity to the majestic tapestry of ecosystems, we unraveled the symphony of existence that harmonizes amidst the verdant canvas of nature. Throughout our expedition, the echoes of urgent challenges reverberated, casting an ominous pall over the natural splendor. The dissonance of habitat loss, climate perturbations, invasive encroachments, and relentless exploitation beckoned us to confront the precipice upon which biodiversity teeters. A stark realization dawned upon us, urging unwavering commitment to fortify the fragile threads that sustain life's grandeur.

As our gaze ventured beyond the horizon, novel frontiers in biodiversity research beckoned with promises of enlightenment and solutions. Advancements in molecular ecology and genomics held the key to deciphering nature's cryptic code, while cutting-edge technology unveiled vistas unseen, empowering us to envision new paradigms of conservation. Yet, this journey of discovery and defense would be incomplete without recognizing the human touch upon the living tapestry. The intricate dance of social and political dimensions demanded inclusion and justice, nurturing a shared sense of responsibility for the intricate legacy we weave.

Our journey does not culminate here, for beyond the words lies the symphony of purpose, where each note of resilience, each chord of conservation, and each crescendo of collaboration reverberate with meaning. Together, we must compose a resolute anthem of biodiversity protection, harmonizing humanity's aspirations with the ancient rhythms of nature. United by purpose, guided by wisdom, and emboldened by innovation, we march toward a sustainable future where biodiversity thrives, and the intricate threads of life shimmer with vitality. In this grand composition, humanity embraces its role as guardians of Earth's enchanting diversity, ensuring that the legacy of life endures for generations yet to come. The tale of biodiversity unfolds, and we stand at the heart of the narrative, tasked with writing its magnum opus in unity and reverence.

References

Abdala-Roberts, L., Puentes, A., Finke, D.L. et al. (2019). Tri-trophic interactions: bridging species, communities and ecosystems. *Ecology Letters* 22 (12): 2151–2167.

Accatino, F., Creed, I.F., and Weber, M. (2018). Landscape consequences of aggregation rules for functional equivalence in compensatory mitigation programs. *Conservation Biology* 32 (3): 694–705.

Akçakaya, H.R., Rodrigues, A.S.L., Keith, D.A. et al. (2020). Assessing ecological function in the context of species recovery. *Conservation Biology* 34 (3): 561–571.

Akoijam, N. and Joshi, S.R. (2022). Conservation metagenomics: understanding microbiomes for biodiversity sustenance and conservation. In: *Molecular Genetics and Genomics Tools in Biodiversity Conservation* (ed. A. Kumar, B. Choudhury, S. Dayanandan, and M.L. Khan), 31–61. Singapore: Springer Nature Singapore.

Albrecht, J., Peters, M.K., Becker, J.N. et al. (2021). Species richness is more important for ecosystem functioning than species turnover along an elevational gradient. *Nature Ecology and Evolution* 5 (12): 1582–1593.

Alsammar, H.F., Naseeb, S., Brancia, L.B. et al. (2019). Targeted metagenomics approach to capture the biodiversity of *Saccharomyces* genus in wild environments. *Environmental Microbiology Reports* 11 (2): 206–214.

Anthem, H., Infield, M., and Morse-Jones, S. (2016). Guidance for the rapid assessment of cultural ecosystem services. *Oryx* 50 (1): 13–13.

Aucone, E., Kirchgeorg, S., Valentini, A. et al. (2023). Drone-assisted collection of environmental DNA from tree branches for biodiversity monitoring. *Science Robotics* 8 (74).

Baag, S. and Mandal, S. (2022). Combined effects of ocean warming and acidification on marine fish and shellfish: a molecule to ecosystem perspective. *Science of the Total Environment* 802: 149807.

Bai, J. and Zhu, K. (2023). China's engagement in Arctic governance for its sustainable development based on international law perspective. *Sustainability* 15 (6): 5429.

Banerjee, P., Stewart, K.A., Dey, G. et al. (2022). Environmental DNA analysis as an emerging non-destructive method for plant biodiversity monitoring: a review. *AoB Plants* 14 (4): plac031.

Bautista, J.A., Manubag, J.J., Sumaya, N.H. et al. (2023). Environmental DNA (eDNA) metabarcoding and fish visual census reveals the first record of Doboatherina magnidentata in the Philippines. *Biodiversitas* 24 (5): 3063–3072.

de Bello, F., Lavorel, S., Hallett, L.M. et al. (2021). Functional trait effects on ecosystem stability: assembling the jigsaw puzzle. *Trends in Ecology and Evolution* 36 (9): 822–836.

Beyer, R.M., Manica, A., and Mora, C. (2021). Shifts in global bat diversity suggest a possible role of climate change in the emergence of SARS-CoV-1 and SARS-CoV-2. *Science of the Total Environment* 767: 145413.

Bezombes, L., Gaucherand, S., Kerbiriou, C. et al. (2017). Ecological equivalence assessment methods: what trade-offs between operationality, scientific basis and comprehensiveness? *Environmental Management* 60 (2): 216–230.

Bieling, C. and Plieninger, T. (2013). Recording manifestations of cultural ecosystem services in the landscape. *Landscape Research* 38 (5): 649–667.

Biggs, C.R., Yeager, L.A., Bolser, D.G. et al. (2020). Does functional redundancy affect ecological stability and resilience? A review and meta-analysis. *Ecosphere* 11 (7): e03184.

Bolam, F.C., Ahumada, J., Akçakaya, H.R. et al. (2023). Over half of threatened species require targeted recovery actions to avert human-induced extinction. *Frontiers in Ecology and the Environment* 21 (2): 64–70.

van den Brandt, A., Jonkheer, E.M., van Workum, D.-J.M. et al. (2023). PanVA: Pangenomic variant analysis. *IEEE Transactions on Visualization and Computer Graphics* 1–15. online ahead of print.

Carlson, C.J., Albery, G.F., Merow, C. et al. (2022). Climate change increases cross-species viral transmission risk. *Nature* 607 (7919): 555–562.

Carlucci, M.B., Brancalion, P.H.S., Rodrigues, R.R. et al. (2020). Functional traits and ecosystem services in ecological restoration. *Restoration Ecology* 28 (6): 1372–1383.

Carscadden, K.A., Emery, N.C., Arnillas, C.A. et al. (2020). Niche breadth: causes and consequences for ecology, evolution, and conservation. *Quarterly Review of Biology* 95 (3): 179–214.

Cavender-Bares, J., Schneider, F.D., Santos, M.J. et al. (2022). Integrating remote sensing with ecology and evolution to advance biodiversity conservation. *Nature Ecology and Evolution* 6 (5): 506–519.

Ceballos, G., Ehrlich, P.R., and Raven, P.H. (2020). Vertebrates on the brink as indicators of biological annihilation and the sixth mass extinction. *Proceedings of the National Academy of Sciences* 117 (24): 13596–13602.

Challender, D.W.S., Cremona, P.J., Malsch, K. et al. (2023). Identifying species likely threatened by international trade on the IUCN Red List can inform CITES trade measures. *Nature Ecology and Evolution* 7: 1211–1220.

Chausson, A., Welden, E.A., Melanidis, M.S. et al. (2023). Going beyond market-based mechanisms to finance nature-based solutions and foster sustainable futures. *PLOS Climate* 2 (4): e0000169.

Cháves-González, L.E., Morales-Calvo, F., Mora, J. et al. (2022). What lies behind the curtain: cryptic diversity in helminth parasites of human and veterinary importance. *Current Research in Parasitology and Vector-Borne Diseases* 2: 100094.

Chua, P.Y.S., Bourlat, S.J., Ferguson, C. et al. (2023). Future of DNA-based insect monitoring. *Trends in Genetics* 39 (7): 531–544.

Cicero, C., Mason, N.A., Jiménez, R.A. et al. (2021). Integrative taxonomy and geographic sampling underlie successful species delimitation. *Ornithology* 138 (2): 1–15.

Cooney, R., Roe, D., Dublin, H. et al. (2017). From poachers to protectors: engaging local communities in solutions to illegal wildlife trade. *Conservation Letters* 10 (3): 367–374.

Cordeiro, A.d.A.C., Klanderud, K., Villa, P.M., and Neri, A.V. (2023). Patterns of species richness and beta diversity of vascular plants along elevation gradient in Brazilian páramo. *Journal of Mountain Science* 20 (7): 1911–1920.

Costanza, J.K. and Terando, A.J. (2019). Landscape connectivity planning for adaptation to future climate and land-use change. *Current Landscape Ecology Reports* 4 (1): 1–13.

Cowie, R.H., Bouchet, P., and Fontaine, B. (2022). The sixth mass extinction: fact, fiction or speculation? *Biological Reviews* 97 (2): 640–663.

Danet, A., Mouchet, M., Bonnaffé, W. et al. (2021). Species richness and food-web structure jointly drive community biomass and its temporal stability in fish communities. *Ecology Letters* 24 (11): 2364–2377.

Daru, B.H., Karunarathne, P., and Schliep, K. (2020). Phyloregion: R package for biogeographical regionalization and macroecology. *Methods in Ecology and Evolution* 11 (11): 1483–1491.

Davies, B.F.R., Gernez, P., Geraud, A. et al. (2023). Multi- and hyperspectral classification of soft-bottom intertidal vegetation using a spectral library for coastal biodiversity remote sensing. *Remote Sensing of Environment* 290: 113554.

Dayer, A.A., Silva-Rodríguez, E.A., Albert, S. et al. (2020). Applying conservation social science to study the human dimensions of Neotropical bird conservation. *Condor* 122 (3): duaa021.

Dembo, M., Radovčić, D., Garvin, H.M. et al. (2016). The evolutionary relationships and age of Homo naledi: an assessment using dated Bayesian phylogenetic methods. *Journal of Human Evolution* 97: 17–26.

DeMiguel, D., Brilha, J., Alegret, L. et al. (2021). Linking geological heritage and geoethics with a particular emphasis on palaeontological heritage: the new concept of 'palaeontoethics.'. *Geoheritage* 13 (3): 69.

Díaz-Ruiz, F., Vaquerizas, P.H., Márquez, A.L. et al. (2023). Unravelling the historical biogeography of the European rabbit subspecies in the Iberian Peninsula. *Mammal Review* 53 (1): 1–14.

Dormann, C.F., Gruber, B., Winter, M., and Herrmann, D. (2010). Evolution of climate niches in European mammals? *Biology Letters* 6 (2): 229–232.

Dou, Y., Yu, X., and Liu, Y. (2021). Rethinking non-material links between people and drylands from a cultural ecosystem services perspective. *Current Opinion in Environment Sustainability* 48: 110–114.

Dzekashu, F.F., Yusuf, A.A., Pirk, C.W.W. et al. (2022). Floral turnover and climate drive seasonal bee diversity along a tropical elevation gradient. *Ecosphere* 13 (3): e3964.

Eisenhauer, N., Bonkowski, M., Brose, U. et al. (2019). Biotic interactions, community assembly, and eco-evolutionary dynamics as drivers of long-term biodiversity–ecosystem functioning relationships. *Research Ideas and Outcomes* 5: e47042.

Elnaiem, A., Mohamed-Ahmed, O., Zumla, A. et al. (2023). Global and regional governance of one health and implications for global health security. *Lancet* 401 (10377): 688–704.

Evangelista, D.A., Wipfler, B., Béthoux, O. et al. (2019, 1895). An integrative phylogenomic approach illuminates the evolutionary history of cockroaches and termites (Blattodea). *Proceedings of the Royal Society B: Biological Sciences* 286: 20182076.

Exposito-Alonso, M., Booker, T.R., Czech, L. et al. (2022). Genetic diversity loss in the Anthropocene. *Science (1979)* 377 (6613): 1431–1435.

Folharini, S.d.O., de Melo, S.N., Ramos, R.G., and Brown, J.C. (2023). Land use and green crime: assessing the edge effect. *Land Use Policy* 129: 106636.

Fontana, V., Guariento, E., Hilpold, A. et al. (2020). Species richness and beta diversity patterns of multiple taxa along an elevational gradient in pastured grasslands in the European Alps. *Scientific Reports* 10 (1): 12516.

Fowler, S.J. and Hope, C. (2007). Incorporating sustainable business practices into company strategy. *Business Strategy and the Environment* 16 (1): 26–38.

Franklin, J. (2023). Species distribution modelling supports the study of past, present and future biogeographies. *Journal of Biogeography* 50: 1533–1545.

de Freitas, A.C., do Nascimento, L.A., de Castro, R.G. et al. (2023). Biodiversity and citizenship in an argumentative socioscientific process. *Sustainability* 15 (4): 2987.

Friedman, R.S., Law, E.A., Bennett, N.J. et al. (2018). How just and just how? A systematic review of social equity in conservation research. *Environmental Research Letters* 13 (5): 053001.

Gallo-Cajiao, E., Lieberman, S., Dolšak, N. et al. (2023). Global governance for pandemic prevention and the wildlife trade. *Lancet Planetary Health* 7 (4): e336–e345.

Gibb, R., Redding, D.W., Chin, K.Q. et al. (2020). Zoonotic host diversity increases in human-dominated ecosystems. *Nature* 584 (7821): 398–402.

Giddens, J., Kobayashi, D.R., Mukai, G.N.M. et al. (2022). Assessing the vulnerability of marine life to climate change in the Pacific Islands region. *PLoS One* 17 (7): e0270930.

Gjerde, K.M. and Rulska-Domino, A. (2012). Marine protected areas beyond National Jurisdiction: some practical perspectives for moving ahead. *International Journal of Marine and Coastal Law* 27 (2): 351–373.

González de Andrés, E. (2019). Interactions between climate and nutrient cycles on forest response to global change: the role of mixed forests. *Forests* 10 (8): 609.

Grande, T.O., Aguiar, L.M.S., and Machado, R.B. (2020). Heating a biodiversity hotspot: connectivity is more important than remaining habitat. *Landscape Ecology* 35 (3): 639–657.

Griffith, D.M., Byrd, K.B., Anderegg, L.D.L. et al. (2023). Capturing patterns of evolutionary relatedness with reflectance spectra to model and monitor biodiversity. *Proceedings of the National Academy of Sciences* 120 (24): e2215533120.

Grimm, M. and Köppel, J. (2019). Biodiversity offset program design and implementation. *Sustainability* 11 (24): 6903.

Hanisch, M., Schweiger, O., Cord, A.F. et al. (2020). Plant functional traits shape multiple ecosystem services, their trade-offs and synergies in grasslands. *Journal of Applied Ecology* 57 (8): 1535–1550.

Hanz, D.M., Cutts, V., Barajas-Barbosa, M.P. et al. (2022). Climatic and biogeographical drivers of functional diversity in the flora of the Canary Islands. *Global Ecology and Biogeography* 31 (7): 1313–1331.

Hardaker, A., Styles, D., Williams, P. et al. (2022). A framework for integrating ecosystem services as endpoint impacts in life cycle assessment. *Journal of Cleaner Production* 370: 133450.

Harlio, A., Kuussaari, M., Heikkinen, R.K., and Arponen, A. (2019). Incorporating landscape heterogeneity into multi-objective spatial planning improves biodiversity conservation of semi-natural grasslands. *Journal for Nature Conservation* 49: 37–44.

Harris, L.R., Holness, S.D., Finke, G. et al. (2022). Practical marine spatial management of ecologically or biologically significant marine areas: emerging lessons from evidence-based planning and implementation in a developing-world context. *Frontiers in Marine Science* 9.

Harvey, B.J., Hart, S.J., Tobin, P.C. et al. (2023). Emergent hotspots of biotic disturbances and their consequences for forest resilience. *Frontiers in Ecology and the Environment* 21: 388–396.

Henry, O.J., Stödberg, T., Båtelson, S. et al. (2023). Individualised human phenotype ontology gene panels improve clinical whole exome and genome sequencing analytical efficacy in a cohort of developmental and epileptic encephalopathies. *Molecular Genetics and Genomic Medicine* 11 (7): e2167.

Hillis, D.M., Chambers, E.A., and Devitt, T.J. (2021). Contemporary methods and evidence for species delimitation. *Ichthyology and Herpetology* 109 (3): 895–903.

Hinsley, A., Willis, J., Dent, A.R. et al. (2023). Trading species to extinction: evidence of extinction linked to the wildlife trade. *Cambridge Prisms: Extinction* 1: e10.

Hoban, S., Bruford, M., D'Urban Jackson, J. et al. (2020). Genetic diversity targets and indicators in the CBD post-2020 Global Biodiversity Framework must be improved. *Biological Conservation* 248: 108654.

Hongo, J.A., de Castro, G.M., Albuquerque Menezes, A.P. et al. (2023). CALANGO: a phylogeny-aware comparative genomics tool for discovering quantitative genotype-phenotype associations across species. *Patterns* 4 (6): 100728.

Hughes, E.C., Edwards, D.P., Bright, J.A. et al. (2022). Global biogeographic patterns of avian morphological diversity. *Ecology Letters* 25 (3): 598–610.

Hughes, A., Auliya, M., Altherr, S. et al. (2023). Determining the sustainability of legal wildlife trade. *Journal of Environmental Management* 341: 117987.

Hulme, P.E. (2020). One biosecurity: a unified concept to integrate human, animal, plant, and environmental health. *Emerging Topics in Life Sciences* 4 (5): 539–549.

Irl, S.D.H., Harter, D.E.V., Steinbauer, M.J. et al. (2015). Climate vs. topography – spatial patterns of plant species diversity and endemism on a high-elevation island. *Journal of Ecology* 103 (6): 1621–1633.

Irwin, A., Geschke, A., Brooks, T.M. et al. (2022). Quantifying and categorising national extinction-risk footprints. *Scientific Reports* 12 (1): 5861.

Jiao, Y., Yeophantong, P., and Lee, T.M. (2021). Strengthening international legal cooperation to combat the illegal wildlife trade between Southeast Asia and China. *Frontiers in Ecology and Evolution* 9.

Johnston, H.R., Keats, B.J.B., and Sherman, S.L. (2019). Population genetics. In: *Emery and Rimoin's Principles and Practice of Medical Genetics and Genomics* (ed. R. Pyeritz, B. Korf, and W. Grody), 359–373. St Louis: Elsevier.

Kacic, P. and Kuenzer, C. (2022). Forest biodiversity monitoring based on remotely sensed spectral diversity – a review. *Remote Sensing* 14 (21): 5363.

Kafkas, Ş., Abdelhakim, M., Uludag, M. et al. (2023). Starvar: symptom-based tool for automatic ranking of variants using evidence from literature and genomes. *BMC Bioinformatics* 24 (1): 294.

Kardos, M., Armstrong, E.E., Fitzpatrick, S.W. et al. (2021). The crucial role of genome-wide genetic variation in conservation. *Proceedings of the National Academy of Sciences* 118 (48): e2104642118.

Kéfi, S., Domínguez-García, V., Donohue, I. et al. (2019). Advancing our understanding of ecological stability. *Ecology Letters* 22 (9): 1349–1356.

Kerry, R.G., Montalbo, F.J.P., Das, R. et al. (2022). An overview of remote monitoring methods in biodiversity conservation. *Environmental Science and Pollution Research* 29 (53): 80179–80221.

Kiessling, W., Smith, J.A., and Raja, N.B. (2023). Improving the relevance of paleontology to climate change policy. *Proceedings of the National Academy of Sciences* 120 (7): e2201926119.

Kohli, M., Borer, E.T., Kinkel, L., and Seabloom, E.W. (2019). Stability of grassland production is robust to changes in the consumer food web. *Ecology Letters* 22 (4): 707–716.

Konietzko, J., Das, A., and Bocken, N. (2023). Towards regenerative business models: a necessary shift? *Sustainable Production and Consumption* 38: 372–388.

Kurland, J., Pires, S.F., McFann, S.C., and Moreto, W.D. (2017). Wildlife crime: a conceptual integration, literature review, and methodological critique. *Crime Science* 6 (1): 4.

Kwok, R. (2019). AI empowers conservation biology. *Nature* 567 (7746): 133–134.

Laffoley, D., Baxter, J.M., Day, J.C. et al. (2019). Marine protected areas. In: *World Seas: An Environmental Evaluation* (ed. C. Sheppard), 549–569. St Louis: Elsevier.

Leal Filho, W., Nagy, G.J., Setti, A.F.F. et al. (2023). Handling the impacts of climate change on soil biodiversity. *Science of the Total Environment* 869: 161671.

Li, Z., Ma, Z., and Zhou, G. (2022). Impact of land use change on habitat quality and regional biodiversity capacity: temporal and spatial evolution and prediction analysis. *Frontiers in Environmental Science* 10.

Liu, M., Wei, H., Dong, X. et al. (2022). Integrating land use, ecosystem service, and human well-being: a systematic review. *Sustainability* 14 (11): 6926.

López-Antoñanzas, R., Mitchell, J., Simões, T.R. et al. (2022). Integrative phylogenetics: tools for palaeontologists to explore the tree of life. *Biology* 11 (8): 1185.

Maclot, F., Candresse, T., Filloux, D. et al. (2020). Illuminating an ecological blackbox: using high throughput sequencing to characterize the plant virome across scales. *Frontiers in Microbiology* 11: 578064.

Marrone, F., Fontaneto, D., and Naselli-Flores, L. (2023). Cryptic diversity, niche displacement and our poor understanding of taxonomy and ecology of aquatic microorganisms. *Hydrobiologia* 850 (6): 1221–1236.

Mehring, M., Mehlhaus, N., Ott, E., and Hummel, D. (2020). A systematic review of biodiversity and demographic change: a misinterpreted relationship? *Ambio* 49 (7): 1297–1312.

Mengist, W., Soromessa, T., and Feyisa, G.L. (2022). Estimating the total ecosystem services value of Eastern Afromontane Biodiversity Hotspots in response to landscape dynamics. *Environmental and Sustainability Indicators* 14: 100178.

Meyerson, L.A., Pauchard, A., Brundu, G. et al. (2022). Moving toward global strategies for managing invasive alien species. In: *Global Plant Invasions* (ed. D. Clements, M. Upadhyaya, S. Joshi, and A. Shrestha), 331–360. Cham: Springer International Publishing.

Mighell, T.L., Thacker, S., Fombonne, E. et al. (2020). An integrated deep-mutational-scanning approach provides clinical insights on PTEN genotype-phenotype relationships. *American Journal of Human Genetics* 106 (6): 818–829.

Miya, M. (2022). Environmental DNA metabarcoding: a novel method for biodiversity monitoring of marine fish communities. *Annual Review of Marine Science* 14 (1): 161–185.

Moilanen, A., Kujala, H., and Mikkonen, N. (2020). A practical method for evaluating spatial biodiversity offset scenarios based on spatial conservation prioritization outputs. *Methods in Ecology and Evolution* 11 (7): 794–803.

Moreno-Mateos, D., Alberdi, A., Morriën, E. et al. (2020). The long-term restoration of ecosystem complexity. *Nature Ecology and Evolution* 4 (5): 676–685.

Mozer, A. and Prost, S. (2023). An introduction to illegal wildlife trade and its effects on biodiversity and society. *Forensic Science International: Animals and Environments* 3: 100064.

Nahrung, H.F., Liebhold, A.M., Brockerhoff, E.G., and Rassati, D. (2023). Forest insect biosecurity: processes, patterns, predictions, pitfalls. *Annual Review of Entomology* 68 (1): 211–229.

Nakamura, G., Rodrigues, A.V., Luza, A.L. et al. (2023). Herodotools: an R package to integrate macroevolution, biogeography and community ecology. *Journal of Biogeography* https://ecoevorxiv.org/repository/view/3714/ (accessed 5 February 2024).

Nelson, T.C., Jones, M.R., Velotta, J.P. et al. (2019). UNVEILing connections between genotype, phenotype, and fitness in natural populations. *Molecular Ecology* 28 (8): 1866–1876.

Nelson, C.E., Wegley Kelly, L., and Haas, A.F. (2023). Microbial interactions with dissolved organic matter are central to coral reef ecosystem function and resilience. *Annual Review of Marine Science* 15 (1): 431–460.

Nishizawa, K., Shinohara, N., Cadotte, M.W., and Mori, A.S. (2022). The latitudinal gradient in plant community assembly processes: a meta-analysis. *Ecology Letters* 25 (7): 1711–1724.

Ntshanga, N.K., Procheş, S., and Slingsby, J.A. (2021). Assessing the threat of landscape transformation and habitat fragmentation in a global biodiversity hotspot. *Austral Ecology* 46 (7): 1052–1069.

de Oliveira Caetano, G.H., Vardi, R., Jarić, I. et al. (2023). Evaluating global interest in biodiversity and conservation. *Conservation Biology* 37: 14100.

Paramesh, V., Ravisankar, N., Behera, U. et al. (2022). Integrated farming system approaches to achieve food and nutritional security for enhancing profitability, employment, and climate resilience in India. *Food and Energy Security* 11 (2): e321.

Pau, S., Wolkovich, E.M., Cook, B.I. et al. (2011). Predicting phenology by integrating ecology, evolution and climate science. *Global Change Biology* 17 (12): 3633–3643.

Penn, J.L. and Deutsch, C. (2022). Avoiding ocean mass extinction from climate warming. *Science (1979)* 376 (6592): 524–526.

Pimiento, C. and Antonelli, A. (2022). Integrating deep-time palaeontology in conservation prioritisation. *Frontiers in Ecology and Evolution* 10.

Piskulova, N. (2023). Challenges for the environmental restructuring of the global economy. In: *Global Governance in the New Era* (ed. Institute of Russian, E. European, and C.A. Studies), 185–192. Singapore: Springer Nature Singapore.

Pitman, R.T., Fattebert, J., Williams, S.T. et al. (2017). Cats, connectivity and conservation: incorporating data sets and integrating scales for wildlife management. *Journal of Applied Ecology* 54 (6): 1687–1698.

Polazzo, F., Hermann, M., Crettaz-Minaglia, M., and Rico, A. (2023). Impacts of extreme climatic events on trophic network complexity and multidimensional stability. *Ecology* 104 (2): e3951.

Pörtner, H. (2008). Ecosystem effects of ocean acidification in times of ocean warming: a physiologist's view. *Marine Ecology Progress Series* 373: 203–217.

Pyć, D. (2023). Global Ocean governance: towards protecting the ocean's rights to health and resilience. *Marine Policy* 147: 105328.

Qiu, J. and Cardinale, B.J. (2020). Scaling up biodiversity–ecosystem function relationships across space and over time. *Ecology* 101 (11): e03166.

Rannala, B. (2015). The art and science of species delimitation. *Current Zoology* 61 (5): 846–853.

Rasmussen, C.M.Ø., Vandenbroucke, T.R.A., Nogues-Bravo, D., and Finnegan, S. (2023). Was the Late Ordovician mass extinction truly exceptional? *Trends in Ecology and Evolution* 38: 812–821.

Rezapouraghdam, H., Akhshik, A., and Ramkissoon, H. (2021). Application of machine learning to predict visitors' green behavior in marine protected areas: evidence from Cyprus. *Journal of Sustainable Tourism* 31: 2479–2505.

Rezende, F., Antiqueira, P.A.P., Petchey, O.L. et al. (2021). Trophic downgrading decreases species asynchrony and community stability regardless of climate warming. *Ecology Letters* 24 (12): 2660–2673.

Rodrigues, R.G., Srivathsa, A., and Vasudev, D. (2022). Dog in the matrix: envisioning countrywide connectivity conservation for an endangered carnivore. *Journal of Applied Ecology* 59 (1): 223–237.

Rodríguez-Ezpeleta, N., Zinger, L., Kinziger, A. et al. (2021). Biodiversity monitoring using environmental DNA. *Molecular Ecology Resources* 21 (5): 1405–1409.

Rogers Van Katwyk, S., Weldon, I., Giubilini, A. et al. (2023). Making use of existing international legal mechanisms to manage the global antimicrobial commons: identifying legal hooks and institutional mandates. *Health Care Analysis* 31 (1): 9–24.

Román-Palacios, C. and Wiens, J.J. (2020). Recent responses to climate change reveal the drivers of species extinction and survival. *Proceedings of the National Academy of Sciences* 117 (8): 4211–4217.

Rosauer, D., Laffan, S.W., Crisp, M.D. et al. (2009). Phylogenetic endemism: a new approach for identifying geographical concentrations of evolutionary history. *Molecular Ecology* 18 (19): 4061–4072.

Santangeli, A., Chen, Y., Kluen, E. et al. (2020). Integrating drone-borne thermal imaging with artificial intelligence to locate bird nests on agricultural land. *Scientific Reports* 10 (1): 10993.

dos Santos, G.M., Linares, M.S., Callisto, M., and Marques, J.C. (2019). Two tropical biodiversity hotspots, two different pathways for energy. *Ecological Indicators* 106: 105495.

Saraswati, P.K. (2022). Geobiology: deep time perspectives. *Journal of the Geological Society of India* 98 (6): 727–730.

Scholl, E.A., Cross, W.F., Guy, C.S. et al. (2023). Landscape diversity promotes stable food-web architectures in large rivers. *Ecology Letters* 26: 1740–1751.

Shivaprakash, K.N., Swami, N., Mysorekar, S. et al. (2022). Potential for artificial intelligence (AI) and machine learning (ML) applications in biodiversity conservation, managing forests, and related services in India. *Sustainability* 14 (12): 7154.

Silvestro, D., Goria, S., Sterner, T., and Antonelli, A. (2022). Improving biodiversity protection through artificial intelligence. *Nature Sustainability* 5 (5): 415–424.

Sink, K.J., Lombard, A.T., Attwood, C.G. et al. (2023). Integrated systematic planning and adaptive stakeholder process support a 10-fold increase in South Africa's marine protected area estate. *Conservation Letters* 16: e12954.

Small, N., Munday, M., and Durance, I. (2017). The challenge of valuing ecosystem services that have no material benefits. *Global Environmental Change* 44: 57–67.

Snoeks, J.M., Driesen, M., Porembski, S. et al. (2021). Contrasting biodiversity and food web structure of three temporary freshwater habitats in a tropical biodiversity hotspot. *Aquatic Conservation* 31 (9): 2603–2620.

Sodré, E.d.O. and Bozelli, R.L. (2019). How planktonic microcrustaceans respond to environment and affect ecosystem: a functional trait perspective. *International Aquatic Research* 11 (3): 207–223.

Streit, R.P., Cumming, G.S., and Bellwood, D.R. (2019). Patchy delivery of functions undermines functional redundancy in a high diversity system. *Functional Ecology* 33 (6): 1144–1155.

Teixeira, J.C. and Huber, C.D. (2021). The inflated significance of neutral genetic diversity in conservation genetics. *Proceedings of the National Academy of Sciences* 118 (10): e2015096118.

Uprety, Y., Chettri, N., Dhakal, M. et al. (2021). Illegal wildlife trade is threatening conservation in the transboundary landscape of Western Himalaya. *Journal for Nature Conservation* 59: 125952.

Van der Jeugt, F., Maertens, R., Steyaert, A. et al. (2022). UMGAP: the Unipept MetaGenomics analysis pipeline. *BMC Genomics* 23 (1): 433.

Van Meerbeek, K., Jucker, T., and Svenning, J. (2021). Unifying the concepts of stability and resilience in ecology. *Journal of Ecology* 109 (9): 3114–3132.

Veloy, C., Hidalgo, M., Pennino, M.G. et al. (2022). Spatial-temporal variation of the Western Mediterranean Sea biodiversity along a latitudinal gradient. *Ecological Indicators* 136: 108674.

Venkatramanan, V. and Shah, S. (2019). Climate smart agriculture technologies for environmental management: the intersection of sustainability, resilience, wellbeing and development. In: *Sustainable Green Technologies for Environmental Management* (ed. S. Shah, V. Venkatramanan, and R. Prasad), 29–51. Singapore: Springer Singapore.

Vieira Nunhes, T., Viviani Garcia, E., Espuny, M. et al. (2021). Where to go with corporate sustainability? Opening paths for sustainable businesses through the collaboration between universities, governments, and organizations. *Sustainability* 13 (3): 1429.

Wake, D.B., Hadly, E.A., and Ackerly, D.D. (2009). Biogeography, changing climates, and niche evolution. *Proceedings of the National Academy of Sciences* 106 (Suppl 2): 19631–19636.

White, L., O'Connor, N.E., Yang, Q. et al. (2020). Individual species provide multifaceted contributions to the stability of ecosystems. *Nature Ecology and Evolution* 4 (12): 1594–1601.

Wiens, J.J. and Donoghue, M.J. (2004). Historical biogeography, ecology and species richness. *Trends in Ecology and Evolution* 19 (12): 639–644.

Wu, D., Xu, C., Wang, S. et al. (2023a). Why are biodiversity-ecosystem functioning relationships so elusive? Trophic interactions may amplify ecosystem function variability. *Journal of Animal Ecology* 92 (2): 367–376.

Wu, B., Guan, X., Deng, T. et al. (2023b). Synthetic denitrifying communities reveal a positive and dynamic biodiversity-ecosystem functioning relationship during experimental evolution. *Microbiology Spectrum* 11 (3).

Wyatt, T. (2021). Canada and the Convention on International Trade in Endangered Species of Wild Fauna and Flora (CITES): lessons learned on implementation and compliance. *Liverpool Law Review* 42 (2): 143–159.

Xiong, F., Shu, L., Zeng, H. et al. (2022). Methodology for fish biodiversity monitoring with environmental DNA metabarcoding: the primers, databases and bioinformatic pipelines. *Water Biology and Security* 1 (1): 100007.

Zhang, K., Zou, C., Lin, N. et al. (2022). The ecological conservation redline program: a new model for improving China's protected area network. *Environmental Science and Policy* 131: 10–13.

Zhao, Q., Van den Brink, P.J., Xu, C. et al. (2023). Relationships of temperature and biodiversity with stability of natural aquatic food webs. *Nature Communications* 14 (1): 3507.

Zvereva, E.L. and Kozlov, M.V. (2021). Latitudinal gradient in the intensity of biotic interactions in terrestrial ecosystems: sources of variation and differences from the diversity gradient revealed by meta-analysis. *Ecology Letters* 24 (11): 2506–2520.

32

Definition, Scope, Characteristics, and Importance of Ecosystems

Udit Jain[1], Faizan ul Haque Nagrami[2], Barkha Sharma[3], Parul[1], and Uma Sharma[2]

[1] *College of Veterinary & Animal Sciences, DUVASU, Mathura, India*
[2] *College of Biotechnology, DUVASU, Mathura, India*
[3] *Department of Veterinary Epidemiology and Preventive Medicine, College of Veterinary Sciences & Animal Husbandry, DUVASU, Mathura, India*

32.1 Definition

The Oxford ecologist and botanist Arthur. G. Tansley first used the word "ecosystem" in 1935. The currently accepted definition of an ecosystem is as follows: "A unit that includes all the organisms, i.e., the community in a given area interacting with the physical environment so that a flow of energy leads to clearly defined trophic structure, biotic diversity, and material cycles, i.e., exchange of materials between living and non-living, within the system" (Odum et al., 1971). Simply said, an ecosystem is the functional and structural unit of ecology where living things interact both with one another and with their surroundings at the same time. An ecosystem, then, is a series of interactions between species and their surroundings.

32.2 Components of Ecosystems

The configuration of biotic and abiotic components determines how an ecosystem is structured. This section discusses the distribution of energy in our environment. It also considers the climate that prevails in that particular environment.

The structure of an ecosystem can be divided into two main components (Figure 32.1):

- biotic components
- abiotic components.

The biotic and abiotic components of an ecosystem are interdependent. The system is open, allowing parts and energy to move freely across boundaries, highlighting the role of biotic and abiotic elements in the structure of the ecosystem.

32.2.1 Biotic Components

The term "biotic component" refers to all forms of life in an ecosystem. Depending on their dietary requirements, biological elements can be classified as

- autotrophs
- heterotrophs
- saprotrophs (or decomposers).

Epidemiology and Environmental Hygiene in Veterinary Public Health, First Edition. Edited by Tanmoy Rana.
© 2025 John Wiley & Sons, Inc. Published 2025 by John Wiley & Sons, Inc.

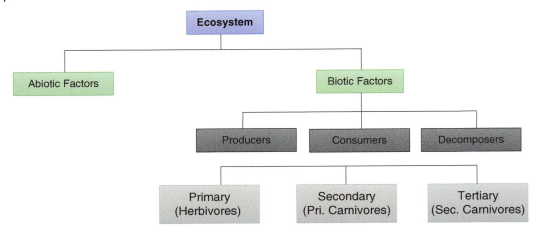

Figure 32.1 Components of an ecosystem.

32.2.1.1 Autotrophs
Plants are referred to as autotrophs because they can produce food through photosynthesis. An organism becomes more reliant on other producers for food as it moves up the food chain.

32.2.1.2 Heterotrophs
Heterotrophs rely on other organisms for food. The majority of consumers are herbivores (primary consumers). Energy is supplied by primary consumers to secondary consumers which can be either omnivores or carnivores. Organisms that rely on secondary consumers for food are referred to as tertiary consumers. Omnivores can also be tertiary consumers. There are quaternary consumers in some food chains. For energy, these organisms feed off tertiary consumers. Additionally, because they lack natural predators, they are frequently at the top of a food chain.

32.2.1.3 Saprotrophs
Saprophytes, such as fungi and bacteria, are decomposers. They rely entirely on dead and decomposing organic matter to survive. Decomposers are crucial to the ecosystem because they assist in recycling nutrients so that plants can use them again.

32.2.2 Abiotic Components

The ecosystem's nonliving components are known as abiotic components, including things like wind, altitude, turbidity, sunlight, water, soil, minerals, temperature, and nutrients.

32.3 Functions of an Ecosystem

The ecosystem serves the following purposes.
- It maintains stability, supports life systems, and controls key ecological processes.
- It also determines how nutrients are transferred between biotic and abiotic components.
- It keeps the ecosystem's various trophic levels in balance.
- Minerals are circulated throughout the biosphere.
- The abiotic components aid in the energy exchange process that results in the synthesis of organic components.

Structural Aspects

1) Inorganic aspects – C, N, CO_2, H_2O.
2) Organic compounds – protein, carbohydrates, lipids – link abiotic to biotic aspects.
3) Climatic regimes – temperature, moisture, light, and topography.
4) Producers – plants.
5) Macroconsumers – phagotrophs – large animals.
6) Microconsumers – saprotrophs, absorbers – fungi.

Functional Aspects

1) Energy cycles.
2) Food chains.
3) Diversity – interlinkages between organisms.
4) Nutrient cycles – biogeochemical cycles.
5) Evolution.

32.4 Food Chains, Food Webs, and Ecological Pyramids

32.4.1 Food Chains

The sun is the primary energy source for the planet. All plant life depends on it for the energy needed to function. Plants use this energy to create food through the process of photosynthesis. Light energy is transformed into chemical energy and transferred through successive levels during this biological process. The term "food chain" refers to the flow of energy from a producer to a consumer and ultimately to an apex predator or a detritivore (Figure 32.2).

The food chain, where plants or producers are solely consumed by primary consumers, primary consumers are solely fed by secondary consumers, and so on, is the best illustration of the flow of energy in an ecosystem. Any food chain has three main trophic levels: producers, consumers, and decomposers. The producers who are able to produce their own food are known as autotrophs. Scavengers break down organic waste and dead and decaying matter into their component parts which are then absorbed by the reducers. After gaining energy, the reducers release molecules into the environment that the producers can use again. Each trophic level has a very low energy efficiency. Therefore, food will be more accessible if the food chain is shorter.

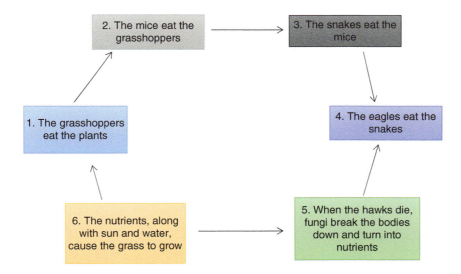

Figure 32.2 A classic example of a food chain in an ecosystem.

In a ground ecosystem, the typical food chain is composed of grass mice, snakes, and hawks. Organisms have more options for food, which helps them survive better. Food webs are more complex and related at different trophic levels. Hawks do not only eat snakes; mice also eat grass and grasshoppers in addition to being eaten by snakes and other animals. A food web is a more accurate representation of an ecosystem's feeding patterns.

32.4.2 Food Webs

In 1927, Charles Elton introduced the idea of the food web, which he called the "food cycle." The concept of a food web was defined by Charles Elton as follows. The herbivores get their energy from the sun. The later carnivores may also be preyed upon by other carnivores. There are chains of animals that are related by food, and all are ultimately dependent on plants. When an animal reaches a point where it has no enemies, it forms the terminus of this food cycle (Figure 32.3).

A food web is a graphical representation of the relationships between species in an ecological community that involve feeding and is made up of all the food chains in that community. The food web is an illustration of the various feeding strategies that connect the ecosystem. It also explains how energy moves through species in a community as a result of their relationships with one another in the food chain.

A food web is made up of all the food chains that are connected to one another and overlap in an ecosystem. Within an ecosystem, there are connections between food chains. One organism may be part of multiple food chains, making these connections extremely complex. A web-like structure instead of a traditional linear food chain results. Because they enable an organism to obtain food from a variety of organisms at lower trophiclevels, food webs are a crucial part of an ecosystem.

32.4.3 Ecological Pyramids

The ecological pyramid shows the various organisms' trophic levels in relation to their ecological functions as producers and consumers. Between the bottom and top of the pyramid, where the food producer is situated, are other trophic levels

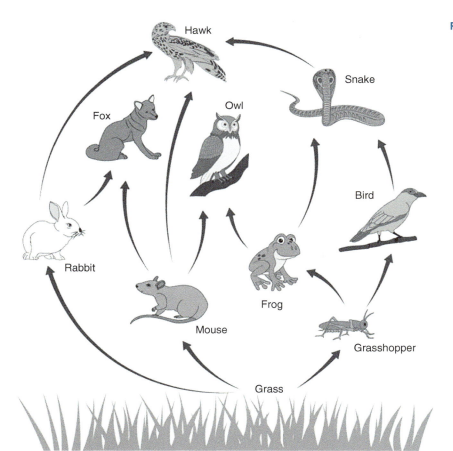

Figure 32.3 Food web.

of consumers. A graphic that illustrates the biomass or bioproductivity at each trophic level in a specific ecosystem is called an ecological pyramid (Figure 32.4). The length of each horizontal bar in the pyramid, which depicts various trophic levels, corresponds to the total number of individuals, biomass, or energy at that trophic level in an ecosystem.

On the ecological pyramid, the trophic levels of various organisms are shown in relation to their ecological functions as producers and consumers. The top of the chain displays the highest level.

Types of pyramids:

- pyramid of numbers
- pyramid of biomass
- pyramid of energy or productivity.

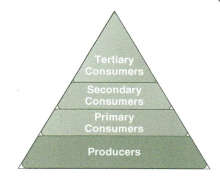

Figure 32.4 Ecological pyramid.

32.4.3.1 Pyramid of Numbers

The total number of entities from various species present at each trophic level is represented by a pyramid of numbers as the trophic level population (Figure 32.5). The pyramid of numbers may be upright or inverted, depending on the number of entities present. The trophic structure of an ecosystem is not entirely defined by the pyramid of numbers because it is very difficult to count all the organisms that are present there.

32.4.3.1.1 Pyramid of Numbers: Upright (Grassland Ecosystem)

The number of organisms in this pyramid decreases as you move up the trophic levels. The pond ecosystem and the grassland ecosystem are two examples of pyramids of numbers. Grass is abundantly found at the base (lowest trophic level) of the grass ecosystem. The primary consumer, or herbivore, is the next higher trophic level (an example would be a grasshopper). The energy level after that is a primary carnivore, like a rat. Rats prey on grasshoppers, so their numbers are lower than those of grasshoppers. Snakes are an example of a secondary carnivore, which is the next highest trophic level. They eat rats as food and rats eaten by hawks to become top carnivores. The number of individuals decreases from lower to higher trophic levels.

32.4.3.1.2 Pyramid of Numbers: Inverted (Tree Ecosystem)

In this type of pyramid, the number of individuals is increased from lower to higher trophic level.

32.4.3.2 Pyramid of Biomass

This is typically determined by gathering the individual organisms that make up each trophic level and figuring out their dry weight (Figure 32.6). All trophic-level organisms are weighed, which will help with the size disparity problem. It is believed that calculating biomass as a percentage of dry weight is more accurate. A standing crop is a particular collection of organisms from each trophic level at a particular moment in time. The standing crop is measured by the mass of living things (biomass), or the number in a specific area.

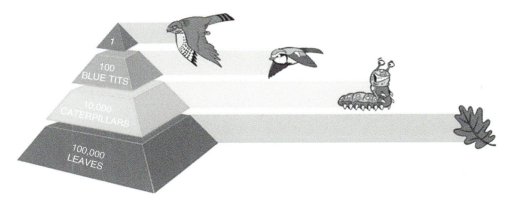

Figure 32.5 Pyramid of numbers.

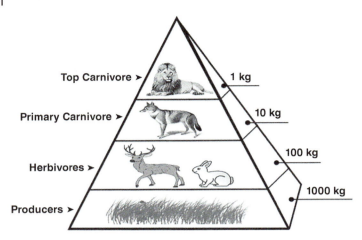

Figure 32.6 Pyramid of biomass.

32.4.3.2.1 Pyramid of Biomass: Upright

The base of the biomass pyramid on land is dominated by primary producers, with a lower trophic level present at the top. Primary consumers, the trophic level above them, have a lower biomass than producers. Secondary consumers, the trophic level above them, have lower biomass than primary consumers.

On the other hand, whereas the pyramid of numbers for aquatic ecosystems is upright, the pyramid of biomass may be present in many aquatic ecosystems in an inverted form. This is because the producers are tiny phytoplankton, which multiply and grow very quickly.

Here, the biomass pyramid is inverted and has a small base relative to the consumer biomass, which is always greater than the producer biomass.

32.4.3.3 Pyramid of Energy

The flow of energy from lower trophic levels to higher trophic levels is represented by the pyramid of energy (Figure 32.7). There is a notable energy loss when energy is transferred from one organism to another. Primary producers, such as autotrophs, have more energy available, while tertiary consumers have the least. As a result, shorter food chains have more energy available, even at the highest trophic level. The most effective way to compare the functional roles of the trophic levels in an ecosystem is thought to be by using an energy pyramid.

An energy pyramid shows how much energy is present at each trophic level and how much energy is lost when moving to a different level. Imagine that an ecosystem receives 1000 cal of light energy each day; most of it is not absorbed by plants; some of it is reflected back to space; green plants use up only a small portion of that energy and of the 1000 cal, only 100 cal (10%) are stored as energy-rich materials.

Let's say an animal consumes a plant that contains 100 cal of food energy, but only 10 of those calories are stored as food energy because the animal uses some of them for its own metabolism. Thus, as energy moves from sunlight to producers, herbivores, and carnivores, usable energy decreases. The energy pyramid will always be upright as a result.

32.5 Types of Ecosystems

An ecosystem can range in size from a few millimeters for a leaf to thousands of kilometers for an ocean. Two types of ecosystems exist.

- Terrestrial (land-based) ecosystem.
- Aquatic (water-based) ecosystem.

32.6 Terrestrial Ecosystems

On the basis of different geological zones on earth, terrestrial ecosystems are of the following types.

- Grassland ecosystems
- Forest ecosystems
- Desert ecosystems
- Tundra ecosystems

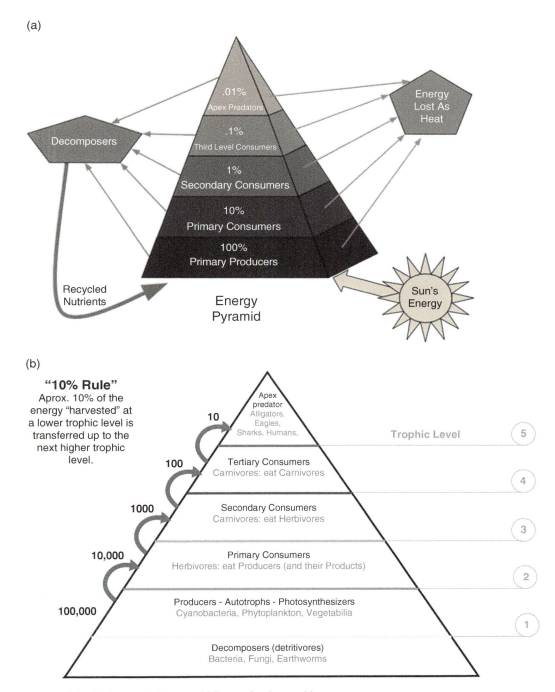

Figure 32.7 (a) Pyramid of energy (b) Enrgy-food pyramid.

32.6.1 Grassland Ecosystem

An ecosystem known as a grassland is one where grasses and other herbaceous (nonwoody) plants predominate (Figure 32.8). It spans 20% of the planet's surface and can be found in both tropical and temperate locations where there is not enough rainfall to support the growth of trees. Except for Antarctica, every continent has grasslands. They cover a percentage of the land at all latitudes and altitudes when the climate, soil, and conditions make it impossible for trees to grow. The growth of grasses and herbs is influenced by the soil, temperature, and locations with low rainfall and poor soil

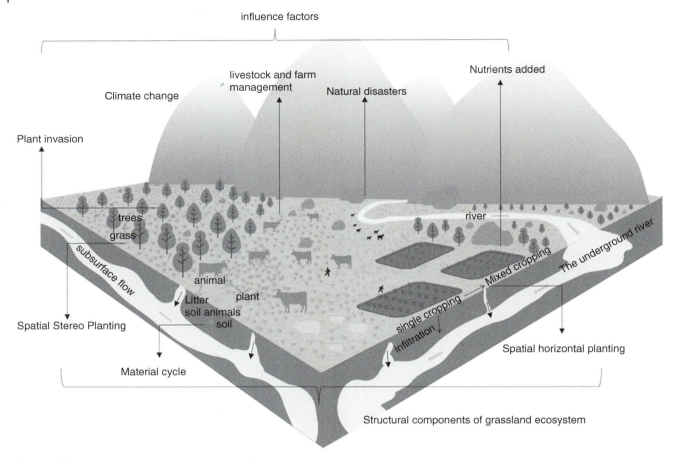

Figure 32.8 Grassland ecosystem.

depth and quality, but the growth of trees is hampered. Prairies, pampas, savannas, and steppes are some of the names of grassland according to geographical region.

Functions of grassland ecosystems include the cycling of nutrients through biogeochemical processes, enhancement of ecosystem production and soil fertility, reduction of mineral leaching as a result of reduced rainfall, and, most significantly, the transfer of energy through the food chain.

32.6.1.1 Living (Biotic) Components of Grassland Ecosystems
Biotic factors include *producers* (grasses, herbs), *consumers* (primary herbivores like cows, goats, sheep, deer, rabbit, buffaloes, termites, etc.), *secondary consumers* (carnivores which feed on primary consumers, such as snakes, birds, foxes, lizards, jackals, etc.), *tertiary consumers* (which feed on secondary consumers, such as hawks and other carnivores), and *decomposers* (bacteria, molds, and fungi that consume decayed organic matter). Decomposers enhance the quality and fertility of the soil by adding and reintroducing minerals, making them accessible to plants.

32.6.1.2 Nonliving (Abiotic) Components of Grassland Ecosystems
In addition to soil nutrients like phosphates, sulfates, nitrates, trace elements, and other macro- and micronutrients, abiotic variables include the atmosphere above the Earth, which contains gases like hydrogen, oxygen, nitrogen, and carbon dioxide. These inanimate components are essential for healthy soil and plant development.

32.6.1.3 Animals (Fauna) of Grassland Ecosystems
Grasslands are the habitat of the majority of large animals in the world. This type of ecosystem is home to a wide variety of creatures, from very small mites, insect larvae, nematodes, and earthworms that live in the world's richest soil at a depth of about 6 cm, to large mammals such as blue wildebeest, American bison, Przewalski's horse, Indian and African elephant, pronghorn, black rhino, white rhino, savanna elephant, swift fox, and one-horned rhino.

32.6.1.4 Trees/Plants/Shrubs/Herbs (Flora) of Grassland Ecosystems

Grassland ecosystems consist of very small grass to large trees which are very important for energy flow via the food chain. This ecosystem includes tall grasses (found in the prairies of North America and grasslands of the African savanna and South America.) woody plants, shrubs, or trees (African savannas). *Quercus robur, Betula pendula, Corylus avellana,* and *Crataegus* are some of the dominant trees of grassland ecosystems. In areas with annual rainfall of 500–900 mm, grasses flourish in large numbers.

32.6.1.5 Economic Importance of Grassland Ecosystems

Rice, corn, and wheat are the three plants mainly grown on grasslands worldwide. Grasslands provide the food source for grazing animals and an efficient system for water absorption. Some grasslands are designated as nature reserves or national parks, which encourages tourism.

32.6.2 Forest Ecosystem

The term "forest ecosystem" refers to the terrestrial system in which people, trees, animals, and insects interact with one another in order to survive (Figure 32.9). It is the planet's largest functional unit, made up of all its geographical features and living things. The temperature and rainfall in the region determine how many different types of forest ecosystems there are. Numerous plants, animals, and microorganisms coexist in harmony with abiotic (environmental) factors in a forest ecosystem. It is the primary carbon sink and a factor in regulating the Earth's temperature. The climatic conditions determine the distribution and number of trees in the forest vegetation.

The three major forest ecosystem classifications are:

- coniferous forest
- temperate forest
- tropical forest.

All these forest biomes are on a gradient from north to south latitude or from high to low altitude in general.

32.6.2.1 Coniferous Forest Ecosystem (Boreal Forest)

Evergreen forests, also referred to as taiga or snow forests, can be found south of the tundra in the northern hemisphere. It is the second largest biome in the world and spans about 20 million hectares in North America, Asia, and Europe.

32.6.2.2 Temperate Deciduous Forest

Because they experience all four seasons and lose their leaves in the autumn and winter, temperate deciduous forests are classified according to their seasonal weather patterns. Deciduous forest biomes are found in the tropics and between regions. As a result, this biome's climate is influenced by air masses from both biomes. Typically, the northern hemisphere, which includes parts of North America, Europe, Russia, China, and Japan, is home to the largest deciduous forests on earth. The southern hemisphere does have deciduous forests, but they are frequently much smaller than those in the north.

32.6.2.3 Temperate Evergreen Forest

The Cenozoic era saw the emergence of temperate evergreen forests. There are temperate evergreen forests in both cold and warm climate zones. Evergreen forests are so tightly packed that the ground never receives any sunlight. They contain a wide variety of heterotrophs and autotrophs. The northern and southern hemispheres are

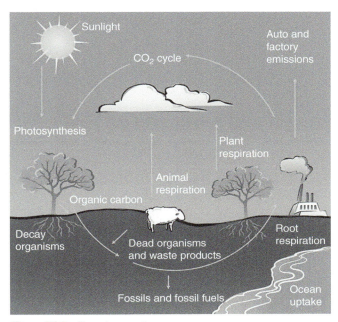

Figure 32.9 Forest ecosystem.

both covered in temperate evergreen forests. Compared to temperate deciduous forests, temperate evergreen forests can be found in milder climates nearer to the equator.

32.6.2.4 Temperate Rainforests
A biome that exists in a temperate climate is known as a temperate rainforest. Simply put, tropical rainforests have higher average temperatures and receive more rain than temperate rainforests. Many temperate regions contain temperate rainforests. The largest temperate rainforests in the world can be found on North America's Pacific coast.

32.6.2.5 Tropical Rainforests
The tropical rainforest is the most complex biome in the world in terms of structure and species diversity. It does best in growing environments which include a lot of rain and warmth all year round. Around 28° north or south of the equator, tropical rainforests can be found in Asia, Australia, Africa, South America, Central America, Mexico, and a number of Pacific Islands. Half of the world's population resides there, and they make up about 6–7% of the planet's surface.

32.6.2.6 Tropical Seasonal Forests
In regions with a protracted dry season, tropical seasonal forests can be found. The amount of defoliation that occurs during the dry season depends on how severe the moisture shortage is. The forest's structure is also less complex than that of the rainforest due to the absence of lush herbaceous and climbing plants as well as fewer tree strata. The distinctive characteristic of seasonal tropical forests is partial or complete leaf loss during the dry season, which occurs only in a few tree species. Other names for them include moist deciduous, semi-evergreen seasonal, tropical mixed, or monsoon forests.

32.6.3 Tundra Ecosystem

Without trees, tundra ecosystems are located in cold climates with little precipitation and are mostly covered in snow throughout the winter. However, the tundra region enjoys a resurgence in the summer when a variety of wildflower species bloom. It is distinguished by arid territory with black soil that is continuously frozen and is home to lichens, mosses, plants, and shrubs (Figure 32.10). The long winter season and brief summer season are the two different seasons in the tundra region, where the lengthy winter season could last up to eight months. Winter months in the tundra region are marked by lengthy nights, whereas summer months are marked by long days.

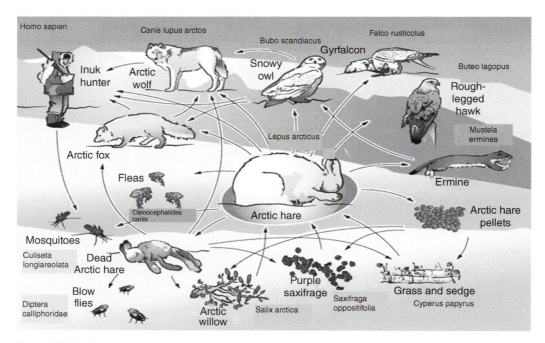

Figure 32.10 Tundra ecosystem.

The tundra environment covers 20% of the Earth's surface and is located in the Arctic and on mountain peaks. It is one of the planet's most unusual ecosystems because of the harsh climatic conditions, such as dry winds, very low precipitation, and extremely cold temperatures. The tundra region's extreme climate makes it challenging for plant and animal species to survive.

32.6.3.1 Arctic Tundra Region

Between the North Pole and the taiga region (a coniferous habitat), there is an area of Arctic tundra. Arctic tundra is characterized mostly by its extreme cold and permanently frozen landscape. North America (northern Alaska, Canada, Greenland), northern Europe (Scandinavia), northern Asia (Siberia), etc. make up the majority of the Arctic tundra habitat.

32.6.3.2 Alpine Tundra Region

Anywhere on the planet, alpine tundra can be found on high mountain peaks above the tree line. Alpine tundra is not permanently frozen like Arctic tundra but is blanketed in snow for the majority of the year. North America (Alaska, Canada, USA, Mexico), northern Europe (Finland, Norway, Russia, Sweden), Asia (southern Asia – Himalayan mountains), Japan (Mount Fuji), Africa (Mount Kilimanjaro), South America (Andes mountains) are all typical places to find Alpine tundra.

32.6.3.3 Tundra Ecosystem Characteristics

32.6.3.3.1 Extreme Climatic Conditions

For most of the year, the tundra ecosystem is extremely cold. The average temperature of the Arctic tundra region ranges from −40 °C to 18 °C. The Alpine tundra, on the other hand, is a little bit warmer, as winter temperatures rarely fall below –18 °C. Due to a brief period of mild temperatures, the living organisms of the tundra ecosystem experience some relaxation in the summer. The Alpine tundra region has a nearly 180-day growing season in the summer, compared to 50–60 days in the Arctic tundra region.

32.6.3.3.2 Permafrost, Poor Vegetation, and Precipitation

Permafrost is the term used to describe the long-lasting frozen layer of soil and other organic material found in the tundra ecosystem, which is a major factor causing the sparse vegetation of the tundra ecosystem. Permafrost can extend hundreds or even thousands of feet beneath the Earth's surface in some areas of the tundra. Surprisingly, this is an essential component of the ecosystem. During the summer, when the permafrost partially melts, small ponds develop on the topmost layer. Only a few plant species can withstand the severe weather of the tundra region, including lichens, sedges, shrubs, mosses, liverworts, and grasses. These plants help the various animal species that live in the tundra to meet their nutritional needs.

The tundra ecosystem is characterized primarily by its extremely low levels of precipitation and its dry climate. Less than 15 in. of precipitation fall on average each year in the tundra region.

32.6.3.3.3 Land of Midnight Sun

In the Arctic tundra, the phenomenon known as the midnight sun frequently occurs, when the sun does not completely set below the horizon in the summer. In the winter, the tundra region experiences a period when the sun never rises above the horizon. Due to this phenomenon, there are 24 hours of daylight during the summer and 24 hours of darkness during the winter. When compared to the equatorial region of the Earth, this phenomenon is very different as organisms living close to the equator experience a nearly constant 12-hour day and night cycle.

32.6.3.4 Tundra Ecosystem Animals (Fauna)

Because of the region's harsh climate, the fauna of the tundra ecosystem has evolved to be resilient. The animals of the tundra ecosystem are active during the summer, in contrast to the winter. For many insect species and animals, the summer is the best time to complete tasks. For instance, the majority of birds migrate north during the summer, various insects lay their eggs in the tundra ecosystem during the summer, and some mammal species come out of hibernation during the summer. For the winter, a small number of animals, such as caribou, migrate south. While some small mammals, like squirrels, protect themselves from the cold by burrowing and hibernating during the bitterly cold and harsh winter months, others, like musk ox, migrate to warmer areas in winter to protect themselves from the cold.

But many species have evolved to do well in tundra environments. Several species, such as the arctic fox, arctic hare, and ermine, among others, change their coat color with the seasons, going from brown in the summer to white in the winter. Other tundra animals, like snowy owls, ptarmigans, and musk oxen, are more active in the winter. In wetland areas of the tundra region, mosquitoes are quite prevalent in the summer.

32.6.3.4.1 Arctic Tundra Animals

The animals of the Arctic tundra ecosystem include snowy owl, reindeer, polar bear, lemming, wolverine, black fly, and white fox.

32.6.3.4.2 Alpine Tundra Animals

Alpine tundra animals migrate to lower elevations in the winter to protect themselves from the cold. Mountain goats, elk, springtails, butterflies, marmots, bighorn sheep, grizzly bears, beetles, and grasshoppers are among the animals that inhabit the Alpine tundra ecosystem.

32.6.4 Desert Ecosystem

Deserts can be found on every continent. There is very little rainfall in these areas, the nights are chilly, and the days are hot. As one of the most significant ecosystems in the world, 17% of the surface of the Earth is covered by desert (Figure 32.11). Nearly every continent contains a desert. Desert ecosystems flourish in regions with extreme temperatures year round and little to no precipitation, less than 50 cm of rain annually. The initial productivity of the desert ecosystem is very low.

A desert ecosystem is defined by species interactions, the environment in which they live, and any other nonliving factors that may have an impact on the habitat. It has less biodiversity because it is the driest terrestrial habitat in the world. The natural lifespan of plants in this desert environment is very short. Within a matter of days, they develop, germinate, and die. Desert plants are able to photosynthesize because of their green, succulent, and waxy stems. Stable high-pressure areas are frequently blamed for the lack of rain in the mid-latitudes; in temperate areas, deserts frequently exist in "rain shadows" or regions where massive mountains block precipitation.

Deserts are of two types namely: hot deserts and cold deserts.

32.6.4.1 Hot/Thar Desert

The Sahara is the largest desert in the world, covering an area of 8.54 million square kilometers, 1000 m above sea level. The climate in this area is very hot and dry, with little to no precipitation throughout the year. In this dry desert, the days are extremely hot. The exposed rocks and sand will become warm during the day when temperatures reach 45–50 °C. Temperatures occasionally fall below 0 °C during the night, making for bitterly cold conditions.

The hot desert covers most of North Africa, including Algeria, Tunisia, Egypt, Mali, Chad, Niger, Sudan, Mauritania, Libya, and Morocco. Around 8 600 000 km^2, or 4800 km east to west and 800–1200 km north to south, make up the entire region.

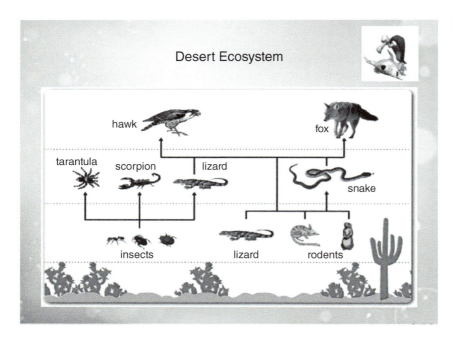

Figure 32.11 Desert ecosystem.

32.6.4.2 Cold/Temperate Desert

The Great Himalayas in eastern Jammu and Kashmir and the western Himalayas in Himachal Pradesh in north India are two temperate regions where cold desert can be found at high altitudes. Due to the high elevation, the climate is unusually chilly and dry.

Due to a lack of moisture in the air to absorb and store the heat produced by the high temperatures during the day, desert nights are frequently cold. Due to extreme temperature swings and extremely low water tables, the desert biome is a difficult geographic mass to inhabit. Temperatures are so extreme throughout the day because there is not enough moisture in the atmosphere to block out the sun's rays. This suggests that the ground absorbs energy from the sun. The earth's surface then heats the air in the immediate vicinity. When the sun sets, the opposite happens. The heated ground and hot air radiate the heat accumulated throughout the day back into the atmosphere, causing a sharp drop in temperature. At night, the temperature may fall below 0 °C.

In comparison to precipitation in cold deserts, precipitation in hot, dry deserts is very different. In hot deserts, there is typically 15 cm of rainfall per year. In contrast, cold deserts typically receive 15–26 cm of rain in the spring, along with a lot of snow.

Seasonal climates in desert ecosystems vary greatly. The summertime temperature ranges between 30 and 49 °C. There is little to no precipitation during the summer. Additionally, evaporation typically occurs faster than precipitation. The wintertime ranges in temperature from 10 to 20 °C.

The type of soil in an ecosystem affects the type of vegetation that grows there. The organic matter, phosphorus, and other nutrients required for plant growth are absent from desert soils. The habitat in the desert is made up of rocky, sandy, and dry soil. There are no large trees because the soil is unsuitable for plant growth.

32.6.4.3 Flora

Low rainfall and large daily temperature swings in desert ecosystems make life challenging for plants. Despite these challenges, this habitat supports a wide variety of plants. The most common plants that thrive in desert biomes include cacti, tiny shrubs, succulents, and grasses. Some examples of desert vegetation include the brittle bush, desert ironwood, chain fruit cholla, joshua tree, palo verde, jumping cholla, ocotillo, pancake prickly pear cactus, soap tree yucca, and Mojave aster.

32.6.4.4 Fauna

Examples of desert creatures include rabbits and wild cats. Bobcats and mountain lions are two of the most prevalent desert wild animals. The desert is also home to a variety of lizards, including tree lizards, banded geckos, and horned lizards. Many desert ecosystems are home to rattlesnakes, coral snakes, and king snakes. The horned lizards, which have horns and spines, only eat ants and beetles. Common desert birds include the vulture, golden eagle, and roadrunner. The Sonoran Desert ecosystem is home to a variety of animals, including Sonoran pronghorn antelopes, coyotes, javelina, desert tortoises, cactus wrens, desert kangaroo rats, thorny devils, desert bighorn sheep, and armadillo lizards.

32.6.4.5 Adaptations in Plants and Animals

To survive in these hostile environmental conditions, desert plants have developed special adaptations. To stop water loss, plants frequently store water in their stems and leaves, coat their leaves with wax, and shed their leaves. Some plants have evolved long taproots to reach water tables. Some plants will go dormant until the next rainy season. For instance, the cactus plant, which can reach a height of 20 ft and has a lifespan of more than 200 years, has successfully adapted to the harsh climatic conditions of desert biomes. The mugma tree is another plant that survives in desert regions. When it rains, the tiny leaves that make up the structure act as a funnel to direct the water to the base of the tree, where shallow roots absorb it. This adaptation generally ensures that the tree gets a lot of water when it rains.

The desert is home to a wide variety of animals which have developed unique cooling and water-saving adaptations. A typical desert animal like the camel may go days without food or water due to the water stored in its hump. Additionally, it has underwool and thick fur to keep warm during the coldest months. If sand is blowing, it can close its nostrils. Camels have large hooves to prevent them from sinking into the sand and two rows of eyelashes to shield their eyes from the sun and wind.

Foxes can escape the oppressive heat of the day by burrowing. Additionally, they have enormous ears which aid in dissipating excess body heat. They are shielded from the chilly nights of the desert by their thick, sand-colored fur. Panting to dissipate heat, seasonal migration, and extended periods of dormancy that last until triggered by moisture and temperature conditions are some of the adaptations that desert animals have developed.

32.7 Aquatic Ecosystems

An aquatic ecosystem is one that exists in and around a body of water, as opposed to terrestrial ecosystems that are based on land. Communities of organisms that depend on one another and their environment make up aquatic ecosystems.
Characteristics of aquatic ecosystems include the following.

- Being submerged in water.
- Being based on water.
- Being a cluster of living things.
- Being a discrete, more or less self-sustained community.

According to how much salt is present, aquatic ecosystems are categorized into the following subgroups.

- Freshwater ecosystems: rivers, lakes, and ponds.
- Brackish water ecosystems: mangroves, estuaries, etc.
- Marine ecosystems: oceans, seas, etc.

32.7.1 Freshwater Ecosystems

The freshwater ecosystem includes lakes, ponds, rivers, streams, and wetlands (Figure 32.12). These have no salt content, in contrast with the marine ecosystem. There are two types of freshwater ecosystems.

32.7.1.1 Lentic Ecosystem
The lentic ecosystem includes all nonflowing waters. Typical examples of the lentic ecosystem are lakes and ponds. These habitats are home to algae, crabs, prawns, and amphibians like frogs and salamanders. It is also known as the still-water or lacustrine ecosystem.

32.7.1.2 Lotic Ecosystem
The lotic ecosystem includes swiftly flowing bodies of water that move in a single direction, like rivers and streams. These environments are home to a wide variety of organisms, such as beetles, mayflies, stoneflies, and different fish species, such as trout, eels, and minnows.

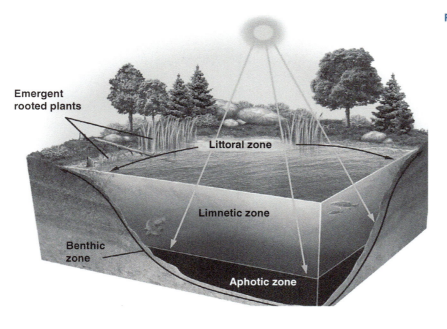

Figure 32.12 Freshwater ecosystem.

32.7.2 Marine Ecosystems

The marine ecosystem includes seas and oceans which have a more substantial salt content and greater biodiversity in comparison to the freshwater ecosystem (Figure 32.13). Water bodies with a salt concentration equal to or higher than seawater (i.e., 35 ppt or above) are referred to as marine ecosystems. The largest aquatic ecosystems on Earth are found in the oceans.

32.7.2.1 Aquatic Biome

Depending on where they are found, aquatic organisms are divided into different groups. Some species, like floating plants, live at the air–water interface. Periphyton are organisms that adhere to the stems and leaves of rooted plants as well as substances that emerge from the mud's surface, such as sessile algae. Plankton are floating microscopic organisms like algae, diatoms, protozoans, and larvae. This category (zooplankton) includes both animals like crustaceans and protozoans as well as microscopic organisms like algae. Due to their weak locomotory abilities, plankton dispersal in aquatic environments is primarily controlled by currents. Nekton are creatures with powerful swimming abilities and can swim against currents. Benthic species are those that reside at the bottom of a body of water.

32.7.2.2 Sunlight

Sunlight penetration quickly declines as it passes through the water column. The depth of a lake's light penetration determines the extent of plant dispersal. Due to suspended particles like clay, silt, phytoplankton, and others, the water turns murky. The amount of light that can enter an area and the potential for photosynthetic activity are both significantly decreased by turbidity. Based on plant distribution and light penetration, they are separated into photic and aphotic zones.

32.7.2.2.1 Photic Zone

The region between the lake's surface and a light level that is 1% of that at the surface is known as the photic (or "euphotic") zone. The depth of this zone depends on how transparent the water is. Both respiration and photosynthesis take plac ein the photic zone.

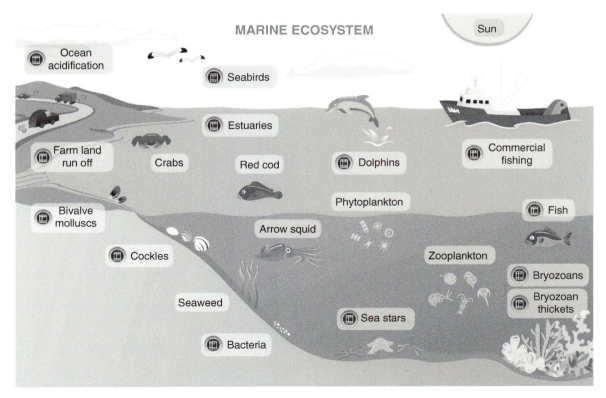

Figure 32.13 Marine ecosystem.

32.7.2.2.2 Aphotic Zone

The aphotic zone is the area of the lake where the light level is less than 1% of that at the surface. Depending on how transparent the water is, this zone can be at any depth.

32.7.2.3 Dissolved Oxygen

Fresh water typically has a dissolved oxygen content of 10 ppm by weight. The oxygen content in the same volume of air is 150 times higher than this. Oxygen enters the aquatic ecosystem through the interaction of air and water and the photosynthetic activity of aquatic plants. Dissolved oxygen leaves the water body through the air–water interface and organism respiration (fish, decomposers, zooplankton, etc.). When the concentration of dissolved oxygen falls below 3–5 ppm, many aquatic organisms perish.

32.7.2.4 Temperature

Because water temperatures are less susceptible to change, aquatic organisms have a limited range of acceptable temperatures. Because of this, they are significantly more vulnerable to even small changes in water temperature than terrestrial creatures are to changes in air temperature.

32.8 Biogeochemical Processes of Nutrient Cycling

Every element on earth is recycled numerous times. Organisms are made up of the major elements, which include oxygen, carbon, nitrogen, phosphorus, and sulfur. The movement of these chemical substances between organisms and their physical environment is referred to as the "biogeochemical cycle." Through processes like respiration, excretion, and decomposition, chemicals ingested by organisms are excreted into the environment, where they enter the food chain and eventually return to the soil, air, and water. As an element progresses through this cycle, it frequently joins forces with other elements to form compounds as a result of natural reactions in the atmosphere, hydrosphere, or lithosphere, as well as metabolic processes in living tissues.

Nutrient cycles are of two types.

- Gaseous
- Sedimentary

The reservoir for gaseous types of nutrient cycles (e.g., nitrogen and carbon cycles) exists in the atmosphere, and for sedimentary cycles (e.g., sulfur and phosphorus cycles), the reservoir is located in the Earth's crust. Environmental factors, e.g., soil, moisture, pH, temperature, etc., regulate the rate of release of nutrients into the atmosphere. The function of the reservoir is to meet the deficit that occurs due to an imbalance in the rate of influx and efflux.

32.8.1 Carbon Cycle

Through the process of photosynthesis, carbon enters the living world in the form of carbon dioxide and carbohydrates (Figure 32.14). Then, the producers pass these organic substances (food) on to the consumers (herbivores and carnivores). The respiration or decomposition of plants and animals by the decomposers ultimately returns this carbon to the surrounding medium. When fossil fuels are burned, carbon is also recycled.

32.8.2 Nitrogen Cycle

Nitrogen is an essential component of protein and is required by all living organisms, including humans. Our atmosphere contains nearly 79% nitrogen, but it cannot be used directly by the majority of living organisms. Broadly, like carbon dioxide, nitrogen also cycles from the gaseous phase to the solid phase and then back to the gaseous phase through the activity of a wide variety of organisms (Figure 32.15). The cycling of nitrogen is vitally important for all living organisms.

There are five main processes which are essential for the nitrogen cycle.

32.8.2.1 Nitrogen Fixation

This process involves conversion of gaseous nitrogen into ammonia, a form in which it can be used by plants. Atmospheric nitrogen can be fixed by the following three methods.

Figure 32.14 Carbon cycle.

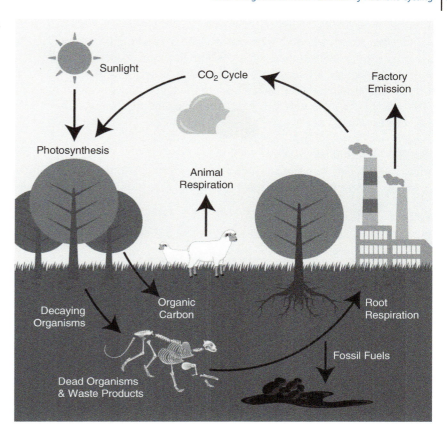

Figure 32.15 Nitrogen cycle.

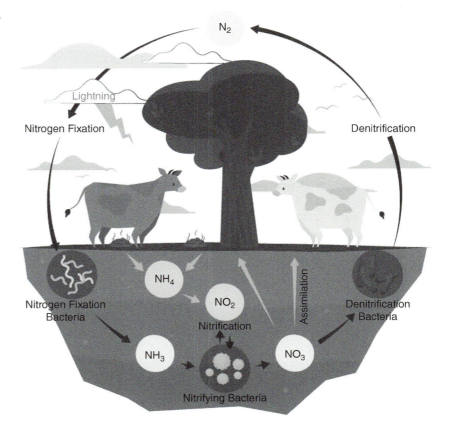

- *Atmospheric fixation*: lightning, combustion, and volcanic activity help in the fixation of nitrogen.
- *Industrial fixation*: at high temperature (400 °C) and high pressure (200 atm), molecular nitrogen is broken down into atomic nitrogen which then combines with hydrogen to form ammonia.
- *Bacterial fixation*: There are two types of bacteria.
    i) Symbiotic bacteria, e.g., *Rhizobium* in the root nodules of leguminous plants.
    ii) Free-living or symbiotic bacteria can combine atmospheric or dissolved nitrogen with hydrogen to form ammonia.

32.8.2.2 Nitrification
Ammonia is transformed into nitrates or nitrites through a process carried out by the bacteria *Nitrosomonas* and *Nitrococcus*, respectively. *Nitrobacter*, a different type of soil bacterium, can convert nitrate to nitrite.

32.8.2.3 Assimilation
In this process, the nitrogen that plants fix in the soil is transformed into organic molecules like proteins, DNA, and RNA. These molecules create the tissue in plants and animals.

32.8.2.4 Ammonification
Urea and uric acid are examples of nitrogenous waste products produced by living things. The bacteria turn these waste materials and the remains of dead organisms back into inorganic ammonia. Bacteria that ammonize aid in this process.

32.8.2.5 Denitrification
Denitrification is the process by which nitrates are transformed back into gaseous nitrogen. Since they prefer an oxygen-free environment, denitrifying bacteria can be found deep in the soil near the water table. The opposite of nitrogen fixation is denitrification.

32.8.3 Water Cycle

Life is dependent on water. Without water, no organism can survive. The only source of water on Earth is precipitation (rain, snow, slush, dew, etc.). The continuous movement of water in the biosphere is known as the water (hydrological) cycle and it results from water vapor produced by direct evaporation and evapotranspiration returning to the atmosphere (Figure 32.16). About two-thirds of the surface of the Earth is covered in water, making it the most water-rich planet in the solar system, but only a tiny portion of this is accessible to animals and plants.

The distribution of water on the Earth's surface is not uniform. The majority of the water on Earth – nearly 95% of it – is chemically bound to rocks and does not cycle. Nearly 97.3% of the remaining 5% is made up of oceans, and 2.1% is made up of polar ice caps. Thus, only 0.6% of the total volume is fresh water, which is found in the form of groundwater and soil water. The driving forces behind the water cycle are gravity and solar radiation.

The two primary processes that contribute to the water cycle are evaporation and precipitation. These two procedures switch off one another. The sun's heat energy causes water in oceans, lakes, ponds, rivers, and streams to evaporate. Additionally, plants transpire a lot of water. Water exists in the air as vapor, forming clouds that float with the wind. Evaporation removes 84% of the water from the surface of the oceans on average. While precipitation contributes 77% of its gains. 7% of the water that flows from land through rivers and into oceans balances the ocean's evaporation deficit. On land, there is 16% evaporation and 23% precipitation.

32.8.4 Phosphorus Cycle

In biological membranes, nucleic acids, and cellular energy transfer mechanisms, phosphorus plays a significant role (Figure 32.17). This element is essential for the production of many animals' shells, bones, and teeth. Rock, which has phosphorus in it as phosphates, is a natural source of phosphorus. Small amounts of these phosphates dissolve in soil solutions during rock weathering and are absorbed by plant roots. The source of this element for herbivores and other animals is vegetation. Phosphate-solubilizing bacteria break down waste materials and dead organisms, releasing phosphorus. There is no respiratory release of phosphorus into the atmosphere, unlike the carbon cycle.

32.8 Biogeochemical Processes of Nutrient Cycling | 383

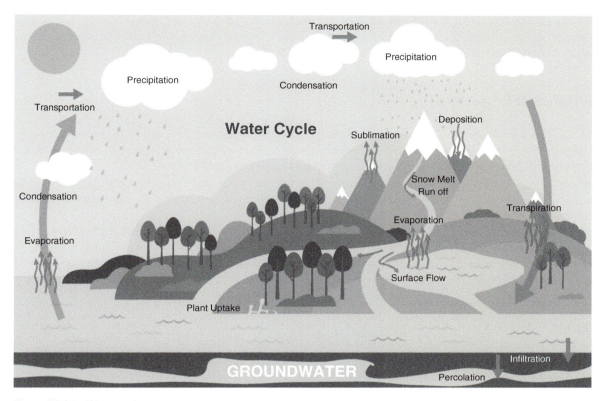

Figure 32.16 Water cycle.

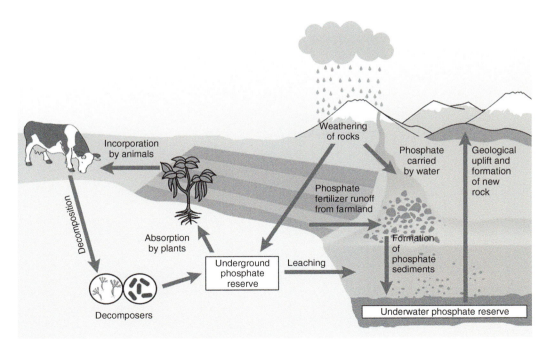

Figure 32.17 Phosphorus cycle.

The other two significant differences between the carbon and phosphorus cycles are, first, that atmospheric inputs of phosphorus through rainfall are significantly less than carbon inputs, and, second, that gaseous exchanges of phosphorus between organisms and their surroundings are hardly ever observed.

32.9 Importance of Ecosystems

In every habitat, an ecosystem is essential. Water, food, sunlight, and all other biotic needs are met by the ecosystem. So, in an ecosystem, crop rotation, afforestation, resource conservation, and wildlife management are essential. All the elements and factors can grow to their full potential in an ecosystem that is stable and prosperous.

Ecological processes are naturally occurring processes that result in the interaction and interlinking of organisms. All the ecosystem's parts are connected by this unbreakable chain, which encourages regulation. Energy flow and biochemical and nutrient cycling are some examples of fundamental ecological processes.

Energy flow is the movement of energy from one organism to another. Examples of energy flow include food chains and webs, where power descends from higher trophic levels. The energy, nutrients, and chemicals that are found in any environment, living or not, are transferred to living things through biochemical and nutrient cycles. The main categories of nutrient cycles are the nitrogen cycle, the carbon cycle, and the water cycle, discussed above.

Further Reading

Kumar, S. (2018). *Fundamentals of Environmental Studies*. New Delhi: Sultan Chand Publications.

Kaushik, A. and Kaushik, C.P. (2018). *Perspectives in Environmental Studies*. New Delhi: New Age International Publishers.

Odum, E.P., Odum, H.T., and Andrews, J. (1971). *Fundamentals of Ecology*. Philadelphia: W.B. Saunders.

Bharucha, E. (2018). *Textbook of Environmental Studies for Undergraduate Courses*. New Delhi: University Grants Commission.

33

Environmental Pollution: Air, Water, Soil, Marine, and Thermal Pollution

Parul, Udit Jain, Barkha Sharma, Anuj Kumar, Renu Singh, and Sanjay Bharti

College of Veterinary & Animal Sciences, DUVASU, Mathura, India

33.1 Introduction

Environmental pollution is a major problem around the globe. Industrial development is one of the main driving factors of pollution. Environmental pollution occurs when pollutants make changes in the physical, chemical, or biological components of the environment. The atmosphere, hydrosphere, and lithosphere are affected by pollutants which gives rise to air, water, and soil pollution (Barletta et al. 2019).

Air pollution is especially a problem of urban areas due to rapid industrialization, urbanization, increased transportation, and overpopulation. Water and soil pollution are interconnected as pollutant discharge in water also pollutes the soil; industrial waste, agricultural waste, and domestic sewage are sources of pollution in water and soil. Marine pollution is a subpart of water pollution where pollutants contaminate the seas and oceans.

There are various ways to understand the nature of pollutants. Primary pollutants are directly emitted from the source while secondary pollutants are byproducts of primary pollutants formed by reactions with other substances. On the basis of degradation ability, pollutants can be biodegradable or nonbiodegradable and on the basis of origin, they can be natural or anthropogenic. Origin can be a unique source (point source) or dispersed sources (nonpoint source).

Human inventions for the comfort and convenience of human beings are great emitters of pollutants (Marlon et al. 2019). Transportation by road, air, and water via automobiles, aeroplanes, and ships is a major source of air pollution. Noxious gases, particulate matter, and harmful substances are released into the air through these sources. Industrialization has resulted in an increase in the manufacture, use, and release into the environment of a wide variety of organic substances.

33.2 Types of Environmental Pollution

Environment is the sum total of all external conditions and influences affecting the life and development of any living being. Environmental pollution is undesirable change in the natural quality of the environment brought about by various physical, chemical or biological agents that may harm human and animal life and plants. Environmental health is affected by different type of pollutants that alter the natural composition of the atmosphere, hydrosphere, and lithosphere and cause air, water and soil, marine, thermal, radiation, nuclear, and plastic pollution (Burroughs Peña and Rollins 2017). The following types of pollution will be discussed in this chapter.

- Air pollution
- Water pollution
- Soil pollution
- Marine pollution
- Thermal pollution

Epidemiology and Environmental Hygiene in Veterinary Public Health, First Edition. Edited by Tanmoy Rana.
© 2025 John Wiley & Sons, Inc. Published 2025 by John Wiley & Sons, Inc.

33.3 Air Pollution

According to the World Health Organization, "Air pollution is contamination of the indoor or outdoor environment by any chemical, physical or biological agent that modifies the natural characteristics of the atmosphere." Many parts of the world suffer from urban air pollution and, despite the vast amount of knowledge about its causes, most countries are slow to implement countermeasures.

33.3.1 Classification of Air Pollutants

Criteria used to classify air pollutants include the nature of the source and chemical properties.

33.3.1.1 Nature of Source
- Major sources
- Minor sources
- Mobile sources
- Natural sources

Major sources are primarily industrial sources (textile, automobile, chemical, fertilizer industries), power stations, refineries, metallurgical plants, incinerators and other industrial plants that emit the air pollutants through chimneys.

Minor sources include indoor sources such as household appliances, domestic cleaning activities, dry cleaners, printing shops, etc.

Mobile sources include automobiles, trains, aeroplanes, helicopters, ships, and other transport vehicles.

Natural sources include forest fires, volcanic erosion, dust storms, avalanches, and agricultural burning.

33.3.1.2 Chemical Properties
Chemical air pollutants include gaseous compounds, CO, CO_2, NO, NO_2, SO_2, SO_3, NH_3, solid dispersed particles, particulate matter, hydrocarbons, pollen grains, microbes, etc. (NEPIS 2017). Most air pollutants are gaseous in nature and on the basis of their effect on human body may be categorized as irritant or nonirritant.

Irritant pollutants are those that cause irritation of mucous membranes in humans and animals; sulfur dioxide and ammonia are irritant gases.

Nonirritant pollutants include particulate matter and carbon monoxide.

33.3.2 Causes of Air Pollution

Dust particles originating from milling, crushing, and grinding activities, especially during road building operations, are responsible for lowering air quality, especially in urban and semiurban areas (Manisalidis et al. 2020).

Other causes include:

- geochemical contamination
- photochemical reactions
- change in climatic conditions
- volcanic eruptions
- gaseous discharge from marshes and swamps
- forest fires
- dust
- fog
- radiation fall-out.

33.3.3 Effects of Air Pollution

Air pollutants, whether gases, particulate matter or air-borne pathogens, exert harmful effects on human, animal, and environmental health. Buildings and monuments are also affected by harmful gases emitted by industries.

33.3.3.1 Effects on Humans

Pollutants differ in their properties and state, thus producing variable toxic effects in various organs of human body. PM10 and PM2.5 particles can penetrate inside the lung tissue when inhaled and produce pneumoconiosis while gaseous compounds either cause irritation to mucosal membranes or affect the nervous and respiratory systems (Kjellstrom et al. 2017). The human respiratory system is especially affected by air pollutants. Gaseous compounds and particles are able to damage lungs and can even enter the bloodstream, leading to the premature deaths of millions of people yearly. Air pollution has various short- and long-term health effects. Short-term exposure to air pollutants is closely related to cough, shortness of breath, wheezing, asthma, and respiratory disease while long-term effects include chronic asthma, chronic obstructive pulmonary disease (COPD), and pulmonary insufficiency.

33.3.3.2 Effects on Animals and Vegetation

Air pollutants also affect animals and plants. Pollutants cause damage to the internal organs of animals, especially the respiratory system. Pollutants tend to decrease production in animals. High atmospheric concentrations of gaseous pollutants like SO_2 and NO_2 may cause acid rain which has a pH less than 5.2. Acid rain causes deleterious effects on vegetation including burning of plant leaves. Notably, soil chemistry can be altered due to acid precipitation by affecting plants and water quality. Moreover, movement of heavy metals is favored by soil acidity (Kankaria et al. 2014).

33.3.4 Control of Air Pollution

Air pollution caused by particulate matter like dust, soot, ash, etc. can be controlled by using settling chambers, fabric filters, wet scrubbers, electrostatic precipitators, cyclone separators, and other mechanical devices (Wu et al. 2020) (Figure 33.1). Particulate matter pollution in industrial plants can be controlled at large scale using the following aids.

33.3.4.1 Settling Chambers

In this process, the particulates settle down by the action of gravitational force and are removed.

33.3.4.2 Fabric Filters

The particulate matter is passed through a porous medium made of fabric. The particulates in the polluted air are collected in the fabric filters, while the gases are discharged. The process of controlling air pollution using fabric filters is called "bag filtration."

33.3.4.3 Wet Scrubbers

These are devices used to trap SO_2, NH_3, and metal fumes by passing the fumes through water.

33.3.4.4 Electrostatic Precipitators

When air containing particulate pollutants is passed through an electrostatic precipitator, it induces an electric charge on the particles which are then precipitated onto electrodes.

33.3.4.5 Cyclone Separators

A cyclone separator has several colloquial names, including "dust separator," "dust collector," "dust extractor," "cyclone extractor," and "cyclone separator." Generally, smaller units are referred to as "dust" separators or extractors, while large-scale industrial separators are referred to as "cyclone separators."

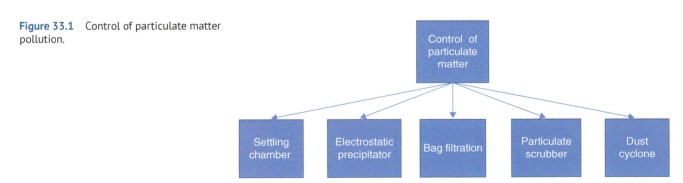

Figure 33.1 Control of particulate matter pollution.

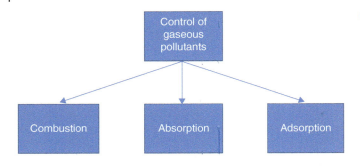

Figure 33.2 Control of gaseous pollutants.

Gaseous byproducts can be removed using the following interventions (Figure 33.2).

- Combustion
- Absorption
- Adsorption

33.3.4.6 Combustion
In this technique, organic air pollutants are subjected to flame combustion or catalytic combustion when they are converted to less harmful carbon dioxide and harmless water.

33.3.4.7 Absorption
Air containing gaseous pollutants is passed through a scrubber containing a suitable liquid absorbent. The liquid absorbs the harmful gaseous pollutants present.

33.3.4.8 Adsorption
In this method, the polluted air is passed through porous solid adsorbents kept in suitable containers. The gaseous pollutants are adsorbed at the surface of the porous solid and clean air passes through.

33.4 Water Pollution

Water pollution has become a worldwide issue mainly resulting from human activities. Overpopulation and industrialization are the leading reasons for pollution of underground as well as surface water. The discharge of industrial effluents, domestic sewage, agricultural waste, and mining effluents into water bodies (rivers, lakes, springs, seas, and oceans) leads to water pollution. Chemical and microbial pollutants change the natural composition of water and also spoil the quality of water. Water pollution affects human, animal, ecosystem, and environmental health (Babuji et al. 2023).

33.4.1 Classification of Water Pollutants

There are various ways to classify water pollutants and many classifications have been proposed. One method is to determine the point of pollution.

33.4.1.1 Point Source Pollution
When the source of pollution is fixed and identified and pollutants are discharged from these points into water bodies or percolate into underground water, this is defined as point source pollution. Examples include outlets of industrial plants and waste water treatment plants pouring waste effluents into water bodies. It is easy to control point source pollution either by sealing the plant or by refinement of effluent discharges before draining into water bodies.

33.4.1.2 Nonpoint Source Pollution
This occurs when the point of pollution is unidentified or not fixed and effluent is discharged into water bodies at various unidentified locations. Effluents can drain into water bodies at places distant from the main source. Storm drainage, agricultural runoff, construction sites, and other land disturbances are classed as nonpoint source pollution, which is difficult to control (Chen et al. 2019).

33.4.2 Causes of Water Pollution

Industrial effluents are the main cause of water pollution; other sources include agricultural activities, natural factors, and insufficient water supply and sewage treatment facilities.

Industries include distilleries, tanneries, pulp and paper, textiles, food, iron and steel, nuclear, etc. Various toxic chemicals, organic and inorganic substances, toxic solvents, and volatile organic chemicals may be released in industrial production. If these wastes are released into aquatic ecosystems without adequate treatment, they will cause water pollution. With the acceleration of urbanization, waste water from industrial production has gradually increased. In addition, water pollution caused by industrialization is also greatly affected by foreign direct investment in less developed countries.

Water pollution is closely related to agriculture, especially pesticides, nitrogen fertilizers, and organic farm wastes.

To sum up, water pollution results from both human and natural factors. Various human activities will directly affect water quality, including urbanization, population growth, industrial production, climate change, and religious activities (Chowdhary et al. 2020). Improper disposal of solid waste, sand, and gravel is another reason for decreasing water quality.

33.4.3 Effect of Water Pollution

Water contamination has long been a serious issue but it is now aggregated with advancements in industrialization and technology. Around the globe, countries are running campaigns regarding water pollution, but it remains a problem due to lack of awareness and violation of rules and policies. Consumption of contaminated water containing harmful chemicals released from industrial effluents, heavy metals and their compounds and radioactive elements exerts harmful effects on health. Growing children and pregnant women have a comparatively higher health risk. Studies show that plastic fiber is present in marine and freshwater bodies as well as groundwater. Consumption of microplastics may lead to cancer (Dwivedi et al. 2018).

Prolonged exposure to polluted water may pose severe health hazards to the digestive, excretory, circulatory, and musculoskeletal systems of the body. Heavy metals, especially mercury, nickel, zinc, cobalt, cadmium, chromium, copper, and lead, may cause toxicity. Minamata disease is a well-known water-borne mercury poisoning arising from consumption of fish containing high concentrations of mercury (Lin et al. 2022) Likewise, cadmium toxicity causes musculoskeletal disorders in human beings.

33.4.4 Control of Water Pollution

To resolve the issue of pollution it should be mandatory that effluents are treated before discharg. Natural and mechanical methods are used for control of water pollution.

33.4.4.1 Natural Bioremediation
A passive type of remediation that uses natural processes to remove contaminants from groundwater. In this process microorganisms modify their natural surroundings until oxygen and levels of nutrients reach acceptable levels. The pollutant is changed through advection, disintegration, cometabolism, adsorption, diffusion, and dispersion. It is less expensive than developed bioremediation and also eco-friendly.

33.4.4.2 Engineered Bioremediation
In engineered bioremediation, natural bioremediation processes are modified to promote rapid activity of microorganisms, as depicted in Figure 33.3.

33.5 Soil Pollution

Soil is the upper layer of the Earth that is produced by weathering of rocks over thousands of years. Soil is a mixture of inorganic minerals and organic compounds. Harmful substances in soil cause severe damage to the quality of soil, adversely affecting agricultural productivity (Brevik et al. 2020).

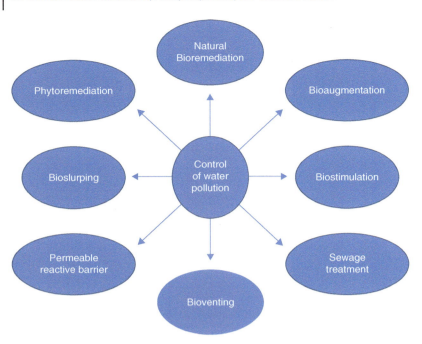

Figure 33.3 Control of water pollution.

33.5.1 Causes of Soil Pollution

- Household/industrial wastes containing organic and inorganic substances, solid wastes, plastics, inorganic chemicals, heavy metals, and toxic chemicals are dumped into soil.
- Domestic waste, sewage, and sludge are major sources of soil pollution in urban areas.
- Large amounts of discarded materials such as concrete, asphalt, paper and rags, leather, plastics, cans, glass and packing materials, etc. are dumped into landfill site.
- Acid rain due to air pollution results in soil pollution, by making the soil acidic and infertile.
- Pesticides, rodenticides, fungicides, and herbicides accumulate in the soil and cause soil pollution.
- Radioactive wastes and nuclear wastes from nuclear reactors and nuclear explosions also cause soil pollution.

33.5.2 Effects of Soil Pollution

The level of toxicity in the soil is increased due to industrial effluents and heavy metal deposition. Fertility is also reduced due to excessive use of chemical fertilizers. In addition, sewage and sludge are a rich source of pathogens, especially typhoid, jaundice, dysentery, and gastroenteritis. Their use as fertilizer may lead to spread of disease in animals and humans (Radomirović et al. 2020).

33.5.3 Control of Soil Pollution

Control of soil pollution can be achieved by using the following practices. Excessive use of chemical fertilizers and pesticides should be avoided and use of biofertilizers and biopesticides should be encouraged. Sewage waste is a big problem in cities but it can be converted into organic manure through composting. Afforestation and bioremediation of soil can reduce soil degradation due to erosion. Leakage of radioactive substances into the soil should be prevented (Gautam et al. 2023).

33.6 Marine Pollution

Release of harmful substances into marine waters can cause damage to the marine ecosystem. Marine pollutants may include industrial waste or toxic chemicals, oil drilling, plastic articles, etc. Pollution results in environmental damage and harms aquatic organisms and exerts a negative effect on the marine ecosystem.

33.6.1 Sources of Marine Pollution

An enormous amount of sewage, garbage, plastic, and agricultural discharge is dumped into river waters which ultimately enter the sea. Oil drilling and shipment cause release of oil and other pollutants in the marine environment and are a prominent factor in marine pollution. Radioactive wastes from nuclear power plants are dumped in deep sea sites. Petroleum refineries, off-shore oil production units, and tankers transporting oil cause significant marine pollution. Shipping industries are also a source of marine pollution.

33.6.2 Effects of Marine Pollution

Aquatic organisms such as phytoplankton, zooplankton, coral reefs, algal species, fishes, birds, and marine mammals are severely affected by marine pollutants. Agricultural pollutants which enter the food chain make fish and other aquatic animals unsuitable for human consumption. Oil spills in the sea affect sensitive aquatic plants and animals by reducing the availability of oxygen and causing the death of marine flora and fauna. Microplastic particles which become embedded in marine animals may be carcinogenic for consumers (Glaucia et al. 2019).

33.6.3 Control of Marine Pollution

- Toxic effluents from industries and sewage treatment plants should not be discharged in coastal waters.
- Developmental activities along coastal areas should be strictly controlled.
- Oil and grease from service stations should be recycled.
- Ecologically vulnerable coastal areas should be protected from oil well drilling.
- Proper treatment of effluents should be undertaken before the discharge and dumping of industrial and radioactive substances.
- Dumping of toxic waste, sewage, and sludge in marine waters should be banned.
- Strict environmental regulations should be implemented for offshore oil wells.
- Public awareness programs should be organized.
- Enforcement of Marine Acts and Coastal Acts.

33.7 Thermal Pollution

Thermal pollution is the change (rise or fall) in temperature of a natural water body caused by human influence. Discharge of hot water to rivers, streams, lakes, and ponds can damage aquatic ecosystems, termed hot water pollution. In contrast, cold water discharge into water bodies causing lowering of temperature is termed cold water pollution (Raptis et al. 2016).

33.7.1 Sources of Thermal Pollution

The main sources of thermal pollution include industrial waste water, thermal power plants, hydroelectric power plants, nuclear power plants, domestic sewage, coal-fired power plants, and urban runoff.

33.7.2 Effects of Thermal Pollution

Thermal pollution mainly affects the aquatic ecosystem, causing a decrease in oxygen levels and denaturation of enzymes, lowering biodiversity and causing a sudden change in temperature of water bodies which may lead to thermal shock in aquatic fauna. Temperature changes disrupt the entire marine ecosystem because changes in temperature cause changes in physiology, metabolism, and biological processes such as respiration rate, digestion, excretion, and development of an aquatic organism.

In cold weather, addition of warm water to water bodies has a less deleterious effect, and thus the aquatic system may be enhanced, in a phenomenon known as thermal enrichment. It is seen more especially in seasonal water bodies.

33.7.3 Control of Thermal Pollution

Heated water from industries should be treated before discharging directly to water bodies. Hot water can be treated by cooling ponds and cooling towers (Thushari and Senevirathna 2020). Artificial lakes are also useful in the control of thermal pollution; in these lakes industries can discharge used or heated water at one end and water for cooling purposes may be withdrawn from the other end so that the heat is eventually dissipated through evaporation.

33.8 Conclusion

Throughout the globe, pollution is a big issue and many policies and laws have been created to curb it. However, we are not achieving our targets, which may be because of ignorance about the rules or not realizing the gravity of the situation. Gradually, all natural resources will be affected by the various pollutants in this world so there is immense need to implement measures to cope with pollutants and pollution and make this Earth safe for all its inhabitants.

References

Babuji, P., Thirumalaisamy, S., Duraisamy, K., and Periyasamy, G. (2023). Human health risks due to exposure to water pollution: a review. *Water* 15 (14): 2532.

Barletta, M., Lima, A.R.A., and Costa, M.F. (2019). Distribution, sources and consequences of nutrients, persistent organic pollutants, metals and microplastics in South American estuaries. *Science of the Total Environment* 651: 1199–1218.

Brevik, E.C., Slaughter, L., and Singh, B.R. (2020). Soil and human health: current status and future needs. *Air, Soil and Water Research* 13: 1178622120934441.

Burroughs Peña, M.S. and Rollins, A. (2017). Environmental exposures and cardiovascular disease: a challenge for health and development in low- and middle-income countries. *Cardiolgy Clinics* 35: 71–86.

Chen, B., Wang, M., Duan, M. et al. (2019). In search of key: protecting human health and the ecosystem from water pollution in China. *Journal of Cleaner Production* 228: 101–111.

Chowdhary, P., Bharagava, R.N., Mishra, S., and Khan, N. (2020). Role of industries in water scarcity and its adverse effects on environment and human health. In: *Environmental Concerns and Sustainable Development* (ed. V. Shuklar and N. Kumar), 235–256. New Delhi: Springer.

Dwivedi, S., Mishra, S., and Tripathi, R.D. (2018). Ganga water pollution: a potential health threat to inhabitants of Ganga Basin. *Environment International* 117: 327–338.

Gautam, K., Sharma, P., Dwivedi, S. et al. (2023). A review on control and abatement of soil pollution by heavy metals: emphasis on artificial intelligence in recovery of contaminated soil. *Environmental Research* 225: 115592.

Glaucia, P.O., Maria, C.T.M., Cassiana, C.M. et al. (2019). Microplastic contamination in surface waters in guanabara bay, Rio de Janeiro, Brazil. *Marine Pollution Bulletin* 139: 157–162.

Kankaria, A., Nongkynrih, B., and Gupta, S. (2014). Indoor air pollution in India: implications on health and its control. *Indian Journal of Community Medicine* 39: 203–207.

Kjellstrom, T., Lodh, M., McMichael, T. et al. (2017). Air and water pollution: burden and strategies for control. In: *Disease Control Priorities in Developing Countries*, 817–832. Washington, DC: World Bank.

Lin, L., Yang, H., and Xu, X. (2022). Effects of water pollution on human health and disease heterogeneity: a review. *Frontiers in Environmental Science* 10: 880246.

Manisalidis, I., Stavropoulou, E., Stavropoulos, A., and Bezirtzoglou, E. (2020). Environmental and health impacts of air pollution: a review. *Frontiers in Public Health* 8: 14.

Marlon, J.R., Bloodhart, B., Ballew, M.T. et al. (2019). How hope and doubt affect climate change mobilization. *Frontiers in Communication* 4: 20.

NEPIS (2017). (National Service Center for Environmental Publications) (Environmental Protection Agency). www.epa.gov/clean-air-act-overview (accessed 15 March 2024).

Radomirović, M., Ćirović, Ž., Maksin, D. et al. (2020). Ecological risk assessment of heavy metals in the soil at a former painting industry facility. *Frontiers in Environmental Science* 8: 560415.

Raptis, C.E., Van Vliet, M.T.H., and Pfister, S. (2016). Global thermal pollution of rivers from thermoelectric power plants. *Environmental Research Letters* 11 (10): 104011.

Thushari, G.G.N. and Senevirathna, J.D.M. (2020). Plastic pollution in the marine environment. *Heliyon* 6 (8): e04709.

Wu, H., Gai, Z., Guo, Y. et al. (2020). Does environmental pollution inhibit urbanization in China? A new perspective through residents' medical and health costs. *Environmental Research* 182: 109128.

34

Environmental Pollution Effect on Animal and Human Health

Goverdhan Singh[1], Balram Yadav[1], and Vivek Agrawal[2]

[1] *College of Veterinary and Animal Science Navania, Vallabhnagar, Udaipur, RAJUVAS, Bikaner, India*
[2] *College of Veterinary Science and Animal Husbandry, NDVSU, Mhow, Indore, India*

34.1 Introduction

The natural environment in which we reside encompasses both living and non-living entities. This intricate system of resources has evolved over millennium through complex evolutionary processes (Patra and Swarup 2000). Numerous physical and chemical elements that interact in different ways make up the environment. Living organisms are fundamentally supported by the physical elements of their natural environment, which include air, water, and land (Swarup et al. 2000). The equilibrium between the reaction of these living organisms and the physical components of the environment is crucial for maintaining harmony between life and the environment. However, in recent decades, human activities have disrupted this balance, resulting in various environmental issues, including pollution (Swarup et al. 2002).

34.1.1 Environment Pollution

Any unfavourable change in the environment that has an adverse effect on flora and fauna is called environmental pollution. When a substance's concentration is higher than its natural abundance and may be linked to either natural or human-caused occurrences, it is classified as a pollutant. Environmental pollution has a long history. The autopsy lesions of an Eskimo lady who died around 1600 years ago show signs of its deleterious consequences, which are similar to those found in coal miners who have black lung disease (Bell et al. 1990).

The twentieth century has seen an exponential rise in pollution levels as a result of fast urbanization, industrialization, and inappropriate use of chemicals like pharmaceuticals and pesticides. Furthermore, an unfavourable habitat for both humans and animals has been produced by the discharge of thousands of synthetic chemicals into the environment. While certain pollutants, like heavy metals, DDT, plastics, and nuclear waste these, take decades to break down and are challenging to eliminate from the environment. Furthermore, Singh and Pandey noted that the dispersal of manure in high animal-density areas can result in water pollution (Singh and Pandey 2005).

34.1.1.1 Effects of Environmental Pollution

Studies have demonstrated that contaminants can start in one place and be carried by wind or water to other locations like that Pollutants are released into the environment as a result of human activity by contaminating the land, water, and air. Decreased crop productivity and detrimental effects on human and animal civilizations can arise from soil pollution, that also has the potential to kill off beneficial microbes and impair fertility. Contaminated water must be purified before consumption, which requires significant resources. Air pollution can cause respiratory diseases and same harm both human and animal health. Plants, animals, and people can all be harmed by the toxicity of pesticides, heavy metals (As, Pb, Hg, Cd), fluorine, and other agrochemicals in the environment.

This assessment seeks to address the consequences of pollution on human and animal health, as well as the environmental effects of pollutants. Scientific literature has documented examples of industrial pollution causing heavy mortality in

Epidemiology and Environmental Hygiene in Veterinary Public Health, First Edition. Edited by Tanmoy Rana.
© 2025 John Wiley & Sons, Inc. Published 2025 by John Wiley & Sons, Inc.

bovines (Sidhu et al. 1994), lead toxicosis (Swarup and Dwivedi 2002), and severe industrial fluorosis in cattle, sheep, and buffaloes (Patra et al. 2001). Environmental pollution has also led to adverse health effects, including cardio-pulmonary diseases in humans and allergic diseases in animals.

Because pollution negatively affects life on Earth, so environmental contamination needs to be minimized and to preserve our survival, it is imperative that the ecosystem must be kept in balance. We must take care to prevent harm to nature and protect the environment, as it can have severe consequences for us.

34.1.1.2 Gaseous Pollutants and Their Health Hazards

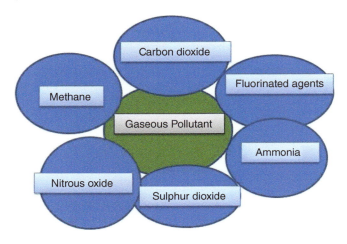

Figure 34.1 Majaor gaseous pollutants of human and animals.

Carbon Dioxide (CO₂)

CO_2 is a primary air pollutant and a greenhouse gas (GHG) that contributes to global warming. The amount of CO_2 increases in the atmosphere by decomposition, respiration, ocean release, photosynthesis, and human activities like burning of fossil fuels, deforestation, and cement production. Within a year, a mature bovine can produce approximately 4000 kg, a pig about 450 kg, a sheep up to 400 kg, and a man up to 300 kg of CO_2 (Figure 34.1).

Methane (CH₄)

In ruminants CH_4 is formed as a result of anaerobic digestion. Their gas production varies from 2 to 12% of their total calorie consumption. Johnson and Johnson (Johnson and Johnson 1995) found that CH_4 has a negative impact on the ozone layer and creates an ecological imbalance in greenhouse environments. Ruminant livestock produce between 250 and 500 litres of CH_4 per day, which could account for 2% of the global warming that could happen in the next 50–100 years. Methane's hazardous effects are over 21 times greater than those of CO_2.

Nitrous Oxide (N₂O)

The third most prevalent greenhouse gas and a "ozone-depleting" chemical is N_2O. Nitric acid (HNO_3) and Nitrous acid (HNO_2) are other kinds of nitrous oxides (NO_x). In 1998, the EPA established NO_2 guidelines of 0.053 parts per million (ppm). The production of acidic products and chemicals, road transportation, agriculture, and power generation are the main sources of N_2O emissions. It is naturally produced by a wide range of biological sources in soil and water, as well as by microbial nitrification and de-nitrification processes. Because it is bacteriostatic and leaves no taste or odour, so it utilized as a mixing and foaming agent in the dairy sector.

Sulphur Dioxide (SO₂)

SO_2 is a colourless, strong odour reactive gas and a significant air pollutant found in cities mainly by sulphur containing materials burning like fossil fuels, smelting ores, and in other industrial operations. Aerosols of sulphuric acid (H_2So_4) are created in the presence of moisture when SO_2 in the atmosphere is further oxidized to sulphur trioxide (SO_3) at a rate of 0.5–10% per hour (WHO 1987). When SO_2 and acid aerosols combine with other pollutants in the form of droplets or solid particles, they create sulphurous smog, which is extremely harmful to human and animal health and can cause respiratory issues such as bronchitis, coughing, asthma attacks, wheezing, and phlegm.

Ammonia (NH₃)

NH$_3$ is a colourless, pungent gas that is a byproduct of mainly agriculture industry and most of the NH$_3$ emitted comes from livestock waste management and fertilizer production. Their elevated levels have negative health impacts on people and livestock. Reduced feed consumption, decrease in egg production, thin-shelled eggs, and low live birth weight are common results of NH$_3$ poisoning in chickens (Miner 1973).

Fluorinated Agents

They have a very high potential for global warming and are compounds that deplete the ozone layer such as hydro-fluoro-carbons (HFCs), sulphur hexafluoride (SF$_6$), per-fluoro-carbons (PFCs), and nitrogen trifluoride (NF$_3$). Fluorine in small amounts is thought to be crucial for preventing dental cavities and osteoporosis in people. Dental fluorosis, on the other hand, exhibits significant osteosclerosis, hypoplasia, hypocalcification, and accelerated tooth wear in addition to mottling of the tooth enamel (Swarup and Singh 1989). Osteoporosis, osteopetrosis, and hyperostosis are the hallmarks of skeletal fluorosis. Fluorosis, or chronic fluorine poisoning, is brought on by consuming excessive amounts of fluorine over time (Swarup et al. 1998). A number of coal-burning and industrial activities like power-generating stations, welding operations and manufacturing or production of metal (steel, iron, aluminum, zinc, phosphorus), glass, chemical fertilizers, cement, bricks, and plastic are generally discharging fluoride in the environment. Bony exostosis, lameness, decreased performance and production, difficulty masticating food, decreased feed conversion efficiency, poor digestibility, and mortality are symptoms of the fluorosis ailment in animals (Swarup and Dwivedi 2002).

34.1.1.3 Heavy Metal Toxicity and Their Health Hazards

Environmental contamination by heavy metals is a major issue in the majority of the world's nations. Toxic heavy metals are released into the environment by a variety of human activities, including burning fossil fuels, mining, metallurgy, industries, and transportation. These heavy metals remain in the environment for a long time and move to many parts of it, including the biotic segment. These toxicants negatively impact both domestic and wild animals by building up in key organs like the liver and kidney (Liu 2003). Altering the properties of soil, contaminating water, and reducing the nutritive value of plants are the main negative impact on environment of heavy metals (Figure 34.2).

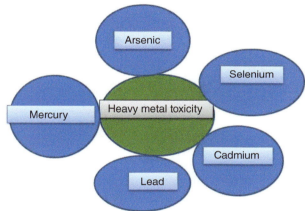

Figure 34.2 Majaor heavy metal toxicity in livestock and human beings.

Arsenic (As)

A common environmental contaminant that discharged into the atmosphere as a result of industrial operations, agricultural use (Ishinishi et al. 2004), through mining, smelting, coal combustion and through weathering of rocks and minerals. In many nations, As poisoning from ground water is a major concern (Rahman et al. 2001; Jin et al. 2004). Only less than 50 ug/l of As is the recommended allowable limit in drinking water (WHO 1993). It has been documented that industrial pollution can cause As poisoning in workers (Kabir and Bilgi 1993). Cattle and pigs who accidentally consumed hazardous amounts of a based growth promoters have been documented to had accidental As poisoning (Ledet et al. 1973; Samad and Chaudhary 1984). Skin disorders such as spotted melanosis, leucomelanosis, hyperkeratosis, and gangrenous extremities are linked to using drinking water contaminated with As. Moreover, splenomegaly, hepatomegaly, and other organ cancers were also seen (Engel and Recover 1993; Rahman et al. 2001). Cattle that are exposed to As poisoning may exhibit neurological or gastrointestinal symptoms. Abdominal pain, restlessness, breathing difficulties, clenching of the teeth, ruminal stasis, and even vomiting is visible in severe cases. Weight loss, irregular eating patterns, mucosal and conjunctival erythema, buccal ulceration, and decreased milk production in cows are all signs of chronic As poisoning. Dehydration, oliguria, and elevated heart rate are typical symptoms of As intoxication. (Radostits et al. 2000).

Mercury (Hg)

Hg pollution is a global concern because it can cycle through the atmosphere, water, and soil. The significant morbidity and death rates are associated with Hg toxicity are a major concern for both humans and animals. Although Hg is not biologically necessary, but employed in many different sectors and discharged into the environment by both man-made and natural processes. Waste disposal, manufacture of non-ferrous metals, and burning of coal are examples of man-made sources. Over the past century, there have been multiple cases of Hg poisoning in Japan, Guatemala, Iraq, and Pakistan as a result of pollution (Dwivedi et al. 2001). The majority of predatory birds and mammals are harmed by methyl mercury, which is the deadly and stable form of the metal Hg. Common clinical manifestations in the human population include kidney disease, blindness, mental retardation in children, deafness, and digestive issues. In India, high Hg levels have been found in a few cities and the neighbourhood's surrounding the paper and chlor-alkali industries (Chandra 1980). In animals cats are the most commonly afflicted by Hg toxicity and the illness is also known as "dancing-cat disease" because of this infected cats may drool, stumble in a zigzag pattern, and eventually collapse.

Lead (Pb)

Pb is an ecological contaminant that is extensively dispersed and lacks a clear biological activity within the body. Plumbriosm can be brought on by a variety of contaminants that can be consumed by grazing ruminants, including paint tins, machinery grease, burned coal, cement manufacturing, the petroleum and power sector, and abandoned batteries. The animals most impacted are those that browse near busy roads and metallurgic complexes. Clinical indications that frequently lead to increased animal mortality include hypersalivation, miscarriages, behavioural issues, head pressing, incoordinated movement, decreased sperm creation, memory loss and learning difficulties, blindness, high blood pressure, and depression. One of the documented reasons of death for vultures in India was Pb poisoning (Oaks et al. 2004). Pb poisoning and mortality in water fowl are caused by blood Pb concentrations above $100\,\mu g/dL$ and liver Pb concentrations of 15–20 ppm on a dry matter basis.

Signs of Pb poisoning in humans include reduced birth weight, adversely impact on nervous system, immune system, cardiovascular system, kidney function, shorter gestation periods, delayed brain development, and early deliveries. Osman 1988 looked into the possibility of Pb poisoning among workers exposed in the Khartoum North industrial sector. According to her report, the average Pb concentrations in the air at the Pb accumulator facility were $329.2\,\mu g/m^3$ in the summer and $305.77\,\mu g/m^3$ in the winter. In August 2006, there were reports of Pb poisoning cases involving humans in Egypt, which were linked with consumption of Pb-contaminated wheat flour and over 100 victims were either morbid or deceased.

Cadmium (Cd)

It is naturally present in the earth's crust and oceans, but through natural and anthropogenic activities it released into the environment, soli, air, and water throughout the electroplating, polymer, battery, and alloy manufacturing processes. It is unwanted and harmful for organisms to possess. The addition of fertilizers, sewage sludge, and other organic wastes to agricultural land raises the amount of Cd in the soil and via food chain it enters into organisms. Cd is a cumulative toxin, that compromises liver and kidney function by long-term absorption, softens animal bones via interferes with calcium metabolism, and reduces productivity. The 30 000 tons of Cd that humans release into the environment each year also include dust and waste water from coal, phosphate rocks, lubricants, and fertilizers, according to Nriagu and Pacyna (Nriagu and Pacyna 1988).

Selenium (Se)

Se poisoning is mostly caused by industries that release fly ash, particularly soft coal. Se overload was identified by Dhillon as one of the major issues impacting the cattle and buffalo population in the Indian subcontinent and contributing to the degnala disease (Dhillon et al. 1990). Symptoms of selenium toxicity are mainly gastrointestinal disturbances (diarrhoea and nausea) and other manifestations include garlic odour from breath, hair loss, fatigue, abnormal nails, dermatitis, irritability, and peripheral neuropathy. In dairy ruminants Se toxicity included foot scaling, baldness and induced infertility in buffaloes. Emaciation, stillbirth, liver degeneration, muscular atrophy, malformed progeny, and significant aberrant feather loss are most prominent signs in birds during Se toxicity (Fleming 1996).

34.1.1.4 Pollution from Industries

The past 15 years have seen a tremendous increase in urbanization and industrialization, especially in emerging nations like India and pollution from these sectors have a major negative impact on livestock and human health. Industries and transportation sector like thermal power plants, oil refineries, pharmaceuticals, petrochemicals, and cement smelters play a major role in pollution in India. In major cities like Delhi, Mumbai, Bangalore, Chennai, and

Calcutta the situation is far worse due to hazardous heavy metals, volatile hydrocarbons, halogen gases, oxidants, and oxides of sulphur, nitrogen, and carbon like industrial pollutants. The type of pollution, the amount of exposure, species, age, and physiology of the affected animals, as well as the presence of interacting chemicals, all affect how severe the pollution is (Swarup and Dwivedi 1998). Animals with poor nutrition are more susceptible to the negative impacts of pollution.

34.1.1.5 Types of Environmental Pollution

Air Pollution

Air pollution is the term used to describe the discharge of contaminants such as biological molecules, gases, and particles into the atmosphere that are hazardous to both the environment, livestock and human health. A specific proportion of gases are present in the atmosphere and it is dangerous for survival if these gasses' composition are changed. This imbalance caused an increase in earth's temperature, that process known as global warming (Figure 34.3).

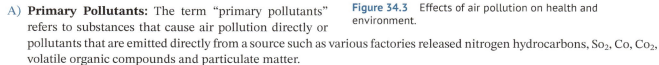

Figure 34.3 Effects of air pollution on health and environment.

Types of Air Pollutants
Mainly two types:

A) **Primary Pollutants:** The term "primary pollutants" refers to substances that cause air pollution directly or pollutants that are emitted directly from a source such as various factories released nitrogen hydrocarbons, So_2, Co, Co_2, volatile organic compounds and particulate matter.

B) **Secondary Pollutants:** Air pollutants that are formed naturally in the environment through chemical reactions between other pollutants such as nitric acid (HNO_3), sulfuric acid (H_2So_4), ozone (O_3), and peroxyacetyl nitrates (PANs) are examples of secondary pollutants that are created when main pollutants mix and react. Same way smog secondary pollutant is produced when fog and smoke combine.

Air Pollution Major Causes

A) **Fossil Fuel Combustion:** Oxides of carbon (Co_2 and Co), nitrogen (NO_2 and N_2O) and sulphur (So_2) are produced in large quantities when fossil fuels are burned that contribute to the formation of smog and acid rain. One of the main causes of carbon monoxide (Co) pollution is incomplete fossil fuel combustion.

B) **Agricultural Practices:** One of the most hazardous gases generated by agricultural practices is NH_3. Livestock buildings, open feedlots, and manure storage facilities are common sources of NH_3 emissions. Fertilizers, insecticides, deforestation for agricultural use, burning agricultural residues and pesticides discharges dangerous substances into the environment that leads to pollution.

C) **Factories and Industries:** Mainly emitted primary pollutants.

D) **Domestic Sources:** Fuel-burning combustion appliances, household cleaning and maintenance products, tobacco products, building and furnishings materials, central heating and cooling systems and humidification devices are the examples of household air pollution. Paints and cleaning supplies for the home also leak toxic chemicals into the atmosphere. Freshly painted walls give out an odor that comes from the chemicals in the paint that affects respiration by contaminating the air.

E) **Automobiles:** Automobile exhaust is a major source of air pollution through gasses released by various vehicles and pollute the environment that are the main causes of human sickness as well as greenhouse gas emissions.

Air Pollution Impacts

A) **Impact on Human:** The direct or indirect impacts of air pollution caused a wide range of respiratory and cardiovascular (heart disease and stroke) conditions to humans that claim countless lives each year. Air pollution more severely affects people who are already ill but vary widely depending on age, location, underlying health of people. In recent decades, lung cancer has become more prevalent and children's who reside close to polluted environments are at an increased risk of asthma and pneumonia like respiratory diseases.

B) **Impact on Animals:** Air pollution negatively impact animal health in many ways, like weakened immune systems, asthma like respiratory diseases, allergies and skin irritations. Air pollution also damages aquatic life by settling on bodies of water and forces animals to abandon their natural homes. In addition to making them stray, this has led to the extinction of numerous animal species.

C) **Other impact:** Acid rain, climate change, haze, ozone depletion, eutrophication and global warming are further effects. PANs, O_3, and oxides of sulphur (So_2) and nitrogen work (N_2O) together to cause lung and skin cancer in both humans and livestock. Rao noted that even at very low concentrations (0.5 mg/kg) of air pollution can cause eyes and respiratory system irritation (Rao 1984). Significant amounts of heavy metals emitted into the atmosphere due to metal smelting, waste incineration, and vehicle smoke caused high pressure atrophy of the bronchial and alveolar ducts, which was followed by mortality (Swarup and Dwivedi 1998).

Water Pollution

The term "water pollution" refers to the contaminating of water bodies (rivers, ponds, and aquifers) mainly by industrial and agricultural effluents that leads any minor or major change in the physical, chemical or biological properties of water and produce a detrimental consequence in any living organism. For many years, the effects of contaminated water are felt and all life forms that depend on water, suffers either directly or indirectly.

Main Water Pollution Sources   Water pollution can be attributed by various factors such as deforestation, west water treatment, urbanization, oil spills, agricultural and industrial runoffs, sewage, and the use of detergents and fertilizers.

Water Pollution Impacts   The kind and quantity of pollutants in the water determine its pollution effects and the position of water bodies also has a significant impact on pollution levels.

A) There is a lot of pollution in near cities because of outcome of commercial and industrial facilities that disposing hazardous waste and chemicals (such as fertilizers, pesticides, heavy metals, nitrates, and fluorides) in nears water bodies.

B) Nutrient pollution that is caused by excess nitrogen and phosphorus in water, is the number-one threat to worldwide water quality, that can also leads to algal blooms.

C) The food chain could be significantly impacted or upset by water pollution. Two hazardous elements, Cd and Pb, can cause further disruption at higher levels in the food chain when they enter through animals (fish).

D) According to a study published in The Lancet water pollution kills1.8 million deaths in 2015. Infectious illness outbreaks, such as cholera outbreaks, are always linked to inadequate treatment of drinking water and polluted water.

E) It also severely impacts human health by causing cancer, respiratory and cardiovascular issues, and reproductive problems.

F) Aquatic life is also significantly impacted by water pollution because dioxin like toxin accumulates in meat, poultry, and seafood that can lead to a number of problems such as cancer and uncontrollably growing cells in the reproductive system. Such chemicals also enter the human body later in life after moving up the food chain.

Karnataka's ground water quality was negatively impacted by the disposal of municipal solid garbage (Ishinishi et al. 2004 & Naik et al. 2007). Another potentially harmful water pollution is cyanide (Cn). The effluent from electroplating units, Chhabra found that ground water samples from the industrial city of Ludhiana had a significant concentration of cyanide (Chhabra 2002). By the overuse of nitrogenous fertilizers, Ray and Bhattacharya study showed that the ground water in districts of Rajasthan, Punjab, Tamil Nadu, and Madhya Pradesh had increased nitrate concentrations (Ray and Bhattacharaya 1989). In cattle, feeding of Napier Bajra hybrid irrigated with wastewater can also lead to acute nitrite poisoning with the clinical signs like anoxic anemia, diarrhea, and respiratory distress.

Soil Pollution

The poisoning of soil with unusually high concentrations of harmful compounds that alter in the natural soil environment is known as soil pollution. The improper disposal of solid, semi-solid, and chemical wastes from mining, radioactive materials, military activities, industrial activity, and agricultural sources (excessive pesticide or fertilizer use) are typically the cause of soil and land pollution. With the various health dangers, it is a serious environmental concern. Among the most harmful soil contaminants are xenobiotics or compounds that are manufactured by humans causes cancer. Leukaemia risk increases, if soil having high quantities of benzene.

34.1 *Introduction* | **399**

Contaminants that Polluted Soil

A) **Heavy Metals:** As, Pb, Hg, chromium (Cr), nickel (Ni), Zinc (Zn), Copper (Cu) and Cd are the main heavy metals that are extremely harmful to humans and livestock when found in soils at abnormally high quantities mainly by mining, agriculture, pesticide, electronic trash, fertilizer, and medical waste are some of the main sources of these metals.

B) **Polycyclic aromatic hydrocarbons** (PAHs): These are organic compounds having numerous aromatic rings and just of carbon and hydrogen two atoms in their structures like anthracene, phenalene, and naphthalene. The extraction of shale oil, car emissions, cigarette smoke, and the manufacturing of coke are all responsible for the soil degradation brought on by PAHs. Many cancer forms, mutations and human cardiovascular disease also have been connected to exposure of PAHs. Grain size, porosity, microbiological diversity, permeability, water-holding capacity, volume, and flexibility of soil can all also be altered by PAHs.

C) **Industrial Waste:** Soil contamination may result from the release of industrial waste into the environment and soil. It is possible for poisonous trash to seep into the soil when it is stored in landfills. Additionally, this garbage may contaminate groundwater.

In India, between 15 and 44.2% of all solid waste is composed of non-biodegradable materials. Additionally, the usage of rubber, and polythene bags by urban society has caused gastrointestinal issues and high death rates in animals that eat a lot, such as cattle because of their indiscriminate eating habits. In ruminants, traumatic pericarditis and traumatic reticulo-peritonitis are frequently result of sharp items like nails and wire, and in addition, some solid wastes, such as abandoned batteries, are the cause of Pb poisoning in dairy cows (Patra and Swarup 2000).

Noise Pollution

"Noise" is the term for undesired sound, and Noise pollution or sound pollution, is the propagation of sound with ranging impacts on the activity of human or animal life. It is an increasing problem of modern societies. WHO defines noise above 65 dB as noise pollution. To be precise, it becomes harmful when it exceeds 75 dB and painful above 120 dB. It is a significant ecological issue with that transportation and industry are the main sources of noise. The typical noise level produced by vehicles is around 70 dB, whereas the noise levels produced by a newspaper press, farm tractor, milling machine, and train whistle are much higher (90–130 dB). Nosal and Bigery found that noise levels greater than 65 dB made a negative impact on lactating cow milk (Nosal and Bigery 2004) and Zhou observed factory's constant noise, which was 73.4 dB, was the main cause of dysphoria, low milk production, and cow abortions (Zhou 1995).

In addition, a range of physiological harms affecting the human and animal CNS and auditory systems are caused by sound pollution such as burning crackers and pyrotechnics, pollutes air and makes animals extremely afraid or scared. Same way airplanes fly produces a supersonic boom that significantly contributes to noise pollution and harms human and animal welfare health. Ship traffic is the source of underwater noise that disturbs typical marine life in the 10–500 hertz band (Shaw 1978).

34.1.2   Impact of Pollution by Radioactive Materials

Radioactive pollution is caused by uncontrolled release of radioactive elements and waste into soil, water, air, or nearby living organisms (environment) and releases ionizing radiation which pollutes its surroundings. The first use of nuclear weapons during World War I (by the United States) started the radioactive material pollution in that people and livestock were negatively impacted for decades due to the extreme severity of radioactive impact. Radioactive materials can induce teratogenicity, cardiotoxicity, leukemia, thyroid cancer, hair loss, and impaired reproduction include uranium (U), radium (Ra), thorium (Th), iodine (I), and plutonium (Pu). These materials are also chemotoxic and by damaging DNA and gene mutations leads to cancer. These days, they are widely employed in the production of nuclear weapons, chemotherapy, electricity production, and hormone estimate. The 1986 Chernobyl nuclear power plant explosion left nations severely radioactively contaminated. Furthermore, to prevent radioactive pollution, radioactive waste should be disposed properly and nuclear tests should be banned, and alternative sources of energy should be used.

34.1.3   Acid Rain

It is currently the most significant types of pollution to the environment that mostly brought on by the combustion of coal and oil in power plants, machinery, and automobiles, which releases sulphur and nitrogen into the atmosphere. NH_3 is another significant substance that contributes to acid rain and it is a typical result of discarding significant amounts of raw manure by animal production systems. In late 1970s saw the first recognition of risks associated with acid rain. According to Hadina, NH_3 upsets the ecological equilibrium, causes acid rain by forming acidic compounds that harms people and animals (Hadina et al. 2001). Acid rain makes the aquatic ecosystem more acidic, which affects fish species thrive ability that is a growing source of public concern.

34.1.4 Pesticide Pollution

In agricultural operations, pesticide chemicals are a crucial tool for pest control. Nonetheless, their widespread application in the agriculture field, coupled with their potentially hazardous nature, implicates them as the primary source of toxicity in both humans and animals (Swarup 2002). Every year, a couple of 25 million workers in underdeveloped nations become poisoned by pesticides (McCauley et al. 2006) and because of their indiscriminate usage in veterinary operations, pesticides (typically insecticides and fungicides) are mostly introduced into animal facilities. Meral and Boghra (Meral and Boghra 2004) have documented elevated pesticide levels in milk and milk products. Stinging eyes, rashes, blisters, blindness, nausea, dizziness, diarrhea and death are acute health effects and reproductive, immunotoxic, cardiogenic effects, and endocrine disrupting are chronic health effect of pesticides (Engel et al. 2000). Furthermore, exposure to pesticides has been linked to neurological diseases, breast cancer (Beseler et al. 2008), depression (Brunstrom et al. 2003), respiratory issues, memory issues, and dermatological disorders (Arcury et al. 2003). Milk samples taken from regions where pesticides were allegedly applied to kill mosquitoes showed pesticide residue levels were 25% higher than the maximum residual limit (Surendranath et al. 2002). The use of pesticide accounts about 6% of total ground level ozone levels. Pesticide pollution still affect aquatic life such as Nile perch fish (Lates niloticus), a resident of Lake Victoria in Africa, Ogwok recently detected increased amounts of total residual endosulfan, dichloro-diphenyl-trichloro-ethane, heptachlor, and aldrin (Ogwok et al. 2009).

34.1.5 Drug Residues

The Swann report's publication (Swann 1969) has brought antibiotic misuse and overuse to the attention of people all around the world. Chemicals and medications for animals are utilized as feed additives to increase growth, improve breeding performance, increase feed acceptability, and serve as for chemotherapeutic and preventative perpose. Worldwide, animal agriculture employs around 300 feed additives, antibiotics, and synthetic hormones (Lee et al. 2001). Antimicrobial residues from food animals that are treated or used to promote growth have toxicological implications for humans and affect the quality of milk and milk products. They could give bacterial pathogens, antibiotic resistance (Honkanen and Suhren 1999), allergy to livestock and humans. Polychlorinated dibenzodioxins, NSAIDs, antidepressants, biphenyls, sulphonamides, furans, and dieldrin are the examples of drug residues.

34.1.6 Greenhouse Effect

The natural warming of the earth that results when gases in the atmosphere trap and heat from the sun that would otherwise escape into space or a natural process that traps sun heat, near the earth's surface and its actually, a result of widespread tree-cutting and air pollution. Heat from the sun enters the earth's atmosphere in a greenhouse and infrared light bounces off from objects and ascends back towards the atmosphere. The atmosphere then lets most of this heat escape while reflecting some of it back. The greenhouse continues to bounce with this heat and because of this continuous prehistoric era, heat was regularly released or held.

By burning fossil fuels, large polluting machinery released Co_2, N_2O, NF_3, HFCs and Co into the atmosphere, which absorbs heat easily. The earth and its atmosphere began to warm as a result of an increase in these gases in atmosphere and causes global warming, ozone layer depletion, ecosystem disruption, food supply disruptions, increased wildfires and climate change. In addition, the presence of trees would lessen the severity of this because trees absorb Co_2 and release O_2 as a byproduct of photosynthesis, that addresses excess Co_2. But now a days trees and forests are being cleared quickly for furniture, paper goods, housing development, and animal grazing. To preserve tree resources for addressing the Co_2 issue, we must employ recycled products and take imperative that we simultaneously curtail our Co_2 emissions in order to maintain stable global temperatures.

34.1.7 Current Patterns and the Requirement for Additional Study

A growing number of scientists are interested in epidemiological studies related to pollution, but there are still several gaps in this field that require critical attention from researchers and all those involved in animal health and industry. There is an urgent need to establish legal regulations and laws for risk assessment and management in order to protect the health of humans and animals. Animal and human health hazards, as well as rising pressures on soil, water, and air like resources in recent years, have focused global attention to find new ways for manage and sustain the ecosystem. For this, biotechnology is a crucial tool that offer fresh perspectives on how to maintain and repair the environment by producing biodegradable products from renewable resources and creating environment friendly production and disposal procedures. Another one is phycoremediation technique that is used for cleaning up soil pollution and creating a green, clean atmosphere. Many plants root also act as a host reservoir for harmful metals. Additionally, recent research also has focused on rumen modifications for lower methane gas eructation.

The growth of green technology will continue, focusing on renewable energy, advanced energy storage, and carbon capture technologies that will also decreases environmental pollution. The term "renewable energy" refers to an energy source that is practically limitless and regenerable. It consists like ocean energy, geothermal energy, sun light and hydropower that sources can be used to generate electricity and heat for industrial processes and buildings, and also as a vehicles fuel. The growing use of renewable energy can help achieve national energy independence, economic and political security, and air pollution reduction by reducing the fossil fuels usages. Reforestation is an additional strategy to stop climate change and for this deforestation can be somewhat decreased if each person grows at least one seedling in their immediate surroundings. Moreover, the installation of contemporary fossil fuel-fired power plants equipped with PCC, IGCC, or NGCC technology can help lower atmospheric Co_2 emissions.

With all that environmental pollution should be studied and researched in order to comprehend environmental challenges, encourage sustainable resource management, set criteria for a healthy environment, and raise environmental consciousness. So, keep addressing the issues in order to make the world clean and ecologically pleasant.

References

Arcury, T.A., Quandt, S.A., and Mellen, B.G. (2003). An exploratory analysis of occupational skin disease among Latin migrant and seasonal farm workers of North Carolina. *Journal of Agriculture Health* 9: 221–232.

Bell, P.A., Fisher, J.D., Baum, A., and Greene, T.C. (1990). *Environmental Psychology*, 3rde. Harcust Porace Jovanovich College publication.

Beseler, C.L., Stallones, L., and Hoppin, J.A. (2008). Depression and pesticide exposure among private pesticide applicators enrolled in the agricultural health study. *Environmental Health Perspectives* 116: 1713–1719.

Brunstrom, B., Axelsson, J., and Halldin, K. (2003). Effect of cadmium modulators on sex differentiation in birds. *Ecotoxicology* 12: 84–95.

Chandra, S. V. (1980). Toxic Metals in Environment: A Status Report of R&D Work done in India. Book, http://library.iiim.res. in:80/cgi-bin/koha/opac-detail.pl?biblionumber=635,65.

Chhabra, A. (2002). Environmental pollution: Challenges ahead to safeguard the animal and human health. In: *Proceedings of the IVth Biennial Conference and Exhibition* (ed. T.K. Mohanty), 84–86. Kolkata: Indian Society for Veterinary Medicine.

Dhillon, K.S., Srivastava, A.K., Gill, B.S., and Singh, J. (1990). Experimental chronic selenosis in buffalo calves. *The Indian Journal of Animal Sciences* 60 (5): 532–535.

Dwivedi, S.K., Swarup, D., Dey, S., and Pata, R.C. (2001). Lead poisoning in cattle and buffalo near primary lead-zinc smelter in India. *Veterinary and Human Toxicology* 43: 93–94.

Engel, R.R. and Recover, O. (1993). Re: "Arsenic ingestion and internal cancers: A review". *American Journal of Epidemiology* 138: 896–897.

Engel, L.S., O'meara, E.S., and Schwartz, S.M. (2000). Maternal occupation in agriculture and risk of limb defects in Washington State. *Scandinavian Journal of Work, Environment & Health* 26: 193–198.

Fleming, W.J. (1996). Fluoride in birds. In: *Environmental Contaminants in Wildlife* (ed. B.W. Nelson, H. Gary, and R. Norwood), 459–471. CRC Press. Inc.

Hadina, S., Vucemilo, M., Tofant, A., and Matkovic, K. (2001). Influence of ammonia on the environment and animal health. *Stocarstvo* 55: 187–193.

Honkanen, B.T. and Suhren, G. (1999). Screening methods used for the detection of veterinary drug residues in raw cow milk – A review. *Bulletin of the International Dairy Federation* 345: 11–12.

Ishinishi, G., Li, X., Li, G. et al. (2004). Study on toxic signs induced by different arsenicals in primary cultured rats. *Toxicology and Applied Pharmacology* 196: 396–403.

Jin, Y., Sun, G., Li, X.G., and Qul, W. (2004). Studies on developmental retardation induced by fluoride toxicity in embryo-larval stages of Bufo raddei. *Toxicology and Applied Pharmacology* 196: 396–403.

Johnson, K.A. and Johnson, D.E. (1995). Methane emissions from cattle. *Journal of Animal Science* 73: 2483–2492.

Kabir, H. and Bilgi, C. (1993). Occupational exposure to chemicals and its effects on health. *Journal of Occupational Medicine* 35: 1203–1207. Winship, 1984.

Ledet, A.E., Duncan, J.R., Buck, W.B., and Ramsey, F.K. (1973). Clinical, toxicological, and pathological aspects of arsanalic acid poisoning in swine. Clinical Toxicology. *Clinical Toxicology* 6: 439.

Lee, M.H., Lee, H.J., and Ryu, P.D. (2001). Public health risks: Chemical and antibiotic residues - Review. Asian-Australasian. *Journal of Animal Sciences* 14: 402–413.

Liu, Z.P. (2003). Lead poisoning combined with cadmium in sheep and horses in the vicinity of non-ferrous metal smelters. *The Science of Total Environment.* 309: 117–126.

McCauley, L.A., Anger, W.K., Kiefer, M. et al. (2006). Studying health outcomes in farm worker populations exposed to pesticides. *Environmental Health Perspectives* 114: 953–960.

Meral, M. and Boghra, V.R. (2004). Pesticide levels in milk and milk products. *Indian Journal of Dairy Sciences* 57 (5): 411–413.

Miner, R. (1973). *Odors from Livestock Production in Gaseous pollutants and odors*, 129–146. American Society of Agricultural Engineers.

Naik, P., Ushamalini, D., and Somashekar, R.K. (2007). Impact of municipal solid waste dumping on ground water quality-A case study in Bangalore district. *Ecology, Environment and Conservation.* 13 (4): 759–760.

Nosal, D. and Bigery, E. (2004). Airborne noise, structure borne sound (vibration) and vacuum stability of milking system. *Journal of Animal Science* 49: 226–230.

Nriagu, J.O. and Pacyna, J.M. (1988). Quantitative assessment of worldwide contamination of air, water and soil by trace metals. *Nature* 333: 134–139.

Oaks, J.L., Gilbert, M., Virani, M.Z. et al. (2004). Diclofenac residues as the cause of vulture population decline in Pakistan. *Nature* 2317: 1–4.

Ogwok, P., Muyonga, E.J.H., and Sserunjogi, E.M.L. (2009). Pesticide residues and heavy metals in Lake Victoria Nile Perch. *Bulletin of Environmental Contamination and Toxicology* 82: 529–533.

Osman, Omayma S. (1988). Risk of lead poisoning among exposed workers as a function of ambient thermal conditions. MSc. Thesis. Institute of Environmental Studies, University of Khartoum, Sudan.

Patra, R.C. and Swarup, D. (2000). Effect of lead on erythrocytic antioxidant defense, lipid peroxide level and thiol groups in calves. *Research in Veterinary Science* 68: 71.

Patra, R.C., Dwivedi, S.K., Bhardwaj, B., and Swarup, D. (2001). Industrial fluorosis in cattle and buffaloes in Udaipur, India. *The Science of Total Environment.* 253: 145–150.

Radostits, O.M., Gay, C.C., Blood, D.C., and Hinchcliff, K.W. (2000). *Veterinary Medicine, A Text Book of The Diseases of Cattle, Sheep, Pigs, Goats and Horses*, 9the (ed. J.H. Arundel, D.E. Jacob, K.E. Leslie, et al.). London: W. B. Saunders Company Ltd.

Rahman, M.M., Chowdhary, U.K., Mukherjee, S.C. et al. (2001). Chronic arsenic toxicity in Bangladesh and West Bengal, India. A Review and Commentary. *Clinical Toxicology* 39: 683–700.

Rao, P.S. (1984). Air pollution and its problems. *Everyman's Science* 19: 22–28.

Ray, P.K. and Bhattacharaya, J.W. (1989). Concerns and management of water pollution in relation to animal and human health. In: *Proceedings of the National Symposium on Emerging Diseases of Livestock Due to Environmental Pollution* (ed. D.N. Verma), 45–56. Izatnagar: IVRI.

Samad, M.A. and Chaudhary, A. (1984). Epizootiology of gastrointestinal nematodes in cattle and buffaloes under rural conditions. *Indian Journal of Veterinary Medicine* 4: 107–108.

Shaw, E.A.G. (1978). Symposium on the effects of noise on wildlife. In: *Effects of Noise on Wildlife* (ed. J.L. Fletcher and R.G. Busnel), 1–5. Academic Press.

Sidhu, P.K., Sandhu, B.S., Singh, J., and Kwatra, M.S. (1994). Lead toxicosis in bovine due to industrial pollution in Punjab. *Indian Journal of Animal Sciences* 64 (12): 1359–1360.

Singh J. and Pandey V. (2005) "Impact of livestock-environment interaction on human life." Proceedings of the 3rd Annual Conference of IAVPHS, PAU Ludhiana, October 28–29, 2005. Published by Indian Association for Veterinary Public Health Specialists, Ludhiana, pp. 52–58.

Surendranath, B., Sarwar Usha, M.A., and Unnikrishnan, V. (2002). Pesticide residues in milk samples. *Indian Journal of Dairy Biosciences* 13: 98–101.

Swann, M. M. (1969). Use of antibiotic in animal husbandry and veterinary medicine. U.K. Joint Committee Report.

Swarup D. 2002. Consequences of industrial pollution on animal health in India. *Proceedings of orientation course of "Industrial Toxicology,"* pp. 124–34 (9–30 September). Ludhiana: Department of Veterinary Pharmacology and Toxicology, PAU.

Swarup, D. and Dwivedi, S.K. (1998). Research on the effects of pollution in livestock. *Indian Journal of Animal Sciences* 68: 814–824.

Swarup, D. and Dwivedi, S.K. (2002). *Environmental Pollution and Effects of Lead and Fluoride on Animal Health*, 46–52. New Delhi: Indian Council of Agricultural Research.

Swarup, D. and Singh, Y.P. (1989). Bovine flourosis in a brick kiln congested zone. *Indian Journal of Veterinary Medicine* 9: 12–14.

Swarup, D., Dwivedi, S.K., Dey, S., and Ray, S.K. (1998). Fluorine intoxication in bovines due to industrial pollution. *Indian Journal of Animal Sciences* 68 (5): 605–608.

Swarup, D., Patra, R.C., Dwivedi, S.K., and Dey, S. (2000). Lead and cadmium content of blood of urban dogs in India. *Veterinary and Human Toxicology* 42: 232–233.

Swarup, D., Dey, S., Patra, R.C. et al. (2002). Clinico-epidemiological observations of industrial bovine fluorosis in India. *The Indian Journal of Animal Sciences* 71: 111–116.

WHO (1993). *A guideline for drinking water quality*, 2nde, vol. I. Geneva, Switzerland: World Health Organization.

WHO (World Health Organization) (1987). *Air Quality Guidelines for Europe*. WHO regional publications European series 23, Denmark.

Zhou, H. (1995). Detrimental effects of noise on dairy cows. *Journal of Veterinary Medicine* 21: 16–17.

35

Rural and Urban Pollution

Mona Abdelghany Nasr[1] and Nourhan Eissa[2]

[1] *Department of Anatomy and Embryology, Faculty of Veterinary Medicine, University of Sadat City, Sadat City, Egypt*
[2] *Department of Animal Hygiene and Zoonoses, Faculty of Veterinary Medicine, University of Sadat City, Sadat City, Egypt*

35.1 Introduction

Pollution is one of the major environmental issues of our times. It has serious impacts on our health, economy, and the environment. Pollution can be of different types, including air pollution, water pollution, and soil pollution (Figure 35.1). Pollution is a worldwide problem that is chiefly impossible to avoid, especially in developing countries (Manisalidis et al. 2020). Although urban areas are usually more polluted than rural areas, pollution can spread to most areas of the world.

Pollution is the introduction of harmful materials into the environment. These materials are called pollutants which according to Whittaker (1975) are classified into radioisotopes, pesticides, heavy metals, and combustion products. These harmful materials can be natural, such as volcanic ash, or they can be created by human activities (Majra, 2011).

In rural areas, the primary source of pollution is often related to agricultural practices, such as the use of fertilizers and pesticides, and the burning of crop residues (Ivanovski et al., 2023). This can lead to air and water pollution, and soil degradation. On the other hand, in urban areas, the sources of pollution are more diverse and concentrated. Vehicle emissions, industrial activities, and the burning of fossil fuels for energy generation all contribute significantly to air pollution. The concentration of population and economic activities in urban areas exacerbates the issue, leading to higher levels of pollution (Balkis, 2012).

Pollution is a growing concern worldwide, affecting both rural and urban areas. It poses a significant threat to the environment and human health. This chapter provides an overview of the factors contributing to pollution in rural and urban areas, the impact of pollution on various ecosystems, and the resulting health risks associated with pollution. Additionally, key research studies conducted on this topic are discussed, offering comprehensive insights into the current state of pollution in both settings.

35.2 Pollution in Rural Areas

Rural areas are often associated with agriculture, livestock production, and natural resource extraction, which can contribute to pollution. Agricultural activities, such as the use of chemical fertilizers and pesticides, can lead to water and soil contamination. The burning of agricultural waste and biomass for cooking and heating purposes releases harmful pollutants into the atmosphere (Charlesworth and Booth, 2019).

According to a study by Dasgupta et al. (2016), rural areas in developing countries commonly experience indoor pollution due to the burning of solid fuels, such as wood and animal dung, for cooking and heating. The study highlights the adverse health effects of indoor pollution, including respiratory and cardiovascular diseases. Furthermore, the indiscriminate disposal of waste, inadequate sewage systems, and industrial activities in rural areas can further exacerbate pollution problems.

Epidemiology and Environmental Hygiene in Veterinary Public Health, First Edition. Edited by Tanmoy Rana.
© 2025 John Wiley & Sons, Inc. Published 2025 by John Wiley & Sons, Inc.

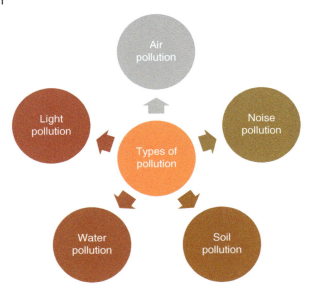

Figure 35.1   Different types of environmental pollution.

35.3   Pollution in Urban Areas

Urban areas are characterized by high population densities, industrial establishments, heavy traffic, and energy consumption, making them particularly vulnerable to pollution. Vehicular emissions, industrial waste discharge, and the burning of fossil fuels for electricity generation contribute to air pollution, resulting in an array of health issues for urban dwellers.

A study conducted by World Health Organization (2016) revealed that for urban areas, air pollution is a significant concern, leading to respiratory diseases, cardiovascular problems, and even premature death. Water pollution is also a significant concern in urban areas due to inadequate wastewater treatment facilities, improper solid waste management, and sewage system failures (Fenger, 1999).

35.4   Impact on Ecosystems

Pollution has devastating effects on ecosystems, in both rural and urban areas. In rural areas, chemical runoffs from agricultural practices can contaminate water bodies, causing eutrophication and leading to the death of aquatic organisms. Additionally, air pollution can negatively impact crop yields, affecting agricultural productivity and food security.

In urban areas, pollution affects biodiversity, particularly through habitat destruction and contamination of water bodies. Aquatic ecosystems suffer from the accumulation of toxins and heavy metals, causing a decline in fish populations and disrupting the food chain. Furthermore, the urban heat island effect, caused by pollution and high-density development, increases temperatures and affects local flora and fauna.

35.5   Health Risks Associated with Pollution

Pollution is sometimes sudden but is usually a gradual process, taking a long period to manifest its effects. This often makes it difficult to treat (Adinna 2003).

Pollution poses severe health risks to individuals residing in both rural and urban areas. Epidemiological studies have linked various forms of pollution to respiratory diseases, such as asthma and bronchitis, cardiovascular problems, including heart attacks and strokes, and cancers. Vulnerable populations, such as children, the elderly, and individuals with preexisting health conditions, are particularly susceptible to the adverse health effects of pollution. For instance, a study by Chen et al. (2017) found a significant association between exposure to particulate matter (PM2.5) and the incidence of childhood asthma. The study emphasized the need for effective pollution control measures to safeguard public health.

Urban centers have become breeding grounds for pollution, due to their insatiable thirst for resources and relentless human activity; the number of urban residents who perceived different types of environmental pollution (air, water, and noise) was higher than rural residents in a study by Yang (2020).

35.6   Air Pollution

Air pollution is one of the most important public health problems related to environmental pollutions. Air pollution in the form of solid particles, liquid droplets or gases has harmful effects on humans, other living organisms, and the environment (Figure 35.2). According to the European Environment Agency (EEA) and the World Health Organization, air pollution has become the second largest environmental issue, after climate change.

Air pollution can result from natural processes such as dust storms, forest fires, and volcanic eruptions, or from human activities such as biomass burning, vehicular emissions, mining, agriculture, and industrial processes. Improved

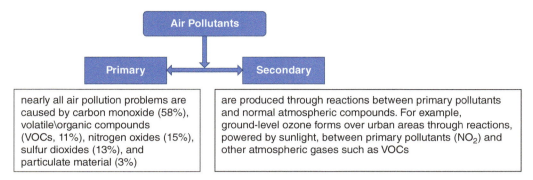

Figure 35.2 Various categories of air pollution, primary and secondary pollutants.

technology and government policies have helped reduce most types of outdoor air pollution in many industrialized countries, including the United States, in recent decades. However, outdoor air quality is still a problem in less industrialized nations, especially in the megacities of rapidly industrializing nations such as China and India. In bustling cities, exhaust fumes from vehicles, emissions from factories, and the burning of fossil fuels create a toxic mix. Several studies have demonstrated the link between air pollution and incidence of respiratory and other air-borne diseases. It is known that 50% of lead pollution enters the blood system through direct inhalation, poisoned food such as exposed or canned foods like those on sale in the streets (Bennett 1981). These pollutants infiltrate people's lungs, causing respiratory illnesses and diminishing quality of life (Adinna 2003). Air pollution in both cities and rural areas was estimated to cause 4.2 million premature deaths worldwide in 2016 (Huang and Liu 2022).

Table 35.1 illustrates the common air pollutants: (1) carbon monoxide; (2) ground-level ozone; (3) nitrogen dioxide; (4) sulfur dioxide; (5) lead; and (6) particulate matter (also known as particle pollutants). Practically all countries have revised their air quality strategies and proposed new regulations according to guidelines published by the WHO in 2021. The guidelines are regularly updated as a result of the growing threat of air pollution.

35.7 Water Pollution

Water pollution is a major problem facing many of our surface and groundwater sources. Contamination of water resources comes in the form of chemical, biological, and physical pollution. It may be natural, due to geological or meteorological events, or anthropogenic (human causes) (Figure 35.3).

Human sources of contamination can be categorized as either point source or nonpoint source (Alley 2007). Point source pollution is water pollution coming from a single point, such as a sewage outflow pipe. Nonpoint source (NPS) pollution is pollution discharged over a wide land area such as agricultural and urban storm water runoff. NPS pollution contamination occurs when rainwater, snowmelt, or irrigation washes off plowed fields, city streets, or suburban backyards and carries pollutants into the water sources. As this runoff moves across the land surface, it picks up soil particles and pollutants, such as nutrients, metals, and pesticides. Incorrect waste disposal systems, industrial discharges, and excessive use of chemicals contribute to the contamination of rivers, lakes, and groundwater sources. This contamination not only endangers aquatic life but also threatens the health of urban dwellers (Ritter and Shirmohammadi, 2000).

35.8 Noise Pollution

In the relentless cacophony of urban existence, noise pollution permeates daily life. The clamor of vehicles, construction sites, and the constant hum of urban activities disrupt sleep patterns, elevate stress levels, and harm overall well-being. Large urban populations are mainly affected by noise pollution, but smaller towns containing industries also experience this problem. The main effects of noise pollution include interference with communication, sleep deprivation and reduced efficiency. Health effects such as deafness and mental failure also occur (Singh and Davar 2004).

Table 35.1 Common air pollutants.

Air pollutant	Characters	Source	Poisonous or toxic health effects
1. Carbon monoxide (CO)	A colorless, odorless gas. CO is considered as an urban pollutant because it is traffic related	Incomplete combustion of fuel; the majority of CO emissions to ambient air come from mobile sources. In addition, oxygenates decrease the emissions of volatile organic compounds (VOCs), which along with oxides of nitrogen are major precursors to the formation of tropospheric O_3	Reducing oxygen delivery to the body's organs (heart and brain) and tissues. Decreases lung function and causes respiratory symptoms, such as coughing and shortness of breath. interfering with hemoglobin's ability to carry oxygen. Hemoglobin absorbs CO about 200 times faster than its absorption rate for oxygen. The CO-carrying protein is known as carboxyhemoglobin and when sufficiently low leads to acute and chronic effects. At extremely high levels, CO can cause death
2. Ground-level ozone (O_3)	A colorless gas with a slightly sweet odor. The pollutant most closely associated with smog is ozone (O_3)	It is not emitted directly into the air but is created by the interaction of sunlight, heat, oxides of nitrogen (NO_x) and VOCs. Emissions from industrial facilities and electric utilities, motor vehicle exhaust, gasoline vapors, and chemical solvents are some of the major sources of NO_x and VOCs	The location of ozone determines whether it is essential or harmful. It is highly reactive with tissues, leading to ecological and welfare effects, such as forest damage and reduced crop production, and human health effects, especially cardiopulmonary diseases. It is likely to reach unhealthy levels on hot sunny days in urban environments. It is increasingly linked to respiratory diseases
3. Nitrogen dioxide (NO_2): found as a compound in fossil fuel	A key atmospheric pollutant. It is one of a group of highly reactive gases known as oxides of nitrogen which include nitrous acid and nitric acid. It is a yellowish-brown to reddish-brown foul-smelling gas that is a major contributor to smog and acid rain. Fuel combustion (e.g., electric utilities, industrial boilers, vehicles, and wood burning)	Nitrogen oxides result when atmospheric nitrogen and oxygen react at the high temperatures created by combustion engines. NO_2 is a traffic-related pollutant and hence emissions are expected to be highest in urban rather than rural areas. Most emissions in the US result from combustion in vehicle engines, electrical utilities, and industrial combustion	Regular exposure to NO_2 is related to an increased occurrence of acute respiratory illness in children and other vulnerable groups. It causes inflammation of the airways at high levels. Aggravates lung diseases leading to respiratory symptoms, hospital admissions, and ED visits; increased susceptibility to respiratory infection. Long-term exposure can decrease lung function and increase the response to allergens
4. Sulfur dioxide (SO_2): one of a group of highly reactive gases known as oxides of sulfur	Colorless gases found in the lower atmosphere. Depending on concentration, these gases can be detected by smell and taste. Found more in urban areas whilst very low levels are recorded in rural areas	The main sources of SO_2 emissions are fossil fuel combustion (especially high-sulfur coal) and electric utilities, and natural sources such as volcanoes. Sources of SO_2 emissions include industrial processes such as extracting metals from their ores, and the burning of high sulfur-containing fuels by locomotives, large ships, and nonroad equipment	Asthma and increased respiratory symptoms. Contributes to particle formation with associated health effects
5. Lead (P): smelters (metal refineries)	A metal found naturally in the environment as well as in manufactured products	In the past, the main sources of lead emissions were fuels in motor vehicles and industrial sources. The major sources of lead emissions today are ore and metal processing and piston-engine aircraft operating on leaded aviation gasoline	Due to continuous urbanization and industrialization, lead poses a threat to human health. It damages the developing nervous system, resulting in IQ loss and effects on learning, memory, and behavior in neonates. Cardiovascular and renal effects in adults and early effects related to anemia
6. Particulate material (PM): PM10, PM2.5	Sometimes known simply as "particulates"; refers to solid particles and liquid droplets suspended in the air we breathe. Made up of a variety of components, including acids (nitrates and sulfates), organic chemicals, metals, soil or dust particles, and allergens	Very diverse and include motor vehicles, fuel combustion and construction work as well as aerosol particles produced by reactions between gases in the air	The size of the particles is directly linked to their potential for causing health problems. PM that are $10\,\mu m$ in diameter or smaller generally pass through the throat and nose and enter the lungs. Short-term exposures can aggravate heart or lung diseases. Long-term exposures can lead to the development of heart or lung disease and premature mortality

35.9 The Shadows of Rural Pollution

While urban areas bear the brunt of some pollutants, rural regions grapple with their own set of challenges (Table 35.2). Often overlooked, the countryside suffers a quieter form of pollution that seeps beneath the surface. Most previous research on pollution has focused on urban areas. Rural populations, however, are potentially exposed to a variety of serious environmental risks from point and nonpoint pollution sources including agricultural activities, industrial facilities, animal containment facilities, mining operations, and others (Farid et al., 2012).

35.9.1 Agricultural Pollution

Rural areas, synonymous with picturesque landscapes and bountiful harvests, can harbor unseen pollutants. Products like fertilizers and pesticides constitute pollutants by joining with the natural system or as residues (Adinna 2003).

Intensive farming practices, excessive fertilizer use, and improper waste management release harmful chemicals and pollutants into the soil and water sources. These pollutants gradually accumulate, posing risks to both human health and the vitality of the ecosystems they support. Exposure to agricultural pesticides has harmful impacts on reproductive health and outcomes including cardiovascular disease, diabetes, and several forms of cancer (Wellenius et al. 2006).

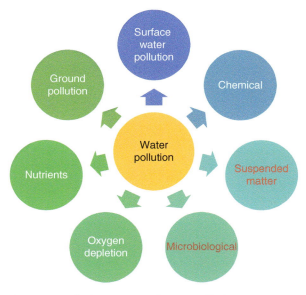

Figure 35.3 Different types of water pollution.

Table 35.2 A comparative study between pollution in rural and urban areas provides insights into the similarities and differences in the types, sources, and impacts of pollution in these two settings.

	Urban areas	**Rural areas**
Region	Places of high populations and high density	Low population and density
Pollution aspect	Urban areas are dangerous and threatening, with pollution from factories and vast amounts of working-class people living in poverty	Rural areas generally experience far less noise and air pollution
Air pollution	Vehicle emissions, industrial activities, power plants	Agricultural practices (e.g., biomass burning, pesticide use)
Water pollution	Industrial discharge, sewage, runoff from roads and parking lots	Agricultural runoff, improper waste disposal
Noise pollution	Traffic, construction activities, densely populated areas	Agricultural machinery, transportation on highways
Light pollution	Excessive use of artificial lighting in buildings, streets, advertising	Agricultural practices, outdoor lighting
Soil pollution	Industrial activities, improper waste disposal	Agricultural practices (e.g., pesticide and fertilizer use)
Health impacts	Respiratory diseases, cardiovascular problems, exposure to pollutants	Respiratory diseases, exposure to pesticides
Environmental impact	Ecosystem disruption, water contamination	Ecosystem disruption, reduced biodiversity, water and soil contamination
Mitigation strategies	Stricter regulations, promotion of clean technologies, public awareness	Improved waste managementl, sustainable agricultural practices

Note: this table is just an example and the specific types and levels of pollution can vary depending on the region and context.

35.9.2 Light Pollution

Away from the glaring city lights, rural areas may seem untouched by urban ills. However, the night skies that once dazzled with celestial wonders dim under the blanket of light pollution. Artificial illumination disrupts natural cycles, confuses wildlife navigation, and obscures the beauty of the stars above, disconnecting humans from the awe-inspiring cosmos.

35.10 Severity of Pollution

The severity of pollution can vary between urban and rural areas due to differences in population density, industrialization, and specific sources of pollution. Generally, urban areas tend to have higher pollution levels compared to rural areas. Here are some factors that contribute to the severity of pollution in each setting.

35.10.1 Urban Areas

- *Population density*: urban areas have higher population densities, leading to increased vehicle emissions, industrial activities, and energy consumption, which contribute to higher pollution levels.
- *Industrial activities*: urban areas are often home to a concentration of industries, factories, and power plants, which release pollutants into the air and water.
- *Transportation*: urban areas experience heavy traffic, resulting in higher levels of air pollution from vehicle emissions.
- *Infrastructure*: urban areas have more built-up infrastructure, such as roads, buildings, and parking lots, which contribute to increased runoff and water pollution.
- *Waste generation*: urban areas generate larger amounts of waste, leading to increased pollution from improper waste disposal and landfill emissions.

35.10.2 Rural Areas

- *Agricultural practices*: rural areas often rely on agricultural activities, which can contribute to pollution through the use of pesticides, fertilizers, and the burning of crop residues.
- *Biomass burning*: in rural areas, biomass burning for cooking, heating, and agricultural purposes can release pollutants into the air.
- *Livestock farming*: rural areas may have a higher concentration of livestock farming, leading to pollution from animal waste and runoff into water sources.
- *Land use changes*: land use changes, such as deforestation or mining, can result in soil erosion and degradation, impacting water quality and ecosystems.
- *Limited infrastructure*: rural areas may have limited waste management infrastructure, leading to improper waste disposal and potential pollution.

35.11 Mitigation and Management Strategies

Managing pollution in both rural and urban areas requires a combination of individual actions, community efforts, and government policies. Here are some strategies that can be implemented.

- *Promote sustainable transportation*: encourage the use of public transportation, car pools, cycling, and walking to reduce vehicle emissions. Develop and maintain proper infrastructure for these modes of transport.
- *Improve waste management*: implement proper waste disposal systems, including recycling and composting programs. Encourage individuals and businesses to reduce waste generation and promote responsible waste management practices.
- *Enhance air quality*: encourage the use of cleaner fuels and technologies, such as electric vehicles and renewable energy sources. Enforce regulations on industrial emissions and promote the use of pollution control devices.
- *Preserve green spaces*: protect and expand green areas in both rural and urban settings. Trees and plants help absorb pollutants and improve air quality. Encourage community gardening and urban farming initiatives.

35.11 Mitigation and Management Strategies | **411**

- *Implement stricter regulations*: enforce regulations on industrial activities, construction sites, and agricultural practices to minimize pollution. Set emission standards and regularly monitor compliance.
- *Increase awareness and education*: educate the public about the impacts of pollution and the importance of sustainable practices. Promote environmental awareness campaigns and provide resources for individuals and communities to take action.
- *Encourage energy efficiency*: promote energy-efficient practices in households, businesses, and industries. This includes using energy-efficient appliances, insulation, and renewable energy sources.
- *Improve water management*: implement proper wastewater treatment systems and promote responsible water usage. Encourage the use of rainwater harvesting and water conservation techniques.
- *Strengthen environmental monitoring*: establish monitoring systems to track pollution levels and identify sources of pollution. Regularly assess air, water, and soil quality to take appropriate actions.
- *Collaborate with stakeholders*: foster partnerships between government agencies, communities, businesses, and non-profit organizations to collectively address pollution issues. Encourage participation and collaboration in finding sustainable solutions.

Managing pollution requires a long-term commitment from individuals, communities, and governments. It is essential to continuously evaluate and adapt strategies to effectively reduce pollution in both rural and urban areas.

Rural areas and urban areas can differ in terms of the sources, types, and impacts of pollution (Table 35.3). Here are some key points to consider.

- *Air pollution*: urban areas are often more affected by air pollution compared to rural areas due to higher population density and industrial activity. A study by the WHO estimated that 91% of the world's population living in urban areas is exposed to air pollution levels above the recommended limits, compared to 56% in rural areas.
- *Water pollution*: while agriculture is a significant source of water pollution in rural areas, urban areas face issues related to industrial discharges, sewage overflows, and storm water runoff. According to the United Nations, around 80% of the world's wastewater is released into the environment without adequate treatment, primarily in urban areas.
- *Noise pollution*: urban areas experience higher levels of noise pollution due to increased traffic, construction activities, and industrial operations. Noise pollution can have adverse effects on human health, including sleep disturbances and increased stress levels.
- *Solid waste generation*: urban areas generate more solid waste compared to rural areas due to higher population density and consumption levels. According to the World Bank, global waste generation is expected to rise by 70% by 2050, primarily driven by urban areas.
- *Urban heat island effect*: cities tend to have higher temperatures than surrounding rural areas due to increased buildings, concrete, and asphalt, known as the urban heat island effect. This can lead to increased energy consumption for cooling, decreased air quality, and health impacts for urban residents.

Table 35.3 General comparison between rural and urban pollution sources.

Pollution source	Rural areas	Urban areas
Agricultural	Chemical fertilizers, pesticides, and herbicides	Limited, but still present
Activities	Livestock farming, animal waste and runoff	Limited, but still present
Biomass burning	Burning of agricultural waste, biomass for cooking and heating	Limited, but still present
Indoor pollution	Burning of solid fuels for cooking and heating	Limited, but still present
Waste disposal	Improper disposal of waste, inadequate sewage systems	Improper waste disposal, emissions from landfills
Vehicular emissions	Limited, but still present	Exhaust gases from cars, trucks, motorcycles
Industrial emissions	Limited, but still present	Discharge of pollutants from factories, power plants
Construction activities	Limited, but still present	Dust and emissions from construction sites
Solid waste management	Limited, but still present	Improper waste disposal, emissions from landfills
Urban heat island effect	Limited, but still present	Increased temperatures due to pollution and high-density development

It is important to note that the extent of pollution can vary significantly depending on the specific location, country, and socioeconomic factors.

35.12 Case Studies

35.12.1 Case Study 1

One aspect of pollution in rural areas is the issue of agricultural pollution caused by the excessive use of fertilizers and pesticides. This case study focuses on the rural farming community in a specific region.

35.12.1.1 Background

The rural area in question is predominantly agricultural, with a significant number of small-scale farms. The farmers rely heavily on chemical fertilizers and pesticides to increase crop yields and protect their crops from pests and diseases. However, the excessive and improper use of these chemicals has led to pollution of the environment, including water bodies and soil.

35.12.1.2 Causes of Pollution
- *Excessive use of fertilizers*: farmers often apply more fertilizers than necessary, leading to the leaching of nitrogen and phosphorus into nearby water bodies. This causes water pollution and the growth of harmful algal blooms.
- *Improper pesticide use*: farmers may misuse or overuse pesticides, leading to the contamination of soil and water. Pesticides can also harm beneficial insects, birds, and other wildlife.
- *Lack of awareness and education*: many farmers may not be aware of the potential environmental impacts of their farming practices. Limited access to information and training on sustainable farming techniques contributes to the problem.

35.12.1.3 Effects of Pollution
- *Water pollution*: the excessive use of fertilizers and pesticides leads to the contamination of nearby rivers, streams, and groundwater sources. This affects the quality of drinking water and aquatic ecosystems, harming fish and other aquatic organisms.
- *Soil degradation*: continuous use of chemical fertilizers and pesticides can degrade soil quality, reducing its fertility and ability to support healthy crop growth. This can lead to long-term damage to agricultural productivity.
- *Health risks*: pollution from agricultural chemicals can pose health risks to farmers and nearby communities. Exposure to pesticides can lead to acute and chronic health issues, including respiratory problems, skin disorders, and even cancer.

35.12.1.4 Solutions
- *Education and training*: provide farmers with access to training programs and workshops on sustainable farming practices. Raise awareness about the potential environmental and health impacts of excessive chemical use.
- *Integrated pest management (IPM)*: promote the adoption of IPM practices, which involve using a combination of cultural, biological, and chemical control methods to manage pests effectively. This reduces reliance on pesticides.
- *Soil and water conservation practices*: encourage farmers to implement soil conservation techniques such as crop rotation, cover cropping, and terracing to prevent soil erosion and nutrient loss. Promote the use of organic fertilizers and compost to improve soil health.
- *Monitoring and regulation*: establish monitoring systems to track the use of fertilizers and pesticides and enforce regulations on their proper use. Regularly assess water and soil quality to identify pollution hotspots and take appropriate actions.
- *Financial incentives*: provide financial incentives and support to farmers who adopt sustainable farming practices. This can include subsidies for organic farming, grants for implementing conservation practices, and access to low-interest loans for purchasing equipment.

By implementing these solutions, the rural farming community can effectively manage and reduce pollution caused by agricultural practices. This will help protect the environment, improve the health of farmers and communities, and ensure the long-term sustainability of agriculture in the region.

35.12.2 Case Study 2

35.12.2.1 Background

The urban area in question is a densely populated city with a high concentration of industries, vehicles, and residential buildings. Rapid urbanization and industrialization have led to increased pollution levels, particularly air pollution.

35.12.2.2 Causes of Pollution

- *Industrial emissions*: the city is home to numerous industries, including manufacturing plants and power plants, which emit pollutants such as particulate matter, sulfur dioxide, nitrogen oxides, and VOCs.
- *Vehicle emissions*: the high number of vehicles contributes to air pollution through the emission of exhaust gases, including carbon monoxide, nitrogen oxides, and particulate matter.
- *Construction activities*: ongoing construction projects release dust and pollutants into the air, contributing to air pollution.
- *Waste management*: improper waste management practices, including open burning and inadequate waste disposal systems, release pollutants into the air.

35.12.2.3 Effects of Pollution

- *Health impacts*: the high levels of air pollution have adverse effects on public health, leading to respiratory problems, cardiovascular diseases, and increased mortality rates. Vulnerable populations, such as children, the elderly, and individuals with preexisting health conditions, are particularly at risk.
- *Environmental degradation*: air pollution contributes to the degradation of the urban environment, including damage to vegetation, soil, and water bodies. It also affects biodiversity and ecosystems.
- *Economic costs*: the health impacts of air pollution result in increased healthcare costs and reduced productivity. Additionally, the city may face economic consequences due to decreased tourism and investment opportunities.

35.12.2.4 Solutions

- *Emission control measures*: implement stricter regulations on industrial emissions, including the installation of pollution control devices and the enforcement of emission standards. Encourage industries to adopt cleaner technologies and practices.
- *Sustainable transportation*: promote the use of public transportation, cycling, and walking to reduce vehicle emissions. Develop and maintain proper infrastructure for these modes of transport. Encourage the adoption of electric vehicles and the expansion of charging infrastructure.
- *Urban planning and design*: incorporate green spaces, parks, and trees into urban planning to improve air quality and provide natural air filters. Implement measures to reduce urban heat island effects, such as using reflective materials and increasing green roofs.
- *Waste management*: improve waste management practices, including recycling and composting programs. Enforce regulations on waste disposal and promote responsible waste management practices to reduce air pollution from open burning and improper waste handling.
- *Public awareness and education*: raise awareness about the impacts of air pollution and the importance of individual actions in reducing pollution levels. Educate the public on sustainable practices, such as energy conservation and responsible waste management.
- *Collaboration and governance*: foster partnerships between government agencies, industries, communities, and nonprofit organizations to collectively address air pollution issues. Develop and implement comprehensive air quality management plans and regularly monitor air quality levels.

By implementing these solutions, the urban area can effectively manage and reduce air pollution, improving public health, protecting the environment, and promoting sustainable development.

35.13 Conclusion

Pollution, an ever-present challenge, manifests differently in rural and urban areas. Urban centers grapple with the visible consequences of industrialization and human activity. In contrast, the countryside harbors hidden pollutants, imperceptible at first glance. Both realms require urgent attention and innovative solutions to preserve the delicate balance of nature.

In urban areas, pollution tends to be more concentrated and diverse. The heavy presence of industries, vehicles, and large population sizes contribute to high levels of air pollution. This leads to increased emissions of pollutants such as nitrogen dioxide (NO_2), sulfur dioxide (SO_2), particulate matter (PM), and VOCs. Urban environments also experience higher levels of noise pollution and light pollution due to the presence of infrastructure and city life.

On the other hand, rural areas may have less air pollution in terms of industrial emissions and vehicular traffic. However, they face pollution challenges of their own. Agricultural activities, especially the use of fertilizers and pesticides, can cause water pollution through runoff. Additionally, waste management practices in rural areas might not be as advanced, leading to issues with improper disposal and contamination of soil and water sources.

In conclusion, pollution is a significant problem in both rural and urban areas, and it requires immediate attention. Strategies should be developed to reduce pollution levels in both regions, and individuals should be educated about the consequences of pollution to encourage them to reduce their pollution footprint. In rural areas, the emphasis should be on sustainable agricultural practices while in urban areas, transportation and waste management systems should be improved. With concerted efforts, it is possible to reduce pollution levels and create a cleaner and healthier environment for everyone.

References

Adinna, E. (2003). Environmental pollution in urban and rural areas: sources and ethical implications. In: *Environmental Pollution and Management in the Tropics* (ed. E.N. Adinna, O.B. Ekop, and V.I. Attah), 298–316. Nigeria: Snaap Press.

Alley, E.R. (2007). *Water Quality Control Handbook*. New York: McGraw-Hill Education.

Balkis, N. (ed.) (2012). *Water Pollution*. Norderstedt: Books on Demand.

Bennett, S.G. (1981). *Exposure, Commitment, Assessment of Environmental Pollution 1*. London: Monitoring and Assessment Research Centre, Chelsea University College.

Charlesworth, S.M. and Booth, C.A. (ed.) (2019). *Urban Pollution: Science and Management*. Hoboken: Wiley.

Chen, Y., Zhan, Y., Chen, H. et al. (2017). Association between ambient air pollution and the prevalence of childhood asthma: a systematic review and meta-analysis. *Environmental Research* 159: 519–530.

Dasgupta, P., Dasgupta, S., Jha, R., and Shukla, P.R. (2016). Indoor air pollution and its health implications in rural India. *Social Indicators Research* 128 (1): 105–122.

Farid, S., Baloch, M.K., and Ahmad, S.A. (2012). Water pollution: major issue in urban areas. *International Journal of Water Resources and Environmental Engineering* 4 (3): 55–65.

Fenger, J. (1999). Urban air quality. *Atmospheric Environment* 33 (29): 4877–4900.

Huang, G. and Liu, F. (2022). Urban/rural differences in air pollution impacts on deaths in Scotland: a comparison study on different pollution data sources. *Spatial Statistics* 52: 100712.

Ivanovski, M., Alatič, K., Urbancl, D. et al. (2023). Assessment of air pollution in different areas (urban, suburban, and rural) in Slovenia from 2017 to 2021. *Atmosphere* 14 (3): 578.

Majra, J.P. (2011). Air quality in rural areas. In: *Chemistry, Emission Control, Radioactive Pollution and Indoor Air Quality* (ed. N. Mazzeo). London: IntechOpen.

Manisalidis, I., Stavropoulou, E., Stavropoulos, A., and Bezirtzoglou, E. (2020). Environmental and health impacts of air pollution: a review. *Frontiers in Public Health* 8: 14.

Ritter, W.F. and Shirmohammadi, A. (ed.) (2000). *Agricultural Nonpoint Source Pollution: Watershed Management and Hydrology*. Boca Raton: CRC Press.

Singh, N. and Davar, S.C. (2004). Noise pollution – sources, effects and control. *Journal of Human Ecology* 16 (3): 181–187.

Wellenius, G.A., Schwartz, J., and Mittleman, M.A. (2006). Particulate air pollution and hospital admissions for congestive heart failure in seven United States cities. *American Journal of Cardiology* 97: 404–408.

Whittaker, R.H. (1975). *Communities and Ecosystem*. New York: Macmillan.

World Health Organization (WHO). (2016). Ambient air pollution: a global assessment of exposure and burden of disease. www.who.int/publications/i/item/9789241511353 (accessed 8 February 2024).

Yang, T. (2020). Association between perceived environmental pollution and health among urban and rural residents – a Chinese national study. *BMC Public Health* 20 (1): 1–10.

36

Global Warming and Green House Effect: Impact of Climate Change, Protocol, Treaties and Convention

Baleshwari Dixit[1], Sulochana Sen[2], and Rajesh Kumar Vandre[2]

[1] Department of Veterinary Public Health & Epidemiology, College of Veterinary Science and Animal Health, 486001, Rewa, Madhya Pradesh, India
[2] Department of Animal Genetics and Breeding, College of Veterinary Science & Animal Health, Rewa, India

36.1 Introduction

Long-term heating of Earth's surface was observed since the pre-industrial period and that phenomenon was termed as Global warming of earth. Global warming is defined as "the increase in the average surface temperature of the earth" because of the increase in the concentration of greenhouse gases (GHGs) such as water vapor, methane, ozone, carbon dioxide, chlorofluorocarbons (CFCs) and nitrous oxide (Environmental Protection Agency/EPA (2010). The main causes of increase of these gases have been associated with the natural sources, like volcanoes, seismic activities, forest fires and human activities involving burning of fossil fuel (Hughes et al., 2017). This term is often confused with the "climate change" however both these terms are linked but not interchangeable climate change is related with the long-term shifts in temperatures and weather patterns spatially and temporally. The causation of both issues may be natural, but after 1800s, the industrial revolution involving over use of natural resources was the main driver of climate change. Since during pre-industrial period, 1°C (1.8° F) increase in Earth's global average temperature have been noted. In corresponds to human activities about more than 0.2°C increase (0.36° F) in temperature per decade is being reported globally and which is continuously proceeding at an unprecedented rate (Houghton et al., 2001).

The greenhouse effect is the process of trapping the heat near Earth's surface by a combination of gases known as GHGs. The greenhouse effect occurs when GHGs in a planet's atmosphere allow the short wave radiation to enter in to the earth's atmosphere which are absorbed by the earth surface and in turn emit long wave radiation which are stopped by the GHGs layer to exit the atmosphere. This process prevent the lowering of temperature of earth in the night. Greenhouse effect is essential to make earth a place to live on comfortably, without GHGs, the earth surface temperature would be too low and so no life will be on earth.

Overuse of fossil fuels as energy resources raises the concentration of the GHGs, such as CO_2, CH_4, N_2O, and water vapor (EA IEA 2017) in the atmosphere to the extent that increases the trapping of more radiation in response and the average surface temperature of the earth rises. Water vapor contributed majorly in the global warming while CO_2 gas is considered as the controlling factor in global warming (Khan et al., 2018). That means the CO_2 level is the critical factor and global warming would not have happened if the concentration of CO_2 did not increase. Studies have indicated that doubling or halving the concentration of CO_2 level in the atmosphere would result in +3.8 C or −3.6 C, changes in average surface temperature of the earth, respectively. However, there are other driving factors which may facilitate the changes like humidity of the air which in return depends on the air's temperature. Other GHGs like CH_4 and N_2O comparatively have more ability to absorb the radiation, but their concentration is low in the atmosphere in comparison to CO_2 that make their contribution in the global warming insignificant (Pedersen et al., 2021).

The Sixth Assessment Report (AR6) of Inter governmental Panel on Climate Change (IPCC) published in 2018, indicated that anthropogenic activities have contributed average temperature increase between 0.8 °C and 1.2 °C (1.4 and 2.2 °F) worldwide, since pre-industrial times and mostly after middle of the twentieth century. Many climate scientists warned that if the global average temperature rise by more than 2 °C (3.6 °F) would result in significant social, economic, and ecological damage. Such damage may include increased extinction of many plant and animal species, shifts in patterns of agriculture, and rising sea levels.

Epidemiology and Environmental Hygiene in Veterinary Public Health, First Edition. Edited by Tanmoy Rana.
© 2025 John Wiley & Sons, Inc. Published 2025 by John Wiley & Sons, Inc.

Global warming is related to the more general phenomenon of climate change, which refers to changes in the totality of attributes that define climate (IPCC, 2009). In addition to changes in air temperature, climate change involves changes to precipitation patterns, winds, ocean currents, and other measures of earth's climate. Normally, climate change is viewed as a result of combined effect of various natural causes occurring in different timescales (IPCC, 2009). With the advent of human civilization the anthropogenic or exclusively human-caused element are directly involved in climate change. Since past two centuries industrial development has contributed immensely in changes of climate along with global warming (Logan, 2010).

36.2 Green House Effect

The greenhouse effect is an essential phenomenon required to the natural warming of the earth which is the trapping of heat of the sun entered in the earth's surface by the atmosphere. The average surface temperature of Earth is regulated by a balance between different forms of terrestrial and solar radiation. The Earth's atmosphere consists of major gases like nitrogen (78.08%), oxygen (20.95%), and argon (0.93%), carbon dioxide (0.04%) and minor gases principally methane, nitrous oxide, and ozone. Beside argon some noble gases, like helium, neon, krypton, and xenon are also present in the air. Water vapor is also an important but variable component of the air which varies in amount as at sea level average around 1% while 0.4% over the entire atmosphere. Apart from these natural gases some synthetic fluorinated gases are also acts as GHGs. Air is the layer of gases which are retained on earth because of its gravity and they forms its planetary atmosphere. However the air composition varies with temperature, and atmospheric pressure that depends upon altitude of area and decrease with high. Earth's atmosphere is divided into five main layers that is called atmospheric stratification. These layers are troposphere that extend up to 12 km from earths, stratosphere (12 to 50 km), mesosphere (50 to 80 km), thermosphere (80 to 700 km), and exosphere (700 to 10 000 km). Air suitable for most of the life is found only in Earth's troposphere. Permanent gases are usually constant in concentration but the concentration of other minor gases like carbon dioxide, nitrous oxides, methane, and ozone is highly variable on daily, seasonally, and annually basis (Venkataramanan, 2011; Composition of the Atmosphere|North Carolina Climate Office n.d.). The special characteristic of GHGs to absorb, trap and reradiate infrared radiation is because of their atoms have internal vibrational modes, differentiating them with other main components of the atmosphere (Roe, 2006).

Of all these GHGs, carbon dioxide is the prime importance, because of its relationship with the greenhouse effect and its role in the human economy. In the earlier decades of industrial age (mid-eighteenth century), the carbon dioxide concentrations were roughly 280 ppm in the atmosphere. At the end of 2022 this concentration had risen to 419 ppm, and, if the responsible anthropogenic activities will continue at this rates, it may reach to 550 ppm a doubling concentrations of carbon dioxide in these years. Different GHGs have different chemical properties and are removed from the atmosphere, over time, by various processes

The earth's average surface and nearby atmosphere temperature is controlled by a balance of terrestrial and solar radiation. Sustainability of life on earth and major determinant of the climate is dependent on solar life (Table 36.1). The solar radiation

Table 36.1 Earths atmospheric composition.

S. No	Gas	Concentration	
		PPM	Percentage
1.	Nitrogen	780 840	78.084
2.	Oxygen	209 460	20.946
3.	Argon	9340	0.9340
4.	Carbon dioxide (April 2022)(C) (Shaheen and Lipman 2007)	417	0.0417
5.	Neon	18.18	0.001818
6.	Helium	5.24	0.000524
7.	Methane	1.87	0.000187
8.	Krypton	1.14	0.000114
9.	Water vapor[D]	0–30 000[D]	0–3%[E]

spectrum have three different ranges of wavelengths including ultraviolet range, visible range and infrared range. Most of the solar radiations are the "shortwave" radiation (high frequencies and the relatively short wavelengths) and terrestrial radiation consists of "long-wave" radiation (low frequencies and long wavelengths). The solar radiation is divided into two types terrestrial and extraterrestrial. When the terrestrial solar radiations passes through the earth's atmosphere some portion get scattered and some of it is absorbed by the atmosphere and only a small fraction is absorbed by the earth. About 30% of incoming radiation is reflected back in to space by atmosphere, clouds, or reflective parts of Earth's surface. The reflective capacity of the earths is termed to as planetary albedo which varies temporally, and depends up on the extent and spatial distribution of reflective portion of the earth like clouds and ice cover etc. The remaining 70 units of solar radiation may be absorbed by the clouds, atmosphere, and the surface of earth (Alley et al. 2005).

Ultraviolet radiation are absorbed by the ozone layer present in the stratosphere of atmosphere and infrared rays are absorbed by the carbon dioxide and methane. As per the maintenance of thermodynamic equilibrium, the same amount of solar radiations reradiated by Earth's surface and atmosphere are returned back in to space. These are infrared radiation of short-wavelength and because of their low temperature in comparison to solar radiation, returning back are again absorbed by the GHGs the atmosphere. Water vapor can absorb a wide range of wave lengths which make it a major component of atmosphere absorbing the solar radiation fall over the earth surface.

36.3 Factors Affect The Global Warming

36.3.1 Natural Factors

The climate of the earth has changed many a times in the past and various natural forces and anthropogenic factors. Before the industrial revolution, changes in earth's climate was occurred due to natural forces and were not related to human activities. The natural forces includes the changes in the amount of solar radiation, volcanic eruptions, and the amount of solar radiation enters in to the earth atmosphere which varies because of milankovitch cycle. Variations in sunlight was the most significant contributor in these changes includes alteration in tiny wobbles in earth's orbit, variations in the Sun itself changes the amount of solar energy reaching earth. Particles generated due to volcanic eruptions reflect the sunlight, brightens the planet and cool down the climate. Volcanic activity has increased the GHGs concentration over millions of years, contributed in global warming to some extent (Riebeek, 2010). Milankovitch cycle is a long-term cycle that occurs every 10000 years, which is known to affect the natural global cooling and warming by three causes: the eccentricity, the precession and the obliquity. Volcanic eruptions also affect the temperature of earth significantly. The eruptions from volcanoes carry concentration of gases and ash into the upper atmosphere and these gases, particularly sulfuric gases, facilitates the formation of clouds which reduces the global temperature (Man et al., 2014). Apart from this these volcanoes also emit large concentration of water vapor, and carbon dioxide and which affects global warming, however, this amount is very small in comparison to anthropogenic emissions (NASA, 2020). As per an estimate the volcanos were found to emit about 130–230 million tons of carbon dioxide per year while this

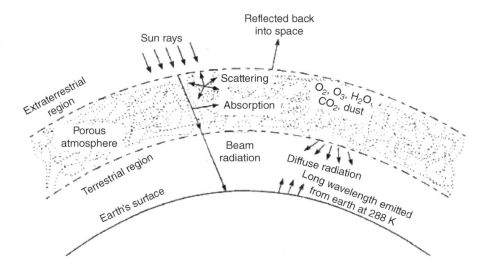

Figure 36.1 Extraterrestrial and terrestrial wavelength spectrum and the characteristics of water vapor and carbon dioxide to absorb radiant energy at short-wave infrared region.

concentration is 26 billion tons per year due to mankind activities which is 100 times more than volcanos. Natural events are still acting but with too small and slow influence on the climate compared with human activity influence (Figure 36.1).

36.3.2 Anthropogenic Factors

Water vapor is abundantly present in the atmosphere which is considered to an important variable for global warming. Water vapor is considered to be responsible for two-third of the global warming. A constant equilibrium is maintained between temperature and water vapor concentration but as the temperature increases to extend a limit this balances get disturbed and which will increase the global warming. The warming ability of water vapor is almost double to the warming caused by carbon dioxide. Warmer climate increases the water vapor in the atmosphere resulting in cloud formation which again affect the global warming. The role of cloud on determining the temperature of earth is highly variable and depending on the size of clouds, it may promote in cooling or even warming the planet. Brighter clouds reflects back the solar radiation resulting in cooling of the planet. In contrast, the ability of clouds to absorb and emit energy, so the low clouds have nearly same temperature of earth surface, so they emitted energy of infrared wave is similar to that earth surface, however the clouds at high distance are more cooler and they absorb the coming energy of lower atmosphere and because of their low temperature, the amount of energy emitted will be low.

Carbon dioxide gas is most significant gas which play a deciding role in increase in green-house effect. Since 1950, a remarkable increase in the concentration of carbon dioxide in the atmosphere has been recorded and of which higher portion was contributed by human's activities. Depending upon the burning of different types of fossil fuel a variable amount of GHGs such as carbon dioxide, nitrous oxides and water vapor are produced. Fossil fuel which are commonly used by anthropogenic activities includes coal, natural gas and oil etc. Coal burning, oil burning and natural gas burning contribute to 45%, 35%, and 20% of CO_2 emissions respectively. Along with the increased emission of CO_2, the anthropogenic activities disturbed the carbon cycle in the nature particularly by deforestation. The destruction of forest ceases the carbon absorption by trees and resulting in increase in concentration of the CO_2 in the atmosphere where it contributed about 25–30% of GHGs emitted yearly. Additionally 50% part of the trees is made up of carbon and burning of these trees will release the stored carbon as CO_2 and that will add in the harmful consequences of the deforestations. The restoration of carbon dioxide takes hundreds of years and so as maintain the balance. With increase in the carbon dioxide concentration the temperature and water vapor levels increases. The CO_2 is also play a role in controlling the amount of water vapor carried by the atmosphere, so due to its diverse role the carbon dioxide, is considered as a controlling factor rather than reacting factor.

Another largest contributing GHGs is Methane which is mainly produced by anthropogenic activities and over the last 150 years the amount of methane emissions have doubled. Anthropogenic methane can be released into the atmosphere during natural gas uses and moreover, notable amounts of methane also released from livestock and agriculture production, disposal of human waste, and sewage landfills. Methane molecule are 10 times more effective than carbon dioxide molecule in absorbing and re-radiation of the energy but more focus is given on the total levels of the concentration rather than the intensity. Carbon dioxide concentration in the atmosphere is about 200 times more than that of methane as well as the more lifetime of CO_2 than the atmospheric methane.

Another important GHG is Nitrous Oxide which is produced by human activities like agriculture, industrial processes, fossil fuel burning, and wastewater disposal which contributes about 40% of the total N_2O emissions. N_2O is a part of nitrogen cycle and it take approximately 114 years to its conversion in to another form which may be by some specific bacteria or it may destroyed by chemical reaction or by ultraviolet radiation. Similar to methane the ability of N_2O to contribute in increase of the temperature is almost 300 times more than that of CO_2 but its concentration is much smaller than CO_2.

36.3.3 Effect of GHGs

Industrial revolution contributed substantially in increase of earth's temperature noted by various international and nation agencies like Goddard Institute for Space Studies (GISS) reported increase in 0.8°C in average earth's surface temperature since 1880. Annual temperature anomalies from 1880 to 2014 was recorded by different agencies like National Aeronautics and Space Administration (NASA) US, the Japan Meteorological Agency, National Oceanic and Atmospheric Administration (NOAA), and the Met Office Hadley Centre United Kingdom which showed same graphical trend and variations. Prediction model based on three CO_2 emissions scenarios, indicate increase of 2–6°C in average surface temperature by the end of twenty-first century. Increase in the global temperature will progress to more disastrous effects on the all the life present on the earth in different ways. Increase in the global temperature will lead to occurrence of more intense, more frequent and widespread extreme weather events like droughts, floods, hurricanes, and heat waves which will adversely affect the humanity. Apart from these warming of climate is causing the melting down of snow and the ice is leading the rise of sea level. This conversion is transforming the snow which are sunlight reflecting surfaces to liquid stage that have sunlight absorbing surfaces, which will further facilitate the trapping of heat in the earth atmosphere (Rohling et al., 2013).

Ocean absorbs substantial amount of CO2 approximately half of the anthropogenic generated CO2 and this process helps in reduction the warming of the climate. However, this process leads to some permanent and serious change in the ocean water chemistry. The absorption of carbon dioxide in water leads to formation of carbonic acidic which lowers the pH of surface water. Over the past 300 million years, pH of oceans' water was 8.2, and over the past two centuries 25% reduction in the acidity was noted and drop in pH to 8.1. Marine lives are highly susceptible to pH of water and this change will adversely affect the life cycle of many marine animals. Heat trapping in the ocean also lead to increase in the heating of which cause the expansion of water and increased temperature also causing melting of ice and snow which further increases the sea water level. The thermal expansion is causing the rise in water level of seas. Since 1990 this sea level rise was recorded at a rate of 0.14 in. per year. At this rate there are possibilities of rise of water level up to 2 m by 2100 that will lead to demolition of thousands of islands and coastal cities as well stronger storm surges in to nearby areas. Furthermore the reduction in percentage of dissolved oxygen due to warming of water will also compromise various marine life as well as it may lead to death of many marine species. Coral bleach is one of example of drastic effect of global warming of sea life because the rise in water temperature is causing the algal death that live inside of coral in symbiosis and it get disturbed which lead to death of the coral.

Global warming is indirectly responsible for the changing of weather conditions and at some place the variation was so unfavorable for the survival of certain species that caused the extinction of these animal and plant species.

Global warming also affect the formation of storm at pole and equators, at tropical areas storms and hurricanes formation depends on the surface's temperature of seas and the humidity contents of air. Temperature rise increases the capacity of atmosphere to hold more moisture particularly at sea surfaces, which increases the possibilities hurricanes forming, intensity storms and more wind speed of these storms. The 0.3 C in temperature of sea water and 4% increase in humidity near surface seawater was reported since 1980.

Other than temperature a change in pattern of precipitations, droughts, and floods is also noticed spatially and temporally in the past decades all over the globe. This difference was directly as well as indirectly associated with global warming. In some areas the intensity of these events have increased due to which the dry regions became drier and wet regions became wetter. Increase in the temperature led to increased capacity of atmosphere to hold more resulted in heavy precipitation. However, with the changes in intensity, the variation in frequency of precipitation over a short period of time contributed to substantial increase in number of floods in twentieth century around the world. Heavy precipitation decreases the soaking of water by soil that increases more runoff of water leading the occurrence of floods.

Another observation consequent to global warming is the changes in the trends of draught particularly in the southern and northern hemispheres. Changes in precipitations events include low to moderate and light rains in some areas and heavy but short precipitations along with early melting of snow were the result of global warming. Globally the very dry areas extended substantially across the world causing the increase in the rate of evaporation from vegetation and soil. Continuous high temperature for a long period of time led to prolongation of hot weather which produces the more heat waves which have significant effects on living beings. On human health, where it causes serious health issues such as heatstroke, fainting, and clams. If the global warming continues at this rate, the occurrence of heat waves may become doubled in the next decade in all over the world.

36.4 Important Environmental Conventions and Protocols on Climate Change

36.4.1 Ramsar Convention

It was named after the Ramsar city of Iran, where it was first signed in 1971.It is also referred as the "Convention on Wetlands" under the auspices of UNESCO. It came into force on 21 December 1975, when it was ratified by a sufficient number of nations. It is an international treaty which was formed for the protection of wetlands of international importance. Earlier it was primarily focused on waterfowl habitat than different wet lands were marked which were also known as Ramsar Sites and this convention provides the conservation and sustainable use of these wet land sites and their resources. In order to protect the wetlands cooperation and action on international and nation level is provided to member countries. Every three years, meeting of representatives contracting parties and the conference of the Contracting Parties (COP), is being held and in which they adopts decisions related to designation of Ramsar sites, resolutions and recommendations are made to administration and implement its objectives.

36.5 Convention on International Trade in Endangered Species of Wild Fauna and Flora (CITES)

It is an international treaty which controls and regulates the international trade of threatened and endangered species of animals and plants. The Convention was adopted in 1973 and entered into force on 1 July 1975. CITES has 184 member parties and It regulates all major markets of trade of over 38 000 species in the world. Under strict supervision and condition an export permits or licences is issued and given the authorization for international trade.

36.5.1 Bonn Convention

It is also known as the Convention on Migratory Species (CMS) and its prime objective was conservation of all ranges of migratory species of wild origin. The agreement was signed in 1979 in Bonn, West Germany, under the patronage of the United Nations Environment Programme and it came in to force in 1983. It has 131 Member States and the depositary is the Government of the Federal Republic of Germany. It is the only global and United Nations-based, intergovernmental organization which was established for the conservation and management of all type of migratory species including terrestrial, aquatic, and avian migratory. The CMS, and its agreements, drafts policies, and provide guidance and assistance on specific issues through their strategies guidelines, action plans, resolutions, and decisions.

36.5.2 Vienna Convention

It is the convention for the Protection of the Ozone Layer is a multilateral environmental agreement which was signed in 1985 at the Vienna Conference of 1985 and entered into force in 1988. These treaties are highly successful and ratified by 198 states as well as the European Union. While not a binding agreement, it acts as a framework for the international efforts for reduction of CFCs which are continuously causing the destruction of the ozone layer. These drafts are providing assistance in international reductions in the formation of hole in ozone layer which will lead to more passage of ultraviolet radiation to earth which is harmful due to increased risk of skin cancer. However, it does not include legally binding reduction goals for the use of CFCs, the Into protect the ozone layer it provide the framework required for regulatory authority and guideline in the form of the Montreal Protocol.

36.5.3 Montreal Protocol

It is an international treaty formed to protect the ozone layer by controlling the production of chemicals that are responsible for ozone depletion. It was signed on 16 September 1987, and came in to action on 1 January 1989 and since then, it has undergone nine revisions. It is one of the successful international agreement, resulting in perhaps slowly but recovering of the ozone hole in Antarctica. Predictive models are indicating the return of the ozone layer to the 1980 levels by 2066 (Cook et al. 2005). Its prime aim was to reduce the production and consumption of substances causing the ozone depletion to the level at which they do not cause any harmful effects, thereby protecting the earth's fragile ozone Layer.

36.5.4 Basel Convention

It is also known as the Basel Convention on the Control of Trans-boundary Movements of Hazardous Wastes and Their Disposal, which was adopted on March 22, 1989 in the Conference of Plenipotentiaries in Basel, Switzerland. It is an international treaty that was signed to reduce the hazardous waste movements between countries, and particularly from developed to developing countries. **Its main objective is to** minimize the toxicity and rate of generation of hazardous wastes in order to protect the human, animal, and environmental health. It provide guidelines and assistance in management of hazardous waste as possible as nearby its source of generation.

36.6 Basel Convention on Biological Diversity (CBD)

The Convention on Biological Diversity (CBD) is a conventions for protection of biological diversity in environment which came in to existence on 29[th]December 1993. It is a legally binding agreement which was signed by 196 countries. Its three main objectives include the CBD, the sustainable use of the components of biological diversity, and the fair and equitable sharing of the benefits arising out of the utilization of genetic resources.

36.6.1 United Nations Framework Convention on Climate Change (UNFCCC)

The convention was adopted on 9 May 1992 in United Nations Conference on Environment and Development (UNCED), also known as the Earth Summit, which was held from 3 to 14 June 1992 in Rio de Janeiro. In order to combat "dangerous human interference with the climate system" with the objective to stabilize the greenhouse gases concentrations in the atmosphere, this framework established an environmental treaty that was signed by 154 states which became effective on 21 March 1994. From 1995 to assess the progress on climate change the parties of convention have met annually in COPs. According to this treaty ongoing scientific research and regular meetings, negotiations, and future policy agreements should consider the processes allow ecosystems to be natural and promote food security and economic sustainable development. Political leaders, scientists, media representatives, diplomats, and non-governmental organizations (NGOs) from signed countries have attended it.

36.6.2 United Nations Convention to Combat Desertification (UNCCD)

It **is** one of the environmental conventions, which was adopted in 1994. The first internationally binding agreement connects sustainable land management to development and the environment. The Convention focuses primarily on the dry-lands, composed of arid, semi-arid, and dry sub-humid regions and is home to some of the most vulnerable ecosystems and populations. To advance the objectives of the Convention and make progress in its implementation, Parties to the Convention meet in COPs every two years as well as in technical meetings throughout the year.

36.6.2.1 Kyoto Protocol

On 1st Conference of the Parties (COP1) it was concluded that parties are unable to stabilize their emissions 2000 was "not adequate" and which given the establishment of Kyoto Protocol in 1997 that ran from 2005 to 2020. The Kyoto Protocol was the first implementation of measures under the UNFCCC which targeted the developed countries for legally binding obligations as per international law directed to reduce their GHGs emissions from 2008 to 2012.

36.6.2.2 The Paris Agreement

It is often regarded as the Paris Accords or the Paris Climate Accords, which is an international treaty designed to control climate change. The agreement was adopted on 2015, which covers mitigation, adaptation, and finance strategies for climate change. During United Nations Climate Change Conference near Paris, France this agreement was negotiated between 195 parties. Of the three UNFCCC member states which have not ratified the agreement, the only major emitter is Iran. In 2020 United States withdrew from this agreement, but rejoined in 2021. The main goal of this agreement was to limit mean global temperature increase well below 2 °C (3.6 °F) above pre-industrial levels, and preferably to 1.5 °C (2.7 °F), considering that this would reduce the effects of climate change. By the middle of the twenty-first century the reduction in emissions should be achieved to reach net zero. To keep the temperature well below 1.5 °C of global warming, it is essential to cut of the emissions by roughly 50% till 2030. This is an aggregate of each country's nationally determined contributions.

36.6.2.3 Rotterdam Convention

This convention was adopted on 10 September 1998 during a Conference of Plenipotentiaries in Rotterdam, Netherlands and ratified on 24 February 2004. Its main goals are to encourage cooperative efforts and shared responsibility among Parties in the international trade of some specific hazardous chemicals in order to protect the human and the environmental health from potential harm. Provide for a national decision-making process on their import and export; and by facilitating information exchange about their characteristics about the convention's goals worldwide.

36.6.2.4 Cartagena Protocol on Biosafety

Cartagena Protocol is conventions on Biosafety which was adopted on 29th January, 2000 and came in to effect on 11th September 2003. The aim of this agreement to ensure the safe transportation, handling and use of living-modified organisms (LMOs) developed from contemporary biotechnology which may cause untoward effects on biological diversity along with their possible risks to human health.

36.6.2.5 Stockholm Convention

The Stockholm Convention, one of the Environmental Conventions, which was adopted during the conference of the Plenipotentiaries, Stockholm on 22nd May 2001 and it came into force on 17th May 2004. It is a global treaty to safeguard the human and environment health from persistent organic pollutants (POPs). POPs are compounds that accumulate in living being particularly in fatty tissue and that may have very persistent long life in the environment and during which time they are unaltered and may impart very harmful effect on people and wildlife.

36.6.2.6 Nagoya Protocol

This protocol was adopted on 29th October 2010, in Nagoya, Japan. During CBD it is a supplementary agreement which has the main objective on access to Genetic Resources and the Equitable and Fair Sharing of Benefits Arising from their Utilization (ABS). It provides a clear legal framework in order to promote the efficient realization of one of the three goals of the CBD that is the equitable and fair sharing of benefits arising from the utilization of genetic resources.

36.6.2.7 Minamata Convention

It is an environmental convention which was adopted in 2013 and came into existence in 2017. It's primary aim was to safeguard the environment and human health from the adverse effects of mercury released from industrial wastes. It restrict the establishment of new mercury mines, the closing of existing ones, the removal or reduction of mercury uses in various objects and procedures, enforcement of control measures for its releases in the atmosphere, land and water, and strict supervision on regulation of the small-scale gold mining and unofficial artisanal industry. The convention emphasizing the supervision on mercury's short-term storage, disposal of waste particularly in mercury-contaminated areas and health concerns (Chesser and Baker, 2006).

36.6.2.8 Kigali Amendment

During 28th October 2016 Meeting of the Parties to the Montreal Protocol, in Kigali, Rwanda, the Kigali Amendment was adopted to the Montreal Protocol on chemicals that are responsible for depletion of Ozone Layer, which calls for the restrict the emission of hydrofluorocarbons (HFCs). As per Kigali Amendment the parties of Montreal protocol are required to gradually reduce their production and consumption of hydrofluorocarbons, or HFCs.

36.7 The United Nations Collaborative Programme on Reducing Emissions from Deforestation and Forest Degradation in Developing Countries (UN-REDD)

It is the platform provided by United Nations on forest solutions to the climate crisis which was launched in 2008 and leverages the technical expertise of food and convening power of the United Nations Environment Programme (UNEP), United Nations Development Programme (UNDP), and Food and Agriculture Organization of the United Nations (FAO).

36.7.1 The United Nations Collaborative Programme on Reducing Emissions from Deforestation and Forest Degradation in Developing Countries + (UN-REDD+)

It is a strategy primarily focused on reducing the global warming which was designed by parties of the United Nations Framework Convention on Climate Change (UNFCCC). It addresses the issue of global warming beyond deforestation and forest degradation, it also focuses the sustainable forest management, forest conservation, and the encouragement promote the storage and sink of forest carbon. It is also known as the Warsaw Framework for REDD+ (WFR), which was officially endorsed in December 2013 at COP 19 in Warsaw.

36.7.2 Adaptation and Mitigation Strategies for Global Warming

If no urgent action taken and this increase in the amount of GHGs in the atmosphere continue it will lead to the life on earth very difficult. The unpreparedness will impact very harsh and then its mitigation in cleaning up the extra GHGs from the atmosphere would be very expensive and very less feasible.

In general meaning adaptation is the process of preparedness and adjustment toward present and future effects of certain change. IPCC defines the adaptation as "the adjustment in nature or human systems in response to actual or expected climatic stimuli or their effects, with moderates harm or exploits beneficial opportunities" Adaptation is the process of anticipating the harmful effects of global warming and being prepared with effective action in order to minimize or reverse of the damage occurred. New and protective techniques required to be developed in order to reduce the impact of global warming (Campisano, 2012). It can be supplemented by adaptation driven government policies and their implementations. However, the adoption strategies have certain limitations including technological, financial, and social factors (Solomon et al., 2007). The critical issues in effectiveness of adaptation process is the resilience of species to the global warming need longer time to make themselves adapt to these strategies (Vijayavenkataraman et al., 2012). To be able to bear the effect of global warming adaptation measures like changes in large-scale infrastructure like construction of such buildings which are robust against any of the disaster conditions, like building of dams particularly at coasts and rivers protect against sea-level rise, or behavioral changes like reduction in food waste.

In contrast mitigation is the process of reducing the impacts of global warming that is possible only by control of atmospheric emission of GHGs. IPCC has defined the mitigation as "an anthropogenic intervention to reduce the source or enhance the sinks of GHGs." Mitigation may be carried by stop emitting or restricting the production or use of sources of these gases and absorption of GHGs from the atmosphere by using some techniques. The atmospheric emission of GHGs can be controlled, by promoting the use of renewable energies; by establishing a cleaner system to absorption or storage systems of these gases such as reforestation because trees can absorb CO_2 from the atmosphere so planting trees can reduce the amount of CO_2 in the atmosphere.

However the most effective way may uses the combination of these two adaptation and mitigations strategies, will have the optimal cost because it will help in limit the emission of greenhouse that will reduce the burden on adaptation strategy in technical and financial matter. It will require an alternative clean energy source or the long-term strategy for prevention of greenhouse emissions. As the carbon dioxide major GHGs responsible for global warming and which is also a controlling factor, so the prime efforts should be taken toward limiting the CO_2 emission as well as the sequestration of CO_2 that will significantly contribute in reduction of consequences of global warming. The major issue in adopting these technologies is economic constraints which make them unfeasible. Energy generation sector are responsible for almost 37.5% of CO_2 emissions so cutting the CO_2 emissions by these sector will be major contributor in controlling of CO_2 in the atmosphere. Renewable energy resources are better option in energy production sectors because renewable energy resources like solar and wind energy are abundant, which are more suitable as an alternative for fossil fuels and their uses are comparatively more affordable and feasible. The energy production with using new techniques or the combination of different approaches can give better option than conventional processes. For example integrated gasification in coal-fired power plant enhances the thermal efficiency up to 45% while the combination of gas turbine with natural gas raises its efficiency by 60%. The use of such combination of technologies in power generation unit, can help in reduction of CO_2 emissions up to 50%.Another major source of CO_2 emission is transportation sector which is responsible for about 22% of the global atmospheric CO_2 emissions. The use of electric, hybrid and the bio-fuel operated vehicles can critically reduce the CO_2 emissions. Apart from this some other efforts in general like more efficient vehicles in utilizing fuels; promotion of hybrid cars; and provision and emphasizing the public transportation system. Furthermore, Building sector is another contributor which is responsible for about 31% of the total CO_2 emissions and in this sector intelligent utilization of energy efficiency in lighting, equipment, and appliances can contribute in cutting the CO_2 emissions significantly. Heating, ventilation and air conditioning systems (HVAC) another component of building operation consuming high level of energy here the insulation of the building's envelope and use of variable refrigerant flow (VRF) HVAC systems can save 82% reduction energy consumption in comparison to conventional means. Industrial sector is also major sector responsible for about 43% of the global CO_2 emissions and use of advanced technologies in recovery of waste heat may substantially lower the energy losses significantly (Dosio et al., 2018). To improve the efficiency in generation of energy the process like promotion of renewable energy resources in place of fossil fuels; and technologies for early capture of carbon from atmosphere can be promoted. Efficient utilization of solar energy is a most promising option for conversion of regular building in to green building i.e. use of solar energy in cooling and heating of building, as fuel for cooking and heating the water etc. some other ways are power and heat recovery; recycle of the materials and substitutions of processes causing more GHGs production with the processes produces less GHGs. In agriculture using the advanced techniques for better utilization of fertilizers with less pollution and less emission of N2O. In animal production system more efficient manure management and its better utilization. Proper waste utilization process including enhanced methane recovery from landfills, minimizing the generation of wastes, and promotion of recycling and provision of heat recovery.

36.8 Conclusion

In current scenario if the consumption of fossil fuel continue with this rate and the GHGs concentrations will continue to rise. On this basis the statistic models predicted in the rise of temperature between 2 °C and 6 °C by the end of the twenty-first century. The catastrophic effects of global warming will be more frequent in terms of extreme weather conditions like hot days and fewer cool days; more intense heat waves; storms; floods; droughts; hurricanes. Anthropogenic activities are the major contributor which are responsible for increase in GHGs in the atmosphere resulted in to global warming. In response to global warming the combination adaptation and mitigation strategies would be effective instead of separate efforts. If no action is taken, the GHGs will be continue with the increasing trends that will have the disastrous impact on the public, animal and plant life with very high economic cost to counteract in response.

References

Alley, R.B. et al. (2005). Ice sheet and sea-level changes. *Science* 310: 456.

Campisano, C. J. (2012). Milankovitch cycles, paleoclimatic change, and hominin evolution, Nature Education Knowledge, 3, 5.
Chesser, R.K. and Baker, R.J. (2006). Growing up with chernobyl. *American Scientist* 94: 542.

Composition of the Atmosphere|North Carolina Climate Office n.d. https://climate.ncsu.edu/edu/Composition (accessed May 19, 2018).

Cook, A.J. et al. (2005). Retreating glacier fronts on the Antarctic Peninsula over the past half-century. *Science* 308: 541.

Dosio, A., Mentaschi, L., Fischer, E.M., and Wyser, K. (2018). Extreme heat waves under 1.5C and 2C global warming. *Environmental Research Letters* 13 (5): 54006.

Environmental Protection Agency (EPA) (2010). *Methane and Nitrous Oxide Emissions from Natural Sources.* Washington, DC: Environmental Protection Agency.

Houghton, J.T., Ding, Y., Griggs, D.J. et al. (2001). Climate change 2001: the scientific basis. In: *Contribution of Working Group I to the Third Assessment Report of the Intergovernmental Panel on Climate Change.* Cambridge, UK: Cambridge University Press.

Hughes, T.P., Kerry, J.T., Alvarez-Noriega, M. et al. (2017). Global warming and recurrent mass bleaching of corals. *Nature* 543: 373–377. https://doi.org/10.1038/nature21707.

IEA IEA (2017). CO2 emissions from fuel combustion 2017 - highlights. *International Energy Agency* 1: 1–162. https://doi.org/10.1787/co2_fuel-2017-en.

IPCC (2009). Climate change 2007: mitigation of climate change. In: *Contribution of Working Group III to the Fourth Assessment Report of the Intergovernmental Panel on Climate Change.* New York: Cambridge University Press.

Khan, A., Mehmood, M., Ganie, S., and Showqi, I. (2018). A brief review on global warming and climate change: consequences and mitigation. *Strategies* 07.

Logan, C.A. (2010). A review of ocean acidification and America's response. *BioScience* 60: 819–828. https://doi.org/10.1525/bio.2010.60.10.8.

Man, W., Zhou, T., and Jungclaus, J.H. (2014). Effects of large volcanic eruptions on global summer climate and east Asian monsoon changes during the last millennium: analysis of MPI-ESM simulations. *Journal of Climate* 27: 7394–7409. https://doi.org/10.1175/JCLI-D-13-00739.1.14.

NASA. NASA Earth Observatory: Global Temperatures. Earth Observatory. 2020. Available online: https://earthobservatory. http://nasa.gov/world-of-change/decadaltemp.php (accessed on 25 November).

Pedersen, J.S.T., Duarte Santos, F., van Vuuren, D. et al. (2021). An assessment of the performance of scenarios against historical global emissions for IPCC reports. *Global Environmental Change* 66: 102199.

Riebeek, H. Global Warming : Feature Articles 2010. https://earthobservatory.nasa.gov/Features/GlobalWarming/ (accessed May 19, 2018). 10. Campisano, C.J. (2012).

Roe, G. (2006). In defense of Milankovitch. *Geophysical Research Letters* 33: 1–5. https://doi.org/10.1029/2006 GL027817.

Rohling, E.J., Haigh, I.D., Foster, G.L. et al. (2013). A geological perspective on potential future sea-level rise. *Scientific Reports* 3: 3461. https://doi.org/10.1038/srep03461.

Shaheen, S.A. and Lipman, T.E. (2007). Reducing greenhouse emissions and fuel consumption. *IATSS Research* 31: 6–20. https://doi.org/10.1016/S0386-1112(14)60179-5.

Solomon, S., Qin, D., Manning, M. et al. (2007). Climate change 2007: the physical science basis. In: *Contribution of Working Group I to the Fourth Assessment Report of the Intergovernmental Panel on Climate Change*. Cambridge, UK: Cambridge University Press https://doi.org/10.1017/CBO 9781107415324.004.

Venkataramanan, S. (2011). Causes and effects of global warming, Indian. *Journal of Science and Technology* 4: 226–229. https://doi.org/10.17485/ijst/2011/v4i3/29971.

Vijayavenkataraman, S., Iniyanm, S., and Goic, R. (2012). A review of climate change, mitigation and adaptation. *Renewable and Sustainable Energy Reviews* 16: 878–897. https://doi.org/10.1016/j.rser.2011.09.009.

n.d. (n.d.b.) 34. Great Barrier Marine Park Authority. Coral bleaching 2014. www.gbrmpa.gov.au/managing-the-reef/threats-tothe-reef/climate-change/what-does-this-mean-for-species/corals/what-is-coral-bleaching (accessed May 19, 2018).

37

Environmental Enrichment and Welfare of Animals

Deepak Nelagonda[1], Ramadevi Pampana[2], and Manoj Kumar Karanam[3]

[1] *Department of Poultry Science, SNK AH Polytechnic College, Anantapur, India*
[2] *Department of Veterinary Parasitology, College of Veterinary Science, Garividi, India*
[3] *Department of Veterinary Surgery and Radiology, College of Veterinary Science, Garividi, India*

37.1 Animal Welfare

The term "animal welfare" refers to the state of an animal's physical and mental well-being, including its ability to experience positive emotions, avoid negative experiences, and exhibit natural behaviors. It involves assessing and addressing the animal's physical health, behavioral needs, and overall quality of life.

An inclusive concept of animal well-being considers a number of elements such as freedom from hunger, thirst, malnutrition, discomfort, pain, anguish, and fear, in addition to the ability to express normal behavior and the possibility of experiencing pleasant mental status.

Animals are sentient beings capable of experiencing pain, sorrow, and joy and hence animal welfare is extremely important in ethical and moral considerations. The notion of animal rights, which is strongly associated with animal care, highlights that these species have rights to be recognized and protected. These include the right to freedom from exploitation, the right to life, and the right to be free from cruelty. Animals should not be regarded as goods or commodities to be utilized by humans, but rather as distinct individuals with inherent value and rights.

The qualities of justice and compassion for all living beings strengthen animal welfare. Since animals have their own interests, they should be considered when making decisions that affect and influence their lives. Furthermore, from a practical standpoint, animal welfare is important as animals with good welfare are healthier, more productive, and more likely to behave in a desirable manner.

For thousands of years, animal welfare has been a concern but not for all people and also not in all circumstances. However, during the last century, concern for animal welfare has become increasingly common and animal abuse is becoming unacceptable.

37.1.1 Improving Animal Welfare

To ensure animal welfare and protect the environment, sustainable farming practices are imperative. Humane treatment, proper living conditions, and access to natural behaviors are all prioritized in these practices. Furthermore, sustainable farming reduces pollution and greenhouse gas emissions while preserving biodiversity and using eco-friendly methods.

Various strategies have been established to enhance the lives of animals in various settings. Key steps to improve animal welfare include the following.

- Analyzing the current situation in animal habitations and identifying welfare constraints.
- Encouraging ethical breeding and population control.
- Creating opportunities for social interaction among animals.

Epidemiology and Environmental Hygiene in Veterinary Public Health, First Edition. Edited by Tanmoy Rana.
© 2025 John Wiley & Sons, Inc. Published 2025 by John Wiley & Sons, Inc.

- Educating and training animal handlers and caretakers.
- Stringent establishment and enforcement of animal welfare laws.
- Environment enrichment and species-specific enrichment.
- Collaborating to conduct research and evaluate enrichment programs.
- Continuous assessment and monitoring of animal welfare.

37.2 Environment Enrichment

Environment enrichment refers to the addition of stimuli or modifications to an animal's environment in order to improve their well-being and promote natural behaviors. It aims to provide animals with opportunities for social interaction, physical and mental stimulation and to facilitate the expression of species-specific behaviors. A wide variety of objects, structures, and activities are provided as part of enrichment to encourage playfulness, exploration, and problem solving. The major emphasis of environment enrichment is to enhance the physical and physiological health of animals and reduce stress and boredom.

Environment enrichment could be implemented in settings ranging from vast enclosures housing numerous animals to wired cages with a single species. Enrichment could be achieved by adding a minor item or material, such as a ball or some straw, or by making a significant modification such as housing animals in a seminatural outdoor enclosure.

37.2.1 Role of Environment Enrichment in the Physical, Mental, and Emotional Well-Being of Animals

- *Enhanced physical health*: the muscle tone, cardiovascular health, and overall fitness of animals can be improved considerably as a result of enrichment, which encourages physical activity, exploration, and natural behaviors.
- *Improved cognitive development*: enrichment stimulates the brain and thereby promotes problem solving, learning, and memory retention.
- *Reduced stress and boredom*: enrichment provides mental stimulation and channels for natural behaviors; it reduces stress and prevents boredom-related issues.
- *Prevention of abnormal behaviors*: enrichment helps to redirect natural behaviors and reduces the occurrence of abnormal behaviors like feather pecking, self-mutilation, etc.
- *Positive social interactions*: enrichment can foster positive social behaviors and reduce aggression among animals.
- *Improved immunological function*: an enrichment program that includes mild stressors can enhance an animal's adaptability and immune function.

Depending on the type of animal, habitat and production system, type of social interaction, etc., the requirements of the animal differ greatly. As a result, the type of enrichment each species requires is also different and hence, environmental enrichment is implemented in a variety of settings.

- Captivity – zoos and wildlife sanctuaries
- Laboratory animal facilities
- Farm animal production systems
- Companion animal environments
- Rehabilitation centers
- Aquariums and marine parks

37.3 Environmental Enrichment in Captivity

Captive animals, including those in zoos, aquariums, and wildlife sanctuaries, are susceptible to a variety of welfare challenges as they are often confined and are not able to express their natural behavior. They face numerous challenges including social isolation, inadequate space, monotonous diet, breeding challenges, health issues, and stress from human interaction.

By restructuring elements of their natural habitats, environmental enrichment can play a vital role in addressing these challenges. This approach also incorporates physical activity and mental stimulation, and encourages species-typical behavior.

37.3.1 Environment Enrichment Techniques in Captivity

In captivity, animals can benefit from various environment enrichment techniques that reduce stereotypical behavior.

- *Providing opportunities for physical exercise and exploration*: this can include the provision of climbing structures, tunnels, and platforms for animals to engage in natural behaviors such as climbing, jumping, and exploring their environment.
- *Offering puzzle feeders or food-dispensing toys*: for animals to access their food, these toys engage them in problem-solving behavior, thereby reducing boredom and redirecting their energy away from stereotypical behavior (Figure 37.1).
- *Providing social interaction and companionship*: animals benefit from interactions with conspecifics or humans. This can include pairing animals together, providing opportunities for social play, or regular interaction with caretakers.
- *Offering sensory stimulation*: this can include the use of scents, sounds, and visual stimuli that mimic the animal's natural environment. For example, providing objects with different textures, scents, or sounds can help engage the animal's senses and reduce stereotypical behaviors.
- *Creating a more complex and stimulating environment*: changing the enclosure layout regularly, introducing new objects or toys, or providing opportunities for animals to engage in natural behaviors such as foraging or nesting (Figure 37.2).
- *Providing hiding places and tunnels*: these create a sense of security for animals and allow them to engage in natural behaviors such as hiding and exploring, reducing stress and promoting natural behaviors.

It is important to note that the effectiveness of specific enrichment techniques may vary depending on the species and individual needs of animals.

37.3.2 Successful Enrichment Programs Implemented in Zoos and Wildlife Sanctuaries

- Cincinnati Zoo's "Gorilla World" exhibit provides climbing structures, trees, and a flowing stream to encourage physical activity and exploration. It has resulted in improved social interactions among the gorillas, increased physical activity, and enhanced well-being for the animals.
- San Diego Zoo's "Polar Bear Plunge" exhibit provides environmental enrichment for polar bears, including a chilled pool, simulated ice, and climbing structures that mimic their natural Arctic habitat.
- At the London Zoo, the lemur walkthrough exhibit encourages natural climbing and exploration behaviors and increases interaction with visitors. The exhibit also provides scents of native plants and novel food items to stimulate their senses.
- Taronga Zoo's "Wild Asia" exhibit features a diverse and complex environment with elements such as waterfalls, rocky outcrops, and natural vegetation. The exhibit has improved the animals' physical and mental well-being.
- Bronx Zoo's "JungleWorld" exhibit provides stimulating and fulfilling living conditions for various species, including primates, birds, and reptiles. The animals' increased activity levels and positive social interactions demonstrate the success of the enrichment program.

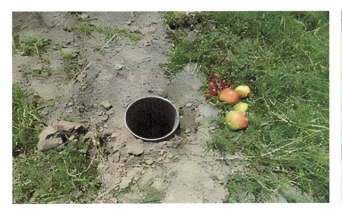 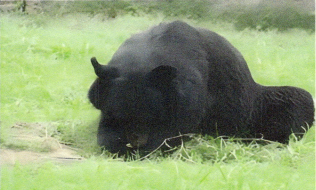

Figure 37.1 Hidden food items in the enclosure. Asiatic black bear digging out food items. *Source:* Central Zoo Authority.

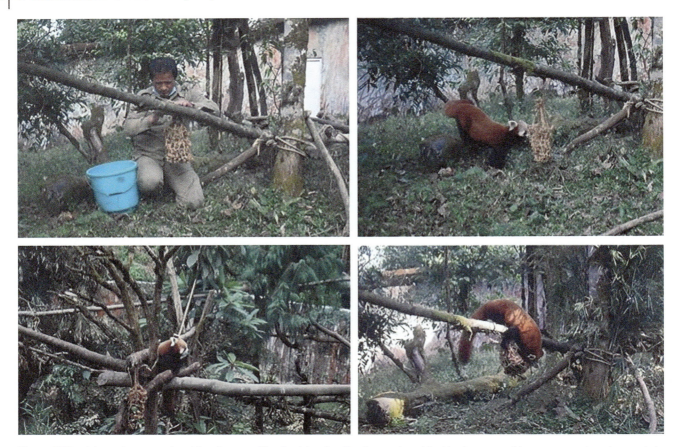

Figure 37.2 Arboreal nets made with coir ropes. The food (apple slices) was placed inside the net and leaves were placed around the nets, so that the animals had to use their skill and cognitive abilities to take out the food items. Arboreal nets were highly successful in increasing foraging behavior. *Source:* Central Zoo Authority.

India has several zoos and wildlife parks that have implemented successful environment enrichment programs for the well-being of animals.

- The Nocturnal House at Nehru Zoological Park is dimly lit to simulate nighttime conditions, and allows visitors to observe the animals' natural behaviors.
- The Arignar Anna Zoological Park's giraffe exhibit provides a spacious enclosure with high structures and platforms that encourage foraging and stretching behaviors.
- The primate enclosure at Assam State Zoo features a stimulating environment with trees, ropes, and climbing structures for various primate species. Enrichment items such as puzzle feeders, hidden treats, and scent trails are provided to encourage natural behaviors and mental engagement.

37.4 Environment Enrichment in Farm Animal Production Systems

It is well known that intensive farming systems have a detrimental effect on animal well-being due to overcrowding, lack of space, and restrictive practices. Keeping animals in crowded environments increases stress and disease transmission and reduces comfort. Additionally, overcrowding hinders natural behaviors and leads to physical deformities. Insufficient space leads to frustration, aggression, and compromised hygiene among animals, and as a result, reproductive issues may also arise. Tethering and intensive confinement cause physical pain and psychological distress to animals, preventing them from expressing their natural behaviors.

To address these issues and to implement animal welfare standards, humane and ethical farming practices must be combined with environment enrichment.

37.4.1 Dairy Animals

The use of environmental enrichment can improve the welfare of indoor-housed cows and calves by reducing stress, promoting positive effects, and improving their biological function. By enriching their environment, animals can cope better with stressors, avoid frustration, and fulfill their behavioral needs. A few basic behavioral requirements, such as social enrichment in the form of contact with conspecifics, are also considered minimum ideals for raising standards of gregarious animals and are outlined in respective state legislations.

There are several ways to provide physical enrichment for dairy cows and calves, such as modifying the size or complexity of their enclosures. There are also accessories that can be added to the enclosure, such as objects, substrates, or permanent structures.

- It has been suggested that giving animals access to alternate enclosures by dividing the space into a number of functional areas could increase the opportunity to explore and patrol, as well as camouflage and hide from predators. Dividing spaces within an enclosure may also effectively reduce antagonistic interactions between calves.
- Allowing dairy cows to graze on pastures for a prolonged time provides them with opportunities for natural behaviors such as grazing, walking, and social interaction.
- Installing scratching brushes or posts in the barn allows cows to engage in natural behaviors such as scratching and rubbing, promoting physical exercise and reducing stress.
- Providing cows with feeders that require their tongues to be used and engage in licking behavior, such as lick wheels and lick mats, can provide mental stimulation and mimic natural feeding habits. Clean, comfortable resting areas and clean, soft bedding allow cows to engage in natural sleeping and resting behaviors and promote physical comfort.
- Hanging chains, balls, or platforms in the barn can encourage exploration, play, and manipulation, providing mental stimulation and reducing boredom.

37.4.2 Poultry Farming

Environmental enrichment and animal welfare are crucial aspects of poultry farming. An enriched environment promotes better health, reduced stress, and increased productivity. In an enhanced environment, poultry can express their natural behaviors like perching, dust bathing, and foraging, which reduces aggression and prevents harmful vices. A welfare-focused and enriching approach to poultry farming is also necessary for regulatory compliance and environmental concerns.

37.4.2.1 Common Welfare Issues Faced by Layers
- *Pecking and cannibalism*: feather pecking is a behavior in which hens peck at the feathers of other birds, causing feather loss, skin damage, and even cannibalism. It is common for this type of behavior to be associated with stress, frustration, and poor environmental conditions.
- *Bone fractures and osteoporosis*: eggshell production requires a large amount of calcium so layers are at risk of bone fractures and osteoporosis. Poor bone health and inadequate calcium intake can affect skeletal health and welfare.
- *Beak trimming*: feather pecking and cannibalism are reduced by trimming beaks in layer hens. However, this can cause pain to birds and compromise their natural behavior and welfare.
- *Confinement in small cages*: in conventional cage systems, hens are restricted in their movements and natural behaviors, which can lead to frustration, stress, and reduced welfare. In addition, overcrowding and a lack of space can increase the risk of aggression and injury.

37.4.2.2 Common Welfare Issues Faced by Broilers
- *Rapid growth rate*: selective breeding for fast growth in broilers can lead to skeletal problems, such as lameness and leg disorders, as well as respiratory and cardiovascular problems. In fast-growing broilers, ascites, or fluid accumulation in the abdominal cavity, is a common welfare concern arising due to cardiac and respiratory problems.
- *Overcrowding*: high stocking densities in broiler houses can lead to poor air quality, increased heat stress, and reduced access to resources, affecting the welfare of the birds.
- *Lack of exercise and behavioral restriction*: many broilers are raised in environments that limit their natural behaviors, such as perching, foraging, and dust bathing, which can lead to frustration and lowered welfare.

37.4.2.3 Enrichment Practices to Improve Welfare of Poultry

- *Perches, nesting areas, and dust bathing*: increasing the complexity of the housing environment by providing perches, nesting, and dust bathing areas allows hens to engage in a wider range of behaviors and promotes their overall welfare (Figure 37.3). By engaging in natural roosting and nesting behaviors, birds improve their skeletal health and natural reproductive instincts. Providing areas with a suitable substrate for dust bathing allows birds to engage in this important behavior for feather maintenance and parasite control.
- *Foraging opportunities*: natural feeding behavior and mental stimulation are stimulated by scattering food or using foraging devices.
- *Light and ventilation*: it is possible to improve the overall health and welfare of hens in cage systems by optimizing the lighting conditions and providing proper ventilation.

37.4.3 Swine Farming

The housing conditions in intensive farming conditions often cause welfare problems for pigs. It is often difficult for pigs to engage in their natural species-specific behaviors in these environments because they lack stimuli. The lack of space and materials to engage in foraging and exploration can lead to damaging oral behaviors such as ear biting and tail biting. Physiological changes and altered immunity can also result from barren housing conditions for pigs. Pigs living in barren conditions may also be more susceptible to lung infections.

Pig behavior, physiology, and cognition can also be negatively affected by adverse early-life experiences. The lack of enrichment during the farrowing phase and limited space before weaning can negatively impact social skills and lead to tail biting in later life. However, environmental enrichment in early life can have beneficial effects on later life functioning, possibly through its effect on brain development and functioning. Pigs reared under enriched conditions show reduced social stress in adulthood and improved cognitive skills.

37.4.3.1 Enrichment Practices to Improve Welfare in Pigs

- *Providing manipulable materials*: it is important to provide pigs with manipulable materials such as straw, wood, or rubber toys to explore, root, and chew (Figure 37.4).
- *Increasing the space allowance*: Providing pigs with more space will enable them to move around more freely, and stress and aggression risks will be reduced.
- *Implementing social enrichment*: natural social behavior is promoted and stress is reduced when pigs are allowed to interact with conspecifics.
- *Providing varied and stimulating feeding methods*: to encourage foraging behaviors and stimulate the mind, puzzle feeders and scatter feeders can be used.

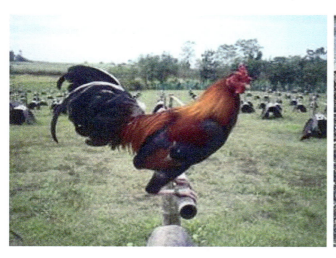
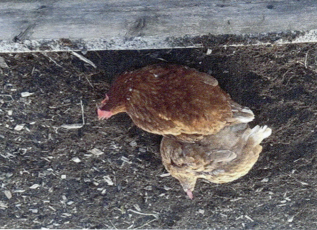

Figure 37.3 Chicken dust bathing and perching. *Source:* Shree Krishna Poultry Farm.

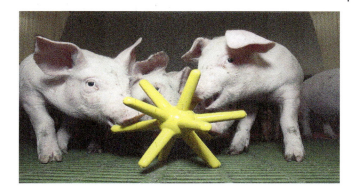

Figure 37.4 Provision of manipulable material as environmental enrichment toys for improving pig welfare. *Source:* Agri & Industrial Rubber Ltd. https://easyfix.com/product-range/enrichment-toys/ (accessed December 05, 2023).

- *Offering environmental complexity*: it is possible to promote exploration and play behavior by providing a complex and stimulating environment that includes platforms, hiding places, and different flooring surfaces.
- *Enhancing sensory stimulation*: pigs require access to fresh air, natural light, and auditory stimulation for their overall well-being.
- *Implementing positive human–animal interactions*: regular positive interaction with caretakers, handling, and positive reinforcement training can improve the pigs' trust and reduce the amount of stress they experience.

37.5 Environment Enrichment in Laboratory Animal Facilities

Confinement and restriction of laboratory animals often cause them to suffer from welfare issues.

37.5.1 Welfare Challenges Faced by Laboratory Animals

- Living in barren cages without environmental complexity leads to boredom and abnormal behavior.
- Some laboratory animals such as mice are housed individually, which causes them stress and anxiety.
- Due to insufficient space, they are restricted in their movement and behavior, leading to physical discomfort.
- The absence of environmental enrichment, in the form of nesting materials and mental stimulation, contributes to boredom and frustration.
- Invasive procedures without proper pain management cause distress, and inadequate veterinary care results in untreated health problems.
- Their well-being is further affected by transportation and stress induced by improper handling.
- Inadequate care, diet, and housing conditions also adversely affect welfare.

To ensure ethical research practices and improve the quality of life of laboratory animals, these challenges must be addressed. Environmental enrichment is important in laboratory animal regulatory toxicology studies because it ensures that animals used to assess the safety of medicines are in a comfortable and stimulating environment. It improves the welfare of experimental animals while balancing the scientific value of a project with its welfare benefits.

37.5.2 Enrichment Techniques in Laboratory Animals

There are several components of environmental enrichment that can be implemented to enhance the well-being of laboratory animals.

- *Addition of physical structures*: physical exercise, exploration, and territorial behaviors can be enhanced by adding structures such as tunnels, platforms, and climbing structures. Various materials can be used to make these structures, including plastic, wood, and metal.
- *Providing nesting materials*: laboratory animals engage in nest-building behaviors when nesting materials such as shredded paper or nesting boxes are provided to them (Figure 37.5). Nesting behaviors are important for maintaining thermoregulation, comfort, and security.

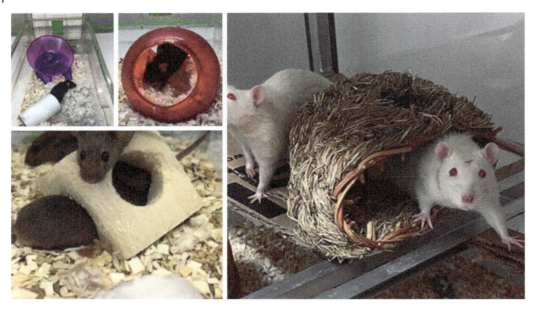

Figure 37.5 Nesting material, refuges, and gnawing items used as enrichment resources for mice and rats. *Source:* NC3Rs. www.nc3rs.org.uk/ (accessed December 05, 2023).

- *Hiding places*: the provision of hiding places, such as shelters or tubes, enables animals to retreat and feel secure when they require privacy or wish to avoid potential stressors. In addition to promoting a sense of safety, hiding places can reduce anxiety.
- *Social interaction*: social companionship is an important aspect of environmental enrichment, especially for the social species. As a result of social interaction, stress can be reduced, natural behavior can be promoted, and the animals' well-being can be enhanced.
- *Sensory stimulation*: it is possible to engage animals via their senses by providing them with sensory stimulation through the use of novel scents, sounds, or visual stimuli. This can stimulate exploration and curiosity.
- *Food enrichment*: natural feeding behavior and mental stimulation can be enhanced by providing food in different formats, such as puzzle feeders or foraging devices. Physical activity and problem solving can be encouraged through food enrichment.

To maintain their effectiveness and address the changing needs of the animals, environmental enrichment strategies should be regularly assessed and modified.

37.6 Environment Enrichment in Companion Animals

There are several welfare issues that affect the physical and emotional well-being of companion animals, including dogs, cats, and small mammals. The most common concerns are inadequate shelter, overcrowding, and unsanitary living conditions, which can lead to stress and disease transmission. Lack of mental stimulation and exercise causes boredom, obesity, and behavioral problems. Insufficient care, such as neglecting grooming and veterinary needs, can negatively impact health and quality of life. Loneliness and behavioral issues can result from social isolation from humans and other animals. Overfeeding and inadequate nutrition can lead to obesity or malnutrition. Irresponsible breeding contributes to overpopulation and homeless animals that may face neglect and ultimately might be euthanized. Stress and anxiety are caused by abandonment and surrender to shelters. In some cases, animals may be subjected to physical abuse or invasive medical procedures without adequate pain management.

Companion animals' well-being can be ensured through responsible pet ownership, education, and enforcement of animal welfare laws. Mental and physical well-being of companion animals can be improved by providing them with an appropriate enriching environment to stimulate their minds, prevent boredom, and reduce behavioral problems.

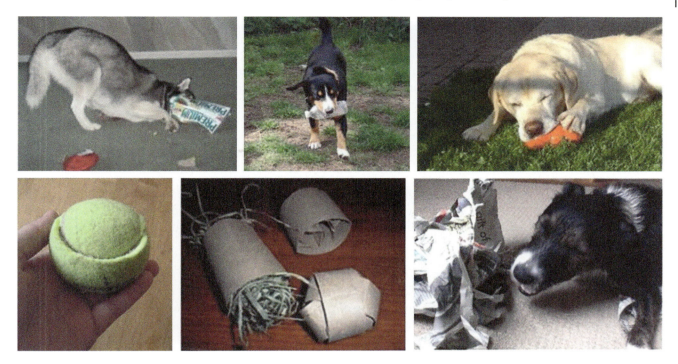

Figure 37.6 Food activity toys for dogs. *Source:* Dogs Trust.

It promotes overall happiness and contentment in the domestic setting, satisfying their natural instincts. Furthermore, environment enrichment can enhance a positive and fulfilling relationship between pets and their owners.

Dogs and other companion animals can benefit from various environmental enrichment procedures.

- *Providing interactive toys*: dogs can be stimulated and entertained by toys that require their mental and physical engagement, such as puzzle or treat-dispensing toys (Figure 37.6).
- *Offering sensory stimulation*: animals can benefit from sensory stimulation when provided with different textures, sounds, and scents. This can be achieved by providing calming music or bedding and scented toys.
- *The social interaction*: socializing with humans and other animals regularly can be enriching for dogs and other companion animals. This can include playtime, training sessions, or just spending time together.
- *Environmental variety*: introducing changes in the environment, such as rearranging furniture or adding new objects, can provide novelty and mental stimulation to animals.
- *Outdoor access*: allowing dogs and other companion animals to spend time outdoors in a safe and secure environment will give them more opportunities to explore and behave naturally.
- *Training and mental stimulation*: training animals or providing mental stimulation, such as scent work or obedience training, can help keep their minds active.

37.7 Factors Affecting the Effectiveness of Environment Enrichment in Animals

Species-specific needs: there are different behavioral and environmental requirements for different animal species. To ensure relevance and effectiveness, enrichment strategies must be tailored to the needs and preferences of each species.

- *Individual differences*: individual animals within the same species may respond differently to enrichment and display different behaviors. Certain enrichment techniques may be more motivating for some individuals than others.
- *Frequency and duration*: the frequency and duration of enrichment activities can affect their effectiveness. Positive behavioral changes are more likely to occur with regular and sustained enrichment.
- *Novelty and variety*: enrichment items and activities with novelty and variety can keep animals engaged and prevent habituation. It is possible to maintain interest and stimulation by regularly introducing new and diverse enrichment.

37 Environmental Enrichment and Welfare of Animals

- _Timing and context_: providing enrichment activities at the right time and in the right context can enhance their effectiveness. For example, natural behaviors can be encouraged by providing food-based enrichment during natural foraging times.
- _Social environment_: animals' responses to enrichment are strongly influenced by their social environment. Group enrichment activities may benefit some species, while some are benefited by individual attention.
- _Training and positive reinforcement_: to encourage active participation and enjoyment in enrichment activities, animals can be trained to interact with enrichment items and positive reinforcement can be used.
- _Health and stress levels_: the overall health and stress level of an animal can affect its response to enrichment. Sick or stressed animals may not be able to participate fully in enrichment activities.
- _Environmental complexity_: depending on the complexity of an animal's environment, enrichment may have a different impact. It is possible to complement specific enrichment activities with an enriched environment that provides opportunities for exploration and interaction.

It is essential to consider these factors when designing and implementing enrichment programs, in order to create experiences that are both effective and meaningful for the animals, thus promoting their physical and mental well-being.

37.8 Evaluating Enrichment Techniques

Evaluating enrichment impact helps prioritize and implement enrichments that best meet animals' needs, ensuring their well-being is optimized in various settings such as zoos, research facilities, and agricultural systems.

When evaluating the effectiveness of environmental enrichments, it is important to consider both short-term and long-term assessments of animal welfare because these assessments provide a comprehensive understanding of the impact of the enrichments on the animal's well-being. To ensure that the basic needs of the animals are met and that enrichment is beneficial for them, these assessments are crucial.

These assessments should be conducted using a combination of behavioral observations, physiological measurements, and other relevant indicators. They help guide the ongoing development and refinement of enrichment strategies to ensure that animals continue to experience improved welfare and quality of life over time.

37.8.1 Short-term Assessment

Short-term assessments focus on immediate improvements in biological functioning and health, such as reductions in injuries, lameness, and disease. These assessments help determine if the enrichments meet the basic needs of the animals and promote their physical well-being. The following are some aspects of short-term assessments.

- _Physical health_: an assessment process for observing changes in the incidence of injuries, diseases, and overall health. A reduction in injuries caused by stereotypical behavior, for instance, could indicate that enrichment has a positive impact.
- _Behavioral changes_: observing changes in behavior patterns, such as increased engagement in natural behaviors, exploration, and social interaction. It is a positive sign if abnormal behaviors like pacing or self-mutilation have decreased.
- _Stress reduction_: stress levels can be assessed using physiological indicators such as cortisol levels, heart rate, and vocalizations. Reduced stress responses indicate that the animals are finding their environment more comfortable and less stressful.

37.8.2 Long-term Assessment

A long-term assessment measures welfare outcomes throughout the animal's entire life cycle or production cycle after the enrichments have been applied. As part of these assessments, factors such as stress resilience and mood are considered, along with long-term satisfaction associated with enrichment use. Aspects of long-term assessments include the following.

- _Emotional well-being_: observing the animals' moods and emotional states over time. It is likely that animals that have access to enrichment that promotes positive emotions will act in a more relaxed and contented manner.
- _Stress resilience_: evaluating how animals cope with environmental stressors and changes. An animal's ability to adapt to new situations and recover from stress should have been enhanced by enrichment.

- *Cognitive skills*: monitoring changes in cognitive abilities such as problem solving, memory, and learning. A mentally challenging environment can improve the cognitive development of animals.
- *Reproductive success*: keeping track of reproductive behaviors and success rates. Breeding success can be positively influenced by enrichment that allows animals to engage in natural mating behaviors and nesting.
- *Social dynamics*: observing changes in social interactions and hierarchy within groups. Enrichment that promotes positive social behaviors can lead to improved relationships among animals.
- *Physical health over time*: monitoring the health, growth, and longevity of animals. In the long run, enrichment that encourages physical activity and reduces stress can lead to healthier animals.

37.9 Limitations of Environment Enrichment

Although environment enrichment has been found to be highly beneficial in improving animal welfare and quality of life, it does have some limitations. For example, researchers found that environmental enrichment improved the welfare of laboratory mice, but their behavior and responses varied. Variability in results has made it more difficult to draw clear conclusions from experimental research. It is important to consider such limitations when implementing environmental enrichment for animals.

- *Cost and practicality*: implementing environmental enrichment can be expensive, especially for large-scale operations. A farm or facility may not be able to afford the additional resources, such as equipment, materials, or labor.
- *Space limitations*: providing adequate enrichment opportunities to all animals can be challenging due to space limitations. Certain enrichment devices cannot be used or natural behaviors engaged due to lack of space.
- *Safety concerns*: to ensure the safety of the animals, environmental enrichment should be carefully designed and monitored. Animals may be injured if enrichment devices are not properly constructed or if they pose a hazard.
- *Habituation and boredom*: over time, animals may become accustomed to or bored with certain enrichment devices. It may be necessary to rotate or introduce new enrichment options regularly to ensure that they remain effective.

The limitations of environmental enrichment can be addressed through a multifaceted approach. Developing practical and cost-effective enrichment strategies can be achieved through collaboration between researchers, animal welfare organizations, and industry professionals. Utilizing natural resources or repurposing recycled materials can provide economically viable solutions. In recognition of the uniqueness of each animal, individualized enrichment plans can be devised based on their preferences and responses.

Enhancement methods should be regularly assessed and adjusted based on animal feedback to ensure sustained effectiveness. Science-based approaches to enrichment programs provide a solid foundation for developing and implementing them. By combining these strategies, one can overcome the challenges presented by environmental enrichment and advance the overall well-being of animals in various environments.

Further Reading

Azevedo, C., Cipreste, C., and Young, R. (2007). Environmental enrichment: a GAP analysis. *Applied Animal Behaviour Science* 102: 329–343.

Baumans, V. (2005). Environmental enrichment for laboratory rodents and rabbits: requirements of rodents, rabbits, and research. *ILAR Journal* 46 (2): 162–170.

Bayne, K. (2018). Environmental enrichment and mouse models: current perspectives. *Animal Models and Experimental Medicine* 1 (2): 82–90.

Beattie, V.E., Walker, N., and Sneddon, I.A. (1996). An investigation of the effect of environmental enrichment and space allowance on the behaviour and production of growing pigs. *Applied Animal Behaviour Science* 48 (3): 151–158.

Bracke, M.B.M. (2011). Review of wallowing in pigs: description of the behaviour and its motivational basis. *Applied Animal Behaviour Science* 132: 1–13.

Brydges, N.M., Leach, M., Nicol, K. et al. (2011). Environmental enrichment induces optimistic cognitive bias in rats. *Animal Behaviour* 81 (1): 169–175.

Campbell, D.L.M., de Haas, E.N., and Lee, C. (2019). A review of environmental enrichment for laying hens during rearing in relation to their behavioral and physiological development. *Poultry Science* 98 (1): 9–28.

Coleman, K., Weed, J., and Schapiro, S. (2017). Psychological environmental enrichment of animals in research. In: *Animal Models for the Study of Human Disease*, 2e (ed. P. Conn), 47–69. St Louis: Elsevier.

Dean, S.W. (1999). Environmental enrichment of laboratory animals used in regulatory toxicology studies. *Laboratory Animal* 33 (4): 309–327.

Donaldson, C., Ball, M., and O'Connell, N. (2012). Aerial perches and free-range laying hens: the effect of access to aerial perches and of individual bird parameters on keel bone injuries in commercial free-range laying hens. *Poultry Science* 91: 304–315.

Giuliotti, L., Benvenuti, M.N., Giannarelli, A. et al. (2019). Effect of different environment enrichments on behaviour and social interactions in growing pigs. *Animals* 9 (3): 101.

Hemsworth, P. and Coleman, G.J. (2010). *Human-Livestock Interactions: The Stockperson and the Productivity and Welfare of Intensively Farmed Animals*. Wallingford: CABI.

Herron, M.E., Kirby-Madden, T.M., and Lord, L.K. (2014). Effects of environmental enrichment on the behavior of shelter dogs. *Journal of the American Veterinary Medical Association* 244 (6): 687–692.

Hutchinson, E., Avery, A., and Vandewoude, S. (2005). Environmental enrichment for laboratory rodents. *ILAR Journal* 46 (2): 148–161.

Lay, D.C., Fulton, R.M., Hester, P.Y. et al. (2011). Hen welfare in different housing systems. *Poultry Science* 90 (1): 278–294.

Mandel, R., Whay, H.R., Klement, E., and Nicol, C.J. (2016). Invited review: environmental enrichment of dairy cows and calves in indoor housing. *Journal of Dairy Science* 99 (3): 1695–1715.

Mason, G.J. and Latham, N.R. (2004). Can't stop, won't stop: is stereotypy a reliable animal welfare indicator? *Animal Welfare* 13 (Suppl): S57–S69.

Newberry, R. (1995). Environmental enrichment: increasing the biological relevance of captive environments. *Applied Animal Behaviour Science* 44: 229–243.

Rampim, L. and Oliva, V.N.L. (2016). Benefits of environmental enrichment in animal welfare: a literary review. *Revista de Ciência Veterinária e Saúde Pública* 3: 60–66.

Schütz, K.E., Rogers, A.R., Poulouin, Y.A. et al. (2010). The amount of shade influences the behavior and physiology of dairy cattle. *Journal of Dairy Science* 93 (1): 125–133.

Shepherdson, D. (2007). Environmental enrichment: past, present and future. *International Zoo Yearbook* 38: 118–124.

Sinclair, M., Fryer, C., and Phillips, C.J.C. (2019). The benefits of improving animal welfare from the perspective of livestock stakeholders across Asia. *Animals* 9 (4): 123.

Swaisgood, R. and Shepherdson, D. (2005). Scientific approaches to enrichment and stereotypies in zoo animals: what's been done and where should we go next? *Zoo Biology* 24: 499–518.

Tarou, L. and Bashaw, M. (2007). Maximizing the effectiveness of environmental enrichment: suggestions from the experimental analysis of behavior. *Applied Animal Behaviour Science* 102: 189–204.

Taylor, P.S., Schrobback, P., Verdon, M., and Lee, C. (2023). An effective environmental enrichment framework for the continual improvement of production animal welfare. *Animal Welfare* 32: e14.

van de Weerd, H. and Ison, S. (2019). Providing effective environmental enrichment to pigs: how far have we come? *Animals* 9 (5): 254.

Wells, D.L. (2009). Sensory stimulation as environmental enrichment for captive animals: a review. *Applied Animal Behaviour Science* 118 (1): 1–11.

Wells, D. and Egli, J. (2004). The influence of olfactory enrichment on the behaviour of captive black-footed cats, Felis nigripes. *Applied Animal Behaviour Science* 85: 107–119.

Whiting, T. (2011). Understanding animal welfare: the science in its cultural context. *Canadian Veterinary Journal* 52 (6): 662.

38

Basics of Water Supply, Quality, and Purification

Nourhan Eissa[1] and Mona Abdelghany Nasr[2]

[1] *Department of Animal Hygiene and Zoonoses, Faculty of Veterinary Medicine, University of Sadat City, Sadat City, Egypt*
[2] *Department of Anatomy and Embryology, Faculty of Veterinary Medicine, University of Sadat City, Sadat City, Egypt*

38.1 Introduction

Water is one of the most prevalent elements on Earth and a chemical essential for life. Water makes up over 70% of both human and animal bodies. Life as we know it would not exist without it. In fact, some academics contend that water is more valuable than silver and gold. The numerous conflicts and disputes worldwide over water reflect its value and significance. Fortunately, most disputes are settled in courtrooms rather than on the battlefield. The fundamentals of water supply, quality, and purification are covered in this chapter (Thomas 2009).

The countless descriptions of water, such as "the essence of life," "blue gold," and "more precious than oil," show how essential it is to life. The specific qualities that are attributed to water's molecular structure are what make it so exceptional and essential to life. The ability to dissolve many polar molecules, cohesive and adhesive qualities, high specific heat capacity, high heat of vaporization, and capacity to dissociate into ions (which generates pH) are only a few of its unique properties (Figure 38.1). We can better understand and appreciate its significance in preserving life on Earth if we are aware of these qualities (EPA 2018).

38.2 Global Water Distribution and Use

The majority of the water on Earth, which makes up around 71% of its surface, is found in oceans and is too salty for human consumption; 97% of all water is salty and the remaining 2% is fresh water stored in ice caps and glaciers. Because of salt (ocean water) and geography (ice caps and glaciers), at least 99% of all water is generally unfit for human use. Only 1.4% of available fresh water is surface water in rivers and lakes, with the majority, 97%, being groundwater that is buried deep beneath the Earth's surface (EPA 2013).

Water is primarily used by the industrial, agricultural, and home sectors. Nonconsumptive usage is defined as the removal of water from its source – such as a river or lake – and its subsequent return to the source. One illustration is the temporary placement of water in cooling ponds for industrial processes before it is eventually returned to the river or lake it originally came from. Consumptive use refers to the removal of water from a source for use by plants, animals, or industrial operations. The water does not return to its source because it evaporates while being used or gets into animal tissue or industrial products. The agricultural sector is by far the largest consumer of water that never returns to its sources (consumptive usage) out of the three sectors (Fetter 2000).

Thermoelectric cooling uses the majority of the water withdrawn in the US. In certain nations, like Egypt, irrigation uses up more than 70% of the water withdrawn. Water is applied through irrigation to support plant growth. In addition to providing protection against frost, irrigation also involves the use of water for chemical application, weed control, field preparation, crop cooling, harvesting, dust suppression, and leaching of salts from the root zone (Howard 2015).

Epidemiology and Environmental Hygiene in Veterinary Public Health, First Edition. Edited by Tanmoy Rana.
© 2025 John Wiley & Sons, Inc. Published 2025 by John Wiley & Sons, Inc.

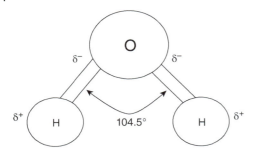

Figure 38.1 A single water molecule is made up of two hydrogen atoms joined by covalent bonds to one oxygen atom (H₂O), where the atoms share electrons and must thus stay together.

Worldwide, water demand is increasing rapidly as a result of industrialization and human population development. According to the Environment Protection Agency (EPA 2013), as more nations become wealthy (rise in industry and standard of living), they use more water than they did in the past.

38.3 The Hydrological Cycle

Oceans, ice caps, glaciers, groundwater, rivers, and lakes make up the majority of the world's water reserves. In the various reservoirs, water remains for varying lengths of time. The volume of water in the reservoir and the speed at which water enters and exits the reservoir are the key variables that determine how long water remains in the reservoir. Water is continuously cycled globally from one reservoir to another as part of the hydrological cycle (also known as the water cycle) (Figure 38.2). The heat energy from the sun, which turns liquid water into water vapor, and the gravitational pull of the Earth, which pulls water to the surface, are the two main forces driving this process (Sipes 2010).

Let's follow a water molecule through the water cycle to obtain a better understanding of it. The water molecule can become a component of the water that is transformed into vapor and enters the atmosphere, starting at the ocean (an arbitrary starting point). Water turns from a liquid to a gas or vapor through the process of evaporation. The main way in which water travels from its liquid state back into the water cycle as atmospheric water vapor is evaporation. Evaporation accounts for around 90% of the moisture in the atmosphere, with transpiration providing the remaining 10%. Through transpiration, moisture is transported from roots to tiny holes (stoma) on the underside of leaves, where it transforms into vapor and is discharged into the atmosphere. The water from evapotranspiration, which is a combination of water transpired from plants and that evaporated from the soil, is carried up into the atmosphere along with the vapor by rising air currents. The vapor rises into the air, where it condenses

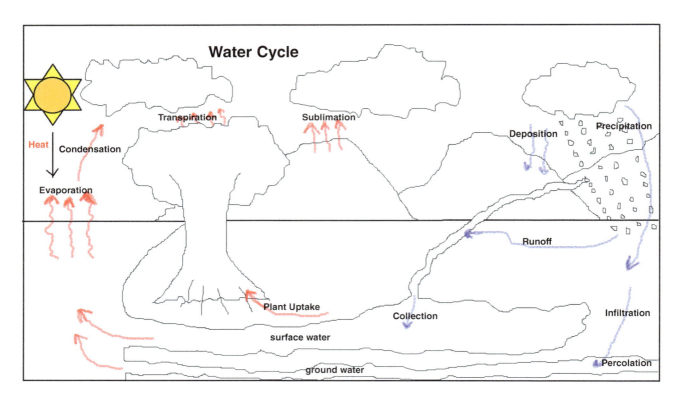

Figure 38.2 The hydrological cycle.

as clouds due to the cooler temperatures. The process by which water vapor is changed from a gaseous state back into a liquid one is called condensation. Eventually, clouds may enlarge and become sufficiently moist to release the water molecule as precipitation. Precipitation is the term used to describe water dropping from clouds in the atmosphere, either as ice (snow, sleet, hail) or liquid (rain, drizzle, etc.). Snow-covered precipitation has the potential to turn into ice caps and glaciers (Hendriks 2010).

Liquid precipitation typically results in surface flow and stream flow. The portion of precipitation that flows over the soil surface and into the adjacent stream channel is known as surface runoff. The flow of a stream is the movement of water in a river or other naturally occurring channel. The majority of precipitation dumps water molecules back into the ocean, where they resume their cycle. The majority of water from surface runoff eventually makes its way back to the ocean via stream flow so it can begin its voyage once more (Horton 1933).

A portion of the water that falls as rain can enter lakes where it can evaporate back into the air, condense into clouds, and then rain again. Aquatic plants have the ability to absorb lake water and release it through transpiration back into the atmosphere. Water that precipitates may sink into the earth and become a component of groundwater. Water enters the subsurface through the process of infiltration under the influence of gravity. Aquifers (saturated subsurface material) are underground reservoirs that can hold vast quantities of fresh water for a very long time. While some groundwater finds openings in the land surface and exits as freshwater springs, some groundwater infiltration remains close to the land surface and can seep back into surface water bodies (including the ocean). Plant roots can collect water that remains in the soil at the surface and leaves can transpire it. However, as time passes, all of this water continues to move, and the majority of it is absorbed by the ocean.

38.3.1 Components of the Hydrological Cycle

38.3.1.1 Atmosphere and Precipitation

Water that has been released from clouds as rain, freezing rain, sleet, snow, or hail is known as precipitation. It is the key link in the water cycle that ensures atmospheric water is delivered to the Earth. Water vapor in an ascending air mass condenses to generate raindrops in the cloud. The transformation of air-borne water vapor into liquid water is known as condensation. Because it causes clouds to form, condensation is essential to the water cycle. Precipitation, which is the main way for water to return to the Earth's surface through the water cycle, may result from these clouds. Evaporation's opposite is condensation, according to Eltahir and Bras (1996).

Rain is the predominant form of precipitation. Frontal, convective, and orographic rain are the three basic types of precipitation. Frontal rainfall is a type of precipitation that develops when two air fronts with varying moisture contents and temperatures come together. Convective rainfall occurs when hot, humid air rises and condenses to create rain clouds as a result of significant localized heating. The clouds would then become overly saturated, resulting in heavy rain. Orographic precipitation forms over mountains. A wet air mass rises and cools when it hits a mountain. Water vapor condenses into rain clouds as it cools, causing rain to fall on the mountain's windward side.

Surface water runoff is how most rainwater is lost. Surface water plays a significant role in the hydrological cycle. It comprises ponds, potholes, rivers and streams, lakes, wetlands, stormwater runoff (overland flow), and the ocean (Tian et al. 2022).

38.3.1.2 Streams and Rivers

Rivers serve as significant water supplies for urban areas. They offer opportunities for recreational pursuits like swimming, fishing, canoeing, and white-water rafting among others. They also house significant biological communities. Given their extensive distribution and accessibility as sources of water, rivers have a significant influence on global settlement patterns. Along rivers are sited major cities, towns, factories, businesses, and power plants. As a result, it is crucial to preserve the integrity and quality of all rivers (Thomas 2009). Sadly, the majority of rivers worldwide are too polluted for some human activities, particularly swimming, fishing, and drinking. In the US, over half of the rivers have been determined to be too dirty for swimming and fishing. Many rivers have also been channelized, narrowed, or dammed, which may limit their capacity to support a variety of biological and human activities (Howard 2015).

Impoundments have the potential to retain stream sediments, which would restrict the amount of material available downstream and enhance accretion behind the dam. Due to a lack of sediment supply, this change in sediment flow has the potential to harm aquatic habitats and worsen stream erosion downstream. Additionally, impoundments can stop some aquatic organisms from migrating upstream or downstream, so reducing their range, decreasing their capacity to withstand environmental changes, and cutting them off from spawning grounds (such as salmon spawning, for example). The local population may be uprooted as a result of the construction of dams, and traditional lands and cultural heritage may be lost to the reservoirs and ponds that often form behind these impoundments (Liu and Zheng 2004).

Over 600 000 river miles have reportedly been dammed in the US. Humans benefit from dams by having a source of water (reservoirs and agriculture ponds), access to recreational waters, and control over local flooding. On the other hand, dams can have detrimental effects on both people and the environment. During periods of heavy rain or when they break, they have the potential to create severe flooding downstream of the dam. A recent example occurred in southern Laos, close to the Cambodian border, on July 23, 2018, when a dam with an estimated project cost of over $1 billion failed (Howard 2015).

38.3.1.3 Lakes, Reservoirs, and Ponds

A body of standing water on the land surface is referred to as a lake, pond, or reservoir. A lake will form if water flows to an area that is surrounded on all sides by higher ground. The lakes that arise when people construct dams to stop rivers from flowing are known as reservoirs. The number of lakes, reservoirs, and ponds in the world is thought to be about 300 million. About 60% of all lakes on Earth are located in Canada. Even though less than 1% of the water on Earth is found in lakes and rivers, the US derives more than two-thirds (70%) of its water from lakes and reservoirs (for drinking, industry, irrigation, and hydroelectric power generation). In addition, lakes serve as the foundation of the US's freshwater fishing business, State tourist industries, and inland water recreation industries (Cardille et al. 2007).

38.3.1.4 Wetlands

A wetland is a place where there is frequently standing water, the soil is frequently saturated, and there are plants that are adapted to survive in floodplains or saturated soils. They serve as crossing points between terrestrial land and aquatic ecosystems like rivers, lakes, and oceans. The three main forms of wetland are bogs (dominated by moss), marshes (dominated by nonwoody plants), and swamps (dominated by trees). Soils (water-saturated soils are present), hydrology (a shallow water table), and vegetation (wetland plants that are adapted to regions that are saturated with water for lengthy periods of time) are the three criteria used to identify wetlands. In terms of biological variety and production, wetlands are crucial, and are also significant because they are the sites of ongoing geochemical and biological cycles and processes. For instance, wetlands are thought to be key sites for carbon sequestration (storage), which affects climate change globally. Prior to entering rivers and lakes, they also serve as filters for stormwater runoff (Bullock and Acreman 2003).

38.3.1.5 Oceans

Because they hold the vast majority of the water on Earth (about 97%), oceans are a crucial part of the hydrological cycle. They receive water from most of the major rivers. The Atlantic, Indian, Pacific, Arctic, and Southern Oceans are the five oceans that make up the Earth's surface. Ocean water makes up around 90% of the water that evaporates into the hydrological cycle. Oceans play a significant role in the hydrological cycle, and they also contain a wide variety of landforms and biological species. Human activities such as pollution and overfishing pose hazards to them.

38.3.1.6 Groundwater

Ninety-seven percent of the fresh water that is readily available is found underground as groundwater. Groundwater is recycled water that is produced by the hydrological cycle. When it rains, some of the water evaporates on the surface and some seeps into the soil. When water travels from the surface, via silt or rocks that are not saturated (unsaturated zone), all the way down to the saturated areas (saturated zone), it transforms into groundwater. The water table, which separates the saturated and unsaturated zones, is located at the top of the saturated area (Winter 2000).

Aquifers, which are rock formations or sediments that retain (and produce) significant volumes of usable water in their pore space, are where most groundwater is found. The porosity and permeability of an aquifer determine its production. The amount of empty space in a rock or sediment body is measured by its porosity. The capacity of a subsurface substance to transfer fluids is known as permeability. The saturated zone of a rock body, where all the pores are full of water, is where groundwater is discovered. It is considered soil moisture instead of groundwater when water is present in the unsaturated zone. A key idea is that groundwater always travels from higher energy (hydraulic head) to lower energy, but surface water always moves from higher elevation to lower elevation (Becker 2006).

Until it becomes a spring or empties into bodies of surface water on land or in the sea, groundwater will continue to flow. There is hardly any stagnant groundwater in the subsoil at any given time. Although rivers are the sources of surface water most often used in the United States and around the world because they are more accessible and dispersed globally, the bulk of fresh water that is available for human use is found in groundwater. Since aquifers are not as widely dispersed as rivers, using groundwater requires specialized equipment to drill into the subsurface in order to retrieve the water (Heath 1998).

38.4 Alternative (Nonconventional) Water Resources

38.4.1 Wastewater Reuse

Water recycling has been shown to be an effective way to increase water availability in many parts of the world, particularly those experiencing water shortage. It can meet agricultural, urban (nonpotable and potable), industrial, and environmental needs while also preserving the environment and human health (Bernacchi et al. 2007). Reusing water is acknowledged as a climate change adaptation strategy (Morote et al. 2019), and it is consistent with the circular economy idea that is strongly supported in industrialized nations (Shen et al. 2020). However, due to frequently strict regulations, socioeconomic concerns, lack of awareness of the potential benefits, and economic constraints created by the need for value chain adaptation and product marketability, water reuse is still not widely implemented in many parts of the world, including the EU (Menegaki et al. 2007).

According to Pazda et al. (2019), wastewater treatment plants (WWTPs), particularly in developed countries, are currently being upgraded with new, more dependable, and energy-sustainable processes, providing high-quality effluent and meeting requirements even for unregulated yet emerging pollutants and agents (pharmaceuticals, antibiotic resistance) and greatly reducing (or even eliminating) threats to the environment and public health (Sabri et al. 2020). Instead of dumping water into surface water bodies, encouraging water recycling for various beneficial uses has many advantages for reducing pollution, preventing the spread of emerging pollutants and antibiotic genes, preserving biodiversity, and enhancing community resilience to climate change.

38.4.2 Rainwater Harvesting (RWH)

In order to fulfill future water needs and maintain/improve the quality of water resources, rainwater collection is a viable alternative water source. In urban and suburban regions, it has been demonstrated to be a cost-effective option (Ghaffarian Hoseini et al. 2016). Growing interest in RWH systems has been observed recently in both developing and developed nations (EU, USA, UK, Japan, South Korea, Australia, Africa), primarily due to their cost-effectiveness and potential advantages for various economic, environmental, water resource, and human health sectors (Suleiman et al. 2020). One comparative advantage of RWH is its adaptability to different types of collection systems, including storm water collection systems from urban, suburban, industrial, and rural areas as well as large-scale structures (multistorey buildings, schools, stadiums, airports, etc.) (Suleiman et al. 2020).

There is still a need for more development in the fields of urban and water planning, economic viability, public health hazards, technology, research, and education (Gwenzi et al. 2015), policy and legal frameworks, and public health risks.

38.4.3 Desalination

Desalination offers a significant alternative water supply, at least locally, to address the increasing water needs of cities. It is a realistic adaptation strategy, especially for urban areas, to climate change and has been employed in expanded agricultural activities to deal with water pollution (Gude 2016). Desalination applications have grown globally as a result of recent technological advances (better membranes, cheaper operating costs, and less energy) (Intelligence 2016). However, a major obstacle to the development of these systems, particularly for poor nations, is the potential environmental effects of desalination procedures (Gude 2016). The use of small-scale desalination plants, the combined use of saltwater and brackish water where possible, and energy recovery during the desalination process are all promising alternatives to current desalination technologies, in addition to their optimization (Voutchkov 2018). Desalination systems may become more popular in the near future as a result of these possibilities, which is supported by the rising demand for alternate water sources and advances in applied technology.

38.5 Quality of Water Resources

Water pollution is a serious problem in intensively farmed areas because of overuse of nutrients and pesticides and the use of unsustainable field management techniques (Evans et al. 2019). According to Schwarzenbach et al. (2010), agricultural watershed pollution may have a serious impact on how well ecosystems function, the quality of water supplies, biodiversity, and human health.

The ecological deterioration of rivers and, consequently, of the derived services has increased as a result of the fast rates of urbanization and industrialization (Dunham et al. 2018). This issue is widespread in China, especially in the northern sections of the country where water availability is limited (Jia et al. 2020). Appropriate reservoir operation, which can repair damaged river ecology, has a crucial role to play in solving these problems.

38.6 Challenges and Opportunities for Improving Water Supply

38.6.1 Growing Population and Urbanization

In the next 30 years, the world's population will pass 10 billion, with a sizeable amount of this expansion occurring in developing nations. More than half of the world's population already resides in metropolitan areas, particularly in densely populated cities; by 2050, this number will rise to more than two-thirds. These metropolitan regions will experience water stress due to the uneven distribution of the world's fresh water supply, which will exacerbate tensions between users, particularly between the urban, agricultural, and industrial sectors (Niva et al. 2020). At the same time, significant effects are anticipated on ecosystem health and derived services (such as food security) (Grimm et al. 2008), availability and quality of water resources (Tam and Nga 2018), soil resource quality (Cui et al. 2017), potential increases in water demand (Singh and Biswal 2019), flood intensity and frequency (Angelakis et al. 2020), and ecosystem functioning. These effects are closely related to one another and are influenced by both human activity and the local environment, including the background climate, land use/cover, geomorphology, and hydrology. The long-term planning of water resources should take these issues into account (Li et al. 2020).

38.6.2 Climate Change (and/or Variability)

Through warming, changes in precipitation patterns, and the increase in extreme weather events (droughts, heat waves, and floods), climate change has already started to have an impact on water resources around the world (Agha Kouchak et al. 2020). These effects are not evenly dispersed but they exhibit significant regional and temporal fluctuations in response to climate change. For instance, the Mediterranean basin has seen warming at a rate much higher than the global average, which is anticipated to have a considerable impact on the amount of water available and the amount needed to deal with the increased frequency of droughts (Dai 2013). Relevant studies show that the global hydrological cycle is either intensifying, as evidenced by increases in both evaporation and precipitation fluxes, or deintensifying, as indicated by variations in precipitation and evaporation patterns and a markedly decreasing trend in global humidity (Durack et al. 2012).

Although there is broad consensus regarding the estimates made by climate models at the global and regional levels, downscaling these projections to levels that allow for planning and efficient management of water resources (such as watershed levels) continues to be a methodological issue. Global climate models and hydrological models continue to have significant levels of uncertainty, even at bigger scales (Wada et al. 2013).

The situation of the domestic sector is comparable. Information on correlations between temperature and water usage is necessary for accurate demand estimation in the future. These correlations were developed by Xenochristou et al. (2020) using a mix of data from smart water meters, household characteristics, and socioeconomic data. They may one day be applied to the planning of water use in the domestic sector. These interactions were intricate, exhibited seasonal and weekly fluctuations, and had a significant impact on household variables, including socioeconomic status and whether or not there were gardens.

38.6.3 Preserving Water Quality

The need for protection is highlighted by the increased necessity for alternate water sources to deal with water scarcity, whether for agricultural use and local irrigation or industrial usage and drinking water. Priority should be given to technological advances in water treatment as well as revising current criteria for various types of reuse to include emerging pollutants (Adegoke et al. 2018). Developing and implementing cost-effective sanitation systems and household-centered sanitation, particularly in rural regions, are essential for developing countries to enhance sanitation and provide the populace with clean drinking water (Schwarzenbach et al. 2010).

Finally, technological innovations and fresh strategies are required to recognize and handle problems created by population growth and climate change. Due to increased rainfall and flooding events, the latter is anticipated to modify the patterns of how pollutants and contaminants travel as well as the frequency of infectious disease outbreaks (Schwarzenbach et al. 2010).

38.7 Drinking Water Purification

Chemical addition, coagulation, flocculation, sedimentation, filtration, and disinfection – typically with chlorine – can all be used in conventional water treatment. Drinking water treatment technologies used in most systems include one or more of these procedures, utilizing a wide variety of adsorbents, filtration techniques, electrical and disinfection methods, and more recent technologies involving nanomaterials, carbon nanotubes, nanocomposites, etc., as shown in Table 38.1.

38.7.1 Filtration Techniques

By inserting a medium that only the fluid can flow through, filtration is a common mechanical or physical process used to separate particles from fluids (liquids or gases). Many different media are used but in recent years, membrane filtration has become more significant (Table 38.2). Membrane filtration is used to provide drinking water through municipal water delivery systems in California, US.

Aerogels are another promising method of water filtration. These are porous, ultralight synthetic materials made from gels in which the liquid portion has been swapped for a gas. Chalcogels are aerogels formed from chalcogens that

Table 38.1 Drinking water purification techniques.

Adsorbent materials	Filtration techniques	Electrical techniques	Disinfection techniques	Polymer and nanotechnology
Diatomaceous earth	Membrane filtration	Electrocoagulation	Chemical treatment	Ion exchange
Zeolites	• Microfiltration	Electrodialysis	Ozonation	Nanomaterials
Activated carbon	• Ultrafiltration	Electroflotation	Ultraviolet radiation	Carbon nanotubes
Activated alumina	• Nanofiltration	Electrochemical methods	Solar energy	Nanocomposites
Ferric hydroxide	• Reverse osmosis		Sonication	Thin films
Ceramics	Membrane distillation		Photocatalysis	Quantum dots
	Aerogels, chalcogels			

Table 38.2 Properties of membrane filtration methods.

Method	Pore size	Molecular weight cutoff	Pressure (bar)	Permeation
Reverse osmosis (RO)	<0.6	<500	30–70	Water
Nanofiltration (NF)	0.6–5	500–2000 Da	10–40	Water, low molecular weight solutes
Ultrafiltration (UF)	5–50	2–500 kDa	0.5–10	Water, low molecular weight solutes, nanomolecules
Microfiltration (MF)	50–5000	>500 kDa	0.5–2	Water, low molecular weight solutes, colloids

Source: Padmaja et al. (2014)/International Journal of Innovative Research in Science, Engineering and Technology.

selectively absorb heavy metals and have the potential to remove mercury, lead, and cadmium from water. Carbon nanotube-graphene hybrid aerogels exhibit highly promising performance in the purification of water, including the capacitive deionization of light metal salts, the removal of organic dyes, and the enrichment of heavy metal ions (Sui et al. 2012). Because they can absorb organic solvents, oils, and other substances 900 times their weight, carbon aerogels are also known as super sponges.

Several electrochemical processes are used to purify drinking water. According to Padmaja et al. (2014), electrocoagulation (EC), electrodialysis, and electroflotation (EF) are a few of the crucial ones. As a result of an applied electric potential, a sacrificial metal anode corrodes in the electrocoagulation process, simultaneously releasing hydrogen at the cathode which is then extracted by flotation. The main benefit of this is that it provides the active cations needed for coagulation without causing the water's salinity to rise (Chaturvedi 2013). Due to its great effectiveness, low cost, and eco-friendliness, this technique is increasingly utilized to treat drinking water. It is primarily used to remove heavy metals from waste water (Padmaja et al. 2014), fluoride ions, etc.

The EC-MF process, which combines electrocoagulation and microfiltration, is a highly efficient method of treating water. The removal efficiencies of total organic carbon (TOC), ammonia-nitrogen (NH_3-N), and oil are influenced by variables such as current density, electrolytic duration, and pH value (Padmaja et al. 2014). As the current density increased, these contaminants became less prevalent. Using EC with iron electrodes and filtering, arsenic can be taken out of drinking water. The oxyhydroxide flocs produced by the EC process are eliminated using a sand filter. According to Ucar et al. (2013), the EC procedure reduces the residual arsenic concentration to less than 10 g/l.

Ions can be transported through semipermeable membranes using the electrodialysis (ED) method of membrane separation. Only charged particles can be removed since the membranes are cation or anion selective. It is a successful method for treating drinking water with a high nitrate content. However, by generating concentrated brines, it merely manages to transfer contamination (Wisniewski et al. 2002). Colloidal particles, oil and grease, and organic contaminants can all be successfully removed from water using EF technology. It has been demonstrated to perform better than impeller flotation (IF), dissolved air flotation (DAF), or sedimentation. Using EF, it is possible to separate the flocculated sludge from the treated water (Padmaja et al. 2014).

38.7.2 Disinfection Methods (Table 38.3)

Table 38.3 Disinfection methods of water.

Specific consideration	Ultraviolet	Ozone	Chlorine
Relative complexity of technology	Low to moderate	Moderate to high	Low to moderate
Relative operational safety concerns	Low	Moderate	Moderate to high
Equipment reliability	Moderate	Low to moderate	Good
Virus effectiveness (>4 log)	Low to moderate	Good	Good
Bacterial effectiveness (>3 log)	Good	Good to high	Good
Efficacy against protozoan cysts (*Giardia* >3 log, *Cryptococcus* >2 log)	Good	Good	Low to moderate
Ease of application, design, and installation	Low to moderate	Moderate to high	Moderate to high
Process control options and flexibility	Low	Moderate	Moderate to good
pH dependency affecting efficacy	None	Low	High
Operation and maintenance level required	Moderate to high	Moderate to high	Low to moderate
Variable flow and/or dose capability	Low	Moderate to high	High
Available and persistent residual	None	None to low	High
Disinfection by-products with potential health concerns	None	Moderate	High

Source: Padmaja et al. (2014)/International Journal of Innovative Research in Science, Engineering and Technology.

38.7.3 Polymer and Nanotechnology (Table 38.4)

Table 38.4 Purification methods and the contaminants removed.

Purification methods	Contaminants removed.	Efficiency and cost-effectiveness
Activated charcoal	Color, pesticides, herbicides, volatile organic compounds (VOCs), foaming agents, polychlorinated biphenyls (PCBs), polycyclic aromatic hydrocarbons (PAHs), trihalomethanes	Very efficient and lower cost
Diatomite	Bacteria, viruses, Fe, Mn, heavy metals	Efficient and cheap
Activated alumina	Fluoride, As, Se, bacteria, viruses	Efficient and cheap
Zeolites	Heavy metal cations and anions and organics	Efficient and cheap
Granular ferric hydroxide	As, Cr, bacteria, viruses	Efficient and cheap
Ceramics	Bacteria, protozoa, microbial cysts	Efficient and slightly costly
Reverse osmosis	Total dissolved salts, organic compounds, pathogens, turbidity, As, Ni, Cu, Cr, Ra, Pb, asbestos, Cd, Hg, Ni, F	Very efficient and cost-effective
Membrane distillation	Salts in water, VOCs, disinfection byproducts, fluoride, and boron	Efficient and slightly costly
Microfiltration	Bacteria, protozoa	Very efficient and costly
Ultrafiltration	Suspended solids, colloids, bacteria, protozoa, viruses, chemicals	Very efficient and costly
Nanofiltration	Bacteria, protozoa, viruses, chemicals divalent cations, organic matter	Very efficient and costly
Electrocoagulation	Heavy metals, colloids, fats, oils, grease, total soluble solids, phosphates, pesticides, organic compounds, radioactivity, fluoride, bacteria	Efficient and cost-effective
Electrodialysis	Organic and inorganic trace contaminants, nitrates, nitrites, fluoride, As, Cd, U, total dissolved solids, PAHs	Efficient and costly
Chemical disinfectants	Bacteria, viruses, germs, pesticides	Efficient and cheap
Ozonation	Protozoa, germs, pesticides, dissolved organics	Efficient and cheap
Solar radiation	Bacteria, viruses, protozoa and worms, dissolved organic carbon, As	Efficient and very cheap
Ultraviolet radiation	Bacteria, viruses, protozoa and worms	Very efficient and very cheap
Sonication	Cyanobacteria, soluble solids, phosphates, Ni, Co	Efficient and low cost
Ion exchange	Harmful metals, cations, anions	Efficient but costly
Carbon nanotubes	Color, organics, heavy metals, bacteria, viruses, cynobacterial toxins, natural organic matter	Very efficient and costly

Source: Padmaja et al. (2014)/International Journal of Innovative Research in Science, Engineering and Technology.

38.8 Conclusion and Future Perspectives

The effects of urbanization and industry on drinking water quality have been worsening dangerously. The availability of clean, uncontaminated water is now a rare occurrence. Every type of treatment has its limitations and to efficiently treat water, a mix of treatments is frequently needed. A multitude of innovative, effective, and affordable techniques for the purification of drinking water have emerged with the development of technology. To provide greater safety of drinking water, purification at the point of entrance and usage more desirable than a centralized system.

References

Adegoke, A.A., Amoah, I.D., Stenström, T.A. et al. (2018). Epidemiological evidence and health risks associated with agricultural reuse of partially treated and untreated wastewater: a review. *Frontiers in Public Health* 6: 337.

Agha Kouchak, A., Chiang, F., Huning, L.S. et al. (2020). Climate extremes and compound hazards in a warming world. *Annual Review of Earth and Planetary Sciences* 48: 519–548.

Angelakis, A.N., Antoniou, G., Voudouris, K. et al. (2020). History of floods in Greece: causes and measures for protection. *Natural Hazards* 101: 833–852.

Becker, M.W. (2006). Potential for satellite remote sensing of ground water. *Groundwater* 44 (2): 306–318.

Bernacchi, C.J., Kimball, B.A., Quarles, D.R. et al. (2007). Decreases in stomatal conductance of soybean under open-air elevation of [CO_2] are closely coupled with decreases in ecosystem evapotranspiration. *Plant Physiology* 143 (1): 134–144.

Bullock, A. and Acreman, M. (2003). The role of wetlands in the hydrological cycle. *Hydrology and Earth System Sciences* 7 (3): 358–389.

Cardille, J.A., Carpenter, S.R., Coe, M.T. et al. (2007). Carbon and water cycling in lake-rich landscapes: landscape connections, lake hydrology, and biogeochemistry. *Journal of Geophysical Research: Biogeosciences* 112 (G2).

Cech, T.V. (2009). *Principles of Water Resources: History, Development, Management, and Policy*, 3e. Hoboken: Wiley.

Chaturvedi, S.I. (2013). Electrocoagulation: a novel waste water treatment method. *International Journal of Modern Engineering Research* 3 (1): 93–100.

Cui, Y., Xiao, X., Zhang, Y. et al. (2017). Temporal consistency between gross primary production and solar-induced chlorophyll fluorescence in the ten most populous megacity areas over years. *Scientific Reports* 7 (1): 14963.

Dai, A. (2013). Increasing drought under global warming in observations and models. *Nature Climate Change* 3: 52–58.

Dunham, J.B., Angermeier, P.L., Crausbay, S.D. et al. (2018). Rivers are social-ecological systems: time to integrate human dimensions into riverscape ecology and management. *Wiley Interdisciplinary Reviews: Water* 5 (4): e1291.

Durack, P.J., Wijffels, S.E., and Matear, R.J. (2012). Ocean salinities reveal strong global water cycle intensification during 1950 to 2000. *Science* 336 (6080): 455–458.

Eltahir, E.A. and Bras, R.L. (1996). Precipitation recycling. *Reviews of Geophysics* 34 (3): 367–378.

Environmental Protection Agency (EPA). (2013). Clean Lakes. https://archive.epa.gov/water/archive/web/html/index-15.html (accessed 21 February 2024).

Environmental Protection Agency (EPA). (2018). Lakes. http://water.epa.gov/type/lakes (accessed 21 February 2024).

Evans, A.E., Mateo-Sagasta, J., Qadir, M. et al. (2019). Agricultural water pollution: key knowledge gaps and research needs. *Current Opinion in Environmental Sustainability* 36: 20–27.

Fetter, C.W. Jr. (2000). *Applied Hydrogeology*, 4e. Upper Saddle River: Prentice Hall.

Ghaffarian Hoseini, A., Tookey, J., Ghaffarian Hoseini, A. et al. (2016). State of the art of rainwater harvesting systems towards promoting green built environments: a review. *Desalination and Water Treatment* 57 (1): 95–104.

Grimm, N.B., Faeth, S.H., Golubiewski, N.E. et al. (2008). Global change and the ecology of cities. *Science* 319 (5864): 756–760.

Gude, V.G. (2016). Desalination and sustainability – an appraisal and current perspective. *Water Research* 89: 87–106.

Gwenzi, W., Dunjana, N., Pisa, C. et al. (2015). Water quality and public health risks associated with roof rainwater harvesting systems for potable supply: review and perspectives. *Sustainability of Water Quality and Ecology* 6: 107–118.

Heath, R.C. (1998). *Basic Ground-Water Hydrology*, vol. 2220. Washington, DC: US Department of the Interior, US Geological Survey.

Hendriks, M.R (2010). *Introduction to Physical Hydrology*. Oxford: Oxford University Press.

Horton, R.E. (1933). The role of infiltration in the hydrologic cycle. *Eos, Transactions of the American Geophysical Union* 14 (1): 446–460.

Howard, P. (2015). The USGS Water Science School. The World's Water. www.usgs.gov/ (accessed 2 February 2024).

Intelligence, G.W. (2016). *IDA Desalination Yearbook 2016–2017*. Oxford: Media Analytics.

Jia, W., Dong, Z., Duan, C. et al. (2020). Ecological reservoir operation based on DFM and improved PA-DDS algorithm: a case study in Jinsha river, China. *Human and Ecological Risk Assessment* 26 (7): 1723–1741.

Li, C., Sun, G., Cohen, E. et al. (2020). Modeling the impacts of urbanization on watershed-scale gross primary productivity and tradeoffs with water yield across the conterminous United States. *Journal of Hydrology* 583: 124581.

Liu, C. and Zheng, H. (2004). Changes in components of the hydrological cycle in the Yellow River basin during the second half of the 20th century. *Hydrological Processes* 18 (12): 2337–2345.

Menegaki, A.N., Hanley, N., and Tsagarakis, K.P. (2007). The social acceptability and valuation of recycled water in Crete: a study of consumers' and farmers' attitudes. *Ecological Economics* 62 (1): 7–18.

Morote, Á.F., Olcina, J., and Hernández, M. (2019). The use of non-conventional water resources as a means of adaptation to drought and climate change in semi-arid regions: South-Eastern Spain. *Water* 11 (1): 93.

Niva, V., Cai, J., Taka, M. et al. (2020). China's sustainable water-energy-food nexus by 2030: impacts of urbanization on sectoral water demand. *Journal of Cleaner Production* 251: 119755.

Padmaja, K., Cherukuri, J., and Reddy, M.A. (2014). Conventional to cutting edge technologies in drinking water purification – a review. *International Journal of Innovative Research in Science Engineering and Technology* 3: 9375–9385.

Pazda, M., Kumirska, J., Stepnowski, P., and Mulkiewicz, E. (2019). Antibiotic resistance genes identified in wastewater treatment plant systems – a review. *Science of the Total Environment* 697: 134023.

Sabri, N., Schmitt, H., Van der Zaan, B. et al. (2020). Prevalence of antibiotics and antibiotic resistance genes in a wastewater effluent-receiving river in the Netherlands. *Journal of Environmental Chemical Engineering* 8 (1): 102245.

Schwarzenbach, R.P., Egli, T., Hofstetter, T.B. et al. (2010). Global water pollution and human health. *Annual Review of Environment and Resources* 35: 109–136.

Shen, K.W., Li, L., and Wang, J.Q. (2020). Circular economy model for recycling waste resources under government participation: a case study in industrial waste water circulation in China. *Technological and Economic Development of Economy* 26 (1): 21–47.

Singh, R. and Biswal, B. (2019). Assessing the impact of climate change on water resources: the challenge posed by a multitude of options. In: *Hydrology in a Changing World: Challenges in Modeling* (ed. S. Singh and C. Dhanya), 185–204. London: Springer.

Sipes, J.L. (2010). *Sustainable Solutions for Water Resources*. Hoboken: Wiley.

Sui, Z., Meng, Q., Zhang, X. et al. (2012). Green synthesis of carbon nanotube–graphene hybrid aerogels and their use as versatile agents for water purification. *Journal of Materials Chemistry* 22 (18): 8767–8771.

Suleiman, L., Olofsson, B., Saurí, D., and Palau-Rof, L. (2020). A breakthrough in urban rain-harvesting schemes through planning for urban greening: case studies from Stockholm and Barcelona. *Urban Forestry & Urban Greening* 51: 126678.

Tam, V.T. and Nga, T.T.V. (2018). Assessment of urbanization impact on groundwater resources in Hanoi, Vietnam. *Journal of Environmental Management* 227: 107–116.

Tian, L., Zhang, B., Chen, S. et al. (2022). Large-scale afforestation enhances precipitation by intensifying the atmospheric water cycle over the Chinese Loess Plateau. *Journal of Geophysical Research: Atmospheres* 127 (16): e2022JD036738.

Ucar, C., Baskan, M.B., and Pala, A. (2013). Arsenic removal from drinking water by electrocoagulation using iron electrodes. *Korean Journal of Chemical Engineering* 30: 1889–1895.

Voutchkov, N. (2018). Energy use for membrane seawater desalination – current status and trends. *Desalination* 431: 2–14.

Wada, Y., Wisser, D., Eisner, S. et al. (2013). Multimodel projections and uncertainties of irrigation water demand under climate change. *Geophysical Research Letters* 40 (17): 4626–4632.

Winter, T.C. (2000). *Ground Water and Surface Water: A Single Resource*. Darby: Diane Publishing.

Wisniewski, C., Persin, F., Cherif, T. et al. (2002). Use of a membrane bioreactor for denitrification of brine from an electrodialysis process. *Desalination* 149 (1–3): 331–336.

Xenochristou, M., Kapelan, Z., and Hutton, C. (2020). Using smart demand-metering data and customer characteristics to investigate influence of weather on water consumption in the UK. *Journal of Water Resources Planning and Management* 146 (2): 04019073.

39

Type, Cause, Effects, Control Methods of Noise Pollution

Baleshwari Dixit[1,2], Sapna Sharma[3], Ranvijay Singh[4], and Serlene Tomar[2]

[1] Department of Veterinary Public Health & Epidemiology, College of Veterinary Science and Animal Health, 486001, Rewa, NDVSU, Jabalpur, Madhya Pradesh, India
[2] Department of Livestock Products Technology, College of Veterinary Science and Animal Husbandry, Rewa, NDVSU, Jabalpur, Madhya Pradesh, India
[3] Department of Public Health & Epidemiology, Post Graduate Institute of Veterinary Education and Research College, 302031, Jaipur, India
[4] Department of Veterinary Public Health & Epidemiology, College of Veterinary Science and A.H., NDVSU 482001, Jabalpur, Madhya Pradesh, India

39.1 Introduction

Any unwanted sound that is unpleasant, loud, or disruptive for hearing is considered as noise. The meaning of noise is highly variable based on different science like biological, physical, chemical etc. In general aspect noise is a pollution that impacts on wellness and health of the living being (Basner et al., 2014)). Prevalence of noise is in increasing trends in terms of magnitude and severity along with economic and social developments. Industrialization, increase travel and trades the various means of noise production sources are increasing. More orientation towards urbanization and the adoption of urban lifestyle with no or inefficient restrictions on noise control along with less emphasis on its harmful effects on population is needed attention. Noise pollution leads to many chronic and socially significant impacts. The negligence or lack of awareness about noise pollution in all over the world, need to be addressed accordingly so its effect can be assessed, recognized and controlled.

The explanation of the meaning of noise in physics indicate no distinction of noise with the desired sound, as both are categorized as the vibrations developed in a medium, like air or water. The difference between noise and desired sound detected by the brain when it receives, and how it process and perceives the signal of a sound. However in the acoustic domain any sound may be detected as a noise whether it is intended (e.g. music or speech) or undeliberate.

In the domain of electronics noise human ear may not hear it and require instruments for its detection. In audio engineering, any unwanted residual electronic signal produce may be considered as acoustic noise which is felt as a hiss. However in experimental sciences, any random fluctuations of data may be considered as a noise that alter the perception of a signal.

In 1859 Florence Nightingale described the noise as a health hazard and stated "Unnecessary noise is the most cruel abuse of care which can be inflicted on either the sick or the well" (Nightingale 1859). Noise pollution is one of the urban territorial phenomenon that is causing serious proportions in every city. The frequency as well as intensity of pollution has been increasing day by day. The word noise is taken from a Latin word "Nausea" that means "unwanted sound" or any unpleasant sound that is comparatively loud and unexpected (Kalisa et al. 2022). Noise may also be defined as any sound that is wrong for people, at the wrong time and in the wrong place. Data from Western Europe (WHO) shows that at least one million healthy life-years are lost per year from traffic-related environmental noise alone. German physician and microbiologist, Robert Koch had predicted that "One day man will have to fight noise as fiercely as cholera and pest." Now it is very essential to realize the social and environmental effects of noise pollution on public health as a priority before it becomes an epidemic.

Noise is any sound that is unwanted and unnecessary form of energy produced by any vibrating object which on reaching to human ear is perceived by brain. However all the sounds produced by vibrating bodies cannot be heard and this limit is different for all the living being. Noise can be perceived either psychologically or physiologically. Physiological perception is recognized subconsciously in which the vibrations of the noise (sound) waves in our physical body however

---

Epidemiology and Environmental Hygiene in Veterinary Public Health, First Edition. Edited by Tanmoy Rana.
© 2025 John Wiley & Sons, Inc. Published 2025 by John Wiley & Sons, Inc.

psychological perception is the event when conscious awareness of a person give attention to that noise rather than letting it ignored. Noise may be of low frequency or of high frequency as well as may be intermittent or continuous which is difficult for normal human hearing and understanding. Different instruments are used to measure and study the sound or noise, some basic instruments are sound level meter that measure the sound intensity in dB. Octave band frequency analyzer expresses the noise in octave bands and the sound spectrum is shown as a plot which indicates the characteristics of the noise in terms of high pitch, low pitch, or variable pitch. Audiometer is the instrument used to measure the hearing capacity of the individual and zero line indicates the normal hearing while dip in the curve is shown in the noise hearing loss.

Atmospheric noise is a radio noise that is caused by natural processes occurring in the atmosphere like lightning during thunderstorms. It occurs primarily due to cloud-to-ground flashes where current passes is stronger compared to cloud-to cloud flashes. Daily 3.5 million lightning flashes (as 40 lightning flashes per second) occur all over the world. The addition of all these lightning flashes constitutes atmospheric noise. Atmospheric noises are often of very low frequency (VLF) and low frequency (LF), and in urban areas mostly manmade noises dominates which are of high frequency (HF), mainly.

Environmental noises are the noise pollution produced by outside sources, particularly by transport systems such as cars, buses, trucks, two/three wheelers, trains, helicopters, aircraft, watercraft, spacecraft along with other recreational activities like music system, instruments performances, sports. Occupational noise are noise that *affect workers* in their work places or job areas that are produced because of work environment, machineries or operations.

39.2   Sources of Noise

Spatially and temporally the most prominent and widespread sources of manmade noise are motor vehicles like cars, trucks, planes and vessels and their traffic of all sorts. Other more intense but normally of short term at local level, repetitive sources of unwanted sound are explosions, seismic surveys, pile driving and military sonar. Highway traffic, shipping lanes, ferry lines, busy airports, construction sites, cleaning machines, motorized recreation, dredging, air conditioners, pumping systems, and industrial generators are some other examples of more long term and lasting sources of noise (Schwela 2021).

Propagation of noise or sound becomes noise pollution, or sound pollution, which imparts number of adverse effects on human or animal life, in various degree harm ranging from unapparent to fatal consequences. Sources of noise pollution are very diverse which vary spatially as well as temporally. Outdoor noise is mainly caused by machines, transport and propagation systems globally. One of the major factor is the poor urban planning that give rise to noise disintegration or pollution, along with no sufficient spatial distance between industrial and residential habitat that *can* result in issue of noise pollution to people of residential areas. Some studies indicated that some developed countries have noise pollution temporally correlated with income and is *highest* in low-income and racial minority neighborhoods (Kalisa et al. 2022). Some other sources of noise pollution in residential areas are various modes of transportation like traffic, airplanes, rail, etc; loud music, construction, electrical generators, explosions wind turbines, lawn care maintenance, and people too. In developing nations, household electricity generators are associated with emerging environmental degradation (Menkiti and Agunwamba 2015). However, it is not related with recent advancement but the problems associated with noise in urban environments had been documented back as far as ancient Rome.

The noise that is distressing, become pollution if it affects the normal wellbeing or harm the physical as well as mental activity of human being and animal life. Recently noise pollution has become a matter of prime concern as it is frequently disrupting the activity or balance of human's way of life. It is unnoticed form of pollution that is increasingly becoming omnipresent and a growing environmental issue in developed countries as well as developing countries.

39.3   Measurement of Noise

Characteristic of noise includes loudness or intensity and frequency of a sound wave, the two parameter use to measure the sound level. The amplitude of a sound is the loudness or maximum displacement of the vibrating particles from their position. The energy in a sound wave or the amplitude of a sound wave is measured, in decibels (dB) or loudness. Decibels are expressed in a logarithmic scale. The frequency of a sound is described by pitch that is measured in hertz (Hz) (Berglund et al. 1999). The decibel (dB) is a relative unit of measurement equal to one tenth of a bel (B). The bel word was given in honor of Alexander Graham Bell, but it is not used commonly. The decibel is most widely used unit of measurement in science, acoustics and electronics etc. The signal noise is commonly measured using A-weighting or ITU-R 468 weighting that is used to represent the sound that humans are capable of hearing at each frequency. Sound level is expressed in terms of dBA and the softest level that a person can hear is of 0 dBA and normal speaking voices are of 65 dBA, heavy street traffic is 60–80 dB while a rock concert may be as high as 120 dBA. The meaning of 65 dB is that sound is 65 dB more intense than the reference sound pressure which is referred to 000.2 microbar or dynes/cm^2. Sound intensity is an average rate of sound energy that is transmitted in a specified direction to a point through a unit area expresses as W/m^2. The tolerable sound limit for human is 85 dB and this dose does not cause any substantial hearing damage. Human ear respond to different sound pressure in a non-uniform way rather than the real loudness of a sound of perceived intensity. This effect is subjective and this perception of intensity or sound emission by normal ear is described as dB(A) sound pressure level conforming to the weighting curve A that is also called curve A. The frequency of sound is expressed as hertz that is the number of sound wave per seconds. One Hz means one wave per second. The audible frequency for human is 20–20 000 Hz and the frequency below 20 is infraaudible and more than 20 000 Hz is ultrasonic (Purves et al. 2001). Some times the level of sound can also be expressed in terms of psychoacoustic that phon. index of loudness which take in to account is intensity and frequency.

The two most commonly used instruments for measuring noise exposures includes the sound level meter and the noise dosimeter. The main instrument used to measure the sound in the air is Sound level meter while some instruments that are used to measure noise in different places include noise dosimeters used in occupational environments, noise monitors that are used to measure environmental noise, and recently smartphone-based sound level meter applications are used to map recreational, crowdsource and community noise.

Sound Level Meter: The sound level meter is the basic measuring instrument for noise exposures. It consists of a microphone, a frequency selective amplifier, and an indicator. At a minimum, it measures sound level in dB SPL.

Noise Dosimeter: A noise dosimeter or noise dosemeter is a sound level meter instrument used to measure the exposure of a person to noise over a period of time. This should preferably be used in working place to measure the exposure of noise of worker to comply with Health and Safety regulations like the Occupational Safety and Health (OSHA) 29 CFR 1910.95 Occupational Noise Exposure Standard (OSHA 1996). It is preferred for measuring a worker's noise exposure when the noise levels are varying or intermittent, when they contain impulsive components, or when the worker moves around frequently during the work shift. The microphone of dosimeter, is put on the worker whose exposure is being measured (Khoza-Shangase et al. 2020). Modern dosimeters have provision to collect data on various parameters like noise dose, sound exposure level, time-weighted average, peak and sound pressure levels (maximum, and minimum). It measures the sound levels and stores the record during an exposure period and analyze the data to calculate the dose in percent and graphical representations of the collected data. If dosimeter recorded the 100% noise dose that means the person has exceeded the permissible noise dose and after that (100% noise dose) hearing damage may occur. To measure all sound levels from 80 to 140 dBA, a noise dosimeter should have an operating range of at least 63 dB and a pulse range of the same magnitude. In contrast, the standard specifies that dosimeters should have an operating range of at least 50 dB and a pulse range of at least 53 dB. Today, noise dosimeters with operating and pulse ranges in excess of 65 dB are quite common. Therefore, NIOSH considers that measuring all sound levels from 80 to 140 dBA with a noise dosimeter is technically feasible (ANSI 1991).

Noise reduction rating (NRR) is a presentation of noise reduction value or attenuation reduced by various types of hearing protectors. These values are single number rating which are generally in the range of 0–30, noise reduces as the value increases. It indicates noise reduction capabilities of the instrument represented in dB that should be mentioned on the label of each hearing protector device.

39.4   Effect of Noise Pollution on Human Health

Any sound becomes nuisance when it start to interfere with normal performance or daily activities such as conversation, sleep, etc. A noise-induced hearing loss is chronic or prolonged exposure to above 85 A-weighted decibels sound frequency noise levels however some time acute or hyper acute noise induced hearing loss may occur due to exposure to very high frequency of sound. Noise pollution may affect various system of body varying from local auditory effects to general systemic issues involving major body systems. Continuous exposure to noise may contribute to hazardous effects on cardiovascular system in humans with an increased incidence of coronary artery disease (Münzel et al. 2018).

Noise pollution affects both physical health and mental health. Duration and level of exposure of noise beyond tolerance may cause or increase the risk of hearing loss, ischemic heart disease, high blood pressure, injuries, sleep disturbances and even decreased efficiency and performance. In humans high degree of noise can affect physiological health associated with tinnitus, hearing loss, high stress levels, sleep disturbances, hypertension, cardiovascular disorders, and other harmful and disturbing effects including faster decline in cognitive activity (Kershaw 2006).

Hearing impairment is typically defined as an increase in the threshold of hearing as clinically assessed by audiometry. Some psychological effects like mental well-being, annoyance and psychiatric disorders have been correlated with continuous exposure to noise (Natarajan et al. 2023). European Environment Agency indicated that in Europe, about hundred million people are exposed to noise levels above 55 decibels (a threshold for human health) mainly by road traffic (WHO 1991). Perhaps it is not clear the concept behind the adoption to noise that describes the tolerance for noise is independent of sound frequency (decibel levels). Nosie may interfere with the normal sleep and can cause visual impairments like narrowing of pupils, visual difficulties, reduced color perception and night vision. Audiogram is a graph showing the result of a pure-tone hearing test. It will show how loud sounds need to be at different frequencies for you to hear them. The audiogram shows the degree, configuration and type of hearing loss. It is a graph of hearing threshold level as it is expressed as the function of frequency. Sounds of frequencies may be infrasonic that is sound with less than 20 Hz and ultrasonics with frequency greater than 20 000 Hz (Musiek et al. 2017; Kileny et al. 2021).

The WHO has documented seven categories of adverse health effects of noise pollution on humans. The guideline provides an excellent, reasonably up-to-date, and comprehensive overview of noise-related issues, as do the other recent reviews on this subject.

39.4.1 Hearing Impairment or Auditory Effect

Auditory fatigue that develop due to exposure to noise of 90 dB and 4000 Hz is characterized by buzzing and whistling in the ears. Noise-induced deafness is highly associated with the occupational exposure and noise exposure at workplace can also contribute to other health issues. In the early stage this pathological condition is mostly unnoticed. It may cause temporary and permanent hearing loss. Temporary hearing loss occurs due to exposure to noise of 4000–6000 Hz and hearing disability appears after 24 hours of exposure. Permanent damage occurs by repeated exposure to noise of 100 dB due to which damage occurs in inner ear like damage in nerve ending or destruction of organ of corti. Exposure to noise of 160 dB can cause the rupture of tympanic membrane leading to permanent loss of hearing (Ryan et al. 2016). Impaired hearing may come from any workplace or from any of the communities, and from a variety of other causes (e.g. trauma, ototoxic drugs, infection, and heredity) (Chloupek et al. 2009). There is general agreement that exposure to sound levels less than 70 dB does not produce hearing damage, regardless of the duration of exposure (Cwynar et al. 2011). There is also general agreement that exposure for more than 8 hours to sound levels in excess of 85 dB is potentially hazardous (Kershaw 2006). Studies suggest that children seem to be more vulnerable than adults to noise induced hearing impairment (Kileny et al. 2021). Noise induced hearing impairment may be accompanied by abnormal loudness perception (loudness recruitment), distortion (paracusis), and tinnitus (Menkiti and Agunwamba 2015). Tinnitus may be temporary or may become permanent after prolonged exposure. The eventual results of hearing losses are loneliness, depression, impaired speech discrimination, impaired school and job performance, limited job opportunities, and a sense of isolation (Münzel et al. 2018).

Occupational setting are one of the most common place of noise exposure which has been identified as a public health issue. A Noise and Hearing Loss Prevention program (NIOSH's) was developed to address these issues. Noise has also been proved an occupational hazard, as noise pollution is the most common work-related pollutant (Musiek et al. 2017). Noise-induced hearing loss, when associated with noise exposure at the workplace is also called occupational hearing loss (Perillo et al. 2017). For example, some occupational studies have shown an association between those who are regularly exposed to noise above 85 decibels to have higher blood pressure than those who are not exposed.

Another cluster includes old age people who become more susceptible to cardiac problems due to noise and children who are more vulnerable to noise, may get a permanent damage. A chronic exposure to noise may pose a serious threat to a child's physical and psychological health and lead to interference in learning and behavioral activities.

39.4.2 Negative Social Behavior and Annoyance

Non auditory effect varies from annoyance to speech loss, decrease in efficiency to serious psychological changes. Annoyance is the first sign of psychological change that develop due to continuous exposure to noise of high intensity particularly at workplace and is shown in the form of frequent agitation, ill temperedness, impatience and irritation. Nosie also affects the working efficiency of workers hence environment of work places related to work with mental concentration should be noise free.

Annoyance is a feeling of displeasure caused by any agent or condition believed by an individual to adversely affect him or her. The term annoyance does not only cover the negative reactions caused by noise pollution but also these include anger, dissatisfaction, disappointment, helplessness, withdrawal, anxiety, depression, distraction, agitation, or exhaustion. Social and behavioral effects of noise exposure are subtle, complex, and indirect.

39.4.3 Interference with Spoken Communication

Speech communication is hindered in the range of 300–500 Hz noise which is commonly seen in places with heavy road traffic. For a good speech its sound should exceed the speech interference level by about 12 dB. Noise pollution interferes with the ability to comprehend normal speech and may lead to a number of personal disabilities, handicaps, and behavioral changes. These include problems with concentration, irritation, uncertainty, misunderstandings, fatigue, stress reactions, lack of self-confidence, decreased working capacity, and disturbed interpersonal relationships.

39.4.4 Sleep Disturbances

Environmental noise is one of the major factor associated with sleep disturbance. When sleep disruption becomes chronic, the results are mood changes, decrements in performance, and other long-term effects on health and well-being. Much recent research has focused on noise from roadways, aircraft, and trains. It is known, for example, that continuous noise in excess of 30 dB disturbs sleep. Apart from various effects on sleep itself, noise during sleep causes increased blood pressure, increased heart rate, increased pulse amplitude, vasoconstriction, changes in respiration, cardiac arrhythmias, and increased body movement. Long-term psychosocial effects have been related to nocturnal noise particularly in high risk groups that include the elderly, night shift workers, persons vulnerable to physical or mental disorders, and sleep disorder patients.

39.4.5 Cardiovascular Disturbances

Noise may also affect the endocrine and autonomic nervous system, leading to indirect effect on cardiovascular system developing a risk factor for cardiovascular disease. These effects begin to be seen with long-term daily exposure to noise levels above 65 dB or with acute exposure to noise levels above 80–85 dB. Cardiovascular affection may include high blood pressure, increased heart rate, and vasoconstriction by altering autonomic responses, shift in electrolytes, and secretion of norepinephrine, epinephrine, and cortisol. Noise pollution due to occupational or environmental conditions associated with exposure of high intensity noise for long duration, increases the heart rate and peripheral resistance, increases blood viscosity, blood pressure and blood lipids. Reflex responses may also evoke by sudden unexpected noise. Night-time noise can never completely be adopted by anyone even in unusual circumstances. Physiologic changes are reversible in temporary noise exposure. However, continuous sudden exposure to high intensity noise for long duration may provoke changes that may not be easily reversed. Even though the noise-induced cardiovascular disease risk is comparatively indirect and small, but considering the number of people at risk and the noise to which they are exposed continue to increase. Children are at high risk as blood pressures and stress-induced hormones levels have noticed to be elevated in children grown in noisy environments.

39.4.6 Disturbances in Mental Health

Noise pollution may cause or contribute to the following adverse effects: stress, nervousness, anxiety, nausea, emotional instability, changes in mood, headache, argumentativeness, sexual impotence, neurosis, increase in social conflicts, hysteria, and psychosis. Noise levels above 80 dB are associated with both an increase in aggressiveness and a decrease in helpful behavior to others. Autistic individuals or patients of Autism Spectrum Disorder (ASD) are generally more sensitive to noise pollution and show hyperacusis, that is a disorder in which a individual have an abnormal sensitivity to sound and react with syndrome of fear and anxiety, and uneasiness in noisy environment which make them to avoid environment with of high sound, results in their separation from community, that negatively affect their quality of life.

39.5 Effects of Noise Pollution on Animal Health

Animal are very sensitive to sound and noise impart direct effects like reproductive physiology or energy consumption as well as indirect effect on dynamics of population by changes in habitat use, parental care courtship and mating,. In animals, noise pollution can cause more severe consequences in terms of increase the danger to life by preventing predator or prey detection and evasion, affecting reproduction and navigation, along with contribute to permanent hearing loss. Aquatic life like water animal also are not left with deleterious effect of noise pollution which is interpreted by number of research on impact of noise on marine animals particularly in mammals, and fishes. This shift has been noticed in the past few years, as scientists are conducting studies on invertebrates and their responses to anthropogenic sounds in the marine environment. A variation in the complexity of their sensory systems between different living systems help scientists to understand range of impact of anthropogenic noise on living organisms with different characteristics (Kershaw 2006).

Farmed animal are exposed to noises produced in animal houses by various sources of noise like routine activities like opening and closing doors, technical devices, push carts, changing pens, washers, workers talk, feed dispensing, mechanical ventilation, animal activities such as climbing and chewing and their vocalizations. In animal houses the sources of noise pollution with more than tolerable threshold, includes feeding (104–115 dB), feed mixing (88–93 dB), high-pressure cleaning (105 dB), and mating (94–115 dB) (Venglovský et al. 2007). In slaughterhouses the noise intensity to which animals and poultry are exposed during slaughter is marginally high, with the range of 80–100 dB (Chloupek et al. 2009). Cattle can hear high-frequency sounds much better in comparison to humans, their high-frequency hearing limit is much higher ie 37 kHz, compared to humans who have only 18 kHz limit (Heffner 1998). In cattle the threshold of noise pollution which may cause discomfort was noted at 90–100 dB, with possible physical damage to the ear may be seen at 110 dB. Auditory range for cattle is 25 Hz to 35 kHz, but they can also detect lower pitched sounds in comparison to other farm animal species. Even in cattle the breed variation indicate that dairy breeds are more sensitive to higher volume than beef breeds. Sheep has auditory range of 125 Hz to 40 kHz with having most sensitivity around 7 kHz (Heffner 1998). The auditory range of pigs is 55 Hz to 40 kHz with more sense of hearing in the range 500 Hz to 16 kHz, particularly at 8 kHz. Although sound present in the environment and anthropogenic noises have different frequency and amplitude they can easily be differentiated. Animals communicate with each other by producing various type of sounds for different purposes of life like for reproduction, navigation, or to alert others from prey or predators. Noises interfere with detection of communicating sounds, affecting overall living of animals particularly wild animals. Almost every species of animals, birds, mammals, amphibians, reptiles, fishes, and invertebrates are affected by noise pollution. The significant morbidity seen as a result of effect of noise pollution is decline in reproduction due not able to find mates and more mortality because of lack of communication and reduced predator detection. Noise can reach undisturbed habitats and can affect the survivability and propensity of different wildlife species (Sordello et al. 2019).

Many birds like European robins habituating in urban environments have been observed to sing at night particularly at more noisy places during the day, suggesting that it may be because of comparable quieter nights in which their sound can clearly be propagated through the environment. High daytime noise is a stronger predictable factor for nocturnal singing than the night-time light pollution. Anthropogenic noise also affects the eco distribution of birds and been noticed for reduced the species richness of birds in Neotropical urban parks (Perillo et al. 2017). Anthropogenic noise also affects the acoustic signals and communication signals in some insects and other animals for example male grasshoppers produce a courtship song to attract female mating partner and in response they produce acoustic signals that is low in amplitude and frequency. However some research has found that noise is affecting this process of mating call. Similarly adverse effect of noise is also seen in sound-producing marine invertebrate processes like behavioral plasticity, behavior perturbation and shifts in population level. Noise producing vehicles like boat have been shown to affect the reproductive efficacy of the sea animals such as embryonic development and survivability of the sea hare. Anthropogenic noise can alter conditions in the environment that have a negative effect on invertebrate survival (Ryan et al. 2016). Although embryos can adapt to normal changes in their environment, evidence suggests they are not well adapted to endure the negative effects of noise pollution. Studies have been conducted on the sea hare to determine the effects of boat noise on the early stages of life and the development of embryos (Schwela 2021). Researchers have studied sea hares from the lagoon of Moorea Island, French Polynesia.

In the study, recordings of boat noise were made by using a hydrophone. In addition, recordings of ambient noise were made that did not contain boat noise. In contrast to ambient noise playbacks, mollusks exposed to boat noise playbacks had a 21% reduction in embryonic development (Sordello et al. 2019). Additionally, newly hatched larvae experienced an increased mortality rate of 22% when exposed to boat noise playbacks.

According to Geber (1966) noise is received by the mother's ear, the different brain cells integrate the signals. The hypothalamus and the hypophysis are activated; the adrenal cortex and medulla are stimulated and secrete their respective hormones (Venglovský et al. 2007). The uterine blood flow, gas-interchange, nutrition and interchange of waste products between fetus and mother are decreased (Sordello et al. 2019). Neural and neuroendocrine systems are possible mechanisms for the effect of noise on feed efficiency. Sound emission at the frequency of 2 kHz in noise of 75 dB, 85 dB, and 95 dB was found to contribute to appetite reduction of animals (Cwynar et al. 2011). Unexpected high intensity noise (above 110 dB), such as low altitude jet aircraft overflights at milking time could reduce effectiveness of the milk ejection reflex, decrease efficiency of milk removal, increase residual milk, and lead to overall reduction in milk yield (Sordello et al. 2019). Noise seems to affect adversely the productive performance of the birds. When poultry are transported to intermittent loud noise, rate of laying eggs and growth rate were decreased and mortality increased (Ryan et al. 2016). Egg productivity was affected at exposure levels as high as 120–130 dB. Noise at 90 dB seemed not to affect productivity and egg quality of laying hens (Purves et al. 2001).

Noise has been demonstrated to induce a variety of physiological changes in mammals, such as changes in the cardiovascular homeostasis and in the secretion of hormones through hearing impulses which are given to the brain stem and the hypothalamus (Perillo et al. 2017). From formatioreticularis the sympathetic nervous system is influenced via the hypophysis, adrenocorticotropic hormone (ACTH), and thyroid-stimulating hormone (TSH) the hypothalamus gives signals to the adrenal medulla and the thyroid gland (Natarajan et al. 2023). The parasympathetic nervous system is also influenced and has a mainly reversed effect compared to the sympathetic nervous system (Musiek et al. 2017). Noise may be a potential stressor causing the organism to react in farm animal husbandry. High noise exposure has also been reported to cause cellular effects. Loud sound is well known for adverse effects on blood pressure and heart rate in humans and animals (Musiek et al. 2017). The most obvious effect is a general stress reaction with higher secretion of ACTH giving an increase of adrenocortical hormones in the blood (Menkiti and Agunwamba 2015). Other effects are sleep disturbances, changes in the glucose metabolism of the liver, changes in the enzymatic activity of the kidneys, an increase of eosinophils percentage in blood, and immunosuppression. Noise intensities of 115 dB were effective in interrupting brooding in hens. Acute noise exposures at 80 and 100 dB in broilers increased corticosterone level after 10 minutes of exposure (Kileny et al. 2021). Noise treatment of both 70 and 80 dB intensities also resulted in a significant elevation of basophil granulocytes. The degree of animal reaction varied with species of animal, age and individual. The character of the behavior reactions observed that domestic animals experience from excessive noise is disturbing their well being (Khoza-Shangase et al. 2020). An understanding of animal response to helicopters or aircrafts is important in predicting the consequences of the disturbance on the ecology, welfare and behavior of exposed free kept farming or wildlife animals. Animals were also reported to tend to be more active in the morning periods than in the afternoon periods tested, which might be related to the arrival of staff and beginning of the working day with a general increase in noise levels (Kalisa et al. 2022). Horses are also very sensitive to noise. Start of noise stimuls horses turned their heads and directed their ears towards the source and then immediately turned their ears away. Sudden, novel sounds seem to affect cattle behavior more than continuous high noise (Chloupek et al. 2009). When the aircraft was 152 m above ground level, the cattle ran for less than 10 m and resumed normal activity within one minute. Unexpected high intensity noise, such as low altitude jet aircraft overflights (above 110 dB), at milking parlor could provoke adverse behavior, such as kicking or stomping (Kalisa et al. 2022). The noise threshold expected to cause a behavioral response by cattle is 85–90 dB. Heifers exposed to the noise from milking parlor show escape type behaviors, consistent with a fear response (Kileny et al. 2021). Noise in the milking facility has direct implications for on-farm efficiency related to improving cow behavior and human-animal interactions (Münzel et al. 2018).

39.6 Control of Noise Pollution

Noise pollution can be effectively controlled by two means includes prevention at the receivers end and control by suppression of noise at source level itself. At receiver's end like for people working in noisy installations, ear-protection aids like headphones, ear-plugs, noise helmets, ear-muffs, etc. can be provided to reduce occupational related exposure. The suppression of noise at source level can be implemented by designing and fabricating the insand using quieter machines to replace the noisy ones. Proper lubrication and better maintenance of machines. Installing noisy machines in sound proof chambers. Covering noise-producing machine parts with sound-absorbing materials to check noise production. Reducing the noise produced from a vibrating machine by vibration damping i.e. making a layer of damping material (rubber, neoprene, cork or plastic) beneath the machine. Using silencers to control noise from automobiles, ducts, exhausts etc. and convey systems with ends opening into the atmosphere. Using glass wool or mineral wool covered with a sheet of perforated metal for the purpose of mechanical protection. Acoustic Zoning: Increased distance between source and receiver by zoning of noisy industrial areas, bus terminals and railway stations, aerodromes etc. away from the residential areas would go a long way in minimizing noise pollution. There should be silence zones near the residential areas, educational institutions and above all, near hospitals. Sound insulation can be utilized in the places involve process of continuous noise production. As sound can travels through the small spaces of cracks remain in-between the door and the wall and these spaces can be filled with the sound absorbing material and fitting the windows with double or triple panes of glass. Acoustical material like acoustic tiles, perforated plywood and hair felt etc. can be fixed on the ceilings, walls, floors to reduce noise. Acoustic ceiling tiles are commonly used to minimize the echo in a noisy room in an effective and easy way. Acoustic ceiling tiles are a type of ceiling improvement that are specifically designed to improve the acoustics of room. They are commonly used in commercial and residential spaces such as sound proof recording rooms, offices, hospitals, and theatres etc. tress and plant are very good absorbents of noise, so planting green trees on road side ways around public places will help in sound absorption to a considerable extent and reduce the deleterious effects. Strict enforcement of legislation for noise pollution should be followed in areas of menace of noise pollution. Loudspeakers and amplifiers uses should be minimum especially near silence zones along with banning pressure horns in automobiles. Personal protective equipment's for sound protection like wear of ear plugs, noise helmets or ear muffs will be helpful considerably to people occupationally involved in industries having noisy areas. People sensitive to noise should maintain distance from high noise areas like industrial area, railway stations, bus terminals, and make their residential area away from these areas. Noise making machine can be installed with specialized sound absorbents like rubber, plastic, glass wool, mineral oil, wool cork or neoprene along with soundproof chambers which can effectively reduce the noise.

References

ANSI (American National Standards Institute) (1991). American national standard: specification for personal noise dosimeters. New York: American National Standards Institute, Inc., ANSI S1.25-1991; ASA 98-1991. Available at https://webstore.ansi.org/preview-pages/ASA/preview_ANSI+ASA+S1.25-1991+(R2017).pdf

Basner, M., Babisch, W., Davis, A. et al. (2014). Auditory and non-auditory effects of noise on health. *The lancet 383* (9925): 1325–1332.

Berglund, B., Lindvall, T., and Schwela, D.H. (1999). *Guidelines for Community Noise*. Geneva: WHO.

Chloupek, P., Voslářová, E., Chloupek, J. et al. (2009). Stress in broiler chickens due to acute noise exposure. *Acta Veterinaria Brno 78* (1): 93–98.

Cwynar, P. and Kolacz, R., Köfer, J., Schobesberger, H. (2011). Animal hygiene and sustainable livestock production. *Proceedings of the XVth International Congress of the International Society for Animal Hygiene*, pp. 1059–1061, Vienna, Austria (3–7 July 2011), Volume 3. Tribun EU.

Geber, W. (1966). Maternal influence on fetal cardiovascular system in sheep, dog and rabbit. *American Journal of Physiology* 202: 653–660.

Heffner, H.E. (1998). Auditory awareness. *Applied Animal Behaviour Science 57* (3–4): 259–268.

Kalisa, E., Irankunda, E., Rugengamanzi, E., and Amani, M. (2022). Noise levels associated with urban land use types in Kigali, Rwanda. *Heliyon 8* (9): e10653.

Kershaw, F. (2006). Noise seriously impacts marine invertebrates. New Science.

Khoza-Shangase, K., Moroe, N.F., and Edwards, A. (2020). Occupational hearing loss in Africa: an interdisciplinary view of the current status. *The South African Journal of Communication Disorders* 67: e1–e3.

Kileny, P.R., Zwolan, T.A., Slager, H.K. et al. (2021). Diagnostic audiology and electrophysiologic assessment of hearing. In: *Cummings Otolaryngology: Head and Neck Surgery*, 7e (ed. P.W. Flint, B.H. Haughey, and V.J. Lund), 2021–2041. Elsevier.

Menkiti, N.U. and Agunwamba, J.C. (2015). Assessment of noise pollution from electricity generators in a high-density residential area. *African Journal of Science, Technology, Innovation and Development 7* (4): 306–312.

Münzel, T., Schmidt, F.P., Steven, S. et al. (2018). Environmental noise and the cardiovascular system. *Journal of the American College of Cardiology 71* (6): 688–697.

Musiek, F.E., Shinn, J., Chermak, G.D., and Bamiou, D.E. (2017). Perspectives on the pure-tone audiogram. *Journal of the American Academy of Audiology 28* (07): 655–671.

Natarajan, N., Batts, S., and Stankovic, K.M. (2023). Noise-induced hearing loss. *Journal of Clinical Medicine 12* (6): 2347.

Nightingale, F. (1859). Notes on nursing: what it is, and what it is not (p. 79). Retrieved from https://archive.org/details/NotesOnNursingByFlorenceNightingale/page/n29

Occupational Safety and Health Administration (OSHA) (1996). OSHA Technical Manual (OTM) Section III: Chapter 5 https://www.osha.gov/otm/section-3-health-hazards/chapter-5

Perillo, A., Mazzoni, L.G., Passos, L.F. et al. (2017). Anthropogenic noise reduces bird species richness and diversity in urban parks. *Ibis 159* (3): 638–646.

Purves, D., Augustine, G., and Fitzpatrick, D. (2001). The Audible Spectrum. In: *Neuroscience*, 2e. Sunderland, MA: Sinauer Associates.

Ryan, A.F., Kujawa, S.G., Hammill, T. et al. (2016). Temporary and permanent noise-induced threshold shifts: a review of basic and clinical observations. *Otology and Neurotology 37*: e271–e275.

Schwela, D. (2021). Environmental noise challenges and policies in low-and middle-income countries. *South Florida Journal of Health 2* (1): 26–45.

Sordello, R., Flamerie De Lachapelle, F., Livoreil, B., and Vanpeene, S. (2019). Evidence of the environmental impact of noise pollution on biodiversity: a systematic map protocol. *Environmental Evidence 8* (1): 1–7.

Venglovský, J., Sasakova, N., Vargova, M. et al. (2007). *Noise in the animal housing environment*, 995–999. Tartu, Estonia: ISAH.

World Health Organization (1991). Report of the Informal Working Group on Prevention of Deafness and Hearing Impairment Programme Planning, Geneva, 18–21 June 1991. Available online: https://apps.who.int/iris/handle/10665/58839

40

Environmental Contamination and Food Chain Bioaccumulation

Kaushik Satyaprakash[1], Annada Das[2], Dipanwita Bhattacharya[1], and Souti Prasad Sarkhel[1]

[1] Faculty of Veterinary and Animal Sciences, Institute of Agricultural Sciences, Banaras Hindu University, Mirzapur, India
[2] Department of Livestock Products Technology, West Bengal University of Animal and Fishery Sciences, Kolkata, India

40.1 Introduction

Population explosion, high demand for food, rapid industrialization and urbanization coupled with enormous anthropogenic activities including indiscriminate use of chemicals have led to contamination of the environment. Environmental contamination refers to "pollution," where the introduction of undesirable substances damages the environment and exerts deleterious effects on ecosystems and human health (Ali and Khan 2017; Hashem et al. 2017). Human exposure and bioaccumulation of environmental contaminants have accelerated since the 1940s and are continuously worsening over the years (Ali et al. 2019; Khan et al. 2004). The Chernobyl nuclear disaster in 1986 in Ukraine, Deepwater Horizon Oil spill in 2010 in the Gulf of Mexico, Minamata disease in the 1950s in Japan involving methyl mercury poisoning, the Bhopal tragedy due to methyl isocyanate (MIC) gas leak in 1984 and the alarming decline in the vulture population in South Asia in the 1990s because of diclofenac use in livestock are some of the many notorious examples highlighting the devastating consequences of environmental contaminants.

Environmental contaminants can be defined as chemical substances that occur in the environment above permissible limits and pose a potential health risk to living beings (Mandaric et al. 2016). In addition to the traditional contaminants, there is concern about "emerging contaminants" including novel pharmaceuticals, personal care products, micro- and nanoplastics, and nanomaterials (Mandaric et al. 2016; Castillo-Zacarías et al. 2021; Margenat et al. 2019; Couto et al. 2022). These contaminants belong to numerous groups including heavy metals/metalloids, persistent organic pollutants (POPs) (e.g., polycyclic aromatic hydrocarbons [PAHs], aldrin, dieldrin, chlordane, hexachlorobenzene [HCB], polychlorinated biphenyls [PCBs], dichlorodiphenyltrichloroethane [DDT], perfluorinated compounds [PFCs]), pharmaceuticals and personal care products (PPCPs), radioactive elements, electronic wastes, microplastics (MPs), nanoparticles (NPs), etc. (Mann et al. 2011; Thompson and Darwish 2019; Sun et al. 2020).

Some of these contaminants occur naturally in the environment and enter the food chain whilst others are produced from anthropogenic activities. These contaminants ultimately contaminate food (crops, livestock, and seafood) (da Araújo et al. 2016; Thompson et al. 2018; Mahmood and Malik 2014) and water (Jin et al. 2003; Enault et al. 2015), thereby exerting adverse effects on public health. Due to the nature of contamination, some foods are contaminated more than others, which may be due to their varying exposure to contaminants or differences in uptake mechanism from the environment (Price et al. 2014; Stasinos et al. 2014). Continuous exposure to toxic contaminants can lead to chronic health problems like cancer, nervous disorders, hormonal imbalances, digestive dysfunction, and mutations (Ubaid ur Rahman et al. 2021; Nieder and Benbi 2022).

Human health risk assessment data are available only after analysis of many food items including foods of plant origin, livestock origin , fishes, and seafoods (Thompson and Darwish 2019). There is a lack of awareness among consumers regarding environmental contaminants, their food chain bioaccumulation and possible adverse health effects. Conducting regular risk assessment studies, monitoring contamination levels, implementation of control measures such as bioremediation and consideration of sociopolitical implications including enactment of policies for mitigation of environmental contaminants will aid in providing safer food globally.

Epidemiology and Environmental Hygiene in Veterinary Public Health, First Edition. Edited by Tanmoy Rana.
© 2025 John Wiley & Sons, Inc. Published 2025 by John Wiley & Sons, Inc.

This chapter explores the intricate relationship between the environmental contamination process, biotransfer, bioaccumulation and biomagnification of contaminants in food chain, and their implications for human and ecological health. It also provides a holistic understanding about the various sources and types of contaminants, pathways of bioaccumulation, deleterious consequences, risk assessment, and bioremediation measures.

40.2 Sources of Environmental Contaminants

The potentially toxic organic and inorganic environmental contaminants originate from a wide range of sources including agricultural practices, industrial activities, improper waste disposal, urbanization, rampant and injudicious use of pharmaceuticals, personal care products, pesticides, microplastics, nanoparticles, electronic gadgets, etc. (Figure 40.1). Industries are the sources of many toxic chemicals, heavy metals and trace elements, volatile organic compounds (VOCs), and POPs (Hashem et al. 2017; Price et al. 2014; Khan et al. 2015). Agricultural practices lead to release of contaminants like pesticides (organochlorines, organophosphorus, carbamates, etc.) and fertilizers, thus contaminating human food (Thompson and Darwish 2019; Sun et al. 2020; Yan et al. 2019; Liu et al. 2019). Indiscriminate drug use (antibiotics, hormones, antidepressants, etc.) in humans and animals further contaminates the food chain ecosystem and ultimately affects public health (Castillo-Zacarías et al. 2021; Koch et al. 2021; Leibson et al. 2018). Improper waste disposal substantially contaminates water bodies, crop fields, groundwater, soil, and air (Sayo et al. 2020; Hsieh et al. 2019). Urban farms and gardens are also the sources of environmental contaminants (Margenat et al. 2019; Taylor et al. 2021; Kohrman and Chamberlain 2014). Additionally, food packaging materials are the major sources of microplastics (Van Raamsdonk et al. 2020; Miller et al. 2020).

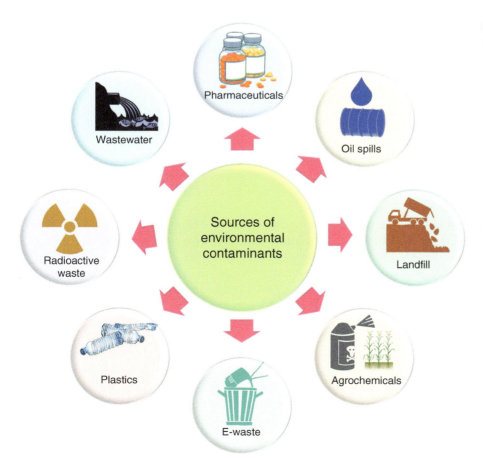

Figure 40.1 Sources of environmental contaminants.

40.3 Types of Environmental Contaminants

40.3.1 Heavy Metals/Metalloids

The "heavy metals or metalloids (semimetals)," better known as "potentially toxic elements" (PTEs), are defined as "the naturally occurring metals/metalloids with atomic number greater than 20 and density greater than 5g/cm^3, that have been associated with contamination and potential ecotoxicity" (Duffus 2002; Ali and Khan 2018; Pourret and Hursthouse 2019). Mining (gold, iron mining, etc.) and industrial processing for extraction of mineral resources and their applications for industrial and economic development have led to most heavy metal contaminations in food chain ecosystems (Pareja-Carrera et al. 2014; Nouri and Haddioui 2016; Xiao et al. 2017). The most hazardous heavy metal and metalloids include Cr, Ni, Co, Cu, Zn, Cd, Pb, Hg, and As (Ali and Khan 2018). Being persistent pollutants, heavy metals accumulate in the environment and the trophic transfer of these elements results in several lethal effects on animal and human health.

40.3.2 Persistent Organic Pollutants (POPs)

The POPs, sometimes known as "forever chemicals," are synthetic organic chemicals that persist in the environment as they are often resistant to chemical, biological, and photolytic degradatio and possess the ability to be biotransported and biomagnified across the food chain and bioaccumulate in human and animal tissues (Olisah et al. 2021; Krithiga et al. 2022). Some of the POPs are used in industry, some are used as pesticides in the agriculture sector, and some are byproducts of combustion processes.

The POPs include pesticides and insecticides like aldrin, dieldrin, chlordane, DDT, hexachlorocyclohexane (HCH), etc., industrial chemicals like HCB, PCBs, PFCs, etc. and unintended byproducts like PAHs, dibenzodioxins, dibenzofurans, etc. (Thompson and Darwish 2019; Olisah et al. 2021). Compounds under POPs are classed as PBTs (persistent, bioaccumulative, toxic) or TOMPs (toxic organic micropollutants) (Kumari et al. 2021). The effect of POPs on human and environmental health was discussed at the Stockholm Convention on POPs at Stockholm, Sweden, in 2001 (Fiedler and Sadia 2021; Fiedler et al. 2023) which was ratified by 152 countries and came into force from May 17, 2004. The POPs typically are halogenated compounds with high lipid solubility which enhances their bioaccumulation in fatty tissues. Some POPs are classified as endocrine-disrupting compounds (EDCs) and are carcinogenic, while others have lethal effects on the immune , reproductive , nervous , digestive, and respiratory systems (Thompson and Darwish 2019; Olisah et al. 2021).

40.3.3 Pharmaceuticals and Personal Care Products (PPCPs)

The PPCPs may include a wide range of emerging contaminants (ECs) that contaminate the environment and enter the food chain, thereby exerting adverse health effects even at very low doses (Couto et al. 2022; Hena et al. 2020). The pharmaceuticals are mostly human and veterinary drugs including antibiotics, antimicrobials, antiinflammatory drugs, cytostatic drugs, beta-blockers, blood lipid regulators, anticonvulsants, hormones, X-ray contrast media, UV filters, etc. Chemicals are used in soaps, shampoos, conditioners, deodorants, toothpastes, sunscreens, insect repellants, body lotions, food preservatives, etc. (Keerthanan et al. 2021; Liu et al. 2020). In 2007, a few common PPCPs including diclofenac, ibuprofen, iopamidol, musk, carbamazepine, clofibric acid, triclosan, and phthalates were added to the European Union's list of priority substances to be removed from surface water (Hena et al. 2020; Ebele et al. 2017). Besides the real threat of inducing antimicrobial resistance, some PPCPs act as carcinogens and EDCs (Thompson and Darwish 2019; Hena et al. 2020).

40.3.4 Radionuclides

Anthropogenic activities including use of nuclear weapons and accidental leakage from nuclear reactors have resulted in environmental contamination by radioactive wastes and increased human exposures over the past years. Effluents from the nuclear industry contain radioactive elements like potassium (^{40}K), uranium (^{238}U, ^{235}U), thorium (^{232}Th), cesium (^{137}Cs), and actinide compounds (Adeola et al 2022; Adebiyi et al. 2021). After a tsunami damaged the nuclear plant in Fukushima, Japan, in 2011, radioactive elements were detected in food and water samples above permissible levels (Hamada et al. 2012). Radionuclides have also been detected in food and water sources in India, Switzerland, and the Balkans (Thompson and Darwish 2019). Short-term and low levels of human exposure to radioactive wastes cause skin allergy, nausea, diarrhea, vomiting, and alopecia. Long-term human exposure to high-level radioactive elements may lead to mutations causing irreparable damage to DNA, skin, lung and thyroid cancers, teratogenic defects, etc.

The tragic incidents in Hiroshima and Nagasaki during World War II are the best examples of the ill effects of radiation exposure, where children born with physical and mental abnormalities due to genetic mutations are still observed even after 75 years (Natarajan et al. 2020).

40.3.5 Electronic Wastes

"Electronic waste (e-waste)" is the term used for unused and discarded electronic or electrical devices like computers, mobile phones, and household appliances (air conditioners, refrigerators, televisions, radio) (Quan et al. 2014). E-wastes produce a huge quantity of environmental pollutants including POPs, heavy metals, plastics, rubber, as well as producing ceramics, glass, cement and some valuable metals (copper, iron, silver, gold, and platinum) (Akram et al. 2019; Han et al. 2019). Developed countries like USA and China produce the maximum e-waste every year, but 80% of e-wastes are transported to developing Asian countries for recycling (Akram et al. 2019; Wu et al. 2008). Improper dumping and crude recycling of e-wastes results in the release of associated pollutants into the environment which ultimately enter the food chain (Akram et al. 2019; Han et al. 2019).

40.3.6 Plastics

Plastic wastes present in the environment are classed as macroplastics (>2 cm size), mesoplastics (0.5–2 cm size), microplastics (<5 mm size), and nanoplastics (<100 nm) (Hu et al. 2022; Krause et al. 2021). Microplastics are emerging as potential environmental pollutants with severe adverse effects on human and animal health. Researchers have identified concentrations of MPs in seafood, fish, milk, vegetables, honey, salt, sugar, drinking water, and breast milk as a consequence of environmental contamination (Van Raamsdonk et al. 2020). Packaging materials and bottled water are considered as the major sources for oral exposure to plastic contaminants (Thompson and Darwish 2019; Van Raamsdonk et al. 2020).

The different types of polymers grouped under plastics are polyethylene (PE), polypropylene (PP), polyvinyl chloride (PVC), polystyrene (PS), polyamide (nylon), polyesters, and polyethylene terephthalate (PET). PE and PP are the most common types of environmental pollutants (Hu et al. 2022).

Depending on the source, plastic contaminants can be classified as primary (manufactured) and secondary. Primary plastics are man-made plastics including microbeads used in products like toiletries, equipment, cosmetics, detergents, and paints, and are discharged to the environment through domestic sewage. Secondary plastics are formed by the degradation of larger plastic particles through physical, microbial, and photochemical action and contribute the most as environmental contaminants (Sun et al. 2020; Krause et al. 2021). Additives from plastic manufacturing processes such as colorants, plasticizers (phthalates), catalysts, and stabilizers also have adverse effects on human health (Thompson and Darwish 2019; Hu et al. 2022). The MPs act as "Trojan horses" carrying other co-contaminants like heavy metals, POPs, pathogens, and nanomaterials (Zhao et al. 2023). The MPs pass the intestinal border and enter the systemic circulation, causing enterotoxicity, disturbing the gut microbiota and lipid metabolism, inducing cancer and oxidative stress (Van Raamsdonk et al. 2020).

40.3.7 Nanoparticles/Nanomaterials

Nanomaterials (NMs) exist naturally and/or can be intentionally or unintentionally produced from anthropogenic sources such as industrial activities (coating, paint, pesticides, pigment, additives, cosmetics), food preservation, bioremediation and scientific research into nanotechnology (Canesi et al. 2015; Saleh 2020). NPs can be defined as materials of 1–100 nm in at least one dimension. One-dimensional NPs include thin films, surfaces and coatings; nanotubes, nanowires and nanofibers are examples of two-dimensional NPs whereas three-dimensional NPs include fullerenes, quantum dots, and dendrimers. The NPs emerging as environmental pollutants are mostly metal oxide based (oxides of silver, gold, iron, titanium, or zinc) and carbon based (fullerene nanotubes) (Saleh 2020). NPs also act as "Trojan horses" carrying other co-contaminants like heavy metals, POPs, pathogens, and microplastics and exert many ecotoxic effects on living organisms (Canesi et al. 2015). The possible adverse effects of NPs include death, cytotoxicity, growth inhibition, disturbed metabolism, and oxidative stress (Davarpanah and Guilhermino 2019).

40.4 Food Chain Bioaccumulation of Environmental Contaminants

Important terminologies associated with bioaccumulation of environmental contaminants are given below.

- *Bioaccumulation* is the gradual accumulation of substances, such as pesticides or other heavy metals, in an organism obtained from the ambient abiotic environment and food at a rate faster than that at which it can be lost by excretion or catabolism. It includes the intake of chemicals by all possible means, including contact, respiration, and ingestion (Yan et al. 2019; Ugulu et al. 2021; Yarsan and Yipel 2013).

$$Bioaccumulation = Bioconcentration + trophic\ transfer - \left(Depuration + biodilution\right)$$

- *Bioconcentration* is the uptake and retention of a substance in an organism entirely by respiration from water in aquatic ecosystems or from air in terrestrial ecosystems (Ali and Khan 2019).
- *Biomagnification* refers to increase in the concentration of a contaminant along the successive trophic level in a food chain. These will reach harmful concentrations at higher trophic levels among top predators (Ali et al. 2019; Sun et al. 2020).
- *Biodilution* is the decrease in the concentration of a contaminant as it progresses up the food chain (Sun et al. 2020).
- *Trophic transfer* is the progress of a contaminant along the food chain from one trophic level to the next. It is also called biotransference (Sun et al. 2020; Ali and Khan 2019).
- *Depuration* is the elimination of chemical contaminant from the organism's body (Mortimer et al. 2021).
- *Trophodynamics* is the study of trophic transfer of contaminants in a food chain (Qadeer et al. 2019).

40.4.1 Quantification of Trophic Transfer of Heavy Metals

Some of the quantitative terms used to quantify the trophic transfer of heavy metals are given below.

- *Trophic transfer factor (TTF)*: the ratio of concentration of heavy metal in an organism's tissue to that in the organism's food (DeForest et al. 2007).

$$TTF = \frac{Metal\ concentration\ in\ organism's\ tissue}{Metal\ concentration\ in\ organism's\ food}$$

- *Transfer factor (TF)*: the ratio of concentration of heavy metal in plant tissue to that in the soil (Cui et al. 2004). In case of plants (especially terrestrial plants), the heavy metals are transferred mostly from the soil.

$$TF = \frac{Metal\ concentration\ in\ plant's\ tissue}{Metal\ concentration\ in\ soil}$$

- *Accumulation factor (AF)*: the ratio of concentration of heavy metal in a plant's edible part to that in the soil (Balkhair and Ashraf 2016).

$$AF = \frac{Metal\ concentration\ in\ plant\ edible\ part}{Metal\ concentration\ in\ soil}$$

- *Bioaccumulation factor (BAF)*: the ratio of concentration of heavy metal in an organism's tissue to that in the abiotic medium (Golam Mortuza and Al-Misned 2015). In case of animals, the heavy metals are transferred from both the abiotic and biotic environment and also from the animal's diet.

$$BAF = \frac{Metal\ concentration\ in\ organism's\ tissue}{Metal\ concentration\ in\ abiotic\ medium}$$

- *Biomagnification factor (BMF)*: the ratio of concentration of heavy metal in an organism to that in the organism's diet (Yarsan and Yipel 2013).

$$BMF = \frac{Metal\ concentration\ in\ organism}{Metal\ concentration\ in\ organism's\ diet}$$

- **Trophic magnification factor (TMF)**: calculated from the slope of logarithmically transformed metal concentrations in organisms plotted against the trophic levels of the organisms in the food web (Conder et al. 2012). TMF value greater than 1 for a contaminant indicates its biomagnification in the given food chain (Ali and Khan 2019).

40.4.2 Pathways of Bioaccumulation

Bioaccumulation occurs through various pathways as pollutants enter the food chain and subsequently accumulate at higher trophic levels. In aquatic ecosystems, contaminants enter natural water sources through runoffs, industrial discharges, and domestic sewage, leading to their atmospheric deposition. The phytoplankton absorb these contaminants, which are subsequently transferred to zooplankton, fish, and other higher organisms. In terrestrial ecosystems, contaminants may be taken up by plants through soil or water absorption and transferred to herbivores and then to carnivores (Khan et al. 2015; Yan et al. 2019; Liu et al. 2019; Ugulu et al. 2021).

Examples of the pathway of bioaccumulation and biomagnification of environmental pollutants in food chains are given below.

40.4.2.1 Minamata Disease – The Case of Mercury Poisoning in Japan

Mercury is a highly toxic metal because it damages the central nervous systems of humans and animals. The Chisso Co. Ltd., a petrochemical and plastic manufacturing company, used mercury as a catalyst in vinyl chloride manufacture. It released methyl mercury (MeHg), a heavy metal waste, into the sea for many years in the 1950s. The mercury compounds bioaccumulated and biomagnified in shellfish and fish in the surrounding water of Minamata Bay and Shiranui Sea for decades.

The inhabitants of the seaside town of Minamata, on Kyushu Island in Japan, observed strange behavior in fishes, birds, cats, and other animals. It was noticed that the cats would exhibit nervous tremors, scream and dance, hence called as "dancing cat fever." Subsequently, the people in that area also experienced syndromes including ataxia, numbness, muscle weakness, impaired vision and speech, hearing damage and in extreme cases paralysis, coma, and death within weeks of symptom onset. The congenital form of the disease also affected fetuses. It is believed that around 5000 people died and perhaps 50 000 people were poisoned by MeHg. This is recognized as Minamata disease, a severe consequence of mercury poisoning (Szynkowska et al. 2017; Budnik and Casteleyn 2019; Yoshino et al. 2020).

In aquatic environments inorganic mercury can be converted through biogeochemical interaction to highly toxic MeHg which is more easily absorbed into the body than inorganic mercury. MeHg is taken up from the water and sediments by plankton, which are subsequently consumed by small fishes over time. Large predatory fishes consume many small fishes. Mercury is tightly bound to the sulfhydryl group of amino acids in proteins (Ruus et al. 2015) and goes on accumulating in large fishes. Consumption of those fishes by humans or other fish-eating animals will lead to bioaccumulation of MeHg in their body tissues. It can cross the blood–brain barrier and placental barrier, leading to impaired reproduction and neurological development (Takahashi et al. 2017).

40.4.2.2 Bioaccumulation and Biomagnification of DDT in an Aquatic Ecosystem

When a water source is sprayed with DDT to control mosquitoes, small amounts of DDT accumulate in the cells of microscopic aquatic organisms, called plankton. Filter-feeders like clams and certain fishes consume the plankton, ingesting the accumulated DDT. The concentration of DDT can be up to 10 times higher in clams compared to the plankton they consume. This bioconcentration process continues up the food chain, leading to higher levels of DDT in organisms at each trophic level. This is because the consumers at each successive trophic level consume more than the preceding ones to fulfill the energy requirement, so DDT goes on accumulating at successive trophic levels at higher concentration. Fish-eating birds can accumulate DDT up to 25 ppm as shown in Figure 40.2 (Skarphedinsdottir et al. 2010; Hellou et al. 2013). A high concentration of DDT disturbs calcium metabolism in birds, leading to thinning of eggshells and their premature breakage which may result in a decline in the bird population (Pandya 2018).

Figure 40.2 Biomagnification of DDT in an aquatic food chain.

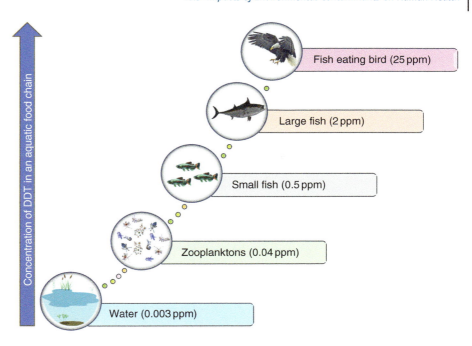

DDT (1,1,1-trichloro-2,2-bis(p-chlorophenyl) ethane) and its primary metabolite DDE (1,1-dichloro-2,2-bis(p-chlorophenyl) ethane) accumulate in adipose tissue (Ishikawa et al. 2015). DDT metabolism occurs mainly in the liver. The half-life of DDE in tissues is longer than that of DDT, hence DDT is cleared from the body more rapidly than DDE. DDT undergoes dechlorination to form DDE or DDD (1,1-dichloro-2,2-bis(p-chlorophenyl) ethylene). This DDD undergoes dechlorination to form DDMU (1-chloro-2,2-bis(p-chlorophenyl) ethane) which further undergoes dechlorination and oxidation to form DDA (2,2-bis(p-chlorophenyl) acetic acid) that is readily excreted in urine as it is water soluble, unlike DDT or DDE (Figure 40.3) (Kirman et al. 2011).

40.5 Impacts of Environmental Contaminants on Human Health

The toxicity of environmental contaminants in an individual depends upon the dietary makeup, route of exposure, age, susceptibility to a particular contaminant, health condition, concentration and duration of exposure (Leibson et al. 2018; Vafeiadi et al. 2015). Vulnerable populations such as pregnant women, infants, older people, immune-deficient and diseased persons are at particularly high risk of toxic effects of environmental contaminants. Persistent human exposure to toxic contaminants through the food chain can lead to chronic health problems including cancer, nervous disorders, hormonal imbalances, digestive dysfunction, and mutations (Ubaid ur Rahman et al. 2021; Nieder and Benbi 2022) as shown in Table 40.1.

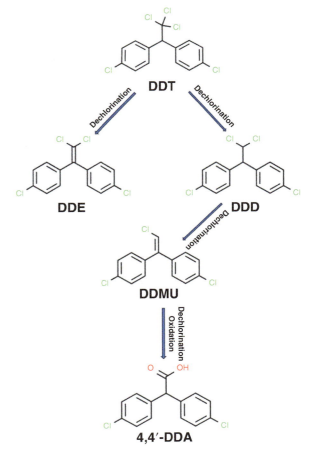

Figure 40.3 Metabolism of DDT. DDT, 1,1,1-trichloror-2,2-bis(p-chlorophenyl) ethane; DDE, 1,1-dichloro-2,2-bis(p-chlorophenyl) ethane; DDD, 1,1-dichloro-2,2-bis(p-chlorophenyl) ethylene; DDA, 2,2-bis(p-chlorophenyl) acetic acid; DDMU, 1-chloror-2,2-bis(p-chlorophenyl) ethane.

40 Environmental Contamination and Food Chain Bioaccumulation

Table 40.1 Possible human health effects of some common environmental contaminants.

Sl. No.	Name of contaminant	Possible human heath effect	References
A. Heavy metals			
1	Arsenic	Dermatological: diffused or spotted hyperpigmentation ("raindrop appearance"), hyperkeratosis, eczematoid lesions, warts, alopecia, gangrenous extremity ("blackfoot disease")	Singh et al. (2015), Mohammed Abdul et al. (2015), Sarkar and Paul (2016)
		GI system: gastroenteritis ("rice water diarrhea")	
		Carcinogenic: basal cell carcinoma, squamous cell carcinoma, lung and bladder cancer	
		Hepatic system: angiosarcoma, hepatomegaly, ascites	
		Cardiopulmonary: hypotension, cough, dyspnea, chest pain	
		Neurological: delirium, seizures, encephalopathy	
2	Lead	Dysfunction of kidney, reproductive system, liver Cardiovascular system	Balali-Mood et al. (2021), Wu et al. (2016), Rehman et al. (2018), Wani et al. (2015)
		Acute and chronic damage to CNS, reduction in cognitive development and intellectual performance	
		Inhibition of hemoglobin synthesis, anemia, high blood pressure	
		Gastrointestinal problems, anoxia, teratogenic effects	
3	Cadmium	Nausea, vomiting, abdominal cramps, muscle weakness	Kumar and Sharma (2019), Zwolak (2020), Genchi et al. (2020)
		Pulmonary effects (dyspnea, pulmonary edema, emphysema, bronchiolitis, alveolitis)	
		Renal tubular dysfunction	
		Cardiac failure, cerebrovascular infarction, osteoporosis, cataract, anosmia	
4	Mercury	Spontaneous abortion, congenital malformation, corrosive esophagitis, hematochezia, acrodynia, gingivitis, stomatitis, congenital malformation	Balali-Mood et al. (2021), Wu et al. (2016), Rehman et al. (2018)
5	Chromium	Allergic dermatitis, increased risk of lung, nasal, and sinus cancer	Balali-Mood et al. (2021)
6	Cobalt	Hearing and visual impairment	Bregnbak et al. (2015), Leyssens et al. (2017)
		Cardiomyopathy, cognitive defect, hypothyroidism, peripheral neuropathy	
B. Persistent organic pollutants			
1	Dieldrin	Linked to Parkinson disease, breast cancer, immunotoxic, neurotoxic with endocrine-disrupting capacity	Ighalo et al., (2022), Islam et al. (2018, 2022), Malhat et al. (2018)
2	Endrin	Neurotoxicity	Ighalo et al. (2022), Islam et al. (2018), Malhat et al. (2018)
3	Heptachlor	Carcinogenic	Islam et al. (2022), Tyagi et al. (2020)
4	Hexachlorobenzene (HCB)	Photosensitive skin lesions, colic, debilitation, porphyria turcica (a metabolic disorder)	Krithiga et al. (2022), Starek-Świechowicz et al. (2017)
5	Toxaphene	Carcinogenic	Carvalho (2017), Hassaan and El Nemr (2020)
6	Polychlorinated biphenyls (PCBs)	Reproductive failure, immunosuppression, developmental delays in children, pigmentation of nail and mucous membranes	Fernández-González et al. (2015), Gupta et al. (2018), Reddy et al. (2019)

Table 40.1 (Continued)

Sl. No.	Name of contaminant	Possible human heath effect	References
7	DDT	Reproductive failure, increased risk of cancer and diabetes, neurological diseases, endocrine disruption	Sifakis et al. (2017), Burgos-Aceves et al. (2021)
8	Dioxins	Carcinogenic, congenital birth defects, disturbances in mental and motor development, stillbirth	Bock (2017), Furue et al. (2021)
C.	Pharmaceuticals and personal care products (PPCPs)	Carcinogenic and endocrine-disrupting compounds (EDCs)	Thompson and Darwish (2019), Hena et al. (2020)
D.	Radioactive elements	Skin allergy, nausea, diarrhea, vomiting, alopecia, mutations causing irreparable damage to DNA, skin, lung and thyroid cancers, teratogenic defects, etc.	Adeola et al. (2022), Natarajan et al. (2020)
E.	Electronic wastes	Carcinogenic, neurotoxicity, hematological disorders	Quan et al. (2014), Akram et al. (2019)
F.	Microplastics and nanoplastics	Enterotoxicity, disturbance of gut microbiota, lipid metabolism, cancer and oxidative stress	Van Raamsdonk et al. (2020), Krause et al. (2021)
G.	Nanoparticles (NPs)	Cytotoxicity, growth inhibition, disturbed metabolism, oxidative stress, death	Canesi et al. (2015), Saleh (2020), Davarpanah and Guilhermino (2019)

40.6 Ecological Consequences

Environmental contaminants and their bioaccumulation have detrimental effects on ecosystems and biodiversity. These contaminants can disrupt reproductive cycles, impair immune systemsn and induce physiological abnormalities in plants and animals, leading to reduced biodiversity. Additionally, bioaccumulation and biomagnification of some toxic environmental contaminants in top predators of the food chain can have a cascading effect, affecting entire ecosystem dynamics (Chormare and Kumar 2022; Guarda et al. 2020).

40.7 Risk Assessment and Monitoring

Risk assessment and monitoring of environmental contaminants are effective processes in evaluating the potential risks posed by various pollutants to human health and the environment. Risk assessment involves identifying, analyzing, and quantifying environmental contaminants, as well as evaluating their potential adverse effects.

The integrated approach of risk assessment and environmental assessment is called environmental risk assessment (ERA) (Chormare and Kumar 2022). The key steps involved in ERA involve "hazard identification" through scientific and toxicological studies; "exposure assessment" through different exposure pathways such as inhalation, ingestion, contact, etc.; dose–response assessment through epidemiological and toxicological studies (animal and nonanimal); "risk characterization" to identify potential risks and sensitive ecosystems; and "risk management" through risk communication, enactment of policies, regulations and control measures to limit exposure to contaminants (Liu et al. 2020; Amiard and Amiard-Triquet 2015). Monitoring aids in continuous assessment and surveillance of contaminants, evaluation of risk management measures, and identification of emerging contaminants.

A monitoring program involves regular sampling from environmental media, sample analysis, data management and analysis through software and risk communication to the public, policy makers, and regulatory agencies. Regular and systemic monitoring also provides information for decision making, policy development, and implementation of control measures to protect human health and the environment (Renaud et al. 2022; Brar et al. 2019).

Risk assessment and monitoring of environmental contaminants by different countries is done mainly by following the core procedure as recommended by the EU with little modification. The agencies concerned with risk assessment and monitoring of environmental contaminants inclue the World Health Organization (WHO), United States Environmental Protection Agency (USEPA), and European Environment Agency (EEA) (Bedi et al. 2015; Sousa et al. 2016; Narsimha and Rajitha 2018). Since 2006, the European Commission has implemented a chemical policy called "REACH" (EC 1907/2006) to identify properties (including toxicities) of chemical environmental contaminants (Amiard and Amiard-Triquet 2015).

40.8 Bioremediation

The process of using living organisms such as bacteria, fungi, and plants to degrade, transform or remove environmental contaminants is called "bioremediation." It is a sustainable and cost-effective measure to remediate the polluted environment (Couto et al. 2022; Natarajan et al. 2020). Some common techniques used in bioremediation are listed below.

- *Microbial or bacterial bioremediation*: genetically modified bacteria capable of degrading complex organic pollutants to simpler, less toxic substances are used in this process. This can be achieved through bioaugmentation (introducing specific microorganisms to enhance degradation) or biostimulation (providing optimal conditions for the growth of naturally occurring microorganisms) (Omokhagbor Adams et al. 2020). *Flavobacterium* spp., *Pseudomonas* spp., *Bacillus* spp., *Corynebacterium* spp., *Mycobacterium* spp., and *Alcaligenes* spp. are used in bioremediation of environmental contaminants like heavy metals, POPs, and PAHs (Verma and Kuila 2019).
- *Phytoremediation*: phytoremediation involves using plants to remove or degrade contaminants from the environment. Different mechanisms include phytoextraction (uptake and extraction of contaminants by plant tissues), rhizofiltration (contaminant filtration by roots), and phytodegradation (contaminant remediation by plant enzymes or associated microbes) (Ancona et al. 2017). Plants with high metal tolerance and faster growth rates like rapeseed (*Brassica napus*), black nightshade (*Solanum nigrum*), Chinese kale (*Brassica oleracea* var. *alboglabra*), and other plant hybrids are commonly used in bioremediation of heavy metals, POPs, and PPCPs (Yu et al. 2014; Wu et al. 2015; Guo et al. 2018).
- *Mycoremediation:* fungi can produce enzymes that degrade contaminants and absorb them into their mycelium. Fungi including *Aspergillus niger*, *A. fumigatus*, *Penicillium* spp., *Mucor* spp., *Trichoderma* spp., white-rot fungi (Deshmukh et al. 2016), extremophilic fungi like *Cryptococcus* spp. from deep sea sediment, and psychrophilic fungi like *Lecanicillium* spp. (Das et al. 2022) are used for bioremediation of various organic contaminants like PAHs, petroleum hydrocarbons, lignin-based compounds, etc.
- *Bioventing:* an *in situ* engineered method of bioremediation that involves introduction of air or oxygen into the contaminated area to stimulate the growth and activity of indigenous soil bacteria, which can metabolize and degrade the contaminants. This technique is mostly used for remediation of soil and groundwater contaminated by petroleum hydrocarbon and heavy metal (Azubuike et al. 2016; Sayqal and Ahmed 2021).
- *Bioleaching:* this method is used for remediation of metal-contaminated soils and water by using certain bacteria and fungi that can solubilize and mobilize metals from solid matrices through metabolic processes (Gu et al. 2018; Phyo et al. 2020).

There are many bioremediation techniques being used by several researchers. Most importantly, the success and effectiveness of any bioremediation technique depend upon the type of contaminant, environmental conditions, and type of microbe.

40.9 Conclusion

The increasing environmental contaminants including ubiquitous microplastics, pervasive "forever chemicals," radionuclides from nuclear fallouts, even e-wastes like old mobile phones, are all evidence that the world is now in the "Anthropocene," or era of humans. These environmental pollutants or contaminants and their subsequent bioaccumulations have become the crux of the sustainability issue. The food chain serves as the primary window for human exposure to environmental contaminants. Persistent human exposure to unwholesome and toxic environmental pollutants through the food chain leads to severe and chronic health problems. Health-conscious consumers are showing increased interest in organic food for reasons related to the health effects of environmental contaminants.

Hence, it is important to understand the diverse sources of contamination and the complex pathways of bioaccumulation, and perform regular risk assessment studies to ascertain the potential public health risks associated with unwholesome environmental contaminants. Improving waste management, adopting safer alternatives to toxic substances, promoting awareness, adopting sustainable practices such as bioremediation techniques, and implementing policy measures are the essential steps toward mitigating the bioaccumulation of environmental contaminants, thereby safeguarding the integrity of food chains for present and future generations.

References

Adebiyi, F.M., Ore, O., Adeola, A. et al. (2021). Occurrence and remediation of naturally occurring radioactive materials in Nigeria: a review. *Environmental Chemistry Letters* 19: 3243–3262.

Adeola, A.O., Iwuozor, K., Akpomie, K. et al. (2022). Advances in the management of radioactive wastes and radionuclide contamination in environmental compartments: a review. *Environmental Geochemistry and Health* 45: 2663–2689.

Ali, H. and Khan, E. (2017). Environmental chemistry in the twenty-first century. *Environmental Chemistry Letters* 15: 329–346.

Ali, H. and Khan, E. (2018). What are heavy metals? Long-standing controversy over the scientific use of the term 'heavy metals'– proposal of a comprehensive definition. *Toxicological and Environmental Chemistry* 100: 6–19.

Ali, H. and Khan, E. (2019). Trophic transfer, bioaccumulation, and biomagnification of non-essential hazardous heavy metals and metalloids in food chains/webs – concepts and implications for wildlife and human health. *Human and Ecological Risk Assessment* 25: 1353–1376.

Ali, H., Khan, E., and Ilahi, I. (2019). Environmental chemistry and ecotoxicology of hazardous heavy metals: environmental persistence, toxicity, and bioaccumulation. *Journal of Chemistry* 25: 1353–1376.

Amiard, J.-C. and Amiard-Triquet, C. (2015). Conventional risk assessment of environmental contaminants. In: *Aquatic Ecotoxicology* (ed. C. Amiard-Triquet, J.C. Amiard, and C. Mouneyrac), 25–49. St Louis: Elsevier.

Ancona, V., Grenni, P., Carraciolo, A. et al. (2017). Plant-assisted bioremediation: an ecological approach for recovering multi-contaminated areas. *Symposium on Soil Biological Communities and Ecosystem Resilience*.

da Araújo, C.F.S., Lopes, M., Ribeiro, M. et al. (2016). Cadmium and lead in seafood from the Aratu Bay, Brazil and the human health risk assessment. *Environmental Monitoring and Assessment* 188: 259.

Azubuike, C.C., Chikere, C., and Okpokwasili, G. (2016). Bioremediation techniques – classification based on site of application: principles, advantages, limitations and prospects. *World Journal of Microbiology and Biotechnology* 32: 180.

Balali-Mood, M., Naseri, K., Tahergorabi, Z. et al. (2021). Toxic mechanisms of five heavy metals: mercury, lead, chromium, cadmium, and arsenic. *Frontiers in Pharmacology* 12: 643972.

Balkhair, K.S. and Ashraf, M.A. (2016). Field accumulation risks of heavy metals in soil and vegetable crop irrigated with sewage water in western region of Saudi Arabia. *Saudi Journal of Biological Sciences* 23: S32–S44.

Bedi, J.S., Gill, J., Aulakh, R. et al. (2015). Pesticide residues in bovine milk in Punjab, India: spatial variation and risk assessment to human health. *Archives of Environmental Contamination and Toxicology* 69: 230–240.

Bock, K.W. (2017). From dioxin toxicity to putative physiologic functions of the human Ah receptor in homeostasis of stem/progenitor cells. *Biochemical Pharmacology* 123: 1–7.

Brar, S.K., Hegde, K., and Pachapur, V. (2019). *Tools, Techniques and Protocols for Monitoring Environmental Contaminants*. St Louis: Elsevier.

Bregnbak, D., Thyssen, J., Zachariae, C. et al. (2015). Association between cobalt allergy and dermatitis caused by leather articles – a questionnaire study. *Contact Dermatitis* 72: 106–114.

Budnik, L.T. and Casteleyn, L. (2019). Mercury pollution in modern times and its socio-medical consequences. *Science of the Total Environment* 654: 720–734.

Burgos-Aceves, M.A., Migliaccio, V., Gregorio, I. et al. (2021). 1,1,1-trichloro-2,2-bis (p-chlorophenyl)-ethane (DDT) and 1,1-Dichloro-2,2-bis (p, p'-chlorophenyl) ethylene (DDE) as endocrine disruptors in human and wildlife: a possible implication of mitochondria. *Environmental Toxicology and Pharmacology* 87: 103684.

Canesi, L., Ciacci, C., and Balbi, T. (2015). Interactive effects of nanoparticles with other contaminants in aquatic organisms: friend or foe? *Marine Environmental Research* 111: 128–134.

Carvalho, F.P. (2017). Pesticides, environment, and food safety. *Food and Energy Security* 6: 48–60.

Castillo-Zacarías, C., Barocio, M., Hidalgo-Vazquez, E. et al. (2021). Antidepressant drugs as emerging contaminants: occurrence in urban and non-urban waters and analytical methods for their detection. *Science of the Total Environment* 747: 143722.

Chormare, R. and Kumar, M.A. (2022). Environmental health and risk assessment metrics with special mention to biotransfer, bioaccumulation and biomagnification of environmental pollutants. *Chemosphere* 302: 134836.

Conder, J.M., Gobas, F., Borga, K. et al. (2012). Use of trophic magnification factors and related measures to characterize bioaccumulation potential of chemicals. *Integrated Environmental Assessment and Management* 8: 85–97.

Couto, E., Assemany, P., Carneiro, G. et al. (2022). The potential of algae and aquatic macrophytes in the pharmaceutical and personal care products (PPCPs) environmental removal: a review. *Chemosphere* 302: 134808.

Cui, Y.J., Zhu, Y., Zhai, R. et al. (2004). Transfer of metals from soil to vegetables in an area near a smelter in Nanning, China. *Environment International* 30: 785–791.

Das, A., Satyaprakash, K., and Das, A.K. (2022). Extremophilic fungi as a source of bioactive molecules. In: *Extremophilic Fungi* (ed. S. Sahay), 489–522. New York: Springer.

Davarpanah, E. and Guilhermino, L. (2019). Are gold nanoparticles and microplastics mixtures more toxic to the marine microalgae Tetraselmis chuii than the substances individually? *Ecotoxicology and Environmental Safety* 181: 60–68.

DeForest, D.K., Brix, K., and Adams, W. (2007). Assessing metal bioaccumulation in aquatic environments: the inverse relationship between bioaccumulation factors, trophic transfer factors and exposure concentration. *Aquatic Toxicology* 84: 236–246.

Deshmukh, R., Khardenavis, A., and Purohit, H. (2016). Diverse metabolic capacities of fungi for bioremediation. *Indian Journal of Microbiology* 56: 247–264.

Duffus, J.H. (2002). "Heavy metals" – a meaningless term? (IUPAC technical report). *Pure and Applied Chemistry* 74: 793–807.

Ebele, A.J., Abdallah, M., and Harrad, S. (2017). Pharmaceuticals and personal care products (PPCPs) in the freshwater aquatic environment. *Emerging Contaminants* 3: 1–16.

Enault, J., Robert, S., Schlosser, O. et al. (2015). Drinking water, diet, indoor air: comparison of the contribution to environmental micropollutants exposure. *International Journal of Hygiene and Environmental Health* 218: 723–730.

Akram, R., Fahad, S., Hashmi, M. et al. (2019). Trends of electronic waste pollution and its impact on the global environment and ecosystem. *Environmental Science and Pollution Research* 26: 16923–16938.

Fernández-González, R., Yebra-Pimentel, I., Martinez-Carballo, E. et al. (2015). A critical review about human exposure to polychlorinated dibenzo-p-dioxins (PCDDs), polychlorinated dibenzofurans (PCDFs) and polychlorinated biphenyls (PCBs) through foods. *Critical Reviews in Food Science and Nutrition* 55: 1590–1617.

Fiedler, H. and Sadia, M. (2021). Regional occurrence of perfluoroalkane substances in human milk for the global monitoring plan under the Stockholm convention on persistent organic pollutants during 2016–2019. *Chemosphere* 277: 130287.

Fiedler, H., Li, X., and Zhang, J. (2023). Persistent organic pollutants in human milk from primiparae – correlations, global, regional, and national time-trends. *Chemosphere* 313: 137484.

Furue, M., Ishii, Y., Tsukimori, K. et al. (2021). Aryl hydrocarbon receptor and dioxin-related health hazards – lessons from yusho. *International Journal of Molecular Sciences* 22: 708.

Genchi, G., Sinicropi, M., Lauria, G. et al. (2020). The effects of cadmium toxicity. *International Journal of Environmental Research and Public Health* 17: 3782.

Golam Mortuza, M. and Al-Misned, F.A. (2015). Heavy metal concentration in two freshwater fishes from Wadi Hanifah (Riyadh, Saudi Arabia) and evaluation of possible health Hazard to consumers. *Pakistan Journal of Zoology* 47: 839–845.

Gu, T., Rastegar, S., Mousavi, S. et al. (2018). Advances in bioleaching for recovery of metals and bioremediation of fuel ash and sewage sludge. *Bioresource Technology* 261: 428–440.

Guarda, P.M., Pontes, A., Domiciano, R. et al. (2020). Assessment of ecological risk and environmental behavior of pesticides in environmental compartments of the Formoso River in Tocantins, Brazil. *Archives of Environmental Contamination and Toxicology* 79: 524–536.

Guo, J.J., Tan, X., Fu, H. et al. (2018). Selection for Cd pollution-safe cultivars of Chinese kale (Brassica alboglabra L. H. Bailey) and biochemical mechanisms of the cultivar-dependent Cd accumulation involving in Cd subcellular distribution. *Journal of Agricultural and Food Chemistry* 66: 1923–1934.

Gupta, P., Thompson, B., Wahlang, B. et al. (2018). The environmental pollutant, polychlorinated biphenyls, and cardiovascular disease: a potential target for antioxidant nanotherapeutics. *Drug Delivery and Translational Research* 8: 740–759.

Hamada, N., Ogino, H., and Fujimichi, Y. (2012). Safety regulations of food and water implemented in the first year following the Fukushima nuclear accident. *Journal of Radiation Research* 53: 641–671.

Han, Y., Tang, Z., Sun, J. et al. (2019). Heavy metals in soil contaminated through e-waste processing activities in a recycling area: implications for risk management. *Process Safety and Environmental Protection* 125: 189–196.

Hashem, M.A., Nur-A-Tomal, M., Mondal, N. et al. (2017). Hair burning and liming in tanneries is a source of pollution by arsenic, lead, zinc, manganese and iron. *Environmental Chemistry Letters* 15: 501–506.

Hassaan, M.A. and El Nemr, A. (2020). Pesticides pollution: classifications, human health impact, extraction and treatment techniques. *Egyptian Journal of Aquatic Research* 46: 207–220.

Hellou, J., Lebeuf, M., and Rudi, M. (2013). Review on DDT and metabolites in birds and mammals of aquatic ecosystems. *Environmental Reviews* 21: 53–69.

Hsieh, H.Y., Huang, K., Cheng, J. et al. (2019). Environmental effects on the bioaccumulation of PAHs in marine zooplankton in Gaoping coastal waters, Taiwan: concentration, distribution, profile, and sources. *Marine Pollution Bulletin* 144: 68–78.

Hu, L., Zhao, Y., and Xu, H. (2022). Trojan horse in the intestine: a review on the biotoxicity of microplastics combined environmental contaminants. *Journal of Hazardous Materials* 439: 139652.

Ighalo, J.O., Yap, P., Iwuozor, K. et al. (2022). Adsorption of persistent organic pollutants (POPs) from the aqueous environment by nano-adsorbents: a review. *Environmental Research* 212: 113123.

Ishikawa, T., Graham, J., Stanhope, K. et al. (2015). Effect of DDT exposure on lipids and energy balance in obese Sprague-Dawley rats before and after weight loss. *Toxicology Reports* 2: 990–995.

Islam, R., Kumar, S., Karmoker, J. et al. (2018). Bioaccumulation and adverse effects of persistent organic pollutants (POPs) on ecosystems and human exposure: a review study on Bangladesh perspectives. *Environmental Technology and Innovation* 12: 115–131.

Islam, M.A., Amin, S., Rahman, M. et al. (2022). Chronic effects of organic pesticides on the aquatic environment and human health: a review. *Environmental Nanotechnology, Monitoring and Management* 18: 100740.

Jin, Y., Liang, C., He, G. et al. (2003). Study on distribution of endemic arsenism in China. *Journal of Hygiene Research* 32: 519–540.

Keerthanan, S., Jayasinghe, C., Biswas, J. et al. (2021). Pharmaceutical and personal care products (PPCPs) in the environment: plant uptake, translocation, bioaccumulation, and human health risks. *Critical Reviews in Environmental Science and Technology* 51: 1221–1258.

Khan, F.U., Rahman, A., Jan, A. et al. (2004). Toxic and trace metals (Pb, Cd, Zn, Cu, Mn, Ni, Co and Cr) in dust, dustfall/soil. *Journal of the Chemical Society of Pakistan* 26: 453–456.

Khan, A., Khan, S., Khan, M. et al. (2015). The uptake and bioaccumulation of heavy metals by food plants, their effects on plants nutrients, and associated health risk: a review. *Environmental Science and Pollution Research* 22: 13772–13799.

Kirman, C.R., Aylward, L., Hays, S. et al. (2011). Biomonitoring equivalents for DDT/DDE. *Regulatory Toxicology and Pharmacology* 60: 172–180.

Koch, N., Islam, L., Sonowal, S. et al. (2021). Environmental antibiotics and resistance genes as emerging contaminants: methods of detection and bioremediation. *Current Research in Microbial Sciences* 2: 100027.

Kohrman, H. and Chamberlain, C.P. (2014). Heavy metals in produce from urban farms in the San Francisco Bay Area. *Food Additives and Contaminants: Part B Surveillance* 7: 127–134.

Krause, S., Baranov, V., Nel, H. et al. (2021). Gathering at the top? Environmental controls of microplastic uptake and biomagnification in freshwater food webs. *Environmental Pollution* 268: 115750.

Krithiga, T., Sathish, S., Renita, A. et al. (2022). Persistent organic pollutants in water resources: fate, occurrence, characterization and risk analysis. *Science of the Total Environment* 831: 154808.

Kumar, S. and Sharma, A. (2019). Cadmium toxicity: effects on human reproduction and fertility. *Reviews on Environmental Health* 34: 327–338.

Kumari, K., Swamy, S., and Singh, A. (2021). Global monitoring plan on persistent organic pollutants (POPs). In: *Persistent Organic Pollutants* (ed. K.S. Kumari). Boca Raton: CRC Press.

Leibson, T., Lala, P., and Ito, S. (2018). Drug and chemical contaminants in breast milk: effects on neurodevelopment of the nursing infant. In: *Handbook of Developmental Neurotoxicology* (ed. W. Slikker, M. Paule, and C. Wang), 275–284. New York: Academic Press.

Leyssens, L., Vinck, B., van der Straeten, C. et al. (2017). Cobalt toxicity in humans—a review of the potential sources and systemic health effects. *Toxicology* 387: 43–56.

Liu, Y.E., Luo, X., Corella, P. et al. (2019). Organophosphorus flame retardants in a typical freshwater food web: bioaccumulation factors, tissue distribution, and trophic transfer. *Environmental Pollution* 255: 113286.

Liu, N., Jin, X., Feng, C. et al. (2020). Ecological risk assessment of fifty pharmaceuticals and personal care products (PPCPs) in Chinese surface waters: a proposed multiple-level system. *Environment International* 136: 105454.

Mahmood, A. and Malik, R.N. (2014). Human health risk assessment of heavy metals via consumption of contaminated vegetables collected from different irrigation sources in Lahore, Pakistan. *Arabian Journal of Chemistry* 7: 91–99.

Malhat, F.M., Loutfy, N., Greish, S. et al. (2018). A review of environmental contamination by organochlorine and organophosphorus pesticides in Egypt. *Journal of Toxicology and Risk Assessment* 4: 1510013.

Mandaric, L., Celic, M.M. et al. (2016). Introduction on emerging contaminants in rivers and their environmental risk. In: *Handbook of Environmental Chemistry*. (ed. M. Petrovic, S. Sabater, A. Elosegi, and D. Barcelo), 3–25. Amsterdam: Springer.

Mann, R.M., Vijver, M., Peijnenburg, W. et al. (2011). Metals and metalloids in terrestrial systems: bioaccumulation, biomagnification and subsequent adverse effects. In: *Ecological Impacts of Toxic Chemicals (Open Access)*. (ed. F. Sanchez-Bayo, P. van den Brink, and R.M. Mann). https://doi.org/10.2174/978160805121211101010043.

Margenat, A., Matamoros, V., Diez, S. et al. (2019). Occurrence and human health implications of chemical contaminants in vegetables grown in peri-urban agriculture. *Environment International* 124: 49–57.

Miller, M.E., Hamann, M., and Kroon, F. (2020). Bioaccumulation and biomagnification of microplastics in marine organisms: a review and meta-analysis of current data. *PLoS One* 15: e0240792.

Mohammed Abdul, K.S., Jayasinghe, S., Chandana, E. et al. (2015). Arsenic and human health effects: a review. *Environmental Toxicology and Pharmacology* 40: 828–846.

Mortimer, M., Kefela, T., Trinh, A. et al. (2021). Uptake and depuration of carbon- and boron nitride-based nanomaterials in the protozoa: Tetrahymena thermophila. *Environmental Science: Nano* 8: 3613–3628.

Narsimha, A. and Rajitha, S. (2018). Spatial distribution and seasonal variation in fluoride enrichment in groundwater and its associated human health risk assessment in Telangana State, South India. *Human and Ecological Risk Assessment: An International Journal* 24: 2119–2132.

Natarajan, V., Karunanidhi, M., and Raja, B. (2020). A critical review on radioactive waste management through biological techniques. *Environmental Science and Pollution Research* 27: 29812–29823.

Nieder, R. and Benbi, D.K. (2022). Integrated review of the nexus between toxic elements in the environment and human health. *AIMS Public Health* 9: 758–789.

Nouri, M. and Haddioui, A. (2016). Human and animal health risk assessment of metal contamination in soil and plants from Ait Ammar abandoned iron mine, Morocco. *Environmental Monitoring and Assessment* 188: 6.

Olisah, C., Adams, J., and Rubidge, G. (2021). The state of persistent organic pollutants in South African estuaries: a review of environmental exposure and sources. *Ecotoxicology and Environmental Safety* 219: 112316.

Omokhagbor Adams, G., Tawari, P., Okoro, S. et al. (2020). Bioremediation, biostimulation and bioaugmention: a review. *International Journal of Environmental Bioremediation and Biodegradation* 3: 28–39.

Pandya, Y. (2018). Pesticides and their applications in agriculture. *Asian Journal of Applied Science and Technology* 2: 894–890.

Pareja-Carrera, J., Mateo, R., and Rodriguez-Estival, J. (2014). Lead (Pb) in sheep exposed to mining pollution: implications for animal and human health. *Ecotoxicology and Environmental Safety* 108: 210–216.

Phyo, A.K., Jia, Y., Tan, Q. et al. (2020). Competitive growth of sulfate-reducing bacteria with bioleaching acidophiles for bioremediation of heap bioleaching residue. *International Journal of Environmental Research and Public Health* 17: 2715.

Pourret, O. and Hursthouse, A. (2019). It's time to replace the term "heavy metals" with "potentially toxic elements" when reporting environmental research. *International Journal of Environmental Research and Public Health* 16: 4446.

Price, P., Zaleski, R., Hollnagel, H. et al. (2014). Assessing the safety of co-exposure to food packaging migrants in food and water using the maximum cumulative ratio and an established decision tree. *Food Additives and Contaminants – Part A* 31: 414–421.

Qadeer, A., Liu, M., Yang, J. et al. (2019). Trophodynamics and parabolic behaviors of polycyclic aromatic hydrocarbons in an urbanized lake food web, Shanghai. *Ecotoxicology and Environmental Safety* 178: 17–24.

Quan, S.X., Yan, B., Lei, C. et al. (2014). Distribution of heavy metal pollution in sediments from an acid leaching site of e-waste. *Science of the Total Environment* 499: 349–355.

Reddy, A.V.B., Moniruzzaman, M., and Aminabhavi, T. (2019). Polychlorinated biphenyls (PCBs) in the environment: recent updates on sampling, pretreatment, cleanup technologies and their analysis. *Chemical Engineering Journal* 358: 1186–1207.

Rehman, K., Fatima, F., Waheed, I. et al. (2018). Prevalence of exposure of heavy metals and their impact on health consequences. *Journal of Cellular Biochemistry* 119: 157–184.

Renaud, J.B., Sabourin, L., Hoogstra, S. et al. (2022). Monitoring of environmental contaminants in mixed-use watersheds combining targeted and nontargeted analysis with passive sampling. *Environmental Toxicology and Chemistry* 41: 1131–1143.

Ruus, A., Overjordet, I., Braaten, H. et al. (2015). Methylmercury biomagnification in an Arctic pelagic food web. *Environmental Toxicology and Chemistry* 34: 2636–2643.

Saleh, T.A. (2020). Trends in the sample preparation and analysis of nanomaterials as environmental contaminants. *Trends in Environmental Analytical Chemistry* 28: e00101.

Sarkar, A. and Paul, B. (2016). The global menace of arsenic and its conventional remediation – a critical review. *Chemosphere* 158: 37–49.

Sayo, S., Kiratu, J., and Nyamato, G. (2020). Heavy metal concentrations in soil and vegetables irrigated with sewage effluent: a case study of Embu sewage treatment plant, Kenya. *Scientific African* 8: e00337.

Sayqal, A. and Ahmed, O.B. (2021). Advances in heavy metal bioremediation: an overview. *Applied Bionics and Biomechanics* 2021: 1609149.

Sifakis, S., Androutsopoulos, V., Tsataskis, A. et al. (2017). Human exposure to endocrine disrupting chemicals: effects on the male and female reproductive systems. *Environmental Toxicology and Pharmacology* 51: 56–70.

Singh, R., Singh, S., Parihar, P. et al. (2015). Arsenic contamination, consequences and remediation techniques: a review. *Ecotoxicology and Environmental Safety* 112: 247–270.

Skarphedinsdottir, H., Gunnarsson, K., Gudmundsson, G. et al. (2010). Bioaccumulation and biomagnification of organochlorines in a marine food web at a pristine site in Iceland. *Archives of Environmental Contamination and Toxicology* 58: 800–809.

Sousa, A.S., Duavi, W., Cavalcante, R. et al. (2016). Estimated levels of environmental contamination and health risk assessment for herbicides and insecticides in surface water of Ceará, Brazil. *Bulletin of Environmental Contamination and Toxicology* 96: 90–95.

Starek-Świechowicz, B., Budziszewska, B., and Starek, A. (2017). Hexachlorobenzene as a persistent organic pollutant: toxicity and molecular mechanism of action. *Pharmacological Reports* 69: 1232–1239.

Stasinos, S., Nasopoulou, C., Tsikrika, C. et al. (2014). The bioaccumulation and physiological effects of heavy metals in carrots, onions, and potatoes and dietary implications for Cr and Ni: a review. *Journal of Food Science* 79: R765–R780.

Sufia, H., Gutierrez, H., and Croue, J. (2020). Removal of pharmaceutical and personal care products (PPCPs) from wastewater using microalgae: a review. *Journal of Hazardous Materials* 403: 124041.

Sun, T., Wu, H., Wang, X. et al. (2020). Evaluation on the biomagnification or biodilution of trace metals in global marine food webs by meta-analysis. *Environmental Pollution* 264: 113856.

Szynkowska, M.I., Pawlaczyk, A., and Mackiewicz, E. (2017). Bioaccumulation and biomagnification of trace elements in the environment. In: *Recent Advances in Trace Elements* (ed. K. Chojnacka and A. Saeid). Hoboken: Wiley.

Takahashi, T., Fujimura, M., Koyama, M. et al. (2017). Methylmercury causes blood–brain barrier damage in rats via upregulation of vascular endothelial growth factor expression. *PLoS One* 12: e0170623.

Taylor, M.P., Isley, C., Fry, K. et al. (2021). A citizen science approach to identifying trace metal contamination risks in urban gardens. *Environment International* 155: 106582.

Thompson, L.A. and Darwish, W.S. (2019). Environmental chemical contaminants in food: review of a global problem. *Journal of Toxicology* 2019: 2345283.

Thompson, L.A., Ikenaka, Y., Yohannes, Y. et al. (2018). Human health risk from consumption of marine fish contaminated with DDT and its metabolites in Maputo Bay, Mozambique. *Bulletin of Environmental Contamination and Toxicology* 100: 672–676.

Tyagi, H., Chawla, H., Bhandari, H. et al. (2020). Recent enhancements in visible-light photocatalytic degradation of organochlorines pesticides: a review. *Materials Today: Proceedings* 49: 3289–3305.

Ubaid ur Rahman, H., Asghar, W., Nazir, W. et al. (2021). A comprehensive review on chlorpyrifos toxicity with special reference to endocrine disruption: evidence of mechanisms, exposures and mitigation strategies. *Science of the Total Environment* 755: 142649.

Ugulu, I., Khan, Z., Safdar, H. et al. (2021). Chromium bioaccumulation by plants and grazing livestock as affected by the application of sewage irrigation water: implications to the food chain and health risk. *International Journal of Environmental Research* 15: 261–274.

Vafeiadi, M., Georgiou, V., Chalkiadaki, G. et al. (2015). Association of prenatal exposure to persistent organic pollutants with obesity and cardiometabolic traits in early childhood: the rhea mother–child cohort (Crete, Greece). *Environmental Health Perspectives* 123: 1015–1021.

Van Raamsdonk, L.W.D., van der Zande, M., Koelmans, A. et al. (2020). Current insights into monitoring, bioaccumulation, and potential health effects of microplastics present in the food chain. *Foods* 9: 72.

Verma, S. and Kuila, A. (2019). Bioremediation of heavy metals by microbial process. *Environmental Technology and Innovation* 14: 100369.

Wani, A.L., Ara, A., and Usmani, J. (2015). Lead toxicity: a review. *Interdisciplinary Toxicology* 8: 55–64.

Wu, J.P., Luo, X., Zhang, Y. et al. (2008). Bioaccumulation of polybrominated diphenyl ethers (PBDEs) and polychlorinated biphenyls (PCBs) in wild aquatic species from an electronic waste (e-waste) recycling site in South China. *Environment International* 34: 1109–1113.

Wu, Q., Leung, J., Huang, X. et al. (2015). Evaluation of the ability of black nightshade Solanum nigrum L. for phytoremediation of thallium-contaminated soil. *Environmental Science and Pollution Research* 22: 11478–11487.

Wu, X., Cobbina, S., Mao, G. et al. (2016). A review of toxicity and mechanisms of individual and mixtures of heavy metals in the environment. *Environmental Science and Pollution Research* 23: 8244–8259.

Xiao, R., Wang, S., Li, R. et al. (2017). Soil heavy metal contamination and health risks associated with artisanal gold mining in Tongguan, Shaanxi, China. *Ecotoxicology and Environmental Safety* 141: 17–24.

Yan, H., Li, Q., Yuan, Z. et al. (2019). Research progress of mercury bioaccumulation in the aquatic food chain, China: a review. *Bulletin of Environmental Contamination and Toxicology* 102: 612–620.

Yarsan, E. and Yipel, M. (2013). The important terms of marine pollution "Biomarkers and Biomonitoring". *Journal of Molecular Biomarkers and Diagnosis* www.researchgate.net/profile/Ender-Yarsan/publication/285610301_The_Important_Terms_of_Marine_Pollution_Biomarkers_and_BiomonitoringBioaccumulation_Bioconcentration_Biomagnification/links/5845703308ae61f75dd789d5/The-Important-Terms-of-Marine-Pollution-Biomarkers-and-Biomonitoring-Bioaccumulation-Bioconcentration-Biomagnification.pdf (accessed 12 February 2024).

Yoshino, K., Mori, K., Kanaya, G. et al. (2020). Food sources are more important than biomagnification on mercury bioaccumulation in marine fishes. *Environmental Pollution* 262: 113982.

Yu, L., Zhu, J., Huang, Q. et al. (2014). Application of a rotation system to oilseed rape and rice fields in Cd-contaminated agricultural land to ensure food safety. *Ecotoxicology and Environmental Safety* 108: 287–293.

Zhao, W.G., Tian, Y., Zhao, P. et al. (2023). Research progress on Trojan-horse effect of microplastics and heavy metals in freshwater environment. *Huan jing ke xue* 44: 1244–1257.

Zwolak, I. (2020). The role of selenium in arsenic and cadmium toxicity: an updated review of scientific literature. *Biological Trace Element Research* 193: 44–63.

41

Principles and Issues of Environmental Protection

Baleshwari Dixit[1], Neelam Kurmi[2], Sapna Sharma[3], Serlene Tomar[4], and Yamini Verma[5]

[1] Department of Veterinary Public Health & Epidemiology, College of Veterinary Science and Animal Health, 486001, Rewa, Madhya Pradesh, India
[2] Department of Animal Husbandry and Dairying, Sagar, India
[3] Department of Public Health & Epidemiology, Post Graduate Institute of Veterinary Education and Research College, 302031, Jaipur, India
[4] Department of Livestock Products Technology, College of Veterinary Science and Animal Husbandry, Rewa, NDVSU, Jabalpur, Madhya Pradesh, India
[5] Department of Veterinary Pathology, College of Veterinary Science & Animal Health, Jabalpur, India

41.1 Introduction

Environmental protection involves taking measures to protect the natural world and is also referred as "environmental preservation." Practices involved in protecting the environment need efforts not only from governments but also groups and individuals. The main objectives of environment protection includes conservation of the existing natural environment, natural resources, repairing damage and reversing changes where possible.

The environment includes all the biological and nonbiological entities in an area along with their interactions. Many environmental issues are growing in size and complexity temporally and threatening the survival of mankind on earth. Ecosystems include all the organisms and interactions in a given habitat and humans are highly dependent on the services provided by various ecosystems. Ecosystems produce natural resources that are often taken for granted such as clean water, agricultural plants, soil, woods, natural gases, minerals, pollination, and clean air; all these services are provided free of cost by ecosystems but are worth trillions of dollars.

Natural resources are of two types: renewable and nonrenewable. Renewable resources are those which are replaced periodically by natural processes like vegetation, water, solar, wind, thermal heat, etc. while nonrenewable resources are those which cannot be replaced once they are exhausted and require millions of years to create, including minerals, fossil fuel, and soil.

Environmental challenges are continuously expanding due to anthropogenic activities and exploitation of natural resources. Factors related to the increase in population include intensive agriculture, urbanization, and rapid industrialization which play key role in environmental degradation. Studies on the environment have pointed out that everything in the environment is interconnected and that there is a limit to environmental activity. Soil is considered as the most neglected part of the ecosystem but it provides critical services like physical and nutritional support for plants, moderating the hydrologic cycle, disposal of waste matter, and regulation of major element cycles. Natural cycles like water, carbon, nitrogen, hydrogen, sulfur, etc. are essential for maintenance of ecosystems, and disruption of these cycles may lead to floods, droughts, pollution, acid rain, extreme weather, and other environmental problems. Indiscriminate use of pesticides, chemicals, fertilizers, and industrial wastes is polluting the air, water, and soil beyond sustainable limits.

Environmental pollution and depletion of natural resources in both developed and developing countries have created difficulties in fulfilling the demands of growing population while controlling degradation of the environment. Natural resources are on the verge of exhaustion; the importance of protection and conservation of our surroundings are recognized globally and serious efforts are being made at national and international levels. The prosperous survival and sustenance of humanity depend on sustainable use of natural resources along with protection of the environment.

Although the idea of protecting the environment is not new and in one form or another efforts have been made in the past. Due to the great acceleration of anthropogenic activities over the past century, pressures on ecosystems have increased which emphasizes the need for systematic environmental protection. Environmental issues like global warming, acid rain,

Epidemiology and Environmental Hygiene in Veterinary Public Health, First Edition. Edited by Tanmoy Rana.
© 2025 John Wiley & Sons, Inc. Published 2025 by John Wiley & Sons, Inc.

478 | *41 Principles and Issues of Environmental Protection*

biodiversity conservation, ozone depletion, and marine pollution indicate the complex nature of the problem. The solution cannot be provided by any one discipline or sector alone but needs an interdisciplinary exposure. For better understanding the complex nature and biotic components of the environment and their interaction, various branches of science including zoology, botany, genetics, microbiology, and biochemistry can be helpful. Knowledge and inputs from other fields such as life sciences, agriculture, public health, medical science, chemistry, physics, and sanitary engineering in the management of environmental issues point to the multidisciplinary nature of the problem.

41.2 Environmental Protection

Population growth, globalization, and industrialization have increased the number of environmental issues that are not restricted by national boundaries but are identified regionally and globally. Significant changes in the utilization of natural resources in one country that have adverse consequences for neighboring countries have escalated transboundary environmental security conflicts. If the issues are of natural origin, like floods or droughts, or they are anthropogenic but not premeditated, like deposits of toxic emissions of industrial waste across the border due to a shift in wind patterns, then the affected countries can share efforts to solve the problem. Transboundary problems related to environmental issues include environmental pollution or degradation, scarcity (shortage), inequitable allocation (misdistribution), and disaster or accident (natural or man-made).

It is very clear that development and modernization aids that have made our lives more comfortable and enjoyable are responsible for most of the current environmental issues. In order to understand how to control and prevent environmental degradation, we need to identify the challenges at the outset. The world is facing various challenges related to protection and management of the environment.

- Prevention, control, and abatement of different kinds of pollution.
- Conservation of natural resources and wildlife.
- Protection and management of forests, water resources, etc.
- Extinction of species and loss of biodiversity.
- Ozone depletion and climate change.
- Access to fresh and potable water.
- Food security and agriculture.
- Eradication of poverty and control of population growth.
- Unplanned urbanization and urban environmental problems.

41.3 Types of Pollution

41.3.1 Chemical, Biological, Radiological, and Nuclear Pollution

Various harmful chemicals produced by anthropogenic activities are released into the environment, thereby contaminating water, air, and soil. Effluents released from chemical factories, indiscriminate use of pesticides, chemical fertilizers, and uncontrolled mining cause chemical pollution of the environment. This has both short-term and long-term health adverse effects on all types of life on Earth. One disastrous example of chemical pollution was the accidental release of methyl isocyanate gas from the Union Carbide plant in Bhopal in 1984, which is considered as one of the worst industrial accidents in history. This incident led to the immediate death of thousands of people (approximate over 8000) along with many disabilities and these continued to affect the exposed population in the following years and even now. The release of toxic gas into the atmosphere from another Union Carbide plant caused illnesses among residents in West Virginia, USA.

In relation to the hazardous effect of Bhopal-like disasters, the Emergency Planning and Community Right-to-Know Act (EPCRA) was enacted in the United States. By this law, companies which handle hazardous waste need to give complete disclosure about their polluting activities, handling and storage facilities, any accidental release of hazardous chemical into the atmosphere above the safe limit, and all necessary action plans to respond to accidental releases. This act led to a substantial reduction in the release of toxic chemicals by the companies who adopted the act and participated in EPCRA disclosures.

Spilled oil pollutes not only land but also water sources. The Exxon Valdez was the most tragic example of this and is considered the worst in reference to the environmental damage it caused. On 24th March 1989, the oil tanker ran aground at Bligh Reef, Alaska, and spilled 11 million gallons of oil into the environment of Prince William Sound. A lack of efficient containment and cleanup protocol compounded the issue and people are still struggling to recover from that damage. In response to the disaster, the Oil Pollution Act (1990) was enacted which, required oil tankers to be double-hulled and gave states more say in their spill prevention standards. The spill response equipment and safeguards at Prince William Sound, a loading terminal for the major tanker route on the Trans-Alaska pipeline system, have been brought up to date.

Nuclear energy is a very controversial issue of our time. At Three Mile Island, Pennsylvania, on March 28, 1979, a partial meltdown of the reactor released radioactivity into the atmosphere, threatening to blow the building and spew radioactivity into an area inhabited by some 3,00,000 people. In 1986, a nuclear explosion in a reactor in Chernobyl, Ukraine, caused cumulative death loss along with many after-effects such as cancer, especially in children. The Three Mile Island accident led to the establishment of the Institute of Nuclear Power Operations (INPO) in the US with the objective of promoting safety in commercial nuclear plants.

The Fukushima nuclear accident occurred due to failure of equipment which caused the release of radioactive materials at the Fukushima nuclear power plant. This accidental disaster was followed by an earthquake of 9.0 magnitude and tsunami on 11 March, 2011.

Radiological weapons may contain any type of radioactive material and disperse variable amount of material contained within the device. Radiological material may be used in medical and industrial equipment and their waste disposal is not controlled in many countries, thus contaminating the environment. The Limited Test Ban Treaty (1963) banned underwater, atmospheric, and outer space testing of nuclear weapons which resulted in the reduction of radioactive contamination of the environment. However, radioactive contamination due to nuclear war is still a threat. The release of nuclear wastes into the atmosphere, particularly in densely populated areas, would not only cause high mortality but the debris clouds can block the sunlight thereby killing plants, destroying the ozone layer, and changing the climate. So it is of utmost importance to prevent such type of environmental disaster *which necessitates governmental cooperation and political action to prevent nuclear war.*

Overuse of chemicals like pesticides, fertilizers, and herbicides that contain nitrates and phosphates are not only a source of water pollution but also pollution of soil. Demolition, construction site mines, landfills and foundries are also sources of soil pollution. These chemicals mix with surface runoff, enter in to lakes, rivers and seep into the groundwater. Industrial emissions are most important cause of water pollution for example paper manufacturers may release mercury in waste water. In water mercury converts in to methyl mercury by the action of bacteria which accumulates in the aquatic flora and fauna and their consumption becomes hazardous. Preventive action at individual and government level should be taken up. At individual level people can adopt simple habits and activities like buying least harmful or hazardous products, mixing and applying pesticides at proper concentration and using alternative fuels

Major sources of chemical pollution include burning of fossil fuels, industries, and motor vehicles. Sulfur dioxide is produced when coal is burned. It is an ingredient of acid rain and can cause lung damage in people who breathe it in large amounts . Nitrogen oxides (NOx) are released from motor vehicles such as cars, trucks, and airplanes and are also an ingredient of acid rain. Other chemicals that cause air pollution include ozone, carbon monoxide, and lead.

Biological agents like exotic plants and animals can be invasive, and agents like microorganisms are capable of causing infectious disease to human population, livestock , or crops. Biological weapons may be produced using small-scale, in-home techniques, or large-scale pharmaceutical or fermentation facilities. In comparison to chemical weapons, the production and proliferation of biological weapons can be challenging to detect and even small amounts may have potentially widespread effects.

41.3.2 Acid Rain

A more accurate term for acid rain is "acid deposition" and is the deposition of wet (rain, sleet, fog, cloud water, snow, and dew) and dry (acidifying compounds and gases) acidic components. Normal rainfall is slightly acidic because of dissolved carbonic acid that is formed by the reaction of water and carbon dioxide in the air. However, gaseous emissions of sulfur dioxide and NOx react with water molecules in the atmosphere to produce acid rain. Sulfur dioxide is produced by volcanic eruptions and oxides of nitrogen are naturally produced by lightning strikes. Sulfur oxides and NOx are chemically converted into sulfuric and nitric acids.

$$SO_2 + H_2O = H_2SO_3$$

$$NO_2 + H_2O = HNO_2 + HNO_3$$

Acid-producing gases are created by biological processes, wildfires, volcanoes that occur on the land, in wetlands, and oceans. Dimethyl sulfide is the major biological source of sulfur. Nitric acid in rainwater is also produced by electrical activity in the atmosphere such as lightning. Anthropogenic activities like factories, electricity generation (coal-fired power plants), and motor vehicles contribute substantially to the generation of oxides of sulfur and nitrogen. Livestock production also plays a major role as animals contributes significantly to sources of ammonia.

The direct effect of acid rain on human health is not commonly seen because acid is too dilute in the rainwater to produce direct adverse effects. However, the particulates present in acid rain (sulfur dioxide and NOx) may cause adverse effects, particularly heart and lung problems including asthma and bronchitis. The adverse impacts of acid rain on forests, freshwater sources, and soils include loss of flora and fauna along with physical damage to buildings and hazardous impacts on human health. For example, pH lower than 5.0 adversely affect the hatching of fish eggs and lower pH can kill adult fish. The US Environmental Protection Agency (EPA) indicated that acid rain cause significant acidity in lakes and streams. Apart from these effects, acid rain also cause changes in the biology and chemistry of soil which not only affect the microbiology of soil but also leach away essential nutrients and minerals such as magnesium and mobilize toxins like aluminum. Forests at high altitude are highly vulnerable because their environment is full of clouds and fog which make it prone to more acidic rain.

Reduction in the anthropogenic emission of oxides of sulfur and nitrogen may help in prevention of acid rain. SO_2 emission can be reduced by the use of flue gas desulfurization (FGD) in coal-fired thermal power plants which can remove sulfur -containing gases from their stack gases. Fitting of autolytic converters to vehicles can reduce the NOx released in automobile emissions. In this regard, a number of international treaties have been signed particularly on the long-range transport of atmospheric pollutants, such as the Sulfur Emissions Reduction Protocol under the Convention on Long-Range Trans-boundary Air Pollution. Most European countries and Canada have signed the treaties. With the Clean Air Act Amendments of 1990 in the United States, the first emissions trading market was established. The overall goal of the Acid Rain Program established by the Act is to achieve significant environmental and public health benefits through reduction in emissions of sulfur dioxide and NOx, the primary causes of acid rain.

41.3.3 Ozone Depletion

Since the late 1970s, two distinct but related phenomena were observed: a decline of the ozone layer in Earth's stratosphere (4% per decade of the total volume) and a much larger decrease in stratospheric ozone in springtime over Earth's polar regions, termed the ozone hole. In addition to these well-known stratospheric phenomena, there are also springtime polar tropospheric ozone depletion events. The polar ozone hole formation process is different from the midlatitude thinning, but the common and most important process is the catalytic destruction of ozone by halogenic compounds. The emission rate of man-made halocarbon refrigerants (CFCs, freons, halons) is associated with ozone depletion. On March 15, 2011, a noticeable loss of ozone layer (about half of the ozone) over the Arctic was observed.

The major function of the ozone layer is to absorb ultraviolet light coming from the sun, and loss of the layer may lead to increased UV levels, which could be potential hazard causing, for example, increases in skin cancer, cataracts, damage to plants, and reduction of plankton populations in the ocean's photic zone. The most common forms of skin cancer associated with increased UV exposure include basal and squamous cell carcinomas, malignant melanoma, and cortical cataracts. An increase in UV radiation would be expected to affect crops.

Depletion of the ozone layer and increase in surface UV also affect a number of economically important plant species, such as rice, which depend on cyanobacteria present on their roots that help in retention of nitrogen. These cyanobacteria are very sensitive to UV light and would be affected by its increase. Depletion of the ozone layer is also associated with an increase in concentration of chlorofluorocarbons. The ozone formed due to photochemical reactions at lower levels naturally has a shorter photochemical lifetime, and cannot compensate for the ozone reduction because it is destroyed before the concentration can reach the required levels, as well as being a health risk for humans.

In 1987, in order to reduce production of ozone-depleting substances (ODS), the Montreal Protocol was signed by various countries. Reduced ozone causes the stratosphere to absorb less solar radiation, thus cooling the stratosphere while warming the troposphere. The increase in ozone concentration particularly in the upper troposphere is a matter of concern because here it acts as a greenhouse gas (GHG), absorbing some of the infrared energy emitted by the Earth. The potency of ozone as a GHG is difficult to determine because of its nonuniform concentrations across the globe. However, the most widely accepted scientific assessments relating to climate change (e.g., the IPCC Third Assessment Report) suggest that the radioactive forcing of tropospheric ozone is about 25% that of carbon dioxide CFCs and other contributory substances are referred to as ODS.

41.3.4 Hazardous Wastes and their Disposal

Wastes are those substances which are required to be disposed of or intended to be disposed of by the provisions of law. Hazardous wastes include various type of products that may be explosive, flammable, or radioactive in nature and are liable to emit flammable gases upon contact with water, combust spontaneously; corrosive, poisonous, infectious, toxic and may be converted into another harmful substance. Waste substances may contain harmful compounds such as mercury, cadmium, arsenic, lead, organic phosphorus, halogenated organic solvents, phenols, and acidic solutions.

Almost all anthropogenic processes may generate different types of waste material. The world is in a phase of fast development in all fields of industrial, commercial, agricultural, construction, medical, and even domestic activities with larger affluent consumption and therefore the production of larger amount of waste. The impact of hazardous wastes on the environment has far-reaching repercussions, particularly on the quality of water and land, so effective regulation of the management and disposal of hazardous wastes requires cooperation at the global level. Mishandling of hazardous wastes could bring about a range of health effects as well as cause severe damage to the environment. Although there is no scientific certainty about the hazards of wastes, they may produce harmful effects in terms of toxicity, corrosivity, carcinogenicity, mutagenicity, and other characteristics harmful to human health and the environment. Concerns about the improper handling, unsafe disposal methods , practices, and adverse effects of hazardous substances are increasing, which has led to the formulation and tightening of regulations and laws. The cost of hazardous waste disposal is high and cheaper methods of waste disposal within the country and across borders in land and water bodies, particularly the sea, are being sought.

41.4 Environmental Management

Environmental management is multidisciplinary academic field dedicated to furthering the human stewardship of natural resources. Environmental studies as a subject encompasses a number of fields, areas and aspects, including environmental pollution and control, natural resources conservation and management, biodiversity conservation and management, social and cultural issues in development and environment, and issues related to increased human population.

Although studies on the environment may be highly specialized, concentrating on technical aspects such as environmental engineering, environmental science, or environment management, some of the basic aspects of environmental studies also have a direct relevance for every section of protection, management, and conservation. Biologists are experts in ecology and have particular interest in flora, fauna, and habitats. Geographers have knowledge of ecology and its relationship with people and their surroundings. Economists evaluate the value of environmental goods and natural services, assess the costs impact of pollution, and calculate mitigation and adoption economics. Engineers can contribute in creating ecotechnology, which may help in restoration of degraded or polluted environments. Political scientists play a major role in the generation and development of environmental policy and regulations. Environmental laws consist of guidelines and legal measures for protection and effective management of the environment. Apart from these, education and mass communication on environmental protection are two important subjects that are instrumental in enhancing environmental awareness.

Some common themes of environmental management are as follows.

- Bilateral and multilateral environmental treaties for transboundary management of environmental issues.
- Design and use of decision support systems for practical utilization of available environmental data and expert systems for environmental management.
- Formulation and enactment of environmental policy.
- Estimation, analysis, and management of environmental risk.
- Formulation of environmental regulations (for dumping of wastes, emission of pollutants, and extraction of resources; monitoring and policing compliance).
- Natural resource conservation (designation of parks, preserves, and other protected areas; designation and protection of wilderness areas in order to provide protection and management of these natural areas).
- Impacts and management of recreation and tourism; promotion of environmentally friendly tourism "ecotourism" programs.

- Environmental economics calculation for justifications for investment in positive impact on environmental protection.
- Promotion of positive environmental values by education and information dissemination.
- Evaluation and management of natural resources.
- "Scoping" and investigation of design of environmental policies, procedures, and norms.
- Strategies, programs, and methods for the rehabilitation of climate change and reduction of adverse environmental impacts.

41.5 Important Conventions, Conferences, Protocols, and Treaties on Environment Protection

41.5.1 Basel Convention

The Basel Convention was the first global legal entity on the disposal and movement of hazardous wastes across boundaries, which was developed under the United Nations Environment Programme (UNEP) and adopted in a conference at Basel in 1989. The Convention has 111 states and the European Community as parties.

The objectives of the Basel Convention are as follows.

- To reduce transboundary movement of hazardous wastes and other wastes to the minimum, consistent with environmental sound management.
- To dispose of generated hazardous wastes and other wastes as close as possible to the source of generation.
- To minimize hazardous wastes generation qualitatively and their hazardous potential.
- To have strict control over transport and movement of hazardous wastes across borders, control and prevent illegal traffic.
- To restrict the shipment of wastes to countries that do not have the legal administrative and technical capacity to manage and dispose of them in an environmentally sound manner.
- To assist developing countries in transition to environmentally sound management of hazardous wastes.

41.5.2 Stockholm Conference, 1972

In 1968, the United Nations General Assembly proposed holding a global conference on environment protection in Stockholm in 1972. In the 1970s, the Organization for Economic Cooperation and Development (OCED) also created a Committee for Environment to look into environmental issues.

The UN Conference on Human Environment was held from 5–16 June 1972, at Stockholm. The Stockholm Action Plan document was a comprehensive effort to identify international environmental issues and provide a roadmap for participating nations to combat those challenges. At that time, the world was still not considering protection of environment as a serious issue. However, the conference produced three important documents including an Action Plan to protect the global environment (106 recommendations for environmental management); the United Nations Environment Program and the related Environment Fund; and the Stockholm Declaration on the Human Environment containing 26 principles. International action was solicited in five major areas as follows.

1) Planning and managing human settlement for environmental quality.
2) Addressing the environmental aspects of natural resources management.
3) Identifying and controlling pollutants of broad international significance.
4) Exploring and strengthening the educational, informational, social and cultural aspects of environmental issues.
5) Addressing the integration of development and environment.

The main purpose of the conference was "to serve as a practical means to encourage, and provide guidelines for, action by Governments and international organizations designed to protect and improve the human environment, and to remedy and prevent its impairment, by means of international cooperation, bearing in mind the particular importance of enabling developing countries to forestall occurrence of such problems."

The Stockholm Declaration on the Human Environment is another visionary document which contained 26 principles of policy that is often referred as the Magna Carta on Human Environment. These principles covered preservation, protection, and improvement of the environment. A number of other organizations were also involved, including UNEP, the

International Maritime Organization, International Union for the Conservation of Nature (IUCN), and UNESCO. Several treaties have been signed at their behest as below.

- Treaties on *transboundary pollution* include the Convention on Long Trans-boundary Air Pollution, 1979; Protocol Concerning Co-operation in Combating Pollution in cases of Emergency, 1981.
- Treaties on *marine pollution* include the Convention on Prevention of Marine Pollution by Dumping of Wastes and other Matter, 1972; Convention on Prevention of Pollution by Dumping from Ship and Aircraft, 1972; International Convention for Prevention of Pollution from Ships, 1973; Protocol relating to the Intervention on High Seas in cases of Pollution by substances other than Oil, 1973; Convention on Prevention of Marine Pollution from Land-based Sources, 1974.
- Treaties on *protection of wildlife and flora and fauna* include the Convention on International Trade in Endangered Species (CITES) of Wild Flora and Fauna, 1973; Agreement on Conservation of Polar Bears, 1973; Bonn Convention Agreement on Conservation of Species of Wild Animals, 1979; Conservation of Wetlands of International Importance, 1971; Protection of World Cultural and Natural Heritage, 1972 (at the initiative of UNESCO); Convention on the Conservation of Wildlife and Natural Habitats, 1979.

41.5.3 Developments Post Stockholm

In 1983, "to re-examine the issues of environment and formulate action plans to deal with them," the UN General Assembly Commission created a "Strategic Document" that has three parts: (i) Common Concerns, (ii) Common Challenges, and (iii) Common Endeavors. This document, entitled *Our Common Future*, recognized the concept of "sustainable development" which was defined as "development that meets the needs of the present without compromising the abilities of future generations to meet their own needs." The concept imposed restrictions on indiscriminate use of resources for the welfare of the present generation, to create balance between development and the environment. The document provided 22 legal principles for environmental protection and sustainable development.

41.5.4 Rio Conference, 1992 (Earth Summit)

The Rio Conference was the continuation of the environmentalism process started at Stockholm in order to further strengthen the concerns about environmental protection and the concept of sustainable development. Its commitment to implement and accept the new "mantra" of environmentalism and development included the following objectives.

- To examine the state of the environment and changes since Stockholm.
- To identify regional and global strategies to address major environmental issues in the socio-economic development processes of all countries within a particular time-frame.
- To recommend national and international measures to protect and enhance the environment, taking into account the specific needs of developing countries.
- To promote further development of international environmental law, taking into account the specific needs of developing countries.

41.5.5 World Summit on Sustainable Development, Johannesburg, 2002

Another landmark was the international environmental law development during the World Summit on Sustainable Development held at Johannesburg, South Africa, from 26 August to 4 September. It was attended by delegates of about 191 countries. At the Summit, Kofi Annan, the UN Secretary General, observed that "the model of development we are accustomed to has been fruitful for few, but flaw for many. A path to prosperity that ravages the environment and leaves a majority of humankind behind in squalor will soon prove to be a dead-end road for everyone."

41.5.6 Agenda 21

This very comprehensive document comprises 40 chapters documenting the future implementation of sustainable development. It is divided into four major sections: (i) Social and Economic Dimensions; (ii) Conservation and Management of Resources; (iii) Strengthening the Role of Major Groups; and (iv) Means of Implementation.

41.5.7 UN Framework Convention on Climate Change, 1992

The object of the UN Framework Convention on Climate Change (UNFCCC) 1992 was "to achieve stabilization of greenhouse gas concentrations in the atmosphere at a level that would prevent dangerous anthropogenic interference with the climate system." The document has 27 Articles, with aims to "stabilize greenhouse gas (GHGs) concentration in the atmosphere at the level that would prevent anthropogenic interference with climate system." As per this framework, each State party was ordered to make national policies and be prepared to take measures on the mitigation of climate change by restricting the emission of GHGs, enhancing and protecting their sinks and reservoirs for GHGs. The Kyoto Protocol of 1997 is part of this Convention suggesting that the conference of the parties may adopt the Protocol. The aim was to achieve such a level of GHGs within a suitable time-frame to allow ecosystems to adapt to climate change naturally, assurance of food production and enablement of sustainable economic development.

41.5.8 Convention on Biological Diversity, 1992

This Convention aimed to develop strategies, plans, and programs for conservation and sustainable use of biodiversity along with providing "*in situ*" and "*ex situ*" conservation processes. It also emphasized the provision of "encourage customary use of biological resources in accordance with traditional cultural practices" that are compatible with conservation or sustainability.

41.5.9 Forest Principles

Forests, the green lungs of the world, have come under severe attack owing to developmental activities which have led to deforestation and desertification. The total forest cover of every nation has decreased. The significance of forests cannot be overstated for ensuring healthy life on the planet. Looking at this scenario, the participating states at the Earth Summit in 1992 adopted a statement of principles for the sustainable management of forests, entitled *Forests Principles: Non-Legally Binding Authoritative Statement of Principles for a Global Consensus on the Management, Conservation and Sustainable Development of all Types of Forests*. It contains 15 principles, of which 13 are merely recommendatory in nature as to what states "should do" to ensure sustainable forestry principles

41.5.10 Conventions on Chemicals and Hazardous Wastes

In 1985, the UNEP issued the Cairo Guidelines and Principles for the Environmentally Sound Management of Hazardous Wastes. In June 1987, the UNEP established a Draft Convention on the Transboundary Shipment of Hazardous Waste and created an *ad hoc* working group composed of legal and technical experts. The Basel Convention on the Control of Transboundary Movement of Hazardous Wastes and their Disposal was adopted in 1989 and enforced on 5 May 1992. The Convention is the response of the international community to the problem caused by the annual worldwide production of 400 million tonnes of wastes which are hazardous to people or the environment because they are toxic, poisonous, explosive, corrosive, flammable, eco-toxic, or infectious.

The main principles of the Basel Convention are as follows.

- Trans boundary movement of hazardous waste should be reduced to a minimum consistent with environmentally sound management.
- Hazardous waste should be treated and disposed of as close as possible to the source of generation.
- Hazardous waste generation should be reduced and minimized at source.

In order to achieve the three main principles, the Convention established its secretariat to control the transboundary movement of hazardous waste, to monitor and prevent illegal traffic, to provide assistance for the environmentally sound management of hazardous waste, to cooperate with party countries or promote cooperation between parties, and to develop technical guidelines for the management of hazardous wastes. The Convention was further modified and decided to reduce exports of hazardous wastes to developing countries, on the grounds that those countries mostly have neither the expertise nor the facilities to manage such wastes.

41.6 Conventions on the Ozone Layer

The UNEP has included the concern of ozone depletion and related issues since 1977. It organized the Convention for the Protection of Ozone Layer in Vienna in 1985. This Convention emphasized the need for commitment of countries for the protection of ozone layer. Cooperation is needed between nations in reference to scientific research in understanding the processes and consequences of ozone depletion. The Convention recommended future protocols and specified procedures for dispute settlement and future amendment.

Following the objectives of this Convention, the Montreal Protocol on Substances that Deplete the Ozone Layer was developed and agreed by nations in 1987. This protocol was further strengthened by five amendments adopted in London (1990), Copenhagen (1992), Vienna (1995), Montreal (1997), and Beijing (1999). The aim of the protocol was to reduce and progressively eliminate the atmospheric emission of ODS. The Vienna Convention and Montreal Protocol are considered highly effective. The Montreal Protocol contains economic incentives to encourage participation and compliance in relation to three provisions: (i) entry into force requirements; (ii) control on trade with nonparties; and (iii) research and technology transfer benefits. The Montreal Protocol also provides a restricted transport and gradual ban on trade with nonparties. The Protocol offers the economic incentives for developing countries to join and comply along with the promotion of technology transfer.

41.7 Conventions on Biodiversity

Although not formally part of the UNCED preparatory process, the Rio Summit provided political impetus for completing the negotiations on the Convention on Biological Diversity (CBD). The CBD aimed to promote the conservation and sustainable use of biodiversity through scientific and technological cooperation, eradicating alien species, formulating protected areas, providing financial resources, and respecting traditional practices and knowledge. The Cartagena Biosafety Protocol 2000 was adopted to address risks associated with cross-border trade and accidental release of living modified organisms.

41.8 International Principles and Doctrines

The above discussed international environmental law developments indicate that one common theme reflected from the Stockholm Declaration 1972 to the Johannesburg Conference 2002 and beyond is the international community's emphasis on "sustainable development." Therefore, it is appropriate to take a holistic look at the features of sustainable development, its contours and their impact on protection, improvement, and management of the environment. The main principles that may be culled from the concept of sustainable development are: the polluter pays principle, precautionary principle, preventive principle, public trust doctrine, and intra/intergenerational equity.

Further Reading

Hamilton, C., Macintosh, A., Patrizi, N., and Bastianoni, S. (2019). Environmental protection and ecology. In: *Encyclopedia of Ecology* (ed. B. Fath), 319–326. St Louis: Elsevier.

Hill, M.K. (2004). *Understanding Environmental Pollution – A Primer*, 2e. New York: Cambridge University Press.

Kotwal, P.C. (2010). *India's Progress Towards Achieving Sustainable Forest Management*. Yokohama: ITTO.

Nagavallemma, K.P., Wani, S.P., Lacroix, S. et al. (2006). *Encyclopedia of Environmental Science and Engineering*, 5e. New York: CRC Press.

Rana, S.V.S. (2005). *Essentials of Ecology and Environmental Sceince*. New Delhi: Prentice-Hall.

Sharma, P.D. (1994). *Ecology and Environment*. Meerut.: Rastogi Publications.

Wildlife Institute of India (2009). *India's Green Book: Forests and Wildlife*. Dehradun: Wildlife Institute of India.

http://www.isaaa.org.

https://blogs.worldbank.org/climatechange/chemical-pollution-next-global-crisis.

https://ehs.psu.edu/environmental-protection.

https://epco.mp.gov.in/uploads/media/PGDEM_2023-24_Prospectus_Syllabus.pdf.

https://oceanservice.noaa.gov/ocean/earthday.html.

www.agbiotechnet.com.

www.agbioworld.org.

www.eea.europa.eu/en/topics/in-depth/climate-change-mitigation-reducing-emissions/current-state-of-the-ozone-layer.

www.environmentalpollutioncenters.org/chemical.

www.greenmountainenergy.com/why-renewable-energy/protect-the-environment.

www.sfc.com/en/glossar/environmental-protection.

42

Challenges of Emergency Animal Management During Disasters

Javed Jameel A[1], Justin Davis K[2], and Athira K[2]

[1] *Department of Veterinary Clinical Medicine, Ethics and Jurisprudence, College of Veterinary and Animal Sciences, Kerala Veterinary and Animal Sciences University, Pookode, India*
[2] *Department of Veterinary Epidemiology and Preventive Medicine, College of Veterinary and Animal Sciences, Kerala Veterinary and Animal Sciences University, Pookode, India*

42.1 Introduction

Disaster is defined by the World Health Organization as "any event that results in damage, economic destruction, human life loss, and deterioration in health and health services on a scale sufficient to warrant an extraordinary response from outside the affected community or area." It is an incident that occurs within a specific timeframe and location, leading to significant social, economic, cultural, and political upheaval, impacting both individuals and communities. No disaster is exactly the same as another and the impact and consequences vary from region to region and community to community. Large-scale disasters might make international news for a few minutes to weeks at the most, yet the effects on the ground last for years. Preparing for and responding to disasters is one of the greatest challenges facing the international community (WHO 2013).

Millions of creatures and their possessors are affected by natural disasters. Numerous major disasters in the past 10 years have increased public awareness of the requirements of animals during emergencies (Heath 2011). Animals are the major source of food and livelihood for the poorest people, and are also companions and valued family members. However, they are frequently left out of response strategies, rehabilitation initiatives, preparedness plans, and efforts to mitigate risks, for several reasons. These include insufficient knowledge and skills, lack of resources, unassigned responsibility, and a lack of organization. Animals are regularly vulnerable to disasters and are not similarly protected when they occur. Consequently, safeguarding animals should be an essential component of efficient emergency preparation and response. Incorporating animal welfare into disaster risk reduction, resilience, and preparedness planning will substantially decrease suffering, expedite recovery, and minimize reliance on postdisaster assistance.

Anthropogenic or natural agents may cause disasters, which are emergencies that affect both humans and animals. Anthropogenic cum technological disasters include fires, environmental pollution, and chemical incidents, as well as disasters resulting from human neglect, misconduct, conflicts, unlawful acts, or acts of terrorism. Natural disasters can be divided into four main groups (Figure 42.1): (i) hydrometeorological-climatological: floods, wave surges, storms, hurricanes, cyclones, landslides, avalanches, fire, droughts, and climate change; (ii) geophysical: tsunamis, earthquakes, and volcanic eruptions; (iii) biological: pandemic diseases, epidemics, and insect infestations; and (iv) extraterrestrial: asteroids, meteoroids, and comets that alter interplanetary conditions that affect the Earth's magnetosphere, ionosphere, and thermosphere (De Paula Vieira 2021).

A disaster takes place when the capacity to foresee and mitigate risks associated with natural or human-made hazards surpasses the typical provisions for health and welfare, leading to a disruption in the usual ability to manage the situation. Disasters can also be classified, according to their impact, as localized, widespread, predictable or unpredictable, and also major or minor. Disasters can have a global, national, or local impact. The beginning of a disaster can be sudden/rapid (fire, flood, avalanche, mudslide, earthquake) or slow (disease, biosecurity breach).

Unfortunately, current international disaster responses have significant gaps and challenges. The COVID-19 outbreak, for example, uncovered a lack of attention to the risks that infected animals and humans pose to public, animal, and

---

Epidemiology and Environmental Hygiene in Veterinary Public Health, First Edition. Edited by Tanmoy Rana.
© 2025 John Wiley & Sons, Inc. Published 2025 by John Wiley & Sons, Inc.

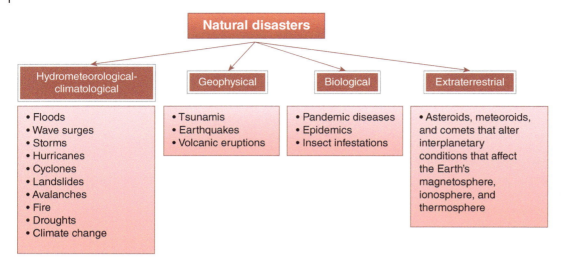

Figure 42.1 Classification of natural disasters.

environmental health. In particular, the FAO guidelines emphasized that disasters not only impact the supply chain (e.g., resulting in animal losses, reduced slaughtering and processing capacity as well as misconceptions regarding animals and animal products being hosts or vehicles of zoonosis that can infect humans) but also the prevention and control capacity of common animal health and welfare services (FAO 2020). These factors encompass a scarcity of labor causing interruptions in the usual animal health and welfare protocols followed by farmers and food processors. Additionally, there are delays and decreased capabilities in testing, diagnostics, and the surveillance and reporting of animal diseases. The impact of a disaster can be categorized as direct, indirect or tertiary.

Besides the public health impacts of disasters, such as the risk of zoonotic diseases and disruptions to the food supply, disasters also result in adverse economic effects, especially in developing nations. In these regions, livestock plays a crucial role by supplying milk, meat, labor for agriculture and transportation, dung, hides, wool, fibers, and more. Additionally, animals serve as a relatively secure investment option and bestow social significance upon their owners.

When animals are impacted by a disaster, the primary issues include:

- contamination or spoilage of their food and/or water sources
- zoonoses
- animal bites
- significant impact on public mental health due to the emotional involvement of the owners with the animals
- reduced dairy and livestock production, due to the scarcity of feed and water, high livestock mortality rates, etc.
- damage to both domestic and wild animal species, due to lack of feed and water and the diseases which spread during and after a disaster.

In most cases, disasters expose underlying systemic vulnerabilities in a community by suddenly opposing chronically unmet needs with equally chronic insufficient resources. The management of animals is crisis driven and transient rather than aimed at long-term and systemic goals by addressing underlying systemic flaws when the solutions to problems impacting animals in disasters are evaluated through the prism of response. Increasing human reliance on animals for survival, including nutrition, food security, health, safety, and livelihood, makes animal disaster management a "wicked problem" (Glassey 2020). Applying the principles of emergency management to the care of animals in disasters results in improvements in public and animal health that are sustainable and can lower the incidence of animal issues arising in disasters.

Human–animal connections, whether they take the form of companionship, support, or guardianship, can have a significant effect on how people make decisions, formulate feelings and attitudes, and behave. Heath et al. (2001a) claim that "companion animal guardianship can be a significant threat to public and animal safety during disasters," calling for greater attention to disaster preparedness regarding companion animals. Therefore, it is crucial to take animal guardianship into account while discussing natural calamities.

Disaster planning, preparedness, response, recovery and mitigation can become extremely complicated when natural disasters occur at a high rate. This can become even more complex due to varying contextual circumstances among affected populations. The needs of animal guardians should be taken into account before, during, and after disasters as a matter of public health and safety. The main reason why this population must be seriously considered by disaster professionals and officials is that guardians often return to disaster sites even when they are not deemed safe for reentry to look for their companion animals.

Animal guardianship can have a significant impact on catastrophe decisions, even at the expense of health and safety (Brackenridge et al. 2012). This can threaten the health and safety of responders who must rescue guardians who fail to evacuate due to refusal to leave their companion animals or due to animal-restrictive policies (Brooks et al. 2016). This can delay rescue for other affected individuals. Abandoned companion animals not only affect the health and well-being of their guardians but can threaten public health and safety of others through needless rescue missions, zoonotic diseases, or aggressive behavior due to anxiety and fright. Disaster experts and policymakers can probably lessen these risks and threats, despite the fact that animal guardianship can influence disaster-relevant decisions (Akhtar 2013).

42.2 Animal Disaster Management

Animal disaster management is a vital aspect of disaster preparedness and response. It encompasses a broad range of activities and considerations aimed at ensuring the safety and well-being of animals during and after disasters. The concept of animal disaster management extends to companion animals and livestock, as well as wildlife in some cases. As disasters become increasingly frequent and severe due to climate change and other factors, addressing the challenges in animal disaster management has become more critical than ever.

Saving lives and guaranteeing that every effort has been made during the planning and response phases to ensure the humane treatment of animals are at the center of animal disaster management. Accordingly, improving critical disaster management issues involves identifying and reflecting on ethical principles, values, and prejudices relevant to disaster management and the plight of animals during disasters. The nature and complexity of the task of animal disaster management suggest that a one-size-fits-all formula is insufficient and that ongoing multilevel ethical assessment, analysis, and deliberation (involving impact on animals) are necessary (Zack 2009).

Disasters in the real world are characterized by the need to act quickly, interrupted coordination and communications, frequent recalibration in the face of uncertainty, imperfect knowledge and inadequate equipment and supplies, and legal sanctions and enforcement. Decisions regarding management and response depend on the context, take into account social and cultural norms, prioritize ethical concerns (such as by analyzing the beliefs, values, and interests of different stakeholders), and take into account practical, legal, and economic aspects. The community's capacity is influenced by whether the disaster is connected to overall preparedness and human culpability and whether legal fault can be assigned (this will affect who pays for response or recovery), local political, topography, and economic factors like resource allocation and wealth distribution and how and which ethical issues are documented, deliberated, weighted, and prioritized. Also, different communities may place different importance on human life and livelihoods, protection of property, risks and harms to human and animal safety, suffering, and fatalities, and community resilience.

Disaster management activities should protect public safety and promote health and welfare to produce desired outcomes consistent with a community's social values. The disaster management goal of minimizing morbidity and mortality among isolated individuals also encompasses safeguarding and enhancing the well-being of the interconnected human–animal–environment community, with a broader perspective (Jennings and Arras 2016; OIE 2016; Heath 1999).

There are five stages in the emergency management lifecycle (Figure 42.2) that emergency managers must consider.

1) Planning
2) Preparedness
3) Mitigation
4) Response
5) Recovery

Animals should be taken into account in all processes. Disasters bring into focus the practical intervention, welfare, public health, civil defense and protection, biosecurity and scientific challenges related to each phase of the disaster management cycle (FAO 2020) as well as the inevitable normative decisions and choices reflecting ethical values that must be made through judicious deliberation regarding our responsibilities to animals (Mepham 2020; Van Herten et al. 2020; Schwartz 2020).

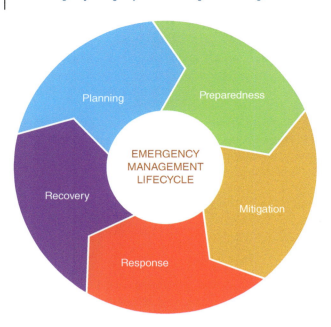

Figure 42.2 Stages of emergency management life cycle.

42.2.1 Planning

Planning affects the entire disaster cycle. A community-centered disaster operations plan should include action and contingency plans and be specific and implementable. The requirements of both animals and their owners should be considered. Such plans should categorize and prioritize realistic threats and delineate the response mission, goals, capabilities and any gaps to meet them such as through the law or descriptive epidemiology, environmental and other disaster-specific data sets. Insufficient planning and training can hinder the coordination and effectiveness of response and recovery teams during emergencies or crises. For shelters to operate effectively, planning efforts can identify appropriate policies for management of animals. This includes determining when shelters will be accessible, the locations for housing animals, the allocation of responsibilities and liabilities among individuals involved, necessary staffing levels, and training of qualified personnel like animal control officers, animal technicians, veterinarians, and volunteers. Additionally, it entails defining the responsibilities of managers and specifying any waivers that owners might need to endorse. By determining the need for training and exercises that improve response capability and by developing a business plan on how to fund, conduct, and evaluate the impact of training, exercises, and real-world events, planning can result in better preparedness. The advance identification of housing and other resources that may be required during a disaster to enable the care of animals is an example of planning to improve response.

In a nutshell, planning for disaster recovery should involve the community at large, community planners, developers, financiers, and subject matter specialists, and should attempt to establish the desired future state of the community.

42.2.2 Preparedness

One of the most significant challenges in animal disaster management is the pervasive lack of awareness and preparedness among pet owners, livestock farmers, and communities at large. Many individuals do not fully comprehend the importance of including animals in their disaster preparedness plans. As a result, they may not have adequate supplies, evacuation plans, or shelters in place for their animals when disasters strike.

Being prepared entails educating the public so that people are equipped to take care of themselves and their dependents, as well as training, testing, and credentialing emergency personnel. Disaster preparedness is important for all animals but is particularly important for livestock because of the size of the animals and the requirements needed to transport and shelter them (Hunt et al. 2012).

The roles of participating officials, stakeholders, and animal welfare and health organizations should all be clearly stated. Working outside the official channels is usually counterproductive when trying to figure out how to manage animals in disasters. A network of operational and public communication methods should be developed, including simulated exercises that take animals into account in all steps and evacuation plans. Vulnerable regions and hazards to animals should also be recognized. As a component of a community's preparedness initiatives, it is advisable to designate a certified volunteer manager in advance for inclusion in the animal emergency response teams. In flood- and cyclone-prone areas, Sastry (1994) advises the construction of multipurpose livestock shelters because they are excellent for protecting animals during floods and cyclones and can also be used as fodder stores, veterinary centers, or government training centers where technical experts can provide advice and training in animal management, vaccine awareness, and disease prevention.

42.2.3 Mitigation

Mitigation involves interventions aimed at lessening the impact or costs of disasters to vulnerable animals ahead of their occurrence through anticipation measures. Classic examples of mitigation include restricting transit routes for hazardous goods to avoid human population centers, implementing suitable building rules for known hazards such as earthquakes and floods, and purchasing specialized equipment needed in the case of a disaster. Legislation, regulations, and their enforcement, as well as other commitments that set minimum standards for the care of animals and make resources available to achieve and maintain those standards during disasters, are all examples of mitigation efforts that lessen negative impacts on the animal health infrastructure, or the public, private, and nongovernment services and facilities in a community that support animal well-being.

Precise disaster technologies and scientific developments can help to alleviate harms for animals and should be encouraged. Examples of situations where the demands of animals in disaster mitigation have fallen short include the need for housing large numbers of stray animals, and external groups leading response efforts rather than local authorities. Local regulations can also mitigate animal disasters by enacting strong animal control laws supported by enforcement. An effective spay-neuter program for dogs and cats would reduce the number of strays in a community, which in turn would reduce the number of stray animals that emerge in the wake of disasters. Regulations limiting the number of animals that people can keep also set expectations for the public to maintain their animal population under reasonable control. Research has indicated a clear link between the quantity of animals in a household and the likelihood of pet owners choosing not to evacuate.

Examples of modifications to the physical environment that lessen disasters for livestock include protection from extreme weather, such as windbreaks for livestock exposed to blizzards, elevated dirt mounds for livestock living in floodplains to move to as flood waters rise, and making sure that sufficient and appropriate feed and water are available to animals exposed to temperature extremes.

Insurance is another mitigation tool that disperses the financial risk resulting from animal disease outbreaks and droughts, to raising livestock during nondisaster times and ensuring adequate funding for response and recovery once disaster strikes.

When individuals keep a larger number of animals than they can adequately attend to or abandon animals during an evacuation, they are placing these animals in hazardous surroundings, which in turn results in neglect of these animals. When people try to provide for too many animals with insufficient resources, they are living on the edge of disaster in which animals could suffer when resources which are already under inadequate supply become further constrained. The persistent lack of adequate funding for animal control agencies represents a shortcoming in mitigation. Because of the poor retention of trained and experienced emergency management personnel that results from low pay for animal control workers, a community's inability to successfully implement all phases of emergency management is further exacerbated.

42.2.4 Response

The response and emergency relief efforts prioritize reducing illness and loss of life, and safeguarding property, thereby laying the foundation for assisting communities in their recovery phase.

The disaster response phase commences upon receiving the initial notification of the disaster. During this phase, preparedness plans (both action and contingency) are implemented in collaboration with various disaster management experts and organizations. This encompasses activities such as search and rescue, veterinary services and care, evacuation, temporary shelter, and ensuring safety and protection. Similar to other aspects of emergency management, the most significant benefit in reducing the adverse consequences of disasters, including impacts on both animal and public health, is achieved through actions taken in the four phases preceding the response phase. Disaster response is characterized by a temporary mismatch between the need to save life and property and the resources available to meet those needs. The need for resources is continuously assessed and gap-analyzed throughout the response, and these processes continue until urgent needs are no longer the predominant reason for resource demand.

High-profile response problems that frequently affect animals during disasters include: (i) lack of clear command and direction; (ii) pet owners who choose not to evacuate because of their animals; (iii) pet owners who evacuate without their animals; (iv) rescue of animals from premises after owners have left them behind; (v) stray animals; (vi) unreliable fund-raising; (vii) mismanaged volunteers. These issues reflect the effectiveness (or lack thereof) of mitigation, planning, and preparedness efforts preceding the disaster.

Lack of distinct leadership and guidance results in contradictory or unclear guidance to the public, such as whether to evacuate with or without animals, the availability of assistance, and information regarding threats and risks to both people and animals. Animal issues are predictably ignored by emergency management officials during a response in communities that have not engaged in adequate planning or mitigation for the needs of animals and their owners. As a result, these communities frequently lack a qualified or experienced person overseeing animal issues during the response to a disaster. Pet relinquishment is a prevalent cultural phenomenon and the underlying cause for the persistent issue of stray animals during disasters. Although much of the literature on animals in disasters is quick to justify the *ad hoc* care of animals under the pretext of emergency management personnel's lack of commitment to animals, this is misleading. While expertise and qualifications cannot be obtained rapidly, the absence of these abilities should not be a deterrent to those eager to provide assistance.

Pet ownership is the single most common factor associated with human evacuation failure that can be positively affected when the threat of disaster is impending (Hunt et al. 2012). Planning efforts should identify pet owners who are at risk, and preparation initiatives should include community-based support networks like buddy systems among neighbors. By providing free cardboard cat carriers and dog leashes when officials go door to door to advertise the need to evacuate with pets, emergency managers can help to limit the number of people who choose not to leave because they have pets. Transportation equipment like carriers, collars, and leashes can be provided as needed through arrangements established between local emergency managers, pet accessory retailers, and other suppliers.

Pet evacuation failure (a form of pet abandonment) occurs when pet owners evacuate and leave their pets at home, and is a fairly common phenomenon in disasters. Inappropriate advice given by emergency management and law enforcement to leave pets behind during disasters can contribute to this. Research findings suggest that the principal reason owners leave their pets behind is because they have weak bonds with pets at the time of (and after) a disaster (Heath et al. 2001b).

One of the outcomes of people leaving their pets behind is their subsequent attempt to rescue their animals after evacuating. This behavior, while rare, is often perilous and draws considerable attention. Most frequently, the desire to rescue a pet arises from peer pressure and media accounts of abandoned pets exposed to danger. Less frequently, it involves owners who were not home when evacuation orders were issued and, despite their efforts, cannot access their residences. In either scenario, the potential threat to human life should be assessed, and if determined to be insignificant, animal rescues are best carried out under the direct supervision of trained emergency response and animal care personnel. These professionals can evaluate whether it is safe to evacuate the animal promptly without risking harm to the responders, owners, or animals involved. Instances of pet evacuation failure and subsequent efforts to rescue pets offer an opportunity for public education that serves as a model for demonstrating proper evacuation behavior.

The abundance of stray animals has been a common concern after major disasters. Cats and dogs found after disasters are more representative of pets surrendered to humane shelters rather than house pets. Common attributes of animals discovered following disasters include being either older or younger (such as puppies and kittens) compared to the typical family pet, lacking identification, displaying signs of chronic illness, and often exhibiting behavioral issues. The quantity of animals found post disaster is similar to what one might encounter among stray animals in the affected region. The animals discovered in disaster areas are primarily a manifestation of the broader problem of pet overpopulation. Throughout disaster response efforts, effective public service announcements (PSAs) can heighten awareness of this concern and garner support for more effective initiatives aimed at pet recovery and mitigation.

Everything must be done to help reconnect animals and owners who have become separated as a result of the calamity. Conscientious pet owners will take all reasonable steps to locate their animals, and they must be given every opportunity to do so, including notification of known animal sighting locations, housing information, and access to searchable web databases to identify and locate their animals. Lack of standardized descriptions, however, makes it difficult to search through databases and reunite lost animals with their owners (Irvine 2009). Animal shelters suffer managerial difficulties when a disaster strikes because they are unable to modify their adoption and euthanasia procedures to accommodate pet owners who require additional time to locate and reunite with their animals. Policies that permit shelters to extend the waiting period for the release of pets for at least an additional three weeks after a disaster should be enacted. In situations where it is impossible to locate the original owner, prospective new owners should be obligated to enter into a fostering agreement for the initial 6–12 months of care. This arrangement ensures that if the original owner reemerges, there will be no ambiguity about who rightfully owns the animal.

Disasters evoke a strong sense of empathy within the public, often resulting in generous donations to various causes, including those aimed at helping animals. When addressing the needs of animals during a disaster response, such as providing shelter, food, necessary equipment, and environmental enrichment, it is crucial to efficiently manage these resources. Requests for assistance conveyed through the media should be well considered and precise, as careless or ill-defined appeals can waste the goodwill of donors and potentially valuable resources. Moreover, there are concerns related to fundraising practices that lack transparency, ranging from fraudulent activities to diverting donated funds to unintended causes or locations. Such unaccountable fundraising can significantly hinder the long-term recovery process.

Fundraising fraud is regrettably common during disasters, and efforts to raise funds for animal care are no exception to this trend. Often, new fundraising websites emerge immediately following a disaster, collecting donations and then disappearing without trace within a matter of weeks. To prevent well-intentioned donors from being misled and to ensure that donations are effectively channeled to the affected communities, it is advisable for communities to proactively identify recipient organizations for potential sponsors before a disaster strikes. Establishing clear agreements in advance on how disaster-related donations will be managed is essential.

In situations where animal disaster triage is required, first responders and relevant experts should possess the ethical decision-making capabilities to optimize resource utilization. Training in triage care should progress to encompass a structured and prompt evaluation for the treatment of severely ill or injured animals, as well as their rehabilitation.

42.2.5   Recovery

The recovery phase becomes apparent as the response phase is subsiding. This phase entails activities that are focused on a desired future or restore a community to a predisaster status quo, including reinstating basic services. Emergency managers start the recovery phase as soon as a disaster occurs but the effectiveness of the early recovery planning often does not emerge until the response is subsiding. Here health, genetic tests, psychological and behavioral rehabilitation measures can be enhanced within suitable animal facilities in preparation for the release and subsequent monitoring of animal populations and wildlife after release. The recovery phase is the lengthiest and most costly, extending over many months or even years.

For communities that take animal issues seriously, the recovery phase is an ideal time to plan and start working toward a better future, such as embarking on a strategy to establish a robust animal health infrastructure that prospers due to the elimination of persistent issues stemming from systemic root causes. Communities that have formulated a comprehensive emergency management strategy, encompassing animal concerns before a disaster occurs, are more likely to achieve their desired future recovery.

In times of disasters, veterinarians play a critical part in maintaining exceptional animal health standards and minimizing animal mortality rates. Veterinarians have a role to play in all stages of disaster mitigation and management, but it is during relief efforts that they can really help to increase the survivability of animals that are victims. Protecting and saving human life is the first priority in disaster relief and protecting property (which includes animals) is the second. Disaster management should be integrated with long-term development planning, and a holistic, rather than a segmented, approach should be taken, with popular participation involving local communities. Development and disaster management planning should go hand in hand and development models must have inbuilt components for disaster reduction, mitigation, and preparedness.

A major challenge of mitigating animal issues is the common approach of treating animal care as a distinct, response-focused matter. However, as numerous emergency managers have learned through difficult experiences, in disasters the connection between people and animals can either disrupt overall response efforts or can be strategically managed to enhance overall operations. Owners can experience a sense of helplessness when they are uncertain about how to handle their pets. However, when they actively participate in community planning, preparedness, and mitigation initiatives, they gain the knowledge and confidence needed to relocate themselves and their animals away from potential dangers. National and local authorities should assume the responsibility of integrating companion animals into their planning processes, rather than depending on international organizations, which may lack familiarity with the social, economic, and cultural context of the disaster, or local NGOs that often face resource constraints and expertise gaps.

Based on worldwide experiences, it has been observed that human fatalities increase when disaster responses fail to include their pets. Furthermore, this exclusion leads to significantly higher negative impacts on animal welfare and animal fatalities. Additionally, it is posited that there may be an uptick in the transmission of zoonotic diseases in the aftermath of disasters.

42.3 Conclusion

Disaster framing is crucial for effective readiness and response. When characterizing disaster management in the context of its objectives, the disaster management team must consider its ethical principles. This entails openly articulating the guiding priorities, values, moral foundations, and rationale behind crisis policies and actions, all while promoting comprehensive crisis coordination across all levels. Disaster management aims can highlight the adequacy of the infrastructure involved in advancing equity, inclusion and community relationships, which will be necessary in mobilizing political will.

The long-term impacts of disasters can affect animals and make those that are already in poor health or welfare more susceptible to both infectious and noninfectious diseases. This susceptibility arises from weakened immune systems, which can result in distress, behavioral issues, and adverse emotional states (FAO 2020). At emergency sites during disasters, there can be a severe shortage of both the quality and quantity of food and water. Additionally, routine management practices like relocating manure, transporting feed and livestock, and automated tasks dependent on energy sources may be disrupted as a result of power failures. Animals are also put at risk by their physical or housing conditions. The way animal facilities are organized and the magnitude of animals housed can result in disastrous consequences for animals and humans alike.

The occurrence of natural disasters has increased significantly in the past 20 years. While the debate continues about the role of climate change, it is predicted that the frequency and intensity of natural disasters will continue to escalate (Thomas et al. 2013). Recognizing the significance of animals in various roles, be it as production animals, working animals, or companions, compels us to make sure that animal protection is an essential component of efficient disaster planning and response.

To summarize, the ethical assessment of whether animals' interests are morally recognized largely depends on the nature and scale of the disaster affecting a community, the perception of animals in relation to human interests and priorities, and the existence of disaster management plans that address the well-being of animals during emergencies. Ensuring the compassionate and dignified treatment of animals in disaster situations necessitates, among other factors, the collaborative efforts of diverse professionals guided by the principles of animal welfare science, along with a reassessment of the attitudes of various stakeholders regarding the ethical consideration of animals.

Ultimately, the goal is to protect and care for all living beings when disaster strikes, fostering a society that values and safeguards the welfare of animals in times of crisis.

References

Akhtar, A. (2013). The need to include animal protection in public health policies. *Journal of Public Health Policy* 34 (4): 549–559.

Brackenridge, S., Zottarelli, L.K., Rider, E., and Carlsen-Landy, B. (2012). Dimensions of the human–animal bond and evacuation decisions among companion animal guardians during Hurricane Ike. *Anthrozoös* 25 (2): 229–238.

Brooks, H., Rushton, K., Walker, S. et al. (2016). Ontological security and connectivity provided by companion animals: a study in the self-management of the everyday lives of people diagnosed with a long-term mental health condition. *BMC Psychiatry* 16 (1): 409.

De Paula Vieira, A., & Anthony, R. (2021). Reimagining human responsibility towards animals for disaster management in the Anthropocene. In B. Bovenkerk & J. Keulartz (Eds.), Animals in our midst: The challenges of co-existing with animals in the Anthropocene (Vol. 33, pp. [226]). Springer. https://doi.org/10.1007/978-3-030-63523-7_13.

Food and Agriculture Organization (FAO) (2020). *Guidelines to Mitigate the Impact of the COVID-19 Pandemic on Livestock Production and Animal Health*. Rome: FAO.

Glassey, S. (2020). Animal Welfare and Disasters. https://doi.org/10.1093/acrefore/9780190228637.013.1528 (accessed 12 February 2024).

Heath, S.E. (1999). *Animal Management in Disasters: A Handbook for Emergency Responders and Animal Owners*, 330. St Louis: Mosby.

Heath, S.E. (2011). Veterinarians in disasters. *Veterinary Record* 169: 185–186.

Heath, S.E., Kass, P.H., Beck, A.M., and Glickman, L.T. (2001a). Human and companion animal- related risk factors for household evacuation failure during a natural disaster. *American Journal of Epidemiology* 153: 659–665.

Heath, S.E., Beck, A.M., Kass, P.H., and Glickman, L.T. (2001b). Risk factors for pet evacuation failure in a slow onset disaster. *Journal of the American Veterinary Medical Association* 218: 1905–1910.

Hunt, M.G., Bogue, K., and Rohrbaugh, N. (2012). Pet ownership and evacuation prior to Hurricane Irene. *Animals* 2: 529–539.

Irvine, L. (2009). *Filling the Ark: Animal Welfare in Disasters*. Philadelphia: Temple University Press.

Jennings, B. and Arras, J.D. (2016). Ethical aspects of public health emergency preparedness and response. In: *Emergency Ethics: Public Health Preparedness and Response* (ed. B. Jennings, J.D. Arras, D.H. Barrett, and B.A. Ellis), 100–103. New York: Oxford University Press.

Mepham, B. (2020). Morality, morbidity and mortality: an ethical analysis of culling nonhuman animals. In: *The End of Animal Life: A Start for Ethical Debate. Ethical and Societal Considerations on Killing Animals* (ed. F.L. Meijboom and E.N. Stassen), 341–362. Wageningen: Wageningen Academic Publishers.

OIE (2016). Guidelines on disaster management and risk reduction in relation to animal health and welfare and veterinary public health. www.woah.org/app/uploads/2021/03/disastermanagement-ang.pdf (accessed 12 February 2024).

Sastry, N.S. (1994). Managing livestock sector during floods and cyclones. *Journal of Rural Development (Hyderabad)* 13 (4): 583–592.

Schwartz, M.E. (2020). *The Ethic of Pandemics*. Peterborough, Canada: Broadview Press.

Thomas, V., Albert, J.R.G., and Perez, R.T. (2013). Climate-Related Disasters in Asia and the Pacific. www.adb.org/sites/default/files/publication/30323/ewp-358.pdf (accessed 12 February 2024).

Van Herten, J., Buikstra, S., Bovenkerk, B., and Stassen, E. (2020). Ethical decision-making in zoonotic disease control: how do one health strategies function in the Netherlands? *Journal of Agricultural and Environmental Ethics* 33: 239–259.

World Health Organization (WHO) (2013). *Emergency Response Framework*. Geneva: WHO.

Zack, N. (2009). The ethics of disaster planning: preparation vs response. *Philosophy of Management* 8: 55–66.

43

Sources of Air Pollution in Animal Houses and Its Consequences

Parul Singh, Barkha Sharma, Udit Jain, Renu Singh, Sanjay Bharti, and Meena Goswami

College of Veterinary & Animal Sciences, DUVASU, Mathura, India

43.1 Introduction

Air pollution inside animal housing is a well-known hazard in intensive systems of animal rearing. Animals used to be kept either separately or in small groups under confinement but now they are oten reared for economic advantage in intensive systems. Industrialization in the animal sector is focused on increased production and decreased labor costs. This intensive system of rearing has its own pros and cons, as it raises the production and financial benefits while pollutants generated in and around animal buildings have deleterious effects on the health of animals, workers, and the environment.

The animal industry produces pollutants including noxious gaseous, waste liquids, and solids. Gaseous pollutants such as carbon dioxide (CO_2), methane (CH_4), nitrous oxide (N_2O), ammonia (NH_3), and hydrogen sulfide (H_2S), particulate matter, odors, volatile organic compounds (VOCs), and bio-aerosols are generated due to animal activities and operations performed in and around animal housing (Guo et al. 2022). Microorganisms in the excretions and secretions of animals also exist inside the buildings and can be transmitted to healthy animals and human workers. Zoonotic bacterial pathogens that may be excreted include *Salmonella*, *E. coli*, viral pathogens including bovine rhinotracheitis and foot and mouth disease virus, avian influenza and Newcastle disease virus, swine fever virus, etc.

Air pollution inside animal houses is due to various extrinsic and intrinsic factors. Feed- and fodder-related operations (chaffing, thrashing), manure storage, solid waste management plants, stationary and mobile sources of pollution are major extrinsic factors. Intrinsic factors are related to the physiology of the animal.

43.2 Sources of Air Pollution inside Animal Housing

43.2.1 Intrinsic Factors

Various animal activities contribute to pollution within animal housing, including respiration, enteric emission of gases, eructation, defecation and urination, saliva, lachrymal, vaginal, and uterine discharges, and release of other pathogens. In intensive livestock units, high stocking density results in the accumulation of various air pollutants that enhance the transmission of disease among the animals. The design of animal housing and ventilation systems also plays a role in the concentrations of air pollutants. Indoor pollution is a bigger issue for pig and poultry farming than other aspects of the animal industry (Kelleghan et al. 2021).

43.2.2 Extrinsic Factors

43.2.2.1 Microbial Decomposition and Spoilage of Remnants

Accumulation of pollutants within farm buildings arises due to microbiological decomposition and spoilage of fecal material, urine, and remnants of feed and fodder. Spoilage of straw, feedstuffs, and bedding materials and decomposition of manure and urine cause a substantial release of harmful gases into the environment. Major gases in this regard include

Epidemiology and Environmental Hygiene in Veterinary Public Health, First Edition. Edited by Tanmoy Rana.
© 2025 John Wiley & Sons, Inc. Published 2025 by John Wiley & Sons, Inc.

ammonia, hydrogen sulfide, methane, and carbon dioxide. Air-borne dust derived from bedding material is also a source of pollution. The accumulation of undesirable odors is an indication of insanitary conditions. Accumulation of manure, urine, and washings within buildings is a potent source of hazardous gases.

43.2.2.2 Stationary Sources of Pollution
Stationary sources of pollution refer to sources that are immovable and stationary in one place. These sources mainly include chemicals and products manufacturing industries. Animals housed near to stationary sources may be exposed to these gases. Small manufacturing industries in nearby areas are also sources of considerable pollution.

43.2.2.3 Mobile Sources of Pollution
Mobile sources include transport vehicles that release noxious air pollutants. Animal buildings situated near roads are continuously exposed to air pollutants emitted by automobiles, one of the most common being SO_2. These animal houses have higher concentrations of air pollutants than houses that are further from the roadside. Besides road transport, waterways (boat, yacht) and air transport (aeroplanes, etc.) also emit air pollutants that may affect the air quality inside animal housing. Sources of air pollution inside animal housing are summarized in Figure 43.1.

The following gaseous and particulate pollutants contribute to air pollution inside animal buildings. See also Figure 43.2.

- Carbon dioxide (CO_2)
- Methane (CH_4)
- Ammonia (NH_3)
- Hydrogen sulfide (H_2S)
- Carbon monoxide (CO)
- Nitrous oxide (N_2O)
- Odor
- Volatile organic compounds (VOCs)
- Particulate matter (PM)
- Bio-aerosols/biological pollutants

43.2.3 Carbon Dioxide

Emission of carbon dioxide inside animal housing is due to respiration. The animal's energy metabolism rate is related to the amount and nutrient composition of the diet and microbial fermentation of manure. Regular cleaning of animal housing, especially removal of manure and washing the floor, reduces the concentration of CO_2. Factors such as deep litter more

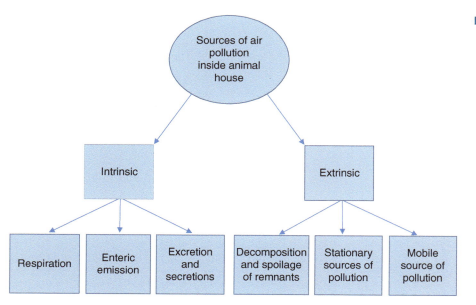

Figure 43.1 Sources of air pollution.

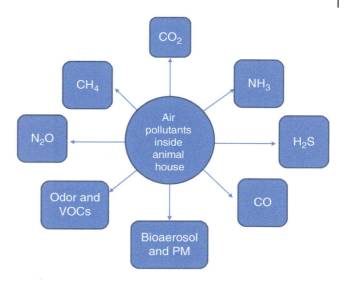

Figure 43.2 Gaseous and particulate pollutants in animal buildings.

than 0.5 m thick produced a considerable amount of CO_2. The following figures are average excretions of CO_2/hour: lactating cow 5.8 cubic feet, horse 3.9 cubic feet, pig 1.3 cubic feet, and sheep 0.55 cubic feet (Pedersen et al. 2008).

Besides respiration and microbial decomposition, another important source of gas emission is enteric fermentation. This is a natural digestive process by which plant biomass, mainly cellulose and hemicellulose, consumed by ruminants is broken down by rumen flora into volatile fatty acids and gaseous waste products carbon dioxide and methane. These gases are expelled from the rumen by the process of eructation (Grossi et al. 2019).

43.2.3.1 Effects of Carbon Dioxide

In animal buildings with a high density of animals and improper ventilation, excessive moisture and gases can accumulate. Carbon dioxide is one of the major greenhouse gases with the capacity to trap heat which may lead to indoor warming. A combination of high moisture and carbon dioxide makes animals uncomfortable and affects production. Studies have shown that a reduction in atmospheric oxygen level up to 10–12% may not prove fatal to animals while an increase of atmospheric carbon dioxide level up to 6.0% may lead to asphyxia and a concentration of 30% for some hours could result in death. In horses, carbon dioxide concentration of 3–5% may cause rapid breathing. Carbon dioxide has a human threshold limit value (TLV) of 0.5% but has been shown to be deleterious to fowl in concentrations above 1.5%.

43.2.4 Methane

Methane is mainly produced by enteric fermentation and manure storage inside animal housing. Methane emission in the reticulorumen is an adaptation that enables the rumen to dispose of hydrogen in the form of methane. Otherwise accumulation of methane inside the animal inhibits carbohydrate fermentation and fiber degradation. The emission of enteric methane varies according to feed intake and digestibility of feed. Fine chopping, grinding, and steam treatment of fodder improve digestibility and can decrease enteric methane production in ruminants (Goglio et al. 2018).

43.2.4.1 Effects of Methane

Methane is also a greenhouse gas and its molecules have more capacity to trap heat in comparison to CO_2. Excessive amounts of methane may cause explosions.

43.2.5 Ammonia

Microbial decomposition of manure is the main source of ammonia. Sewage treatment plants also release ammonia. It can be produced in relatively high concentrations from microbial decomposition of poultry manure because of its high uric acid content (Kim and Ko 2019).

43.2.5.1 Effects of Ammonia

Ammonia is a gas that is frequently found in dirty animal housing and a concentration between 0.04% and 0.5% causes irritation of mucous membranes. The continuous presence of NH_3 causes various conditions such as:

- central paralysis
- liver disease
- asphyxia and death.

43.2.6 Hydrogen Sulfide

This is a colorless gas with a strong and generally objectionable rotten egg odor. It is produced in anaerobic environments by microbial decomposition of sulfur-containing organic matter in manure.

43.2.6.1 Effects of Hydrogen Sulfide

A concentration of 0.01–0.14% of hydrogen sulfide is associated with irritation of eyes, throat and nose, and lung edema. Accumulation of hydrogen sulfide in animal housing may lead to (Kim and Ko 2019):

- paralysis
- digestive disturbances
- liver diseases.

43.2.7 Carbon Monoxide

Carbon monoxide, an organic pollutant and a gas that is toxic to humans and animals, can be generated during aerobic digestion of organic waste. Biowaste treatment is the major source of emissions and vehicles also emit the gas. Animal buildings near roads are continuously exposed to emission of this gas from mobile sources (Stegenta-Dabrowska et al. 2019).

43.2.7.1 Effects of Carbon Monoxide

Carbon monoxide is a silent killer which binds to the iron atoms in hemoglobin, with an affinity 200–250 times that of oxygen. It impairs the oxygen-carrying capacity of blood and causes hypoxia. Neurological effects of CO include headaches, dizziness, weakness, nausea, vomiting, disorientation, visual confusions, collapse, and coma (Talaiekhozani et al. 2018).

43.2.8 Nitrous Oxide

Manure is a source of this gas and the emission is related to environmental conditions, type of management and composition of the manure and nitrogen content of excreta. Therefore, when manure is handled as a solid (dung) or deposited on pastures, nitrous oxide production increases while little or no methane is emitted. Nitrous oxide is generated through both the nitrification and denitrification processes of the nitrogen contained in manure, which is mainly present in organic form (e.g., proteins) and in inorganic form as ammonium and ammonia (Grossi et al. 2019).

43.2.8.1 Effects of Nitrous Oxide

The molecular mechanism of toxicity caused by N_2O exposure is related to vitamin B12 insufficiency and it is believed to interact with folate metabolism and subsequently causes methionine synthase inhibition, mitochondrial dysfunction, and DNA damage. These micro-changes may be linked to adverse health effects observed in populations exposed to N_2O such as genotoxicity, neurotoxicity, and teratogenicity (Menon et al. 2021).

43.2.9 Odor

According to the US Environmental Protection Agency, an "odorous substance" is a chemical product responsible for generating an odor sensation, while "odor" is defined as any gaseous emanation perceptible through the sense of smell.

The growing interest in air quality has led to the recognition of annoying odors as atmospheric pollutants, defining as "odor pollution" their negative impact on the surrounding environment and exposed population.

Odor emissions from livestock farms are related to animal diet, spilled feed, urine, and manure. In animal housing, if feces and urine are present for a long time then the organic matter of feces starts to volatilize and ferment on the surface to generate odor. Many compounds that contain either nitrogen or sulfur cause odor. Thus ammonia and hydrogen sulfide are odorous pollutants while carbon dioxide, methane, and nitrous oxide are odorless gases present inside animal buildings. In livestock farming, odors are a big problem and are sometimes so pungent and toxic that they create health problems in animals and workers. Complaints regarding odors are also made by people living around the animal industry. Odor emissions from livestock farms can be reduced by management practices related to cleaning, sanitation, and feeding plan of animals (Zhang et al. 2021).

43.2.9.1 Health Hazards of Odor

Emission of odors seriously affects human and animal health. The ecological environment gas pollutants ammonia, hydrogen sulfide, and VOCs are the major odorous substances emitted by livestock production and long-term exposure can reduce animal production performance (Cao et al. 2023).

43.2.10 Volatile Organic Compounds

Volatile organic compounds are emitted as gases from solids or liquids. VOCs include a variety of organic compounds that vaporize very easily and spread in the environment under normal conditions. VOCs are mobile and resistant to degradation and can spread long distances in the environment (David and Niculescu 2021). Organic chemicals like cleaning and disinfecting agents are widely used in animal housing. Fuels are made up of organic chemicals. All these products can release organic compounds while in use and, to some degree, when they are stored. Concentrations of many VOCs are consistently higher indoors (up to 10 times higher) than outdoors.

43.2.10.1 Health Hazards of Volatile Organic Compounds

Volatile organic compounds adversely affect the environment and human and animal health. They evaporate at room temperature and under normal pressure and can be present in both closed and open spaces. Volatility may vary among compounds; some are more volatile than others and evaporate faster and may have more effects on health.

The main sources of VOCs are biofuels, cooking oils, bioethanol, incinerators, and biomass combustion, especially from forests and agricultural wastes; complete combustion results in carbon dioxide and water while incomplete combustion results in a variety of VOCs. Some substances in VOCs, such as benzene and acetaldehyde, are also carcinogenic and hazardous, and can directly enter an animal's body through the respiratory tract, skin, and other routes, seriously damaging the liver and nervous system and causing irritation of the throat and eyes (Konkol et al. 2022). NH_3, H_2S, and VOCs released into the atmosphere can not only harm the respiratory organs and nervous systems of humans and animals but also lead to serious environmental problems.

43.2.11 Particulate Matter

According to the CDC, particulate matter (PM) is defined as particles (tiny pieces) of solids or liquids that are present in the air, also known as particle pollution. According to the EPA, particulate matter is defined as a mixture of solid particles and liquid droplets found in the air. These particles vary in size; some particles are big enough to be seen by the naked eye while some are detected by microscope only. These particles may include dust, dirt, soot, smoke, and drops of liquid.

On the basis of particle diameter, PM is categorized as follows.

- *PM10*: includes particles with a diameter of 10 μm or less.
- *PM2.5*: particles with a diameter of 2.5 μm or less. These include a complex mixture of aerosols such as combustion products, biogenic aerosols, secondary aerosols, and tropospheric (i.e., ground-level) ozone (O_3), a secondary pollutant that results when emissions of nitrogen oxides and VOCs (e.g., motor vehicles, oil and gas, biomass burning, and petrochemical industry) react in the presence of sunlight.

43.2.11.1 Sources of Particulate Matter

These particles come in many sizes and shapes and can be made up of hundreds of different chemicals. Some are emitted directly from a source, such as construction sites, unpaved roads, fields, smokestacks or fires. Most particles form in the atmosphere as a result of complex reactions of chemicals such as sulfur dioxide and nitrogen oxides, which are pollutants emitted from power plants, industries, and automobiles. The biological sources of PM from inside animal houses are numerous, including feces, urine, dander, feeding and bedding material, skin, and hair of the animals (Sang et al. 2022).

43.2.11.2 Health Hazards of Particulate Matter

Particulate matter contains microscopic solids or liquid droplets that are so small that they can be inhaled and cause serious health problems. Some particles less than $10\,\mu m$ in diameter can get deep into the lungs and some may even get into the bloodstream. Of these, particles less than $2.5\,\mu m$ in diameter, also known as fine particles or PM2.5, pose the greatest risk to health. Microbes attaching to PM can expose animals and workers to infectious and allergic diseases, including pneumonia, asthma, rhinitis, and bronchitis (Kim and Ko 2019).

43.2.12 Bio-aerosols

Bio-aerosols are microscopic air-borne contaminants of biological origin (viruses, bacteria, fungi, pollen grains) with diameters in the range $0.5–50\,\mu m$. A variety of microbes are carried by air and the variation in concentration depends on temperature, humidity, and amount of particulate and gaseous pollutants. The microbes are adsorbed on dust particles and carried over long distances under favorable weather conditions (high wind velocity), especially during disease outbreaks.

A large number of organisms (many of them pathogens) can be transmitted through the air in an area. Biological contaminants include viruses, bacteria and molds, carried and transmitted by animals and people, and many of these biological contaminants are small enough to be inhaled. Microorganisms spread from animal to animal by direct contact, indirect contact (e.g., on walls or floors), on equipment and people, and by air-borne dust and droplets. In dry air-borne dust, most of the infectious organisms die quickly but their toxins (e.g., endotoxins) can still be harmful when inhaled (Bai et al. 2022). Aerosol droplets containing organisms dry out rapidly at low humidity and the organisms die. At the middle range of humidities the droplets do not dry out and the organisms remain viable and infective. At very high humidities (>90%), droplets and dust pick up water, increase in size, and are precipitated out of the air.

Microbes released by animal and human sources survive in the environment for varying lengths of time. While some organisms may not survive for more than few minutes (*Leptospira* in dry atmosphere), others can resist adverse environmental conditions for as long as 28 years (spores of *Bacillus anthracis* in soil). Brucellae can survive in soil for about one month. Exposure to sunlight causes destruction of many environmental microorganisms (*Mycobacterium* spp). In soil, however, *Mycobacteria* can survive for up to six months.

Various species of air-borne bacteria can occur in buildings housing animals; studies suggest that air-borne bacteria in animal housing are mostly Gram positive whereas Gram-negative bacteria are generally present at very low concentrations. Gram-negative *E. coli* and *Enterobacter* of the Enterobacteriaceae and Gram-positive bacterial species like *Staphylococcus*, *Streptococcus*, and *Bacillus* are most numerous.

Furthermore, the material used in livestock housing also affects the concentration of microorganisms in the air. Hay on the floor may increase the propionic bacteria and *Lactobacillus*, the use of sand increases the number of *Streptococcus*, and the use of sawdust increases the level of coliforms and *Klebsiella* in the animals.

43.2.12.1 Effect on Health

Animals suffering from respiratory diseases discharge the microorganisms during sneezing and coughing. In humans, it is estimated that a sneeze can release 10 000–1 000 000 droplets.

Some biological contaminants trigger allergic reactions in animals as follows.

- Hypersensitivity pneumonitis
- Allergic rhinitis
- Asthma
- Sneezing
- Watery eyes

- Coughing
- Shortness of breath
- Dizziness
- Lethargy
- Fever
- Digestive problems

43.3 Control of Air Pollution in Farm Buildings

Air pollution inside animal buildings can be mitigated by the following management practices.

43.3.1 Balanced Ventilation

Ventilation is used to control temperature and humidity and other internal factors (Figure 43.3). The concentration of air pollutants is comparatively low in well-ventilated animal buildings. If possible, the building should have both natural and artificial ventilation. Automatic mechanical ventilation systems are often fitted in buildings to promote the productivity of animals through control of temperature and humidity parameters. However, buildings are often not equipped with adequate ventilation technology suitable for local climatic conditions in order to minimize management costs.

43.3.2 Best Management Practices (BMPs)

Best management practices refer to use of appropriate production methods, technologies, and waste management practices to prevent or control air pollutant in agricultural operations. Emissions of odors and gases from livestock production facilities arise from buildings, manure storage, and land application. There are various BMPs that can be implemented to reduce gas emissions and odor from dairy operations.

The accumulation of manure in buildings will result in an increase in gaseous air pollution, particularly if it is left where disturbance by the stock can promote gaseous release. In the case of cow housing and piggeries, manure is mainly deposited on concreted areas from where it can be easily removed daily by flushing with water or by mechanical scrapers. In the case of poultry, however, this is not possible with typical systems of management. With broilers, feces are deposited on the litter, in caged layers it is deposited in pits under the cages, and in layers, kept on semi-littered floors, it is deposited in pits or lagoons under the wire or slatted floors, on which the perches, drinkers, and feeders are usually placed. In the case of pits and lagoons, these are only emptied infrequently.

43.3.3 Monitoring Levels of Air Pollution

Many reliable methods of identifying and estimating the concentration of gaseous pollutants in the air are available so monitoring of air pollutants inside animal buildings should be done routinely. Monitoring of theAir Quality Index (AQI) is a effective approach to determine the air pollution and presence of air-borne pathogens.

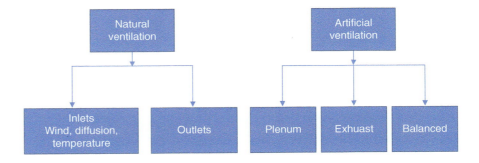

Figure 43.3 Types of ventilation.

43.4 Conclusion

The quality of air within animal buildings has a direct bearing on the health of animals and their productivity. The switch from extensive housing systems to intensive ones, especially in regard to dairy cattle, poultry, and piggeries, has significantly altered the priorities of livestock management programs. Pollutants emitted from sources inside and around the building can be controlled by balanced ventilation and management practices. To increase the effectiveness of these practices, intense monitoring should established inside the animal housing. In order to optimize animal health and productivity, the ambience inside the animal housing should be fresh and clean.

References

Bai, H., He, L.Y., Wu, D.L. et al. (2022). Spread of airborne antibiotic resistance from animal farms to the environment: dispersal pattern and exposure risk. *Environment International* 158: 106927.

Cao, P.T., Zheng, Y., and Dong, H. (2023). Control of odor emissions from livestock farms: a review. *Environmental Research* 225: 115545.

David, E. and Niculescu, V.C.C. (2021). Volatile organic compounds (VOCs) as environmental pollutants: occurrence and mitigation using nanomaterials. *International Journal of Environmental Research and Public Health* 18: 13147.

Goglio, P., Smith, W.N., Grant, B.B. et al. (2018). A comparison of methods to quantify greenhouse gas emissions of cropping systems in LCA. *Journal of Cleaner Production* 172: 4010–4017.

Grossi, G., Goglio, P., Vitali, A., and Williams, A.G. (2019). Livestock and climate change: impact of livestock on climate and mitigation strategies. *Animal Frontiers* 9: 1), 69–76.

Guo, L., Zhao, B., Jia, Y. et al. (2022). Mitigation strategies of air pollutants for mechanical ventilated livestock and poultry housing – a review. *Atmosphere* 13: 452.

Kelleghan, D.B., Hayes, E.T., Everard, M., and Curran, T.P. (2021). Predicting atmospheric ammonia dispersion and potential ecological effects using monitored emission rates from an intensive laying hen facility in Ireland. *Atmosphere Environment* 247: 118214.

Kim, K.Y. and Ko, H.J. (2019). Indoor distribution characteristics of airborne bacteria in pig buildings as influenced by season and housing type. *Asian-Australian Journal of Animal Science* 32: 742–747.

Konkol, D., Popeila, E., Skrzypczak, D. et al. (2022). Recent innovations in various methods of harmful gases conversion and its mechanism in poultry farms. *Environmental Research* 214: 113825.

Menon, J.M.L., Luijk, J.A.K.R.V., Swinkels, J. et al. (2021). A health-based recommended occupational exposure limit for nitrous oxide using experimental animal data based on a systematic review and dose-response analysis. *Environmental Research* 201: 111575.

Pedersen, S., Blanes-Vidal, V., Joergensen, H. et al. (2008). Carbon dioxide production in animal houses: a literature review. https://edepot.wur.nl/22415 (accessed 12 February 2024).

Sang, S., Chu, C., Zhang, T. et al. (2022). The global burden of disease attributable to ambient fine particulate matter in 204 countries and territories, 1990–2019: a systematic analysis of the Global Burden of Disease Study 2019. *Ecotoxicology and Environmental Safety* 15 (238): 113588.

Stegenta-Dabrowska, S., Drabczyński, G., Sobieraj, K. et al. (2019). The biotic and abiotic carbon monoxide formation during aerobic co-digestion of dairy cattle manure with green waste and sawdust. *Frontiers in Bioengineering and Biotechnology* 7: 283.

Talaiekhozani, A., Nematzadeh, S., Eskandari, Z. et al. (2018). Gaseous emissions of landfill and modeling of their dispersion in the atmosphere of Shahrekord, Iran. *Urban Climate* 24: 852–862.

Zhang, Y., Ning, X., Li, Y. et al. (2021). Impact assessment of odor nuisance, health risk and variation originating from the landfill surface. *Waste Management* 126: 771–780.

44

Farm Waste and Sewage Disposal

Jaysukh B. Kathiriya[1] and Bhavesh J. Trangadia[2]

[1] *Department of Veterinary Public Health & Epidemiology, College of Veterinary Science & Animal Husbandry, Kamdhenu University, Junagadh, India*
[2] *Department of Veterinary Pathology, College of Veterinary Science & Animal Husbandry, Kamdhenu University, Junagadh, India*

44.1   Introduction

Livestock waste includes livestock excreta, bedding material, rain or other water, soil, hair, feathers or other debris normally included in animal waste handling operations. According to the 19th Livestock Census, the livestock population in India is 512.05 million which produces 1095 million MT dung per year (Prasad et al. 2014). Waste from the livestock and poultry industry includes a mixture of excreta (manure), bedding material or litter (e.g., wood shavings or straw), waste feed, dead animals/birds, broken eggs, feathers, and farm sweepouts.

Animal husbandry specialists used to be concerned about how the effect of environment on animals can be mitigated. But more recently, there is talk of livestock and livestock industries themselves polluting the environment in general. In fact, like any other production activity, livestock and climate have mutual positive as well as negative interactions of different intensities. Indian livestock methane production estimated using the dry matter intake approach was 10.08 Tg (1 trillion grams = 1 ton) methane due to enteric fermentation in the year 2010, in which crossbred cattle, indigenous cattle, buffaloes, goats and sheep, and other livestock emitted about 4.6%, 48.5%, 39%, 4.7%, 1.8%, and 1.4%, respectively. Amongst states, methane emission was highest in Uttar Pradesh followed by Madhya Pradesh and Bihar due to their larger livestock population.

The early method of handling livestock wastes was very simple. The manure from livestock on pasture was not even recovered but left to become integrated in the soil. However, with the advent of modern livestock production, considerable attention is being given to alternative uses and treatments of livestock wastes to recover fertilizer, feed, and fuel and at the same time achieve pollution control. All these properties of animal waste will be available only if they are carefully managed. If not, they might cause detrimental effects on climate and human beings.

44.2   Importance of Livestock Waste Management

The most common concern with animal waste is that it releases large quantities of CO_2 and ammonia, which might contribute to acid rain and the greenhouse effect. It could also pollute water sources and be instrumental in spreading infectious diseases. If the disposal of water is not properly planned, it might create social tension owing to the release of odors and contamination of water sources.

Proper management of livestock waste is required due to following reasons.

- Livestock manure helps to maintain soil fertility in soils lacking organic content. Adding manure to the soil increases the nutrient retention capacity, improves the soil's physical condition by increasing its water-holding capacity, and improves soil structure.
- Animal manure helps to create a better climate for microflora and fauna in soils.
- Dung is used as fuel.

Epidemiology and Environmental Hygiene in Veterinary Public Health, First Edition. Edited by Tanmoy Rana.
© 2025 John Wiley & Sons, Inc. Published 2025 by John Wiley & Sons, Inc.

- Waste manure and other organic materials from livestock farms could be an important source of energy production.
- Livestock waste can be used in resource management, in crop and livestock production, and in the reduction of postharvest losses (FAO, 2009).
- Livestock waste management plays an important role in the livelihoods of many rural dwellers in India.
- Bioenergy sources are increasingly gaining attention as a sustainable energy resource that may help to cope with challenges like increasing demand for energy and rising fuel prices by providing substitutions for expensive fossil fuels.
- Biogas from livestock waste and residues provides renewable and environmentally friendly sources that support sustainable agriculture. Additionally, the byproducts of the "digesters" provide organic waste of superior quality (Arthur and Baidoo, 2011).
- Reduces sources of infection for animal and human population.
- Reduces sources of methane emission (0.28–1.95 g/d).
- Reduces causes of bad odor.
- Reduces fly nuisance.
- Helps in proper nutrient management practices (reduced loss of organic matter).
- Helps in controlling vectors and fomites.
- Reduces environment pollution.
- Reduces illegal discharge of waste which can pose a direct threat to the quality of soil and water system.
- Nitrogen in manure is tied up in its organic state. Until, through decomposition, it is converted to a soluble form (ammonium nitrate). When ammonium nitrate is mixed with soil, it improves soils fertility.

44.3 Types of Livestock Waste

44.3.1 Solid Waste

- *Dung*: also known as cow pats or cow manure, this is the waste product of bovine animal species. Cow dung is the undigested residue of plant matter, which has passed through the animal gut. The resultant fecal matter is rich in minerals.

Cow dung contains:

Moisture	77%
Organic matter	20%
Nitrogen	0.32%
Phosphorus	0.14%
Potassium	0.30%
Calcium	0.40%

- *Wasted feeding material*: food that is discarded or lost or uneaten.
- *Soiled bedding material*: straw, sawdust, wood shavings, paper-based bedding materials, etc.

44.3.2 Liquid Waste

- Urine (Table 44.1).
- Washed water (Table 44.2).

44.4 Collection of Livestock Waste

Because of the management system, which allows grazing during the day and kraaling at night, a substantial amount of feces is deposited on crop fields and grazing land. These components of wastes are not usually collected but rather go directly to fertilize the soil. For those deposited within enclosed structures such as the animal house and poultry buildings, they must be removed to avoid health hazards.

Table 44.1 Dung and urine production by different species.

| Animals | Quantity of dung (kg/day/animal) | | Urine (ml/kg bwt/day) |
	Range	Average	Range
Horse	9–18	13.50	3–18
Cattle	18–30	24.00	17–45
Buffalo	25–40	32.50	3–18
Sheep and goat	1–25	1.25	10–40
Pigs	3–5	4.00	5–30
Poultry (100 birds)	2.5–3.5	3.00	—

Table 44.2 Water requirement for washing.

Species	Water requirement for washing (liters)/animal/day
Cattle and buffalo	45–70
Horse	36
Pigs	25–28

44.4.1 Separate Collection

Solid and liquid manure are separated and a special pit has to be constructed to allow the solid waste to decompose. The pit should be far away from water sources, animal and human habitations to avoid fly menace and spread of diseases. When planning for construction of a pit, due attention should be given to the labor required in transporting and the mode by which the manure will be shifted to the pit.

44.4.1.1 Collection of Solid Waste

By means of wheelbarrow and shovel, waste deposited in a pit for decomposition. Such manure will return 75% of its fertilizing value to the soil. Manure pits should be at least 200 m away from buildings. The production of manure from each dairy cow is about 24 kg/d. The volumetric capacity of fresh manure is 700–900 kg/m^3. Frequency of collection should be twice a day.

44.4.1.2 Collection of Liquid Waste

Flushing of liquid waste can be done by the drain channel up to the storage tank, or it can drain directly in the main drain channel of the area.

44.4.2 Flushing of Both Wastes

Manure along with other waste is flushed together. In these types of animal sheds, a U- shaped gutter or drain should be located longitudinally to the long axis of the shed. Outside the shed the liquid manure from each shed can be connected to a main closed drain. The main drain leads the liquid water to a liquid storage tank from where it can be pumped to agricultural lands for manuring (Sastry and Thomas 2015).

44.4.3 Semiautomatic Cow Dung Cleaning Machine

This semiautomatic machine runs on electricity and is a small trolley with four wheels, fork, and brush. The brush rotates with the help of a gear motor with belt drive and pulley arrangement.

44 Farm Waste and Sewage Disposal

Advantages of the machine include:

- Low power consumption
- Frequent cleaning gives better hygiene and better cow health
- Easy installation
- Smart equipment features

44.5 Traditional Method of Livestock Waste Management

- *Dung cake*: the only use for manure other than as fertilizer is in underdeveloped countries, where cow manure is gathered by hand and placed on suitable racks to sun-dry for use as fuel for cooking and heating. In north Indian states, cow dung cake is the major fuel for cooking (Rawal and Saha 2012).
- *Dumping into heaps or pits*: the most common and traditional method of waste management.
- *Composting*: an accelerated biooxidation of organic matter passing through a thermophilic stage (45–65 °C) where microorganisms (mainly bacteria, fungi, and actinomycetes) liberate heat, carbon dioxide, and water. The heterogeneous organic material is transformed into a homogeneous and stabilized humus-like product through turning or aeration. Composting is the aerobic degradation of biodegradable organic waste. It is a relatively fast biodegradation process, taking typically 4–6 weeks to reach a stabilized material. The composted material is odorless and fine-textured with low moisture content and can be used as an organic fertilizer.

Composting biological waste with poultry manure can be an effective means of conserving the nitrogen in the manure, which not only improves the fertilizer value but also reduces the potential for ammonia to contribute to environmental pollution (Mahimairaja et al. 1994).

44.5.1 Disadvantages

Disadvantages include loss of nitrogen and other nutrients during composting, equipment cost, labor, odor and requirement of land. Moisture (60%) and carbon/nitrogen (C/N) ratio (20:1) have a major influence on a successful composting process (Table 44.3). For poultry waste, a low C/N ratio contributes to large ammonia losses. High moisture content of more than 75% inhibits a quick start to the composting process.

44.6 Methods of Composting

Farm compost is made by placing farm wastes in trenches of suitable size (4.5–5.0 m long, 1.5–2.0 m wide, 1.0–2.0 m deep). Farm waste is placed in the trenches layer by layer. Trenches are filled to a height of 0.5 m above the ground. The compost is ready for application within 5–6 months. There are various methods of composting.

Table 44.3 Factors affecting composting.

Factors	Range	References
Temperature	52–60 °C	Miller (1992)
Moisture content	50–60%	Gajalakshmi and Abbasi (2008)
pH	5.5–6.8	Miller (1992)
C/N	25:1 to 35:1	Bishop and Godfrey (1983)
Aeration (oxygen)	15–20%	Miller (1992)

44.6.1 Coimbatore Method

Composting is done in pits of different sizes depending on the type of waste material available. A layer of waste materials is first laid in the pit. It is moistened with a suspension of 5–10 kg cow dung in 2.5–5.0 l of water and 0.5–1.0 kg fine bone meal sprinkled over it uniformly. Similar layers are laid one over the other till the material rises to 0.75 m above ground level. It is finally plastered with wet mud and left undisturbed for 8–10 weeks.

44.6.2 Indore Method

Organic wastes are spread in the animal shed to serve as bedding. Urine-soaked material along with dung is removed every day and formed into a layer about 15 cm thick at suitable sites. Urine-soaked earth scraped from animal sheds is mixed with water and sprinkled over the layer of wastes twice or thrice a day.

44.6.3 Bangalore Method

Dry waste material of 25 cm thick is spread in a pit and a thick suspension of cow dung in water is sprinkled over for moistening. A thin layer of dry waste is laid over the moistened layer. It is turned, plastered with wet mud and left undisturbed for about five months or until required.

44.7 Benefits of Compost

- Compost adds organic matter, improves soil structure, reduces fertilizer requirements, and reduces the potential for soil erosion.
- Composting reduces the weight and moisture content and increases stability of manure. Compost is easier to handle than manure and stores well without odors or fly problems, thus lowering the risk of pollution and nuisance complaints.
- Composted manure is less susceptible to leaching and further ammonia losses.
- Composting high-carbon manure/bedding mixtures lowers the C/N ratio to acceptable levels for land application.
- Proper temperature within the compost pile will reduce pathogens.

44.8 Advanced Methods of Livestock Waste Management

44.8.1 Solid Waste Management

44.8.1.1 Biogas Production

Biogas is a clean environment-friendly fuel that can be obtained by anaerobic digestion of animal residues and domestic and farm wastes, abundantly available in the countryside. Biogas is created by bacterial conversion of organic matter into gases under anaerobic conditions. Biogas generally comprises of 55–65% methane, 35–45% carbon dioxide, 0.5–1.0% hydrogen sulfide, and traces of water vapor. The average calorific value of biogas is 20 MJ/m^3 (4713 kcal/m^3). One estimate indicates that India has a potential of generating 6.38×10^{10} m^3 of biogas from 980 million tons of cattle dung produced annually. The heat value of this gas amounts to 1.3×10^{12} MJ (Jiang et al. 2011). In addition, 350 million tons of manure would also be produced along with the biogas.

There are various advantages of biogas production.

- Biogas provides an environmentally friendly process that supports sustainable agriculture.
- It is one of the simplest sources of renewable energy and can be derived from sewage; liquid manure from hens, cattle, and pigs; and organic waste from agriculture or food processing (Table 44.4).
- The byproducts of the "digesters" provide organic waste of superior quality.
- Biogas is particularly well suited to household energy needs as it improves both soil conditions and household sanitation (Table 44.5).

510 | 44 Farm Waste and Sewage Disposal

Table 44.4 Potential of gas production from different wastes.

Type of waste	Gas yield/kg (m^3)	Normal manure availability per animal per day (kg)	Gas yield per day (m^3)
Cattle dung	0.036	10.00	0.360
Buffalo dung	0.036	15.00	0.540
Pig manure (approx. 50 kg wt)	0.078	2.25	0.180
Chicken manure (approx. 2 kg wt)	0.062	0.18	0.011
Human excreta (adult)	0.070	0.40	0.028

Table 44.5 Quantities of biogas consumed for various applications.

Use	Specifications	Quantities of gas consumed
Cooking	Per person per day	$0.24 \, m^3/d$
Lighting of lamp	100 candle power lamp	$0.13 \, m^3/h$
Dual fuel engine	75–80% replacement of diesel oil per BHP	$0.50 \, m^3/h$
Electricity	1 kwh	$0.21 \, m^3/h$

Source: Adapted from Khandelwal and Mahdi (1986).

- Manure-based biogas digester systems are considered ecological since the technology captures and utilizes methane directly, thereby limiting total greenhouse gas emissions from livestock.
- By using bioenergy resources and nonpolluting technology, biogas generation serves a triple function: waste removal, environmental management, and energy production.
- Biogas is now widely integrated with animal husbandry and can become a major means of manure treatment in the agricultural sector and environmental protection (Figure 44.1).

44.8.1.1.1 Types of Biogas Digester

Biogas digesters are generally sized on the basis of local energy requirements and the cattle dung production of the farm. Two main designs of biogas plant exist: fixed dome type (Figure 44.2) and floating drum type (Figure 44.3).

- The fixed dome biogas plant is placed underground. The plant is constructed with local materials and has an estimated lifetime of 25 years. The family size biogas plant ranges from 1 to 10 cubic meters, depending on the resources available and gas utilization. The average cost of a $2 \, m^3/d$ fixed dome biogas plant is Rs. 21,500/-.
- The floating drum biogas plant is relatively simple in construction but costly as compared to the fixed dome type for the same size plant. The average cost of a floating drum type biogas plant of $2 \, m^3/d$ capacity is around Rs. 35,000/-. The gas drum is installed above the digester in the ground. The inlet tank is installed higher than the outlet tank and connected to the digester with an asbestos cement pipe. The biogas produced in the digester is stored in the floating drum which is connected to the gas burner with GI/PVC tubing. The cattle dung is mixed with water in 1:1 ratio in the input tank and fed into the digester after proper mixing for biogas production. After complete digestion, the digested slurry comes out from the digester and is stored in an outlet tank for use as organic fertilizer for crop production.

44.8.1.1.2 Biogas Production Process

The biogas production process (anaerobic digestion) is a two-stage process (Figure 44.4).

- In the first stage, complex components, including fats, proteins, and polysaccharides, are hydrolyzed and broken down to their component subunits. This is facilitated by facultative and anaerobic bacteria, which then subject the products of hydrolysis to fermentation and other metabolic processes, leading to the production of simple organic compounds. This first stage is commonly referred to as acid fermentation and in this stage organic material is simply converted to organic acids, alcohols, and new bacterial cells.

Figure 44.1 Multiple benefits from integration of waste flows for energy production.

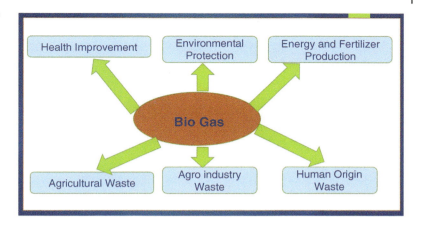

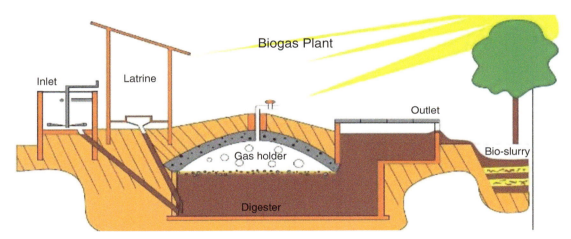

Figure 44.2 Fixed dome type biogas plant.

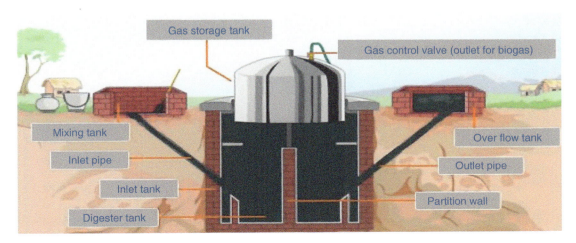

Figure 44.3 Floating drum type biogas plant.

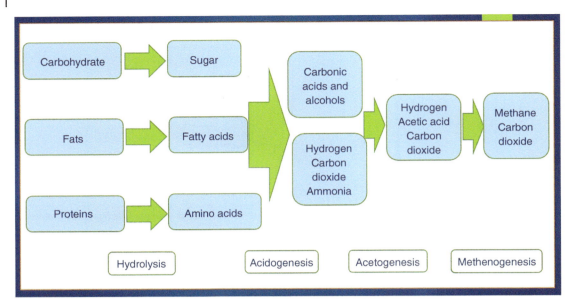

Figure 44.4 Bio gas production.

- The second stage involves the conversion of the hydrolysis products to gases (mainly methane and CO_2) by several species of strictly anaerobic bacteria and is referred to as methane fermentation. Anaerobic digestion results in the production of biogas and also stabilizes raw slurry and reduces a substantial proportion of its polluting power in terms of biochemical oxygen demand and chemical oxygen demand. The readily degraded organic components are removed and the resulting materials are more uniform, more liquid, and much easier to mix. Some of the fibers are partially degraded and the solid fraction can be separated from the liquid portion, sorted in a heap, and utilized for land application. The odor is reduced and much of the original nitrogen is retained in the liquid fraction.

44.8.1.1.3 Factors Affecting Optimum Biogas Production
- Temperature (35–37 °C mesophilic condition).
- C/N ratio (optimum between 25:1 and 30:1).
- pH (optimally pH between 6.8–7.2).
- Solid material that is toxic or harmful to bacteria should not be used in the digester.
- Hydraulic retention time (30, 40, 55 days).
- Loading rate.

44.8.1.1.4 Utilization of Biogas
Biogas can be used in a specially designed burner for cooking. A biogas plant of 2 cubic meters capacity will provide the cooking fuel needs of a family of about five persons (Lantz et al. 2007).

Biogas is used in silk mantle lamps for lighting. The requirement of gas for powering a 100 candle lamp (60 W) is 0.13 cubic meter per hour.

Biogas can be used to operate a dual fuel engine to replace up to 80% of diesel oil. Diesel engines have been modified to run 100% on biogas. Petrol and compressed natural gas engines can also be easily modified to use biogas.

After removal of carbon dioxide, hydrogen sulfide, and water vapor, biogas can be converted to natural gas quality for use in vehicles.

44.8.1.1.5 Compressed Biogas (CBG)
Compressed biogas is produced by compressing 40% by volume of carbon dioxide and fraction of hydrogen sulfide (Figure 44.5). Using a scrubbing system enriched with about 95% methane, it makes gas moisture free by passing it through filters. Gas is compressed up to 200 bar pressure using a three-stage gas compressor and stored in high-pressure steel cylinders (Table 44.6) (Vijay et al. 2011).

Figure 44.5 Process flowchart of biogas enrichment and compression.

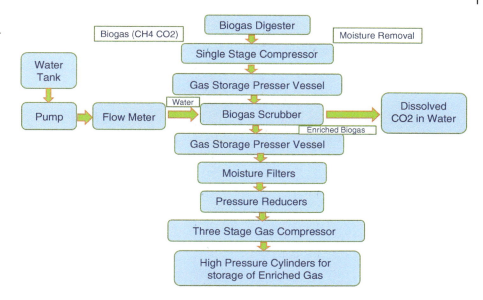

Table 44.6 Estimate for 1000 m³ biogas to CBG bottling plant.

	Amount
Waste required	20 tons cattle dung
Biogas production	1000 m³/d
Cost	Rs. 60 lakhs
Purified gas quantity	375 kg
Purified gas composition	CH_4 95%, H_2S <25 ppm, moisture <20 ppm
Annual profit	Rs. 34.125 lakhs

It can be used:

- To power motor vehicles
- As fuel for cooking
- For indoor lighting.

44.8.1.1.6 Electricity from Biogas

Methane produces 600–800 Btu/ft³ heat, which can be used in a generator to produce electrical power. Gas turbines and internal combustion diesel engines can be used to convert gas into power (Figure 44.6). It can produce maximum 15 kw power and fuel consumption is 1 m³ of biogas per kwh output. Cost Rs. 20 K–25 K per installation (Govil 2010).

44.8.1.1.7 Rotary Drum Composter

A drum is mounted on four metal rollers attached to a metal stand, which is rotated by a 7.5 MW motor twice a day. Rotation adds oxygen and releases heat and gaseous products of decomposition. Maximum particle size in the mixed waste is 1 cm (Khandelwal and Mahdi 1986).

Advantages of this system are:

- Composting time is drastically reduced to 2–3 weeks
- It can be placed at the site of organic waste generation.

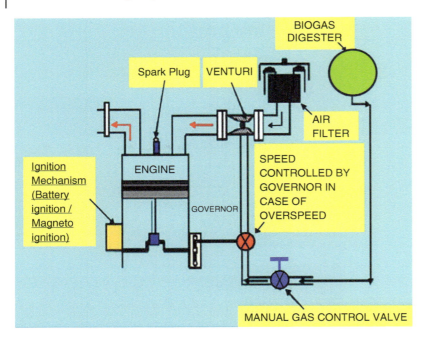

Figure 44.6 Schematic diagram for conversion of diesel engine to biogas.

44.8.1.2 Vermicomposting

In this system, earthworms eat the organic matter and excrete pelleted material called vermicompost. During vermicomposting, important plant nutrients, such as N, P, K, and Ca, present in the organic waste are converted into forms that are more soluble and available to the plants. Vermicompost also contains biologically active substances such as plant growth regulators. Moreover, the worms themselves provide a protein source for animal feed. It increases NPK content 3–4 times and composting time is reduced to 60–75 days.

44.8.1.2.1 Types of Earthworms

There are different species of earthworms such as *Eisenia foetida*, *Perionyx excavatus*, etc. The red earthworm is preferred because of its high multiplication rate, which converts organic matter into vermicompost within 45–50 days. Since it is a surface feeder, it converts organic materials into vermicompost from the top. Its conversion rate is 2 quintal/1500 worms/two months.

44.8.1.2.2 Methods of Vermicomposting

Vermicomposting is done by various methods; the bed and pit methods are most common.

Bed Method Composting is done on a pucca/kachcha floor by making a bed (6 × 2 × 2 feet) of organic mixture (Figure 44.7). This method is easy to maintain and to practice.

Pit Method Composting is done in cemented pits of size 5 × 5 × 3 feet (Figure 44.8). The unit is covered with thatch grass or other locally available materials. This method is not preferred due to poor aeration, waterlogging at the bottom, and higher cost of production.

44.8.1.2.3 Process of Vermicomposting

- The vermicomposting unit should be in a cool, moist, and shady site.
- Cow dung and chopped dried leafy materials are mixed in the proportion of 3:1 and kept for 15–20 days. A layer of 15–20 cm of chopped dried leaves/grasses should be kept as bedding material at the bottom of the bed.
- Beds of partially decomposed material of 6 × 2 × 2 feet should be made.

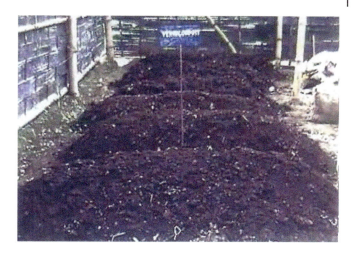

Figure 44.7 Bed method of composting (red earthworms, *Eudrilus eugeniae*, night crawler).

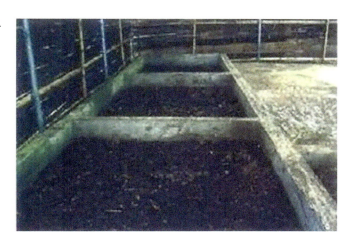

Figure 44.8 Pit method of composting.

- Each bed should contain 1.5–0.2 quintal of raw material and the number of beds can be increased in relation to raw material availability and requirement.
- Red earthworms (1500–2000) should be released on the upper layer of the bed.
- Water should be sprinkled daily and covered with gunny bags.
- The bed should be turned once after 30 days to maintain aeration for proper decomposition.
- Compost is ready in 45–50 days.

The finished product will be three-quarters of the raw materials used.

44.8.1.2.4 Harvesting

When raw material is completely decomposed, it appears black. Watering should be stopped when the compost is ready. After two days the compost can be separated and sieved for use. An optimum moisture level of 30–40% should be maintained and temperature should be 18–25 °C. The C/N ratio of vermicompost should be 11.88, total nitrogen should be 1.2%, total phosphorus should be 0.30%, total potassium should be 0.24%, and calcium and magnesium should be 0.17% and 0.06%, respectively.

The doses for field crops should be 4.5–5 t per hectare and for fruit crops 3–5 kg per plant.

44.8.1.3 Pyrolysis

This is a thermochemical process, in which waste is chemically decomposed in a closed system at 400–1472 °F. Pyrolysis is the chemical decomposition of condensed organic materials by heating in a reactor, largely in the absence of oxygen. It mainly uses straw, branches, sawdust, and other agricultural and forestry waste as raw material and through high temperature and pressure transforms the raw materials into a variety of products. Manure may be pyrolyzed by subjecting it to a temperature of 480–1830 °F in an oxygen-deficient atmosphere. The products are gases, oil, and ash. The gases include H_2, H_2S, CH_3, CO, and ethylene. Dairy feces produced the most gas per unit of dry solids, followed by chicken, beef, and swine feces (White and Taiganides 1971).

44.8.1.4 Soldier Fly Breeding
Black soldier fly (BSF) larvae are uniquely suited to treat livestock waste. BSF adults only live for a few days, their larvae can live for several weeks, and during that time they can consume huge quantities of food waste or manure. There are two useful byproducts of this process: the residue or castings which can be used as a soil enrichment, and the larvae themselves which represent an excellent source of food for many types of animals including fish, birds, reptiles, amphibians, etc.

44.8.1.5 Litter Management
Poultry litter includes excreta, bedding, wasted feed, and feathers. Bedding may consist of wood shavings, sawdust, straw, peanut hulls or other fibrous materials. Most poultry litter is produced by broiler production. The litter may be from one crop of broilers or accumulated over several crops of birds. The litter usually contains 20–25% moisture.

Poultry litter fed mainly to beef cows and stocker cattle. Broiler litter contains 25–50% crude protein and 55–60% total digestible nutrients (TDN), dry matter basis, and is rich in essential minerals. Thus, the nutritional value is similar to or higher than good-quality legume hay. Poultry litter instead of being a problem of waste, it should be a source of energy and nutrients.

Poultry farms in India exist in clusters and the quantity of litter available is not high enough to encourage investors to opt for power generation using combustion. Therefore, gasification (thermal degradation) appears to be the economically viable solution for the effective disposal of waste with revenue generation (Kirubakaran et al. 2006).

44.8.2 Liquid Waste Management

44.8.2.1 Ammonia Recycling
Recycling ammonia from livestock waste water by using gas-permeable membranes is a common method (Vanotti and Szogi 2011). This membrane is waterproof and allows only the passage of gases. Passage of gaseous ammonia through a microporous hydrophobic membrane helps to capture and concentrate gases in a stripping solution. Membranes used for filtering include polypropylene and polyurethane. The average removal rate is 45–153 mg of ammonia per liter per day. Ammonia recovery is 1.2% per hour when manure pH is 8.3 and 13% per hour when pH is 10.

44.9 Carcase Disposal

44.9.1 Traditional Methods

44.9.1.1 Burial
This is the most common method of carcase disposal. A pit of about 8–9 ft depth is dug, the width and length depending upon the size of carcase. The carcase is laid on its back with feet upward in the pit. Bedding used for the dead animal, its excreta, leftover feed, and the top 5 cm of soil from the place where the dead animal was lying should be buried along with the carcase. The carcase is covered with a thick layer of quicklime and the pit is then filled with soil. The pit can be fenced if required. The area surrounding the burial pit can also be sprayed with suitable disinfectant.

Select burial sites with care to avoid groundwater contamination.

- The pit must be five feet above the seasonal high-water table.
- Keep away from lakes, rivers, streams, ditches, etc.
- Cover immediately with enough soil to keep scavengers out (3 ft is sufficient).
- Avoid sandy or gravelly soil types.
- Maintain at least 10 ft vertical separation from bedrock.
- After burial, the site must be covered by at least 3 ft of soil, with at least the top 1 foot capable of sustaining vegetative growth.

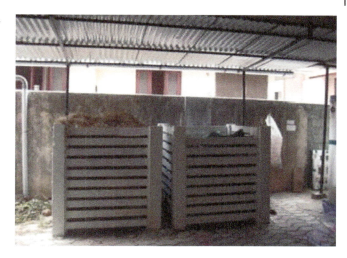

Figure 44.9 Ferrocement Thumburmuzhy model.

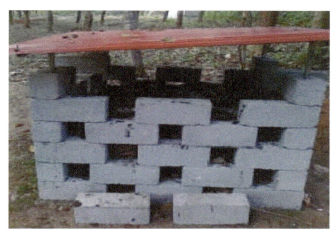

Figure 44.10 Concrete brick masonry.

44.9.1.2 Burning

In this method, 7 ft long trenches crossing each other are dug. The trenches are made 15″ wide and 18″ deep in the center and shallow towards the ends. The trench is first filled with wood, tree branches, straw, etc. before adding the carcase. Sufficient kerosene is sprinkled over the entire material and then the straw is ignited by firing the wood so that the carcase and all the infectious materials will be completely burnt.

Carcases can also be burnt in electric incinerators. This is economical and safe for cremating large numbers of carcases by a single trained operator in less time without risk of infection.

44.9.2 Advanced Methods of Composting Carcases

The Thumburmuzhy model is used to compost animal carcases. In this method a ferrocement tank 4 ft × 4 ft × 4 ft is constructed of concrete bricks with air holes in the side (Figures 44.9 and 44.10). Six-inch layers of fresh cow dung, dry leaves/straw, and organic waste are layered over the base of the bin, with the first layer acted as the bacterial consortium, the second layer as the carbon source (Epstein 1997), and the third layer is the carcase. Curing time is 90 days.

44.10 Sewage Disposal

Processes involved in sewage treatment include treating and screening of the sewage. This also involves disposing of the sewage in such a way that it does not cause any hazard or harm to nature and the human health.

Waste generation is one of the most inescapable and natural activities of the human lifestyle. Water is essential for human life to perform various activities including domestic tasks, industrial manufacturing, services like railways, restaurants, etc. All these uses generate a large amount of wastewater. Even though natural water reservoirs replenish periodically, the resource is not unlimited. As the human population is increasing day by day, so the use of water for various functions is increasing, so in order to protect water supplies for future generations, it is vital to reuse water if possible.

Thus, sewage management methods can help to recycle used wastewater to avoid adverse situations such as scarcity or drought in future.

44.10.1   Methods of Sewage Treatment

Sewage treatment is a process that can eliminate impurities from household sewage and industrial wastewater. Four main methods of sewage water treatment are available: physical, biological, chemical, and sludge water treatment. Using these methods, wastewater is disinfected and converted into treated water that is safe for both human usage and the environment.

- *Physical method*: this is the process of removing floating and suspended solids from sewage through processes of sedimentation and filtration. First, the suspended or floating particles are removed by filtration. The filtrate is then kept in large open tanks where the suspended impurities are allowed to settle down.
- *Biological method*: human waste or other degrading wastes are treated by bacteria and microbes that convert the sewage waste into byproducts such as sludge.
- *Chemical method*: in this method, chemicals are used to sterilize the wastewater so that it does not transmit any kind of infection.
- *Activated sludge method*: this method uses microorganisms to feed on the organic components of the wastewater. This process in turn produces a purified effluent. This solution is injected and supplied with a large amount of air to meet the oxygen demand of the microorganisms.

This entire containment removal process occurs before impure used water reaches natural water bodies such as lakes, rivers, oceans, and estuaries. As the availability of pure water is scarce, the difference between clean and polluted water is completely based on impurity concentration and intent of usage.

In other words, water is considered polluted when it is not fit for any specific purpose like drinking, fishing, swimming, etc. Water contamination primarily happens due to drainage of impure wastewater into groundwater or surface water.

44.10.2   Types of Sewage

44.10.2.1   Domestic Sewage
Domestic wastewater includes all used water from households. This type of wastewater is also known as sanitary sewage.

44.10.2.2   Industrial Wastewater
Industrial wastewater carries contaminated water from chemical or manufacturing processes. Various pollutant chemicals can be present in the sewage. As this wastewater mainly comes from industries, it can be toxic and contaminated with heavy metals.

44.10.2.3   Storm Sewage
Storm water is the runoff sewage that comes from the atmosphere in the form of water particles collected in open channels. This can include rain, drizzle, snow, etc. Above 99.9% of the entire wastewater comes from domestic sewage. Even though the principal contaminants are described as plant nutrients and organic materials, domestic wastewater also contains harmful microbes. This wastewater contains the nutrients that can be collected after sewage treatment.

44.10.3   Major Pollutants

44.10.3.1   Organic Substances
The quantity of perishable or biodegradable organic materials in wastewater is calculated by biochemical oxygen demand (BOD). BOD is the oxygen amount required by microbes to decompose these organic substances in wastewater. It is one of the most vital criteria for the operation and design of sewage management methods.

44.10.3.2 Suspended Solids

The amount of sludge generated in a water treatment plant depends on the entire suspended solids included in the wastewater. Storm and industrial sewage carry a larger volume of suspended solids than domestic wastewater.

44.10.3.3 Plant Nutrients

Primarily, domestic wastewater carries chemical elements like phosphorus and nitrogen, which are the fundamental nutrients for plant growth. If these elements are excessively present in surrounding water bodies like lakes, it can boost the growth of algae. This may accelerate the natural aging of these water bodies.

44.10.3.4 Microbes

Domestic wastewater also carries various microbes that come from the intestinal tract of human beings, in which, Coliform bacteria are found in high concentrations. By sewage treatment methods, these pollutants are removed from the sewage water so that it can be reused.

44.11 Sewage Treatment Methods

By employing various wastewater treatment methods, contaminants like chemicals and sewage can be eliminated from wastewater which is recycled for further use. There are main four methods of sewage treatment that are listed below.

44.11.1 Physical Treatment

- Several physical processes, like sedimentation, skimming, and screening are employed to eliminate solid wastes.
- By sedimentation, heavy or insoluble particles can be separated.
- Another effective method is aeration to circulate air (oxygen) through wastewater.
- Filtration is applied to filter out all containments and make the water usable.
- Most importantly, no chemical is applied in the physical treatment of wastewater.

44.11.2 Biological Treatment

- Different biological processes are involved in decomposing the organic substances present in sewage like human waste, food, oil, etc.
- An aerobic process involves bacteria that can break down these organic materials and transfer them into CO_2. In this process, O_2 is produced.
- An anaerobic process involves fermentation of waste material at high temperature. In this process, O_2 is not generated.
- Composting is a specific kind of aerobic process which uses various carbon sources to treat the sewage.

44.11.3 Chemical Treatment

- In this process, several chemicals are used to treat water.
- Chlorine is a common oxidizing agent that eliminates germs and bacteria in water.
- Ozone is also used as an oxidizing agent to purify wastewater.
- By adding base or acid, wastewater is treated to keep the pH neutral. This is known as neutralization.

44.11.4 Sludge Treatment

- One of the most effective solid–liquid separation methods.
- This requires the least possible remaining moisture in solid phase.
- It needs the lowest possible remaining solid molecules in isolated liquid phase.

44.12 Sewage Disposal Methods

Sewage disposal methods are the basic components of a sewage management system. The following are some well-known sewage disposal methods practiced around the globe.

44.12.1 Municipality Systems

In the municipal wastewater system, treatment plant connected to the source of wastewater. By treating the used water, this plant efficiently removes nearly 95% of impurities. Then using an anaerobic process, the sludge is treated again to ensure that the water is safe to use.

44.12.2 Off-site Sewage System

Due to increasing urbanization, the off-site sewage system has becomre more popular. In urban areas, houses are built on plots and each plot is connected to a wastewater line. These wastewater lines collect waste from various households and flow toward a community sewage treatment plant. Here, excess water is directed toward a nearby river or irrigation area once the treatment is complete.

44.12.3 On-site Sewage System

This disposal system is composed of a septic tank where the sewage can be settled and treated. In this process, the wastewater is disposed of and treated in natural ways. Usually, an on-site system comprises a septic tank and disposal field for soil absorption. The wastewater slurry is carried out to this leach field, where microorganisms can decompose it over time. These sewage disposal methods are reliable, hygienic, economical, and efficient.

44.12.4 Full Wastewater System

In a full wastewater disposal system, the sewage water is collected from households and then directed to various sewer pipes. During this process, all solid wastes go through multiple sharp blades or macerators which helps to decrease the dimension of solid waste before further processing.

44.12.5 Lagoons

Lagoons are large open ponds that can collect wastewater from households. These water bodies contain a large number of microorganisms that decompose the waste. Sunlight and wind act as catalysts in this process by accelerating the decomposition process. Algae also assist in the breeding process of bacteria in waste. Due to the presence of algae, these lagoons appear greenish.

44.12.6 Pit Latrines

Pit latrines are age-old sewage disposal methods found in most human civilizations. In the modern day, they are found in rare places with restricted water supply. This disposal system includes a borehole, trench latrines, and ventilated improved pit. Shallow trench latrines are used by large gatherings for a shorter time and once they are nearly full, closed with soil.

44.13 Methods of Sewage Collection

A sewage system is typically designed with underground channels to carry wastewater discharged by localities. The collection system is configured with pipes, manhole drains, holding basins, catch basins, inlets, and pump stations that can move sewage from the collection point to discharge. The pipe systems and other appurtenances are primary methods of sewage collection in urban places.

44.13.1 Combined System

A combined collection system carries both storm and domestic wastewater. This system is typically constructed with pipelines or tunnels of wide diameter. However, in rainy seasons, this system sometimes fails as water treatment plants cannot treat a heavy volume of storm sewage.

44.13.2 Separate System

In relatively newer cities, wastewater systems that carry domestic and storm wastewater separately are found. The surface runoff sewage or stormwater is disposed of in open water streams like a river. Small holding basins or catch basins can be installed for heavy water flow during wet seasons. However, domestic wastewater is directed to a treatment plant.

44.14 Conclusion

Livestock production systems produce a large quantity of animal manure. The management of manure as a resource can offer benefits to livestock producers. Livestock waste management helps to maintain soil fertility in soils lacking organic content. Efficient management of livestock waste helps to increase socioeconomic status of developing countries and also reduce the chances of spreading disease.

References

Arthur, R. and Baidoo, M.F. (2011). Harnessing methane generated from livestock manure in Ghana, Nigeria, and Burkina faso. *Biomass and Bioenergy* 35 (11): 4648–4656.

Bishop, P.L. and Godfrey, C. (1983). Nitrogen transformation during sludge composting. *Food and Agriculture Organization of the United Nations* 24 (4): 34–39.

Epstein, E. (1997). *The Science of Composting*. Boca Raton: CRC Press.

Food and Agriculture Organization (FAO) (2009). *Analysis of the Value Chain for Biogas in Tanzania Northern Zone. Pisces Report*. Rome: FAO.

Gajalakshmi, S. and Abbasi, S.A. (2008). Solid waste management by composting: state of art. *Environmental Science and Technology* 38 (5): 311–400.

Govil, G.P. (2010). Conversion kit of diesel engine into 100% biogas engine. *Biogas Forum- India E-News Letter* 1: 21–24.

Jiang, X., Sommer, S.G., and Christonsent, K.V. (2011). A review of the biogas industry in China. *Energy Policy* 39 (10): 6073–6081.

Khandelwal, K.C. and Mahdi, S.S. (1986). *Biogas Technology: A Practical Handbook*, 2e. New Delhi: Tata McGraw-Hill.

Kirubakaran, V., Sivaramakrishnan, V., Premalatha, M., and Subramanian, P. (2006). Establishing auto-gasification of poultry litter using thermo gravimetric analysis. *Advances in Energy Research* 11: 2–9.

Lantz, M., Svensson, M., Bjornsson, L., and Borjesson, P. (2007). The prospects for an expansion of biogas system in Sweden: incentives, barriers and potentials. *Energy Policy* 35 (9): 1830–1843.

Mahimairaja, S., Bolan, N.S., and Hedley, M.J. (1994). Denitrification losses of nitrogen from fresh and composted manures. *Journal of Science Direct* 27 (9): 1223–1225.

Miller, F.C. (1992). Composting as a process based on the control of ecologically selective factors. *Soil Microbial Ecology* 2: 5–16.

Prasad, C.S., Prasad, G., Singh, R. et al. (2014). *Handbook of Animal Huabandry*, 4e. New Delhi: Indian Council of Agricultural Research.

Rawal, V. and Saha, P. (2012). Women's Employment in India. https://archive.indianstatistics.org/misc/women_work.pdf (accessed 12 February 2024).

Sastry, N.S.R. and Thomas, C.K. (2015). *Livestock Production Management*, 5e. Uttar Pradesh: Kalyani Publishers.

Vanotti, M. and Szogi, B. (2011).Use of gas permeable membranes for removal and recovery of ammonia from high strength livestock waste water. *Proceedings of the water Environment Federation, Nutrient Recovery, and Management*.

Vijay, V.K., Subramanian, K.A., Mathad, V.C., and Subbarao, P.M.V. (2011). Comparative evaluation of emulsion and fuel economy of an automatic spark ignition vehicle fuelled with methane enriched biogas and CNG using chasis dynamometer. *Applied Energy* 105: 17–29.

White, R.K. and Taiganides, E.P. (1971). Pyrolysis of livestock wastes. *Proceedings of the International Symposium of the American Society of Agricultural Engineers*.

45

Biomedical Waste Management

Gungi Saritha

Department of Veterinary Medicine, Sri Venkateswara Veterinary University, Tirupati, India

45.1 Introduction

It is a well-established fact that hospital waste is a potential health hazard to healthcare workers, the public, and local flora and fauna. The interaction and integration of the macro surroundings and the micro environment determine the health status of the local community. A serious imbalance could have serious results for the health of the country. To raise living requirements and promote a healthy society, a balance must consequently be preserved (Neema and Gareshprasad 2002; Murthy et al. 2011).

Medicinal waste products include prescription drugs, particularly those utilized in veterinary medicine. Due to its ability to injure anyone who comes into contact with it, clinical waste produced in veterinary establishments is considered as regulated waste. Personnel need to receive training in the correct management and disposal of biomedical waste.

Veterinarian medicines include any substance or combination of substances used in the analysis, treatment, or prevention of animal illness. They also include biological products, sanitary items, and products used to treat internal and external parasites and disease-transmitting vectors. Every year, the worldwide manufacturing and use of pharmaceuticals increases substantially. Concern regarding those chemical substances' destiny and environmental effects has multiplied along with this growth (Friends of the Earth 2008). Traces of pharmaceutical chemical compounds are regularly detected in ground and surface waters. Even though pharmaceutical ambient concentrations are generally lower than effective doses, they are still concerning.

45.2 Biomedical Waste Definition

Biomedical waste is defined as any waste generated during the process of diagnosis and treatment or immunization of humans or animals or in research activities contributing to the biological production or testing. The waste materials generated in hospitals and other healthcare facilities are called biomedical waste (BMW). BMW comprises infectious or potentially infectious materials including medical, research, or laboratory waste. BMW can also be classified into general, radioactive, chemical, infectious, sharps, pharmaceuticals, and pressurized wastes (Bansod and Deshmukh 2023). It is the duty of every person who has control over an institution or its premises to take the required steps to ensure that waste generated is handled without any adverse effect to human health and the environment.

The negative effects of biomedical waste produced by healthcare centers have to be minimized and for this a common biomedical waste treatment facility (CBWTF) has to be set up. This can minimize occupational hazards to the sanitation and medical examiners who are regularly exposed to BMW. A CBWTF treats biomedical waste produced by several healthcare facilities to minimize negative outcomes.

Epidemiology and Environmental Hygiene in Veterinary Public Health, First Edition. Edited by Tanmoy Rana.
© 2025 John Wiley & Sons, Inc. Published 2025 by John Wiley & Sons, Inc.

45.3 Types of Waste

Waste streams may be divided into two categories: hazardous waste and nonhazardous waste (Figure 45.1). Waste can take many forms and can be characterized by various methods. Bodily states (solid, liquid, and gaseous), bodily attributes, reuse potential, biodegradable potential, and source of introduction are some methods of categorization.

45.4 Sources of Biomedical Waste

Biomedical waste control is a major problem for hospitals and other healthcare facilities. The amount of biomedical waste produced is affected by numerous variables, including waste control strategies, the type of healthcare unit, affected person load, and unit specialization, as well as the use of reusable items and the provision of sources and infrastructure. Biomedical waste and its disposal are a humanitarian issue (Figure 45.2).

45.5 Veterinary Scientific Wastes

Plastic, paper, glass, cardboard, sharp instruments, chemical and biological waste make up the waste produced by veterinary facilities. The significance of veterinary medicines which persist in the bodies of animals, which provide food for tens of millions of humans, is highlighted. A marked rise in antimicrobial utilization has occurred due to the intensifying production of animal protein and the absence of clear legal guidelines and controls on their use (Oliveira et al. 2019).

Similar to other scientific specialties, waste generated in veterinary medicine can be divided into three categories: medical waste, nonhazardous waste, and hazardous waste. Clinical waste consists of sharps (inclusive of needles and syringes) and discarded surgical instruments, animal tissues and specimens, and other discarded substances which can harm the environment and human health.

The primary goals of biomedical waste control are to prevent disease transmission from one patient to another, from patients to healthcare workers and vice versa, and to avoid injury to healthcare personnel. In turn, this aids in decreasing publicity about the damaging outcomes of the cytotoxic, genotoxic, and chemical wastes produced in hospitals. When achieved efficaciously, waste management can be a practice that is moderately effective and efficient and is related to compliance (Pasupathi et al. 2011).

According to a World Health Organization (WHO) document, clinic wastes are made up of 85% nonhazardous materials; the remaining 15% of wastes are divided into infectious (10%) and noninfectious but unsafe (5%) classes. In a country like India, this may range from 15% to 35%.

Biomedical waste control is now considered to be a humanitarian problem on a global scale. Dangerous and inadequate biomedical waste management affects both human and animal health as well as the environment (Sharma and Chauhan 2008; Mathur et al. 2012).

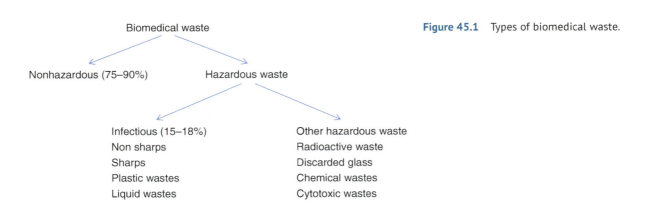

Figure 45.1 Types of biomedical waste.

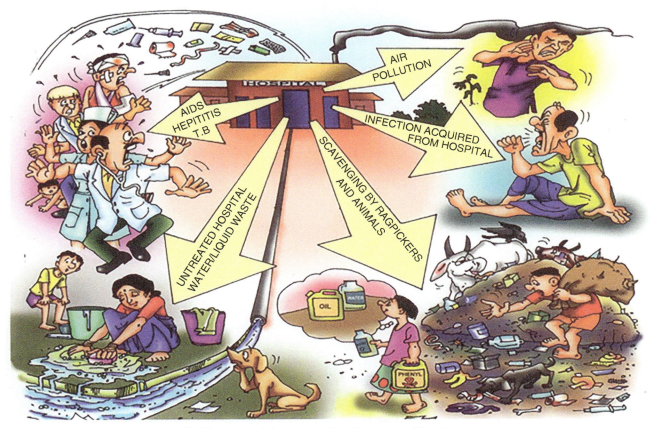

Figure 45.2   Some effects of biomedical waste.

45.6   Medical Solid Wastes and Their Risks

Drug wastes pose a significant risk to human health and environmental integrity. Studies have detected medical residues in sewage, treated wastewater, river sediment, surface waters, and drinking water (Oliveira et al. 2019).

Improper medical solid waste (MSW) disposal and management cause all types of pollution: air, soil, and water. Indiscriminate dumping of wastes contaminates surface and groundwater. In city areas, MSW clogs drains, creating stagnant water for insect breeding and floods during the wet seasons. Uncontrolled burning of MSW and incorrect incineration contribute to urban air pollution. Greenhouse gases are generated from the decomposition of natural wastes in landfills and untreated leachate pollutes surrounding the soil and water. Insect and rodent vectors are attracted to the waste and can spread disease. The use of water polluted by MSW for bathing, irrigation, and drinking can also expose people to infective organisms and other contaminants (Alam and Ahmade 2013).

45.7   Effect of Waste in Soil and Water

The incorrect disposal of unused medicines from homes and healthcare facilities is a major source of prescribed drugs in water. Many individuals put them in the garbage or flush them down the toilet (Dar et al. 2019). Pharmaceutical residues are detected in most water sources at trace levels but even these low concentrations – between one element in one trillion and one component in a thousand million – have dangerous outcomes (Bruno et al. 2016).

45.8 Dangers to Human and Animal Health

The breeding of disease vectors, broadly speaking flies and rats, poses indirect health risks to the general population (Alam and Ahmade 2013). Drug-resistant bacteria pose a critical hazard to public health because of the overuse of excessive and subtherapeutic antimicrobial dosages in animal production and the flawed disposal of animal healthcare provider waste (Oliveira et al. 2019).

The relationship among MSW and commercial effluents containing heavy metals discharged to drainage and/or open dumping results in a vicious cycle in which there is the danger of concentration of heavy metals in the food chain. The following are a few of the possible results: low birth weight, cancer, congenital malformations, neurological ailments, nausea and vomiting, mercury toxicity from ingesting fish with excessive levels of mercury, and plastics ingested by animals and birds.

Workers in this profession are at maximum risk of direct health outcomes and therefore it is essential to protect them from contact with wastes as much as possible. In many locations, protection for trash workers and pickers from direct contact and harm is uncommon, and the codisposal of dangerous and clinical wastes with MSW constitutes an extreme health hazard (Alam and Ahmade 2013). Pharmaceutical wastes are detected in increasing quantities in groundwater or rivers used for human supply and effluents may additionally have significant effects on human health if they are not properly dealt with in treatment plants (Oliveira et al. 2019).

45.9 Environment-related Risks

It can be difficult to eliminate unneeded or outdated medicinal drugs in an environmentally responsible manner (Pharmaceutical Society of Ireland 2017). The disposal method has an instantaneous impact on environmental health and protection. One frequent source of local environmental degradation is the breakdown of waste into its component parts (Alam and Ahmade 2013). The principal ways in which veterinary drugs enter the environment are via the urine and feces of medicated animals, soil fertilization by animal waste, incorrect packaging disposal, sharp item disposal, disposal of leftover and expired tablets in urban solid waste, and direct release of medication used in aquaculture into the water (Oliveira et al. 2019).

45.10 Classification of Organic Wastes

45.10.1 Nonhazardous Wastes

Approximately 85% of the waste produced by healthcare centers is nonhazardous. This includes food scraps, wash water, paper cartons, packaging, and so forth.

45.10.2 Hazardous Wastes

Hazardous wastes include regulated wastes from scientific facilities as well as infectious and contagious wastes, medical and organic wastes, dangerous and purple bag wastes, and contaminated and infectious clinical wastes. Although the terminologies used in regulation are usually defined in a more precise manner, all of these classes essentially discuss the same varieties of waste.

45.11 Policies and Schedules for the Management of Biomedical Waste

Disposal of biomedical waste is a difficult problem. The Biomedical Waste (Management and Handling) Rules took effect in India in 1998. Every "inhabitant" must comply with the Rules and shall take all reasonable measures for proper disposal (Table 45.1).

Table 45.1 Categories of waste and their treatment.

Waste category	Treatment
Human anatomical waste (human tissues, organs, body parts)	Incineration, deep burial
Animal waste (animal tissues, organs, body parts carcases, fluids, blood, experimental animals used in research, waste generated by veterinary hospitals and colleges, discharge from hospitals, animal houses)	Incineration, deep burial
Microbiology and biotechnology waste (wastes from laboratory cultures, stocks or specimens of microorganisms, live or attenuated vaccines, human and animal cell culture used in research and infectious agents from research and industrial laboratories, wastes from production of biologicals, toxins, devices used for transfer of cultures)	Local autoclaving, microwaving, incineration
Waste sharps (needles, syringes, scalpels, blades, glass, etc. that may cause puncture and cuts. This includes both used and unused sharps)	Disinfection (chemical treatment, autoclaving, microwaving, shredding)
Discarded medicines and cytotoxic drugs (outdated, contaminated, and discarded medicines)	Incineration and drugs disposal in secured landfills
Soiled waste (items contaminated with blood and body fluids including dressings, soiled plaster casts, linens, beddings, other material contaminated with blood)	Incineration, autoclaving, microwaving
Solid waste (wastes generated from disposable items other than sharps such as tubing, catheters, intravenous sets, etc.)	Disinfection by chemical treatment, autoclaving, microwaving and shredding
Liquid waste (waste generated from laboratory and washing, cleaning, house-keeping and disinfecting activities)	Disinfection by chemical treatment and discharge into drains
Incineration ash (ash from incineration of any biomedical waste)	Disposal in municipal landfill
Chemical waste (chemicals used in production of biologicals, chemicals used in disinfection, as insecticides, etc.)	Chemical discharge into drains for liquids and secured landfill for solids

45.12 Limitations of Biomedical Waste Control

Biomedical waste law is currently inadequate as it is unable to prevent healthcare centers adopting an incorrect and careless approach to waste disposal. Streams have become polluted because of the mixing of clinic waste with other wastes. This leads to environmental pollution, an offensive odor, and an increase in pests, amongst other matters. It also gives rise to ailments like typhoid, cholera, hepatitis, and AIDS via wounds resulting from infected sharps. The increase in pests facilitates the transmission of diseases such as plague and rabies.

45.13 Waste Management Strategies

The steps to be taken for the proper control of biomedical wastes are outlined below.

45.13.1 Segregation of Waste

A key issue of any waste control approach is segregation. Colored bins should be used to separate and store different waste types until disposal. Waste to be buried deeply or burned needs to be collected in a yellow plastic bag or box. Waste which needs to be autoclaved, microwaved, or dealt with chemically dealt should be collected in a red or blue container. Sharps must be collected in a suitable receptacle (Figure 45.3, Table 45.2).

Items that need disinfection, destruction, or shredding should be collected in a white, translucent container that is puncture proof. This container will then be sealed or can be recycled. When disposed of in landfill, chemical waste, expired medications, and cytotoxic materials have to be placed in a black container labeled "cytotoxic." All packing containers and bags must have a biohazard label, except black packing containers and bags which need to have a cytotoxic label attached (Friends of the Earth 2008).

Auto-Disable Syringes

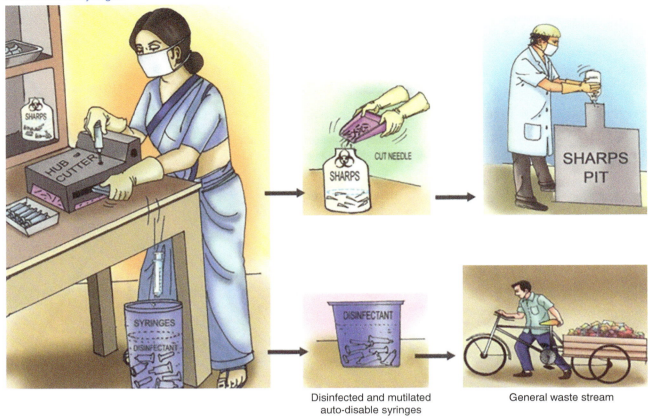

Figure 45.3 Segregation of biomedical waste.

Table 45.2 Color coding for different waste types.

Color	Type of container	Waste categories
Yellow	Plastic bags	Cat 1 Human anatomical waste
		Cat 2 Animal waste
		Cat 3 Microbiological waste
		Cat 6 Solid waste
Red	Disinfected containers, plastic bags	Cat 3 Microbiological waste
		Cat 6 Soiled dressings
Blue/white	Plastic bags, puncture-proof containers	Cat 4 Waste sharps
		Cat 7 Plastic disposables
Black	Plastic bags, puncture-proof containers	Cat 5 Discarded medicines
		Cat 9 Incineration ash
		Cat 10 Chemical waste

The management of wastes of diverse types in different containers allows possible reuse, recycling, and reduction. Reusing chemical substances, medical elements, and instruments can create financial savings. Recycling certain materials, which includes plastic that has been wiped clean and shredded, helps by reducing waste and therefore waste disposal charges.

Separation of waste helps to prevent the transmission of infection, lowering the chance of infection for medical employees. Do not mix glass, plastic, or biological wastes with combustible wastes, chemical wastes with organic wastes, or particular laboratory wastes.

45.13.2 Waste Disposal

The Biomedical Waste (Management and Handling) Rules 1998 stipulate that the wastes should be saved consistent with their specifications. Before they can be competently disposed of, biological wastes can be temporarily held under refrigeration. Storage areas should be placed near garbage treatment centers. Floor drains should not be used for spill containment; rather, liquids should be stored in recessed areas. It is also necessary for floors and walls to be impervious to liquids and to make cleaning methods simple to use.

45.13.3 Packing Containers and Labeling

If treatment is executed chemically and thermally, nonleak bins must be used in conjunction with adequate labeling. Biohazardous substance containers need to be sealed. Chemical substances must be stored in containers which can withstand thermal and chemical treatment and are leak-evident. Steel sharps must be disposed of in rigid bins that can take a strain of 40 psi without rupturing and are puncture proof. For nonhazardous items, heavy-duty plastic bags or bins must be utilized labeled with the biohazard symbol. Biohazard bags of crimson or orange coloration must not be used for materials which can be nonhazardous.

Pasteur pipettes and broken glassware need to be stored in inflexible, puncture-evident containers made from heavy-duty plastic that can be autoclaved. There is no need for labeling unless there is a chance that the waste may be recycled, in which case the container needs to be marked "Do not recycle." Every container of medical waste needs to have an adhesive label containing information about the generator of the waste.

Every untreated box of biohazardous waste has to be simply identified and well classified with the biohazard emblem.

45.13.4 Shipping

Biomedical wastes must be collected and transferred in a way that prevents any risk to the environment or human health. Only operatives who have received the necessary training may handle biohazardous waste that has not been treated. While handling these wastes, it is very important to minimize the threat of needlestick accidents and infections. Biomedical waste should not be mixed with other types of rubbish. Untreated waste should be moved from the place that generated it to some other treatment facility and untreated medical waste must be disposed of right away (Kautto and Melanen 2004; Marinkovic et al. 2005).

When transporting biomedical waste, the following factors should be taken into account.

- The personnel area of the transporting vehicle and the biomedical waste cabin need to be completely separate from each other.
- The waste cabin base must be free from leaks.
- The cabin's layout should make it simple to disinfect iand make it possible to store waste boxes in tiers.
- Decrease water stagnation as much as possible; the interior of the cabin should be sufficiently smooth.
- Sufficient structures should be provided to make it easy to load or offload waste packing containers.
- The vehicle must be labeled with the biohazard image.

45.14 Techniques of Treatment and Disposal

Biological wastes must be mutilated or shredded to ensure against unlawful reuse. Chemical treatment makes use of hypochlorite in a 1% solution. However, there is no pretreatment involved in the incineration method. Most effective in towns with a human population of fewer than five lakhs is deep burial. Additionally, waste needs to be treated as near as possible to the place of its production.

45.14.1 Systems for Eliminating Clinical Waste

Pharmaceutical waste may be competently and correctly processed, even though it is related to several risks (Boxall et al. 2003). To prevent infectious materials from contaminating or spreading to other places, different types of medical waste necessitate different disposal strategies. A small amount of well-identified medical waste may be dumped in landfill. Some types need specialized care, such as a scientific incinerator. To ensure that all viruses and bacteria are eliminated, the great majority of clinical waste needs to be burned.

45.14.2 Return to Manufacturer or Donor

Returning unused medications to the producer can be safe. These medications even have the capacity to be reused by the manufacturer if they are properly separated and have not reached their expiry date. Returns to the maker or donor need to go through significant chemical processing before they can be sold again (Bruno et al. 2016).

The possibility of returning unused medications to the producer for safe disposal must be investigated, mainly for medicinal drugs that pose disposal problems, like antineoplastics. It should also be possible to send back undesirable or unrequested donations to the donor or manufacturer for destruction, especially if they arrive near or after their expiry date.

45.14.3 Transfer of Pharmaceutical Waste Across Borders

Damaged or out-of-date medications are classified as unsafe waste and therefore they may be controlled by the Basel Convention on the Control of Transboundary Movements of Hazardous Wastes and Their Disposal. This involves following strict rules to gain authorization to transport waste to other countries, a process which may require many months.

45.14.4 Landfill

Although it has the capability to be quite dangerous, the most effective method is to take waste to landfill (Boxall et al. 2003). This is the traditional approach to disposing of solid waste and it is also the most cost-effective solution as long as natural decomposition takes place.

However, unscheduled landfill is a common practice for waste disposal in many developing nations (Alam and Ahmade 2013). The use of landfill for pharmaceutical waste management should always be the last resort because of the possibility of allowing prescribed drugs to enter waterways through runoff and therefore affect the environment. The use of landfill for scientific waste is only safe if the sites are placed a long way from bodies of water or are particularly set up to contain risky waste. Most landfills used nowadays are designed to include household waste but not to prevent pharmaceutical waste from leaching out into the water supply (Bruno et al. 2016). Controlled nonengineered landfill can be used for drug waste (FMHACA 2011). However, untreated waste discharged into an uncontrolled, nonengineered open landfill does not safeguard the local environment and should not be used (FMHACA 2011). Untreated waste prescription drugs need to preferably be discharged after immobilization (see below) by way of encapsulation or inertization.

45.14.4.1 Designed Landfill

This carries certain safeguards to guard against chemical leakage into aquifers. Discharging immobilized pharmaceutical waste into this type of landfill is more appropriate than direct depositing of prescription drugs.

45.14.4.2 Advanced-excellent Sanitary Landfill

This type of landfill has facilities for leachate treatment, groundwater tracking, and landfill gas extraction, all of which are supervised by trained employees. It entails depositing MSW in thin layers, compacting it to the smallest extent feasible, and protecting it with soil.

To protect the environment, aquifers, watercourses, and the air, engineered sanitary landfills should follow environment impact assessment (EIA) guidelines and be built effectively.

An evacuated pit that is above the water table and remote from watercourses constitutes a properly built sanitary landfill. To prevent water from leaching into the environment and gaseous emissions into the open air, the base of the construction needs to be sealed and closed with impermeable materials (Hegde et al. 2007). The anaerobic breakdown of natural materials in solid waste results in the production of methane (rich biogas) (Alam and Ahmade 2013). An engineered, sanitary landfill needs to include areas for leachate treatment, groundwater monitoring, and fuel extraction. The gas extraction facility should have the option of turning collected fuel into power or burning it.

Liquid waste from municipalities can be disposed of at landfills which have been properly constructed and maintained.

Conservation of aquifers is of primary importance. Residual waste is compacted and protected with soil. A facility that is properly located, constructed, and managed is known as a "safe sanitary landfill."

45.14.5 Waste Encapsulation and Immobilization

To prevent chemical substances from leaking into the environment, it is common practice to partly fill a plastic (or metallic) drum with medicines before filling it with concrete or some comparable substance (Bruno et al. 2016) as a solid block to immobilize the medicines. Drums should be thoroughly wiped clean before use and should not have previously held explosive or dangerous agents.

The drums are packed with solid and semisolid prescription drugs to a level of 75%, with the final area being packed with cement (cement-lime mixture), plastic foam (bituminous sand), and so on. The combination of lime, cement, and water is added in the ratio of 15:15:5 (by weight). Extra water can be added to achieve a proper liquid consistency. Then, the tops of metal drums must be reshaped and sealed, ideally by a seam or spot welding. The sealed drums are positioned at the base of the landfill, after which stable municipal waste is introduced.

The drums can be set on pallets for ease of shipping, which could then be positioned on a pallet transporter. The method for encapsulating most anticancer drugs is slightly different.

45.14.6 Inertization

Inertization is a type of encapsulation in which the drugs are removed from their packaging. The drugs are then crushed, then water, cement, and lime are blended to create a homogenous paste. As there can be a dust hazard, employee protection in the form of protective clothes and masks is essential. The paste is then delivered to a landfill in a concrete mixer truck in liquid form and decanted into the ordinary city garbage. The procedure can be completed with the use of existing equipment and is reasonably cheap. Pharmaceutical waste (65%), lime (15%), cement (15%), and water (5% or extra to make a good liquid consistency) are the approximate weight ratios required.

45.14.7 Sewer

After being properly diluted and controlled, treatment waste is flushed into the sewer system (FMHACA 2011). There are some liquid medications (syrups and IV fluids) that may be diluted with water and flushed into the sewers without causing public health or environmental issues. It is also possible to flush small amounts of properly diluted liquid medications or antiseptics into swiftly moving waterways. In instances where sewers are broken or damaged, the help of a hydrogeologist or sanitary engineer may be needed.

45.14.8 Open Field Burning

Given that harmful contaminants could be released into the air while burning pharmaceuticals at low temperatures in open bins, this approach should no longer be used. If they cannot be recycled, paper and cardboard packaging can be burned, but not plastic. Burning pharmaceutical waste is a common disposal choice even if it is not encouraged. It is strongly advised to dispose of waste medicinal drugs in this way in only very modest quantities.

45.14.9 Incineration

Incineration is a less complicated approach to dealing with pharmaceutical waste. It involves burning drugs at temperatures as high as 1200 °C. The principal advantage of this technique is that waste is not released into water sources but burning waste can be an expensive disposal method (Boxall et al. 2003). It involves a managed combustion process for generating gases and residue by way of burning solid wastes at high temperatures of around 1000 °C and above in the presence of extra air (oxygen). Incineration is a hotly contested issue worldwide, partially because of its unfavorable outcomes for the environment.

45.14.9.1 Incineration at Medium Temperature

There are not many nations that have high-temperature, two-chamber incinerators that can burn greater than 1% halogenated chemical compounds. Strict emissions regulations, which include those outlined by the EU, can be met with the aid of those incinerators. However, most medical waste disposal will be dealt with in simple furnaces and incinerators with a middle-temperature range.

With a minimal operating temperature of 850 °C and a minimum combustion retention duration of 2 seconds within the chamber, a two-chamber incinerator may be used to get rid of unused drugs in emergencies. The use of this method as a stopgap treatment instead of much less safe alternatives, including inadequate disposal to landfill, is recommended because many older municipal waste incinerators are medium-temperature only.

45.14.9.2 High-Temperature Incineration

Foundries, coal-fired thermal electricity plants, cement kilns, and other high-temperature industries usually have furnaces that perform at temperatures much above 850 °C, have lengthy combustion retention capacity, and distribute exhaust. Many countries lack complex chemical waste disposal centers or are unable to justify them financially. Therefore, using an existing business facility provides a practical and cheaper solution.

Prescription drugs that have reached the end of their shelf-life, chemical waste, spent oil, and other garbage can all be disposed of in cement kilns. Cement kilns are best for disposing of prescription drugs due to numerous traits. Whilst burning, the materials used for cement attain temperatures of 1450 °C, and the combustion gases can reach 2000 °C. All organic waste additives are efficaciously decomposed under these conditions. Potentially harmful or toxic combustion products are eliminated within the heat equipment or absorbed into the cement clinker product.

A thermal process calls for high temperature and managed waste combustion conditions to transform the waste into gases and inert materials. Three simple kinds of incinerators are normally used to burn medical institution waste: controlled air types, rotary kilns, and multiple fireplace types (Gravers 1998). Incinerators used to burn medical waste produce dangerous air pollutants and poisonous ash residues, which are the principal environmental sources of dioxins. The potential exists for the unsafe ashes which might be disposed of in landfill to seep into groundwater.

Crimson bags should not be burned as they may contain cadmium which can produce toxic emissions. Additionally, if a crimson bag is full of items containing mercury, the mercury will contaminate the infectious wastes and the environment.

45.14.10 Nonincineration Treatments

Nonincineration treatment includes four essential techniques: thermal, chemical, irradiative, and biological. In the majority of nonincineration techniques, thermal and chemical procedures are used. The primary aim of this treatment technology is the decontamination of wastes via microbial annihilation. Facilities must be provided to fulfill the region's disinfection requirements (Thornton et al. 1996).

Disposal of various forms of wastes is enabled through plasma-generated high temperatures. Pyrolysis of medical wastes into carbon monoxide and hydrogen, caustic soda, and hydrochloric acid is one method that ensures the adequate disposal of scientific wastes.

45.14.11 Chemical Disintegration

If a suitable incinerator is not available, landfill ought to be utilized first, then chemical decomposition in line with the producer's instructions. However, this system is not recommended. Chemical inactivation is hazardous and time-consuming and therefore this technique is probably suitable only for disposing of a tiny quantity of anticancer drugs. Chemical breakdown is not suitable for large volumes of waste.

The numerous strategies for disposing of clinical waste are outlined below

- Landfill, biodigestion, or incineration of animal carcasses and body parts.
- Animal waste (along with bedding and manure).
  - Biohazardous animal waste needs to be handled chemically or thermally for combustion and disinfection.
  - Composting or use of nontoxic animal feces as fertilizer.

- Chemical waste: for proper disposal, 1% sodium hypochlorite or other chemical agent of equal strength must be used. After treatment, liquids can be discharged into drains and solids to landfill (Gupta and Boojh 2006).
- When discarding genetically changed organisms or substances containing recombinant DNA, local institutes of health (NIH) guidelines should be followed.
- Infected human body parts and excrement.
  - Dead bodies with identifiable bodily components must be cremated or buried for disposal.
  - Solids need to be burned or disinfected before being discarded. Body fluids must be thermally or chemically disinfected before being discharged into the drainage.
- Metal sharps must be disposed of with encapsulation to prevent harm to laboratory, transport, and landfill workers. Even after sterilization or capping and whilst kept in proper containers, needles, knives, and other objects pose a biohazard. If autoclaving is necessary, a tape strip with an autoclave indication must be located within the container. Gas chromatography needles must be rinsed to remove dangerous materials after which they can be disposed of with broken, noncontaminated glassware (Patil and Pokhrel 2004).
- Microbiological waste: thermal or chemical treatment is essential before discharge into the sewer.
- Even if materials are nonhazardous, autoclaving or chemically treating all microbiological products is required for proper laboratory practice.
- Disinfection by thermal, chemical, or encapsulating treatment is required for plastic debris, pipettes, and damaged glassware infected with biohazardous materials. Plastics and glassware should not be burned.
- Radioactive waste: radioactive animal corpses should be stored at temperatures below freezing (FMHACA 2011). A health physics/radiation protection application should be created, especially for steel sharps that have been infected with radioactive materials. Federal and state governments additionally require the packaging and transportation of carcases containing long-lived radionuclides to a repository site where nuclear materials are authorized. The overall rule for radiation safety when disposing of radioactive wastes is that the quantity of radiation exposure for the waste treatment plan as an whole should not exceed the following values: an effective dose of 0.01 mSv per year. A responsible individual who can discharge radioactive material into the sewer system or environment is obligated to prepare a waste treatment plan.

45.14.12 Other Disposal Strategies

Other strategies of disposal which might be used for medical wastes include on-site, off-site, and mailback disposal. On-site treatment requires expensive technology, and only very large hospitals have the capacity to provide this. For off-site treatment, waste removal companies which have trained personnel are hired to remove clinical trash in distinct packing containers. Treatment occurs in a facility designed to house an enormous amount of clinical waste. Mailback disposal of medical wastes is similar, with the exception that the wastes are shipped through postal services as opposed to hauliers.

45.15 Waste Reduction

One crucial approach for handling waste is waste reduction. Waste output may be reduced by optimizing manufacturing methods and materials in industrial settings. The reduction of waste is important for businesses and decreases costs. Reusing second-hand items, repairing broken items in preference to purchasing new ones, and being able to replenish and reuse them are some approaches to reduce costs.

45.16 Accumulation and Storage of Wastes

Waste accumulation and storage take place between the point of waste production and the places that process waste. Any waste that is kept offsite is also taken into consideration to be saved. Spills have to be contained and ground drains need to be recessed. Flooring and drains must be constructed in order that liquid may be contained effortlessly and cleansing is made easy. In the case of putrifiable wastes, refrigeration is required for long-term storage. Relevant warning signs must also be posted in the storage and treatment areas (Hegde et al. 2007).

45.17 Measures to Prevent the Risks of Clinical Wastes

To ensure that hazardous waste does not harm the environment or create further problems, proper waste control is essential.

The manufacturing of products that generate little waste after use must be encouraged, in addition to materials recycling; plastic recycling identity codes and labels must be used to make sorting and recycling of plastic packaging simpler; and municipalities should improve the level of service they provide to the public concerning waste sorting.

Animal medications on the farm should be properly organized in order to prevent excess purchases. The farm worker should buy only what is needed and can be used before the product expiry date. Refuse samples provided by veterinarians if they are no longer needed and if existing products have expired, assess all options for disposal before throwing them in the garbage.

References

Alam, P. and Ahmade, K. (2013). Impact of solid waste on health and the environment. *International Journal of Sustainable Development and Green Economics* 2 (1): 165–168.

Bansod, H.S. and Deshmukh, P. (2023). Biomedical waste management and its importance: a systematic review. *Cureus* 15 (2): e34589.

Boxall, A.A., Kolpin, W.D., Sorensen, B., and Tolls, J. (2003). Are veterinary drug treatments causing environmental risks? *Environmental Technology and Era* 37: 286A–294A.

Bruno, J., Eaton, S., Hemingway, J., Towle, E. (2016). Pharmaceutical waste disposal: current practices in Tirana, Albania. BSc thesis, Worcester Polytechnic Institute.

Dar, M.A., Maqbool, M., and Rasool, S. (2019). Pharmaceutical wastes and their disposal practice in routine. *International Journal of Information and Computing Science* 6: 78–92.

Food, Medicine and Healthcare Administration and Control Authority of Ethiopia (FMHACA) (2011). Medicines Waste Management and Disposal Directive. https://forsslund.org/StandardHealthFaclitiy/Medicines%20Waste%20Management%20 &%20Disposal%20Directive%20-%20Final%20prin.pdf (accessed 21 February 2024).

Friends of the Earth (2008). Mechanical biological treatment. https://foe.cymru/sites/default/files/mchnical_biolo_treatmnt.pdf (accessed 22 February 2024).

Gravers, P.D. (1998). Management of hospital wastes – an outline. Proceedings of National Workshop on Management of Hospital Waste, Jaipur.

Gupta, S. and Boojh, R. (2006). Report: biomedical waste management practices at Balrampur Hospital, Lucknow, India. *Waste Management and Research* 24: 584–591.

Hegde, V., Kulkarni, R.D., and Ajantha, G.S. (2007). Biomedical waste control. *Journal of Oral and Maxillofacial Pathology* 11 (1): 5–9.

Kautto, P. and Melanen, M. (2004). How does industry respond to waste policy instruments – Finnish experiences. *Journal of Cleaner Production* 12 (1): 11.

Marinkovic, N., Vitale, K., Afric, I., and Janev, H.N. (2005). Hazardous medical waste management as a public health issue. *Arhiv za Higijenu Rada i Toksikologiju* 56 (21): 32.

Mathur, P., Patan, S., and Shobhawat, A.S. (2012). Need of biomedical waste management system in hospitals – an emerging issue – a review. *Current World Environment* 7 (1): 117–124.

Murthy, P.G., Leelaja, B.C., and Hosmani, S.P. (2011). Biomedical waste disposal and management in some major hospitals of Mysore City, India. *International NGO Journal* 6 (3): 71–78.

Neema, S.K. and Ganeshprasad, K.S. (2002). Plasma pyrolysis of scientific waste. *Current Science* 83: 271–278.

Oliveira, K.S., Morello, L., Oliveira, V.S. et al. (2019). Disposal of animal healthcare services waste in southern Brazil: One Health at risk. *Saude Debate* 43: 78–93.

Pasupathi, P., Sindhu, S., Ponnusha, B.S., and Ambika, A. (2011). Biomedical waste management for the health care industry. *International Journal of Biological and Medical Research* 2 (1): 472–486.

Patil, G.V. and Pokhrel, K. (2004). Biomedical solid waste management in an Indian hospital: a case study. *Waste Management* 25: 592–599.

Pharmaceutical Society of Ireland (2017). Guidelines for the disposal of medicinal products for a retail pharmacy business. www.thepsi.ie/Libraries/Folder_Pharmacy_Practice_Guidance/01_5_Disposal_of_Medicinal_Products_for_Retail.sflb.ashx (accessed 22 February 2024).

Sharma, S. and Chauhan, S.V.S. (2008). Assessment of biomedical waste control in three apex government hospitals of Agra. *Journal of Environmental Biology* 29 (2): 159–162.

Thornton, J., Tally, M.C., Orris, M.C., and Wentreg, J. (1996). Hospitals and plastic Dioxin prevention and medical waste incineration. *Public Health Reports* 1: 299–313.

46

General Hygiene, Sanitation, and Disinfection of Animal Housing and Hospital Environment

Jay P. Yadav[1], Sivakumar Mani[2], and Maninder Singh[1]

[1] *Department of Veterinary Public Health and Epidemiology, College of Veterinary Science, Guru Angad Dev Veterinary and Animal Sciences University, Rampura Phul, India*
[2] *Department of Veterinary Public Health and Epidemiology, Veterinary College and Research Institute, Tamil Nadu Veterinary and Animal Sciences University, Theni, India*

46.1 Introduction

The term "hygiene" is derived from the Greek word "hygieinos" which means "beneficial to health" and includes a variety of measures (Heinemann 2020). Proper hygiene and sanitation in animal houses and associated environments are essential to prevent survival and transmission of disease-causing pathogens between animals and humans.

According to the International Society on Animal Hygiene, the term "animal hygiene" is defined as "interaction between abiotic and biotic factors of environment and domestic animals, especially food animals, with the aim to prevent diseases and to promote animal health and to ensure species-specific health and welfare needs of such animals" (Thielen 2000). The main purpose of animal hygiene is not to cure animals that are already diseased, but to provide preventive health measures and create optimal environmental conditions to maintain a high standard of health and welfare (Hoy et al. 2016). The importance of cleaning and disinfection in livestock production increases with the rising numbers of animals per area and per barn (Müller et al. 2011). Therefore, sanitation is an integral part of modern intensive farm animal housing.

Many animals enter shelters in poor health, malnourished, stressed, and with no history of vaccination. Some animals intermittently shed harmful pathogens, with or without showing any clinical signs of disease. However, the occurrence of disease in a particular host depends on various factors, such as condition of the host (exposed or unexposed with infected animals), virulence of the pathogen, pathogen load, and environmental factors affecting the level of exposure (Hurley and Baldwin 2012). The amount of pathogen present and the duration of exposure can be controlled through proper cleaning and disinfection. Effective shelter and hospital environment sanitation prevents illness in both animals and humans and creates pleasant environmental conditions (Karsten 2021).

The goal of a sanitation plan is not only to sterilize an environment but to reduce the pathogen load to a level that minimizes the risk of disease transmission between animals and humans. The standard of care at every veterinary hospital should include a high level of hygiene, awareness about the category of infectious agents and their mode of transmission, and reducing the risk of infection wherever possible. Such infection control procedures are necessary to prevent the introduction and spread of infectious diseases within a group of patients and their human caregivers, thereby protecting human, animal, and environmental health against biological threats.

The following terms are generally used in sanitary practices of animal shelters and associated environments.

- *Cleaning*: a process of removing foreign material (e.g., contaminants, including dust, soil, chemical residues, pyrogens, large numbers of microorganisms) and the organic matter protecting them. It is normally accomplished using water with detergents or enzymatic products. Thorough cleaning is required before high-level disinfection and sterilization, because inorganic and organic materials remaining on surfaces interfere with the effectiveness of disinfectants and sterilizers.
- *Pathogen*: a disease-causing agent (such as, bacteria, virus, fungus, parasite, prions, rickettsia, chlamydia).
- *Detergent*: a cleansing agent; synthetic water-soluble or liquid organic preparations that are chemically different from soaps but are able to emulsify oils, hold dirt in suspension, and act as wetting agents.

Epidemiology and Environmental Hygiene in Veterinary Public Health, First Edition. Edited by Tanmoy Rana.
© 2025 John Wiley & Sons, Inc. Published 2025 by John Wiley & Sons, Inc.

- *Disinfectant*: a chemical that destroys vegetative forms of harmful microorganisms (such as bacteria and fungi), especially on inanimate objects.
- *Disinfection*: the process of reducing the number of vegetative forms of most pathogenic microorganisms on a surface, usually with the use of a chemical product to minimize the risk of infection for animals and humans who come into contact with those surfaces directly or indirectly.
- *Soap*: a cleansing and emulsifying agent made usually by the action of alkali on fat or fatty acids and consisting essentially of sodium or potassium salts of such acids.
- *Antisepsis*: a special category of disinfection, referring to the inhibition or destruction of pathogenic microbes on the skin and mucous membranes.
- *Biocides*: chemical substances that are distinct from disinfectants in that they are intended to destroy all forms of life, not just microorganisms.
- *Fomite*: any object or substance that is able to carry infectious organisms and transfer them from one individual to another.
- *Sanitation*: reduction of the number of bacterial contaminants to a safe level. It is the promotion of hygiene and prevention of disease by maintenance of sanitary conditions such as cleaning and disinfection.
- *Terminal cleaning*: process carried out after a patient under isolation has been discharged, end of the day cleaning in areas such as operating rooms, or end of procedure cleaning in areas in which a patient known to be infected with a contagious disease has been.
- *Sterilization*: process of removing all forms of microorganisms using physical or chemical agents.

46.2 Steps in the Sanitation Process

Cleaning and disinfection of animal houses and hospital environments should be carried out in a three-step process.

1) *Mechanical removal of visible organic matter and dust*: this is the first and foremost step in the sanitation process. Most detergents and disinfectants are either partially or completely inactivated in the presence of organic matter such as food, dung, urine, saliva or soil. Therefore, removal of visible contamination before cleaning with detergent or disinfectant is essential, followed by drying of the surfaces (Russell and Hugo 1987; Steneroden 2012).
2) *Cleaning with disinfectant or detergent and hot water*: cleaning with soap or detergent and hot water in combination with mechanical removal of visible organic matter and dust will remove 90% of environmental pathogens (Morgan-Jones 1987) and is the most important component in determining the outcome of disinfection activities (Kahrs 1995).
3) *Disinfection*: disinfectants must be applied to clean surfaces, because many of them are inactivated by the presence of organic matter, soap or detergent left on a surface. In addition, disinfectants must be used in the appropriate concentrations, left on a surface for a specified period of time, and should have proper methods of preparation, storage, application, disposal, and safety. They should be labeled for use against particular pathogens based on concentration and contact time (Steneroden 2012; Karsten 2021).

46.3 Important Aspects of a Sanitation Plan

Effective sanitation requires knowledge, a plan of action, and evaluation (Grow 1995; Kahrs 1995). Having a written protocol for cleaning and disinfection will greatly help in the training of new employees and provides a reference for evaluation of the effectiveness of the plan. A clearly written and well-understood sanitation plan is the cornerstone of a shelter's infection control strategy.

46.3.1 Avoiding Disease Spread

The goal of cleaning and disinfection activities is to improve the cleanliness of the environment and thereby lessen disease spread. However, without proper knowledge and training, there is a chance that those performing sanitation activities may spread disease by the use of contaminated equipment, clothing or hands. Separate sanitary supplies such as mops, rags, and buckets should be provided for each section of the shelter to prevent spreading of disease. Spreading or aerosolizing disease particles during cleaning should be avoided by using damp mops, electrostatic mops, or dust mops rather than vigorous cleaning with brooms and high-pressure hoses. Staff should change outer clothing and gloves and wash hands before and after cleaning. Wearing of designated clothes during cleaning that can be changed before handling animals will help to reduce the possibility of disease spread.

46.3.2 Order of Cleaning

In order to decrease the further risk of spreading disease while cleaning, staff should be instructed to proceed from areas housing healthy animals to areas of housing with suspected or infected animals. It is important to avoid revisiting areas containing healthy animals after cleaning an area with unhealthy ones. Cleaning should be performed first in areas with young animals; then healthy adoptable animals; healthy stray animals; animals in quarantine; and sick animals in isolation last. It is also important to evaluate the health of animals in a particular room or area prior to cleaning. If any animals housed in the same area with healthy animals have clinical signs of infectious disease, they should be moved to isolation or handled last after the healthy animals. When cleaning a particular area or room, start with the highest point and work downward to avoid dripping dirty water onto a just cleaned surface (Kahrs 1995).

46.3.3 Minimizing Animal Stress

The cleaning process can be very disruptive and stressful to shelter animals; care should be taken to minimize noise, unnecessary animal handling, and animal movement. Animals should be confined while cleaning their cages and not allowed to run loose, which may agitate other caged animals and spread the infectious agents. Performing sanitation chores at the same time of day with the same staff can also help reduce stress.

A method such as spot cleaning (where a cage is spot cleaned on a daily basis but disinfected less often) is useful in areas containing cats. A guillotine door system is ideal for cleaning dog kennels, so that dogs can move freely to the adjacent clean cage while their cage is being cleaned. Cages should never be hosed with animals still in them and care should be taken to dry kennels prior to returning the animals. It is also important to maintain good ventilation while cleaning to decrease the possibility of irritating the mucous membranes of humans and animals by the use of sanitizing agents.

46.3.4 Product Preparation

It is important to follow the manufacturer's instructions for product preparation, as disinfectants must be used at the correct concentration to be effective. Sanitation protocols should include clear instructions on how to dilute, apply, store, and discard all products in use. Measuring equipment should be readily available, as evaluating disinfectants by smell, color, simple visualization or otherwise guessing is not acceptable. In addition to written protocols and instructions, staff must be given hands-on training on how to prepare, apply, store, and discard the product safely.

The following are important considerations when developing any shelter sanitation plan.

- Whichever disinfectant and cleaning products are used, they should not be mixed together unless directed by the manufacturer or supported by research.
- Whenever mixed randomly, disinfectants and detergents can cancel each other's efficacy or even create toxic fumes (e.g., bleach with ammonia or undiluted accelerated hydrogen peroxide).
- The expiry date, which indicates the time the disinfectant will lose its efficacy after dilution, must be considered (efficacy for accelerated hydrogen peroxide is 90 days, bleach stored in an open container should be remixed daily, and the efficacy of diluted potassium peroxymonosulfate is usually a week).
- Storage temperature and method can also affect stability. For instance, bleach stored in a light-proof, sealed container retains its bacterial efficacy for at least a month, while it is more rapidly inactivated when stored in transparent containers (Rutala et al. 1998).

46.3.5 Contact Time

Many, but not all, disinfectants require 10 minutes of wet contact time for effectiveness, especially against the hardiest pathogens (e.g., parvoviruses). However, it may be prudent to leave a disinfectant in contact for an hour or more when organic contamination cannot be removed or at very low environmental temperatures. Some disinfectants, such as accelerated hydrogen peroxide, will be substantially effective in as little as one minute under ideal conditions (Omidbakhsh and Sattar 2006). However, factors such as low temperature, pH, the hardness of the water, and contamination with organic matter will increase the amount of time needed for any disinfectant. It is also important to note which products require rinsing after the appropriate contact time. Failure to rinse the products before drying can result in caustic residues that can be harmful if they come in contact with skin or are ingested.

It is also important to note that some pathogens, such as parvovirus or *Microsporum* (e.g., *M. canis*), can exist in the environment and on objects for months to years under certain conditions (e.g., away from direct sunlight, in organic material or after inadequate disinfection) (Greene and Decaro 2012). Thus, it is not appropriate or practical to close sanitation areas when a known or suspected case of disease involving these pathogens is diagnosed. Waiting for the pathogen to be inactivated with the passage of time does not increase the protocol's effectiveness. One recommendation is to clean and disinfect three times with a product that has efficacy against both organic material and unenveloped viruses (e.g., potassium peroxymonosulfate or accelerated hydrogen peroxide) at the correct dilution for the necessary contact time to help ensure that all surfaces have been sufficiently covered. All three cycles can be completed in one day and animals can be allowed access to the housing unit or area again.

46.3.6 Application Systems

The method of application and use of proper equipment are as important as the choice of disinfectant. Outbreaks of disease or disinfectant toxicity have been traced to defective disinfectant dispensers. The use of mops and buckets in animal shelters should be avoided, if possible, as they can contribute to the spread of dirt and pathogens. For small cleaning operations, bottles with "squirt tops" rather than spray tops are ideal to decrease the amount of disinfectant aerosolized into the environment, thus helping animal and human respiratory health. If a spray bottle is used for spot cleaning, the rag or paper towel should always be sprayed instead of the surface to help decrease aerosolizing and splashing of the disinfectant.

Different products such as Rescue® may also be available as disinfectant wipes for small clean-up operations; however, the active ingredients and contact time must be noted to ensure that the product is effective against the pathogens of concern. For example, Clorox® wipes do not contain bleach and the label states that contact time for it to be virucidal is four minutes. All bottles should be clearly labeled with the identity of the disinfectant, all required safety information, the expiry date of the solution, and the date and initials of the person who made up the solution. This is required by the Occupational Health and Safety Administration (OSHA) and will permit accountability and retraining in case of faulty disinfectant formulation.

46.3.7 Drying

Whatever disinfectant and method of application are used, the final decontamination step should be drying of the environment. Most pathogens will survive for longer in moist conditions and some that are not particularly resilient in the environment (e.g., *Giardia* cysts) may persist for hours or days in a damp area. Some fatal pathogens can persist in moist and damp environments, even in the presence of disinfectant. For instance, *Streptococcus equi* subsp. *zooepidemicus*, associated with a fatal outbreak in dogs (Pesavento et al. 2008), was isolated from pools of water remaining in kennels that had been completely cleaned and disinfected.

Drying is especially important if the surface to be cleaned is uneven and likely to retain pools of water or in humid climates where effective air drying may not be possible. Therefore, awareness and training on usage of drying tools (e.g., squeegees, towels, paper towels) must be provided to accompany all sanitation protocols. Quiet floor fans can be used on low to expedite drying when needed. Care should be taken to ensure fans are not blowing directly onto animals. Minimizing humidity in animal housing areas will also assist in drying. Again, animals should neither get wet during the sanitation process nor be returned to enclosures that are still wet.

46.3.8 Importance of Animal Housing/Facility Design

Consideration of animal housing design is an essential component of an effective sanitation plan. Good housing design, along with proper use, facilitates effectiveness and efficacy of sanitation. Conversely, poor housing or inappropriate use of good housing can compromise the staff's ability to adequately clean and care for animals, which can result in process inefficiencies. This in turn can result in the need for more staff, increased cleaning and disinfectant product use, and higher disease rates, which contribute to increased costs and decreased welfare.

Individual animal housing should meet the basic physical and behavioral needs of the animal, allow effective and efficient cleaning without the need to remove the animal from the housing unit, and limit animal exposure to cleaning procedures. Appropriately sized double-compartment housing (kennels or cages) is generally used for short lengths of stay (up to about two weeks) of individually housed small animals (such as dogs and cats). In case of limited number of double-compartment housing, the highest priority for use of these enclosures should be given to new intakes, juveniles, and dangerous animals as well as all animals housed in isolation areas.

For sanitation reasons, simple sealed concrete is not recommended in most shelter facilities where heavy animal traffic occurs. A more durable, cleanable material for high-traffic areas is roughly polished sealed concrete (colored or not). Resinous epoxy and urethane coating surfaces over concrete generally meet kennel flooring needs. Other more expensive materials such as nonporous, nonslippery tiles with epoxy grout can be used, but cost often precludes this in animal shelter facilities. Before construction of shelters, owners need to consult with contractors who are familiar with the various challenges in the selection of the best materials for use in animal housing areas.

To allow quick and adequate drying, high water use areas such as dog kennels must have proper drainage. This includes an appropriately sloped floor to a correctly placed drain with adequate flow; properly sized drainpipes to avoid backflow; appropriate drain covers to protect animals from injury, and proper plumbing to avoid clogging. Individual kennel drains or properly designed and covered trench drains prevent cross-contamination from kennel to kennel. Drains should be provided both within the housing unit and in the corridor or walkway.

People and animals should not have to walk through one animal housing area to get to another. To further help disease control, all animal rooms should be designed such that daily cleaning and care can be provided with minimal staff movement into and out of the room. Each animal room should be fitted with its own dedicated cleaning supplies and equipment (identified for use in that room only) and have storage space for them to reduce unnecessary clutter.

46.3.9 Population Management

When designing a comprehensive shelter healthcare plan, consideration of the composition, size, and management of the population is as important as the sanitation protocols and the design of the shelter building itself. The most thorough sanitation program and best building cannot compensate for the negative consequences suffered when a population is not well managed. Clinical experience and research have shown that the longer an animal remains in the shelter, the more likely it is to develop clinical signs of disease, so shelters must always strive to manage the population so each animal's length of stay (LOS) will be as short as possible for the desired outcome (Edinboro et al. 2004; Dinnage et al. 2009). Various strategies such as managed or diverted intake, daily population rounds, identifying and addressing delays in flow-through, and removing barriers to adoption can all help with reducing LOS.

When a shelter is crowded, not only is the LOS increased but the likelihood of direct and indirect contact between animals is increased. This leads to higher pathogen loads in shelters, and animals experience greater stress that negatively impacts their immune system and productivity. Additionally, shelter staff are frequently overwhelmed and unable to provide adequate daily care, making it difficult to both monitor and implement good sanitation practices. This can all result in an inability to meet the physical and behavioral needs of the animals which, in turn, can lead to increased health and/or behavioral concerns, diminished quality of life, and longer LOS.

46.4 Sanitation Procedures in Animal Shelters

Sanitation can be achieved by chemical means (soaps, detergents, disinfectants) or physical means (heat including steam, ultraviolet [UV] light, radiation, desiccation). In shelters, for the most part, chemicals are relied upon to clean and disinfect. In some circumstances, UV light and desiccation may be utilized as an aid to sanitation (e.g., in dry, sunny parts of the country, laundry may be hung outside or cages cleaned and put in the sun to dry).

The choice of products to use for cleaning and disinfection will depend on the particular shelter and the infectious diseases of concern, but will include soap or detergent for cleaning, disinfectant to kill hazardous microorganisms, and a degreaser to use periodically to penetrate layers of dried-on greasy debris. Cleaning and disinfection products must always be used at their proper concentrations. If the same product is being used to both clean and disinfect, it is important to follow the manufacturer's instructions for product preparation for each function. A disinfectant's efficacy claim against a particular pathogen is determined by testing it under specific concentrations and contact times. If these concentrations and contact times are not followed in practice, product efficacy is unknown. Accurate measurement with measuring devices is necessary to ensure proper concentrations are obtained. Some products are labeled for use at different concentrations but in general, a stronger concentration will not necessarily kill more organisms and may actually harm animals and the humans performing the cleaning operations (Coppock et al. 1988; Bello et al. 2009).

Different products used in sanitization should never be mixed together unless specifically approved by the manufacturer. For instance, quaternary ammonium compounds (QACs) are inactivated by soaps and detergents (Jeffrey 1995), and mixing bleach with ammonia can result in toxic vapors. Cleaning products should be stored away from food and under appropriate heat and light conditions in order to remain effective. Training on the safe use of cleaning products must be an integral part of shelter staff and volunteer training.

However, certain cleaning products should be used with caution or not at all in animal shelters. Phenolic compounds should be avoided in cat shelters because cats are highly sensitive to these products (Petersen et al. 2008). Aldehydes can be carcinogenic to humans and should be avoided. Biguanides such as chlorhexidine, Nolvasan®, and Virosan® are toxic to fish and should be avoided due to environmental concerns.

46.4.1 Characteristics of an Ideal Disinfectant

Broad spectrum: it should have a wide antimicrobial spectrum (including sporicidal) to kill pathogens that are the common cause of shelter-and hospital-acquired infections (HAIs).

- *Fast acting*: it should have high germicidal activity, rapid kill and short kill/contact time listed on the label.
- *Remains wet*: surfaces stay wet long enough to meet listed kill/contact times with a single application.
- *Not affected by environmental factors*: disinfectants should be stable and effective in the presence of organic matter (e.g., blood, feces, sputum, urine, etc.).
- *Chemical compatibility*: it should be compatible with soaps, detergents, and other chemicals encountered in use, such that the effectiveness of neither chemical is affected and mixing does not result in toxicity, increased corrosiveness, or other reactivity.
- *Nontoxic*: it should not be irritating to users, other staff, clients, or patients. It is also important that it does not cause induction of allergies (especially asthma and dermatitis). Disinfectant products with the lowest toxicity rating should be chosen.
- *Surface compatibility*: it should be capable of penetration without destruction, and compatible with common surfaces and equipment found in veterinary settings.
- *Persistence*: it should have sustained antimicrobial activity or residual postapplication antimicrobial effect.
- *Easy to use*: it should be easily available in multiple forms (e.g., wipes, sprays, concentrates) and simple to use.
- *Acceptable odor*: odor and esthetics should be acceptable to users and others.
- *Economical*: it should be economical for end users and when considering the costs of disinfectant product capabilities, the cost per compliant use should also be considered.
- *Solubility*: it should be soluble in water.
- *Stability*: it should be stable in concentrate form and when diluted for a specific period of time.
- *Cleaner*: it should have good cleaning properties.
- *Nonflammable*: it should be nonflammable and the flash point should be higher than 65.5 °C (150 °F).

There are numerous chemical agents available to disinfect animal shelters and healthcare facilities. These agents are mostly liquid based and fall into nine broad categories: acids, alcohols, aldehydes, alkalis, biguanides, halogens (hypochlorites and iodine-based iodophors), oxidizing agents, phenolics, and QACs. Accelerated hydrogen peroxide products (e.g. Accel®), which claim virucidal, bactericidal, fungicidal, and tuberculocidal activity, have been introduced for disinfection of noncritical environmental surfaces and equipment. In addition, there are some newer disinfectant combinations that have synergistic actions (e.g., Siloxycide®); a combination of hydrogen peroxide plus silver nitrate claims increased efficacy compared with products containing individual component and is approved for use in healthcare settings. Characteristics of commonly used disinfectants in veterinary settings are given in Table 46.1.

Table 46.1 Characteristics of different disinfectants used in veterinary settings.

Category	Mechanism of action	Suitable applications	Efficacy with organic material	Efficacy with detergents/ soap	Efficacy with hard water	Residual activity	Advantages	Disadvantages	Effective against
Acids (acetic acid, citric acid, lactic acid)	Precipitate proteins, disrupt nucleic acid	Specifically used for disinfection in large animal settings and not recommended for general use	Poor/ reduced	ND	ND	Some	Nontoxic, nonirritating at specific concentrations	Hazardous at high concentrations, corrosive, toxic, change environmental pH	G (P), G (N), EV, SNV, Fungi, Spores
Alcohols (ethanol, isopropanol, methanol)	Precipitate proteins, denature lipids and cause cell lysis	Topical antiseptic, hand sanitizers, but limited surface disinfection	Poor/ reduced	ND	ND	No	Fast acting, no residual effect, overall low toxicity	Cause irritation to injured skin, flammable and evaporate rapidly	G (P), G (N), Mycobacteria, EV, LNV, SNV, Fungi, Spores
Aldehydes (formaldehyde, glutaraldehyde, orthophthalaldehyde)	Denature proteins and alkylate nucleic acid	Surface disinfection, fumigant (F), sterilization (G), high-level disinfectant (OPA)	Moderate/ reduced	Reduced	Reduced	ND	Relatively noncorrosive and inexpensive, sporicidal in alkali solution and have broad spectrum activity	Irritating to mucous membranes and tissues, recommended to use in well-ventilated areas, toxic to fish and having carcinogenic risk (F)	G (P), G (N), EV, LNV, SNV, Fungi, Spores
Alkalis (sodium hydroxide, calcium hydroxide, sodium carbonate, ammonium hydroxide)	React with membrane lipids and damage it	Used as environmental disinfectants but not recommended for general use	High (sodium hydroxide) to moderate	ND	ND	ND	Effective against coccidial oocysts (ammonium hydroxide) and prion destruction (sodium hydroxide)	Corrosive to metals, toxic to aquatic life, highly caustic and ammonium hydroxide have intense pungent fumes	G (P), G (N), Mycobacteria, EV, LNV, SNV, Fungi, Spores
Biguanides (chlorhexidine diacetate and gluconate)	Alter cell membrane permeability	Used as topical antiseptic and surface disinfectants	Very poor (rapidly inactivated)	Inactivated	ND	Yes (skin)	Relatively low toxicity, have broad spectrum of activity against bacteria	Functions only in narrow pH range (5–7), limited activity against viruses, toxic to fish (environmental concern) and cause keratitis	G (P), G (N), EV, LNV, SNV, Fungi
Chlorine-releasing agents (sodium hypochlorite, calcium hypochlorite and chlorine dioxide)	Denature proteins	Acts as surface disinfectants and chlorine dioxide functions in fumigation and gas sterilization	Very poor (rapidly inactivated), except chlorine dioxide (moderate activity)	Inactivated	Effective	No	Inexpensive, sporicidal at higher concentration, have broad spectrum of activity and short contact time	Irritating to mucous membranes and skin, reduced activity at high pH and low temperatures, inactivated by sunlight and some metals, corrosive to metals (not stainless steel) and some other materials, discolors fabrics and mixing with acids release toxic chlorine gas	G (P), G (N), Mycobacteria, EV, LNV, SNV, Fungi, Spores

(Continued)

Table 46.1 (Continued)

Category	Mechanism of action	Suitable applications	Efficacy with organic material	Efficacy with detergents/soap	Efficacy with hard water	Residual activity	Advantages	Disadvantages	Effective against
Iodine (iodine solutions and tinctures) and iodophors (povidone iodine, betadine)	Denature proteins and disrupt nucleic acid	Topical antiseptics and acts as surface disinfectants	Very poor (rapidly inactivated)	Effective	ND	Some	Stable in storage, relatively safe to use and have broad spectrum of activity	Corrosive, inactivated by QAC, stains clothes, some surfaces and plastics; have contact sensitivity and frequent application needed	G (P), G (N), Mycobacteria, EV, LNV, SNV, Fungi, Spores
Oxidizing agents (hydrogen peroxide, accelerated hydrogen peroxide, peroxyacetic acid and peroxymonosulfate)	Denature proteins and lipids	Topical antiseptics, acts as surface disinfectants, HP helps in vapor sterilization, PAA in fumigation and PMS in aerosol fumigation	Variable (HP- low, AHP- moderate, PMS and PAA- high)	ND	ND	Yes (hydrogen peroxide)	Fast acting, broad spectrum, considered environmentally friendly, sporicidal	Damaging to metals, concrete, and some other surfaces (PMS and PAA), discolor fabrics and cause eye irritation	G (P), G (N), Mycobacteria, EV, LNV, SNV, Fungi, Spores
Phenolic compounds (2-phenylphenol, benzylphenol, 4-chloro-3,5-dimethylphenol)	Alter cell wall permeability and denature proteins	Acts as surface disinfectants	High (effective)	Effective	Effective	Yes	Noncorrosive, stable in storage, effective over large pH range and have broad spectrum of activity	Irritating to skin and eye, have unpleasant odor, toxic to animals, particularly cats and pigs and not recommended for food surfaces	G (P), G (N), Mycobacteria, EV, LNV, SNV, Fungi
Quaternary ammonium compounds (cetalkonium chloride, cetyl pyridinium chloride, benzalkonium chloride, benzethonium chloride, tetraethylammonium bromide, cetyl trimethylammonium bromide, and domiphen bromide)	Denature proteins, disrupt cell membrane and inactivate enzymes	Surface disinfectants	Poor to moderate, reduced	Inactivated	Inactivated	Some	Generally nonirritating to skin, effective at high temperatures and pH range (9–10), stable in storage and broad spectrum of activity	Reduced activity at pH <3.5 and low temperatures and toxic to fish	G (P), G (N), Mycobacteria, EV, Fungi

G (P), Gram positive; G (N), Gram negative; EV, enveloped viruses; LNV, large nonenveloped viruses; SNV, small nonenveloped viruses; F, formaldehyde; G, glutaraldehyde; HP, hydrogen peroxide; OPA, orthophthalaldehyde; HP, hydrogen peroxide; AHP, accelerated hydrogen peroxide; PAA, peroxyacetic acid; PMS, peroxymonosulfate; ND, not determined.

46.5 Sanitation of Animal-related Items

46.5.1 Bowls, Toys, Litter Boxes, and Animal Handling Products

Items such as bowls, toys, resting platforms, and litter boxes are high-contact surfaces that can readily become contaminated with pathogens. Therefore, these items must be thoroughly cleaned and disinfected regularly. High-quality stainless steel is the preferred material for food and water bowls because it is nonporous and durable and can be easily cleaned and disinfected. However, with the availability of new products with good penetration into porous surfaces (e.g., accelerated hydrogen peroxide), other materials such as plastic may be acceptable even though they are less durable over time.

The items should be cleaned with a detergent to remove all visible debris and then soaked in a disinfectant at the appropriate dilution for the necessary contact time. Articles should be rinsed and allowed to dry completely before reuse. The disinfectant dip should be changed periodically whenever necessary and visibly dirty. Ideally, bowls and toys should be handled in an area separate from litter boxes, and whenever possible they should not be handled in the same sink at the same time. The use of commercial dishwashers or sanitizers is also effective to clean/disinfect these items. All cleaning and disinfecting activities should take place away from areas where human food is handled, consumed or stored. Equipment used for handling animals, such as catch poles, muzzles, and leather gloves, should be sanitized regularly using appropriate disinfectant in proper concentration and contact time.

46.5.2 Laundry

Soiled hospital laundry and animal bedding may be considered a potential source of infection to both staff and patients and may cause cross-contamination of the environment. All reusable linens and bedding that have been contaminated with blood, urine, feces, or any other bodily fluids or exudates must be subjected to a decontamination process (McDonald and Pugliese 1999; Hoffman 2009). During laundering, microbial decontamination is achieved by an interaction between physical removal (such as mechanical action in the wash and rinse cycles), as well as chemical and thermal inactivation during laundering to achieve effective sanitization. Laundry detergents that contain perborate or percarbonate together with a bleach activator release active oxygen in contact with water in a temperature-dependent manner. The primary purpose of including activated oxygen bleach (AOB) in the detergent is to enhance stain removal and chemical inactivation of pathogens.

All workers involved in the collection, transport, sorting or washing of soiled bedding must be appropriately trained and wear required personal protective equipment (PPE), including gloves of a sufficient thickness to minimize sharps injuries, face mask, and eye protection.

When necessary (e.g., when handling bedding or materials suspected of being contaminated with zoonotic pathogens), cover any exposed broken skin or lesions. There should be access to hand-washing facilities. Every effort should be made to eliminate inadvertent harmful objects, such as sharps or instruments. Additionally, animal bedding must be carefully shaken free of all loose debris and fecal matter before processing. All soiled materials should be transported in bins or bags impervious to liquids. Also, clean and dirty laundry must have separate transport and storage facilities.

46.5.3 Transport Carriers

The cleaning and disinfection of transport carriers and vehicles used for animals are of extreme importance in the sanitation plan. This includes removal of fecal materials, dirt, and other organic debris. Application of disinfectant (e.g., potassium peroxymonosulfate or accelerated hydrogen peroxide) with efficacy against nonenveloped viruses and in the presence of organic matter at the proper concentration for the correct contact time is also important. After cleaning, the surface should be thoroughly dried.

46.5.4 Other Equipment

Equipment that is reused by medical staff, such as endotracheal (ET) tubes and breathing circuits, also require a sanitation protocol. Soaking them in either a chlorhexidine gluconate or accelerated hydrogen peroxide solution for at least five minutes or spraying all tube surfaces with accelerated hydrogen peroxide and letting them sit for at least five minutes and then rinsing is an effective method for sanitation of endotracheal tubes (Crawford and Weese 2015). However, chlorhexidine has limited efficacy against nonenveloped viruses (Karsten 2021).

46.6 Personal Sanitation

46.6.1 Hand Sanitation

Hand hygiene is the single most important measure in healthcare settings to help prevent direct or indirect transmission of pathogens between patients, staff, and the environment (Mathur 2011). There are three methods for managing hand hygiene in healthcare settings: washing with soap and water, applying hand sanitizers, and wearing gloves.

46.6.1.1 Hand Washing
Frequent hand washing is recommended, especially after handling animals or their waste, handling garbage, blowing one's nose, sneezing, using the toilet and before handling food (Steneroden 2012). Proper hand washing has a significant advantage over hand sanitizers as it helps to remove even the most resistant pathogens (WHO 2009). For the best hand-washing results, guidance provided by the Centers for Disease Control and Prevention (CDC) is that hands should be wet with warm water, soap applied, and hands rubbed together for at least 20 seconds to create a lather over the entire surface of the hands, between fingers and under nails, rinsed thoroughly under running water, and dried with a clean towel or air-dried (CDC 2015).

46.6.1.2 Hand Sanitizers
Hand sanitizers play an important role but cannot take the place of thorough hand washing with running water and soap. It should be considered as an option for hand sanitation between handling healthy animals. Hand sanitizers do not work effectively if hands are contaminated with visible dirt or organic debris or in the presence of pathogens such as parvovirus, calicivirus, and ringworm. It is recommended that hand sanitizers should contain at least 60% alcohol to kill microorganisms by denaturing proteins and disrupting the cell membrane.

46.6.1.3 Gloves
Wearing gloves can help to prevent disease transmission, provided they are put on, taken off, and changed at the appropriate time interval, i.e., while handling animals that may be infected with environmentally resilient and zoonotic pathogens, or during any outbreak of disease. Before putting on and after removing gloves, hands should always be carefully washed, especially in case of handling an infected animal or contaminated surfaces (Karsten 2021).

46.6.2 Clothing

Clothing plays an important role in disease transmission in both human and veterinary medicine. In veterinary practices, disease transmission through clothing is enhanced by an animal's propensity to shed hair, which may be contaminated with pathogens from a variety of sources, such as dermal, salivary, and environmental. Some pathogens may even cluster around hair follicles, facilitating the spread of diseases such as ringworm and feline calicivirus infection.

One of the most important and reasonably easy infectious disease control procedures in shelters is to provide separate uniforms or clothing for staff to wear when cleaning, disinfecting, and handling diseased and healthy animals. In order to prevent the transmission of disease from the shelter to the home, clothing and shoes worn in the shelter should not be worn at home. It is also recommended that staff should frequently change their clothing or wear protective garments while cleaning and treating sick animals. Scrub tops or protective smocks can be used while interacting with a potentially infectious or high-risk animal (such as juveniles and ringworm-infected animals).

An instrument designed to measure adenosine triphosphate (ATP) levels is used to assess the relative cleanliness of the clothes of animal healthcare workers or caretakers. This instrument is based on the principle that ATP is the energy source in all living cells, so the amount present provides an indirect measurement of the relative quantity of contamination of surfaces by microorganisms.

46.6.3 Footbaths

Footbaths are commonly used as an attempt to provide foot sanitation. However, there are limitations of using footbaths and they should not be relied upon as an adequate means of preventing fomite transmission from contaminated footwear. The common disinfectants used in footbaths and foot mats are bleach, QAC, potassium peroxymonosulfate, and 1% trifectant solutions. In canine and feline parvovirus outbreaks, bleach and trifectant are more effective than QAC.

To be effective, footbath or foot mat solutions must be changed regularly. Frequency of changing the disinfectant will depend on turbidity of solution due to debris, qualities of the disinfectant used, location, and amount of foot traffic. In areas with heavy fecal or organic matter contamination, the soles of footwear must be scrubbed with brushes prior to stepping in the footbath.

Disinfectant footbaths are often kept at insufficient depth and used without prior removal of gross organic matter contamination present on shoes, making the chemicals ineffective. All disinfectants used in footbath solutions require some amount of contact time for an optimal effect, and this will not be achieved merely by brief submersion in a footbath. Therefore, considering the difficulty of maintaining the footbath solution correctly, it may create additional risk in disease transmission and it is not recommended to use them in animal shelter areas. The use of shoe/boot covers or dedicated shoes is recommended in animal shelters where necessary, particularly in areas housing animals under quarantine or undergoing treatment for highly transmissible pathogens such as parvoviruses and *M. canis* (Karsten 2021).

46.7 Sanitation Training

For the shelter sanitation program to be effective, every staff member, including veterinarians, veterinary technicians, shelter staff including directors and managers, kennel staff and volunteers, must receive proper education and training to follow all protocols and guidelines. Staff input should be considered during development of the sanitation plan to ensure that it is realistic for staff to meet the expectations. Most importantly, the sanitation plan must be communicated effectively to all staff and volunteers. Whenever possible, those performing sanitation chores should be encouraged to suggest improvements to increase staff compliance and safety (Petersen et al. 2008).

In addition to discussing the established sanitation plan, its importance and potential hazards, essential training points may also be included for the identification of signs of infectious diseases, their routes of transmission, and the impact of zoonotic diseases in communities. The sanitation plan should be reevaluated periodically to ensure that it is functioning properly. Regular evaluation allows for updates and reinforces the shelter's mission and goals.

Sanitation protocols may appear cumbersome and time-consuming to staff, particularly if they do not have input into the process and do not understand the importance of the specific procedures. Staff should be observed periodically while cleaning to ensure their adherence to protocols and offered opportunities for retraining whenever problems are anticipated or observed.

Failure of a sanitation plan may occur for a variety of reasons, including lack of a realistic plan; failure to update the plan to accommodate new techniques; overcrowding that does not permit staff members sufficient time to clean; shortage of staff; damaged or nonfunctional equipment; wrong product selection; poor shelter design, etc. The involvement of all individuals in development of asanitation plan, regardless of their roles, helps to create an overall infection control culture within the shelter.

46.8 Healthcare-Associated Infections and Environmental Contamination in Veterinary Hospitals

In veterinary medicine, specific numbers and incidence of HAIs are not well documented. However, there is more than enough evidence to indicate that, as in human medicine, HAIs in veterinary hospitals are part of the world in which we live. Although certain issues, the principal pathogens, and thus the control measures may differ, it is nonsensical to imagine that veterinary medicine is any different from human medicine, in that HAIs exist and must be subject to control measures (Traverse and Aceto 2015).

Two studies were carried out to estimate the occurrence of HAIs in clinical settings at veterinary teaching hospitals (VTHs) using the standardized syndromic surveillance (Ruple-Czerniak et al. 2013, 2014). Ruple-Czerniak et al. (2013) reported that among a total of 1535 dogs and 416 cats hospitalized in a critical care unit (CCU), 16.3% (confidence interval [CI] 14.3–18.5) of dogs and 12% (95% CI 9.3–15.5) of cats had at least one nosocomial event. Similarly, among the 297 hospitalized horses admitted for gastrointestinal disorders, 19.7% (95% CI 14.5–26.7) were reported to have at least one nosocomial event (Ruple-Czerniak et al. 2014). In both small animals and horses, the most commonly reported syndrome was surgical site inflammation, with urinary tract inflammation and intravenous catheter site inflammation being the second most common syndromes in small animals and horses, respectively. In addition, in surveys conducted by biosecurity experts at 38 VTHs, 82% hospitals reported the occurrence of a nosocomial disease outbreak in the five years before the survey (Benedict et al. 2008; Scheftel et al. 2010). Although most of these outbreaks were associated with large animal facilities, there are reports of HAIs and outbreaks in small animal clinics also (Greene 2006; Weese and Stull 2013).

Many of the pathogens associated with HAIs in humans are found in VTHs and can cause infections in animals. Due to paucity of data on veterinary HAIs, the relationship of environmental contamination with most of these pathogens to HAIs is not well defined. Nevertheless, as with human medicine, the link between HAIs and the environment of veterinary clinics is becoming clearer. There are numerous descriptions of environmental contamination associated with HAIs in large animal hospitals (Ewart et al. 2001; Burgess et al. 2004; Dunowska et al. 2007; Dallap Schaer et al. 2010; Ekiri et al. 2010; Traverse and Aceto 2015). In addition, documented methicillin-resistant *Staphylococcus aureus* (MRSA) events in veterinary settings showed that environmental contamination ranged from 1% to 12% (Weese et al. 2004; Loeffler et al. 2005; Heller et al. 2009; Hoet et al. 2011) and there are reports of contamination of the environment and equipment in small animal hospitals with enterococci, many of which were multidrug resistant (MDR) (Ghosh et al. 2012; KuKanich et al. 2012).

KuKanich et al. (2012) investigated the hypothesis that cage doors, stethoscopes, thermometers, and mouth gags used in participating hospitals would have bacterial contamination that could contribute to HAIs. This investigation was accomplished by determining the prevalence of surface contamination with enterococci at 10 different veterinary hospitals. Because the locations within the hospitals that were sampled had direct patient contact, it is perhaps not surprising that they all yielded enterococci. To compare cleaning protocols with bacterial contamination, a veterinarian at each hospital was asked to complete a questionnaire. Results showed that only half of the hospitals had written standard operating procedures for hospital cleaning, and the wide variety of disinfectants used precluded examination of any relationship between cleaning and contamination. Moreover, five out of 10 veterinarians surveyed reported almost never cleaning their stethoscopes, and there were also deficiencies in the cleaning of cage doors, thermometers, and mouth gags at some hospitals.

Despite the relative paucity of data, it should be apparent that veterinary hospitals are inherently contaminated and that any number of bacterial, viral, or fungal organisms may be harbored in the hospital environments. The nature of animals and the challenges they pose in terms of hygiene and containment almost guarantee contamination of a space. The range of species that may require hospitalization is large and varied, and each species may have distinct flora and different susceptibility risks.

As our understanding of HAIs in veterinary medicine increases, medical staff and administrators alike are coming to realize the acute threat that HAIs pose to hospitalized veterinary patients and are looking toward proactive preventive measures rather than reactive damage control. The additional financial burden (e.g., increased length of hospital stay, increased treatment costs, possible indemnification and legal costs, loss of future business) that HAIs in general and outbreaks in particular can impose on a hospital is undoubtedly another motivating factor (Kim et al. 2001; Dallap Schaer et al. 2010; Ekiri et al. 2010). The fact that many of the pathogens of importance to the health of hospitalized animals are also zoonotic is an equally important consideration, and all infection control programs should include measures to protect human health (Scheftel et al. 2010). In common with human medicine, it is becoming clear that the hospital environment is an important target of these proactive measures (Traverse and Aceto 2015).

46.9 Conclusion

A well-planned and systematic effort to minimize animal stress, limiting the transmission of disease, and proper training and education of staff members are essential to maintaining shelter sanitation. Designing and implementing a thorough, well thought out shelter sanitation plan helps in the good health, welfare and increased productivity of the animals. Similarly, the standard of care at every veterinary hospital should include a high level of hygiene and sanitation, awareness of the route of transmission of infectious agents between animals and humans, and ways to reduce infection risk wherever possible. Development of well-understood protocols and schedules for cleaning and disinfection, waste disposal, and environmental maintenance is essential for proper sanitation in the animal shelter and hospital environment. Training and education of stakeholders such as veterinarians, veterinary technicians, shelter staff, and volunteers are needed for maintenance of high standards of cleaning and disinfection in these settings.

Acknowledgment

The authors thank Guru Angad Dev Veterinary and Animal Sciences University and Tamil Nadu Veterinary and Animal Sciences University administrations for providing the necessary facilities for undertaking this work.

References

Bello, A., Quinn, M.M., Perry, M.J., and Milton, D.K. (2009). Characterization of occupational exposures to cleaning products used for common cleaning tasks– a pilot study of hospital cleaners. *Environmental Health* 8 (1): 1–11.

Benedict, K.M., Morley, P.S., and Van Metre, D.C. (2008). Characteristics of biosecurity and infection control programs at veterinary teaching hospitals. *Journal of the American Veterinary Medical Association* 233 (5): 767–773.

Burgess, B.A., Morley, P.S., and Hyatt, D.R. (2004). Environmental surveillance for Salmonella enterica in a veterinary teaching hospital. *Journal of the American Veterinary Medical Association* 225 (9): 1344–1348.

Centers for Disease Control (CDC) (2015). When & How to Wash your Hands. www.cdc.gov/handwashing/when-how-handwashing.Html (accessed 26 October 2023).

Coppock, R.W., Mostrom, M.S., and Lillie, L.E. (1988). The toxicology of detergents, bleaches, antiseptics and disinfectants in small animals. *Veterinary and Human Toxicology* 30 (5): 463–473.

Crawford, S. and Weese, J.S. (2015). Efficacy of endotracheal tube disinfection strategies for elimination of Streptococcus zooepidemicus and Bordetella bronchiseptica. *Journal of the American Veterinary Medical Association* 247 (9): 1033–1036.

Dallap Schaer, B.L., Aceto, H., and Rankin, S.C. (2010). Outbreak of salmonellosis caused by Salmonella enterica serovar Newport MDR-AmpC in a large animal veterinary teaching hospital. *Journal of Veterinary Internal Medicine* 24 (5): 1138–1146.

Dinnage, J.D., Scarlett, J.M., and Richards, J.R. (2009). Descriptive epidemiology of feline upper respiratory tract disease in an animal shelter. *Journal of Feline Medicine and Surgery* 11: 816–825.

Dunowska, M.A.G.D.A., Morley, P.S., Traub-Dargatz, J.L. et al. (2007). Comparison of Salmonella enterica serotype Infantis isolates from a veterinary teaching hospital. *Journal of Applied Microbiology* 102 (6): 1527–1536.

Edinboro, C.H., Ward, M.P., and Glickman, L.T. (2004). A placebo-controlled trial of two intranasal vaccines to prevent tracheobronchitis (kennel cough) in dogs entering a humane shelter. *Preventive Veterinary Medicine* 62: 89–99.

Ekiri, A.B., Morton, A.J., Long, M.T. et al. (2010). Review of the epidemiology and infection control aspects of nosocomial Salmonella infections in hospitalised horses. *Equine Veterinary Education* 22 (12): 631–641.

Ewart, S.L., Schott, H.C. II, Robison, R.L. et al. (2001). Identification of sources of Salmonella organisms in a veterinary teaching hospital and evaluation of the effects of disinfectants on detection of Salmonella organisms on surface materials. *Journal of the American Veterinary Medical Association* 218 (7): 1145–1151.

Ghosh, A., KuKanich, K., Brown, C.E., and Zurek, L. (2012). Resident cats in small animal veterinary hospitals carry multi-drug resistant enterococci and are likely involved in cross-contamination of the hospital environment. *Frontiers in Microbiology* 3: 19232.

Greene, C.E. (2006). Environmental factors in infectious disease. In: *Infectious Diseases of the Dog and Cat*, 3e (ed. C.E. Greene), 991–1013. St Louis: Saunders Elsevier.

Greene, C.E. and Decaro, N. (2012). Canine viral enteritis. In: *Infectious Diseases of the Dog and Cat* (ed. C.E. Greene), 67–79. St Louis: Saunders Elsevier.

Grow, A.G. (1995). Writing guidelines to require disinfection. *Revue Scientifique et Technique* 14 (2): 469–477.

Heinemann, C. (2020). Hygiene management in farm animal housing: assessment of hygiene indicators and critical points in sanitation. Doctoral dissertation, Rheinische Friedrich-Wilhelms-Universität, Bonn.

Heller, J., Armstrong, S.K., Girvan, E.K. et al. (2009). Prevalence and distribution of meticillin-resistant Staphylococcus aureus within the environment and staff of a university veterinary clinic. *Journal of Small Animal Practice* 50 (4): 168–173.

Hoet, A.E., Johnson, A., Nava-Hoet, R.C. et al. (2011). Environmental methicillin-resistant Staphylococcus aureus in a veterinary teaching hospital during a nonoutbreak period. *Vector-Borne and Zoonotic Diseases* 11 (6): 609–615.

Hoffman, P. (2009). Laundry, kitchens and healthcare waste. In: *Ayliffe's Control of Healthcare-Associated Infection: A Practical Handbook*, 5e (ed. A.P. Fraise and C. Bradley), 107–149. London: Hodder Arnold.

Hoy, S., Gauly, M., and Krieter, J. (2016). *Nutztierhaltung und – Hygiene*, 2e. Stuttgart: Ulmer.

Hurley, K.F. and Baldwin, C.J. (2012). Prevention and management of infection in canine populations. In: *Infectious Diseases of the Dog and Cat* (ed. C.E. Greene), 1124–1130. St Louis: Saunders Elsevier.

Jeffrey, D.J. (1995). Chemicals used as disinfectants: active ingredients and enhancing additives. *Revue Scientifique et Technique* 14 (1): 57–74.

Kahrs, R.F. (1995). General disinfection guidelines. *Revue Scientifique et Technique* 14 (1): 105–122.

Karsten, C. (2021). Sanitation. In: *Infectious Disease Management in Animal Shelters* (ed. L. Miller, S. Janeczko, and K. Hurley), 166–190. Hoboken: Wiley.

Kim, L.M., Morley, P.S., Traub-Dargatz, J.L. et al. (2001). Factors associated with Salmonella shedding among equine colic patients at a veterinary teaching hospital. *Journal of the American Veterinary Medical Association* 218 (5): 740–748.

KuKanich, K.S., Ghosh, A., Skarbek, J.V. et al. (2012). Surveillance of bacterial contamination in small animal veterinary hospitals with special focus on antimicrobial resistance and virulence traits of enterococci. *Journal of the American Veterinary Medical Association* 240 (4): 437–445.

Loeffler, A., Boag, A.K., Sung, J. et al. (2005). Prevalence of methicillin-resistant Staphylococcus aureus among staff and pets in a small animal referral hospital in the UK. *Journal of Antimicrobial Chemotherapy* 56 (4): 692–697.

Mathur, P. (2011). Hand hygiene: back to the basics of infection control. *Indian Journal of Medical Research* 134 (5): 611–620.

McDonald, L.L. and Pugliese, G. (1999). Textile processing service. In: *Hospital Epidemiology and Infection Control*, 2e (ed. C.G. Mayhall), 1031–1034. Philadelphia: Lippincott Williams & Wilkins.

Morgan-Jones, S. (1987). Practical aspects of disinfection and infection control. In: *Disinfection in Veterinary and Farm Animal Practice* (ed. A.H. Linton, W.B. Hugo, and A.D. Russell), 144–167. Oxford: Blackwell Scientific Publications.

Müller, W., Schlenker, G., and Zucker, B.-A. (2011). *Kompendium der Tierhygiene* (ed. B.-A. Zucker). Berlin.: Lehmanns Media.

Omidbakhsh, N. and Sattar, S.A. (2006). Broad-spectrum microbicidal activity, toxicologic assessment, and materials compatibility of a new generation of accelerated hydrogen peroxide-based environmental surface disinfectant. *American Journal of Infection Control* 34 (5): 251–257.

Pesavento, P.A., Hurley, K.F., Bannasch, M.J. et al. (2008). A clonal outbreak of acute fatal hemorrhagic pneumonia in intensively housed (shelter) dogs caused by Streptococcus equi subsp. zooepidemicus. *Veterinary Pathology* 45 (1): 51–53.

Petersen, C., Dvorak, G., and Spickler, A. (ed.) (2008). *Maddie's Infection Control Manual for Animal Shelters*. Ames: Center for Food Security and Public Health.

Ruple-Czerniak, A., Aceto, H.W., Bender, J.B. et al. (2013). Using syndromic surveillance to estimate baseline rates for healthcare-associated infections in critical care units of small animal referral hospitals. *Journal of Veterinary Internal Medicine* 27 (6): 1392–1399.

Ruple-Czerniak, A.A., Aceto, H.W., Bender, J.B. et al. (2014). Syndromic surveillance for evaluating the occurrence of healthcare-associated infections in equine hospitals. *Equine Veterinary Journal* 46 (4): 435–440.

Russell, A.D. and Hugo, W.B. (1987). Chemical disinfectants. In: *Disinfection in Veterinary and Farm Animal Practice* (ed. A.H. Linton, W.B. Hugo, and A.D. Russell), 12–42. Oxford: Blackwell Scientific Publications.

Rutala, W.A., Cole, E.C., Thomann, C.A., and Weber, D.J. (1998). Stability and bactericidal activity of chlorine solutions. *Infection Control & Hospital Epidemiology* 19 (5): 323–327.

Scheftel, J.M., Elchos, B.L., Cherry, B. et al. (2010). Compendium of veterinary standard precautions for zoonotic disease prevention in veterinary personnel: National Association of State Public Health Veterinarians Veterinary Infection Control Committee 2010. *Journal of the American Veterinary Medical Association* 237 (12): 1403–1422.

Steneroden, K. (2012). Sanitation. In: *Shelter Medicine for Veterinarians and Staff* (ed. L. Miller and S. Zawistowski), 37–47. Hoboken: Wiley.

Thielen, M.J.M. (2000). Animal hygiene: the key to healthy animal production in an optimal environment. *Proceedings of the Xth International Congress on Animal Hygiene, Maastricht*.

Traverse, M. and Aceto, H. (2015). Environmental cleaning and disinfection. *Veterinary Clinics of North America: Small Animal Practice* 45 (2): 299–330.

Weese, J.S. and Stull, J. (2013). Respiratory disease outbreak in a veterinary hospital associated with canine parainfluenza virus infection. *Canadian Veterinary Journal* 54 (1): 79–82.

Weese, J.S., DaCosta, T., Button, L. et al. (2004). Isolation of methicillin-resistant Staphylococcus aureus from the environment in a veterinary teaching hospital. *Journal of Veterinary Internal Medicine* 18 (4): 468–470.

World Health Organization (WHO) (2009). *Guidelines on Hand Hygiene in Health Care*. Geneva: World Health Organization.

47

Management of Stray, Fallen Animals and Carcass Disposal

Poornima Gumasta, Narendra Kumar, Mahmuda Malik, and Diptimayee Sahoo

College of Veterinary and Animal Sciences, Bihar Animal Sciences University, Patna, Bihar, India

47.1 Introduction

Poultry, cattle farming including stray animals inevitably results in mortality. Animals in India, where there is a sizable population of animals perish from various diseases, mishaps, and natural calamities (Blake 2004). Deaths are typically dumped into rivers, farms, and roadways, which results in a variety of threats to the environment. In order to maximize the effectiveness of reaction, strategies for disposing of carcasses, especially on a larger scale, require preparation well in advance of a disaster. The best disposal or carcass management plans will be those that take full advantage of all appropriate and accessible disposal choices, no matter what those options may be. The disposal technique must to be low-cost, feasible, safe, and make use of mortality rates – a crucial component of biosecurity (Ahuja, 2011).

It is imperative that decision-makers gain a thorough understanding of all the disposal technologies at their disposal in order to arm themselves with an extensive knowledge base. This kind of awareness entails knowing a wide range of information about each technology, such as its working principles, logistical requirements, manpower needs, expected costs, environmental factors, disease agent considerations, benefits and drawbacks, and lessons learned.

Traditionally, animal carcasses are disposed of by burning, incinerating, rendering, composting, or burial. However, the employment of these conventional technologies on a broader scale has been largely prohibited due to the installation of many environmental and social rules (Pollard et al., 2008). Every one of these approaches has certain drawbacks. The act of burying deceased birds in a pit may contaminate groundwater. In addition to being costly, incineration may contaminate the air. Transportation costs and limitations on the movement of infected birds from one place to another limit the amount of deceased birds that can be rendered into by-product meal. Land availability and restrictions on the transit of infected carcasses affect land filling. In general, these various approaches have additional drawbacks such as labor intensity, cost, pollution of the environment, and offensive odor. Innovative and non-traditional disposal techniques are a solid choice for environmentally responsible mortality disposal.

In the following chapter the traditional carcass disposal methods will be discussed with different biosecurity, environmental and economic issues related to them (Figure 47.1).

47.1.1 Burial

It involves disposing of the carcass in trenches, graves, or mortality pits – open-bottomed containers. Because of the introduction of infectious pathogens into the human food chain and environmental contamination, this approach is prohibited in the majority of developed countries. Mass burial in various tragedies may result in the introduction of diseases and chemical breakdown products into surface and ground water. The most critical variables affecting how long it takes for animal carcasses to decompose in the ground are temperature, moisture content, and burial depth. Other variables include soil type and drainability, animal species and size, humidity and dryness, rainfall, and other variables. Compared to the burial of ordinary mortalities, mass burial of carcass presents noticeably higher dangers to the environment and biosecurity. The concentrations of *E. coli* and cryptosporidium in surface and ground water were greater because fewer carcasses

---

Epidemiology and Environmental Hygiene in Veterinary Public Health, First Edition. Edited by Tanmoy Rana.
© 2025 John Wiley & Sons, Inc. Published 2025 by John Wiley & Sons, Inc.

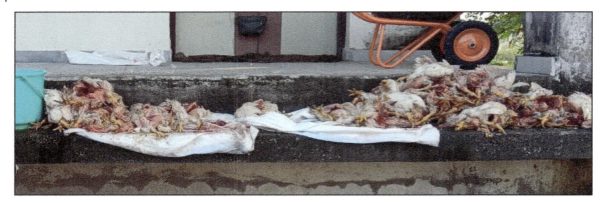

Figure 47.1 Dead poultry carcasses, waiting for disposal.

were buried than because of animal waste. Variations in soil type, permeability, water table depth, and rainfall all have a major impact on the viruses' ability to travel from disposed of carcasses through soil to groundwater.

There are no studies in the literature that relate the burial of animal carcasses to harmful effects on the health of humans or animals; nevertheless, there have been cases of contaminated groundwater when humans have been buried near a water table. Thirteen the effective reduction of pathogen survival has been achieved with the use of hydrated lime (Ca(OH)2) in burial. In contaminated abattoir waste treated with lime at a rate of 10 g of CaO lime per kg of trash, Avery et al. (2015) discovered no viable *E. coli* cells. Overuse of lime can hinder the growth of all microorganisms and hence slow down the decomposition process, both in the building and maintenance stages of burial sites.

Even while the burial of carcasses seldom results in the contamination of drinking water, the decomposition of the carcasses leaves behind some infectious material, such as prions or anthrax spores, in the soil. This could result in animals consuming contaminated soil and infectious agents, which could then cause the return of anthrax or the development of neurological diseases (such Bovine spongiform encephalopathy (BSE) or scrapie in the case of prions). In order to reduce the likelihood of infectious pathogens returning to the surface, burial sites should be placed far from animal farms and human locality (Johnson et al., 2007).

47.1.2 Burning

The practice of burning farm carcasses on pyres is widespread, especially in underdeveloped nations. There have been reports of carcasses being burned during disease outbreaks like Foot and mouth disease (FMD) and anthrax. The evidence of soil contamination from pyres, groundwater contamination from ash burial, and air emissions from pyres did not substantially impact the environment outside of the immediate neighborhood, despite the possibility that pollution could result from the mass burning of carcasses (Sharp and Roberts, 2006). Studies reveal that it was extremely unlikely for the FMD virus to spread through burning smoke plumes.

Since open-air combustion is unlikely to achieve a high enough temperature for incineration, biosecurity risks resulting from transmissible spongiform encephalitis (TSE) during burning persist. It is extremely unlikely that TSEs from animal carcass could be transferred by air or ground ash, according to Brown et al. (2004). When enough work, air, and fuel are available, the carcass will completely burn for a safe disposal. Aside from direct smoke inhalation and physical burns, incomplete combustion of carcasses releases dioxins, which pose a concern to human health. Dioxins and furans are known carcinogens that have detrimental effects on human development, reproduction, and immune systems. Despite the fact that burning has been demonstrated to have no effect on the environment, there have been significant social concerns raised about odor, unsightliness, etc. Since there isn't much data to support or disprove the practice of burning carcasses on farms, further research is needed to validate popular theories such elevated dioxin levels and groundwater contamination (Vinten et al., 2008).

47.1.3 Incineration

Burning animal carcass to inorganic ash at temperatures above 8500° C is known as incineration. All infectious agents are eliminated by the treatment. Only 1–5% of the initial carcass volume is made up of ash, though this will vary depending on the kind of incinerator, the procedure, the fuel, and the kind of animal. Ash originating from specified risk material (SRM) – such as the brain and spinal cord – is then transported to approved landfill sites in developed nations like the United States and the European Union. The main issue with burning dead bodies is the gaseous emissions, which account for 60.2% of all air emissions.

Adopting best practices, such as using afterburners, has greatly reduced the amount of dangerous gases, such as polycyclic aromatic hydrocarbons. Additional health risks associated with incineration include the production of dioxins and furans, which are produced by incomplete combustion, can settle in the vicinity of carcass incinerators and may enter the food chain through human eating of contaminated carcass or grazing animals. On the other hand, incinerators equipped with afterburners can significantly lower the possibility of emitting harmful emissions. It is widely acknowledged that, except from alkaline hydrolysis, burning kills prion proteins more efficiently than other techniques for getting rid of animals.

Regarding the health of humans and animals, the high temperature of incineration also totally eliminates animal and zoonotic infections, including hardy spore-forming bacteria like *Bacillus anthracis* (anthrax). Transportation of dead livestock between farms is one of the main perceived risks associated with off-farm incineration; vehicles may travel considerable distances between farms while carrying the carcasses of diseased animals, which has caused the livestock industry to express serious concerns. By using appropriate biosecurity procedures, such as cleaning collecting vehicles and wearing protective gear in between sites, as well as by using sealed containers that are inaccessible to cattle and rodents and through which fluids cannot escape, these dangers can be decreased. It is evident that additional research is required to assess the dangers of disease transmission through the movement of carcass within and across farms (Baba et al., 2017).

47.1.4 Rendering

In order to produce usable goods like meat and bone meals and tallow, rendering involves crushing carcass into small, homogeneous pieces, heating the particles, and removing the fat, proteinaceous material, and water. One excellent source of organic materials is livestock mortality (Avery et al., 2009). About 32% of a fresh carcass is made up of dry matter, of which 41% is fat, 52% is protein, and 6% is ash. Safe and valuable final products are produced when rendering processes run smoothly. The heat treatment used in rendering procedures lengthens the shelf life of final goods by eliminating raw material-borne germs and eliminating moisture, which is necessary for microbial activity.

Because the infection persists after the carcass is heated, rendering practices are discouraged in TSE and prion-infected cases. Rendering tallow is used as a lipid in the chemical industry, in soaps, and in cosmetics. Its high fat content allows it to be burned to produce energy, lowering the process's overall environmental impact. The primary environmental issues related to rendering are the emissions of petrol and odors. Ninety percent of smells in rendering can be eliminated by employing scrubbers, afterburners, and biofilters along with cold water washing. In order to avoid releasing wastewater into water bodies that have a high biological and chemical oxygen demand, rendering factories must restrict the discharge of certain effluents, such as oils, greases, and suspended particulates. Efficient wastewater filtering, reuse, and usage, as well as more thorough wastewater treatment at sewage treatment plants on- or off-site, can lower the risk of pollution (Casagrande, 2002).

According to NABC9, rendering effectively eliminates the majority of germs, however handling, storing, and shipping the finished product can re-contaminate it, especially with Salmonella. For those who have access to a central collecting service, it still represents a well-established method of disposing of cattle, even though the biosecurity concerns around the collection and transportation of carcasses for rendering still exist. There is a growing shortage of commercial rendering facilities as a result of industry-wide economic pressures. Farmers have historically been compensated for the deaths of their animals, but in many regions of the world, the method has not been able to eradicate TSEs, which has resulted in a decline in marketable goods. Rendering, however, remains and is probably going to remain the best option for handling mortalities; ideally, it will be used in conjunction with incineration and a pathogen surveillance programme.

47.1.5 Composting

In the composting process, carcasses are layered between layers of carbon-rich substrate, such as sawdust, straw, or rice husks, and then the entire pile is covered with a final layer of carbon-rich substrate (Sivakumar et al., 2007). Poultry, wild birds and other avian can be layered, but larger carcasses are usually arranged in single layers; the compost piles are then stirred or aerated. The waste material may break down into a valuable product that can be used as a soil amendment at rates as high as 1–2 kg/day, depending on the carcass weights. The process basically happens in two stages: a primary phase that is thermophilic (generating temperatures as high as 70 °C for several weeks) and a secondary phase that is mesophilic (usually generating temperatures between 30 and 40 °C for several months). Small-scale composting of mortalities has been demonstrated to contaminate the surrounding soil when an impermeable substrate is not employed. This is because the compost piles lose high-ionic-strength leachate, especially during periods of significant rainfall.

Composting facilities shouldn't be situated next to livestock production facilities from a biosecurity standpoint, and all operating vehicles should be thoroughly cleaned and disinfected before every trip. The location should have a limited or attractive view for nearby residents or passing cars, be downwind from residential areas, and perhaps have a nice look and landscaping. According to McGahan (2002) runoff from a compost pile of carcasses may contain organic substances that could deteriorate the quality of adjacent surface or ground water. All runoff from the composting plant needs to be gathered and processed via a filtering area or filter strip in order to prevent this. In the same drainage area, the compost facility should be situated at least 300 ft (90 m) away from streams, ponds or lakes, and at least 3 ft (1 m) above the high water table level.

Composting should be done on an impermeable basis (such as a hard surface or plastic liner) with a bulking agent (such as sawdust) used to absorb surplus liquids produced by the decomposing carcasses in order to reduce the danger of pollution (i.e., leaching and runoff). By conducting the composting process indoors or beneath gas-permeable covers to stop rainwater from getting into the compost piles, the risk can be further decreased. In addition to stopping runoff and nutrient leaching, this precaution should lower ammonia emissions. When compared to manure-related facilities, the odor levels from composting carcasses are thought to be lower in terms of gaseous emissions. It has been demonstrated that the temperatures produced during the thermophilic phase of carcass composting efficiently lower the populations of helminthes, viruses, bacteria, and protozoa. But as the composting process approaches its conclusion, certain bacteria, like Salmonella, might re-colonize the material if the pile has not been sufficiently rotated or aerated, or if temperatures drop. If insufficient temperatures are obtained, it is also possible that opportunistic pathogens will colonize the compost pile.

According to Schwarz et al. (2008) after a year, the number of bacterial indicator species in deer carcass composting was almost completely eliminated. However, they advise exercising caution and using the compost in places where there is little to no human contact, like road verges, to further reduce any risks. Research indicates that the avian influenza virus can be rendered inactive within a week at room temperature (15–20 °C) or in about 15 minutes when combined with chicken manure at 56 °C – temperatures that are easily attained in composting piles (Guan et al., 2009). Furthermore, composting quickly gets rid of the viruses that cause Newcastle According to Glanville et al. (2006) compost piles carrying vaccine strains of the Newcastle Disease virus and avian encephalomyelitis could not infect sentinel birds if a 45–60 cm layer of clean material was placed over cattle carcasses.

Regarding the fate of spore-forming bacteria like *Bacillus anthracis* or prions during carcass composting, not much is known. In their investigation with scrapie-infected lambs, Huang et al. (2007) did discover some initially encouraging data, with prion removal in one experiment and prion decrease (but not elimination) in the second. A pathogen monitoring programme, a maximum mass of carcasses to be disposed of, stringent regulations to restrict subsequent land spreading to specific soil types, and good composting practices (e.g. using clean and fresh carbon substrate) would all work together to further reduce perceived risks. Geographic information systems and groundwater vulnerability maps can be used to locate ideal composting sites.

47.1.6 Economic Aspects of Disposing of Carcass

A comprehensive and multifaceted approach is required to organize the disposal of animal deaths. Disposing of a lot of animal carcasses in an economical, socially and environmentally responsible way is a crucial component of that plan. Planning needs to take into account both the financial implications and the resources available for corpse disposal. To find the optimal option, a thorough cost-benefit analysis of several disposal strategies for distinct scenarios is required.

It's also necessary to identify the main economic aspects and their ramifications and to evaluate and contrast the various disposal solutions. It is also necessary to assess and quantify the effects on the environment, land values, public opinion, and general economic issues. Economics should be considered while making decisions, but it cannot and should not be the only consideration. The state authorities may view the most cost-effective disposal technique as unsound if economically appealing methods fail to meet regulatory standards. It is advisable to bargain in advance with technology providers to reduce the costs associated with various disposals. The ultimate goal is to improve the process of decision-making on the large-scale disposal of carcasses. The scientific community should conduct more research on each disposal technology so that companies and the government may better prepare for any large-scale carcass disposal event.

47.2 Conclusion

While there are a variety of conventional ways for disposing of carcass, such as landfilling, rendering, incineration, and burial, each has drawbacks. Ground water pollution results from the burial of carcasses; air pollution and higher capital costs are associated with incineration. Transportation costs are related to carcass rendering. The mobility of carcasses and the availability of land are limitations for landfilling. There are also other drawbacks, such as the spread of diseases like TSE and prions, which are not entirely eliminated by many of these techniques, which limits their applicability in the evolving legal landscape.

Due to various regulatory requirements that farmers must meet, there has been significant non-compliance, which may have increased the danger of environmental contamination from unlawful dumping and other activities. Farmers prefer to dispose of mortalities on-site due to the advantages it offers in terms of biosecurity, economy, practicality, and the environment. Because of the potential benefits of their final products, processes like rendering and compositing have become more and more popular worldwide. It is imperative that new techniques for disposing of carcasses be developed and approved in accordance with various laws. Systems for disposing of dead bodies must be grounded in a practical strategy in order to be secure from the perspectives of biosecurity and the environment. Future research should focus on a few areas, including the usage of end products and the extraction of precious materials. The economic effects of disposal systems also require more investigation in order to determine their applicability both on and off farms. Therefore, both large and small size animal farms and processing units would profit from the development of a technically and economically effective technology for this purpose. In this sense, a crucial waste management tool for maintaining a lucrative and healthy livestock farming operation is the early disposal of animal carcasses using an effective technique.

References

Ahuja, S.M. (2011). Cost effective solution for carcass disposal in India. *International Journal of Environmental Sciences* 1 (6): 1–6.

Avery, L.M., Williams, A.P., Killham, K. et al. (2009). Heat and lime-treatment as effective control methods for *E coli* (O157:H7) in organic wastes. *Bioresource Technology* 100 (10): 2692–2698.

Baba, I.A., Banday, M.T., Khan, A.A. et al. (2017). Traditional methods of carcass disposal: a review. *Journal of Dairy, Veterinary and Animal Research* 5 (1): 21–27.

Blake, J.P. (2004). Methods and technologies for handling mortality losses. *World Poultry Science Journal.* 60 (4): 489–499.

Brown, P., Rau, E.H., Lemieux, P. et al. (2004). Infectivity studies of both ash and air emissions from simulated incineration of scrapie-contaminated tissues. *Environmental Science and Technology* 38: 6155–6160.

Casagrande, R. (2002). Biological warfare targeted at livestock. *BioScience* 52 (7): 577–581.

Glanville, T.D., Richard, T.L., Harmon, J.D. et al. (2006). *Environmental Impacts and Biosecurity and Composting for Emergency Disposal of Livestock Mortalities.* USA: Iowa State University.

Guan, J., Chan, M., Grenier, C. et al. (2009). Survival of avian influenza and Newcastle disease viruses in compost and at ambient temperatures based on virus isolation and real-time reverse transcriptase PCR. *Avian Diseases* 53 (1): 26–33.

Huang, H., Spencer, J.L., Soutyrine, A. et al. (2007). Evidence for degradation of abnormal prion protein in tissues from sheep with scrapie during composting. *Canadian Journal of Veterinary Research* 71 (1): 34–40.

Johnson, C.J., Pedersen, J.A., Chappell, R.J. et al. (2007). Oral transmissibility of prion disease is enhanced by binding to soil particles. *PLoS Pathogens* 3 (7): e93.

Mc Gahan, E. (2002). *Pig Carcass Composting.* Australia: Queensland Government Department of Primary Industries.

Pollard, S.J.T., Hickman, G.A.W., Irving, P. et al. (2008). Exposure assessment of carcass disposal options in the event of a notifiable exotic animal disease: application to avian influenza virus. *Environmental Science and Technology* 42 (9): 3145–3154.

Schwarz, M., Harrison, E., and Bonhotal, J. (2008). *Pathogen Analysis of NYSDOT Road Killed Deer Carcass Compost Facilities; Temperature and Pathogen Final Report.* USA: Cornell Waste Management Institute/Cornell University.

Sharp, R.J. and Roberts, A.G. (2006). Anthrax: the challenges for decontamination. *Journal of Chemical Technology and Biotechnology* 81 (10): 1612–1625.

Sivakumar, K., Kumar, R.S.V., and Mohamed, A.M. (2007). Composting of poultry carcass with farm yard manure in summer. *Research Journal of Agriculture and Biological Sciences* 3 (5): 356–361.

Vinten, A., Smith, H., Watson, C. et al. (2008). *Assessment of Risks of Water Contamination with E coli, Salmonella and Cryptosporidium from Burial of Animal Carcasses Using Artificially Drained Field Burial Plots.* UK: Macaulay Institute.

48

Vector and Reservoir Control in Veterinary Public Health

Jitendrakumar Nayak[1], Santanu Pal[2], Pranav Anjaria[1], and Varun Asediya[3]

[1] *College of Veterinary Science and Animal Husbandry, Kamdhenu University, Anand, India*
[2] *ICAR-Indian Veterinary Research Institute, Izatnagar, Bareilly, India*
[3] *M. B. Veterinary College, Dungarpur, India*

48.1 Introduction

In India, livestock plays a vital role in farming as approximately 65–70% of the human population relies on agriculture and related sectors, particularly animal husbandry, creating a greater risk of transmission of zoonotic diseases from animals to humans (Kulkarni and Reddi 2018). The recognition of emerging infectious diseases increased in the late 1980s following the occurrence of significant outbreaks worldwide, such as the Hantaan virus in the United States (Löscher and Prüfer-Krämer 2009). Subsequently, multiple emerging diseases have been reported in various countries, posing significant risks to human health and potential economic impacts, including severe acute respiratory syndrome (SARS), bovine spongiform encephalopathy (BSE), avian influenza, and Nipah virus (McMichael and Weiss 2004). The increase in zoonotic diseases, whether new or existing, can be attributed to several key factors, including expansion and shift in populations, behavior pattern variations, urbanization, overcrowding, ecological and environmental changes, the rise of novel microbial strains, and insufficiency of public health support (Rahman et al. 2020).

Vector-borne zoonotic diseases have become the predominant emerging diseases worldwide affecting both humans and animals, caused by viruses, bacteria, and parasites (WHO 2012). As per the WHO's brief on vector-borne diseases in 2014, it is estimated that these diseases account for one-sixth of the global burden of illness and disability, with currently over half of the world's population at risk of developing them. Additionally, over 1 billion global cases of vector-borne diseases are reported annually, causing approximately 1 million deaths (Gubler 2009).

Vectors, such as mosquitoes, ticks, fleas, and flies, can carry and transmit various pathogens, while reservoirs, comprising various domestic and wild animals and birds, harbor and propagate these pathogens. The close interaction between humans and animals and with their surroundings, particularly in developing countries, poses a great risk of development of zoonotic diseases (Rahman et al. 2020). The key determinants influencing the emergence of vector-borne diseases include climate change, urbanization, global travel, resistance to control measures, and pathogen evolution (Chala and Hamde 2021). Additionally, the role of socioeconomic factors and migration in facilitating disease transmission is examined. The impact of vector-borne diseases is most severe on the vulnerable segments of urban, periurban, and rural communities living in poor conditions, specifically with limited access to adequate housing, safe drinking water, and proper sanitation (WHO 2014). Understanding these factors is crucial in formulating effective prevention and control strategies, which necessitate collaboration between public health authorities, environmental agencies, and local communities.

There are no vaccines available for many vector-borne illnesses, and drug resistance is a growing hazard to public health. Therefore, in the field of veterinary public health, effective control strategies for vectors and reservoirs are crucial to mitigate transmission and prevent outbreaks of these diseases and safeguard the well-being of both animal populations and human communities (Upadhyay et al. 2018).

Traditionally, vector control strategies have aimed at eliminating mosquitoes using various insecticides. Environmental management, involving the reduction or elimination of mosquito breeding sites, has frequently been employed along with chemical or biological ovicides, larvicides, and pupicides (Benelli 2015). The use of synthetic insecticides leads to the

---

Epidemiology and Environmental Hygiene in Veterinary Public Health, First Edition. Edited by Tanmoy Rana.
© 2025 John Wiley & Sons, Inc. Published 2025 by John Wiley & Sons, Inc.

48 Vector and Reservoir Control in Veterinary Public Health

development of insecticide resistance and concerns about environmental damage and effects on nontarget organisms. Due to widespread insecticide resistance in numerous mosquito species, there is an increasing demand for innovative, cost-effective, and dependable mosquito control strategies (Ranson and Lissenden 2016). Efforts have been made to explore environmentally friendly alternatives, aiming to alleviate the selection pressure for insecticide resistance. The diverse bio-control strategies include the use of parasitoids, predators, and pathogens which target various stages of the mosquito lifecycle, aiming to be environmentally safe and sustainable (Benelli et al. 2016).

Recently, genetic control strategies have emerged as promising approaches for managing vector-borne diseases by targeting populations of disease-transmitting vectors. Advances in genetic technologies and their potential impact on vector population dynamics include the use of genetically modified vectors, gene drives, and *Wolbachia*-based approaches (Wang et al. 2021). While these innovative approaches hold great promise for mitigating vector-borne diseases, their successful implementation hinges on collaborative efforts among scientists, policy makers, and affected communities.

Prevention and control of vector-borne diseases continue to be challenging in public health endeavors worldwide. The multifaceted challenges encountered in combating vector-borne diseases include the emergence of insecticide resistance, climate change impacting vector distribution, and the complexities of integrated vector management. There are limitations to current preventive measures, such as bed nets and vaccines, along with the need for research and development of novel interventions. Additionally, the role of community engagement, health system strengthening, and international cooperation in addressing these challenges is crucial. Effective control of vector-borne diseases demands a comprehensive and adaptive approach, integrating innovative technologies and collaborative efforts, to protect communities from these persistent threats and achieve sustainable health outcomes.

48.2 Overview of Vector-borne Diseases

Vector-borne diseases are a group of infectious illnesses caused by various pathogens, including bacteria, viruses, and parasites, that are transmitted from one host to another through the bites of vector organisms. Vectors are living carriers, often arthropods such as mosquitoes, ticks, fleas, and flies, that act as intermediaries between infected and susceptible hosts. These diseases are a significant global health concern, affecting millions of people and animals every year (WHO 2014). Understanding the overview of vector-borne diseases is essential for effective prevention, control, and public health measures.

Vector-borne diseases occur in various parts of the world, with prevalence influenced by factors such as climate, geography, socioeconomic conditions, and public health infrastructure (Lemon et al. 2008). Many vector-borne diseases are more prevalent in tropical and subtropical regions due to the abundance of suitable vectors and hosts. These diseases can cause a wide range of symptoms, from mild to severe, and can lead to significant morbidity and mortality. Some vector-borne diseases are particularly dangerous, with high fatality rates if left untreated. They can affect people of all ages and demographics but vulnerable populations, such as children, pregnant women, and the elderly, are often at a higher risk of severe outcomes.

The transmission of vector-borne diseases often exhibits seasonal patterns, with higher incidence during specific times of the year when vector populations are more active. For instance, mosquito-borne diseases may peak during the rainy season when mosquito breeding sites proliferate. Climate change can impact the distribution and transmission patterns of vector-borne diseases. Rising temperatures and altered rainfall patterns can expand the geographic range of certain vectors and pathogens, potentially exposing new populations to these diseases (Campbell-Lendrum et al. 2015). New vector-borne diseases can emerge due to changes in human behavior, urbanization, deforestation, and international travel. Additionally, some diseases that were previously under control have resurfaced due to factors such as insecticide resistance, weakened public health infrastructure, and environmental changes.

Some of the diseases are briefly discussed below to enhance understanding of their vectors, host range, epidemiology, and geographical distribution patterns (Table 48.1).

48.2.1 Leishmaniasis

Leishmaniasis, also known as "dom-dom fever," is a protozoan disease of significant medical and veterinary importance which is transmitted to susceptible hosts through infected female *Phlebotomus* sand flies (Dantas-Torres 2006, 2007). Visceral leishmaniasis exhibits a wide prevalence, extending across tropical and subtropical regions in Africa, Asia, the Mediterranean, and South and Central America (Samad 2011). Zoonotic visceral leishmaniasis (ZVL) is a growing public

Table 48.1 Significant threats of pathogen introduction include spread to new regions and extensions within endemic areas – probable sources and pathways.

Vector-borne diseases	High-risk areas	Endemic zones	Routes of entry
Japanese encephalitis virus	Americas	Asia	Infected livestock
Rift Valley fever virus	Americas, southern Europe	Africa, Asia	Infected livestock
Venezuelan equine encephalitis virus	Europe, Asia, Africa	America	Infected livestock
Chikungunya virus	Europe, America, Australia	Africa, Asia	Infected people
Zika virus	Europe, America	Africa, Asia	Infected people
Crimean-Congo hemorrhagic fever	North Africa, east Asia, central and western Europe	Africa, Asia, and Europe	Infected livestock
Dengue virus	Southern Europe	Southern hemisphere	Infected people
West Nile virus	Central Europe, Turkey	Africa, Asia, Europe, and Australia	Migratory or dispersing birds

Source: Kilpatrick and Randolph (2012).

health concern primarily due to demographic and ecological factors. Rodents, wild canids, ruminants, and several other unidentified carrier animals have the potential to transmit the disease, making it essential to consistently monitor the incidence and carrier status of leishmaniasis.

48.2.2 Malaria and Dengue Fever

Malaria is another significant zoonotic vector-borne parasitic disease transmitted by infected female *Anopheles* mosquitoes that primarily bite mammalian hosts between sunset and sunrise. Over 60 species of anophelines are identified globally as biological vectors of malaria (WHO 2010). Dengue is the most widely spreading viral disease transmitted by mosquitoes worldwide. *Aedes aegypti*, the primary vector for dengue, is known for its preference to bite during the daytime. Over the past five decades, the incidence of dengue has surged significantly, with a 30-fold increase. The disease has expanded its geographic reach, affecting new countries, from urban to rural areas. Presently, over 2.5 billion people worldwide are at risk of dengue infection (Mukhtar 2013).

48.2.3 Japanese Encephalitis

Japanese encephalitis (JE) is a severe viral zoonotic disease transmitted by *Culex* and *Anopheles* mosquitoes with the potential for epidemics and a high mortality rate. It is the predominant cause of viral encephalitis in children worldwide, leading to approximately 50 000 cases and 10 000 deaths annually (Solomon et al. 2003). Pigs (amplifying host) and birds as the primary reservoirs for the disease can carry a high virus titer to mosquitoes. Then mosquitoes act as vectors, transmitting the disease from these reservoirs to humans and cattle.

48.3 Factors Influencing the Emergence of Vector-Borne Diseases

The emergence of vector-borne diseases is influenced by a complex interplay of various factors, involving a combination of environmental, socioeconomic, and human factors (Figure 48.1). Addressing these factors requires a multifaceted approach, including research, surveillance, public health interventions, and international collaboration to effectively prevent and control the spread of vector-borne diseases.

Some of the key factors influencing the emergence of vector-borne diseases include the following.

- *Climate change*: changes in climate patterns can significantly impact the distribution and abundance of vectors and the pathogens they carry. Rising temperatures, altered precipitation patterns, and changes in humidity can create more favorable conditions for vectors to breed and thrive, expanding their geographic range into new areas. This can lead to the introduction of vector-borne diseases to populations that were previously unaffected.

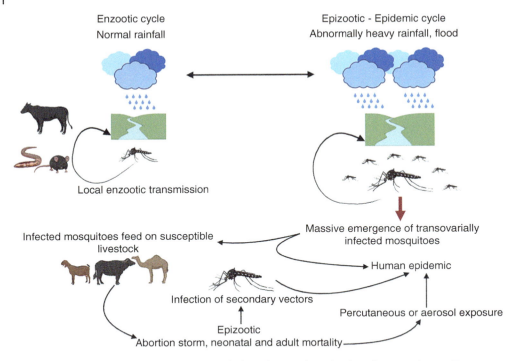

Figure 48.1 Factors influencing the transmission of enzootic and epizootic vector-borne diseases.

- *Urbanization and deforestation*: rapid urbanization and deforestation can disrupt natural ecosystems and force vectors and reservoir hosts into closer contact with humans. As urban areas expand, suitable habitats for vectors may increase, leading to a higher risk of disease transmission to urban populations.
- *Global travel and trade*: increased international travel and trade facilitate the movement of vectors and infected individuals, allowing pathogens to be introduced to new regions. Infected individuals traveling to areas with susceptible populations can trigger outbreaks of vector-borne diseases.
- *Vector control challenges*: the development of insecticide resistance in vectors and the difficulty in implementing effective vector control measures can contribute to the resurgence of vector-borne diseases. Inadequate resources and infrastructure for vector control in some regions can further exacerbate the problem.
- *Pathogen evolution*: vector-borne pathogens have the potential to evolve and adapt to changing environments and hosts. Genetic mutations in the pathogen may lead to new strains that are more virulent or have altered transmission patterns, making them more difficult to control.
- *Socioeconomic factors*: socioeconomic factors, such as poverty, limited access to healthcare, and inadequate sanitation, can increase the vulnerability of populations to vector-borne diseases. Impoverished communities may lack the resources to protect themselves from vectors or seek timely medical care, leading to a higher incidence of infections and more severe disease outcomes.
- *Ecological changes*: human-induced ecological changes, such as irrigation projects, land-use changes, and dam construction, can create new breeding sites for vectors or alter the dynamics between vectors and their reservoir hosts, potentially leading to disease emergence.
- *Zoonotic reservoirs*: many vector-borne diseases are zoonotic, meaning they can be transmitted between animals and humans. Changes in the behavior or distribution of reservoir hosts can influence the prevalence and spread of these diseases.
- *Public health infrastructure*: the effectiveness of surveillance, diagnosis, and response to vector-borne diseases is influenced by the strength of a country's public health infrastructure. Strong surveillance systems and early detection can help contain outbreaks and prevent further spread.
- *Human behavior*: human behavior, such as outdoor activities, outdoor sleeping habits, and water storage practices, can affect exposure to vectors and the risk of infection.

48.4 The Role of Vectors and Reservoirs in Disease Transmission

Vectors are living organisms, typically arthropods like mosquitoes, ticks, fleas, and flies, that can carry disease-causing pathogens from one host to another (Figure 48.2). These pathogens can be bacteria, viruses, parasites, or other microorganisms. Vectors act as intermediaries between the reservoir (the natural environment where the pathogen persists) and the susceptible host (a person or animal that can become infected). Mosquitoes, for example, are well-known vectors for diseases like malaria, dengue fever, Zika virus, and West Nile virus; ticks can transmit Lyme disease and various other tick-borne illnesses (Table 48.2).

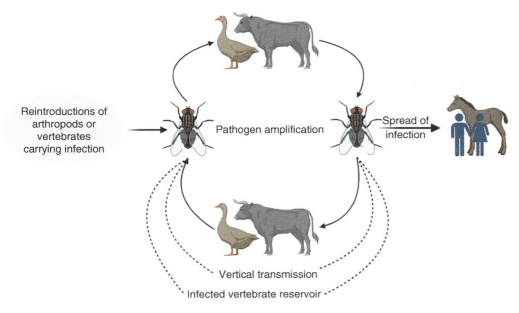

Figure 48.2 Role of vectors and reservoirs in disease transmission to the susceptible host.

Table 48.2 Important vectors and disease transmission mechanisms.

Vector	Mechanism	Diseases
Houseflies	Mechanical	Diarrheal diseases, worms, food poisoning, infective hepatitis
Aedes aegypti	Biological	Dengue, yellow fever, chikungunya, Zika virus
Aedes albopictus	Biological	Chikungunya, dengue, West Nile virus
Culex quinquefasciatus	Biological	Lymphatic filariasis
Anopheles (more than 60 known species can transmit diseases)	Biological	Malaria, lymphatic filariasis (in Africa)
Louse	Biological	Typhus fever, relapsing fever, dermatitis
Mite	Biological	Scabies, chigger
Sandflies	Biological	Leishmaniasis
Blackflies	Biological	Onchocerciasis
Tsetse fly	Biological	Sleeping sickness (trypanosomiasis)
Bedbug	Biological	Dermatitis, Chagas disease
Ticks	Biological	Crimean-Congo hemorrhagic fever, tick-borne encephalitis, typhus, Lyme disease
Fleas	Biological	Plague, murine typhus/endemic typhus
Freshwater snail	Biological	Schistosomiasis

Source: Adapted from Khan (2015).

Vector-borne diseases can be transmitted through:

- *direct contact*: vectors transmit the pathogen directly to a different host by close contact, e.g., scabies and pediculosis
- *mechanical transmission*: pathogens are transported on the contaminated legs, wings, or excreta without developing within the vector, e.g., mechanical transmission of diarrhea, dysentery, typhoid, and food poisoning by a housefly (Khan 2015; Kilpatrick and Randolph 2012).
- *biological transmission*: infectious agents complete their development cycle within the vectors before infecting the hosts.

When a vector bites an infected host, it ingests the pathogen along with the blood meal. The pathogen then undergoes development and multiplication within the vector's body (Weaver and Barrett 2004). Once the pathogen reaches maturity or a certain stage of development, it can be transmitted to a new host through the vector's bite. Three types of biological transmission are possible.

- *Propagative*: the pathogen multiplies inside the vector's body without undergoing any cyclic changes, e.g., plague bacteria in rat fleas.
- *Cyclopropagative*: the cyclical changes and multiplication of the pathogen occur inside the body of the vector, e.g., malaria parasites in the anopheline mosquito.
- *Cyclodevelopmental*: when the pathogen undergoes only cyclical changes without multiplying inside the body of the arthropods, e.g., filarial parasite inside *Culex* mosquitoes.

Reservoirs are natural environments where pathogens can persist and maintain their infectious state without the need for ongoing transmission between hosts. The reservoirs can be either living organisms, such as animals, birds, or insects, or nonliving environmental sources like soil or water (Kilpatrick and Randolph 2012). In some cases, the reservoir species may not exhibit any symptoms of the disease or show only mild symptoms, but they can still carry and transmit the pathogen to other susceptible hosts. These individuals are called carriers. An example of a disease with a wildlife reservoir is the rabies virus, which is often carried by various mammalian species, such as bats, raccoons, and foxes (WHO 2012). In these cases, the virus remains prevalent within the wildlife population and can spill over into domestic animals and humans through bites or scratches.

48.5   Prevention and Control of Vector-borne Diseases

The prevention and control of vectors and reservoirs are essential components of efforts to combat vector-borne diseases and reduce their impact on human and animal populations. Public health authorities can effectively mitigate the spread of these diseases by targeting the sources of infection and transmission. Here are some key strategies for preventing and controlling vectors and reservoirs.

48.5.1   Vector Control Strategies

48.5.1.1   Insecticide Application
The strategic application of insecticides can be an effective method for controlling vector populations. A diverse array of insecticides, classified into the organochlorine, organophosphorus, and carbamate groups , are accessible for vector control (Knols et al. 2010). Indoor residual spraying (IRS) targets the resting places of vectors like mosquitoes, while insecticide-treated bed nets (ITNs) can protect individuals from nighttime bites.

48.5.1.2   Environmental Management
Modifying or eliminating vector breeding sites can help reduce their population and is the best control strategy as the effects show a permanent solution (McMichael and Weiss 2004). Stagnant water, such as in puddles, containers, and discarded tires, is a common breeding ground for mosquitoes. Regular cleaning, draining, or covering these areas can disrupt the breeding cycle. To achieve this, comprehensive health education programs for the public along with political support are very much required.

48.5.1.3   Biological Control
Introducing natural predators, parasites, or pathogens that target vector species can be a sustainable approach to reducing their population. Several fish species, such as *Gambusia affinis*, *Aplochilus panchax*, and *Paecilia holbrooki*, have proven to

be effective predators of anopheline mosquitoes (Chandra et al. 2008). Several omnivorous copepods, i.e., aquatic cyclopoid crustaceans such as *Cyclops vernalis* and *Megacyclops formosanus*, can target young mosquito larval stages (Marten et al. 1989). *Bacillus thuringiensis* and *B. sphaericus* are notable examples of predator bacteria (Lacey 2007). One extensively studied fungus is *Coelomomyces* (Scholte et al. 2007). Due to their primary focus on adult mosquitoes and the various toxins they produce during infection that are lethal to mosquitoes, entomopathogenic fungi are expected to exert less intense selection pressure for resistance compared to rapidly acting insecticides (Knols et al. 2010). *Nosema algerae*, *Thelohania*, and *Vorticella* are examples of predator protozoa (Benelli et al. 2016).

48.5.1.4 Integrated Vector Management

Integrated vector management (IVM) in veterinary public health is a comprehensive approach to control and manage vector-borne diseases that affect animals and humans (Beier et al. 2008). It involves the coordinated use of various strategies to minimize the transmission of diseases carried by vectors. Those include a combination of surveillance and monitoring of vector populations, identification of specific vectors, habitat management to disrupt breeding sites, biological control using natural enemies, judicious use of insecticides, reservoir control in livestock and wildlife areas, community engagement, continuous research, and innovation (WHO 2004). By integrating these methods, IVM aims to achieve effective and sustainable disease control while minimizing the impact on the environment and nontarget organisms.

48.5.1.5 Genetic Control

Genetic manipulation techniques, such as the release of genetically modified vectors, are being explored to reduce vector populations or make them less competent at transmitting pathogens. Transgenic technology enables the precise manipulation of an insect's genome through the direct insertion of DNA into its germline (Lees et al. 2014). This approach presents a novel possibility to harness genes and gene contents across species barriers, introducing specific sequences without disrupting the genome as seen in traditional cross-breeding methods. Transgenic technology helps in controlling vector-borne diseases, for example by inducing insecticide susceptibility and temperature sensitivity in vectors (Figures 48.3 and 48.4).

48.5.1.6 Other Control Methods

Novel vector control methods, involving the release of mosquitoes, are designed to decrease the population of vectors (Figure 48.5). In the sterile insect technique (SIT), male insects are subjected to irradiation or sterilizing chemicals inducing significant random damage to their chromosomes or the induction of dominant-lethal mutations in their sperm on a large scale. Once released into the wild population, these males mate with wild females, resulting in a significant reduction in the vector population size due to the scarcity of viable offspring being produced (Lees et al. 2014).

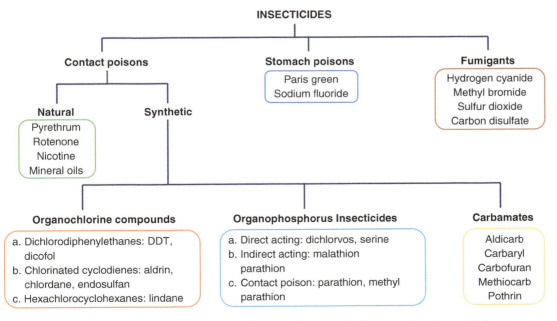

Figure 48.3 Different types of insecticides applied as chemical control of vectors of public health importance.

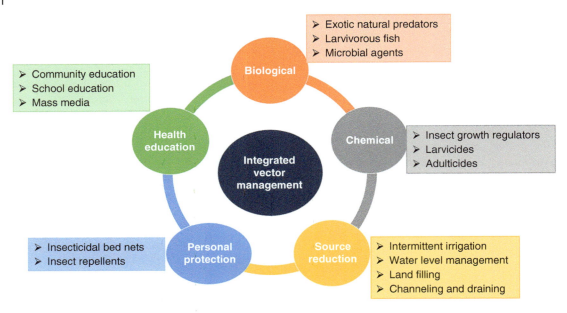

Figure 48.4 Integrated vector management approaches to control vector population.

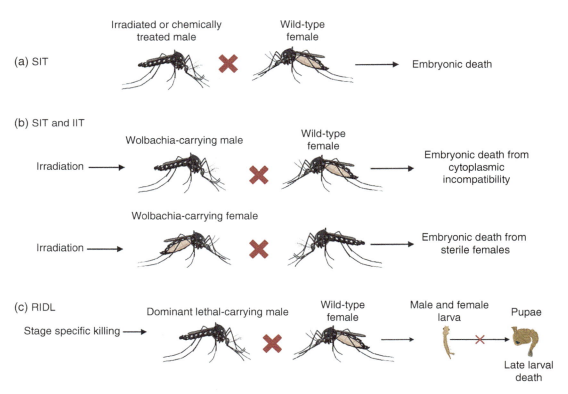

Figure 48.5 Modification of vectors for population reduction. (a) Sterile insect technique (SIT) approach, (b) Incompatible insect technique approach (IIT) and a combination of SIT and IIT. (c) Release of insects with dominant lethality (RIDL).

The incompatible insect technique (IIT) approach involves the stable introduction of a *Wolbachia* strain into a colony of a mosquito species (Brelsfoard and Dobson 2011). In this approach, only *Wolbachia*-infected males are released. When these males mate with females that do not carry the same *Wolbachia* strain or do not have *Wolbachia* at all, it leads to the death of their offspring due to cytoplasmic incompatibility. IIT and SIT techniques can be employed in combination to reduce mosquito populations effectively. *Wolbachia*-infected mosquitoes are subjected to low-level irradiation. As with IIT alone, *Wolbachia*-infected males mating with wild females will not produce viable offspring. Additionally, if there are accidental female releases, these irradiated females become sterile and cannot reproduce with either wild or *Wolbachia*-infected males.

Release of insects with dominant lethality (RIDL) is a suppression strategy that involves releasing males carrying a transgene-inducing late-acting lethality into the open field. These males mate with wild-type females and their offspring perish before reaching the pupal stage (Harris et al. 2012).

48.5.2 Reservoir Control Strategies

Targeted vaccination: vaccinating reservoir animals against specific diseases can help prevent the spread of pathogens. This approach is commonly used in controlling diseases such as rabies, where vaccination campaigns target both domestic and wild animal reservoirs.

- *Culling and surveillance*: in some cases, culling or controlling the population of reservoir species may be necessary to prevent disease transmission. Regular surveillance of reservoir populations helps identify outbreaks and implement control measures promptly. Poison baiting and trapping have been extensively utilized as effective measures to control reservoir hosts. Rodent control strategies include environmental cleanliness, use of rodenticides, and fumigation.
- *Wildlife management*: controlling zoonoses in wildlife presents significant challenges, and eradicating them is often unattainable. Currently, there is no specific treatment for West Nile virus (WNV), and vaccines are only approved for administration in horses, not wild animals or humans (Saiz 2020). Despite various successful approaches in developing WNV vaccines, which have notably decreased its occurrence among horses in the US, none have advanced to phase III clinical trials for other animals. However, significant efforts are required before these vaccines can be implemented as effective tools on a larger scale. In areas where wildlife serves as reservoir hosts, management strategies can be employed to reduce contact between wildlife and domestic animals. This can involve implementing fencing, habitat modifications, or targeted wildlife population control methods.
- *Public education and awareness*: educating the public about the importance of reservoir control measures, such as responsible pet ownership and wildlife interaction, is vital. Raising awareness about the risks associated with specific reservoirs can encourage behavior changes that minimize disease transmission.

48.6 Challenges in the Control of Vector-borne Diseases

Controlling vector-borne diseases presents various challenges due to the complex nature of these diseases and the involvement of vectors and reservoirs in their transmission. Here are some of the key challenges.

- *Vector complexity*: vector-borne diseases involve intricate interactions between the pathogen, vector, and host. Understanding the biology and behavior of these vectors is crucial for effective control measures, but their lifecycles and habits can be quite complex and vary among species.
- *Pathogen diversity*: different vector-borne diseases are caused by a wide range of pathogens such as viruses, bacteria, and parasites. Each pathogen may require unique control strategies, making it difficult to adopt a one-size-fits-all approach.
- *Climate sensitivity*: vector distribution and behavior are highly influenced by climate factors, such as temperature and humidity. Climate change can expand the geographic range of vectors and the diseases they transmit, making control efforts more challenging.
- *Insecticide resistance*: relying solely on insecticides for vector control is no longer entirely effective, as direct resistance has already emerged in more than 100 species of arthropods that are of significant public health concern. This reduces the effectiveness of insecticides and demands the development of new, sustainable methods (Ranson and Lissenden 2016). The combination of insecticide resistance with the risk of environmental contamination has resulted in the limited use of many insecticides in certain countries. Due to the lack of alternate control methods that are as efficient and economical as insecticides, it is postulated that many developing countries will continue to rely on organochlorine pesticides for vector control in the coming future.
- *Urbanization*: rapid urbanization creates conducive environments for vectors to thrive, leading to increased disease transmission. Urban planning needs to incorporate vector control measures to address this issue effectively.

- *Global travel and trade*: international travel and trade facilitate the movement of infected vectors and hosts, enabling the rapid spread of vector-borne diseases across borders.
- *Socioeconomic factors*: poverty, lack of access to healthcare, and inadequate sanitation facilities can exacerbate the spread of vector-borne diseases in certain regions, making it challenging to implement control measures effectively.
- *Diagnostic challenges*: early diagnosis of vector-borne diseases can be challenging, as symptoms may mimic other common illnesses. This often leads to delayed treatment and increased disease transmission.
- *Vaccine development*: while vaccines exist for some vector-borne diseases, the development of effective vaccines for others remains a challenge due to the complexity of the pathogens and the lack of suitable animal models for testing.
- *Community engagement*: successful vector-borne disease control requires active participation and cooperation from local communities. Educating and involving the public in control efforts can be difficult, especially in remote or marginalized areas.
- *Surveillance and reporting*: establishing efficient surveillance systems to monitor vector populations and disease prevalence is crucial for early detection and rapid response. However, limited resources and infrastructure can hinder surveillance efforts.
- *Integrated approach*: implementing an integrated vector management approach that combines various control methods, such as insecticides, biological control, environmental modifications, and community participation, can be logistically challenging to coordinate and sustain.

48.7 Conclusion

Over the last three decades, among the global resurgence of infectious diseases affecting both humans and animals, vector-borne diseases remain on top. These diseases have demonstrated an alarming increase in the frequency of epidemic transmission, and have exhibited a concerning trend of crossing geographic barriers with ease. Therefore, effective vector and reservoir control is crucial for mitigating the impact of vector-borne diseases on public health. In developing countries, financial and technological challenges continue to hinder efforts in diagnosing and controlling diseases, particularly where they remain most prevalent, whereas limited knowledge about vector-borne diseases prevents populations in developed countries from taking necessary action to minimize the effects of these diseases.

Veterinary public health professionals play a key role in implementing integrated strategies that target both vectors and reservoirs. By understanding the biology and behavior of vectors and reservoir hosts, employing various control approaches, and embracing a One Health approach, we can enhance our ability to prevent and control vector-borne diseases. Biological control methods, utilizing natural enemies and symbiotic microorganisms, have overcome the problem of insecticide resistance and shown promise in reducing vector populations sustainably and without causing harm to the environment. The utilization of genetic technologies to modify vector populations and disrupt their ability to transmit pathogens also offers a powerful tool in disease control.

Integrated vector management, incorporating biological control alongside other innovative novel approaches, has emerged as a comprehensive and effective means of vector-borne disease prevention. However, ongoing research, collaboration, and innovation are essential to tackle emerging challenges and develop sustainable solutions in vector and reservoir control.

References

Beier, J.C., Keating, J., Githure, J.I. et al. (2008). Integrated vector management for malaria control. *Malaria Journal* 7: 1–10.

Benelli, G. (2015). Plant-borne ovicides in the fight against mosquito vectors of medical and veterinary importance: a systematic review. *Parasitology Research* 114 (9): 3201–3212.

Benelli, G., Jeffries, C.L., and Walker, T. (2016). Biological control of mosquito vectors: past, present, and future. *Insects* 7 (4): 52.

Brelsfoard, C.L. and Dobson, S.L. (2011). Wolbachia effects on host fitness and the influence of male aging on cytoplasmic incompatibility in Aedes polynesiensis (Diptera: Culicidae). *Journal of Medical Entomology* 48 (5): 1008–1015.

Campbell-Lendrum, D., Manga, L., Bagayoko, M., and Sommerfeld, J. (2015). Climate change and vector-borne diseases: what are the implications for public health research and policy? *Philosophical Transactions of the Royal Society B: Biological Sciences* 370 (1665): 20130552.

Chala, B. and Hamde, F. (2021). Emerging and re-emerging vector-borne infectious diseases and the challenges for control: a review. *Frontiers in Public Health* 9: 715759.

Chandra, G., Bhattacharjee, I., Chatterjee, S.N., and Ghosh, A. (2008). Mosquito control by larvivorous fish. *Indian Journal of Medical Research* 127 (1): 13–27.

Dantas-Torres, F. (2006). Leishmune® vaccine: the newest tool for prevention and control of canine visceral leishmaniosis and its potential as a transmission-blocking vaccine. *Veterinary Parasitology* 141 (1–2): 1–8.

Gubler, D.J. (2009). Vector-borne diseases. *Scientific and Technical Review of the Office International des Epizooties* 28: 583–588.

Harris, A.F., McKemey, A.R., Nimmo, D. et al. (2012). Successful suppression of a field mosquito population by sustained release of engineered male mosquitoes. *Nature Biotechnology* 30 (9): 828–830.

Khan, M.A.H.N.A. (2015). Important vector-borne diseases with their zoonotic potential: present situation and future perspective. *Bangladesh Journal of Veterinary Medicine* 13: 1–14.

Kilpatrick, A.M. and Randolph, S.E. (2012). Drivers, dynamics, and control of emerging vector-borne zoonotic diseases. *Lancet* 380: 1946–1955.

Knols, B.G., Bukhari, T., and Farenhorst, M. (2010). Entomopathogenic fungi as the next-generation control agents against malaria mosquitoes. *Future Microbiology* 5 (3): 339–341.

Kulkarni, V.P. and Reddi, L.V. (2018). A cross-sectional study of knowledge, attitude, and practices regarding zoonotic diseases among agricultural workers. *Public Health Review: International Journal of Public Health Research* 5: 71–76.

Lacey, L.A. (2007). Bacillus thuringiensis serovariety israelensis and Bacillus sphaericus for mosquito control. *Journal of the American Mosquito Control Association* 23 (sp2): 133–163.

Lees, R.S., Knols, B., Bellini, R. et al. (2014). Improving our knowledge of male mosquito biology about genetic control programmes. *Acta Tropica* 132: S2–S11.

Lemon, S.M., Sparling, P.F., Hamburg, M.A. et al. (2008). *Vector-borne Diseases: Understanding the Environmental, Human Health, and Ecological Connections*. Washington, DC: National Academies Press.

Löscher, T. and Prüfer-Krämer, L. (2009). Emerging infectious diseases and re-emerging infectious diseases. In: *Modern Infectious Disease Epidemiology* (ed. A. Kramer, M. Kretzschmar, and K. Krickeberg). New York: Springer.

Marten, G.G., Astaiza, R., Suarez, M.F. et al. (1989). Natural control of larval Anopheles albimanus (Diptera: Culicidae) by the predator Mesocyclops (Copepoda: Cyclopoida). *Journal of Medical Entomology* 26 (6): 624–627.

McMichael, A.J. and Weiss, R.A. (2004). Social and environmental risk factors in the emergence of infectious diseases. *Nature Medicine* 10 (12): 70–76.

Mukhtar, M. (2013). Integrated vector management (IVM): best way forward to control dengue in Pakistan. *Bayer Public Health Journal* 24: 1–7.

Rahman, M.T., Sobur, M.A., Islam, M.S. et al. (2020). Zoonotic diseases: etiology, impact, and control. *Microorganisms* 8 (9): 1405.

Ranson, H. and Lissenden, N. (2016). Insecticide resistance in African anopheles mosquitoes: a worsening situation that needs urgent action to maintain malaria control. *Trends in Parasitology* 32 (3): 187–196.

Samad, M.A. (2011). Public health threat caused by zoonotic diseases in Bangladesh. *Bangladesh Journal of Veterinary Medicine* 9 (2): 95–120.

Scholte, E.J., Takken, W., and Knols, B.G. (2007). Infection of adult Aedes aegypti and Ae. albopictus mosquitoes with the entomopathogenic fungus Metarhizium anisopliae. *Acta Tropica* 102 (3): 151–158.

Solomon, T., Ni, H., Beasley, D.W. et al. (2003). Origin and evolution of Japanese encephalitis virus in southeast Asia. *Journal of Virology* 77 (5): 3091–3098.

Upadhyay, A.K., Maansi, P.T., Singh, P., and Pathak, A.P. (2018). Vector-borne zoonotic diseases. *Journal of Animal Health and Behavioural Science* 2: 1–6.

Wang, G.H., Gamez, S., Raban, R.R. et al. (2021). Combating mosquito-borne diseases using genetic control technologies. *Nature Communications* 12 (1): 4388.

Weaver, S.C. and Barrett, A.D. (2004). Transmission cycles, host range, evolution and emergence of arboviral disease. *Nature Reviews Microbiology* 2 (10): 789–801.

World Health Organization (WHO) (2010). Treatment of severe P. Falciparum malaria. In: *Guidelines for the Treatment of Malaria*, 2e, 35–47. Geneva: World Health Organization.

World Health Organization (WHO) (2004). *Global Strategic Framework for Integrated Vector Management*. Geneva: World Health Organization.

World Health Organization (2012). *Handbook for Integrated Vector Management*. Geneva: World Health Organization.

Dantas-Torres, F. (2007). The role of dogs as reservoirs of Leishmania parasites, with emphasis on Leishmania (Leishmania) infantum and Leishmania (Viannia) braziliensis. *Veterinary Parasitology* 149 (3-4): 139–146.

World Health Organization (2014). *A Global Brief on Vector-borne Diseases*. Geneva: World Health Organization.

Saiz, J.C. (2020). Animal and human vaccines against West Nile virus. *Pathogens* 9 (12): 1073.

49

Principles of General Disease Prevention and Control Measures

Jitendrakumar Nayak, Manasi Soni, Pranav Anjaria, and Manubhai N. Brahmbhatt

College of Veterinary Science and Animal Husbandry, Kamdhenu University, Anand, India

49.1 Introduction

The World Health Organization (WHO) defines disease as any adverse variation from an organism's normal structural and functional condition, typically accompanied by a variety of signs and symptoms and distinct from physical harm. It includes a wide range of environmental and social initiatives meant to improve and safeguard everyone's health and standard of living by addressing and avoiding the root causes of ill health rather than merely concentrating on treatments and cures (WHO 1986). These can assist people in controlling their psychological and physical ailments, enhancing their quality of life and social, familial, and individual well-being. Additionally, they lengthen healthy life expectancy globally and cut waste and unnecessary medical costs (Omenn 1990).

Effective prevention of infectious diseases can also be carried out at the individual level through behavioral interventions that minimize contact with pathogens. These include isolating or cohorting infected individuals in separate rooms, using protective clothing like masks or gowns, applying insect repellents, and practicing regular handwashing with antiseptic agents (Fraise et al. 2012). Interventions are targeted at various stages of disease development with the goal of eradicating, eliminating, or reducing its effects or, if none of these options are practical, delaying the onset of illness and incapacity.

49.2 Levels of Disease Prevention

Measures that aim to prevent the development of disease (including injury), prevent its progression, and minimize its effects if it has already occurred are referred to as disease prevention. There are various levels of disease prevention.

- Primordial prevention
- Primary prevention
- Secondary prevention
- Tertiary prevention
- Quaternary prevention

49.2.1 Primordial Prevention

In 1978, a new approach to prevention called primordial prevention was introduced. The term was first mentioned in a 1982 report by the WHO. Primordial prevention focuses on reducing risk factors across an entire population by addressing social and environmental conditions. Typically, such measures are promoted through laws and national policies. Since primordial prevention is the earliest form of prevention, it often targets children to minimize their exposure to risks.

The goal of primordial prevention is to address the underlying social conditions that contribute to the onset of diseases. Its objective is to prevent the emergence and establishment of environmental, economic, social, and cultural factors that are

---

Epidemiology and Environmental Hygiene in Veterinary Public Health, First Edition. Edited by Tanmoy Rana.
© 2025 John Wiley & Sons, Inc. Published 2025 by John Wiley & Sons, Inc.

known to increase disease risks. Recognizing that individuals face various constraints, primordial prevention primarily relies on intersectoral action to empower people to make healthy choices. For instance, improving access to safe sidewalks in urban neighborhoods can promote physical activity, reducing risk factors for obesity, cardiovascular disease, type 2 diabetes, and other related conditions.

The significance of primordial prevention has become more pressing due to accelerated and widespread societal changes, rising inequalities, and global processes such as the expansion of international travel and trade. Additionally, worsening environmental conditions, such as pollution and the use of harmful chemicals, along with deforestation and the ongoing destruction of the natural environment leading to reduced biodiversity, further emphasize the need for immediate attention to primordial prevention.

49.2.2 Primary Prevention

Primary prevention encompasses measures that specifically target a susceptible population or individual. Its primary objective is to prevent the occurrence of a disease altogether, focusing on individuals who are already in good health. This type of prevention typically involves activities that either minimize the exposure to risk factors or enhance the immunity of individuals at risk, thereby preventing progression of a disease from a susceptible individual to a subclinical state. Immunizations serve as an example of primary prevention.

The decline of infectious diseases can be attributed to public health improvements such as the provision of clean drinking water and the implementation of safe sewage disposal systems. Measures aim to reduce or eliminate the causative agent from the environment, subsequently reducing exposure (Kisling and Das 2022). Another example is reducing *Cryptosporidium* spp. transmission by limiting animal density on farms and minimizing contact between personnel, calves, and other herds, keeping young animals or susceptible hosts that have high risk of infection separated from adult animals, and maintaining a short calving period which may decrease the opportunities for *Cryptosporidium* spp. to spread within animal herds (Hoar et al. 2001; Pumipuntu and Piratae 2018).

49.2.3 Secondary Prevention

Secondary prevention targets healthy-appearing people with subclinical disease states and emphasizes early disease identification. Diseases with quantifiable risk factors or an aberrant condition that existed before the onset of the disease are the focus of secondary prevention. The purpose of secondary prevention is to take action before the onset of the disease by either lowering risk factors or treating the underlying problem. Subclinical disease comprises pathological changes but no overt symptoms that can be diagnosed during a doctor's visit.

Screening is a common technique of secondary prevention. It can be used only when the natural history of a disease includes an early period when it is easily identified and treated, thereby allowing interruption of progression to a more serious stage. It relies on safe and precise ways to detect disease, preferably in its early stages, and effective methods of treatment. It reduces risk in those who are most at risk but have not yet developed the disease (Hobbs 2004). Examples include screening for early detection of cervical cancer and breast cancer (Basu et al. 2018).

49.2.4 Tertiary Prevention

Tertiary prevention focuses on the clinical and outcome stages of disease. It is administered to symptomatic persons with the goal of reducing both the severity of the illness and any possible after-effects. It is aimed at reducing the impact of the disease once it has been established in a person, whereas secondary prevention aims to prevent the beginning of illness. Rehabilitation initiatives are frequently used as tertiary preventive strategies, the main objective being to lessen the impact of established disease by eliminating or lowering disability, minimizing suffering, and maximizing possible years of quality life (Dekker and Sibai 2001; Jacobsen and Andrykowski 2015). Tertiary prevention, in terms of epidemiology, tries to lessen the incidence and/or severity of complications.

49.2.5 Quaternary Prevention

Quaternary prevention, according to the WONCA International Dictionary for General/Family Practise, is "action taken to identify patient at risk of overmedicalization, to protect him from new medical invasion, and to suggest to him interventions, which are ethically acceptable." When Marc Jamoulle first introduced this idea, the major objectives were individuals who were ill but did not have a recognisable condition. "Action done to safeguard humans (persons/patients) from medical operations that are likely to cause more harm than good," according to a recent change, is now the term (Martins et al. 2018; Kisling and Das 2022).

49.3 Blocking Routes of Transmission

These methods fall into two categories: direct and indirect (Osterholm and Hedberg 2015) (Figures 49.1 and 49.2). The most frequent method is the direct and quick transmission of an infectious agent to a receptive portal of entry, which allows for the establishment of human infection. This kind of direct contact transmission happens via touching, kissing, or sexual activity. It can also happen when an infected host directly sprays droplets (droplet spread) into the conjunctiva or mucous membranes of another host's nose or mouth. The second type of direct transmission occurs when host-susceptible tissue is exposed to the agent, such as through the bite of a rabid animal or contact with soil or decaying matter in which the agent leads a saprophytic existence (e.g., systemic mycosis).

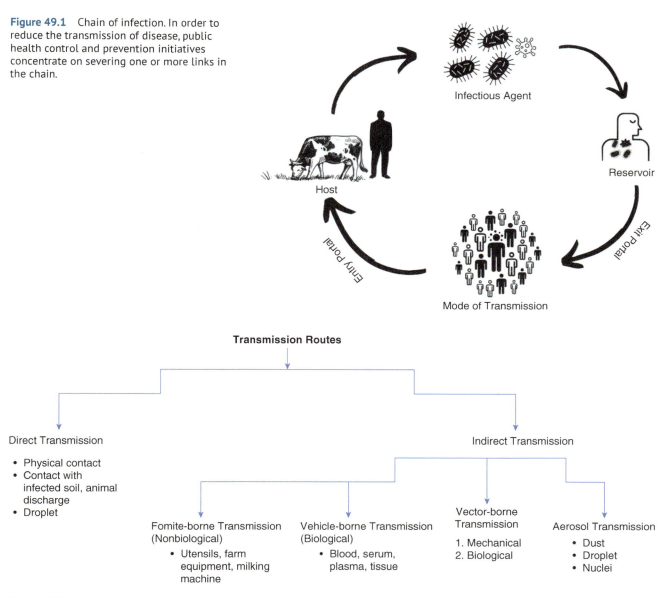

Figure 49.1 Chain of infection. In order to reduce the transmission of disease, public health control and prevention initiatives concentrate on severing one or more links in the chain.

Figure 49.2 Routes of transmission.

The four primary mechanisms of indirect agent transmission are fomite (nonbiological) vehicle borne, vector borne, and air borne. Fomite transmission involves nonbiological objects capable of transmitting an infectious agent. Vehicle-borne transmission occurs when any nonliving material serves as an intermediate means (usually of biological origin) by which an infectious agent is transported or introduced into the susceptible host through a suitable portal of entry. These materials may include water, food, biological products such as blood, serum, plasma, tissues, and organs. It is not necessary that the agent multiply or develop in or on the vehicle before it is transmitted.

The third method of indirect transmission is vector-borne transmission, which may be mechanical or biological. Mechanical transmission occurs when an insect carries an infectious agent through the soiling of its feet or proboscis or through carriage in its gastrointestinal tract. Transmission occurs in the agent without multiplication or development of the organism. In contrast, biological vector-borne transmission occurs when propagation (multiplication), cyclic development, or a combination of these events (cyclopropagative) is required before the arthropod can transmit the infected form of the agent to humans, i.e., strongyloidosis.

The fourth type of indirect transmission is air borne, involving the dissemination of aerosols with infectious agents to a suitable portal of entry into a host, usually the respiratory tract. These aerosols are suspensions of particles in the air that consist partially or wholly of infectious agents. The particles are in the range of 1–5 μm. Air-borne transmission does not include droplets and other large particles that promptly settle out, which result in direct transmission, e.g., influenza, tuberculosis, foot and mouth disease (FMD). Some infections transmitted by the air-borne route may be carried great distances from their sources, For this reason, there is particular concern that agents such as *B. anthracis* and *Yersinia pestis* could be used as weapons of mass destruction in a civilian bioterrorism event (Dennis et al. 2001; Inglesby et al. 2000, 2002).

Direct transmission can be blocked by:

- avoiding physical contact
- proper care of wounds, cuts, injuries, and scars
- avoiding contact with infected animals.

Blocking of indirect transmission includes:

- good ventilation
- dust control (damp dusting, vacuum sweeping)
- hygiene in slaughtering, safety of animal products
- withdrawal or treatment of contaminated products
- controlling risk factors associated with water, personnel, environment etc.

49.4 Diagnosis

In order to treat patients appropriately and conduct preventive and control surveillance operations, accurate disease diagnosis is necessary. Sensitivity and specificity are two crucial factors that should be taken into account for any diagnostic test that is used.

Sensitivity describes a test's capacity to accurately identify people who are infected with an agent (or who are "positive in disease"). Those with the disease (and possibly some without) are more likely to be detected by a very sensitive test; there will not be many false negatives in a highly sensitive test. Specificity is a measure of a test's ability to correctly identify people who are not infected by a certain agent (who are "negative in health"); high specificity suggests a low number of false-positive results. Often, confirmatory tests are more focused (to obviate false-positive screening tests) whereas screening tests are extremely sensitive (to detect any potential instances) (van Seventer and Hochberg 2017).

Diagnostic reasoning may be based heavily on the known frequency of potential causative agents in the age group of the patient, the specific geographic or physical setting, the season, and epidemic behavior. It includes the following.

- Brief description.
- Identify the etiological agent.
- Measure frequency of distribution by factors such as age and geography.
- Occurrence in the population (Kaslow 2014).

Various diagnostic methods are shown in Figure 49.3.

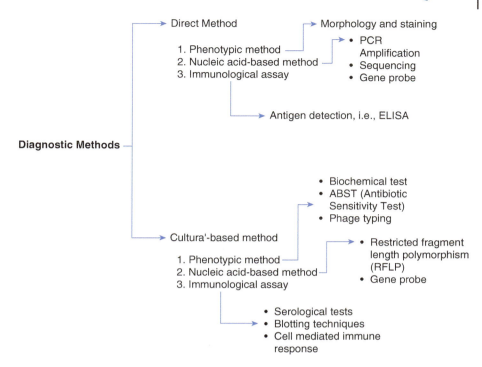

Figure 49.3 Different diagnostic techniques.

49.5 Isolation

This is the oldest communicable disease control measure. It is defined as "separation for the period of communicability of infected persons and animals from others in such places and under such conditions as to prevent and limit the direct or indirect transmission of the infectious agent from those infected to those who are susceptible or who may spread agent to others" (http://ecoursesonline.iasri.res.in/mod/page/view.php?id=20675). This involves physical isolation of the case or carrier and if necessary, treatment until free from disease. Types of isolation include standard isolation, strict isolation (utilized to stop the spread of all highly communicable diseases that spread by contact or air borne, e.g., chickenpox, rabies), protective isolation, and high security isolation.

Individuals must be isolated if they meet the following criteria.

- Known or suspected communicable infection/disease, e.g., pulmonary tuberculosis, chickenpox.
- Unexplained rash if considered to be of an infectious cause.
- Multiresistant organisms, e.g., methicillin-resistant *Staphylococcus aureus* (MRSA), extended-spectrum beta-lactamase (ESBL)-producing coliforms.
- Multiresistant *Acinetobacter baumannii* (MRAB).
- Diarrhea and/or vomiting until microbiologically proven negative or symptoms subside.
- *Clostridium difficile*.
- Symptoms of influenza.

49.6 Quarantine

The WHO defines "quarantine of persons" as the act of restricting activities or separating individuals who are not ill but may have been exposed to an infectious agent or disease (Table 49.1). The main purpose of quarantine is to monitor symptoms and promptly detect cases. The effectiveness of quarantine in curbing the spread of contagious diseases is widely acknowledged and undisputed.

Essentially, the concept relies on the existence of an incubation period between the time a person is exposed to a contagious illness and the moment they become contagious to others if infected. By ensuring that exposed and infected individuals do not come into contact with others during this contagious phase, infection transmission can be halted. Health

Table 49.1 Differences between isolation and quarantine.

Quarantine	Isolation
People are kept separate from others because they have been exposed to contagious disease	Isolation is the procedure used to keep individuals who are sick with a contagious disease separate from other individuals
Healthy individual	Affected individual
Purpose: to monitor potentially exposed individuals during the incubation period of the disease	Purpose: to prevent infected individuals from spreading the disease to others who are not affected
Individuals should be free after their quarantine period is over	After recovery, some tests may be performed
Done at healthcare facilities	Done at home or other locations, away from others

authorities can apply quarantine measures on various modes of transportation such as ships, airplanes, railways, and automobiles, or other means to prevent the spread of the disease, its reservoirs, or vectors (Patel et al. 2020; Calonge et al. 2020).
Quarantine may be active or passive.

- *Active quarantine*: animals are maintained in a secluded area for a set amount of time. During and after the quarantine period, either the isolated population or specific pathogen-free (SPF) sentinel animals in nearby cages are included. They are tested for various microbial infections during and after the quarantine period with different technologies like bacterial culture, serological testing, fecal examination, and histological examination.
- *Passive quarantine*: newly acquired animals are housed in a secluded area and are not subjected to experimental manipulation for a set amount of time. They undergo a clinical evaluation to look for symptoms of illnesse throughout this time.

49.7 Epidemiological Control

Epidemiological control involves collaborative efforts of healthcare professionals, public health agencies, governments, communities, and international organizations in a proactive and multifaceted approach to protect the health of populations and minimize the impact of infectious diseases. The frequency, transmission, manifestation, and distribution of infections and diseases in communities, as well as the variables influencing these aspects, are the focus of infectious disease epidemiology.

49.7.1 Host, Agent, and Environment

One method for determining the reasons for infectious disease outbreaks is to consider the factors of hos, agent, and environment (Noone 2008). These three key elements determine the occurrence and characteristics of infections: the agent (Virus) itself, the host (individual), and the environment (Figure 49.4). The virus must be in the appropriate state and present in sufficient quantity to infect the host. Depending on the virus's infectivity, different amounts of viral inoculum are required to start an infection. The infection is established after the minimum inoculum is introduced, successfully attaches to, and penetrates its target cells. The virus then induces a reaction that may or may not be clinically evident, again depending on numerous characteristics of the agent, host, and environment.

Once infection is established, the virus triggers a response that may or may not cause clinical symptoms. The ability of a virus to elicit a response from the host's immune system is called its immunogenic potential. This refers to the virus's capacity to generate an immune response that can protect the host from reinfection or significant disease upon preexposure. Some viruses are highly immunogenic and confer lifelong immunity, while others can avoid generating highly neutralizing antibodies, leading to persistent or chronic infections.

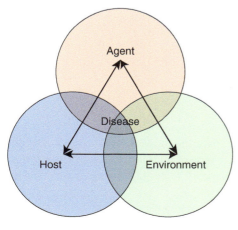

Figure 49.4 Interaction of host, disease, and environment.

In the context of immunization, immunogenicity refers to how well a vaccine can provide a level of protection similar to that achieved through natural infection. It has frequently been successful in replicating high levels of reducing antibodies or lifelong protection in vaccines against highly immunogenic illnesses. When the agents responsible for noninfectious diseases are consistently nonspecific, determining causal factors becomes challenging, as host susceptibility cannot be evaluated and the environment exhibits multiple interconnected layers of influence. Agent, host, and environment explanations have substantial limits in these situations (McDowell 2008).

49.8 Occurrence

Occurrence depends on properties such as the efficiency of spread from cell to cell, either by direct involvement of contiguous cells or by transport via body fluids to other susceptible cells; the number of cells infected; and the consequences of viral multiplication on the cell itself and on the organism as a whole. Further biochemical and physiological details of these cellular processes can be gleaned from basic science texts.

In the public health context, *incidence* may refer to new infections or new cases of existing disease. Incidence is the number of new events (e.g., instances of infection or cases of disease) occurring in a particular time interval. Generally, the *incidence rate* is the number of new events divided by the number of people at risk. The incidence rate may be expressed more specifically as the number of events per unit of population per unit of time or as the number of events in a fixed total population during a fixed total time period.

Prevalence is the number of persons with infection or cases of disease existing at a designated time or in a time interval. The *prevalence rate* is the number of such cases divided by the population at risk, a measure used most commonly for chronic diseases. Prevalence of infection is usually measured by a test for the presence of a substance (e.g., antibody, antigen, fragment of nucleic acid, or other component) in biological fluid or tissue samples from a given population. More specifically, the prevalence of infection or disease is determined by the duration of incident cases: the longer the duration of an incident condition, the higher the number of prevalent cases of that condition. That proportionality can be represented as prevalence = incidence × duration.

Disease at population level can happen randomly or in a pattern which includes secular, periodic, and seasonal trends (Table 49.2).

49.9 Therapy and Chemoprophylaxis

The development of antiviral agents involves focusing on vulnerable points in a virus's replicative cycle, ideally targeting areas distinct from any pathways in the human host's synthetic processes. There are now numerous candidate drugs with proven clinical antiviral efficacy, and advances in computer programs allow for precise *in silico* design of new compounds by modeling protein–protein interactions and predicting their biological effects.

Despite these promising developments, achieving the ideal antiviral agent remains challenging. Limitations include the poor correlation between predicted effects from *in silico*, *in vitro*, or animal studies and actual observations in humans. Additionally, different virus strains may respond differently to treatments, and resistance to antiviral drugs can emerge

Table 49.2 Disease occurrence pattern.

Secular	Periodic	Seasonal
Long time trend to disease occurrence	Temporary interruption of the general trends of secular variation	Cyclic variation of disease frequency by time and year
Numbers may rise or fall depending on natural factors	Waves of new cases every 2–4 years depending on how fast new susceptible individuals are introduced into a population	Fluctuation in environment factors, occupational and recreation activities
Local populations experience gradually declining rates of a particular strain of respiratory virus as population-level immunity develops following repeated exposures	Human migration may account for periodicity that is predictable but might not occur every year in the same season	Characteristic of many viral infections in the absence of widespread vaccine-induced immunity

49.9.1 Immunization

Immunization is a powerful public health tool that helps protect individuals and communities from infectious diseases. It is essential to ensure that vaccination programs are accessible, well implemented, and supported by accurate information to maximize their effectiveness in preventing and controlling diseases. Vaccines have been proven safe and effective, and widespread immunization is a vital component of public health efforts to safeguard communities and enhance global health outcomes. Traditional vaccines have used immunization processes to protect an individual against potential future exposure to an infectious agent. Even when the process is not 100% efficacious, a sufficient proportion of the population is protected and "herd immunity" is created. In such a case, the population is protected against subsequent infections of individuals and endemic persistence of the infectious agent. When an infectious agent infects one individual, another susceptible host is not encountered in the immediate environment and transmission of the organism cannot occur before the transmissible stage of the lifecycle of the infection is passed.

49.9.1.1 Active Immunization
Active vaccines are administered with the goal of stimulating antibody production by the host to provide a high degree and long duration of protection but with no or minimal accompanying illness.

49.9.1.2 Passive Immunization
Passive immunization with an immunoglobulin (Ig) preparation is a useful approach for short-term prevention, especially when administered soon after exposure, ideally within hours. For this method to be effective, the Ig preparation should contain a high concentration of antibodies that can effectively combat the specific agent causing the disease. These Ig preparations can be obtained from different sources, including individuals who have recovered from the disease (convalescent), individuals hyperimmunized against the disease, or donors with high antibody titers (Centers for Disease Control and Prevention 2002). Passive immunization is typically limited to specific scenarios, such as well-defined exposures to the rabies virus, or in cases where patients have a weakened immune system (immunocompromised) and are susceptible to certain viruses like hepatitis A virus, hepatitis B virus, varicella-zoster virus, cytomegalovirus, and vaccinia (which is unlikely without smallpox immunization, but potentially useful if vaccinia virus becomes accepted as a carrier for other antigens).

Many diseases exist for which there is no effective preventive vaccine. Several additional strategies are currently being used to produce vaccines for infections against which traditional vaccines have not been successful. Examples of strategies used to induce effective immunity without adverse consequences include subcomponent vaccines, peptide-based vaccines, recombinant DNA vaccines, chimeric vectors, and alternative routes of administration.

49.10   Disease Eradication and Elimination

Eradication is defined as "permanent reduction to zero of the worldwide incidences of infection caused by a specific agent as a result of deliberate efforts; intervention measures are no longer needed" (Dowdle 1998) (Table 49.3). Smallpox was the first and so far only disease to have been officially declared eradicated from the Earth. From the moment of that historic accomplishment in 1977, this success of the WHO eradication program has inspired initiatives to replicate it with other diseases. In 1979, Rotary International began its remarkable commitment to polio eradication and for three decades, through its worldwide chapters, it performed tireless vaccine campaign work that captured the attention of major news organizations (Dayan et al. 2008). By 2006, polio was present in only four countries as significant progress had been made in controlling the disease.

49.10.1   Biological Control

Numerous infectious diseases are transmitted between hosts through an intermediary carrier, known as a vector. The rate of disease transmission is closely connected to the frequency of encounters between vectors and hosts, which in turn relies

Table 49.3 Diseases identified as potential candidates for global eradication by the International Task Force for Disease Eradication (Kaslow 2014; Carter Center International Task Force for Disease Eradication 2024).

Diseases	Primary challenges for eradication	Conclusion
Measles	Lack of suitably effective vaccine for young infants	Potentially eradicable
Poliomyelitis	Addressing insecurity; low vaccine coverage; enhanced national commitment needed	Eradicable
Rubella	Lack of data on impact in developing countries; difficult diagnosis	Potentially eradicable
Mumps	Lack of data on impact in developing countries; difficult diagnosis	Potentially eradicable

on the density of vectors. Vector-borne diseases can impact humans, livestock, and crops, making their eradication crucial for economic and public health reasons.

One effective method to control such diseases is by introducing biological enemies (biocontrol agents) of the vectors. The use of biological control for vectors is increasingly recognized as a promising approach to manage a range of disease-causing agents, including well-known human illnesses like malaria, Chagas disease, trypanosomiasis, and Lyme disease, as well as crop diseases like the tomato leaf curl virus in India and the cassava mosaic virus in sub-Saharan Africa (Okamoto and Amarasekare 2012).

49.10.2 Early Warning System

An early warning system gives the local government time to implement control measures that will lower the cost of healthcare for the neighborhood (Figure 49.5). Early warning systems are frequently described as instruments for anticipating and detecting hazards, but this definition leaves unclear if the information provided by the warnings is truly used to lower risks.

An early warning system should be viewed as an information system created to assist decision making by pertinent national and local institutions and to enable vulnerable individuals and social groups to take action to mitigate the effects of an impending hazard in order to fulfill an effective risk reduction function. Improved coordination among relevant parties, including scientific organizations that forecast hazard events, national and local management agencies that assess risk and develop response strategies, and public communication channels used to disseminate warning information, must be a priority in addition to better hazard monitoring and prediction.

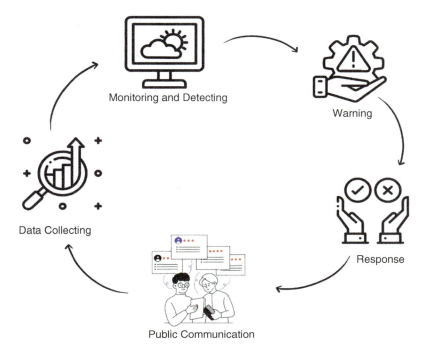

Figure 49.5 Harnessing the power of an early warning system.

An effective early warning system includes the following aspects.

49.10.2.1 Epidemiological Surveillance
Continuous and systematic monitoring of disease incidence, including changes in vector populations, using standardized routines and timely dissemination of information. Ecologically based surveillance systems are employed to monitor St Louis encephalitis and western equine encephalomyelitis in California (Reisen et al. 1992, 2000; Novello et al. 2000).

49.10.2.2 Environmental Observations
Since the effects of weather or climate events frequently depend on prior circumstances, systematic climate observations are a crucial feature of an early warning system. For example, whether heavy rainfall causes flooding depends on the recent history of rain in that area. To predict disease outbreaks, the system will use advanced technology to monitor things like how wet the soil is, how much vegetation there is, and the temperature of the ocean all around the world. This helps us better understand and prepare for possible disease threats.

49.10.2.3 Vulnerability Assessment
Vulnerability refers to a population's sensitivity to a hazard, as well as its ability to cope with the hazard, considering factors like nutrition, shelter, sanitation, and access to healthcare. The development of disease control measures and the evaluation of the potential for outbreaks depend heavily on vulnerability assessment and public health surveillance.

49.10.2.4 Risk Analysis
Risk analysis is a process used to calculate the chances of a potential hazard causing specific impacts. It involves considering various factors like the type of hazard, vulnerabilities, possible effects of the hazard, and the ability of communities to handle and recover from those effects. Risk patterns are constantly changing due to factors such as urbanization, economic changes, population growth, migration, environmental degradation, and armed conflict. However, in many places, risk analysis is still limited because outdated cartographic and census information does not reflect the real risk levels. To improve risk analysis, it is essential to monitor dynamic changes in risk patterns more accurately, with detailed information about spatial and temporal aspects, so that we can better understand the potential impact of a hazard in a specific area.

49.10.2.5 Preparedness/Response
Warning systems should be developed in coordination with local, national, or regional responders, especially in areas that are highly vulnerable. Often, scientific advances in predicting hazards do not lead to improved ways of using this warning information effectively.

It is crucial to create response strategies based on the specific needs and priorities of the community. Response plans that go against the coping methods of vulnerable groups are unlikely to be successful. Preventing or controlling disease outbreaks can be expensive, especially for resource-limited countries, and may burden their resources significantly. If the costs of implementing a recommended response plan outweigh the health benefits, it can reduce the credibility of the early warning system. Additionally, the implementation of certain control measures, like widespread insecticide spraying, may face active public resistance.

To avoid potential issues and ensure success, response plans need to be carefully assessed, considering cost–benefit factors and tailored to match the local community's priorities, needs, and capacity.

49.10.2.6 Public Communication
To ensure that warning information and recommended response strategies are heeded by the populations at risk, effective public communication strategies must be developed (National Research Council (US) Committee on Climate 2001). These strategies should identify and prioritize specific audience groups, deliver accurate and science-based messages from credible sources, and use familiar channels to reach the intended recipients. Credibility and trust are crucial factors to consider in communication efforts. If the warning authority lacks respect in the area or has a history of strained relationships with local communities, the warnings may not be taken seriously. Moreover, excessive or inconsistent warnings in the past can undermine the credibility of future warnings.

To prevent unnecessary panic, early disease warnings should provide clear explanations of the actual level of risk and highlight the vulnerable groups that are most at risk. By considering these aspects, public communication can effectively enhance preparedness and response to potential hazards.

49.10.3 Education and Training

Professionals specializing in zoonotic diseases should be properly trained. It is crucial to expand medical knowledge among those who might encounter the initial cases of zoonoses in either animal or humans. Likewise, acquiring expertise in molecular epidemiology will enable us to gain deeper insight into the various pathogens involved and their specific sources, and ultimately improve our capacity to manage and prevent infections.

49.11 Failure of Disease Prevention and Control in South Asia

The failure of disease prevention and control in South Asia is a significant concern, and several factors contribute to this issue.

- *Limited resources*: many countries in South Asia face challenges in allocating sufficient resources to healthcare systems. This limitation hinders the implementation of comprehensive disease prevention and control programs.
- *Overburdened healthcare systems*: rapid population growth and limited healthcare infrastructure result in overburdened healthcare systems. This strain makes it difficult to effectively manage and control the spread of diseases.
- *Inadequate access to healthcare*: large segments of the population in South Asia have limited access to healthcare services due to factors like geographical remoteness, poverty, and lack of awareness.
- *Poor sanitation and hygiene*: inadequate sanitation and poor hygiene practices contribute to the spread of communicable diseases, making prevention and control efforts more challenging.
- *Antibiotic resistance*: misuse and overuse of antibiotics in the region have led to an increase in antibiotic-resistant infections, making it harder to treat diseases effectively.
- *Climate change and environmental factors*: South Asia is vulnerable to the impacts of climate change, which can lead to the spread of vector-borne diseases and other health hazards.
- *Political and socioeconomic factors*: political instability, social inequality, and economic disparities can hinder the implementation of effective disease prevention and control strategies.
- *Limited health awareness and education*: lack of health awareness and education among the population can result in delayed or inadequate responses to disease outbreaks.

Addressing these challenges requires collaborative efforts from governments, international organizations, and local communities. Investments in healthcare infrastructure, improved access to healthcare services, health education, and disease surveillance systems are essential to strengthen disease prevention and control measures in South Asia.

References

Basu, P., Mittal, S., Vale, D., and Kharaji, Y. (2018). Secondary prevention of cervical cancer. *Best Practice and Research: Clinical Obstetrics and Gynaecology* 47: 73–85.

Calonge, N., Brown, L., and Downey, A. (2020). *Evidence-Based Practice for Public Health Emergency Preparedness and Response.* Washington, DC: National Academies Press.

Carter Center International Task Force for Disease Eradication. (2024). www.cartercenter.org/health/itfde/index.html (accessed 14 February 2024).

Centers for Disease Control and Prevention. (2002). Recommendations of the Advisory Committee on Immunization. www.cdc.gov/vaccines/acip/recommendations.html (accessed 14 February 2024).

Dayan, G.H., Quinlisk, M.P., Parker, A.A. et al. (2008). Recent resurgence of mumps in the United States. *New England Journal of Medicine* 358 (15): 1580–1589.

Dekker, G. and Sibai, B. (2001). Primary, secondary, and tertiary prevention of pre-eclampsia. *Lancet* 357: 209–215.

Dennis, D.T., Inglesby, T.V., Henderson, D.A. et al. (2001). Tularemia as a biological weapon: medical and public health management. *JAMA* 285: 2763–2773.

Dowdle, W.R. (1998). The principles of disease elimination and eradication. *Bulletin of the World Health Organization* 76 (Suppl. 2): 22.

Fraise, A., Maillard, J., and Sattar, S. (2012). *Russell, Hugo and Ayliffe's Principles and Practice of Disinfection, Preservation and Sterilization.* Hoboken: Wiley.

Hoar, B., Atwill, E., Elmi, C., and Farver, T. (2001). An examination of risk factors associated with beef cattle shedding pathogens of potential zoonotic concern. *Epidemiology & Infection* 127: 147–155.

Hobbs, F. (2004). Cardiovascular disease: different strategies for primary and secondary prevention? *Heart* 90: 1217–1223.

Inglesby, T., Dennis, D., Henderson, D. et al. (2000). Plague as a biological weapon: medical and public health management. *JAMA* 283: 2281–2290.

Inglesby, T.V., O'Toole, T., Henderson, D.A. et al. (2002). Anthrax as a biological weapon: updated recommendations for management. *JAMA* 287: 2236–2252.

Jacobsen, P. and Andrykowski, M.A. (2015). Tertiary prevention in cancer care: understanding and addressing the psychological dimensions of cancer during the active treatment period. *American Psychologist* 70: 134–145.

Kaslow, R.A. (2014). Epidemiology and control: principles, practice and programs. In: *Viral Infections of Humans: Epidemiology and Control* (ed. R.A. Kaslow, L. Stanberry, and J. Le Duc), 3–38. New York: Springer.

Kisling, L. and Das, J. (2022). *Prevention Strategies*. Treasure Island: StatPearls.

Martins, C., Godycki-Cwirko, M., Heleno, B., and Brodersen, J. (2018). Quaternary prevention: reviewing the concept. *European Journal of General Practice* 24 (1): 106–111.

McDowell, I. (2008). From risk factors to explanation in public health. *Journal of Public Health* 30: 219–223.

National Research Council (US) Committee on Climate (2001). Toward the development of disease early warning systems. In: *Under the Weather: Climate, Ecosystems, and Infectious Diseases*. Washington, DC: National Academies Press.

Noone, P. (2008). Agent, host and environmental interactions. *Occupational Medicine* 58: 594.

Novello, A., White, D., Kramer, L. et al. (2000). Update: West Nile Virus activity – Eastern United States. *Morbidity and Mortality Weekly Report* 49: 1044–1047.

Okamoto, K. and Amarasekare, P. (2012). The biological control of disease vectors. *Journal of Theoretical Biology* 309: 47–57.

Omenn, G.S. (1990). Prevention and the elderly: appropriate policies. *Health Affairs* 9 (2): 80–93.

Osterholm, M. and Hedberg, C.W. (2015). Epidemiologic principles. In: *Mandell, Douglas, and Bennett's Principles and Practice of Infectious Diseases* (ed. J. Bennett, R. Dolin, and M. Blaser), 146–157. St Louis: Elsevier.

Patel, A., Patel, S., Fulzele, P. et al. (2020). Quarantine an effective mode for control of the spread of COVID19? A review. *Journal of Family Medicine Primary Care* 9 (8): 3867.

Pumipuntu, N. and Piratae, S. (2018). Cryptosporidiosis: a zoonotic disease concern. *Veterinary World* 11 (5): 681–686.

Reisen, W., Milby, M., Presser, S.B., and Hardy, J. (1992). Ecology of mosquitoes and St. Louis encephalitis virus in the Los Angeles Basin of California, 1987–1990. *Journal of Medical Entomology* 29: 582–598.

Reisen, W.K., Lundstrom, J.O., Scott, T.W. et al. (2000). Patterns of avian seroprevalence to western equine encephalomyelitis and Saint Louis encephalitis viruses in California, USA. *Journal of Medical Entomology* 37 (4): 507–527.

van Seventer, J.M. and Hochberg, N.S. (2017). *Principles of Infectious Diseases: Transmission, Diagnosis, Prevention, and Control*. St Louis: Elsevier.

World Health Organization (WHO) (1986). Ottawa Charter for Health Promotion. www.who.int/teams/health-promotion/enhanced-wellbeing/first-global-conference (accessed 14 February 2024).

50

Accident Prevention for Animal Well-being

Abbas Rabiu Ishaq

Paws and Claws Specialist Veterinary Clinic, Riyadh, KSA

50.1 Introduction

An accident is any event that causes bodily injuries and can occur due to many animal/human interactions (Runyan 2003; Woodward 2013). An accident is an unforeseen event that occurs especially due to ignorance or carelessness.

50.2 Accident Investigation

This can be achieved by the sequential timed events plotting (STEP) procedure (Hendrick and Benner 1986). Animal restraint and handling are major risk factors for personnel and livestock accidents on the farm (Grandin 2008). Agriculture falls among occupations that have numerous reported accidents globally (WHO 2018), with up to 170000 being reported annually from the European Union (McNamara et al. 2018).

Farms are mostly located in the countryside, equipped with infrastructure, buildings, livestock, machinery/equipment (such as motor vehicles, milking machines, generators, incubators, incinerators, etc.) and numerous chemicals, all of which have potential for inducing accidents (Field and Tormoehlen 2005).

50.3 Accident Categories

Accidents can broadly be personnel associated or livestock associated (Doyle and Conroy 1989) (Figure 50.1). Personnel injuries come from riding horseback, sorting/penning cattle, and livestock handling equipment (Boyle et al. 1997). This is mostly seen among cattle/livestock raisers and cattle dealers (Douphrate et al. 2009). Personnel injuries are mostly scrapes/abrasions, cuts/lacerations, fractures, and contusions. These frequently affect the head/skull and the hand/wrist/fingers. The majority of farm animal-inflicted personnel injuries are from horses or cattle, less so for pigs, dogs, etc. (Rivara 1997). McNamara et al. (2019) categorized farm accidents as relating to machinery/vehicles, organizational, livestock, slurry related, trips, falls, buildings related, and electrical based on their possible causes.

50.3.1 Occupational/Personnel Accidents

Occupational/personnel accidents occur more often in agriculture compared to construction projects (Horsburgh et al. 2001) (Figure 50.2). This can include loss of control of the machine, transport/handling equipment, hand-held tools, animal inflicted, objects breaking, bursting, splitting, slipping, falling, and collapsing (Javadi and Rostami 2007).

Epidemiology and Environmental Hygiene in Veterinary Public Health, First Edition. Edited by Tanmoy Rana.
© 2025 John Wiley & Sons, Inc. Published 2025 by John Wiley & Sons, Inc.

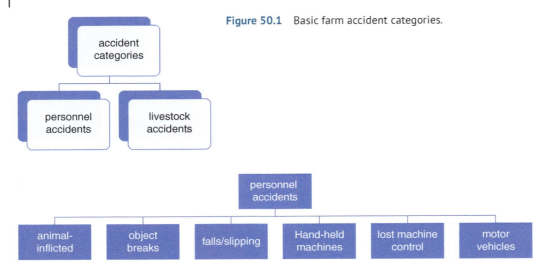

Figure 50.1 Basic farm accident categories.

Figure 50.2 Causes of farm personnel accidents.

50.3.2 Livestock Accidents

Livestock accidents occur on the farm or during transit (Valadez-Noriega et al. 2018). Transit of livestock to auctions, feedlots, abattoirs or other farms is essential for production (Gilkeson et al. 2016). This may adversely affect the need for protection and management of animal welfare at all levels (Thomson et al. 2015).

Livestock transportation can expose animals to several forms of accidents ranging from adverse weather conditions, morbidity (Grandin 2014), fatigue, loading/unloading injuries, severe noise stress, thermal stress, mortality, immunity suppression, and infections (Cernicchiaro et al. 2012; Miranda-De La Lama et al. 2014). Bertocchi et al. (2018) indicated that housing and management factors such as inadequate or slippery flooring, poor bedding materials, poor planning for trimming and inspection processes expose livestock to hazards on the farm. Valadez-Noriega et al. (2018) stated that breaches of animal welfare were precursors for farm animal accidents. Animal welfare is the humane and responsible treatment of animals by humans in charge of them, in relation to breeding, feeding, medical care, and other aspects such as transportation (Kumar et al. 2022).

50.4 Types of Accidents

Accident types, possible causes, frequencies, and various methods of prevention are presented below (Figures 50.3 and 50.4).

50.4.1 Transport Vehicle Accidents

Woods and Grandin (2008) published a research paper on livestock transport accidents in the United States and Canada between 1994 and June 2007. They collected data such as time of day, month of the year, animal species involved, gross/percentage losses, truck type/part affected, and immediate cause of accident. With respect to the time of the day, about 59% of these accidents occurred during the early hours, that is 12 midnight to 9 a.m., mostly due to driver error (Woods and Grandin 2008). McCartt et al. (2000) emphasized that most accidents occur during late nights and early mornings and are related to driver sleep deprivation during long-haul journeys. This is in line with the findings of Mitler et al. (1997). With respect to species and truck types, two-deck trucks loaded with cattle have more accidents (Mitler et al. 1997; Woods and Grandin 2008). Single drivers carrying livestock over long distances for periods up to 20 hours have more accidents compared to two drivers taking turns, attributed to fatigue (Hartley et al. 1994).

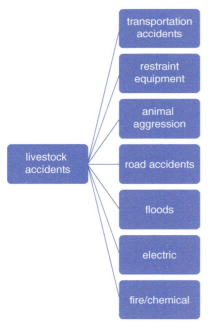

Figure 50.3 Sources of livestock accidents.

50.4.2 Road Accidents

Besides accidents during animal transport as mentioned above (McCartt et al. 2000), animals can escape from farms and get hit by passing road traffic. This is mostly seen in newly introduced bulls that try to return to their previous homes (Smith et al. 1989).

50.4.3 Animal Handling/Restraint Accidents

Handling fearful animals can lead to severe injuries for the animals and the handlers (Grandin 1999) (Figure 50.5). Fear is a survival extinct seen in all animals (Boissy 1998; Grandin 1997). An understanding of animal behavior especially during handling will reduce the chances for injury of personnel and animals. Most animal handling accidents arise from male aggression, faulty equipment, maternal aggression, fear, and agitation (Grandin 1999).

50.4.4 Faulty Facility Injuries

Grandin (1999) assessed restraint facilities such as manual squeeze chutes and hydraulic-powered chutes. About 20% of animal/personnel injuries occur around the squeeze chutes on a farm (Huhnke et al. 1997). Manual squeeze chute accidents occur due to ratchet loosening, hip entanglement on the headgate, and chocking of animal/personnel on the headgate (Grandin 1980b). On the other hand, injuries during use of hydraulic-powered chutes arise because of failure of pressure relief valves, making them safer than the manual ones (Grandin 1999).

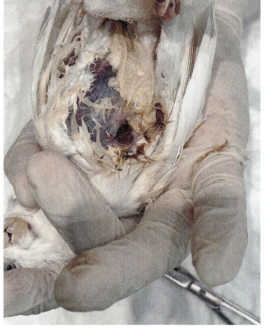

Figure 50.4 A psittacine bird attacked by a cat. The bird sustained four massive wounds around the keel muscles and under the wing. *Source:* Dr Farida Abubakar (DVM).

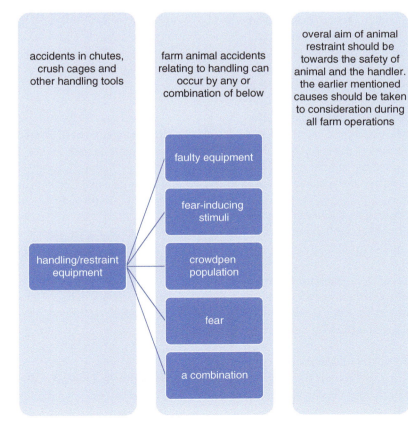

Figure 50.5 Possible causes of injuries on farm animals during handling.

50.4.4.1 Precautionary Measures to Avoid Machinery Injuries

Provision of adequate lighting for enclosed restraint facilities as animals are commonly afraid of dark places (Grandin 1982; Van Putten and Elshoff 1978).

- Removing any form of distraction that can cause an animal to deviate from target restraint such as people approaching, water splashes, rapid air movements, banging sounds of metals, metallic light reflections, and dripping water (Grandin 1996).
- Use of solid-sided loading ramps with single file around the squeeze and crowd pens (Grandin 1980a).
- Constructing man-gates for personnel escape, nonslip flooring, anti-backup gates, equipment maintenance, and noise reduction (Grandin 1999).

50.4.5 Fear as a Source of Animal Accidents During Restraint

Fear is a conditioned reflex in upper animals (vertebrates) in general (LeDoux and Phelps 1993), involving the brain (Davis 1992). Grandin (1997) observed that animals being put into squeeze chutes or corral systems for the first time exhibit high levels of fear and that avoidance of painful manipulations will help. Grandin (1999) conducted research on understanding fear responses in animals during handling, as follows.

50.4.5.1 Hearing Patterns

There is species variation in sound pitch perception (Grandin 1999). Horses tend to be disturbed at 1000–16 000 Hz (Heffner and Heffner 1983), cattle are more sensitive at 8000 Hz, sheep at 7000 Hz (Ames and Arehart 1972; Heffner and Heffner 1983), and pigs 8000 Hz (Talling et al. 1996).

50.4.5.2 Sight Perception

Cattle and horses are not color blind as some used to claim (Gilbert and Arave 1986), except that the ability to differentiate green colors in horses is weaker (Pick et al. 1994). Grazing animals have wider angles of view that can go beyond 300°, except for the blind spots that are directly behind their bodies (Prince 1977). Ruminants perceive depth by standing still and lowering the head (Lemmon and Patterson 1964). Injuries are prevented with respect to sight by taking account of blind spots of animals and not approaching them from that angle (Grandin 1999).

50.4.5.3 Animal Behavior Patterns

Understanding fear-induced behavioral changes in animals will reduce the chances of accidents (Huhnke et al. 1997). Animals separated from the herd tend to be afraid and can do anything to get back to the herd, thereby increasing the chances of harm to themselves or personnel by sudden movements (Grandin 1987). Key behavioral factors to be considered when handling animals are discussed below.

50.4.5.3.1 Movement Patterns

The easiest and safest way to move animals is by taking note of their point of balance, which is an imaginary line near the shoulder (Pas et al. 1998). Standing behind the point of balance makes the animal move forward, while standing in front makes the animal move backwards (Grandin 1998; Kilgour and Dalton 1984). Previously agitated animals will usually return to normal when allowed to rest for some minutes, making them easier to handle (Stermer et al. 1981).

50.4.5.3.2 Crowd Pen Population

Overstocking the crowd pens increases aggressive behavior in larger animals. Bovines and equines should be moved in smaller groups, while ovines can be a bit more densely packed (Grandin 1999).

50.4.5.3.3 Fear-inducing Stimuli

Most farm animals exhibit some level of agitation and fear when they are subjected to unfamiliar stimuli (Dantzer and Mormède 1983; Grandin 1997). This undesired response leading to potential accidents can be minimized by careful handling and training the animals (Grandin 1999).

50.4.5.3.4 Flight Zone

The flight zone is the range of space around which the animal feels safe in the presence of handlers or other animals and can increase/decrease with respect to the individual animal's temperament and level of domestication (Grandin 1980a).

An understanding of these flight zones by handlers and veterinarians is crucial (Grandin 1987, 1994; Grandin and Deesing 2022). Riding horses and show horses have no flight zones compared to cattle that only occasionally see humans (Grandin 1980b).

50.4.5.3.5 History of Previous Handling

Young animals, especially calves, when raised under supervision tend to be more easily handled at maturity (Pascoe 1986; Rushen 1986). However, this can be difficult in cases where the animals were handled in a cruel manner because some animals have good memories of past events (Grandin et al. 1986; Hutson 1985).

50.4.5.3.6 Habituation of Animal toward a Routine

Some farm animals easily habituate to certain levels of nonpain-associated procedures (Alam and Dobson 1986; Crookshank et al. 1979; Peischel et al. 1980) such as being moved gently through squeeze chutes (Grandin and Deesing 2022). It is difficult to habituate animals that have high levels of fear even with several attempts (Lanier et al. 1995).

50.4.5.3.7 Animal Aggression

Farm animal aggression toward handlers and veterinarians varies by species, sex, and purpose of keeping, for example male and maternal aggression (Price and Wallach 1990). Male aggression is more commonly seen in dairy bulls than in beef bulls, while maternal aggression is seen in animals with newborns (Grandin 1999). Early male castration reduces aggression toward handlers (Pas et al. 1998).

50.4.5.4 Floods

Flooding is an extensive spread of water across a geographical location due to heavy rainfall, dam failure or inadequate drainage systems (Gardiner 1995). Collins et al. (2014) put floods into four categories (Figure 50.6).

- Flash floods that last for a few hours.
- Single event floods, with long duration.
- Multiple event floods.
- Seasonal floods occurring mostly during the rainy months.

Floods can also be classified based on source.

- Rainfall.
- Dam failure.
- Ice melt.
- Tidal/sea surge floods (Gautam and Van Der Hoek 2003).

Damage caused by floods can be direct or indirect (Smith et al. 1989). Morphological changes seen along riverbanks form the basis of assessing the impacts of floods (Gardiner 1995). One of the environmental threats seen with floods is dispersal of environmental wastes, increasing the risk of animal infections (Montz and Tobin 2008).

Schmidt (2000) reported a massive number of deaths of cattle, pigs, chickens, and turkeys as a result of a hurricane flood.

50.4.6 Electric Accidents

Electric accidents come from electric fences, earthing faults or faulty underground wiring. Any voltage more than 1 affects milk/beef production, while higher voltages up to 25 can cause death (Baker 2000). Electric fencing is a safe and economical way of demarcating animal farms but the use of poorly designed fencing poses a risk of animal electrocution (Dalziel 1950).

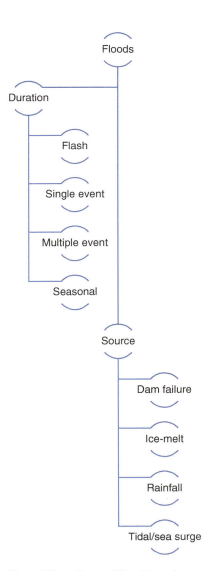

Figure 50.6 Types of flood based on duration and possible sources.

50.4.7 Fire and Chemical Accidents

Livestock can be subject to fire hazards, hydrocarbon (organic/petrochemical) poisoning (Moussa and Devarakonda 2014), and heavy metals poisoning (Mandal 2017). Moussa and Devarakonda (2014) analyzed the chances of fire outbreaks, oil spillages, explosions, and noxious release of gases from chemical storage plants. Chemicals posing accident risks to animals can be corrosive, toxic, reactive, or flammable. Gross incidences have direct relation with storage temperatures (Wilkinson 1991). Farm animals are at higher risks, owing to the common proximities of farms to these storage plants in the countryside (Lead 1995). Fire outbreaks are the most frequent of all chemical storage accidents (Chang and Lin 2006). These storage fire outbreaks occur due to overfilling of tanks, release of chemicals during maintenance, release during operation, leakages of tanks, fire engulfment or drastic tank failure (Moussa and Devarakonda 2014). Risks associated with these fire outbreaks and chemical exposure can be assessed based on the following scales: time factor, exposure factor, inventory factor damage/injury intensity, and energy factor (Lees 2012).

Prevention of these accidents can be achieved by building farms away from storage facilities (Moussa and Devarakonda 2014), building dike walls/bunds to demarcate storage tanks (Wilkinson 1991), and maintenance of fire extinguishers (Rains 2009).

Heavy chemical/mineral poisoning in animals can arise from grasses, contaminated drinking water, vegetables, and feed additives (Mandal 2017). The emission of these heavy metals occurs by air, surface water, and soil (Mazumder 2008). Exposure of monogastric animals to chemicals such as thallium, copper, arsenic, and phenol causes nervous signs, toxemia, and dysentery (Smith et al. 2006).

Arsenic can be organic or inorganic; inorganic forms are associated with contaminated drinking waters while organic forms are seen in aquatic animals such as fish (WHO 2003). Once an animal is exposed to an items contaminated with arsenic (Guha Mazumder 2003), it is absorbed and retained in blood, feces, urine, tissues, hair, and skin. When the dung is used as manure, it increases the circulation of this agent (Pal et al. 2007). Of all the possible sources, contaminated groundwater is the most common means of exposure, which when prolonged can cause cancer (of lungs, urinary bladder, and skin) (Kadirvel et al. 2007), liver fibrosis, anemia, skin hyperpigmentation, toe gangrene, hepatomegaly, lung disease, and neuropathy (Guha Mazumder 2003; Mazumder 2008). Arsenic exposure in beef cattle lead to anorexia, lethargy, diarrhea, ataxia, and death (Faires 2004). Clinical reports in goats revealed that most ingested arsenic is deposited in the liver, spleen, and kidney, while excretion is chiefly via urine and feces (Selby et al. 1974). Chronic arsenic poisoning in cattle (Mandal 2017) brings about fibrosis, manifested as joint stiffness and asymmetrical enlargement of limb joints such as the hock (Smith et al. 2006). Diarrhea, stiff gait, lameness, tremor, convulsions, coffee-colored urine, ruminal amotility, drooling saliva, hindquarter paresis, increased heart/respiratory rate, and congested mucosae are seen in acute/per-acute experimentation of arsenic poisoning. Chronic experimental arsenic exposure in goats manifested as polyuria, coffee-colored urine, congested mucosae, and loss of weight (Biswas et al. 2000).

Arsenic has been used as a feed additive for livestock since the 1940s in many countries (Mazumder 2008). Regulated amounts of 2 mg/kg for all species and 10 mg/kg for fishes and fur animals are acceptable (Radostits et al. 1994; Bampidis et al. 2013). Depending on exposure dose, absorbed arsenic targets the erythrocytes and binds to the globin part of hemoglobin (Radostits et al. 1994; Järup 2003) before being passed to the skin and hair due to its high affinity for the sulfur incorporated in the proteins of these tissues (NRC 1999).

Arsenic exists as either trivalent or pentavalent forms, with the first being more damaging (Mizumura et al. 2010). It suppresses mitochondrial enzymatic reactions thus resulting in impairment of tissue respiration (Singh and Rana 2010). Other effects include altered mitochondrial membrane potential, leading to apoptosis (Paul et al. 2008; Obinaju 2009), release of reactive oxygen species (Lewińska et al. 2007; Colognato et al. 2007), and suppression of DNA replication (Miller Jr et al. 2002; Paul et al. 2008).

50.4.7.1 Controlling Arsenic Poisoning

This can be achieved through control of drinking water quality (Merck 2005; NRC 2001; WHO 2010). Ascorbic acid reduces mitochondrial membrane damage under experimental conditions (Bampidis et al. 2013; Singh and Rana 2010).

50.4.7.2 Lead Poisoning

Farm animal lead poisoning occurs mostly by oral ingestion of lead-containing products, contaminated water, and pastures (Oskarsson et al. 1992) (Figure 50.7). It occurs less frequently from skin penetration from lead-containing skin applications and inhalation (Lemos et al. 2004). Sources of lead include grease, car lubricants, lead accumulators, pipes, and paints (Traverso et al. 2004). Lead poisoning susceptibility is higher in cattle (Traverso et al. 2004; Guagnini et al. 2005; Marçal 2005)

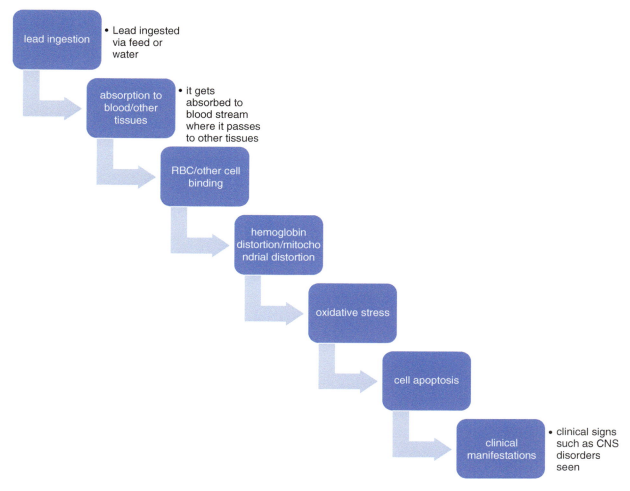

Figure 50.7 Pathogenesis of lead poisoning in livestock.

than in birds (Mazliah et al. 1989), small animals (Morgan 1994), goats (Borelli et al. 2013), horses (Palacios et al. 2002), and sheep (Liu 2003).

Lead poisoning in farm animals, especially cattle, is evidenced by teeth grinding, muscle tremors, blindness, nasal discharges, head pushing toward objects (Lemos et al. 2004), tongue atony, excessive salivation, inappetence, labored breathing, proprioceptive disorders (Barbosa et al. 2014), and death (Traverso et al. 2004). Poultry lead poisoning mostly manifests as a drop in egg production, due to interference with calcium and zinc absorption, leading to vitamin D metabolism defects (Lead 1995). Pathological changes, though rare, include kidney tubular necrosis in chicken and mild cortical astrocytosis in calf brain (Krametter-Froetscher et al. 2007). Traverso et al. (2004) reported pathological changes such as gliosis, neuronal necrosis, cerebrocortical malacia, and renal convoluted tubular inclusion bodies.

50.4.7.3 Organophosphate Poisoning Accidents

Organophosphate chemicals such as terbufos cause acute poisoning in farm animals, manifested as salivation, diarrhea, dyspnea, rumen amotility, etc. (Khan 2001). Poisoning can be reversed when noticed early with high doses of atropine sulfate (Boermans et al. 1984)

References

Alam, M.G. and Dobson, H. (1986). Effect of various veterinary procedures on plasma concentrations of cortisol, luteinising hormone and prostaglandin F2 alpha metabolite in the cow. *Veterinary Record* 118 (1): 7–10.

Ames, D.R. and Arehart, L.A. (1972). Physiological response of lambs to auditory stimuli. *Journal of Animal Science* 34 (6): 994–998.

Baker, D. E. (2000). How to prevent electrical accidents. https://mospace.umsystem.edu/xmlui/handle/10355/50854?show=full (accessed 15 February 2024).

Bampidis, V.A., Nistor, E., and Nitas, D. (2013). Arsenic, cadmium, lead and mercury as undesirable substances in animal feeds. *Scientific Papers: Animal Science & Biotechnologies* 46 (1): 17–22.

Barbosa, J.D., Bomjardim, H.D.A., Campos, K.F. et al. (2014). Lead poisoning in cattle and chickens in the state of Pará, Brazil. *Pesquisa Veterinária Brasileira* 34: 1077–1080.

Bertocchi, L., Fusi, F., Angelucci, A. et al. (2018). Characterization of hazards, welfare promoters and animal-based measures for the welfare assessment of dairy cows: elicitation of expert opinion. *Preventive Veterinary Medicine* 150: 8–18.

Biswas, U., Sarkar, S., Bhowmik, M.K. et al. (2000). Chronic toxicity of arsenic in goats: clinicobiochemical changes, pathomorphology and tissue residues. *Small Ruminant Research* 38 (3): 229–235.

Boermans, H.J., Black, W.D., Chesney, J. et al. (1984). Terbufos poisoning in a dairy herd. *Canadian Veterinary Journal* 25 (9): 335.

Boissy, A. (1998). Fear and fearfulness in determining behavior. In: *Genetics and the Behaviour of Domestic Animals* (ed. T. Grandin), 67–111.

Borelli, V., Salete Wisser, C., Emmerich, T. et al. (2013). Intoxicação por chumbo em bovinos em santa Catarina. *Archives of Veterinary Science* 18: 3.

Boyle, D., Gerberich, S.G., Gibson, R.W. et al. (1997). Injury from dairy cattle activities. *Epidemiology* 8 (1): 37–41.

Cernicchiaro, N., Renter, D.G., White, B.J. et al. (2012). Associations between weather conditions during the first 45 days after feedlot arrival and daily respiratory disease risks in autumn-placed feeder cattle in the United States. *Journal of Animal Science* 90 (4): 1328–1337.

Chang, J.I. and Lin, C.C. (2006). A study of storage tank accidents. *Journal of Loss Prevention in the Process Industries* 19 (1): 51–59.

Collins, M.J., Kirk, J.P., Pettit, J. et al. (2014). Annual floods in New England (USA) and Atlantic Canada: synoptic climatology and generating mechanisms. *Physical Geography* 35 (3): 195–219.

Colognato, R., Coppede, F., Ponti, J. et al. (2007). Genotoxicity induced by arsenic compounds in peripheral human lymphocytes analysed by cytokinesis-block micronucleus assay. *Mutagenesis* 22 (4): 255–261.

Crookshank, H.R., Elissalde, M.H., White, R.G. et al. (1979). Effect of transportation and handling of calves upon blood serum composition. *Journal of Animal Science* 48 (3): 430–435.

Dalziel, C.F. (1950). Electric fences – their hazards, types, regulations, and safe application. *Transactions of the American Institute of Electrical Engineers* 69 (1): 8–15.

Dantzer, R. and Morméde, P. (1983). Stress in farm animals: a need for reevaluation. *Journal of Animal Science* 57 (1): 6–18.

Davis, M. (1992). The role of the amygdala in fear and anxiety. *Annual Review of Neuroscience* 15 (1): 353–375.

Douphrate, D.I., Rosecrance, J.C., Stallones, L. et al. (2009). Livestock-handling injuries in agriculture: an analysis of Colorado workers' compensation data. *American Journal of Industrial Medicine* 52 (5): 391–407.

Doyle, Y. and Conroy, R. (1989). The spectrum of farming accidents seen in Irish general practice: a one-year survey. *Family Practice* 6 (1): 38–41.

Faires, M.C. (2004). Inorganic arsenic toxicosis in a beef herd. *Canadian Veterinary Journal* 45 (4): 329.

Field, W.E. and Tormoehlen, R.L. (2005). Education and training as intervention strategies. In: *Agricultural Medicine: A Practical Guide* (ed. J. Lessenger), 42–52. New York: Springer.

Gardiner, J. (1995). Developing flood defence as a sustainable hazard alleviation measure. In: *Defence from Floods and Floodplain Management* (ed. J. Gardiner, O. Starosolszky, and Y. Yevjevich), 13–40. Dordrecht: Springer Netherlands.

Gautam, K.P. and Van Der Hoek, E.E. (2003). *Literature Study on Environmental Impact of Floods*. Netherlands: Delft Cluster.

Gilbert, B.J. Jr. and Arave, C.W. (1986). Ability of cattle to distinguish among different wavelengths of light. *Journal of Dairy Science* 69 (3): 825–832.

Gilkeson, C.A., Thompson, H.M., Wilson, M.C.T., and Gaskell, P.H. (2016). Quantifying passive ventilation within small livestock trailers using computational fluid dynamics. *Computers and Electronics in Agriculture* 124: 84–99.

Grandin, T. (1980a). Good cattle-restraining equipment is essential. *Veterinary Medicine Small Animal Clinician* 75 (8): 1291–1296.

Grandin, T. (1980b). Observations of cattle behavior applied to the design of cattle-handling facilities. *Applied Animal Ethology* 6 (1): 19–31.

Grandin, T. (1982). Pig behavior studies applied to slaughter-plant design. *Applied Animal Ethology* 9 (2): 141–151.

Grandin, T. (1987). Animal handling. *Veterinary Clinics of North America: Food Animal Practice* 3 (2): 323–338. http://dx.doi.org/10.1016/S0749-0720(15)31155-5.

Grandin, T. (1994). Solving livestock handling problems. *Veterinary Medicine* 89 (10): 989–998.

Grandin, T. (1996). Factors that impeded animal movement at slaughter plants. *Journal of the American Veterinary Medical Association* 209: 757–759.

Grandin, T. (1997). Assessment of stress during handling and transport. *Journal of Animal Science* 75 (1): 249–257.

Grandin, T. (1998). Handling methods and facilities to reduce stress on cattle. *Veterinary Clinics of North America: Food Animal Practice* 14 (2): 325–341.

Grandin, T. (1999). Safe handling of large animals. *Occupational Medicine* 14: 195–212.

Grandin, T. (2008). *Humane Livestock Handling*. New York: Storey Publishing.

Grandin, T. (2014). Animal welfare and society concerns finding the missing link. *Meat Science* 98 (3): 461–469.

Grandin, T. and Deesing, M.J. (2022). Genetics and behavior during handling, restraint, and herding. In: *Genetics and the Behavior of Domestic Animals*, 131–181. Cambridge: Academic Press.

Grandin, T., Curtis, S.E., Widowski, T.M., and Thurmon, J.C. (1986). Electro-immobilization versus mechanical restraint in an avoid-avoid choice test for ewes. *Journal of Animal Science* 62 (6): 1469–1480.

Guagnini, F.D.S., Corrêa, A.M.R., Colodel, E.M. et al. (2005). Intoxicação por chumbo em bovinos em área de treinamento militar. *Actae Scientiae Veterinariae* 46: 253.

Guha Mazumder, D.N. (2003). Chronic arsenic toxicity: clinical features, epidemiology, and treatment: experience in West Bengal. *Journal of Environmental Science and Health, Part A* 38 (1): 141–163.

Hartley, L.R., Arnold, P.K., Smythe, G., and Hansen, J. (1994). Indicators of fatigue in truck drivers. *Applied Ergonomics* 25 (3): 143–156.

Heffner, R.S. and Heffner, H.E. (1983). Hearing in large mammals: horses (Equus caballus) and cattle (Bos taurus). *Behavioral Neuroscience* 97 (2): 299.

Hendrick, K. and Benner, L. (1986). *Investigating Accidents with STEP*, vol. 13. Boca Raton: CRC Press.

Horsburgh, S., Feyer, A.M., and Langley, J.D. (2001). Fatal work related injuries in agricultural production and services to agriculture sectors of New Zealand, 1985–94. *Occupational and Environmental Medicine* 58 (8): 489–495.

Huhnke, R.L., Hubert, D.J., and Harp, S.L. (1997). *Identifying Injuries Sustained on Cow Calf Operations in Oklahoma*. St Joseph: American Society of Agricultural Engineers.

Hutson, G.D. (1985). The influence of barley food rewards on sheep movement through a handling system. *Applied Animal Behaviour Science* 14 (3): 263–273.

Järup, L. (2003). Hazards of heavy metal contamination. *British Medical Bulletin* 68 (1): 167–182.

Javadi, A. and Rostami, M.A. (2007). Safety assessments of agricultural machinery in Iran. *Journal of Agricultural Safety and Health* 13 (3): 275–284.

Kadirvel, R., Sundaram, K., Mani, S. et al. (2007). Supplementation of ascorbic acid and α-tocopherol prevents arsenic-induced protein oxidation and DNA damage induced by arsenic in rats. *Human & Experimental Toxicology* 26 (12): 939–946.

Khan, O. (2001). Organophosphate poisoning in a group of replacement heifers and dry cows. *Canadian Veterinary Journal* 42 (7): 561–563.

Kilgour, R. and Dalton, C. (1984). Farrowing pens and behaviour. In: *Livestock Behaviour: A Practical Guide* (ed. R. Kilgour), 150–191. London: Routledge.

Krametter-Froetscher, R., Tataruch, F., Hauser, S. et al. (2007). Toxic effects seen in a herd of beef cattle following exposure to ash residues contaminated by lead and mercury. *Veterinary Journal* 174 (1): 99–105.

Kumar, P., Singh, A., Rajput, V.D. et al. (2022). Role of artificial intelligence, sensor technology, big data in agriculture: next-generation farming. *Bioinformatics in Agriculture* 625–639.

Lanier, E.K., Friend, T.H., Bushong, D.M. et al. (1995). Swim habituation as a model for eustress and distress in the pig. *Journal of Animal Science* 73 (Suppl. 1): 126.

Lead, I.I. (1995). *Environmental Health Criteria 165*, vol. 38, 93–99. Geneva: World Health Organization.

LeDoux, J.E. and Phelps, E.A. (1993). Emotional networks in the brain. *Handbook of Emotions* 109: 118.

Lees, F. (2012). *Lees' Loss Prevention in the Process Industries: Hazard Identification, Assessment and Control*. Oxford: Butterworth-Heinemann.

Lemmon, W.B. and Patterson, G.H. (1964). Depth perception in sheep: effects of interrupting the mother–neonate bond. *Science* 145 (3634): 835–836.

Lemos, R.A., Driemeier, D., Guimarães, E.B. et al. (2004). Lead poisoning in cattle grazing pasture contaminated by industrial waste. *Veterinary and Human Toxicology* 46 (6): 326–328.

Lewińska, D., Arkusz, J., Stańczyk, M. et al. (2007). Comparison of the effects of arsenic and cadmium on benzo (a) pyrene-induced micronuclei in mouse bone-marrow. *Mutation Research/Genetic Toxicology and Environmental Mutagenesis* 632 (1–2): 37–43.

Liu, Z.P. (2003). Lead poisoning combined with cadmium in sheep and horses in the vicinity of non-ferrous metal smelters. *Science of the Total Environment* 309 (1–3): 117–126.

Mandal, P. (2017). An insight of environmental contamination of arsenic on animal health. *Emerging Contaminants* 3 (1): 17–22. http://dx.doi.org/10.1016/j.emcon.2017.01.004.

Marçal, W.S. (2005). Intoxicação por chumbo em gado bovino em zona rural próxima a indústria metalífera. *Veterinária Notícias* 11 (1): 87–93.

Mazliah, J., Barron, S., Bental, E., and Reznik, I. (1989). The effect of chronic lead intoxication in mature chickens. *Avian Diseases* 33: 566–570.

Mazumder, D.G. (2008). Chronic arsenic toxicity and human health. *Indian Journal of Medical Research* 128 (4): 436–447.

McCartt, A.T., Rohrbaugh, J.W., Hammer, M.C., and Fuller, S.Z. (2000). Factors associated with falling asleep at the wheel among long-distance truck drivers. *Accident Analysis & Prevention* 32 (4): 493–504. http://dx.doi.org/10.1016/S0001-4575(99)00067-6.

McNamara, J., Leppälä, J., van der Laan, G. et al. (2018). 1768 Safety culture and risk management in agriculture (sacurima). *Occupational and Environmental Medicine* 75: A462.2–A462.

McNamara, J., Griffin, P., Phelan, J. et al. (2019). Farm health and safety adoption through engineering and behaviour change. *Agronomy Research* 17: 1–7.

Miller, W.H. Jr., Schipper, H.M., Lee, J.S. et al. (2002). Mechanisms of action of arsenic trioxide. *Cancer Research* 62 (14): 3893–3903.

Miranda-De La Lama, G.C., Villarroel, M., and María, G.A. (2014). Livestock transport from the perspective of the pre-slaughter logistic chain: a review. *Meat Science* 98 (1): 9–20.

Mitler, M.M., Miller, J.C., Lipsitz, J.J. et al. (1997). The sleep of long-haul truck drivers. *New England Journal of Medicine* 337 (11): 755–762.

Mizumura, A., Watanabe, T., Kobayashi, Y., and Hirano, S. (2010). Identification of arsenite- and arsenic diglutathione-binding proteins in human hepatocarcinoma cells. *Toxicology and Applied Pharmacology* 242 (2): 119–125.

Montz, B.E. and Tobin, G.A. (2008). Livin' large with levees: lessons learned and lost. *Natural Hazards Review* 9 (3): 150–157.

Morgan, R.V. (1994). Lead poisoning in small companion animals: an update (1987–1992). *Veterinary and Human Toxicology* 36 (1): 18–22.

Moussa, N. A. and Devarakonda, V. (2014). Prediction of toxic emissions from chemical fire and explosion. Fire Safety Science – Proceedings of the Eleventh International Symposium.

National Research Council (1999). *Arsenic in Drinking Water*. Washington, DC: National Academies Press.

National Research Council (2001). *Nutrient Requirements of Dairy Cattle: 2001*. Washington, DC: National Academies Press, National Academies Press.

Obinaju, B.E. (2009). Mechanisms of arsenic toxicity and carcinogenesis. *African Journal of Biochemistry Research* 3 (5): 232–237.

Oskarsson, A., Jorhem, L., Sundberg, J. et al. (1992). Lead poisoning in cattle – transfer of lead to milk. *Science of the Total Environment* 111 (2–3): 83–94.

Pal, A., Nayak, B., Das, B. et al. (2007). Additional danger of arsenic exposure through inhalation from burning of cow dung cakes laced with arsenic as a fuel in arsenic affected villages in Ganga–Meghna–Brahmaputra plain. *Journal of Environmental Monitoring* 9 (10): 1067–1070.

Palacios, H., Iribarren, I., Olalla, M.J., and Cala, V. (2002). Lead poisoning of horses in the vicinity of a battery recycling plant. *Science of the Total Environment* 290 (1–3): 81–89.

Pas, T.G., Oldfield, J.E., and Boyd, L.J. (1998). Reducing handling stress improves both productivity and welfare. *Professional Animal Scientist* 14 (1): 1–10.

Pascoe, P.J. (1986). Humaneness of an electroimmobilization unit for cattle. *American Journal of Veterinary Research* 47 (10): 2252–2256.

Paul, M.K., Kumar, R., and Mukhopadhyay, A.K. (2008). Dithiothreitol abrogates the effect of arsenic trioxide on normal rat liver mitochondria and human hepatocellular carcinoma cells. *Toxicology and Applied Pharmacology* 226 (2): 140–152.

Peischel, A., Schalles, R.R., and Owenby, C.E. (1980). Effect of stress on calves grazing Kansas Hills range. *Journal of Animal Science* 51 (Suppl. 1): 245.

Pick, D.F., Lovell, G., Brown, S., and Dail, D. (1994). Equine color perception revisited. *Applied Animal Behaviour Science* 42 (1): 61–65.

Price, E.O. and Wallach, S.J. (1990). Physical isolation of hand-reared Hereford bulls increases their aggressiveness toward humans. *Applied Animal Behaviour Science* 27 (3): 263–267.

Prince, J.H. (1977). The eye and vision. In: *Dukes Physiology of Domestic Animals* (ed. M. Swenson). New York: Cornell University Press.

Radostits, O.M., Blood, D.C., and Gay, C.C. (1994). *Veterinary Medicine. A Textbook of the Diseases of Cattle, Sheep, Pigs, Goats and Horses*, 8e. London: Baillière Tindall.

Rains, G. C. (2009). Accident extrication procedures for farm families and employees. https://extension.uga.edu/publications/detail.html?number=C860&title=accident-extrication-procedures-for-farm-families-and-employees (accessed 15 February 2024).

Rivara, F.P. (1997). Fatal and non-fatal farm injuries to children and adolescents in the United States, 1990–3. *Injury Prevention* 3 (3): 190–194.

Runyan, C.W. (2003). Introduction: back to the future – revisiting Haddon's conceptualization of injury epidemiology and prevention. *Epidemiologic Reviews* 25 (1): 60–64.

Rushen, J. (1986). Aversion of sheep for handling treatments: paired-choice studies. *Applied Animal Behaviour Science* 16 (4): 363–370.

Schmidt, C.W. (2000). Lessons from the flood: will Floyd change livestock farming? *Environmental Health Perspectives* 108 (2): A74–A77.

Selby, L.A., Case, A.A., Dorn, C.R., and Wagstaff, D.J. (1974). Public health hazards associated with arsenic poisoning in cattle. *Journal of the American Veterinary Medical Association* 165 (11): 1010–1014.

Singh, S. and Rana, S.V.S. (2010). Ascorbic acid improves mitochondrial function in liver of arsenic-treated rat. *Toxicology and Industrial Health* 26 (5): 265–272.

Smith, S.R., Bouton, J.H., and Hoveland, C.S. (1989). Alfalfa persistence and regrowth potential under continuous grazing. *Agronomy Journal* 81 (6): 960–965.

Smith, A.H., Marshall, G., Yuan, Y. et al. (2006). Increased mortality from lung cancer and bronchiectasis in young adults after exposure to arsenic in utero and in early childhood. *Environmental Health Perspectives* 114 (8): 1293–1296.

Stermer, R.A., Camp, T.H., and Stevens, D.G. (1981). *Feeder Cattle Stress During Handling and Transportation*. St Joseph: American Society of Agricultural Engineers.

Talling, J.C., Waran, N.K., Wathes, C.M., and Lines, J.A. (1996). Behavioural and physiological responses of pigs to sound. *Applied Animal Behaviour Science* 48 (3–4): 187–201.

Thomson, D.U., Loneragan, G.H., Henningson, J.N. et al. (2015). Description of a novel fatigue syndrome of finished feedlot cattle following transportation. *Journal of the American Veterinary Medical Association* 247 (1): 66–72.

Traverso, S.D., Loretti, A.P., Donini, M.A., and Driemeier, D. (2004). Lead poisoning in cattle in southern Brazil. *Arquivo Brasileiro de Medicina Veterinária e Zootecnia* 56: 418–421.

Valadez-Noriega, M., Estévez-Moreno, L., Rayas-Amor, A. et al. (2018). Livestock hauliers' attitudes, knowledge and current practices towards animal welfare, occupational wellbeing and transport risk factors: a Mexican survey. *Preventive Veterinary Medicine* 160: 76–84.

Van Putten, G. and Elshoff, W.J. (1978). Observations on the effect of transport and slaughter on the well-being and lean quality of pigs. *Animal Regulation Studies* 1: 247–271.

Wilkinson, A. (1991). *Bund Overtopping – The Consequences Following Catastrophic Failure of Large Volume Liquid Storage Vessels*. London: HMSO.

Woods, J. and Grandin, T. (2008). Fatigue: a major cause of commercial livestock truck accidents. *Veterinaria Italiana* 44 (1): 259–262.

Woodward, G.C. (2013). *The Rhetoric of Intention in Human Affairs*. Lanham: Lexington Books.

World Health Organization (WHO) (2010). *Hardness in Drinking-Water: Background Document for Development of WHO Guidelines for Drinking-Water Quality*. Geneva: World Health Organization.

World Health Organization (WHO) (2003). *Arsenic in Drinking-Water: Background Document for Development of WHO Guidelines for Drinking-Water Quality*. Geneva: World Health Organization.

World Health Organization (WHO) (2018). *Occupational Safety and Health in Public Health Emergencies: A Manual for Protecting Health Workers and Responders*. Geneva: World Health Organization.

51

Maintenance of Industrial Hygiene

Mona Abdelghany Nasr[1] and Nourhan Eissa[2]

[1] *Department of Anatomy and Embryology, Faculty of Veterinary Medicine, University of Sadat City, Sadat City, Egypt*
[2] *Department of Animal Hygiene and Zoonoses, Faculty of Veterinary Medicine, University of Sadat City, Sadat City, Egypt*

51.1 Introduction

Industrial hygiene is the practice of identifying, evaluating, and controlling workplace hazards that can affect the health and well-being of workers. It involves monitoring and analyzing hazard exposure, implementing engineering solutions, and enforcing workplace controls to maintain a safe and healthy work environment (DiNardi 2003).

Industrial hygiene has been defined as "that science and art devoted to the anticipation, recognition, evaluation, and control of those environmental factors or stresses arising in or from the workplace, which may cause sickness, impaired health and well-being, or significant discomfort among workers" (Spellman 2017).

Industrial hygiene, also known as occupational hygiene, is the science and art of recognizing, evaluating, and controlling workplace conditions that may cause injury, illness, or discomfort to workers (Jacobs and Donham 1994).

The maintenance of industrial hygiene is crucial for promoting the health and safety of workers in various industries. By ensuring that workplace conditions are free from hazards and potential risks, organizations can protect their employees from injuries, illnesses, and discomfort (Dawson et al. 2021).

This chapter provides a comprehensive overview of the importance of maintaining industrial hygiene, discusses various strategies for maintenance, and presents relevant evidence-based practices. We will explore the importance of effectively maintaining industrial hygiene, the challenges organizations may face, and the strategies they can employ to ensure the ongoing maintenance of a safe work environment.

The challenges organizations may face in maintaining industrial hygiene include complexity and diversity of workplace hazards, changes in technology or processes, budget constraints, and lack of awareness or knowledge about occupational health and safety practices.

In today's fast-paced industrial world, ensuring the safety and well-being of workers is of vital importance. Industrial hygiene plays an important role in achieving this goal. It involves the anticipation, recognition, evaluation, and control of environmental factors that may cause physical or psychological harm or discomfort to workers (Figure 51.1). To effectively maintain industrial hygiene, it is vital to implement proactive measures, regular inspections, proper training, and continuous monitoring.

51.2 Industrial Hygiene Principles: Anticipation, Recognition, Evaluation, Control, and Confirmation

51.2.1 Anticipation of Health Hazards

The first step toward maintaining good industrial hygiene is the anticipation and recognition of potential hazards. This typically requires a survey of the workplace design, operations, processes, work tasks, materials, and worker population. A current inventory of chemicals and their safety data sheets will quickly identify all the chemical hazards in the workplace. This requires a thorough understanding of the work processes, materials used, and potential risks associated with

---

Epidemiology and Environmental Hygiene in Veterinary Public Health, First Edition. Edited by Tanmoy Rana.
© 2025 John Wiley & Sons, Inc. Published 2025 by John Wiley & Sons, Inc.

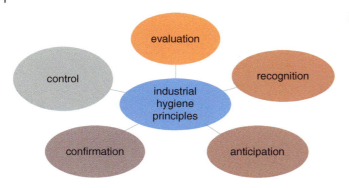

Figure 51.1 Industrial hygiene principles.

various tasks. Employers should identify possible health hazards related to exposure to chemicals, physical agents (such as noise or vibration), biological agents, ergonomic factors, and psychosocial stressors. By identifying these hazards, appropriate control measures can be put in place (Spellman 2017).

51.2.2 Recognition of Health Hazards

Recognition of health hazards is the second principle of industrial hygiene. It is important to recognize and understand the potential hazards of the work environment, internal processes, and job tasks, including chemical and physical hazards. For example, do some employees have greater exposure to occupational hazards because they work in an area with poor ventilation? Do their work tasks generate a lot of dust and are their work shifts or tasks longer? This also includes individual work tasks and how they affect adjacent work activities that could create exposure to hazards for other workers in the facility, also called simultaneous operations. Another step in recognizing health hazards is to determine if there are occupational exposure limits (OELs) or restrictions for the hazardous products identified in the chemical inventory.

51.2.3 Evaluation of Exposure

Evaluation of exposure is the third principle in industrial hygiene. Engineering, work practice, and administrative controls are the primary means of reducing employee exposure to occupational hazards. After anticipating and recognizing the health hazards, the risk of exposure should be evaluated through an occupational exposure assessment. Traditionally, evaluation means workplace monitoring. Due to the complexity of the work environment and the measuring instruments, monitoring should only be done by a qualified professional such as an industrial or occupational hygienist.

51.2.3.1 Industrial Hygiene Monitoring

Industrial hygiene monitoring captures the exposure level of a population of workers during their work activities at a certain time. This measurement can be conducted on those with the highest potential exposure, or a representative exposure; measurements can also refer to a similar exposure group (SEG), including workers who perform the same tasks at the same frequency, with similar materials.

Industrial hygiene monitoring measures a specific physical, biological or chemical agent where the exposure occurs. Monitoring also needs to consider variations in exposure during different work shifts or facility maintenance activities like turnaround. Monitoring will have a defined purpose or question it is trying to answer; generally, it is trying to determine if exposures are safely below or over the OELs for the hazardous product.

Qualitative and quantitative analysis of data gained from monitoring is used to determine if exposure results are acceptable, unacceptable, or uncertain. Coming to this conclusion requires a knowledge of the OEL in the relevant jurisdiction. OELs for long-term and short-term exposure to a hazardous substance vary by province, state, and country. Not all substances in commerce have OELs developed for them.

51.2.4 Control Over Worker Exposure

This is the next principle of industrial hygiene. When hazardous exposure is determined to be unacceptable, controls need to be implemented to protect workers. They should be used to guide decisions on a multifaceted approach to exposure

Table 51.1 The fundamental elements of industrial hygiene.

Anticipation/Recognition	Evaluation	Control
• Commitment	• Hazard identification	• Examination
• Planning	• Exposure assessment	• Substitution
• Design	• Monitoring studies	• Engineering
• Training	• Observation	• Administration
		• Protective equipment

control. Although people instinctively think of personal protective equipment (PPE) first, it should be the last control applied once elimination, substitution, engineering controls, and administrative practices have been considered.

51.2.5 Confirmation of Control Measures

Confirmation is the last principle of industrial hygiene. This step highlights the importance of assessing the performance of hazard control measures and subsequent worker exposures. Investigating existing or potential issues and applying corrective actions are also part of confirming that the industrial hygiene program is effective. Maintaining data and reports is also key to track and trend the success of the industrial hygiene program to prevent injury, illness, or negative effects to the well-being of workers.

51.2.6 Develop an Industrial Hygiene Program with CHAMP

The principles of industrial or occupational hygiene are dynamic and require continual evaluation and reassessment as new hazards are introduced to the workplace and facilities change. Following these principles will protect a workplace's most valuable asset: its people. Chemscape's Chemical Hazard Assessment Management Program, also known as CHAMP, has the tools to identify and effectively manage the chemical hazards in the workplace (Table 51.1).

51.3 Maintenance Strategies for Industrial Hygiene

51.3.1 Routine Inspections and Assessments

Regular inspections and assessments are essential for identifying potential hazards and monitoring workplace conditions. This strategy involves conducting walkthroughs, evaluating processes, and reviewing documentation to identify areas of improvement and implement necessary controls.

Routine inspection and assessment strategies can vary depending on the specific context and industry.

51.3.1.1 Steps of Routine Inspection
- *Planning*: define the purpose and objectives of the inspection or assessment. Determine the scope, frequency, and areas/activities to be inspected or assessed.
- *Documentation*: establish a record-keeping system to document the inspection/assessment findings. This may include checklists, forms, photos, and other relevant documents.
- *Preinspection/preassessment activities.*
  - Review relevant regulations, standards, policies, and procedures.
  - Identify potential hazards, risks, and compliance requirements related to the area or activities being assessed.
  - Ensure necessary equipment, tools, and resources are available for the inspection or assessment.
- *Execution.*
  - Conduct a physical inspection or assessment of the identified area or activities. This may involve visual inspections, measurements, sampling, interviews, and review of records.
  - Observe and evaluate the condition, performance, and compliance of equipment, processes, facilities, or systems.
  - Identify and document any noncompliances, deficiencies, hazards, or risks.

- *Analysis.*
  - Review and interpret collected data, observations, and information.
  - Assess the significance, seriousness, and potential impacts of identified noncompliances or deficiencies.
  - Identify root causes of issues and potential corrective or preventive actions.
- *Reporting and communication.*
  - Prepare a written report summarizing the inspection or assessment findings, including any noncompliances, deficiencies, and recommendations for corrective actions.
  - Communicate the results to relevant stakeholders, such as management, employees, regulators, or clients.
  - Ensure that clear follow-up plans and deadlines are established for addressing any identified issues.
- *Follow-up actions.*
  - Monitor the implementation of corrective actions.
  - Track the progress and effectiveness of actions taken.
  - Conduct periodic reviews or reassessments to ensure ongoing compliance and improvement.

51.3.2 Hazard Identification and Risk Assessment

Systematic hazard identification and risk assessment enable industrial hygienists to determine the likelihood and severity of potential hazards. This process involves evaluating potential chemical, physical, biological, ergonomic, and psychosocial hazards to prioritize controls accordingly.

51.3.3 Engineering Controls

Engineering controls aim to eliminate or minimize hazards through design modifications. Examples include installing local exhaust ventilation systems, implementing noise reduction measures, and using safer equipment and machinery (OSHA 2019).

51.3.4 Administrative Controls

Administrative controls focus on the implementation of policies, procedures, and practices to minimize worker exposure to hazards. This strategy may involve training workers, implementing rotation schedules, and establishing safe work practices and emergency procedures.

51.3.5 Personal Protective Equipment (PPE)

When engineering or administrative controls are not feasible or sufficient, the use of PPE becomes crucial. PPE should be selected based on the identified hazards and include items such as respirators, gloves, safety glasses, and hearing protection (NIOSH 2022).

51.4 Evidence-Based Practices

The evidence-based practice strategy in industrial hygiene involves using scientific research and data to guide decision making and implement effective interventions to protect workers from occupational health and safety hazards. It is based on the principle that recommendations and practices should be grounded in rigorous scientific evidence, rather than relying on anecdotal experience or personal opinion (Sackett et al. 1996).

Here are the key steps involved in the evidence-based practice strategy of industrial hygiene.

1) *Research question formulation*: identify the specific issue or problem that needs to be addressed in the workplace. This could be related to exposure to harmful substances, physical hazards, ergonomic issues, or any other occupational health and safety concern.
2) *Literature review*: conduct a comprehensive search for existing scientific literature and studies related to the research question. This involves accessing databases, journals, and other sources to gather relevant information and evidence.
3) *Critical appraisal*: evaluate the quality and credibility of the identified research studies. Assess factors such as study design, reliability of data, sample size, and statistical significance.

51.4.1 Exposure Monitoring

Regular monitoring is essential to accurately assess worker exposure levels and validate the effectiveness of implemented controls. Monitoring can be conducted through air sampling, biological monitoring, or noise dosimetry, among others.

51.4.2 Health Surveillance

Health surveillance involves regularly monitoring the health status of workers to identify and manage potential work-related health issues. This practice encompasses medical examinations, clinical assessments, and biological monitoring to detect early signs of occupational diseases and take appropriate action (World Health Organization 1995).

51.4.3 Training and Education

Ensuring workers are well informed and trained in industrial hygiene practices is vital. Training programs should focus on hazard recognition, control methods, proper use of PPE, and emergency response procedures. Additionally, ongoing education and communication campaigns can help maintain awareness and reinforce safe work practices.

51.5 Conclusion

The significance of maintaining industrial hygiene cannot be overstated. When workplaces are not properly managed and maintained, workers can be exposed to a wide range of hazards that can have both short-term and long-term health implications. These hazards may include chemical and biological agents, physical hazards such as noise, vibration or radiation, ergonomic risks, and psychosocial factors. The consequences of such exposures can lead to acute injuries, chronic illnesses, reduced productivity, increased healthcare costs, and potential legal liabilities.Organizations may face challenges in maintaining industrial hygiene due to various factors, including the complexity and diversity of workplace hazards, changes in technology or processes, budget constraints, and lack of awareness or knowledge about occupational health and safety practices. These challenges highlight the importance of having a systematic approach to industrial hygiene management.

Maintenance of industrial hygiene is an ongoing process that requires a systematic approach to identify, evaluate, and control workplace hazards. By implementing strategies such as routine inspections, hazard identification, and engineering controls, organizations can provide a safe and healthy work environment for their employees. Evidence-based practices, including exposure monitoring, health surveillance, and proper training, further contribute to the effective maintenance of industrial hygiene.

References

Dawson, B.J., Cih, C., Faiha, K.B.D. et al. (2021). Occupational and industrial hygiene as a profession: yesterday, today, and tomorrow. In: *Patty's Industrial Hygiene*, vol. 1 (ed. V. Rose and B. Cohrssen), 3. Hoboken: Wiley.

DiNardi, S.R. (2003). *The Occupational Environment: Its Evaluation, Control, and Management*, vol. 111, 18–27. Fairfax: AIHA Press (American Industrial Hygiene Association).

Jacobs, R.R. and Donham, K.J. (1994). Industrial hygiene principles. In: *Organic Dusts Exposure, Effects, and Prevention* (ed. R. Rylander and R. Jacobs), 267. Boca Raton: CRC Press.

National Institute for Occupational Safety and Health (NIOSH). (2022). Industrial Hygiene: Concepts and Practice. www.cdc.gov/niosh/index.htm (accessed 5 February 2024).

Occupational Safety and Health Administration (2019). Industrial Hygiene. www.osha.gov/sites/default/files/training-library_industrial_hygiene.pdf (accessed 15 February 2024).

Sackett, D.L., Rosenberg, W.M., Gray, J.A. et al. (1996). Evidence-based medicine: what it is and what it isn't. *BMJ* 312 (7023): 71–72.

Spellman, F.R. (2017). *Industrial Hygiene Simplified: A Guide to Anticipation, Recognition, Evaluation, and Control of Workplace Hazards*. Lanham: Bernan Press.

World Health Organization (WHO) (1995). *Global Strategy on Occupational Health for All: The Way to Health at Work*. Geneva: World Health Organization.

52

Environmental Planning, Monitoring, and Management

Jaysukh Kathiriya[1] and Bhavesh J. Trangadia[2]

[1] *Department of Veterinary Public Health & Epidemiology, College of Veterinary Science & Animal Health, Kamdhenu University, Junagadh, India*
[2] *Department of Veterinary Pathology, College of Veterinary Science & Animal Health, Kamdhenu University, Junagadh, India*

52.1 Introduction

An environment management plan (EMP) represents the key mitigation and enhancement measures for major impacts, which are translated into concrete action programs/projects and define the institutional framework and mechanisms for ensuring their appropriate implementation. It also provides estimated investment requirements and commitments/guarantees to carry out the proposed plan.

The EMP is composed of the following components:

- design and construction management program
- social development and institutional plans
- environmental monitoring plan.

52.2 Design and Construction Management Program

Careful planning and adequate engineering design as well as observance of proper construction practices are expected to address the impacts predicted to occur during the construction and operation phases of the Competent Authority for Land Acquisition (CALA) project in India. The Department of Public Works and Highways (DPWH) or its consultants shall prepare the appropriate engineering studies/plans and implement the construction program. To ensure that the roles and responsibilities of the DPWH and its contractors in relation to the environment aspects are properly carried out, the Terms of Reference for such contracts should contain specific provisions pertaining to design criteria, safety considerations, and observance of pertinent laws and regulations for civil works, safety, and environment. Environmental provisions and conditionalities must be adequately stipulated in the DPWH's manual of operation and the contractors' tender documents and construction activities. Compliance with these conditions will be closely monitored by the DPWH in coordination with the Department of Environment and Natural Resources (DENR).

The critical component covered by the program refers to construction management since the key impacts are those generated during this phase of work. During construction, the following should be closely observed.

- Location and set-up of construction quarters near the project site (for migrant workers only). These shall be provided with power and water supply and sanitary toilet and washing facilities.
- Provision of stockyard for construction materials such as aggregates, cement, reinforcing bars, among others.
- Identification of appropriate areas where excavated materials will be temporarily stockpiled.
- Coordination with local government units (LGU) and DENR authorities in the identification of the disposal site for solid waste materials.
- Programming of land clearing and excavations during the dry season where practicable.
- Inevitable removal and cutting of trees must be undertaken with permit duly authorized by the DENR.

Epidemiology and Environmental Hygiene in Veterinary Public Health, First Edition. Edited by Tanmoy Rana.
© 2025 John Wiley & Sons, Inc. Published 2025 by John Wiley & Sons, Inc.

600 | *52 Environmental Planning, Monitoring, and Management*

- Construction of temporary erosion ponds and silt traps as necessary around the work areas.
- Strict observance of proper cut-and-fill procedures to avoid or minimize any wastage or removal of excavated materials from the work areas.
- Placing of material stockpiles and spoil dumps as far away as possible from the waterways and provision of proper and adequate containment.
- Reduction of storage time of construction spoils and materials in the work areas.
- Observance of proper operational procedures in the use of heavy equipment for transporting, hauling, and moving earth spoils from one area to another so as to avoid spills into rivers or nearby waterways.

The DPWH must require its contractors to implement a waste management program, which will include regular collection and disposal of wastes at designated sites approved by the DENR. This program should include the following waste management practices.

- Provision of waste bins in various strategic points within the construction area for the workers to dispose their wastes. Wastes from these containers will be collected regularly to be disposed at a designated dumpsite by the LGU.
- Placing of recyclable materials at local material recovery facilities (MRF).
- Thorough orientation of workers on proper waste disposal practices.
- Reuse of excess excavated materials as aggregate or fill.
- Regular hauling of construction debris to the designated dumping area to prevent accumulation on site.
- Equipment/vehicle clean-up and maintenance as far away as possible from work areas and waterways. Collection of spent and placement of used oil placed in sealed containers and their proper disposal or sale to other users.
- Post construction clean-up and disposal of construction debris shall be a contractor responsibility.

The following measures shall be observed by the contractor to reduce the incidence of project-related accidents.

- Designation of a safety engineer or equivalent at the construction site at all times.
- Provision of rubber boots, safety gloves, dust masks, high-visibility clothing, and other equipment for all workers as deemed necessary.
- No admittance of technical staff or construction workers to work areas without the use of appropriate safety apparel.

Contractors working with the DPWH should be required to source most of their labor from the locally available and qualified labor force. Where practicable, construction and other materials and supplies should be locally sourced to provide business and livelihood to the host barangays, municipality, and province.

The formulation of an emergency response plan applies to projects whose failure will translate to loss of life and property. In the case of the CALA road project, the risk is essentially limited to vehicular accidents. Mitigation of these events shall be part of the implementation of traffic rules and regulations as required by the DPWH and the Department of Transportation and Communications (DOTC).

The required rehabilitation plan shall be under the regular road maintenance activities which include among others the monitoring/maintenance of embankments, drainage systems, and bridge abutments.

52.3 Social Development Program (SDP)

The SDP addresses the key socioeconomic issues/concerns raised during the household and perception surveys and focus group discussions (FGD). It consists of the following components.

- Information, education, and communication
- Land acquisition and resettlement.
- Employment and livelihood development.

52.3.1 Information, Education, and Communication (IEC)

The IEC will be undertaken to encourage the participation and cooperation not only of affected households but a broader sector of stakeholders and facilitate the establishment of support linkages in the implementation of the project. The IEC consists of the following.

- Information dissemination on the results of the environmental impact assessment (EIA).

- Information on the final design of the proposed road alignments based on the detailed engineering study and consultation with the affected households.
- Information on project implementation and monitoring.

52.3.1.1 Information on Project Design and EIA Results

This will be done by means of a public presentation or distribution of information materials during the preconstruction phase of the project, to include the following information.

- Brief description of the project showing the proposed road alignment including a sketch map of the project location and vicinities.
- The environmental issues/concerns raised during the surveys and FGDs and the potential environmental impacts during the preconstruction, construction, and operation/maintenance phases of the project.
- The recommended mitigation/enhancement measures that will address both negative and positive impacts, especially those related to right-of-way (ROW) acquisition.
- The participation/roles of the stakeholders in the implementation of the project.

The information materials will be in the form of flyers, fact sheets, posters, and pamphlets.

52.3.1.2 IEC During Project Implementation and Monitoring

IEC will be undertaken during project implementation to generate participation and support of the community, especially affected families, in the following activities.

- ROW acquisition.
- Project monitoring.
- Employment of local labor and livelihood promotion.

While information dissemination was already conducted during consultations with LGU officials, from the municipal to the barangay levels, and the FGDs conducted in all the affected barangays, a more intensive campaign will be undertaken for the directly affected households, especially in barangays where many households were still apprehensive about the project and were thus hesitant to participate in the sharing of information, such as those related to ROW acquisition, during the surveys.

The distribution of IEC materials will be done, therefore, to complement the continuing consultation with affected households and other stakeholders in the project area. The IEC will be crucial in finalizing the Land Acquisition and Resettlement Plan (LARP), especially the compensation scheme and entitlements for directly affected households.

The estimated cost of the IEC component of the SDP is P2.25 million, at an average of P0.25 million per municipality/city.

52.3.2 Land Acquisition and Resettlement

52.3.2.1 Preparation/Finalization of the LARP

The detailed LARP will be prepared and finalized to provide appropriate and acceptable measures for mitigating the loss of land and other properties as well as income opportunities of project-affected families and persons (PAFs/PAPs). To be finalized through consultations with the PAFs/PAPs during the detailed engineering phase of the project, the LARP will be comprehensive and provide details on the process and mechanics for the identification and profiling of PAFs/PAPs, inventory of losses (land, houses, other assets, income), valuation procedures and appraisal, estimation of costs and budget, resolution of complaints and grievances, and the different relocation stages and process (if relocation is considered as an alternative compensation package instead of cash compensation for loss of residential land and house).

52.3.2.2 Entitlements and Compensation Scheme

The DPWH and PAFs/PAPs will jointly determine and agree on the appropriate compensation in accordance with the following compensation scheme.

52.3.2.3 Productive Lands and Crops

PAFs/PAPs losing more than 20% or all of their agricultural land, or in cases when the remaining assets are not economically viable, are entitled to[1]:

---

1 *Resettlement refers* to all measures taken to mitigate any and all adverse impacts of the project on PAFs/PAPs property and/or livelihood, including compensation, relocation, and rehabilitation, where applicable.

- full compensation at replacement cost of the entire asset either through provision of equivalent land of equal productive capacity (if available and so desired by the displaced person) or through cash compensation
- displaced persons who will lose their income will be provided opportunities for livelihood, job matching or business development assistance in the project area
- appropriate transfer and subsistence allowances will be given during the transition phase.

PAFs/PAPs losing less than 20% of their productive assets, where the remaining assets remain viable for continued use, are entitled to cash compensation at replacement cost for the affected asset.

Replacement of damaged or lost crops will be compensated at full replacement cost for their net loss of income and/or damaged assets.[2]

PAFs/PAPs whose land is temporarily taken will be compensated at full replacement cost for their net loss of income and/or damaged assets.

Verification of land titles and tax payments will be undertaken before land replacement or cash compensation.

52.3.2.4   Residential Land, Houses, and Other Structures

Full compensation at replacement cost of the entire asset either through provision of equivalent land of equal productive capacity (if available and so desired by the displaced person) or through cash compensation, and cash compensation reflecting full replacement cost of the structures, without depreciation.

- If the PAF/PAP so wishes and the remaining land is still a viable residential lot, cash compensation at full replacement cost will be provided.
- If after acquisition, the residential land and/or house are sufficient to rebuild the residential structure lost, then at the request of the PAF/PAP the entire residential land and structure will be acquired at full replacement cost, without depreciation.
- Tenants who have leased a house for residential purposes will be provided with a cash grant of three months' rental fee at the prevailing market rate in the area, and will be assisted in identifying alternative accommodation.

52.3.2.5   Loss of Business

The provision of alternative business site of equal size and accessibility to customers, satisfactory to the displaced PAF/PAP.

- Cash compensation for the lost business structure reflecting full replacement cost without depreciation.
- Cash compensation for the loss of income and opportunity during the transition phase.

52.3.2.6   Voluntary Land Donations

Voluntary donation of land from community members who wish to do so in exchange for project benefit or for the sake of the community will be accepted. However, procedures will be in place to ensure that all donations are voluntary and freely given, that the donor is the legitimate owner of the land, and that the donor is fully informed of the nature of the project and the implications of donating the property.

The following safeguards must be applied, depending on their appropriateness to the cases encountered.

- An assessment that the supposed donor does not suffer a substantial loss affecting his/her economic viability as a result of the donation.
- Certification from the LGUs and the DPWH that the land is free of claims or encroachments from any third party.
- Deed of donation to the DPWH, as witnessed by LGU/government officials and notarized by a registered lawyer, with copies of donation papers sent to the office of the municipal Assessor and the provincial Register of Deeds.
- Waiver of rights/quit claim (for plants, trees, houses, structures claimed by tenants or informal settlers).

52.3.2.7   Costs and Budget

The LARP will include detailed costs of compensation and other entitlement, with a breakdown of replacement or rehabilitation costs for agricultural and residential land houses and other structures, business and other assets, public facilities and services, and utilities. The cost estimates will make adequate provisions for continuous consultation and information dissemination, surveys, and project supervision under contingencies.

---

2 *Replacement cost* refers to the value determined to be fair compensation for real property based on its productive potential, replacement cost of houses and structures (as reckoned on current market price of building materials and labor without depreciation or deductions for salvaged building materials), and the market value of residential land, crops, trees, and other commodities.

52.3.2.8 Complaints and Grievances

Complaints and grievances relative to any aspect of the resettlement entitlements and/or activities, including the determined areas and price of the lost asset, will be managed as follows.

- Grievances will be filed by the PAF/PAP with the Complaints and Grievance Committee (CGC) to be established by the project at barangay level to hear complaints and grievances regarding the acquisition of land and other assets, compensation, relocation, rehabilitation, and other entitlements. Members of the CGC include the Barangay Captain, Barangay Secretary, a member of the Barangay Justice, as well as formal and informal representatives of the community, where applicable.
- The complaint, grievance and appeal shall have the following levels.
  - *Level 1*: PAF/PAP lodges complaints and grievances with the CGC. The CGC will document its investigation of the facts presented and provide a written response to the PAP within fifteen (15) calendar days from receipt of the complaints.
  - *Level 2*: If the PAF/PAP is not satisfied with the decision of the CGC, the PAF/PAP may appeal the case to the DPWH Project Management Office (PMO) within fifteen (15) calendar days from receipt of the written decision/s from the CGC. The decision of the PMO shall be rendered within thirty (30) calendar days from receipt of the appeal after validating the facts of the complaints.
  - *Level 3*: If the PAF/PAP is not satisfied with the decision of the PMO, the PAF/PAP may appeal the case to the DPWH Secretary, through the DPWH Regional Office, within fifteen (15) calendar days from receipt of the written decision from the Office of the Secretary. The said decision shall be rendered within thirty (30) calendar days from receipt of the appeal after validating the facts of the case.

PAFs/PAPs will be exempted from paying all administrative and legal fees. Resorting to courts without using this complaint and grievance process will make the appellant's action dismissible on the ground of nonexhaustion of administrative remedies.

52.3.2.9 Implementation Arrangements, Supervision, and Monitoring

The DPWH will implement the LARP in coordination with and with the assistance of the respective LGUs and national agencies concerned such as the National Health Authority (NHA) and the National Police. The DPWH will be fully responsible for the preparation of the asset inventories and the compensation plans in consultation with the PAFs/PAPs, and the implementation of the LARP until the entire requirement has been completed.

Implementation of the LARP will be regularly supervised and monitored by the DPWH Project Office. Internal monitoring and supervision will include the following.

- Verification that the baseline information of all PAFs/PAPs has been established and that the valuation of lost or damaged assets and provision of compensation and other entitlements have been carried out in accordance with the policies and procedures adopted by the project.
- Record all grievances and their resolution and ensure that complaints are dealt with in a timely manner.

Payment of compensation for ROW acquisition will have to be completed as planned and issues pertaining to it likewise be resolved in accordance with the policies and guidelines governing acquisition of land for ROW. The DPWH cannot proceed to the construction phase of the project unless these are accomplished.

52.3.2.10 Relocation Phases and Processes

If relocation is considered as an alternative mode of compensation preferred by PAFs/PAPs, the activities will be incorporated in the final LARP. It will be divided into three phases and undertaken in accordance with the humane approach as spelled out in RA 7279 and its applicable implementing guidelines.

52.3.2.11 Pre-relocation Phase

This phase will consist of the following preparatory activities.

- Forging of interagency agreement, through a Memorandum of Agreement (MOA), among agencies that may be involved in the undertaking, namely, the DPWH, respective LGUs, and the NHA, and creation of a relocation committee and action teams composed of representatives of these agencies.
- Selection, acquisition, and development of the relocation site, which are among the first concerns of the committee and action teams.
- Conduct of social preparation activities, namely consultations with community leaders and social preparations for PAFs/PAPs active participation in the various relocation processes.
- Conduct of socioeconomic survey, census, and tagging.

52.3.2.12 Actual Relocation Phase

The actual relocation phase will include the following activities.

- Preparations prior to dismantling of houses and other structures.
- Dismantling of houses and other structures.
- Loading and transporting of families, dismantled and reusable housing materials, and other items to the relevant site.
- Assignment of home lots and/or housing units.

52.3.2.13 Postrelocation Phase

The activities to be undertaken after the actual relocation are the following.

- Establishing interaction linkages between relocated families and the host community.
- Facilitating job placement of PAFs/PAPs in the project or their engagement in available livelihood and business opportunities therein, subject to the employment and livelihood promotion policies and procedures adopted by the DPWH as discussed in the next topic.

52.3.3 Employment and Livelihood Promotion

In order to facilitate employment of qualified local labor to fill the work requirements during the construction phase of the project and, at the same time, enable the residents to enjoy the livelihood and business opportunities that will be generated by the project, a manpower placement and livelihood promotion committee will be organized for this purpose by the DPWH in each of the nine municipalities/city. It will be composed of representatives from the LGUs (municipality and barangay), affected households, and the DPWH, and will undertake the following with support from the respectively represented offices/groups.

- Identify the job requirements of the project that can be filled by local labor through proper representation with the contractors, and match this with the skills of the existing labor force in the locality for subsequent placement.
- Identify the livelihood and business opportunities to be generated by the project and promote these to the residents of the area and, if necessary, extend assistance to those who are interested in terms of establishing contacts with clients/customers as well as suppliers.

52.4 Institutional Plan

An environmental group exists within the DPWH which is responsible for the compliance of the agency to existing environmental rules and regulations. The same group shall be responsible for the overall implementation of the EMP which will include, among others:

- overall planning and management of environmental mitigation, enhancement, and monitoring measures
- overseeing the finalization and implementation of the various proposed plans such as the LARP and Social Development Program
- organization of the Multipartite Monitoring Team (MMT) and secretariat support to the various committees of the MMT
- coordination with DENR, LGUs, irrigators' associations and the Federation of Irrigators' Associations (FIA), and local communities concerning implementation of the various management plans
- regular checking of the operation of the construction contractors regarding compliance with environmental clauses/conditionalities in their contracts.

52.5 Environmental Monitoring Program

Environmental monitoring shall be undertaken to:

- ensure that the recommended mitigation and enhancement measures as embodied in the EMP and environmental compliance certificate (ECC) conditionalities are being implemented

52.5 Environmental Monitoring Program | **605**

- undertake regular monitoring of specific parameters in compliance with existing environmental quality standards
- determine the effectiveness of the EMP and make recommendations for any corrective or additional mitigating measures.

52.5.1 Monitoring Plan

A monitoring plan shall be developed based on the mitigation/enhancement measures identified for significant environmental impacts and those that are moderately significant but can have critical effects if not mitigated. The environmental monitoring plan proposed, including the key parameters to be monitored, is presented in Table 52.1. This covers both the preconstruction/construction and operation stages.

The key parameters to be closely monitored are the following.

- Soil erosion and sedimentation of water bodies during construction.
- Changes in water quality during construction.
- Air quality and noise impacts during construction and operation.
- Tree planting and revegetation of critical areas.

Based on the anticipated impacts, the frequency of monitoring by the DPWH and MMT will be more constant and rigid during the construction phase. Monitoring during the operation phase will be closely coordinated with the regional office of the DENR. The baseline information generated during the EIA will generally serve as the benchmark data. Additional measurements shall be made at stations near the proposed final alignment on the final road position as determined in the feasibility study.

52.5.2 Implementation Monitoring

In compliance with the guidelines of DAO 96-37, a MMT will be established to take charge of the preparation of the final monitoring program and annual monitoring plan, including the conduct of monitoring activities. The MMT is to be composed of the following.

- DPWH representative
- DENR representatives (DENR Regional Environmental Management Bureau and/or Provincial Environment and Natural Resources Office/City Environment and Natural Resources Office)
- LGU designated representative(s)
- Nongovernment organizations (NGO)/PO designated representative
- Barangay designated representatives

The constituted/organized MMT shall review and validate, among others, the following:

- coverage of monitoring
- frequency of monitoring
- standard procedures/method of monitoring
- schedule of monitoring
- manpower requirements
- logistics.

The MMT shall implement the environmental monitoring action plan. A monitoring evaluation and reporting system shall be established to enable stakeholders to participate in the process. Where necessary, the system shall be reviewed and updated in relation to actual construction and site conditions.

This system may include the following elements.

- A system to properly coordinate, support, and enhance the various monitoring activities of the MMT as well as its manner of information exchange for monitoring and evaluation.
- Identify institutional and other implementation issues or problem areas and identify processes/mechanisms in resolving such issues/problems.
- Identify capability building mechanisms to be able to sustain and institutionalize project monitoring.

Table 52.1 Environmental monitoring plan.

Project phase	Method and scope	Parameter	Location	Frequency	Responsibility	Cost (P)
1. Preconstruction/construction period						
Physical						
• Right of way acquisition	• Monitoring of earth-moving activities	• Contractor's material handling program	• Construction sites especially at bridge sites	Once a week during construction	DPWH	Part of DPWH supervision cost
• Vegetation clearing/tree cutting	• Engineering geological assessment of slopes	• Slope profile and signs of instability	• Abutments of bridge crossings, steep and high cuts	Once a week during construction or after heavy rains or earthquake event	Construction contractor	Part of CC cost
• Excavation works	• Water quality tests (DENR Administrative Order No. 34 [1990])	• River water quality – DOH, pH, TSS, BOD, total and fecal coliform	• Within 50 m downstream of bridge sites (only at the point where river water is used for some purpose downstream)	Monthly during active construction periods	DPWH/DENR/MMT	P750 000/year ~ P 9000 per point
• Foundation works	• Geo-hazard assessment	• Erosion and siltation	• Waterways near construction sites	Weekly	DPWH/DENR/MMT	P240 000/year
	• Measurement of ambient concentrations (1999 Philippine Clean Air Act)	• TSP, SOx, NOx	• Construction areas near built up areas (12 points)	Monthly during active construction period	DPWH/DENR/MMT	P1 400 000/year ~ P7500 per point
	• Measurement of ambient level (1978 NPCC Rules and Regulations)	• Noise	• Construction areas near built up areas (12 points)	Monthly during active construction period	DPWH/DENR/MMT	P1 400 000/year
	• Monitoring of solid waste disposal	• Presence or absence of dumps, waste bins, collection system	• Construction sites and temporary quarters of workers	Monthly	Contractor	
Biological						
	• Site inspection	• Tree cutting/balling	• Vegetated areas with ROW	Before construction	DPWH/DENR/MMT	P240 000
Socioeconomical						
	• Site inspection	• Worker health and safety	• Construction areas, workers' camp	Weekly	Contractor	
	• Site inspection	• Waste management	• Project site, workers' camp	Daily	Contractor	
2. Operation and maintenance period						
Physical						
• Operation and Maintenance of roads	• Measurement of ambient concentrations (1999 Philippine Clean Air Act)	• TSP, SOx, NOx	• Selected sections of the completed roads (12 points)	Yearly	DPWH/DENR/MMT	
	• Measurement of ambient level (1978 NPCC Rules and Regulations)	• Noise	• Selected sections of the completed roads (12 points)	Yearly	DPWH/DENR/MMT	
Biological						
		• Tree planting, revegetation	• Critical areas along ROW	Weekly		

DOH, Department of Health; BOD, Board of Directors; TSS, total suspended solids; TSP, total suspended particulates.

- A system of reporting and utilizing monitoring and evaluation results for information dissemination and for consequent action.
- Capacity building and strengthening for those staff who will be responsible for the implementation of the EMP.

The initial cost of the establishment of the MMT and finalizing the monitoring plan is estimated at P100 000. Monitoring during construction and operation is initially placed at about P500 000 and P700 000 annually, respectively.

52.6 Overall EMP Implementation and Resource Requirement

The overall EMP summary, including mitigation/enhancement measures, schedule of implementation, estimated investment requirements, institutional responsibilities, and guarantees/agreements, is shown in Table 52.2. The cost computations are rough estimates and need to be verified/validated during the plan finalization.

52.7 Environmental Guarantees, Commitments, and Agreements

52.7.1 Environmental Guarantees

To ensure the protection of the environment during the project, environmental guarantees, commitments, and agreements for the implementation of the proposed EMP are provided by the proponent along with the stakeholders of the project.

A MOA was entered into by DENR and DPWH in 1999, setting down the rights and obligations of both agencies for the protection of the environment and conservation of the country's natural resources. It is here that the Environmental Guarantee Fund (EGF), which is the usual provision of a fund source by the proponent for any work required to address damages brought about by projects, was replaced. This is stipulated in the MOA as follows.

> 10. As a replacement to EGF, the DPWH shall ensure that Contractor's All Risk Insurance (CARI) is provided to cover expenses for the following: indemnification/compensation of damage to life and property that may be caused by the implementation of the projects and abandonment/decommissioning of the project facilities related to the prevention of possible negative impact.

Likewise, an environmental monitoring fund shall no longer be established by the DPWH to support the operation of the MMT and its various monitoring activities since the undertaking of monitoring activities shall be carried out through a "Bayahihan" approach. This is also stipulated in the MOA as follows.

> 12. The Multipartite Monitoring Team (MMT) will be formed through Bayanihan Approach, since there are no funds available for Environmental Monitoring Fund (EMF). The MMT will be formed on a voluntary basis (bayanihan) with members coming from the EIAPO, Planning Service, EIARO (DPWH Regional Offices), CENRO, PENRO, Local Government Units (LGU), Non Government Units (NGO), POs experts and other cause oriented environmental groups. In this regard, expenses of members of MMT in the performance of their official duties will be charged to appropriate funds of their respective offices.

52.7.2 Project Commitments, Affirmations, and Agreements

The commitment of the stakeholders responsible for the implementation of the environmental management plan is essentially bound by the ECC conditionalities that shall be issued by the DENR. This ECC shall be complemented by the contract which shall contain the appropriate environmental management provisions and the MOAs which may be forged among the contractor, LGU, and MMT.

Table 52.2 Environmental management plan.

Project activities	Predicted environmental impacts	Degree/type of impact	Mitigation/enhancement measure	Cost	Responsible institution	Guarantees/ agreements
1. Preconstruction/construction period						
A. Physical environment						
Land						
• Detailed engineering design; clearing within ROW area; site grading, excavation, backfilling, bored piling at bridge areas, hauling/ stockpiling of excavated and construction materials	Terrain modification, soil and weathered rock displacement Erosion, siltation of local waterways particularly at bridge crossings	S, P (negative) S, T (negative)	• Clearing and excavation works to be planned during dry season where practicable and scheduled so as to allow speedy concreting/backfilling of excavated sections • Use of temporary siltation ponds[a] • Excavated materials be placed on appropriate dumpsites or spoils area at some distance from structure sites and provided with adequate containment; re-use soil spoils for backfilling • Stockpiles of sand and gravel be fenced or so located to reduce transport of sediments during heavy rains including reducing storage time in work areas • Observance of proper materials handling and heavy equipment operations for transport, hauling and moving earth spoils to minimize spills into rivers and 4 • nearby waterways • Immediate revegetation of exposed areas which will not be occupied by road structures • Strict observance of proper cut and fill procedures and materials balance to minimize wastage of excavated materials from work areas • Restoration or dredging of silted waterways upon completion of construction activities • Use of temporary sumps for detention of bentonite used in drilling bored piles • Use of tarpaulins or equivalent to cover exposed stockpiles of excavated and construction materials • Monitor river quarrying for construction materials within the project area. Sources of construction materials for the project will be identified and approved for quarrying by the Mines and Geosciences Bureau and/or the concerned LGU. • Monitoring of earthmoving activities by a qualified geotechnical engineer or engineering geologist	• Part of construction cost	• Contractor, DPWH, DENR, MMT	• Part of constructor's contract and as input to the feasibility study

Slope destabilization at new cuts	MS, T (negative)	• Undertake slope stability analysis supported by adequate geologic mapping, field tests and laboratory analysis for sections which will involve large cuts. Drilling accompanied by appropriate laboratory test may be undertaken. This is an option to be taken by the contractor should his designer require subsurface data for the proposed slope stabilization measure • Install as necessary slope protection measures such as shotcreting, rock bolts or soil nails. A soil nail anchors soil-like materials which are likely to fail into more stable strata located farther into the slope	• Part of design cost • Part of construction cost	• Contractor and DPWH • Contractor, DPWH, DENR, MMT	• Part of contractor's contract and as input into the design stage • Part of contractor's contract
Degradation of national and provincial roads used for hauling construction materials and for movement of heavy equipment	MS,T (negative)	• Regular road maintenance, restoration of roads original conditions after construction activities. As practiced, the roads used by the contractors that are degraded by the passage of heavy equipment are restored or repaired at the end of the project or upon completion of construction activities in the particular area	• Part of construction cost	• Contractor, DPWH, DENR, MMT	• Part of contractor's contract
Increased generation of solid wastes	NS, T (negative)	• Provision of waste bins in various strategic points within the construction area for the workers to dispose their wastes. Wastes from these containers will be collected (dump truck of the contractor) regularly to be disposed at a designated waste disposal site • Reuse and recycling of scrap materials and containers such as bottles, cans, boxes, and plastics as much as practicable or selling them to scrap buyers • Conduct of a thorough orientation of workers on proper waste disposal practices • Reuse construction spoils as aggregate or filling materials where practicable • Regular hauling of construction debris to the designated disposal area to prevent accumulation on site resulting in negative effects on the landscape • Conduct of equipment/vehicle clean-up and maintenance in only one designated area located as far away as possible from waterways. Spent and used oil should be collected and placed in sealed containers and disposed of properly or sold to used oil recyclers/buyers to prevent draining into waterways	• Part of construction cost	• Contractor and DPWH	• Part of contractor's contract

(Continued)

Table 52.2 (Continued)

Project activities	Predicted environmental impacts	Degree/type of impact	Mitigation/enhancement measure	Cost	Responsible institution	Guarantees/agreements
			• Efficient housekeeping practices including the use of covered receptacles for refuse generated by workers and construction scrap/debris will ensure the proper handling and disposal of solid wastes • In order to minimize the need to dispose of earth materials, the contractor shall make use of excavated materials as much as possible for filling and as part of construction materials. For nonsuitable materials, these are placed in low areas where the possibility of erosion is limited			
Air	Increase in particulates and gaseous emissions and noise levels	MS, T (negative)	• Sprinkle water in exposed areas on regular basis especially during dry and windy periods • Speed of vehicles used for construction should be regulated to minimize stirring up of loose materials • Sinks for dusts/spoils • Proper handling and storage of spoil materials • Proper maintenance of engines for efficient fuel burning to lessen gaseous emissions • Schedule construction activities during daytime • Installation of silencers or mufflers for as many vehicle engines and heavy equipments as possible	• Part of construction cost	• Contractor, DPWH, DENR, MMT	• Part of contractor's contract
	Increased traffic at road intersections leading to construction areas	MS, T (negative)	• Contractor to assign traffic aides at key road sections to assist in traffic management	• Part of construction cost	• Contractor, DPWH	• Part of contractor's contract
Water	Changes in river water quality	S, T (negative)	• Refer to mitigation measures on soil displacement, erosion and siltation of waterways • Locate gravel crushing, screening areas and concrete batching operations as far away as possible from waterways • Undertake regular monitoring of water quality focusing on DO, BOD, TSS, and TDS • Provide adequate temporary sanitary facilities with proper drainage to prevent leaching and wash water from reaching water courses, use of portalets • Contractors to prepare and implement a materials handling program for construction spoils and solid waste management • Contractor to observe proper equipment maintenance and operation to minimize spillage of oil and grease into waterways	• Part of construction cost	• Contractor, DPWH, DENR, MMT	• Part of contractor's contract

B. Biological environment

Terrestrial

• Vegetation clearing, excavation and grading and other construction activities	Loss, disturbance and damage to existing vegetation; habitat degradation of dependent species	MS, T (negative)	• For every tree cut, the required replacements must be made • Secure necessary permit from DENR for tree cutting • Implement tree balling where practicable • Immediate revegetation	• Part of construction cost	• DPWH	• Part of ECC requirement

Fresh water

	Local aquatic habitat alteration and temporary displacement of species	NS, T (negative)	• Same mitigation for the control of soil erosion and sedimentation			

C. Socioeconomic environment

• Detailed engineering design; clearing within ROW area; site grading, excavation, backfilling bored piling at bridge areas, hauling/ stockpiling of excavated and construction materials including ROW acquisition	Total or partial loss of land/farm area, properties and crops, dislocation and loss of income due to ROW acquisition	S, P (negative)	• Negotiate with PAFs/PAPs for an acceptable compromise on valuation and compensation • Finalize the RAP incorporating therein the agreements reached during public consultations	NA	• DPWH	• Commitment of DPWH via MOA
	Increase in employment opportunities	MS, T (positive)	• Require contractors to source workforce from qualified locals • Contractors to orient workers on desirable working relationship, especially if there are nonresident workers	NA	• Contractor, DPWH	• Part of contractor's contract
	Increase in livelihood and business opportunities	MS, T (positive)	• Priority to be given to local subcontractors • Priority to be given to local suppliers of construction materials and equipment • Supply of food and catering to be preferentially awarded to local suppliers	NA	• Contractor, DPWH	• MOA of LGU with contractor
	Potential health, sanitation and safety problems	NS, T (negative)	• Contractor to provide temporary housing facilities for workers equipped with adequate water and sanitation facilities • Contractors to implement proper solid waste management in the work site, workers will be oriented to observe proper hygiene and sanitation practices and provided with appropriate protection gear while working • Construction areas to be enclosed as necessary and provided with appropriate signage to avoid accidents			

(Continued)

Table 52.2 (Continued)

Project activities	Predicted environmental impacts	Degree/type of impact	Mitigation/enhancement measure	Cost	Responsible institution	Guarantees/ agreements
D. Land use						
Land use and zoning						
	Change in land value	S, P (positive)	• Property appraisal by the local government unit before construction			
2. Operations and maintenance period						
A. Physical environment						
Land						
	Erosion at major discharge points of the road's storm drains	NS, T (negative)	• Installation of dissipators at major discharge points of the road's storm drains	• Dissipators: P1 481 000		
Air						
• Operation and maintenance of roads	Increase in particulates and gaseous emissions	MS, P (negative)	• IEC to road users on the proper maintenance of engines for efficient fuel burning and minimization of gaseous emissions • Tree planting along the roads • Regular road cleaning activity such as regular water sprinkling	• Tree planting: P158,090 000	• DPWH, tollway operator	• Part of ECC requirement
	Increase in noise levels	MS, P (negative)	• Traffic controls (e.g., speed limits and traffic volume restrictions) and vehicle controls along the highway (e.g., truck bans) • Tree planting along the roads • Noise barrier panel should be installed along the roads which pass sensitive areas such as hospitals and schools	• Tree planting: P158 090 000 • Sound barrier: P6 459 000		
B. Socioeconomic environment						
• Operation and maintenance of roads	Lessened traffic congestion and improved access to public utilities and services	MS, P (positive)	• Enhance accessibility by providing appropriate signage to guide traveling public to use shortest and most convenient route to reach the interior places from the highway via the existing access roads and vice versa	• Part of operations cost	• DPWH, tollway operator	• Part of ECC requirement and standard operation procedures
	Increased livelihood and business opportunities, and revenues for LGUs	MS, P (positive)	• Encourage LGUs to use part of the increased revenues for expanding business operations and establishing new livelihood activities, by maintaining peace and order and improving basic services and infrastructure and utilities	NA	• Initiative of LGU	• Initiative of LGU
	Increased migration and population	MS, P (negative)	• Concerned LGUs (barangay and municipal/city) to regulate encroachment in watershed areas (forest land) through proper zoning and enforcement	NA	• Initiative of LGU	• Initiative of LGU

			• LGUs to adequately plan/provide for social services and infrastructures including health services, waste management and facilities and road network • Encourage LGUs to regulate or prevent the establishment of squatter colonies by strictly enforcing RA 7279 or the Urban Development Housing Act			
	Regional severance	S, P (negative)	• In order not to disturb human flow between communities, measures for crossing the road should be installed such as flyover, underpass, at grade intersection, and service road	• Part of construction cost	• Contractor, DPWH	• Part of contractor's contract and as input into the design stage
	Increased accidents	MS, T (negative)	• Intersection signal and sign board installation	• Part of construction cost	• Contractor, DPWH	• Part of contractor's contract and as input into the design stage
	Damage of landscape	MS, P (negative)	• Revegetation of exposed areas • Tree planting along the roads	• Tree planting: P158 090 000	• Contractor, DPWH	• Part of contractor's contract and as input into the design stage
C. Land use						
Land use and zoning						
	Change in land value	S, P (positive)	• Regular property appraisal by the local government			

S, significant impact; MS, moderately significant impact; NS, nonsignificant impact; T, temporary impact; P, permanent impact; negative, negative impact; positive, positive impact.

[a] *Siltation ponds* correspond to sumps which temporarily detain water pumped out of excavations. Detention will facilitate the settlement of sediments from the water prior to eventual release into nearby waterways.

Further Reading

BMG (1982). *Geology and Mineral Resources of the Philippines*, Geology, vol. 1. Manila: Bureau of Mines and Geosciences, Ministry of Natural Resources.

Canter, L.W. (1996). *Environmental Impact Assessment*. New York: McGraw-Hill.

Cardwell, R.K., Isacks, B.L., and Karig, D.E. (1980). The spatial distribution of earthquakes, focal mechanism solutions and subducted lithosphere in the Philippines and Northeastern Indonesian Islands. In: *The Tectonic and Geological Evolution of Southeast Asian Seas and Islands* (ed. D.E. Hayes), 1–35. Washington, DC: American Geophysical Union.

Department of Environment & Natural Resources (2000). Implementing Rules and Regulations of the Philippine Clean Air Act of 1999.

Fitch, T.J. (1972). Plate convergence, transcurrent faults, and internal deformation adjacent to Southeast Asia and the Western Pacific. *Journal of Geophysical Research* 77 (23): 4432–4460.

Hamburger, M., Cardwell, R.K., and Isacks, B.L. (1983). Seismotecnics of the Northern Philippine Islands arc. In: *The Tectonic and Geologic Evolution of Southeast Asian Seas and Islands. Part 2* (ed. D.E. Hayes), 1–22. Washington, DC: American Geophysical Union.

Lichel Technologies Inc. (2006). Environmental Baseline Study for the Feasibility Study and Implementation Support on the Cavite-Laguna (CALA) East-West National Road Project.

Ludwig, W.J., Hayes, D.E., and Ewing, J.I. (1967). The Manila Trench and West Luzon Trough – I. Bathymetry and sediment distribution. *Deep Sea Research* 14: 533–544.

Masters, G. (1985). *Introduction to Environmental Science & Engineering*. New York: McGraw-Hill.

Taylor, B. and Hayes, D.E. (1983). Origin and history of the South China Sea Basin. In: *The Tectonic and Geologic Evolution of Southeast Asian Seas and Islands. Part 2* (ed. D.E. Hayes), 23–56. Washington, DC: American Geophysical Union.

Wark, K. and Warner, C.F. (1976). *Air Pollution: Its Origin and Control*. New York: Harper & Row.

Index

Note: Page numbers followed by *f* and *t* indicate figures and tables.

a

aardvarks (*Orycteropus afer*) 86
abiotic components 366
abiotic resources 329
absorption 388
accidental host 70
accidents 581
  animal handling/restraint accidents 583
  categories 581–2, 582*f*
  causes of injuries on farm animals during handling 583*f*
  electric accidents 585
  faulty facility injuries 583–4
  fear as source of animal accidents during restraint 584–5
    animal behavior patterns 584–5
    floods 585, 585*f*
    hearing patterns 584
    sight perception 584
  fire and chemical accidents 586–7
    controlling arsenic poisoning 586
    lead poisoning 586–7, 587*f*
    organophosphate poisoning accidents 587
  investigation 581
  livestock accidents 582, 582*f*
  occupational/personnel accidents 581, 582*f*
  precautionary measures to avoid machinery injuries 584
  reducing incidence of project-related 600
  road accidents 583
  transport vehicle accidents 582
  types of 582–7
accumulation factor (AF) 465
accuracy and precision, of diagnostic test 202, 202*f*
Acidithiobacillus ferrooxidans 334
acid rain 387, 390, 399–400, 479–80
acquired immunodeficiency syndrome 118
active data collection 111
active immunization 576
active quarantine 574

active surveillance 7
acute infectious diseases 245
adaptation 423
adenosine triphosphate (ATP) 546
adsorption 388
adult mortality rate 133
Advanced Very High Resolution Radiometer sensor (AVHRR) 139
Aedes aegypti 559
aerial monitoring techniques 90
aerogels 445
African animal trypanosomiasis (AAT) 255
African buffalo (*Syncerus caffer*) 87
African elephant (*Loxodonta africana*) 90
African swine fever (ASF) 4, 57*t*, 74, 163*t*, 185
Agenda 21 483
agent 22–3, 574–5
agent-based microsimulation (ABM) model 249
agent determinants 37, 48–50
  of animal disease 37*f*
  gradient of infection 49, 49*t*
  outcome of infection 49–50
  virulence and pathogenicity 37, 48–9
agent-environment interaction 23
age-specific death rates 132
agricultural pollution 409
air-borne pollutants/air contaminants 316–17
air-borne transmission 72, 572
air pollution 334, 386–8, 406–7, 411
  air pollutants 408*t*
  inside animal housing 497–503
    extrinsic factors 497–8
    intrinsic factors 497
    microbial decomposition and spoilage of remnants 497–8
    mobile sources of pollution 498, 499
    stationary sources of pollution 498

Epidemiology and Environmental Hygiene in Veterinary Public Health, First Edition. Edited by Tanmoy Rana.
© 2025 John Wiley & Sons, Inc. Published 2025 by John Wiley & Sons, Inc.

Index

air pollution (*cont'd*)
  categories of 407*f*
  causes 386
  classification 386
    chemical properties 386
    nature of source 386
  control
    balanced ventilation 503, 503*f*
    best management practices (BMPs) 503
    in farm buildings 503
    of gaseous byproducts 388, 388*f*
    monitoring levels of pollution 503
    of particulate matter pollution 387, 387*f*
  effects 386–7
    on animals and vegetation 387
    on health and environment 397*f*
    on humans 387
  gaseous and particulate pollutants in animal
      buildings 498, 499*f*
    ammonia 499–500
    bio-aerosols 502–3
    carbon dioxide 498–9
    carbon monoxide 500
    hydrogen sulfide 500
    methane 499
    nitrous oxide 500
    odors 500–1
    particulate matter 501–2
    volatile organic compounds 501
  impacts 397–8
  major causes 397
  primary pollutants 397
  secondary pollutants 397
  sources of 498*f*
  types 397
Air Quality Index (AQI), monitoring of 503
alcohol-based disinfectants 152
alkaline hydrolysis 150
alpine tundra
  animals 376
  region 375
Amblyomma variegatum infestation 255
American College of Veterinary Preventive Medicine 339
ammonia (NH$_3$) 382, 395, 397, 399–400, 499–500, 505, 516
ammonification 382
anaerobic digestion 150
analytical epidemiology 5–6, 191, 207
  common methods in 5–6
    case-control studies 5–6
    cohort studies 6
    disease intervention 5

    evaluating interventions 6
    evidence-based decision-making 5
    preventing outbreaks 6
    statistical modeling 6
  understanding 5
"AND" operator 234
Animal and Plant Health Inspection Service (APHIS),
    USDA's 293
animal disaster management 489–94
  emergency management lifecycle 490*f*
  mitigation 491
  planning 490
  preparedness 490–1
  recovery 493–4
  response 491–3
animal disease alerts and forecasting
  disease prognosis, in India 140–1
  early warning 136
    initiatives for 136
    system development 137
  Geographical Information System (GIS) 140
  Global Early Warning and Response System
    (GLEWS) 138–40
  purpose of forecasting 135–6
animal diseases
  advances in estimating cost of outbreaks 169, 171
    OutCosT 171
    vector error correction model 169, 171
  basic economic model 157–8, 157*f*
    direct losses 158
    indirect losses 158
  climate change impact on 263–4
  common modeling techniques
    in animal health economics 158–9, 159*f*
    definitions, and indications 160*t*
  costs of 157*f*
  differences between economic and animal health
    approach 156*f*
  economic impact on 155–72
  economics of 156–60
  estimation of economic losses due to 165–9
    climate-sensitive diseases 169
    loss from mortality 165
    loss in milk yield 166
    transboundary animal diseases 166–9
    treatment costs 166
  Global Burden of Animal Diseases (GBADs)
    program 164–5
    approach to evaluating burden of animal diseases 165*f*
    key components of 164*f*
  global strategies for control/eradication of 305

network for surveillance of   141
outbreaks, monitoring and managing   7
prevention and treatment of   264–5
strategies for controlling   104–5
surveillance   108
TADs. *See* transboundary animal diseases (TADs)
animal guardianship   488–9
animal handling/restraint accidents   583
animal health
accident prevention for   581–7
biomedical waste and   526
common modeling techniques in   158–9, 159*f*
delivery, at herd level   256
economics   155
functions of mathematic models   158*f*
noise pollution on   456–7
See also air pollution; environmental pollution
Animal Health Codes   101, 104
Animal Health Law   183
animal hygiene   537
animal productivity, factors influencing   39–40
animal-related functions, of veterinarians   301
animal shelters
sanitation procedures in   541–4
See also sanitation
Animals Quarantine Rules 1968   178
Animals (Import) Rules 1968   178
animal vaccinations   271. *See also* vaccines and vaccination
animal welfare   427–8
improving   427–8
Annan, Kofi   483
annoyance   455
anthrax   57*t*, 85, 101, 146*t*, 147*t*, 148*t*, 285, 340, 552
anthropogenic noise   456
anthropogenic threats to biodiversity
biological invasions and global trade   355
climate change and biodiversity   354
habitat loss and fragmentation   354
overexploitation and illegal wildlife trade   355
antibiotics, reduction in need for   275
antigens   272
antimicrobial resistance (AMR)   62, 342
building global governance on   305
Global Action Plan on (GAP-AMR)   305, 307
Global Antimicrobial Resistance and Use Surveillance
System (GLASS)   307
global initiatives to fight   305
Gonococcal Antimicrobial Surveillance Program
(GASP)   308
antimicrobials   284
aphotic zone   380

Aplochilus panchax   562
aquatic (water-based) ecosystems   378–80
characteristics of   378
freshwater ecosystems   378, 378*f*
marine ecosystems   379–80, 379*f*
arbitrator   236
arboviruses   82
arctic tundra
animals   376
region   375
area data   15
Arignar Anna Zoological Park's giraffe exhibit   430
Aristotle   302
arithmetic mean   220
arsenic (As)   395, 468*t*, 586
arsenic poisoning, controlling   586
artificial intelligence (AI)   26, 357
Aspergillus fumigatus   76
Assam State Zoo   430
Assistance to States for Control of Animal Diseases
(ASCAD)   182
association, causation and   6
ATHENS   233
atmosphere and precipitation   441
atmospheric noises   452
atmospheric stratification   416
"attack rate"   129
attenuated vaccines   272–3
attributable fraction   194
audiogram   454
audiometer   452
auditory effect   454
Aujeszky disease   57*t*, 273
authors, contacting   238, 242
autoregressive integrated moving average (ARIMA)   247*t*
autoregressive model (AR)   247*t*
autoregressive moving average (ARMA)   247*t*
autotrophs   366
avian influenza (AI)   23, 57*t*
crisis   139

b

babesiosis piroplasmosis   146*t*
baboons   89
Bacillus anthracis   502, 553, 554, 572
Bacillus sphaericus   563
Bacillus thuringiensis   563
backward citation searching   237
bacterial biofilms   76
bag filtration   387
Bang, Bernhard   300

Index

barrier vaccination   148
Basel Convention on Biological Diversity (CBD)   421
Basel Convention on the Control of Transboundary
     Movements of Hazardous Wastes and Their
     Disposal   420–1, 482, 484, 530
benzalkonium chloride   152
benzene   314
Berlin Principles   302
best management practices (BMPs)   503
Betula pendula   373
Bhopal tragedy (1984)   461, 478
bias   126
  assessing   243
  associated with epidemiological studies   195
big data   216–19
  acquiring   216–17
  approaches to overcome errors in handling of
    eliminating incidental endogeneity   218
    Hadoop/core Hadoop   219
    impacts of big data   219
    impacts on infrastructure demands   219
    independence screening of variables   218
    MapReduce   219
    penalized quasi-likelihood   218
    using sparest solution in independence set   218
  architecture of HDFS   219
  challenges/constraints of   217
  economics and finance   217
  genomics   217–18
  goals of analyzing   217
  hidden characteristics
    heterogeneous nature   218
    incidental endogeneity   218
    noise accumulation   218
    spurious correlation   218
  impacts on computation   219
  neurological sciences   217
  other applications   218
  preprocessing technique   219
  small data storage   219
  storage techniques   219
  uses/applications   217–19
biguanides   542
bioaccumulation   465, 469
  and biomagnification of DDT in aquatic
    ecosystem   466–7, 467*f*
  pathways of   466–7
bioaccumulation factor (BAF)   465
bio-aerosols   502–3
biochemical oxygen demand (BOD)   518
bioconcentration   465
biodegradation   326

biodilution   465
biodiversity
  advancing conservation design and management   355
  anthropogenic threats to biodiversity   354–5
  biological invasions and global trade   355
  climate change and   354
  conceptualizing   349–51
  conservation strategies   355–6, 356*f*
  corporate biodiversity stewardship   356
  different types of conservation strategies for   354*f*
  ecological significance of   353
  ecosystem diversity   350–1
  ecosystem functioning   353
  ecosystem services and biodiversity   353
  elevational biodiversity patterns   352, 352*f*
  genetic diversity   349–50
  habitat loss and fragmentation   354
  integrating into land use planning and corporate
    sustainability   356
  latitudinal gradients   351–2
  linking to ecosystem functioning   350
  molecular ecology and genomics, advancements in   357
  offsets and compensatory mitigation   355–6
  overexploitation and illegal wildlife trade   355
  patterns of   351–3
  research and conservation   357
  social and political dimensions of biodiversity
    conservation   357
  and social equity   357
  spatial planning for   356
  species diversity   350, 351*f*
  technology for conservation   357
  temporal biodiversity dynamics   352–3
  and trophic interactions   353
biofilms   76
biogas production   509–13
  advantages of   509–10
  biogas digester, types of   510, 511
  compressed biogas (CBG)   512–13, 513*t*, 513*f*
  conversion of diesel engine to biogas   514*f*
  from different wastes   510*t*
  electricity from   513, 514*f*
  factors affecting optimum   512
  multiple benefits from waste flows, for energy
    production   511*f*
  process   510, 512, 512*f*
  quantities, consumed for various applications   510*t*
  rotary drum composter   513
  utilization   512
biogeochemical cycle   380
bioleaching method   470
biological hazards, prevention and control of   323

biological invasions and global trade
  invasion pathways and hotspots   355
  invasive species on native biodiversity and
    ecosystems   355
biological threat reduction, global initiatives for   305
biological transmission   562
biomagnification   465
  of DDT, in aquatic food chain   466–7, 467f
biomagnification factor (BMF)   466
biomass, pyramid of   369–70, 370f
biomedical functions, of veterinarians   301
biomedical research   293
biomedical waste (BMW)
  classification of organic wastes   526
  common biomedical waste treatment facility
    (CBWTF)   523
  control   524
  dangers to human and animal health   526
  definition   523
  effects of   525f
  environment-related risks   526
  hazardous wastes   524, 526
  limitations of control   527
  management   523–34
    categories of waste and their treatment   527t
    color coding for different waste types   528t
    packing containers and labeling   529
    policies and schedules for   526–7
    segregation of waste   527–9, 528f
    shipping   529
    strategies   527–9
    waste disposal   529
  measures to preventing risks of clinical wastes   534
  medical solid wastes and their risks   525
  negative effects of   523
  nonhazardous wastes   524, 526
  and pharmaceuticals   314–15
  in soil and water   525
  sources of   524
  techniques of treatment and disposal   529–33
    advanced-excellent sanitary landfill   530–1
    chemical disintegration   532–3
    designed landfill   530
    incineration   531–2
    inertization   531
    landfills   530–1
    nonincineration treatments   532
    open field burning   531
    other disposal strategies   533
    returning unused medications to producer   530
    sewer   531
    systems for eliminating clinical waste   530

  transfer of pharmaceutical waste across borders   530
  waste encapsulation and immobilization   531
  types of   524, 524f
  veterinary scientific wastes   524
  waste accumulation and storage   533
  waste reduction   533
bioremediation   325–6, 470
  applying genetically engineered strains to clean up
    environment   325–6
  biodegradation   326
  biotechnological approaches   325
  rain water harvesting   326
  recharge to groundwater   326
biosecurity measures
  factors responsible for spreading disease   153f
  slaughter process   151
  strategies of disease management   152–3
biosecurity, primary hazards to   100t
biotic components, of ecosystem   365–6
  autotrophs   366
  heterotrophs   366
  saprotrophs   366
biotic resources   329
biotransference. See trophic transfer
bioventing   470
black quarter   146t, 147t
black soldier fly (BSF) larvae   516
blanket culling   151
blanket vaccination   145
bloat   146t
blood tests   148
bluetongue   57t, 107, 147t, 264
Bonn Convention   420
boreal forest   373
Borrelia burgdorferi   272
Botswana, diseases of animals acts in   179–80
  Declaration of Foot and Mouth Disease (Infected Area)
    Order 2003   180
  Disease of Stock Regulations 1926   179
  Diseases of Animals (Inoculation) Order 1952   179
  Diseases of Animals (Muzzling) Order 1954   179
  Diseases of Animals (Declaration of Stock-Free Zones)
    Order 1982   180
  Diseases of Animals (Prohibition of Use of Anabolic
    Hormones and Thyrostatic Substances) Regulations
    1987   180
  Diseases of Animals (Stock Feed) Regulations 2004   180
  Diseases of Animals (BSE Control [Removal of Specified
    Risk Material]) Regulations 2004   180
  Diseases of Animals (Animal Information and Traceability
    System) Regulations 2018   180
  Diseases of Stock (Poultry) Regulations 1941   179

620 | *Index*

Botswana, diseases of animals acts in (*cont'd*)
  Foot-and-Mouth Disease (Conveyance of Products) Order
    1960   179
  Movement of Stock (Restriction) Order 1960   179
  Prohibition of Sale of Imported Cattle to the Botswana
    Meat Commission for Export to the European Union
    Regulations 1998   180
  Stock Diseases (Semen) Regulations 1968   179
bovine alimentary papillomas   51
bovine brucellosis   57*t*, 168
bovine leukosis   288
bovine spongiform encephalopathy (BSE)   111, 282, 284
bovine viral diarrhea (BVD)   107
Brucella abortus eradication program   275
brucellosis   146*t*, 147*t*, 168–9, 170*t*, 254, 275
brush-tailed possum (*Trichosurus vulpecula*)   90
buffalopox   147*t*
burial method, of carcase disposal   516, 551–2
burial sites   149
burning method, of carcase disposal   150, 517, 552

C

cadmium (Cd)   396, 468*t*
  toxicity   389
Cairo Guidelines and Principles for the Environmentally
    Sound Management of Hazardous Wastes   484
calf health   149
Campylobacter infections   304
campylobacteriosis   60
canarypox-vectored vaccines   273
Candida albicans   77
Candida neoformans   77
canine melanomas   48
Cape buffalo (*Syncerus caffer*)   90
carbon cycle   380, 381*f*
carbon dioxide (CO_2)   394, 415, 416, 419, 498–9, 505
  effects of   499
  emission   418, 423
carbon monoxide (CO)   317, 408*t*, 500
  pollution   397
carbon sequestration   324–5
  geological   324
  ocean   325, 326*f*
  terrestrial   324, 325*f*
carcase disposal   149–50, 516–17
  advanced methods of composting   517, 517*f*
  economic aspects of   554
  traditional methods
    burial   516, 551–2
    burning   517, 552
cardiovascular disturbances, and noise   455
carnivores   368, 369

carriers   70, 78
carrier state   34, 50
Cartagena Biosafety Protocol 2000   485
Cartagena Protocol on Biosafety   422
case–control study   120, 120*f*, 193–4, 266
  in analytical epidemiology   5–6
  calculation of odds ratio in   194*f*
  design   193*f*
case fatality   131
case reporting   10
categorical variables   13
causation, in veterinary epidemiology   6
caves   86
Centers for Disease Control and Prevention (CDC)   293
Central Disease Diagnostic Laboratory (CDDL)   141
central tendency, measures of   219–20
Centre for Animal Disease Research and Diagnosis
    (CADRAD)   141
Centre for Reviews and Dissemination (CRD)   233
chalcogels   445–6
chemical air pollutants   386
chemical/fire accidents   586–7
Chemical Hazard Assessment Management Program
    (CHAMP)   595
chemical hazards, prevention and control of   323
chemical pollution   478–9
chemoprophylaxis   150, 575–6
chemotherapy   150
Chernobyl nuclear disaster (1986)   399, 461, 479
chikungunya virus   559*t*
child mortality rate   132
chlorine-based disinfectants   152
chlorofluorocarbons   480
chromium   468*t*
chronic arsenic poisoning   586
chronic disease   34
chronic infectious diseases   245
citation searching   237–8
classic swine fever (CSF)   148*t*, 170*t*
Classic Swine Fever Control Program (CSF-CP)   183
class intervals   216
Clean Air Act Amendments of 1990   480
climate change
  adapting to emerging diseases and   16
  biodiversity and   354
  effects on frequency and distribution of disease   38
  effects on health   59
  environmental conventions and protocols on   419–20
  global warming and   415, 416
  impact on animal diseases   263–4
  impact on non-vector-borne diseases and livestock
    diseases   59–60

impact on water resources   444
   natural resources and   337
   vector-borne diseases and   559
climate sensitive livestock diseases   59–60, 62, 169
clinical and subclinical disease   33–4
clinical heterogeneity   241
clinical infection   49t
clinical trials   197–202
   assessment of outcome   201
   case definition   197–8
   cluster randomized trials   200
   community trials   200
   cross-over design   200
   designing of   199f
   external and internal validity of   197, 198f
   factorial designs   200
   follow-up and compliance   200–1
   inclusion and exclusion criteria   199–200
   informed consent and other ethical considerations   201
   limitations of   201–2
   masking/blinding   201
   multicenter trials   200
   in practice   202
   selecting the controls
      historical controls   198–9
      random allocation   199
      simultaneous nonrandomized controls   199
      stratified randomization   199
   specifying the intervention   199
   superiority, equivalence, and noninferiority trials   200
   See also randomized controlled trials (RCTs)
clinical wastes
   measures to preventing risks of   534
   strategies for disposing of   532–3
   systems for eliminating   530
Clorox® wipes   540
Clostridium botulinum   86
clothing, role in disease transmission   546
cluster randomized trials   200
cluster sampling   11
cobalt   468t
coccidioidomycosis (valley fever)   288
Cochliomyia hominivorax   264
Cochrane Collaboration   229
Cochrane Qualitative and Implementation Methods
      Group   230
Cochrane Risk of Bias tool   243
Codex Alimentarius Commission (CAC, Codex)   187, 188,
      205, 304
Coelomomyces   563
cohort life tables   91, 92
cohort studies   122, 123f, 191–3

in analytical epidemiology   6
calculation of relative risk in   192, 193f
design   192f
prospective cohort study   191–3
retrospective cohort study   191–2, 193
cold/temperate desert   377
cold water pollution   391
combination vaccines, for animals   274
combustion   388
common-source outbreaks   53
common vehicle   53
communicable diseases   67
community ecology   83
community trials   124–5, 200
   limitations of   125
companion animals, environment enrichment in   434–5
compartmental models   18
Competent Authority for Land Acquisition (CALA) project,
      in India   599
compliance   201
composting procedure/methods   150, 508–9
   Bangalore method   509
   bed method of   514, 515f
   benefits of   509
   carcases   517, 553–4
   Coimbatore method   509
   factors affecting   508t
   Indore method   509
   pit method of   514, 515f
Comprehensive Metaanalysis (CMA)   243
compressed biogas (CBG)   512–13, 513t
Compulsory Reporting of Cattle Deaths Notice 1925   177
condensation   441
confidence intervals   244
confounding   51, 126–7, 195, 266
   control of   127
   situations   127f
coniferous forest ecosystem   373
CONSORT statement   212
contact spread/transmission   53, 74, 101
contagious bovine pleuropneumonia (CBPP)   57t, 111, 170t
contagious ecthyma   147t
continuous biosecurity   153
continuous data   15
continuous variables   13
Contractor's All Risk Insurance (CARI)   607
control
   of environmental hazards   323–4
   and eradication of zoonoses   283–4
   strategies of disease management   150–2
      chemoprophylaxis   150
      chemotherapy   150

622 | Index

control (*cont'd*)
  disinfection   152
  of internal parasites by deworming   151–2
  slaughter   150–1
Control and Diseases of Animals Act–Malawi   177
Control and Diseases of Animals (Prohibition of Importation of Animals) Order 1990   178
Control and Diseases of Animals (Veterinary Services Fees) Rules 1973   178
Control and Diseases of Farm Animals Rules 1968   178
controlled trials   197
Control of Dogs Rules 1969   178
convalescent carrier   70
convective rainfall   441
Convention on Biological Diversity (CBD)   421, 484, 485
Convention on International Trade in Endangered Species of Wild Fauna and Flora (CITES)   420, 483
Convention on Long-Range Trans-boundary Air Pollution   480
Convention on Migratory Species (CMS)   420
Convention on Wetlands   419
Conventions on Chemicals and Hazardous Wastes   484
Conventions on the Ozone Layer   485
Coordinated Programme for the Control of Ticks and Tick-Borne Diseases   254–5
Coronavirus Disease 2019 (COVID-19)   56*f*, 71, 487
corporate biodiversity stewardship   356
correlational studies. *See* ecological studies
Corylus avellana   373
cost–benefit analyses (CBAs)   159, 160*t*
cost–benefit assessment (CBA) methods   169
COVID-19 pandemic, statistical modeling for   249–50
cow pats/cow manure   506
cox proportional hazards model   13, 15
Crataegus   373
Crimean-Congo hemorrhagic fever   56*f*, 559*t*
cross-over design   200
cross-sectional studies   120, 194–5, 194*f*, 208, 210
crude mortality rate   131
crude rates   51
Cryptococcus neoformans   77
Cryptosporidium spp.   570
Ctenocephalides felis   87
Culex mosquito   68–9
Culicoides imicola   263
cultural ecosystem services   353
cumulative incidence   131
cutaneous squamous cell carcinoma   48
cyanide (Cn)   398
cyanobacteria   480
cyclone separators   387

Cyclops vernalis   563
cysticercosis   255
cytotoxic T cells   272

d

dampening down vaccination   148
"dancing-cat disease"   396, 466
data
  analysis   219–20
  extraction   232
  meaning of   215
  nature of   216–19
  synthesis   232
  See also big data
data collection   215–16
  and analysis technologies   26
  case reporting   10
  challenges of   11
    access to populations   11
    data management and security   11
    ensuring accuracy and reliability   11
    ethical issues   11
    legal compliance   11
    resource constraints   11
  focus group   215
  importance of
    research and policy development   10
    surveillance and early detection   10
    understanding disease dynamics   10
  interviews   216
  introduction   9
  methods of   10–11
  MOSS method   111–12
  observation   216
  sampling   10–11
  scope and relevance   9–10
  in veterinary epidemiology   9–10
data curation   215
data extraction, in systematic review   238–40
  description of exposure and outcome measurements   239
  participant description   239
  statistical data/results   239
  study description   239
dead-end hosts   70
death rates   131
decibels (dB)   452–3
Decision Support Systems (DSS)   20
  supporting policy and management decisions   20
  technological advances   20
decision tree analysis   160*t*

Declaration of Diseases of Animals 1969 178
decomposers 366
Deepwater Horizon Oil spill (2010) 461
definitive host 69
deforestation 332–3, 332*f*
  causes of 333
  and desertification 484
  major effects of 333
  risk of disease transmission 560
dengue virus 56*f*, 559, 559*t*
denitrification 382
Department of Animal Husbandry, Dairying and Fisheries
    (DADF) 141
Department of Environment and Natural Resources
    (DENR) 599, 600
Department of Public Works and Highways (DPWH)
    599, 600, 603, 605
Department of Transportation and Communications
    (DOTC) 600
depletion of ozone layer 480
depuration 465
desalination 443
descriptive epidemiology 4–5
  as essential for multitude of reasons 4
    characterizing affected populations 4
    early detection of outbreaks 4
    identifying temporal trends 4
    mapping the geographic distribution 4
  significance of 4
  tools in 5
    disease mapping 5
    spatial analysis 5
descriptive statistics 12, 13
descriptive studies 118
desert ecosystem 376–7, 376*f*
  adaptations in plants and animals 377
  cold/temperate desert 377
  fauna 377
  flora 377
  hot/thar desert 376
desertification 336
determinants of disease 35–9, 41–51
  agent determinants 37, 37*f*, 48–50
  classic epidemiological triad 46*b*
  classification of determinants 42*b*
  environmental determinants 37–9, 50–1, 50–1*t*
  extrinsic determinants 42*b*, 43, 44–5*t*, 44*b*
  host determinants 36–7, 36*f*, 47–8
  intrinsic determinants 42*b*, 43, 44–5*t*, 44*b*
  primary determinants 42, 42*b*, 43*f*
  secondary determinants 42, 42*b*, 43*f*

  triad 36*f*, 43
deterministic models 18
deworming
  frequency of 152
  methods and medications 151
  schedule for pigs 152
  schedule for sheep and goats 152
  schedule recommended for buffalo calves 151*t*
diagnostic testing 202–4
  in practice 204
  quality of test
    accuracy 202
    negative predictive value 203
    parallel testing 203
    positive predictive value 203
    precision 202
    sensitivity 203
    serial testing 203–4
    specificity 203
  reliability of tests
    interobserver variation 204
    intraobserver variation 204
    intrasubject variation 204
diarrheal ailments 67
dichlorodiphenyltrichloroethane (DDT) 312, 314
  bioaccumulation and biomagnification, in aquatic
      ecosystem 466–7, 467*f*
  metabolism of 467*f*
  possible human health effects 469*t*
dieldrin 468*t*
dimethyl sulfide 480
dioxins 469*t*
  and furans 552
direct costs 157–8
direct standardization method 52
direct transmission 71
  blocking of 572
  of diseases 24, 562, 571
Disability-Adjusted Life Year (DALY) 60, 62
disaster 487–8. *See also* animal disaster management
discrete variables 13
disease 145
  definition of 99–100
  early diagnosis of 148–9
  external factors causing illness 100*t*
  forecasting, approaches 140
  frequency, measuring 128
  incidence patterns 101–2, 101*f*
  mapping 5
  monitoring 108
  prognosis, in India 140–1

624 | Index

disease (cont'd)
  prognosticating and forecasting 140
  See also determinants of disease; livestock diseases;
    specific entries
disease causation triad 22–3
disease, consequences of 77*f*
  active disease
    clinical/overt 78
    inapparent 77
    subclinical 77
  carrier stage 78
  chronic stage 78
  death 78
  latency 78
  recovery 78
disease control and prevention
  quarantine measures 8
  vaccination programs 8
  in veterinary epidemiology 8
disease control program (DCP) 108
disease dynamics
  burden pyramid of infectious disease 58–9
    and epidemiological severity parameters 58*f*
  current trends in distribution of infectious diseases of
    animals 57–8*t*
  drivers of change in 57*f*
  examples of epidemic periods
    associated with different eras of human
      transportation 55*f*
  major diseases of animal-origin affecting human health 56*f*
  major trends in 54–9
disease ecology 81
  and factors in emergence 81–5
  population ecology, genetics, and emergence disease 82–5
disease emergence, factors and determinants of 62, 63*f*
disease eradication
  biological control 576–7
  early warning system 577–8
    environmental observations 578
    epidemiological surveillance 578
    harnessing the power of 577*f*
    preparedness/response 578
    public communication 578
    risk analysis 578
    vulnerability assessment 578
  education and training 579
  and elimination 576–9, 577*t*
  program (DEP) 108
  strategy for
    at continental level 254
    global initiatives for 304–5
    at global level 253–4

disease, factors affecting spread of
  agent factors 69
  effective contact 69
  host factors 68–9
disease management, strategies of
  biosecurity measures 152–3, 153*f*
    continuous biosecurity 153
    locational biosecurity 152–3
    operational biosecurity 153
    structural biosecurity 153
  control 150–2
    chemoprophylaxis 150
    chemotherapy 150
    disinfection 152
    of internal parasites by deworming 151–2
    slaughter 150–1
  prevention 145–50
    animal comfort 149
    calf health 149
    disposal of carcase 149–50
    early disease diagnosis 148–9
    host movement 149
    improvement in environment, husbandry, and
      feeding 149
    quarantine 148
    tools of epidemiology 149
    udder health 149
    vaccination programs 145–8, 147–8*t*
  See also disease prevention, and control measures
disease outbreaks
  advances in estimating cost of 169, 171
  early detection and containment of 3, 135
  investigating 9, 104
  monitoring 7
  See also animal diseases
disease prevention, and control measures
  blocking routes of transmission 571–2, 571*f*
  diagnosis 572, 573*f*
  disease occurrence pattern 575, 575*t*
  epidemiological control 574–5
  failure, in South Asia 579
  immunization 576
  incidence/prevalence rate 575
  isolation 573
  levels of 569–71
  primary prevention 570
  primordial prevention 569–70
  quarantine 573–4
  quaternary prevention 570–1
  secondary prevention 570
  tertiary prevention 570
  therapy and chemoprophylaxis 575–6

disease's level, finding
  example A
    accumulated occurrence 102
    density of incidence 102
    prevalence 103
  example B
    period prevalence 103
    point prevalence 103
    rate of attack 103
Diseases of Animals Act Botswana 179
Diseases of Animals Rules 1923 177
Diseases of Animals (Cattle) Rules 1942 177–8
Diseases of Animals (Stock Route) Rules 1958 178
disease surveillance 108
  and ICAR 141
  and outbreak investigation 293
  system 139–40
disease tracking list (DTL) 139
disease transmission
  through clothing 546
  direct transmission 24, 562, 571
  indirect transmission 24, 571, 572
  vectors and reservoirs in 561–2, 561*f*
  See also transmission
disinfection, as control measure for disease
        management 152
disinfection methods of water 446*t*
dissolved oxygen 380
DNA plasmid vaccines 272
"dom-dom fever". *See* leishmaniasis
domestic sewage 518
dose-response relationship 6
double-blind study 201
Draft Convention on the Transboundary Shipment of
        Hazardous Waste 484
drainage 86
drinking water purification 445–7
  disinfection methods 446*t*
  filtration techniques 445–6, 445*t*
  polymer and nanotechnology 447*t*
  techniques 445*t*
droplet transmission 24
drug residues 400
drug wastes 525
dung 506
  and urine production 507*t*

e

early detection and containment of disease outbreaks, in
        animal populations 3
early warning systems 136, 577–8
  environmental observations 578

epidemiological surveillance 578
EWS components 139–40
harnessing the power of 577*f*
initiatives for 136–7
preparedness/response 578
public communication 578
risk analysis 578
system development 137
vulnerability assessment 578
Earths atmospheric composition 416*t*
Earth Summit (1992), Rio de Janeiro 321, 322*f*, 421, 483
earthworms 514
Ebola virus disease 56*f*, 60, 279
ecological fallacy 119
ecological monitoring
  Global Information System (GIS) 90
  ground sampling 89–90
  practical application of veterinary data acquired by 90–1
  remote sensing 90
  systematic reconnaissance flights 90
  techniques 85, 89–90
ecological pyramids 368–70, 369*f*
  pyramid of biomass 369–70, 370*f*
  pyramid of energy 370, 371*f*
  pyramid of numbers 369, 369*f*
ecological release 84
ecological studies 118–19
ecological system of living things 83*f*
economic losses, due to animal diseases
  climate-sensitive diseases 169
  estimation of 165–9
  loss from mortality 165
  loss in milk yield 166
  transboundary animal diseases 166–9
  treatment costs 166
ecosystem
  abiotic components 366
  aquatic ecosystems 378–80
    freshwater ecosystems 378, 378*f*
    marine ecosystems 379–80, 379*f*
  biotic components 365–6
    autotrophs 366
    heterotrophs 366
    saprotrophs 366
  components of 365–6, 366*f*
  definition of 365
  ecological pyramids 368–70, 369*f*
    pyramid of biomass 369–70, 370*f*
    pyramid of energy 370, 371*f*
    pyramid of numbers 369, 369*f*
  food chains 367–8
  food webs 368, 368*f*

Index

ecosystem (cont'd)
functions of 366–7
impact on 406
importance of 384
nutrient cycling, biogeochemical processes of 380–4
carbon cycle 380, 381*f*
nitrogen cycle 380–2, 381*f*
phosphorus cycle 382–4, 383*f*
water cycle 382, 383*f*
terrestrial ecosystem 370–7
desert ecosystem 376–7, 376*f*
forest ecosystem 373–4, 373*f*
grassland ecosystem 371–3, 372*f*
tundra ecosystem 374–6, 374*f*
types of 370
ecosystem diversity 350–1
ecosystem typology 350
functional redundancy and complementarity 351
trophic interactions and food webs 351
ecosystem functioning
biodiversity-ecosystem functioning experiments 353
role of biodiversity in nutrient cycling, and productivity 353
ecosystem services and biodiversity
cultural ecosystem services 353
quantifying 353
ecosystem stability and resilience, biodiversity loss on 353
edge effects and fragmentation 354
effective contact 69
electric accidents 585
electrocoagulation (EC) 446
electrodialysis 446
electroflotation (EF) 446
electronic wastes. *See* e-waste
electrostatic precipitators 387
elevational biodiversity patterns
biogeographical drivers 352, 352*f*
species richness and turnover 352
Eliminate Yellow Fever Epidemics (EYE) Strategy
(2017–2026) 307
Elton, Charles 368
EMBASE 233
Emergency Planning and Community Right-to-Know Act
(EPCRA) 478
Emergency Prevention System (EMPRES)
for Animal Health (EMPRES-AH) 251
goal of EMPRES-i 137
initiative for early warning 137
for Transboundary Animal and Plant Pests and
Diseases 253
emergency vaccination 145
emerging and exotic diseases, control of 275
emerging diseases, identifying 8

emerging infectious diseases (EIDs) 25, 41, 62
employment and livelihood promotion 604
endangered species, identifying threats to 355
endemic diseases, control of
animal health delivery at herd level 256
brucellosis 254
contribution of isotopic and nuclear techniques 259
diagnosis 257–8
enabling domains 257
information 257
insect-borne diseases 255–6
non-infectious and production diseases 256
tick-and tick-borne diseases 254–5
vaccines 258
veterinary sciences 258–9
endemic diseases, incidence of 102
endotoxins 272
endrin 468*t*
energy, pyramid of 370, 371*f*
engineered bioremediation 389
Enhanced Gonococcal Antimicrobial Surveillance Program
(EGASP) 308
enterohemorrhagic *Escherichia coli* (EHEC) 284
enterotoxemia 147*t*
environment 321
environmental contaminants
air-borne pollutants 316–17
biomedical wastes and pharmaceuticals 314–15
bioremediation 470
defined 461
ecological consequences 469
e-waste 317–18, 464
and food chain bioaccumulation 465–7
healthcare-associated infections and 547–8
heavy metals/metalloids 312–13, 463
impacts on human health 467–9
microplastics 315–16
nanoparticles/nanomaterials 464–5
pathways of bioaccumulation 466–7
persistent organic pollutants (POPs) 313–14, 463
pesticides 310–12
pharmaceuticals and personal care products (PPCPs) 463
plastics 464
possible human health effects of 468–9*t*
radionuclides 463–4
risk assessment and monitoring 469–70
solvents 314
sources and hazardous effects of 309–18, 311*t*, 462, 462*f*
types 463–5
environmental determinants 37–9, 50–1
of animal disease 37*f*
classification of 50–1*t*

climate 38
climate change 38
husbandry 38
location 38
stress 38–9
environmental DNA (eDNA) and metabarcoding
techniques 357
Environmental Guarantee Fund (EGF) 607
environmental hazards 323
environmental hygiene
advances in 324–6
bioremediation 325–6
applying genetically engineered strains to clean up
environment 325–6
biodegradation 326
biotechnological approaches 325
rain water harvesting 326
recharge to groundwater 326
carbon sequestration 324–5
geological 324
ocean 325, 326f
terrestrial 324, 325f
definition 321–2
general aspects of 321–8
objectives of 323–4
prevention and control
of biological hazards 323
of chemical hazards 323
of physical hazards 323
sociological and psychological hazards 324
scope of 322–3
environmental impact assessment (EIA) 600, 601
environmental management, themes of 481–2
environmental monitoring program 604–7
implementation monitoring 605, 607
monitoring plan 605, 606t
environmental noises 452, 455
environmental pollution 337
acid rain 399–400
air pollution 386–8
causes 386
classification 386
control 387–8, 387f, 388f
effects 386–7
effects on health and environment 397f
impacts 397–8
major causes 397
primary pollutants 397
secondary pollutants 397
types 397
current patterns and requirement for additional study 401
different types of 406f

drug residues 400
effect on animal and human health 393–401
effects of 393–4
gaseous pollutants 394–5
greenhouse effect 400
heavy metal toxicity 395–6, 395f
impact of pollution by radioactive materials 399
marine pollution 390–1
control 391
effects 391
sources 391
noise pollution 399
pesticide pollution 400
pollution from industries 396–7
soil pollution 389–90, 398–9
causes 390
control 390
effects 390
thermal pollution 391–2
control 392
effects 391
sources 391
types of 385, 397–9
water pollution 398
causes 389
classification 388
control 389, 390f
effect 389
environmental preservation. See environmental protection
environmental protection 478
conventions/treaties on 482–5
international principles and doctrines 485
principles and issues of 477–85
types of pollution 478–81
Environmental Protection Agency (EPA) 292, 480
environmental risk assessment (ERA) 469
environment enrichment 428
in animals, factors affecting effectiveness of 435–6
in captivity 428–30
in companion animals 434–5
enrichment practices
to improving welfare in pigs 432–3
to improving welfare of poultry 432
enrichment programs
in zoos and wildlife sanctuaries 429–30
evaluating enrichment techniques 436–7
long-term assessment 436–7
short-term assessment 436
in farm animal production systems 430–3
dairy animals 431
poultry farming 431–2
in laboratory animal facilities 433–4

environment enrichment (*cont'd*)
limitations of 437
role in physical/mental/emotional well-being of
animals 428
swine farming 432–3
techniques in captivity 429
environment, in host-agent interaction 23, 574–5
environment management plan (EMP) 599
design and construction management program 599–600
environmental guarantees 607
environmental monitoring plan 604–7
implementation and resource requirement 607, 608–13*t*
project commitments, affirmations, and agreements 607
social development and institutional plans. *See* social
development program (SDP)
enzootic bovine leucosis (EBL) 111
enzyme-linked immunosorbent assay (ELISA) 149, 258
epidemic diseases
eradication versus control 252–3
incidence of 102
epidemics and their investigation
investigation of outbreak 53–4
pathogenesis of outbreak 53
steps in epidemic investigations 54*t*
epidemiological studies 117
biases associated with 195
classification of 118*t*, 192*f*
comparative 191–5
experimental study 195
systematic reviews in 229–44
assessing bias 243
citation searching 237–8
components 233*f*
contacting authors 238
data extraction 238–40
diagrammatic representation 230*f*
gray literature in 234
guidelines 232–3
handling search results 234–5
metaanalysis 241–4
methods section of protocol 231–2, 231*f*
narrative synthesis 240–1
primary goal of 229
process 229–30
PROSPERO 230
protocol for 232
results synthesis 240–4
risk of bias assessment 240
screening search result 235–7
searching databases 232*t*, 233–4
sensitivity analysis 243
See also experimental epidemiology; observational studies

epidemiological triads
determinants associated with 42*b*
of disease 22, 82*f*
for Kyasanur Forest disease (KFD) and winter
diarrhea 68*f*
epidemiologic triangle. *See* triad of disease causation
epidemiology 41, 245
and environmental health in veterinary medicine 339–42
and risk analysis 187–8
tools of 149
See also analytical epidemiology; descriptive epidemiology;
experimental epidemiology; nutritional epidemiology;
veterinary epidemiology
Epi-InfoTM (Analysis Project on Livestock Disease
Forecasting/Forewarning) 141
epizootic diseases, outbreaks of 89
"equimarginal principle" 156
equine abortion 148*t*
equine herpesvirus 1 148*t*
equine influenza 148*t*, 171*t*
equivalence studies 200
eradication, defined 576
Eradication of East Coast Fever Rules 1969 178
Escherichia coli 44, 304, 325, 497, 551
Escherichia coli O157:H7 101, 112, 275, 290
ethanol 152
ethical criteria for controlled trials 201
ethical issues, in data collection 11
evergreen forests 373
evidence-based practice, in industrial hygiene 596–7
e-waste 317–18, 464, 469*t*
exosphere 416
experimental epidemiology 118, 123
adult mortality rate 133
age-specific death rates 132
case fatality 131
community trials 124–5
limitations of 125
confounding 126–7
control of 127
situations 127*f*
cumulative incidence 131
death rates 131
external validity 128
field trials 124
incidence 129, 130
infant mortality 132
internal validity 128
matching 127
maternal mortality rate 132
measurement bias 126
measuring disease frequency 128

mortality 131
population at risk 129
potential errors in epidemiological 125
prevalence 129–30, 130f
proportionate mortality 132
random error 125
randomization 127
randomized controlled trials (RCTs) 124, 124f
restriction 127
sample size 125
selection bias 126
stratification and statistical modeling 127–8
systematic error 126
validity 128, 128f
experimental population research 212
experimental study 195
exposure/outcome model 231
extended host range 76
external validity 128, 197, 244
extraterrestrial and terrestrial wavelength spectrum 417f
extrinsic determinants 42b, 43
of canine pruritus 44t
causes of haemolysis 45t
character of 44b
extrinsic incubation period 68
Exxon Valdez 478

f

fabric filters 387
facility-based sentinel surveillance system 140
factorial designs 200
false-color techniques 90
farm animal production systems, environment
enrichment in 430–3
farming methods 281
farm waste 505–21
carcase disposal 516–17
See also livestock waste management; sewage disposal
fauna 377
faunal factors 88–9
fecal examination 149
fecal–oral route 74
fecundity schedule 92, 93
Federal Select Agent Program (FSAP) 293
field trials 124
fire 89
fire and chemical accidents 586–7
controlling arsenic poisoning 586
lead poisoning 586–7
organophosphate poisoning accidents 587
fixed dome type biogas plant 510, 511f
floating drum type biogas plant 510, 511f

floods 85, 585, 585f
flora 377
flue gas desulfurization (FGD) 480
fluorinated agents 395
fMRI 217
focus group data collection, advantages/disadvantages of 215
folate 266
follow-up
and compliance 200–1
and incidence studies. *See* cohort studies
fomite 70, 71
transmission 572
Food and Agriculture Organization (FAO) 99, 137, 156, 257,
261, 302, 303
Animal Health Service 259
Animal Production and Health Division 303
biotechnology networks at 258
Early Warning System for Global Avian Influenza
Monitoring 139
FAO/World Health Organization Food Standards
Program 99
Field Programme 255
Global Rinderpest Eradication Programme (GREP) 253
livestock programme 256
role 252
Technical Cooperation Programme (TCP) 255, 256
WHO Expert Committee on Veterinary Public Health 301
Food and Drug Administration (FDA) 292
food-borne diseases 62, 289, 304
transmission 24
food chain bioaccumulation
of DDT in aquatic ecosystem 466–7, 467f
of environmental contaminants 465–7
Minamata disease 466
pathways of bioaccumulation 466–7
quantification of trophic transfer of heavy metals 465–6
food chain, in ecosystem 367–8, 367f
food production chain 281
food safety 4, 99, 188
global initiatives for 304
inspection programs 293
methods of ensuring 283f
risk analysis 205
food webs 368, 368f
foot and mouth disease (FMD) 102, 103, 146t, 147t, 148t,
156, 163t, 166–8, 170t, 185, 254, 263, 288
components of losses due to 167t
on fertility of cattle 193
global economic impact 168f
global impact due to vaccination costs and production
losses 168t
impacts 167f

foot diseases 262
forecasting 135
  purpose of 135–6
foregone revenues 158
forest ecosystem 373–4, 373f
  coniferous forest ecosystem 373
  temperate deciduous forest 373
  temperate evergreen forest 373–4
  temperate rainforests 374
  tropical rainforests 374
  tropical seasonal forests 374
Forest Principles 484
forest resources 331–3
  abuses 332–3
  deforestation 332–3, 332f
    causes of 333
    major effects of 333
  ecological uses 332
  esthetic uses 332
  overexploitation of forests 332
  productive uses 331
  protective uses 331
  regulative uses 331–2
forever chemicals. *See* persistent organic pollutants (POPs)
forward citation searching 237
fossil fuel
  combustion 397
  overuse of 415
fowlpox 288
fowlpox virus and herpesvirus recombinant vaccines 273
fragmentation, habitat loss and 354
Framingham study 122
Francisella (Pasteurella) tularensis 86
frank clinical reaction 49t
free-text terms 231, 232t, 234
frequency distribution 216
freshwater ecosystems 378, 378f
  lentic ecosystem 378
  lotic ecosystem 378
frontal rainfall 441
fruit bats (*Pteropus* spp.) 74, 87
Fukushima nuclear accident 479
full-text screening 236
full wastewater sewage disposal system 520
functional complementarity 351
functional redundancy 351

g

Gambusia affinis 562
gaseous byproducts 388, 388f
gaseous pollutants
  ammonia (NH_3) 395, 499–500

in and around animal housing 497
bio-aerosols 502
carbon dioxide (CO_2) 394, 498–9
carbon monoxide 500
fluorinated agents 395
of human and animals 394f
hydrogen sulfide 500
methane (CH_4) 394, 499
nitrous oxide (N_2O) 394, 500
odor 500–1
particulate matter 501–2
sulfur dioxide (SO_2) 394
and their health hazards 394–5
volatile organic compounds 501
gastroenteritis 60
gastrointestinal nematodes 89
gene-deleted vaccines 273
Gene Expression Omnibus (GEO) 217
generalizability 128, 197
generation time 95
genetic determinants 47
genetic diversity 349–50
  genomic approaches 349
  phylogenomics 350
  population genetics 350
genetic manipulation techniques 563
genetic predispositions 25
genetic variability 83
genomics
  big data in 217–18
  integration with conservation biology 357
genotype, of host 47
Geographical Information System (GIS) 7, 15, 101, 135, 140, 255
geological sequestration 324
gerbil (*Meriones shawi*) 87
glanders 57t
Global Action Plan on Antimicrobial Resistance (GAP-AMR) 305, 307
Global Antimicrobial Resistance and Use Surveillance System (GLASS) 307
Global Burden of Animal Diseases (GBADs) program 164–5
  approach to evaluating burden of animal diseases 165f
  key components of 164f
Global Burden of Disease (GBD) study, for human health 164
Global Early Warning and Response System (GLEWS) 138–40
  aims of 138
  combined risk assessment for zoonotic diseases 138
  GLEWS Management Committee (GMC) 138
  method for treating highly pathogenic avian influenza (HPAI) 139

national and regional networks support   138
   Rift Valley fever (RVF) and   139
global governance and conservation   357
global health, future challenges   63
Global Influenza Surveillance and Response System
   (GISRS)   307
Global Information System (GIS)   90
Global Outbreak Alert and Response Network
   (GOARN)   137
Global Rinderpest Eradication Programme (GREP)
   253, 271
Global Surveillance and Early Warning System
   (GLEWS)   285–6
global warming   397
   adaptation and mitigation strategies for   423
   anthropogenic factors   418
   defined   415
   effect of GHGs   418–19
   factors affecting   417–19
   natural factors   417–18
Global Yellow Fever Elimination Strategy (GYFES)   307
gloves, wearing   546
goat pox   147t
Goddard Institute for Space Studies (GISS)   418
Gonococcal Antimicrobial Surveillance Program
   (GASP)   308
"Gorilla World" exhibit   429
gradient of infection   49, 49t
grassland ecosystem   369, 371–3, 372f
   animals (fauna) of   372
   economic importance of   373
   living (biotic) components of   372
   nonliving (Abiotic) components of   372
   trees/plants/shrubs/herbs (flora) of   373
gray literature   234
greenhouse effect   400, 415–17
greenhouse gases (GHGs)   415, 416, 418–19, 480, 484, 525
ground-level ozone (O_3)   317, 408t
ground sampling   89–90
groundwater   442

h

habitat fragmentation   83–4
habitat loss and fragmentation
   edge effects and fragmentation   354
   land use change and habitat conversion   354
Hadoop/core Hadoop   219
Hadoop distributed file system (HDFS)   217
   architecture of   219
Haemaphysalis spinigera   68
haemolysis, causes of   45t
HANDISTATUS   257

Handistatus II System   137
handling search results   234–5
hand sanitation   546
   gloves   546
   hand sanitizers   546
   hand washing   546
Hantaan virus   557
hantaviruses   88, 282
hazard analysis critical control point (HACCP) method
   281, 284, 343
hazard identification   205
hazardous air pollutants (HAPs)   317
hazardous waste   524, 526
   and disposal   481
health   145, 279
   and hygiene   322f
   integrated systems for monitoring   340f
   surveillance   597
   See also animal health; human health; public health
healthcare-associated infections
   and environmental contamination in veterinary
      hospitals   547–8
health hazards
   anticipation of   593–4
   recognition of   594
health risks, associated with pollution   406, 412
health schemes and its importance   251–9
Health Technology Assessments (HTA) database   234
healthy carriers   70
hearing impairment   454
heat stress   263
heavy metals   312–13, 389, 393, 399, 463, 468t, 586
   quantification of trophic transfer of   465–6
heavy metal toxicity
   arsenic (As)   395
   cadmium (Cd)   396
   lead (Pb)   396
   mercury (Hg)   395–6
   selenium (Se)   396
   and their health hazards   395–6, 395f
hedgehogs (Erinaceus europaeus)   88
Hemispheric Programme for Eradication of Food and Mouth
      Disease   254
hemorrhagic fever with renal syndrome (HFRS)   88
hemorrhagic septicemia (HS)   146t, 147t, 148t
Hendra virus disease   56f, 69, 87
heptachlor   468t
herbivores   368, 369
Herd Health and Production Programme (HH&PP)
      protocol   256
herd immunity   34–5
hertz (Hz)   453

Index

heterogeneity
  assessment 243
  and subgroup analyses 244
heterogeneous nature, of big data 218
heterotrophs 366
hexachlorobenzene (HCB) 468t
highly pathogenic avian influenza H5N1 (HPAI H5N1)
    56f, 88, 100, 139, 170–1t, 285
Hippocrates 302
Histoplasma capsulatum 77
historical biogeography 351
historical cohort studies 122
historical control studies 198
hit and run strategy 75
HIV/AIDS 56f
hog cholera 146t
homogeneity of studies 241
hookworms (*Ancylostoma* spp.) 87
horizontal transmission 35, 71, 101
hormonal determinants 47
hospital-acquired infections (HAIs), in veterinary
    hospitals 547–8
host determinants 36–7, 47–8
  age 36, 47
  of animal disease 36f
  behavior 36, 48
  coat color 37, 48
  genotype 47
  other determinants 48
  sex 36, 47
  size and conformation 37, 48
  species and breed 36, 47–8
host-environment interaction 23
hosts 23, 59, 574–5
  accidental host 70
  definitive host 69
  movement of 149
  parasites and 83
  paratenic host 70
  primary/natural/maintenance host 69
  secondary host 69
hot/thar desert 376
human health
  acid rain effect on 480
  assessing risks to 19–20
  biomedical waste and 526
  environmental contaminants impacts on 467–9
  Global Burden of Disease (GBD) study for 164
  major diseases of animal-origin affecting 56f
  noise pollution on 453–6
  veterinarians in 300–1
  See also environmental pollution

husbandry
  diet 38
  housing 38
  management 38
hydatidosis 255
hydrofluorocarbons (HFCs) 400, 422
hydrogen cyanide 88
hydrogen peroxide 152
hydrogen sulfide 500
hydrological cycle 440–2, 440f
  components
    atmosphere and precipitation 441
    groundwater 442
    lakes/reservoirs/ponds 442
    oceans 442
    streams and rivers 441–2
    wetlands 442
hygiene 537
  defined 326–7
  UNICEF scenario on 327–8
  World Health Organization scenario on 327
hypomagnesemia 50–1
hyraxes (*Procavia capensis*) 86

i

I2 value 243
iatrogenic transmission 74
illegal wildlife trade 355
immune status, of host 25
immune suppression 76
immunization 576
  active 576
  passive 576
immunogenicity 575
immunoglobulin (Ig) preparation 576
inapparent (silent) infection 49t
incidence and prevalence 101f, 117, 129, 130, 575
  correlation between 103
  differences between 129t
incidence density 102
incidental endogeneity 218
incineration 531–2, 552–3
  high-temperature 532
  at medium temperature 532
  nonincineration treatments 532
  process 150
incompatible insect technique approach (IIT)
    564, 564f
incubation period 35, 68
incubatory carrier 70
independent variable screening 218
in-depth/unstructured interviews 216

India
  Assistance to States for Control of Animal Diseases (ASCAD)   182
  Biomedical Waste (Management and Handling) Rules in   526, 529
  call centers   183
  Classic Swine Fever Control Program (CSF-CP)   183
  disease prognosis in   140–1
  Existing Veterinary Hospitals and Dispensaries (ESVHD) establishment and strengthening of   183
  livestock wastes   505
  Mobile Veterinary Units (MVUs)   183
  Peste des Petits Ruminants Eradication Program (PPR-EP)   183
  pesticide production   310
  regulations in   182–3
  zoos and wildlife parks   430
indirect costs   158
indirect standardization method   52
indirect transmission   71–2
  blocking of   572
  of diseases   24, 571
industrial emissions   413
industrial hygiene
  defined   593
  evidence-based practices   596–7
    exposure monitoring   597
    health surveillance   597
    training and education   597
  fundamental elements of   595t
  maintenance of   593–7
  maintenance strategies for
    administrative controls   596
    engineering controls   596
    hazard identification and risk assessment   596
    personal protective equipment (PPE)   596
    routine inspections and assessments   595–6
  principles   593–5, 594f
    anticipation of health hazards   593–4
    confirmation of control measures   595
    control over worker exposure   594–5
    developing program, with CHAMP   595
    evaluation of exposure   594
    industrial hygiene monitoring   594
    recognition of health hazards   594
industrial waste, and soil pollution   399
industrial wastewater   518
industries, pollution from   396–7
inertization   531
infant mortality   132
infection, maintenance of   75–7
  biofilm   76

extended host range   76
hit and run strategy   75
hit and stay/persistence within host   76
no environmental stage   76–7
resistant form   76
infectious bovine rhinotracheitis (IBR)   111, 147t
infectious diseases   62, 67, 99, 145, 245, 264
infectiousness   68
infectivity of agent   69
inferential statistics   12
Influenza A virus subtype H1N1   56f
information, education, and communication (IEC)   600–1
informed consent   201
infrared radiation   417
ingestion, method of transmission   74
inhalation, method of transmission   74
injectible dewormers   151
inoculation, method of transmission   74
insect-borne diseases   255–6
insecticides application, for controlling vector populations   562, 563f
insecticide-treated bed nets (ITNs)   562
insolation   88
Institute of Nuclear Power Operations (INPO)   479
institutional plan   604
integrated pest management (IPM)   312, 412
integrated vector management (IVM), in veterinary public health   563, 564f
intent-to-treat analysis   201
Interagency Coordination Group on Antimicrobial Resistance (IACG)   305
Inter-American Meeting   282
Intergovernmental Panel on Climate Change (IPCC)   59
internal parasites by deworming, control   151–2
internal validity   128, 197
International Plant Protection Convention (IPPC)   188
International Statistical Classification of Diseases and Related Health Problems (ICD)   131
international trade, benefits and barriers of   185
international travel and trade, in animals and animal products   281
interobserver variation   204
interquartile range   220
intervention studies   195. *See also* experimental epidemiology
interviews (in-depth/unstructured interviews)   216
intraobserver variation   204
intrasubject variation   204
intrinsic determinants   42b, 43
  of canine pruritus   44t
  causes of haemolysis   45t
  character of   44b

Index

intrinsic rate of increase 95–6
investigation of outbreak 53–4, 54t
invisible losses 158
iodine-based disinfectants 152
irritant pollutants 386
isolation 573
  and quarantine 574t
isopropyl alcohol 152
isotopic and nuclear techniques, contribution of 259

j

Jamoulle, Marc 570
Japanese encephalitis (JE) virus 70, 559, 559t
Jenner, Edward 300
Johne's disease 57t, 86
Joint Centre for Zoonotic Diseases and Antimicrobial
    Resistance 252
Joint FAO/OIE/Pan-American Health Organization (PAHO)
    Conference 254
"JungleWorld" exhibit 429

k

Kaplan-Meier estimators 15
Keys, Ancel 266
Kigali Amendment 422
Kikuyu grass (*Pennisetum clandestinum*) 88
Knox test 101
Koch, Robert 451
Kyasanur Forest disease (KFD) 68, 68f
Kyoto Protocol 421, 484

l

laboratory animal care 293
laboratory animal facilities
    enrichment techniques in laboratory animals 433–4
    welfare challenges 433
lagoons 520
lakes/reservoirs/ponds 442
lameness 262
Lancini 302
Land Acquisition and Resettlement Plan (LARP) 601
    See also social development program (SDP)
land use change and habitat conversion, on biodiversity 354
land use planning and corporate sustainability, biodiversity
    integration within 356
Lassa fever 56f
latent disease 34
latent infections 50
latitudinal gradients, in biodiversity 351–2
    contemporary explanations 352
    historical biogeography 351
lead (Pb) 396, 408t, 468t

lead poisoning 586–7, 587f
Leishmania aethiopica 86
leishmaniasis 87, 558–9
lentic ecosystem 378
Leptospira 502
life expectancy 94
life table technique and application 91–6, 93f
    calculating key parameters 93–4
        age-specific survivorship 94
        life expectancy 94
        standardized survival schedule 93
        survivorship curves 94, 94f
    cohort life tables 91, 92
    key parameters 92–3
    parameters 92–6
    population growth or decline 94–6
        generation time 95
        intrinsic rate of increase 95–6
        net reproductive rate 94–5
    reproductive value 96
    static life tables 91, 92
    varieties 91
lifetime prevalence 130
light pollution 410
Limited Test Ban Treaty (1963) 479
liquid precipitation 441
liquid waste 506, 507t
    collection of 507
    flushing of 507
    management 516
livestock accidents 582, 582f
Livestock Disease Control Act 1994, in Victoria 180–2
livestock diseases
    carrier state 34
    clinical and subclinical disease 33–4
    economic and social impacts of 156
    factors influencing 33–5
    herd immunity 34–5
    incubation period 35
    international laws and regulations on controlling 177–83
    modes of transmission 35
    outbreaks 155, 156
    pathways through pathogenic pathogens causing 100–1
livestock models, classification of 159f
livestock sensitive diseases
    key challenges and knowledge gaps in control of 62
        complexity of disease dynamics 62
        joint occurrence of climate sensitive diseases 62
        multi-host disease systems 62
        paucity of information 62
livestock waste management
    advanced methods of 509–16

collection 506–8
  flushing 507
  of liquid waste 507
  semiautomatic cow dung cleaning machine 507–8
  separate collection 507
  of solid waste 507
composting methods 508–9
importance of 505–6
liquid waste 506, 507*t*
  ammonia recycling 516
  management 516
solid waste 506
solid waste management
  biogas production 509–13
  litter management 516
  pyrolysis 515–16
  soldier fly breeding 516
  vermicomposting 514–15
traditional method of 508
  disadvantages 508
locational biosecurity 152–3
locoweed (*Oxytropis* spp.) 88
logistic and Poisson regression models 13
lotic ecosystem 378
lumpy skin disease (LSD) 57*t*, 169, 171*t*
Lyme disease 84, 272

m

machine learning
  algorithms, in predictive modeling 18–19
  artificial intelligence and 357
  and deep learning 26
  in epidemiology 14
macroclimate 38
Magna Carta on Human Environment 482
malaria 559
mammal productivity 88–9
Manhattan Principles 302
Mannheimia haemolytica 273
MapReduce 219
Marburg virus 56*f*, 86, 279
marine biodiversity, understanding effects on 354
marine ecosystems 379–80, 379*f*
  aphotic zone 380
  aquatic biome 379
  dissolved oxygen 380
  photic zone 379
  sunlight 379–80
  temperature 380
marine pollution 390–1
  control 391
  effects 391

sources 391
  treaties on 483
marmots (Marmota bobac) 88
masking (or blinding) 201
matching 127
maternal mortality rate 132
mathematical modeling 17–18
  agent-based models 18
  deterministic versus stochastic models 18
  differential equations 17
  overview of 17–18
  types of 18
  See also statistical and mathematical modeling
mean (arithmetic mean) 220
measles 82, 577*t*
measurement bias 126
measures of central tendency 219–20
  interquartile range 220
  mean (arithmetic mean) 220
  median 220
  mode 220
  range 220
  standard deviation 220
median 220
medical or healthcare waste 314–15
medical solid waste (MSW) disposal 525
MEDLINE 233
Megacyclops formosanus 563
membrane filtration 445, 445*t*
Mendelian inheritance 36, 47
meningeal worm (*Parelaphostrongylus tenuis*) 87
mercury (Hg) 313, 395–6, 466, 468*t*, 479
MeSH (Medical Subject Headings) terms 231, 232*t*, 233
mesosphere 416
metaanalysis 241–3
metagenomics 349
metalloids 463
Metawin 243
methane (CH_4) 394, 415, 418, 499, 505
methicillin-resistant *Staphylococcus aureus* (MRSA) 548
methyl isocyanate (MIC) gas 461, 478
methyl mercury (MeHg) 313, 396, 461, 466, 479
microbes 519
microbial/bacterial bioremediation 470
microbial traffic 62
microbiological waste 533
microclimate 38
microplastics (MPs) 315–16, 389, 462, 464, 469*t*
Microsoft Excel, conducting metaanalyses in 243
Middle East respiratory syndrome (MERS) 56*f*, 57*t*, 60
midnight sun, land of 375
Milankovitch cycle 417

milk fever 146t
milk testing 149
Minamata Convention 422
minamata disease 389, 461, 466
mineral resources 333–4
  abuses 334
  environmental impact 334
  remedial measures 334
  uses 333
mitigation 423
  control costs 158
  disaster 491
mobile sources of pollution 498, 499
Mobile Veterinary Units (MVUs) 183
mode 220
modeling and simulation, in veterinary epidemiology 16–22
  applications of 19
  challenges and limitations 19–21
    adaptive modeling and advances 21
    complexity and assumptions 21
    data limitations and quality 20
    ethical considerations 21
  Decision Support Systems (DSS) 20
  definition and purpose of 16–17
  disease spread and dynamics 19
  evaluating control measures 19
  future trends 21–2
    advancements in computational power 21
    integration of molecular epidemiology 21
    interdisciplinary collaboration 22
  historical evolution and significance 17
    computational era 17
    interdisciplinary integration 17
    pre-computational era 17
  mathematical modeling 17–18
  predictive modeling 18–19
  public health and zoonotic disease modeling 19–20
  relationship with traditional epidemiology 17
  transmission patterns 19
molecular ecology and genomics, advancements in
  environmental DNA and metabarcoding 357
  genomics and conservation 357
molecular epidemiology, integration of 21
monitoring 108
monitoring and surveillance system (MOSS) 109
  data collection method 111–12
  trade regulation change on MOSS planning and
    implementation 112–14
Montreal Protocol 420, 480, 485
MOOSE, guideline for conducting metaanalyses 233

mortality 117, 131
  during 2003 heat wave 119f
  pits 149
Movement of Farm Animals Rules 1968 178
moving average (MA) 247t
multicenter trials 200
multidrug-resistant *Salmonella typhimurium* 279, 284
Multipartite Monitoring Team (MMT) 604, 605, 607
multivariate analysis 12
mumps 577t
municipal wastewater system 520
Musca domestica 70, 72
Mycobacterium spp 502
Mycobacterium tuberculosis 74, 76
mycoremediation 470

n

NADRES (National Animal Disease Referral Expert
  System) 141
Naegleria fowleri 48
Nagoya Protocol 422
nanoparticles/nanomaterials 464–5, 469t
nanoplastics 469t
narrative synthesis, in systematic review 240–1
National Agricultural Technology Programme 141
National Center For Biotechnology Information (NCBI) 217
National Oceanic and Atmospheric Administration
  (NOAA) 135
natural bioremediation 389
natural disasters 487
  classification of 488f
  occurrence of 494
natural resources
  abiotic resources 329
  biotic resources 329
  conservation of 337
  cultural importance 337
  definition of 329
  economic importance 336
  environmental importance 336
  forest resources 331–3
    abuses 332–3
    uses 331–2
  importance of 336–7
  mineral resources 333–4
    abuses 334
    environmental impact 334
    remedial measures 334
    uses 333
  nonrenewable 330f, 331

renewable   329–31, 330*f*

soil resources   334–6

abuses   334–6

desertification   336

soil erosion   334, 335*f*

threats to   337

climate change   337

environmental pollution   337

overpopulation   337

types of   329, 330*f*

water resources   336

abuses   336

uses   336

negative predictive value (NPV)   203

neglected tropical diseases (NTDs)   60, 61*f*

nekton   379

nested case-control studies   123, 123*f*

net reproductive rate   94–5

network metaanalysis (NMA)   242

neural tube abnormalities (NTDs)   266

neuroimaging techniques   217

newcastle disease   171*t*

New World Screw worm (NWS)   255, 279–80

Nightingale, Florence   451

Nipah virus disease   56*f*, 58*t*, 60, 87, 285

Nipah virus encephalitis   74, 75*f*

nitric acid   480

Nitrobacter   382

Nitrococcus   382

nitrogen cycle   380–2, 381*f*

ammonification   382

assimilation   382

denitrification   382

nitrification   382

nitrogen fixation   380, 382

nitrogen dioxide (NO_2)   408*t*

nitrogen oxides (NOx)   317, 479

Nitrosomonas   382

nitrous oxide (N_2O)   394, 415, 418, 500

Nocturnal House at Nehru Zoological Park   430

nodes   219

noise

accumulation   218

dosimeter   453

meaning of   451

measurement of   452–3

sources of   452

Noise and Hearing Loss Prevention program   454

noise pollution   334, 399, 407, 411

cardiovascular disturbances   455

control of   457–8

disturbances in mental health   455–6

effect on animal health   456–7

effect on human health   453–6

hearing impairment   454

interference with spoken communication   455

negative social behavior and annoyance   455

sleep disturbances   455

noise reduction rating (NRR)   453

nonconventional water resources

desalination   443

rainwater harvesting (RWH)   443

wastewater reuse   443

nonhazardous waste   524, 526

noninfectious and production diseases   256

noninfectious diseases   145

noninferiority trial   200

nonirritant pollutants   386

nonliving vaccines, for animals   271–2

antigens generated by gene cloning   272

DNA plasmid vaccines   272

subunit vaccines   272

nonmigratory mammals, distribution of   87

nonpoint source pollution   388, 407

nonrenewable natural resources   330*f*, 331, 477

non-tsetse-transmitted animal trypanosomiasis (NTTAT)   255

normalized difference vegetation index (NDVI)   139

norovirus   71

Nosema algerae   563

notifiable animal diseases   112

"No Time to Wait: Securing the Future from Drug-Resistant Infections" report   305

Nufer, Jacob   301

numbers, pyramid of   369, 369*f*

nutrient cycling, biogeochemical processes of   380–4

carbon cycle   380, 381*f*

nitrogen cycle   380–2, 381*f*

phosphorus cycle   382–4, 383*f*

water cycle   382, 383*f*

nutritional epidemiology

in determination of causality   265–6

in development of policy   266

research plan hierarchy in   265*f*

O

observational studies   117–18, 191–5, 207–13

case–control study   120, 120*f*, 193–4, 193–4*f*

cases and controls, selection of

cohort studies   122, 123*f*

exposure   121

observational studies (*cont'd*)
  historical cohort studies 122
  nested case-control studies 123, 123*f*
  odds ratio 121–2
 cohort study 191–3
  calculation of relative risk in 192, 193*f*
  design 192*f*
  prospective cohort study 193
  retrospective cohort study 193
 cross-sectional study 120, 194–5, 194*f*, 208, 210
 descriptive studies 118
 design 208
 ecological fallacy 119
 ecological studies 118–19
 experimental population research 212
 randomized controlled trials 210–12
 STROBE statement 207–13, 209–10*t*
observation bias 195
observation data collection, advantages/
  disadvantages of 216
occupational determinants 47
Occupational Health and Safety Administration
  (OSHA) 540
occupational hygiene. *See* industrial hygiene
occupational noise 452
occupational/personnel accidents 581, 582*f*
Occupational Safety and Health (OSHA) 453
ocean carbon sequestration 325, 326*f*
oceans 442
ocean warming and acidification 354
odds ratio 121–2
 calculation in case–control study 194, 194*f*
odors 500–1
 health hazards of 501
Office International des Épizooties (OIE) 99, 101, 104, 137,
  156, 163, 252, 257, 302, 303
 Aquatic Animal Health Code 188
 building global governance on AMR 305
 and Codex 187, 304
 EBO-SURSY Project 306
 Fifth Strategic Plan (2011–2015) 305
 global initiatives
  for biological threat reduction 305
  for disease eradication 304–5
  to fight antimicrobial resistance 305
  for food safety 304
  in One Health 306
 initiatives 304–6
 internal standards/guidelines for animal and aquatic
  health 186–7
 role in global trade in animals and animal products 185–9
 Specialist Commissions 188

 SPS Agreement 186–7
 standards 188
 steps in OIE framework 205
 Terrestrial Animal Health Code 188
 trade-facilitating approach for OIE-listed diseases 188–9
 WTO role and 186
Office of the State Veterinarian 294
off-site sewage system 520
OIE. *See* Office International des Épizooties (OIE)
Oil Pollution Act (1990) 479
Old World screw worm (*Chrysomya bezziana*, OWS) 88, 255
One Health approach 16, 23, 26, 41, 46, 46*f*, 62, 252,
  285*f*, 301–3
 animal, environmental, and human interactions 291*f*
 building capacity to managing zoonotic disease risks 306
 collaboration 306
 global initiatives in 306
 history of 302–3
 international collaboration in 302–3
 strengthening surveillance systems 306
 training health professionals in 306
 triad 302*f*
One Health High-Level Expert Panel (OHHLEP), creation
  of 302–3, 303*f*
"One Medicine" approach 279, 280, 302
"One World, One Health" concept 280, 285
"one world–one medicine" phrase 341, 341*f*
on-site sewage system 520
operational biosecurity 153
organic solvents 314
organic wastes, classification of
 hazardous wastes 526
 nonhazardous wastes 526
organism's infectious potential 37
Organization for Economic Cooperation and Development
  (OCED) 482
organophosphate poisoning accidents 587
Ornithodorus ticks 87
orographic precipitation 441
"OR" operator 234
ortho-phenylphenol (OPP) 152
Osler, William 280
OspA 272
osteosarcoma 48
Our Common Future document 483
outcome measures 241
OutCosT (OUTbreak COSting Tool) 171
overexploitation and illegal wildlife trade
 combating wildlife trafficking 355
 identifying threats to endangered species 355
overexploitation of forests 332
overmatching 127

overpopulation 337
OVID 233
ozone-depleting substances (ODS) 480
ozone depletion 480

p

Paecilia holbrooki 562
paleontological perspectives 352
Pan-African Rinderpest Campaign (PARC) 254, 258
Pan African Veterinary Vaccine Centre (PANVAC) 258
PANAFTOSA 257
Pan American Health Organization (PAHO) 282
pandemic diseases, incidence of 102
parallel testing 203
parasitic endemic diseases 60
parasitism 51
paratenic host 70
Paris Agreement 421
partial budgeting 160t
participant observation 216
particle pollution 501
particulate matter (PM) 316, 408t, 501–2
  health hazards of 502
  sources of 502
passive immunization 576
passive quarantine 574
passive surveillance 7, 104, 105
Pasteurella multocida 273
Pasteur, Louis 271
pathogenesis of outbreak 53
pathogenicity 69
  and virulence 37, 48
pathogen infection, cycle of 83f
per capita fecundity 92
period prevalence 103
periphyton 379
permafrost 375
permeability 442
per-protocol analyses 201
persistent organic pollutants (POPs) 309, 313–14, 422,
    463, 468–9t
personal hygiene 326
personal protective equipment (PPE) 545, 595, 596
person-time incidence rate 130
peste des petits ruminants (PPR) 147t, 163t, 171t, 183
  Eradication Program (PPR-EP) 183
pesticide pollution 400
pesticides 310–12, 412, 462
pharmaceuticals and personal care products
    (PPCPs) 463, 469t
pharmaceuticals/biomedical wastes 314–15, 526, 530, 531
phenolic compounds 152

Phlebotomus pedifer 86
phosphorus cycle 382–4, 383f
photic zone 379
phycoremediation technique 401
phylogenetic diversity 350, 351f
phylogenomics 350
physical hazards, prevention and control of 323
phytoplankton 466
phytoremediation 470
pilot testing 238–9
pit latrines 520
placebo 201
plague (*Yersinia pestis*) 87
planetary albedo 417
plankton 379, 466
planning for disaster recovery 490
Plasmodium spp. 69
plastic contaminants 464
plastic production, increase of 315
point data 15
point prevalence 103
point-source outbreaks 53
point source pollution 388, 407
"Polar Bear Plunge" exhibit 429
polio 576
poliomyelitis 577t
polychlorinated biphenyls (PCBs) 468t
polycyclic aromatic hydrocarbons (PAHs) 399
polymer and nanotechnology 447t
polymerase chain reaction (PCR) 7, 149
population approach, in veterinary epidemiology
  reasons for 6–7
    disease control 6
    preventive measures 7
    public health 7
population at risk 129
population genetics 350
positive predictive value (PPV) 203
potentially toxic elements (PTEs) 463
poultry farming 431–2
povidone-iodine 152
prairie dogs (*Cynomys leucurus*) 87
precipitation 441
precision 202, 202f
precision livestock farming (PLF)
  commercial concerns 345–6
  examples of commercializing PLF technologies and
      guiding principles 345
  as facilitator of progress 346
  and its advantage to environment 343–7
  limiting circumstances for commercialization 345–6
  observations and suggestions 347

precision livestock farming (PLF) (*cont'd*)
  primary responsibility of 344
  scientific problem 343–5
  scientific theories and PLF principles 343–4
  technical and scientific advancements 345
  traceability in 344
preclinical disease 34
predictive modeling, in veterinary epidemiology
  benefits 19
  challenges and considerations 19
  data quality and availability 19
  dynamic nature of diseases 19
  early warning systems 19
  machine learning algorithms 18–19
  resource allocation 19
  spatial modeling 19
  techniques and approaches 18–19
  time series analysis 18
preemptive slaughter technique 151
preslaughter management 150
prevalence 101*f*, 103, 117, 129–30, 129*t*, 130*f*, 575
prevalence studies. *See* cross-sectional studies
prevention
  disease control and 8
  of environmental hazards 323–4
  and eradication of zoonoses 283–4
  levels 146*t*
  strategies of disease management 145–50
  transboundary animal diseases (TADs) 162, 162*f*,
    163*t*, 164*f*
  and treatment of animal diseases 264–5
Prevention and Control of Infectious and Contagious
    Diseases in Animals Act 2009 177
Prevention of Rabies Rules 1969 178
Prevention of Trypanosomiasis Rules 1968 178
primary air pollutants 397
primary and secondary microplastics 316, 464
primary determinants 42, 42*b*
  characteristics 42*b*
  of disease 43*f*
primary/natural/maintenance host 69
primary prevention 570
primordial prevention 569–70
principal component analysis (PCA) 14
PRISMA, guideline for reporting systematic reviews 233
production environments and disease transmission, climate
    change effects on 262–3
Programme for the Control of African Animal
    Trypanosomiasis and Related Development 255
Programme for the Eradication of *Amblyomma
    variegatum* 255

Prohibition of Treatment except by Veterinary Officers
    1928 177
Project Directorate on Animal Disease Monitoring and
    Surveillance (PDADMAS) 140, 141
propagated/progressive outbreaks 53
PROPEXAN initiative 257
proportionate mortality 132
prospective cohort study 191–3. *See also* cohort studies
protection of wildlife and flora and fauna, treaties on 483
Psammomys, habitats of 87
Pseudomonas aeruginosa 76
Pteropus fruit bats 74, 87
publication bias 241, 243–4
public health 279, 299–300
  pesticides used in 311
  program management and leadership 293
  surveillance 296
  veterinarians in current practice of 340–2
  and zoonotic disease modeling 19–20
    assessing risks to human health 19–20
    intervention strategies 20
public health functions 295–8, 301
  competent and well-trained healthcare
    workforce 295, 297
  developing policies and plans 295, 297
  educating people about health issues 295, 296
  investigating health problems and hazards 295, 296
  laws and regulations enforcement 295, 297
  link people to needed health services 295, 297
  mobilizing community partnerships to solve health
    problems 295, 296
  monitoring health status 295, 296
  quality of personal and population-based health services,
    evaluating 295, 298
  research for new insights and innovative solutions to
    health problems 295, 298
public hygiene 326
public service announcements (PSAs) 492
pyramid
  of biomass 369–70, 370*f*
  of energy 370, 371*f*
  of numbers 369, 369*f*
pyrolysis 515–16

q

Q-statistic tests 243
quality assessment 240
quarantine 573–4, 574*t*
quarantine measures, in veterinary epidemiology 8
quaternary ammonium compounds (QACs) 152, 542
quaternary ammonium hydrogen peroxide (QAC-HP) 152

quaternary prevention 570–1
Quercus robur 373

r

rabies 58*t*, 69, 70, 76, 85, 163*t*, 168, 170*t*, 300
rabies vaccine 271
radioactive contamination 479
radioactive materials/elements 399, 469*t*
radioactive wastes 391, 533
radionuclides 463–4
rainwater harvesting (RWH) 326, 443
Ramsar Convention 419–20
random allocation 199
random error 125
randomization 127
randomized controlled trials (RCTs) 124, 124*f*, 195, 202,
        210–12, 265
random mixing 35
random sampling 11
range 220
REACH (chemical policy) 470
recall bias 195
recombinant vaccinia-vectored rabies vaccines 275
recovery phase, in animal disaster management 493–4
reemerging diseases, drivers of 342*f*
reference management software 235
reforestation 84, 401
Regional Immunization Technical Advisory Group
        (RITAG) 307
regulations, in India 182–3
relative risk 192
    calculation, in cohort study 193*f*
release of insects with dominant lethality (RIDL) 565
remote sensing 90
    applications, in biodiversity research and monitoring 357
rendering processes 553
renewable energy 401, 423
renewable natural resources 329–31, 330*f*, 477
replacement cost 602
reproductive failure, in pigs 44
reproductive value 96
Rescue® 540
reservoirs/vectors 70, 442
    control strategies 565
    role in disease transmission 561–2, 561*f*
respiratory tract infections 67
response and emergency relief efforts 491–3
retrospective cohort study 191–2, 193
reverse causality 265
RevMan (Review Manager) 243
Rhipicephalus appendiculatus 264

Rift Valley fever (RVF) 56*f*, 58*t*, 139, 169, 279, 559*t*
rinderpest 58*t*
ring vaccination 145
Rio de Janeiro Earth Summit (1992) 321, 322*f*, 421, 483
risk
    of bias assessment 232, 240
    definition of 204–5
risk analysis 187, 204–6, 578
    components of 205–6, 205*f*
        acceptable level of risk 206
        hazard identification 205
        qualitative/quantitative assessment 206
        risk assessment 205
        risk communication 206
        risk management 206
    definition of risk 204–5
    in practice 206
risk assessment and monitoring, of environmental
        contaminants 469–70
risk factors, in disease occurrence 24–5
risk ratio 192
rivers 441–2
road accidents 583
rotary drum composter 513
Rotary International 576
rotavirus diarrhea 67
Rotterdam Convention 421–2
rubella 577*t*
rural and urban pollution 405–6
    agricultural pollution 409
    air pollution 406–7, 408*t*, 411
    case studies 412–13
    comparative study 409*t*
    general comparison between 411*t*
    health risks associated with 406
    impact on ecosystems 406
    light pollution 410
    mitigation and management strategies 410–12
    noise pollution 407, 411
    severity of 410
    solid waste generation 411
    urban heat island effect 411
    water pollution 407, 409*f*, 411

s

"safe sanitary landfill" 531
Salmon, Daniel 300
Salmonella 304
Salmonella enteritidis 275, 279, 284
Salmonella typhi 70, 76
Salmonella typhimurium 341

salt licks 87
sample size 125
sampling 10–11
  challenges in conducting 11
  cluster 11
  overview of methods 11
  principles of sampling design 10
  random 11
  stratified 11
Sanitary and Phytosanitary Measures (SPS)
    Agreement 112–13, 186–7, 304
  core principles of 186
  importance of transparency 187
  obligations in 187
  scientific justification 187
  specific trade concerns of 187
sanitary sewage 518
sanitation
  animal-related items
    bowls/toys/litter boxes 545
    laundry 545
    other equipment 545
    transport carriers 545
  characteristics of ideal disinfectant 542
    in veterinary settings 543–4t
  clothing 546
  footbaths 546–7
  hand sanitation 546
    gloves 546
    hand sanitizers 546
    hand washing 546
  important aspects of plan 538–41
    animal housing design, importance of 540–1
    application systems 540
    avoiding disease spread 538–9
    contact time 539–40
    drying 540
    minimizing animal stress 539
    order of cleaning 539
    population management 541
    product preparation 539
  personal sanitation 546–7
  procedures in animal shelters 541–4
  sanitary practices of animal shelters 537–8
  three-step process 538
  training 547
saprotrophs 366
satellite imagery 90
scabby mouth 147t
Schwabe, C.W. 280, 302
screening search result 235–7
screening technique 570

Screw worm Emergency Centre for North Africa (SECNA) 255
searching databases 233–4
  approaches to 231, 232t
seasonal autoregressive integrated moving average
    (SARIMA) 247t
Sea Turtle Egg Fusariosis (STEF) disease 46
secondary air pollutants 397
secondary determinants 42, 42b
  characteristics 42b
  of disease 43f
secondary host 69
secondary prevention 570
second epidemiological transition 54
segregation of biomedical waste 527–9, 528f
selection bias 126, 195
selenium (Se) 396
semiautomatic cow dung cleaning machine 507–8
semipermanent environmental attributes 86–8
  distribution of nonmigratory mammals 87
  ephemeral or seasonal environmental attributes 87–8
  human settlements, villages, roads, farms, and ranches 87
sensitivity 203, 572
sensitivity analysis, in metaanalysis 243, 266
sentinel network 112, 139
sequential timed events plotting (STEP) procedure 581
serial testing 203–4
severe acute respiratory syndrome (SARS) 56f, 285, 341
sewage disposal 517–19
  collection methods 520–1
    combined system 521
    separate system 521
  major pollutants
    microbes 519
    organic substances 518
    plant nutrients 519
    suspended solids 519
  methods
    full wastewater system 520
    lagoons 520
    municipality systems 520
    off-site sewage system 520
    on-site sewage system 520
    pit latrines 520
  sewage treatment methods
    biological treatment 518, 519
    chemical treatment 518, 519
    physical treatment 518, 519
    sludge treatment 518, 519
  types of sewage
    domestic sewage 518
    industrial wastewater 518
    storm sewage 518

Index | 643

sewer system 531

sex biases 25

sex-influenced inheritance 47

sex-limited inheritance 47

sex-linked inheritance 47

sheep and goat plague. *See* peste des petits ruminants (PPR)

sheep pox 58*t*, 147*t*

SI (susceptible to infected) model 247, 248*f*

simultaneous nonrandomized controls 199

single-blind study 201

single nucleotide polymorphism (SNP) analysis 349

SIR (susceptible-infected-recovered) model 248–9, 249*f*

of disease transmission 109

SIS model (no immunity model) 247–8, 248*f*

Sixth Assessment Report (AR6)

of Intergovernmental Panel on Climate Change (IPCC) 415

slaughter techniques, minimizing risk of infection 150–1

sleep disturbances, and environmental noise 455

small data 216

storage 219

smallpox 576

social and ethological determinants 47

social and political dimensions, of biodiversity conservation 357

social development program (SDP) 600–4

employment and livelihood promotion 604

information, education, and communication (IEC) 600–1

information on project design and EIA results 601

during project implementation and monitoring 601

land acquisition and resettlement

actual relocation phase 604

complaints and grievances 603

costs and budget 602

entitlements and compensation scheme 601

implementation arrangements/supervision 603

loss of business 602

post-relocation phase 604

preparation/finalization of LARP 601

pre-relocation phase 603

productive lands and crops 601–2

relocation phases and processes 603

residential land, houses, and other structures 602

voluntary land donations 602

social equity, biodiversity and 357

sociological and psychological hazards, prevention and control of 324

sodium hypochlorite (bleach) 152

soft ticks (*Ornithodorus moubata*) 86, 87

soil-borne transmission 24

soil conservation techniques 412

soil contamination 309

soil degradation 412

soil erosion 334, 335*f*

soil pollution 389–90, 398–9, 479

causes 390

control 390

effects 390

soil resources 334–6

abuses 334–6

desertification 336

soil erosion 334, 335*f*

soils 85–6

solar radiations 416–17

soldier fly breeding 516

solid waste 506

collection of 507

flushing of 507

generation 411

management 509–16

solvents 314

sore mouth 147*t*

sound level meter 453

South American Commission for the Control of Foot-and-Mouth Disease 254

South Asia Rinderpest Eradication Campaign (SAREC) 254

spatial analysis 5

spatial and temporal analysis, in veterinary epidemiology 14–16

adapting to emerging diseases and climate change 16

applications in real-world epidemiology 15

challenges in spatio-temporal analysis 15

combining spatial and temporal dimensions 15

defining spatial analysis 15

developing expertise in 16

emerging techniques and tools 15

ethical implications 15

fundamentals, in epidemiology 15–16

global disease monitoring and epidemiological networks 16

implementing analysis in field settings 15–16

informing policy and public health decision making 16

introduction 14

One Health approach and integrative analysis 16

promoting interdisciplinary collaboration 16

spatial data types and sources 15

spatial statistics and modeling techniques 15

technological advancements and data integration 16

temporal analysis, in epidemiology 15

time-to-event data, analyzing 15

spatial biosecurity. *See* locational biosecurity

species and breeds, roles in spread of disease 36

Index

species diversity
  functional traits and community ecology 350
  phylogenetic diversity 350, 351f
  species discovery and delimitation 350
species survival and biogeography, implications for 354
specificity 203, 572
sporadic diseases, incidence of 101
spurious correlation 218
stability 69
stamping out method of slaughter 151
standard deviation 220
Standardized Mortality Ratio (SMR) 52–3
Standard Operating Procedures (SOPs) 344
state public health veterinarians (SPHVS) 294
static life tables 91, 92
stationary sources of pollution 498
statistical analysis
  application of statistics in veterinary epidemiology 13–14
    advanced statistical methods 14
    data quality and management 14
    disease prevalence and incidence analysis 13
    epidemiological modeling 13
    risk factor analysis 13
    survival analysis 13–14
  challenges and future directions 14
  data visualization and communication 14
  ethical considerations in data analysis 14
  importance of 12
    enhancing disease surveillance and response 12
    establishing relationships 12
    informing decision-making 12
    interpreting data 12
    unveiling patterns and trends 12
  key statistical methods and applications 12
    descriptive statistics 12
    inferential statistics 12
    multivariate analysis 12
  spatial and temporal analysis 14–16
  statistical software and tools 14
  variables 13–14
    categorical 13
    choosing the right statistical test 13
    continuous 13
    discrete 13
    time-to-event 13
    types 13
statistical and mathematical modeling 245–50
  assumptions for 246
  for COVID-19 pandemic 249–50
  differences between 246
  importance in epidemiology 245–6
  SI (susceptible to infected) model 247, 248f

SIR (susceptible-infected-recovered) model
  248–9, 249f
  SIS model (no immunity model) 247–8, 248f
  time series regression (TSR) model 247
statistical heterogeneity 241
statistical modeling, in analytical epidemiology 6
statistical packages, for metaanalysis 242–3
statistical software and tools, in veterinary epidemiology 14
Steele, James H 302
Sterile Insect Technique (SIT) 255, 563, 564f
still-water/lacustrine ecosystem 378
stochastic models 18
Stockholm Conference (1972) 482–3
Stockholm Convention, on Persistent Organic
  Pollutants 313, 422, 463
storm sewage 518
stratification and statistical modeling 127–8
stratified randomization 199
stratified sampling 11
stratosphere 416, 480
streams and rivers 441–2
strengthening the reporting of observational studies in
  epidemiology (STROBE)
  limitations and consequences of 212–13
  objectives and application of 207–12
  statement 208, 209–10t
Streptococcus uberis 44
stress 38–9
structural biosecurity 153
subclinical infection 49t
subcutaneous (SC)/intramuscular (IM) injection 273
subunit vaccines 272
sulfur dioxide (SO_2) 317, 394, 408t, 479
Sulfur Emissions Reduction Protocol 480
superiority trials 200
super sponges 446
surface runoff 441
surveillance
  of animal diseases 7–8
  and culling 565
  and early detection 10
  epidemiological 578
  flow of information in 109f
  identifying emerging diseases 8
  and monitoring 108
  monitoring disease outbreaks 7
  system's configuration, survey of potential methods for
    examining 109–11
  types
    active surveillance 7
    passive surveillance 7
    syndromic surveillance 7

survey 108
survivorship schedule 92, 93
susceptibility 68
susceptible-infected-recovered (SIR) model 18, 248–9, 249f
susceptible-infectious-susceptible (SIS) (no immunity) model 247–8, 248f
sustainable development 483, 485
Sustainable Development Goals (SDGs) 251
swamps 86
swine farming 432–3
  enrichment practices to improving welfare in pigs 432–3
swine fever 183, 285
Swine Fever Rules 1968 178
swine vesicular disease 58t
syndromic surveillance 7, 104
systematic error 126
systematic reconnaissance flights 90
systematic vaccination 145
systems ecology 82
systems simulation 160t

t

taiga/snow forests 373
Tansley, Arthur G. 365
targeted strategies 8
targeted surveillance 112
targeted vaccination 145, 565
temperate deciduous forest 373
temperate evergreen forest 373–4
temperate rainforests 374
temporal analysis, in epidemiology 15
temporal biodiversity dynamics
  historical context 352–3
  paleontological perspectives 352
terbufos 587
termite mounds 86
Terrestrial Animal Health Code 104, 105
terrestrial carbon sequestration 324, 325f
terrestrial (land-based) ecosystem 370–7
  desert ecosystem 376–7, 376f
  forest ecosystem 373–4, 373f
  grassland ecosystem 371–3, 372f
  tundra ecosystem 374–6, 374f
terrestrial solar radiations 417
tertiary prevention 570
theileriosis 147t
Thelohania 563
thermal enrichment 391
thermal pollution 391–2
  control 392
  effects 391
  sources 391

thermosphere 416
Three Mile Island accident 479
three Rs, to conserve natural resources 337f
Thumburmuzhy model, composting carcases 517, 517f
tick-borne diseases (TBDs) 169, 254–5, 264
time series analysis, in predictive modeling 18
time series models, classification and description of 247t
time series regression (TSR) model 247
time series studies 119
time-to-event variables 13
title and abstract screening 236
tolerance 76
toluene 314
topography 85–6
  caves 86
  drainage, waterholes, and swamps 86
  soils 85–6
  static animal features 86
toxaphene 468t
Toxoplasma gondii
  horizontal and vertical transmission of 71
  life cycle of 72f
Toxoplasma infections 74
traceability in livestock management 344
transboundary animal diseases (TADs) 137
  brucellosis 168–9
  context and sources of impact of 162f
  defined 161
  economic impact of 160–3, 161t, 169, 170–1t
  foot and mouth disease 166–8
    components of losses, in different species 167t
    global economic impact 168f
    global impact due to vaccination costs and production losses 168t
    impacts 167f
  lumpy skin disease (LSD) 169
  major diseases of livestock 160f
  prevention and control interventions 162
    average annual cost of disease control programs 163t, 164f
    costs and benefits 162f, 163t
  rabies 168
  WOAH global animal disease control and eradication strategies 163t
transboundary pollution, treaties on 483
trans fatty acids (TFAs) 266
transfer factor (TF) 465
transgenic technology, in controlling vector-borne diseases 563
transmissible spongiform encephalitis (TSE) 171t, 552

646 | Index

transmission
  air-borne 72, 572
  biological 562
    via vector 72
  blocking routes of 571, 571f
  chain of 70–1
    for rabies virus 71f
  contact spread 53, 74, 101
  of diseases 24
  droplet 24
  fomite 572
  food-borne diseases 24
  horizontal/vertical 35, 71, 101
  iatrogenic 74
  mechanical 562, 572
  methods of 74
    contact 74
    iatrogenic 74
    ingestion 74
    inhalation 74
    inoculation 74
    venereal 74
  modes of 35, 71–2
    direct transmission 71
    indirect transmission 71–2
    of infectious agent 73f
    Nipah virus 74, 75f
    of pathogens 73t
  patterns 19
  soil-borne 24
  of vector-borne diseases 558, 562
  vehicle-borne 572
  vehicular 101
  venereal 74
  waterborne pathogen 24
  See also direct transmission; indirect transmission
transport vehicle accidents 582
tree ecosystem 369
triad of disease causation 22–3
Trichinella spiralis 49, 76, 302
trichinellosis 255
triclosan 152
triple-blinded trial 201
trophic magnification factor (TMF) 466
trophic transfer 465
  of heavy metals 465–6
trophic transfer factor (TTF) 465
trophodynamics 465
tropical rainforests 374
tropical seasonal forests 374
troposphere 416
Trypanosoma evansi 255

Trypanosoma species 76
Trypanosoma vivax 255
Trypanosomiasis equiperdum 255
trypanosomosis 169
tuberculosis (TB) 58t, 101, 306
tundra ecosystem 374–6, 374f
  alpine tundra region 375
  animals (fauna) 375–6
    alpine tundra animals 376
    arctic tundra animals 376
  arctic tundra region 375
  characteristics
    extreme climatic conditions 375
    land of midnight sun 375
    permafrost 375
Typhoid Mary 70

u

udder health 149
ultraviolet radiation 417
UNICEF scenario on hygiene 327–8
United Nations Collaborative Programme on Reducing
    Emissions from Deforestation and Forest Degradation
    in Developing Countries (UN-REDD) 422–4
  adaptation and mitigation strategies for global
    warming 423
  UN-REDD+ 422
United Nations Conference on Environment and
    Development (UNCED) 421
United Nations Conference on Human Environment 482
United Nations Convention to Combat Desertification
    (UNCCD) 421
United Nations Environment Programme (UNEP) 252, 302,
    482, 484, 485
United Nations Framework Convention on Climate Change
    (UNFCCC) 421, 422, 484
United States Department of Agriculture (USDA)
    266, 292, 293
United States Department of Health and Human Services
    Dietary Guidelines Advisory Committee 266
United States Public Health Service (USPHS) 295
urban areas
  pollution in 406
  severity of pollution 410
  See also rural and urban pollution
urban heat island effect 411

v

vaccines and vaccination 258, 271–6
  advances in vaccinology 275–6
  attenuated vaccines 272–3
  combination vaccines, for animals 274

control of emerging and exotic diseases 275
control of zoonotic diseases 275
and food production 275
gene-deleted vaccines 273
modified live vaccines for animals 272–3
nonliving vaccines for animals 271–2
objectives of 271
programs 8, 145–8
reduction in need for antibiotics 275
risk factors for 274
route of administration, in animals 273–4
routine prophylactic schedule for cattle and
    buffalo 147*t*
schedules
  for animals 274
  for equines 148*t*
  for pig 148*t*
  for sheep and goats 147*t*
targeted 145, 565
veterinary vaccines, importance of 275
virus-vectored vaccines 273
validity 128
external 128
internal 128
and reliability 128*f*
van Leeuwenhoek, Antonie 76
variables 13–14
variant Creutzfeldt–Jakob disease (vCJD) 282
vector autoregressive (VAR) 217
vector-borne diseases 59, 68, 82, 135, 169
challenges in control of 565–6
factors influencing emergence of 559–60, 560*f*
Japanese encephalitis 559
leishmaniasis 558–9
malaria and dengue fever 559
overview of 558–9, 559*t*
prevention and control of 562–5
reservoir control strategies
  culling and surveillance 565
  public education and awareness 565
  targeted vaccination 565
  wildlife management 565
Rift Valley fever (RVF) and GLEWS approach 139
transmission of 24, 558, 562
vector control strategies
  biological control 562–3
  environmental management 562
  genetic control 563
  insecticide application 562, 563*f*
  integrated vector management 563, 564*f*
  modification of vectors for population reduction 564*f*
  other control methods 563–5

vector error correction model (VECM) 169, 171
vectors and reservoirs 70, 71
control strategies 565
role in disease transmission 561–2, 561*f*
vehicle-borne transmission 572
vehicle emissions 413
vehicular transmission 101
venereal transmission 74
venezuelan equine encephalitis virus 559*t*
ventilation 503, 503*f*
vermicomposting 514–15
earthworms, types of 514
harvesting 515
methods 514
  bed method 514, 515*f*
  pit method 514, 515*f*
process 514–15
vertical transmission 35, 71, 101
veterinarians
addressing public health issues 339
in current practice of public health 340–2
in disaster mitigation and management 493
educating the public about health-related
    risks 291
engaging in community outreach and education
    initiatives 292
examples of public health activities 287
in government and legislative roles 293–4
health education 291–2
holistic approach to public health 290*f*
in human health 300–1
international collaboration and reference centers,
    role 289
maintenance of laboratory animal facilities and diagnostic
    laboratories 289
managing zoonoses and nonzoonotic communicable
    diseases 288
multifaceted roles of 288*f*
oath 339
in regulatory process 292–3
role in public health 287–99
safeguarding health across species 295*f*
at state level 294
within USDA 293
veterinary epidemiology 341
agent, host, and environment 22–4
  ecological perspectives 23–4
  triad of disease causation 22–3
aims and scope of 7–9
analytical epidemiology 5–6
  common methods in 5–6
  understanding 5

648 *Index*

veterinary epidemiology (*cont'd*)
  causation and association 6
    consistency 6
    dose-response relationship 6
    strength of association 6
    temporality 6
  challenges and future trends 25–6
  components of 22–5
  data collection 9–11
    and analysis technologies 26
    case reporting 10
    challenges of 11
    importance of 10
    introduction 9
    methods of 10–11
    sampling 10–11
    scope and relevance 9–10
  definition of 3
  descriptive epidemiology 4–5
    as essential for multitude of reasons 4
    significance of 4
    tools in 5
  disease control and prevention 8
    quarantine measures 8
    vaccination programs 8
  disease transmission
    direct transmission 24
    indirect transmission 24
  emerging infectious diseases (EIDs) 25
  importance, in safeguarding animal and public
      health 3–4
    assessment of veterinary interventions 4
    early detection and containment of disease outbreaks 3
    economic impact and livestock industry 3–4
    ensuring food safety 4
    preventing zoonotic diseases 3
  methods in 9–22
  modeling and simulation
    applications of 19
    challenges and limitations 19–21
    Decision Support Systems (DSS) 20
    definition and purpose of 16–17
    future trends 21–2
    historical evolution and significance 17
    mathematical modeling 17–18
    predictive modeling 18–22
    public health and zoonotic disease modeling 19–20
    relationship with traditional epidemiology 17
  One Health approach 16, 23, 26
  population approach 6–7
    disease control 6
    preventive measures 7

    public health 7
    reasons for 6–7
  principles of 4–7
  research and investigation 9
    identifying risk factors 9
    investigating disease outbreaks 9
  risk factors 24–5
  statistical analysis
    application of statistics 13–14
    challenges and future directions 14
    data visualization and communication 14
    ethical considerations in data analysis 14
    importance of 12
    key statistical methods and applications 12
    spatial and temporal analysis 14–16
    statistical software and tools 14
    variables 13–14
  surveillance of animal diseases 7–8
    identifying emerging diseases 8
    monitoring disease outbreaks 7
    types of surveillance 7
  understanding disease patterns 4–6
veterinary medicine 299, 311, 523
  environmental health in 339–42
veterinary public health (VPH) 300
  administration of 282–3
  aims of 280
  challenges and its future trends 285
  core domains 280–1
  defined 279, 340
  domains of 280–2
  emerging domains in 281
  importance of 283–5
    prevention, control, and eradication of zoonoses 283–4
    protection and preservation of environment 284, 285*f*
    protection of food 284
  initiatives in 304–8
  international agencies in 303–4
  leadership 284
  other contributions of 281–2
    emerging and reemerging zoonotic diseases 282
    farming methods 281
    food production chain 281
    interactions between humans and animals 281
    natural and man-made disasters 282
    pace of change 282
    reduced resources 282
    trade, travel, and movement 281
  role of 280*f*
  scope of 280
  section at Centers for Disease Control (1947) 302
  vector and reservoir control in 557–66

WHO initiatives 306–8

See also Office International des Épizooties (OIE); vector-borne diseases

veterinary sciences 258–9

veterinary vaccines, importance of

control of emerging and exotic diseases 275

control of zoonotic diseases 275

reduction in the need for antibiotics 275

safe and efficient food production 275

Victoria, regulations in

Livestock Disease Control Act 1994 180–2

Livestock Disease Control Regulations 1995/2006/2017 181–2

Vienna Convention 420, 485

Virchow, Robert 280

Virchow, Rudolf 302

virulence 37, 48, 69

virus-vectored vaccines 273

visceral leishmaniasis 89, 558

visible losses 158

volatile organic compounds (VOCs) 317, 501

health hazards of 501

Vorticella 563

vulnerability assessment 578

W

wallows 87

Warsaw Framework for REDD+ (WFR) 422

warthogs (*Phacochoerus aethiopicus*) 86

waste

accumulation and storage 533

disposal 529

hazardous/nonhazardous 524, 526

management 153, 322, 410, 413, 600

organic 526

reduction of 533

segregation of 527–9, 528*f*

See also biomedical waste (BMW)

wastewater reuse 443

wastewater treatment plants (WWTPs) 443

water 439, 440*f*

alternative (nonconventional) resources 443

challenges and opportunities for improving water supply 444–5

climate change 444

growing population and urbanization 444

preserving water quality 444–5

consumptive/nonconsumptive usage 439

contaminants 309

desalination 443

distribution and use 439–40

drinking water purification 445–7

disinfection methods 446*t*

filtration techniques 445–6, 445*t*

polymer and nanotechnology 447*t*

quality of water resources 443–4

rainwater harvesting (RWH) 443

vapor 418, 441

wastewater reuse 443

water cycle 382, 383*f*. *See also* hydrological cycle

waterborne pathogen transmission 24

waterholes 86

water pollution 334, 398, 407, 411, 412, 443, 479

causes 389

classification

nonpoint source pollution 388

point source pollution 388

control 389, 390*f*

engineered bioremediation 389

natural bioremediation 389

effect 389

impacts 398

main sources 398

in urban areas 406, 409*f*

water resources 336, 342

abuses 336

uses 336

Western Asia Rinderpest Eradication Campaign (WAREC) 254

West Nile virus (WNV) 282, 285, 288, 559*t*, 565

wetlands 442

wet scrubbers 387

"Wild Asia" exhibit 429

wildebeest (*Connochaetes taurinus*) 88

wildlife–livestock interface, diseases at 60, 61*f*, 61*t*

wildlife trafficking, combating 355

winter diarrhea 67, 68*f*

Wolbachia strain 564

World Acaricide Resistance Reference Centre, in Berlin 255

World Animal Health Information Database (WAHID) Interface 137

World Animal Health Information System (WAHIS) 137

World Antimicrobial Awareness Week (WAAW) 305

World Health Assembly 282, 307

World Health Organization (WHO) 62, 137, 156, 252, 282, 291, 302, 304

on air pollution 386

AMR Surveillance and Quality Assessment Collaborating Centres Network 307

on biomedical waste 524

on disaster 487

on disease 569

effects of noise pollution on humans 454

World Health Organization (WHO) (*cont'd*)
  Eliminate Yellow Fever Epidemics (EYE) Strategy (2017–2026) 307
  eradication program 576
  Global Action Plan on Antimicrobial Resistance (GAP-AMR) 305
  Global Antimicrobial Resistance and Use Surveillance System (GLASS) 307
  Global Influenza Surveillance and Response System (GISRS) 307
  Global InfoBase 120
  Gonococcal Antimicrobial Surveillance Program (GASP) 308
  guide for determining sample size 125
  initiatives 306–8
  scenario on hygiene 327
  Thirteenth General Programme of Work of the WHO (GPW13) 307
  on veterinary public health 299, 340
  WHO 1+1 initiative 306
World Organization for Animal Health (WOAH, OIE). *See* Office International des Épizooties (OIE)
World Summit on Sustainable Development, in Johannesburg (2002) 321, 483
World Trade Organization (WTO) 112, 186, 304

x
xylene 314

y
yearling disease (rinderpest) 88
yellow fever outbreaks, eradicating 307
Yersinia pestis 572

z
Zika fever/virus 56*f*, 559*t*
zoonoses
  defined 280, 302
  and other negative effects 264
zoonotic diseases 99, 101
  control of 275
  direct/indirect costs in 158
  early research 81
  emergence of 84
  emerging and reemerging 282
  GLEWS combined risk assessment for 138
  as global health threats 62
  impacts on economy 156
  management 294
  and nonzoonotic diseases 136*t*
  preventing 3, 7
  public health and 19–20
  rise of 14
  transmission of 280*f*
  See also vector-borne diseases; *specific entries*
zoonotic visceral leishmaniasis (ZVL) 558–9

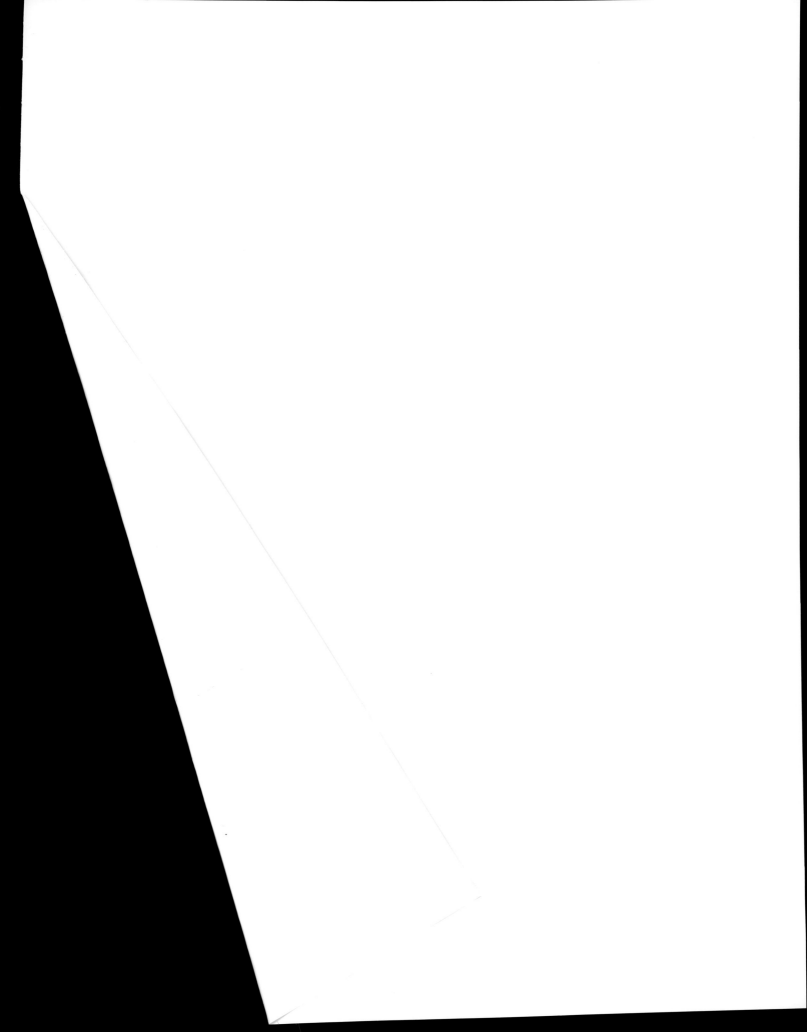

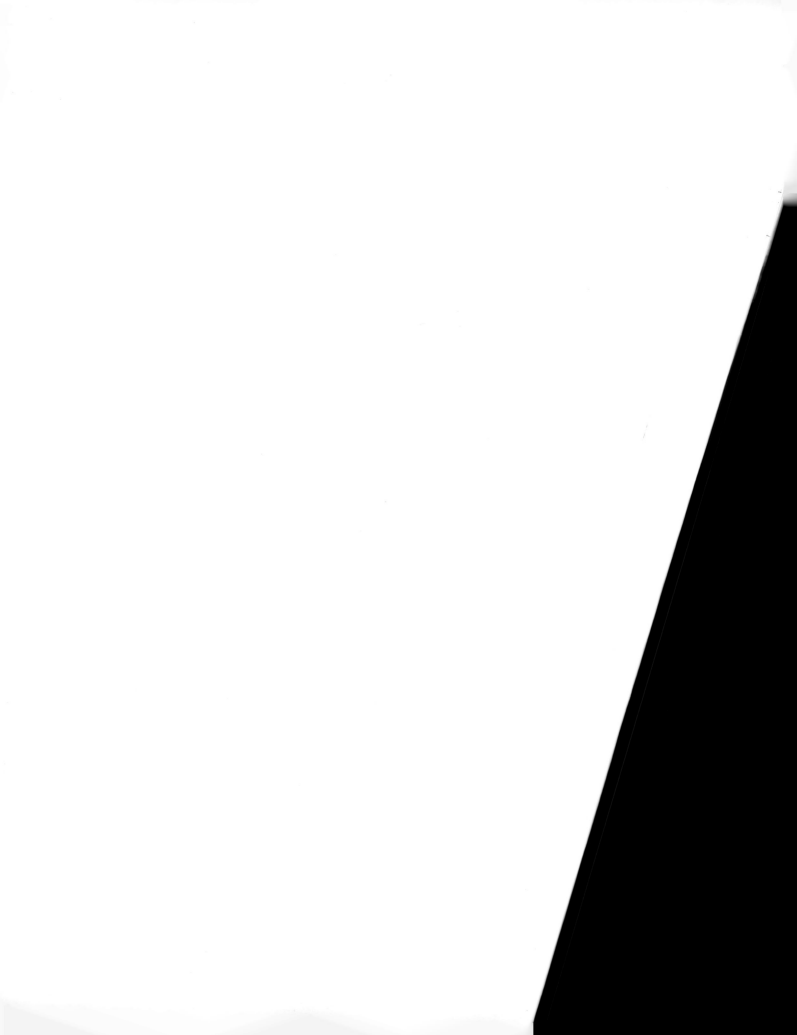